Cleveland Clinic Colorectal Case Studies

James S. Wu • Michelle D. Inkster
Editors

Cleveland Clinic Colorectal Case Studies

Volume I

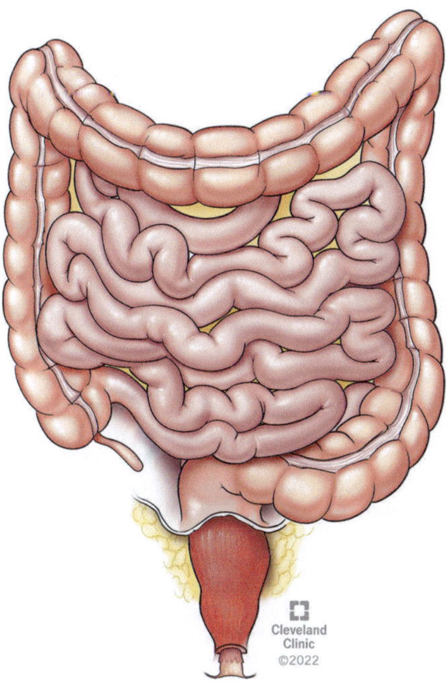

Springer

Editors
James S. Wu
Department of Colon and Rectal Surgery
Cleveland Clinic
Cleveland, OH, USA

Michelle D. Inkster
Department of Gastroenterology
Cleveland Clinic
Cleveland, OH, USA

ISBN 978-3-031-39882-7 ISBN 978-3-031-39880-3 (eBook)
https://doi.org/10.1007/978-3-031-39880-3

This Springer imprint is published by the registered company Springer Nature Switzerland AG
The registered company address is: Gewerbestrasse 11, 6330 Cham, Switzerland

Paper in this product is recyclable.

To our daughter, Margaret, the light of our lives.

Foreword

Dr. Wu and Dr. Inkster have written and recruited respected clinical and academic physicians to contribute to this work on colon and rectal surgery. Anatomy, pathology, radiology, endoscopy, and medical illustrations support a collection of case studies selected from decades of clinical experience. The presentations are arranged distal to proximal starting at the perianal and anal areas then move in sequence to the rectum, the colon, and finally the small intestine. The cases are a mixture of the common and the unusual reflecting their origin from a tertiary medical center. The intention of the book is the introduction of fundamental principles to those who are beginning their journey. Each clinical presentation is followed by a discussion centered on history, especially on contributions of early practitioners who not only did but also recorded what they did for the benefit of generations that would follow long after they were gone. Included are not only their words but also their visual impressions preserved from woodcuts, engravings, and pen/ink drawings. Chronologically, the discussions end short of the present. The "latest and the greatest" is not the point. How we got here and who led us here is. Notable is the inclusion of cases that most would recognize as failures or complications. By including these, we are reminded, sometimes painfully, that the results of our decisions and our actions do not always end the way we would like.

The book is dedicated to my friend and colleague, Vic Fazio. He preceded me from Australia to work with Dr. Rupert Turnbull in the early 1970s. Both of us never left. We, like others, came here because of the Cleveland Clinic's reputation for excellence in intestinal surgery. Dr. Tom Jones in the 1940s achieved the lowest mortality rate for abdominoperineal resection for his time. Dr. Turnbull came on as Dr. Jones' Fellow. In that role, although he assisted in hundreds of operations, he only performed one himself. Following Dr. Jones' untimely passing in 1949, Dr. Turnbull performed almost 100 operations in one year, achieving the same low mortality as his mentor. Dr. Turnbull was a world authority on ulcerative colitis, Crohn's disease, colorectal cancer, ostomy surgery, and nursing ostomy education. Under his guidance, the specialty of colorectal surgery blossomed slowly at first then inexorably. Among his first recruits were Drs. Frank Weakley, Victor Fazio, and David Jagelman. In 1951, with Dr. George "Barney" Crile, he championed subtotal colectomy and ileostomy for toxic ulcerative colitis resulting in reduced mortality. In 1953, he described an operation to prevent ileostomy dysfunction. In the same year, he introduced Karaya as a barrier to protect the skin of ostomates. In the 1950s and

60s, he advocated the "no-touch" isolation technique for the operative treatment of colon cancer. In 1958, a former patient, Ms. Norma Gill, became the Clinic's first full-time "enterostomal" therapist. The School of Enterostomal Therapy subsequently was created and produced its first graduates in 1961. The Department of Colorectal Surgery was formed in 1968 with Dr. Turnbull serving as its chairman from 1968 to 1975. Those of us who trained with him learned operative techniques that we used our entire careers. We in turn shared this information with many Fellows and trainees whom we have had the honor of teaching. I have been told that there is a "Cleveland" way of doing certain things that if seen in the operating room even from a distance identifies the operator as having passed through here. Many of these techniques are represented in this work. I expect that, like everything, some things will last because they continue to be useful while others will fall by the wayside as they are replaced by something better. For the moment, I think what is presented here still has merit. Hopefully, that will continue to be the case for a while longer.

The book ends with recollections written by the nurses, secretaries, and staff who kept Vic's practice afloat. Their memories emote feelings of dedication, respect, pride, and love.

Congratulations to Dr. Wu and Dr. Inkster and the contributing authors.

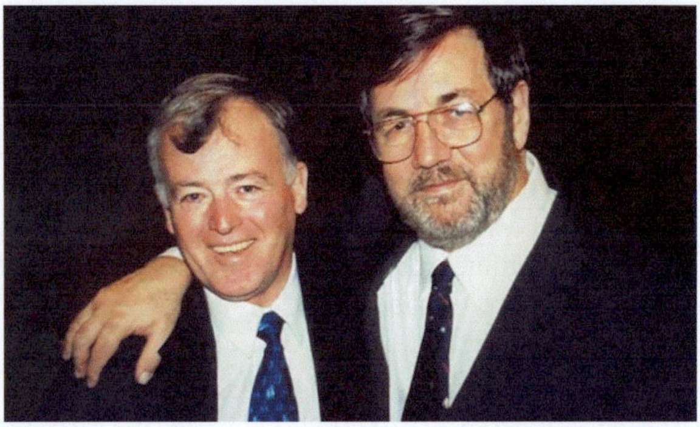

Drs. Ian Lavery and Victor Fazio at the 21st Annual Turnbull Symposium on the occasion of Dr. Fazio's 25th anniversary as Chairman of the Department of Colon and Rectal Surgery.[1]

[1]Access to this photo was provided by Ms. Joyce Balliet.

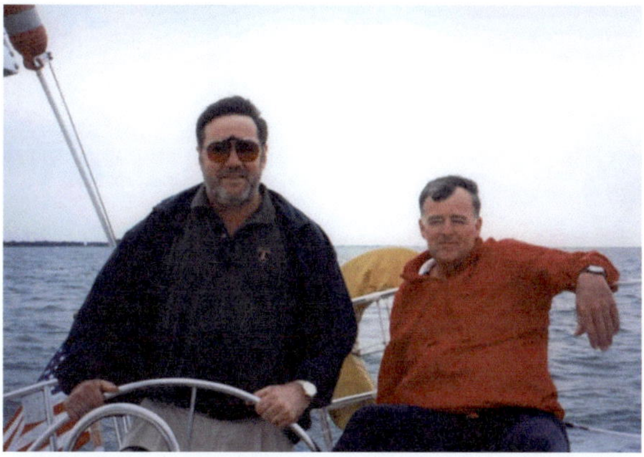

Aussies on the water.[1]

Cleveland, OH, USA
March, 2023

Ian C. Lavery

Preface

This work is dedicated to Dr. Victor W. Fazio, formerly the Chairman of the Department of Colon and Rectal Surgery, who served as a mentor to a generation of physicians and surgeons from around the world. The book introduces colorectal surgery and gastroenterology concepts using a case study format. All cases were contributed by practitioners associated with the Cleveland Clinic. Operative photographs, radiographs, endoscopic images, histology, illustrations, and historical perspective are emphasized. Also included are sections on anatomy, embryology, intestinal anastomoses, and surgical instruments. The intended audience is students and residents. Each case contains a teaching point. The artwork, created under the direction of the Cleveland Clinic medical illustration team, provides cohesion to the whole.

This project began in 2005, when one of us (MDI) suggested that we should collect cases that we encounter during our daily practices at the Cleveland Clinic for publication at some future date for the purpose of education regarding disease, diagnostic evaluation, management, and complications of therapy. A few of these are presented for the benefit of students and trainees, current and future.

The presentations are followed by comments that emphasize historical origins as much as possible. In 1985, a medical school classmate (of JSW) presented a case of breast cancer to Dr. Samuel A. Wells, Jr, Chairman of the Department of Surgery at Washington University in St. Louis. The student referred to Dr. William Halsted. Dr. Wells stopped the presentation and asked, "Who was Halsted?" The message to us in the audience was clear: you have to know where you come from. Our decision to avoid editorialization when possible follows the approach of Mr. Harlow Giles Unger, preeminent author of American historical biographies, who states: "As a former reporter, I never editorialize (when writing historical biographies). I let the characters speak for themselves."

Reference

1. Unger Harlow G., The Taft School, *Taft Bulletin;* Fall 2019. https://www.taftschool.org>bulletin>fall-2019. p. 42–47; published Nov 25, 2019. We thank Mr. Unger for his permission to quote him and Ms. Linda Hedman Beyus, Editor of the Taft School Bulletin, The Taft School Alumni Office, for her kind introduction to Mr. Unger.

Warrensville Hts, OH, USA — James S. Wu
Cleveland, OH, USA — Michelle D. Inkster

Origins

During World War I, three surgeons, Drs. Frank Bunts, George Crile Sr., and William Lower all served at the U.S. Army's Base Hospital No. 4 (the Lakeside Unit) at Rouen, France. They were joined by Dr. John Phillips, an internist, who during the war had served as a Captain in the medical corps. At war's end, following the military model, these four citizen-soldiers conceived a unified practice that would encompass all medical and surgical specialties. The Cleveland Clinic was incorporated on February 5, 1921.

What is now termed General Surgery was the parent of all the surgical departments. George Crile, Sr. was famous for thyroid surgery, particularly for goiters, and that was what kept the Clinic flourishing for its first 20 years. As chiefs of surgery, Dr. Crile and later Dr. Thomas Jones established standards that allowed the Clinic as a whole to achieve surgical mortality that was among the lowest in the country. Although gastroenterology was practiced at the Clinic from the beginning as part of internal medicine, a formal department was not officially founded until 1936. The first chairman was Dr. Everett Collins, who originally came here in 1931 as a radiologist and who was very interested in gastrointestinal disease. Having observed his interest, the founders asked him to start a specialized gastroenterology program. Within that department, he emphasized inflammatory bowel diseases. Rigid endoscopy, practiced by Dr. R. J. F. Renshaw in the 1930s was followed by flexible fiberoptic endoscopy by Dr. Benjamin Sullivan in the 1960s. Intestinal surgery was practiced as part of general surgery from the clinic's inception. However, it was Dr. Jones who showed that surgery for colon and rectal cancer could be achieved with consistently low mortality.

Over the next half-century, Drs. Edgar Achkar, Charles Brown, George Crile, Jr., Richard Farmer, Thomas Jones, George Rankin, Eugene Winkelman, Rupert Turnbull, and Frank Weakley set the cornerstones of an institutional focus on inflammatory bowel disease and colorectal cancer. Following the untimely death of Dr. Jones in 1949, Dr. Turnbull continued his legacy, becoming the first Chairman of a separate Colon and Rectal Surgery Department in 1968. Dr. Turnbull's contributions focused on intestinal stomas, colon cancer, and inflammatory bowel disease. In 1961, with Ms. Norma Gill, a former patient, Dr. Turnbull created a school dedicated to the discipline of enterostomal therapy. This program has benefited ostomy patients worldwide. Dr. Victor Fazio succeeded Dr. Turnbull as Chairman of the Department of Colon and Rectal Surgery in 1975. Dr. Fazio's team partnered with, recruited, and trained like-minded surgeons, physicians, and specialists from around the world to meet the needs of the ever-expanding discipline of colon and rectal surgery. The clinic motto, "To act as a unit," continues to guide and to inspire us today [1, 2].

Comment

The Cleveland Clinic was founded based on the military experience of its founders in France during WWI. It was there that Dr. George Crile coined the Clinic's motto, "To act as a unit." That is, out of battlefield necessity, to act as a unit for the benefit of many. A few of Dr. Crile's recollections from that conflict are presented [3].

Paris, September 16th [4]

"Military surgery has its shadows and its highlights. The highlights are romantic, for in a brief season, whole areas of the body are conquered; great principles are worked out; foundation stones laid.

Patients come in volleys. The surgeon is barraged with fractures, shelled with broken heads: bombed with bellies; gassed with wounds.

Mobile Hospital No. 5, October 4th [5]

This morning our troops went over. The war goes on. Off with peace! Roads are all but impassable; automobiles are mired everywhere; wreckage is on every side. Guns are booming; mile of convoys, ammunition and food are going up; trains of wounded are coming down. The Argonne forest is sprouting wooden crosses.

Mobile Hospital No. 5, October 17th

Everything is overflowing with patients. Our divisions are being shot up; the wards are full of machine gun wounds.

I have been operating on 12-hour shifts here. One hundred and twenty cases are waiting for operation this morning. In one night I had sixty deaths.

Rain, rain; mud, blood; blood, death! All day, all night we hear the incessant tramp of troops—troops going in, wounded coming back, Even in our dreams we hear it. If it ceases for a few hours it is so insistent in our conditioned brain that the incessant rhythmic tramp continues.

Autumn in the beautiful Argonne! Rolling hills, green meadows, shepherd dogs, sheep, lazy cows, brown oak leaves, yellow linwood, red gum, grey and velvety beeches, the rocks and the ground brilliantly blotched with blood—all color blending with the dying and the dead!

C.C.S. 17, September 30th [6, 7]

Ed Lower and I are convinced from our experience with war wounds that there exists no basic distinction between the war patient and the civilian patient; between the man exhausted of days and weeks of intensive fighting waiting, dirty, wet, hungry, and thirsty, and the starved patient exhausted by the ravages of disease.

No. 9, August 27th [8, 9]

Frank Bunts came today to be the C.O. in the place of Ed who has returned to the United States. Frank will make a good C.O. I am more delighted that I can express to have him here, for I have missed Ed sorely. What a remarkable record Bunts,

Crile and Lower have had all of these years. We have been rivals in everything, yet could differ in opinion about anything and through all the vicissitudes of personal, financial, and professional relations we have been able to think and act as a unit" [10].

References

1. Clough JD, Studer PG, Szilagyi S, editors. To act as a unit. The story of the Cleveland Clinic. 5th ed. Cleveland, OH: Cleveland Clinic Foundation; 2011.
2. We are indebted to Mr. Frederick K. Lautenzenheiser and Mr. John E. Bowen, Cleveland Clinic Archivists, for providing us with access to and direction towards the individuals mentioned above.
3. Crile GW. George Crile. An autobiography, edited with sidelihts, by Grace Crile. Philadelphia, PA: J.B. Lippincott Company; 1947.
4. Crile GW. George Crile. An autobiography, edited with sidelights, by Grace Crile. Philadelphia, PA: J.B. Lippincott Company; 1947. p. 312.
5. Crile GW. George Crile. An autobiography, edited with sidelights, by Grace Crile. Philadelphia, PA: J.B. Lippincott Company; 1947. p. 350–351.
6. Crile GW. George Crile. An Autobiography, edited with sidelights, by Grace Crile. Philadelphia, PA: J.B. Lippincott Company; 1947. p. 337; C. C. S 17 refers to Casualty Clearing Center No. 17.
7. Crile GW. George Crile. An Autobiography, edited with sidelights, by Grace Crile. Philadelphia, PA: J.B. Lippincott Company; 1947. p. 315.
8. Crile GW. George Crile. An Autobiography, edited with sidelights, by Grace Crile. Philadelphia, PA: J.B. Lippincott Company; 1947. p. 344.
9. Crile GW. George Crile. An Autobiography, edited with sidelights, by Grace Crile. Philadelphia, PA: J.B. Lippincott Company; 1947. p. 326; No 9 refers to General Hospital No. 9.
10. These excerpts were taken from a copy of Dr. Crile's two volume autobiography that was given to Dr. Inkster by one of her patients.

James S. Wu
Michelle D. Inkster

Vesalius-The intestines

Brevis intestinorum historia enumeratio.

Intestina invicem variant, omnia tamen inter ventriculum, et qua excrementa egerimus.

Andreas Vesalius

De Humani Corporis Fabrica [1]

Brief account of the intestines

The intestines follow one after another but all [are located] between the stomach and where we discharge the excrements.

Andreas Vesalius

On the Fabric of the Human Body

Revised Version of 1555 [2, 3]

References

1. Vesalius A. De Humani Corporis Fabrica, A Facsimile of the revised version of 1555, Vol II of II. Leopold Publishing; 2014. p. 135.
2. This translation was by Transperfect. www.transperfect.com.
3. Richardson WF, Carman JB. ON THE FABRIC OF THE HUMAN BODY. A translation of De Humani Corporis Fabrica Libri Septem. Book V. The Organs of Nutrition and Generation. Novato, CA: Norman Publishing; 2007. p. 87.

Chinese Proverb

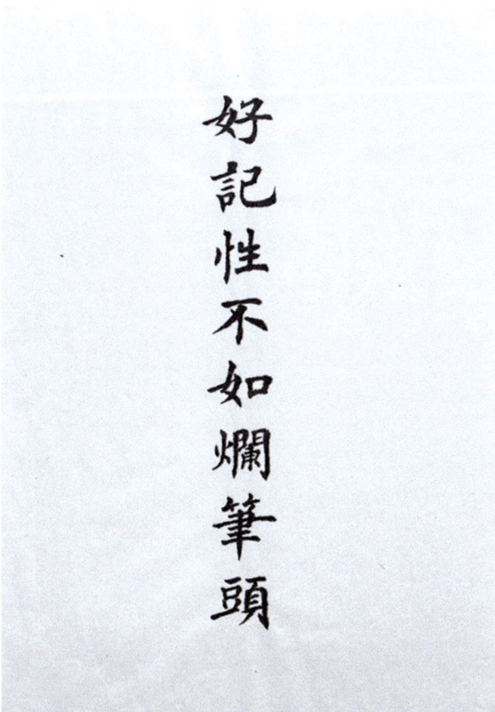

好記性不如爛筆頭
Hǎo jì xìng bù rú làn bǐtóu
"The palest ink is more powerful than the sharpest memory."
Chinese proverb
Calligraphy by: Jian Ma, mamin@frontier.com

In Remembrance

Victor Warren Fazio, A.O., M.B.M.S., F.R.A.C.S., F.R.C.S., Eng (Hon), F.R.C.S., Edin (Hon), F.A.C.S., F.R.A.C.S. (Hon), M.D. Lodz (Hon), F.R.C.S.I. (Hon)

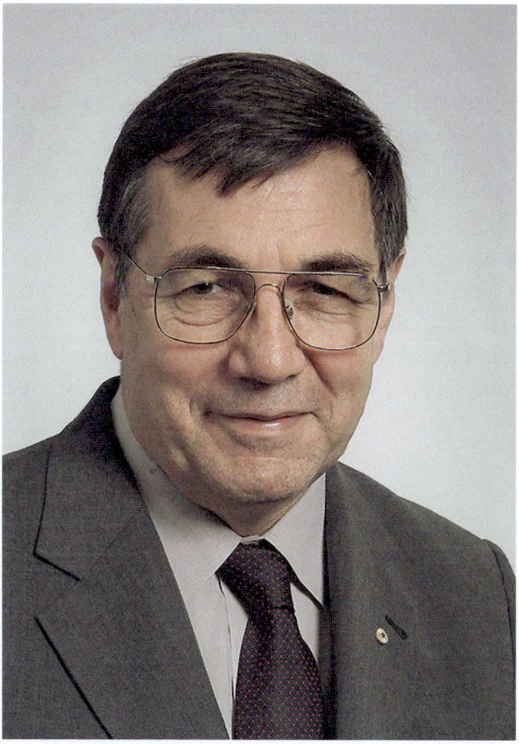

Victor Warren Fazio, A.O., M.B.M.S.
Master surgeon, preeminent educator and pioneer in the field of Colon and Rectal Surgery
Victor Warren Fazio
1940 Born in Sydney, New South Wales

- Secondary School-St. Joseph's College, Hunter's Hill

  1965 M.B.B.S., University of Sydney

- Postgraduate training at St. Vincent's Hospital, Sydney

  under the direction of Dr. Noel C. Newton

- Additional training with Sir E. S. R. Hughes

1970 Fellow Royal Australasian College of Surgeons (F.R.A.C.S.) by examination
1971 Service in Bien Hoa (Vietnam) under Dr. Fred Collins
1972 Lahey Clinic, Hepatobiliary service of Dr. Ken Warren;
Colorectal Surgery service of Dr. Malcolm Veidenheimer
1973 Cleveland Clinic, Colorectal service of Dr. Rupert Turnbull, Jr.
1974 Cleveland Clinic, Staff Surgeon
1975 Cleveland Clinic, Chairman, Colon & Rectal Surgery
1995 Master of Surgery (honoris causa)
The University of Sydney
2004 Order of Australia, Officer (A.O.) in the General Division
2013 Emeritus Professor of Surgery

Awards, Short List

Honorary Fellowship European Surgical Association, April 2007 -Fifth N.E.C.R.S. Distinguished Recognition Award, 2006 -Cleveland Clinic Teacher of the Year Award Winner, 2005-6 -Distinguished Alumnus Award Cleveland Clinic Foundation, June 2005 -America's Top Doctors 2004 (Castle Connolly Ltd. Peer Nomination), June 2004, June 2002 -Officer, Order of Australia (Services to colorectal surgery), January 2004 -Al and Norma Lerner Humanitarian Award, October 2002 -Creation of the Victor W. Fazio Endowed Chair in Colorectal Surgery.

Acknowledgments

First and foremost, we thank the Cleveland Clinic for its unreserved support of this work. We express our heartfelt gratitude to the Cleveland Clinic Library staff for providing access to the world literature for more than 20 years. We thank the Cleveland Clinic Department of Medical Art and Photography for extraordinary artwork. Mr. Joe Pangrace and his staff, Mr. Tony Christovich, Ms. Gwen Fuller, Ms. Emily Hromi, Mr. Ken Kula, Ms. Amanda Mendelsohn, Ms. Maribel Ruiz, and Ms. Erika Woodrum, created illustrations that communicate that which words alone are inadequate to express. We thank Ms. Kathy Miller for preparing and then teaching us to prepare for ourselves digital images suitable for publication. We thank Mr. Fred Lautzenheiser and Mr. John Bowen of the Cleveland Clinic Archives for teaching us Cleveland Clinic History. We thank Professors Richard Drake and Jennifer McBride for co-writing the chapters on anatomy. We gratefully acknowledge Dr. John Goldblum, Chairman of the Cleveland Clinic Department of Anatomic and Surgical Pathology, and members of his staff, present and former, including: Ms. Kathleen Ranney, Drs. Daniela Allende, Ana Bennett, Michael Cruise, Mohamed El Hag, Clifton Fulmer, Ilyssa Gordon, Scott Kilpatrick, James Lapinski, Kelsey McHugh, Mark Melaragno, Rish Pai, Melissa Piliang, Scott Robertson, Erica Savage, Sebouh Setrakian, Charles Sturgis, Jacob Sweeney, Ralph Tuthill, and Jing-Jing Yang. In particular, we thank Drs. David Hernandez Gonzalo, Keith Lai, Homer Wiland, Eric Willis, and Catherine Forse, who, when Fellows in the department, volunteered to provide the majority of the histopathologic images used in this book. They performed this work during their own time before and after regular hours. We acknowledge their generosity and collegiality. We thank Dr. Carolyn Power, Research Fellow in the Department of Colon and Rectal Surgery, for her dedicated and selfless contribution to this book over two years. We thank Drs. Abraham Ahmed, Joseph Azok, Mark Baker, Ajay Bhardwaj, Sean Carlson, Michael Christian, Mark Cohen, Bradley Cole, David Einstein, Ihab Haddadin, Paul Janicki,

Leonard Kahn, Paresh Mahajan, Patrick O'Keefe, Charles O'Malley, Jr., Arthur Parsee, Erick Remer, Samuel Ruskin, Todd Stultz, and Ryan Ward of the Radiology Institute for selection and description of diagnostic images. We thank Ms. Joyce Balliet, medical photographer, for photographing Dr. Fazio's operations and preserving the details of each operation in 35 mm and digital formats. We thank Mr. Apollo Draco for technical expertise in the preparation of videos. We thank Drs. Tracy Hull, Scott Steele, Conor Delaney, and Matthew Walsh of the Digestive Diseases and Surgery Institute for their continuous support. We thank the case contributors. Without their experience, generosity, and commitment to education, this book would not have been possible. We thank Dr. Ian Lavery for reviewing this work and writing its foreword. We thank Mr. Robert Yonchak, Esq., Mr. Michael Michetti, Esq., Ms. Rose Wenstrup, Esq, and Mr. Gregory Stein, Esq. for guiding this work to publication. We thank the Springer Nature Publishing Company and our project editors, Mr. Richard Hruska, Ms. Anila Vijayan, Ms. Shaik Jainul Safha, Ms. Jananee Ravichandran, Ms. Patricia Gutierrez, Mr. Dhanapal Palanisamy, and Mr. Kristopher Spring for putting this book into print. Finally, we thank Drs. Kenneth Bennett, Robert Fry, and Ira Kodner, surgeons at the Washington University School of Medicine, all prior Fellows of the Cleveland Clinic, for mentorship and friendship over many years.

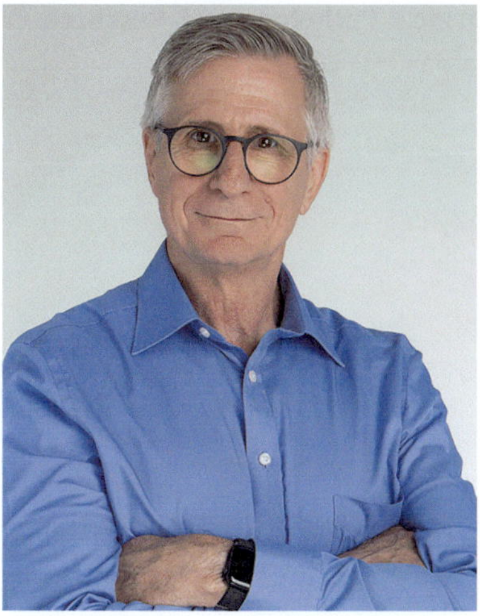

For the past 37 years, Mr. Joseph A. Pangrace has applied his knowledge and skill as a medical illustrator for the Cleveland Clinic. He began working at the Cleveland Clinic immediately following his graduation from the Medical Illustration Program at the Cleveland Institute of Art. Mr. Pangrace's work has been published in medical journals, textbooks, and atlases. In 2005, he was awarded the Medical Illustrator's Max Bröedel prize for continuous-tone illustration. He currently acts as the Medical Illustration Section Leader for the Center for Medical Art and Photography and Medical Art Director for the Cleveland Clinic Journal of Medicine.

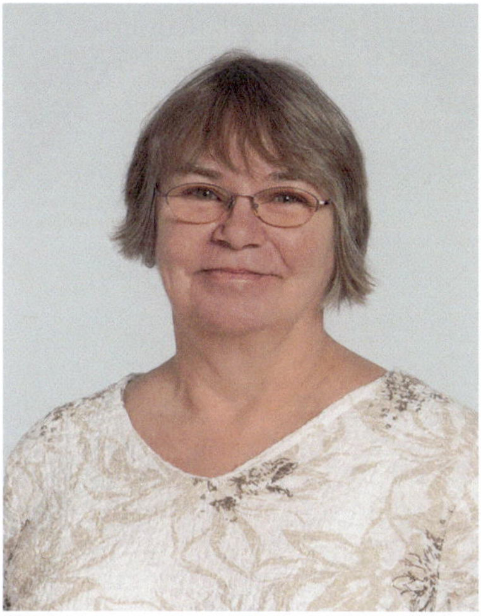

Ms. Kathleen Miller, Digital Technologist, Cleveland Clinic Department of Medical Art and Illustration, prepared the majority of photographs and illustrations used in this work for publication. This work was done with painstaking attention to detail, with many revisions, over many years. Her steadfast commitment to this book is warmly acknowledged.

Cleveland Clinic Surgical Pathology and Research Fellows

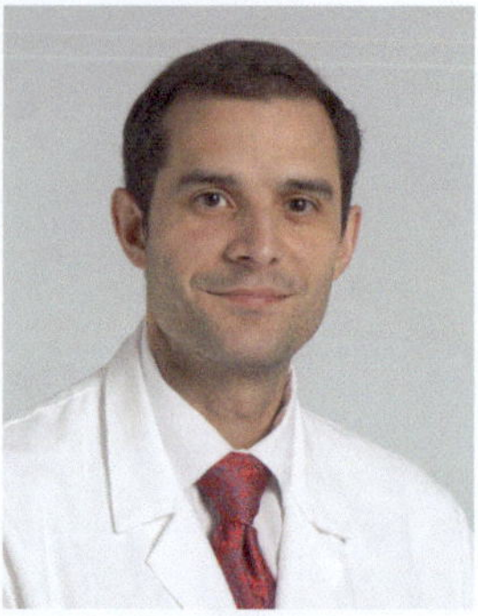

David Hernandez Gonzalo, MD

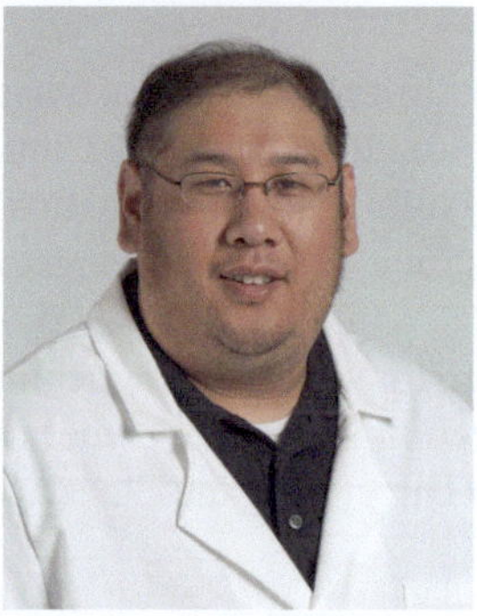

Keith K. Lai, MD

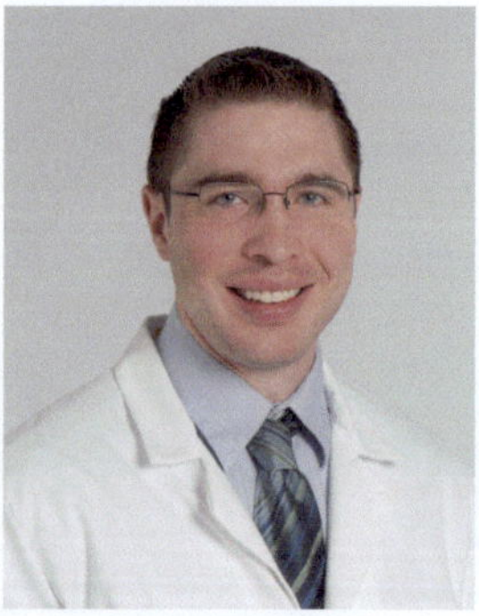

Homer O. Wiland, MD

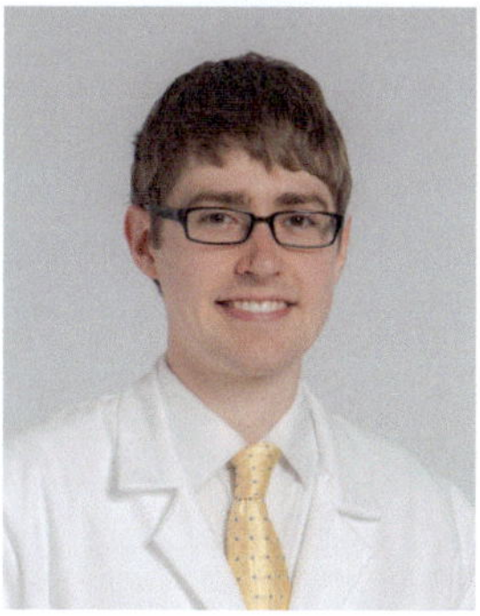

Eric W. Willis, MD

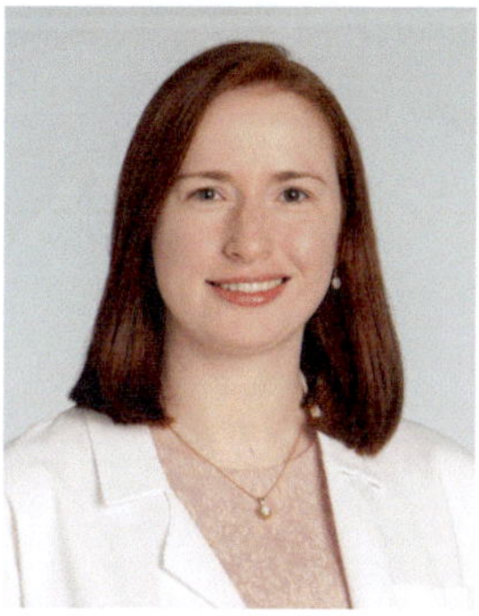

Catherine L. Forse, MD

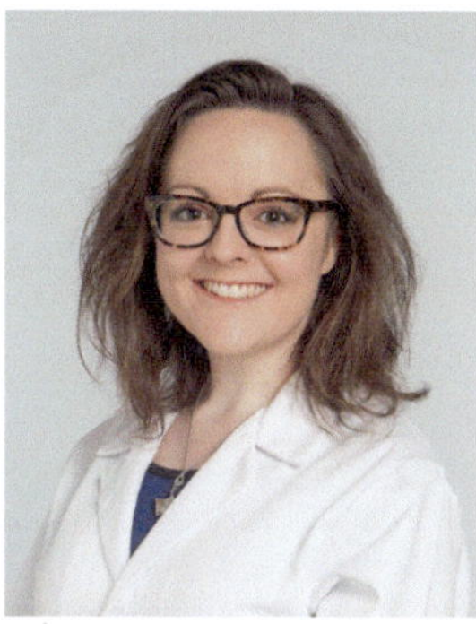

Carolyn L. Power, MD

Cleveland Clinic Library Staff (1994–2025)
"Without whom, this work would not have been possible."
Previous Staff
Gretchen Hallerberg
Jodith Janes
Kevin Kennedy
Javan Jackson
Devera Kastner
Marian Simonson
Marlene Englander
Cindy Avallone
Barb Anderson
Brian Hanna
Doug Bazdar
Antoinette Bolden
Mina Chercourt
Lorelei Woody
Kate Kretschmann
Evone Jeffries
Laura Migneco-Fretnzko
Jill Moorman
Kim Brady
Current Staff
Rosa Blackburn
Latoya Lee
Matt Weaver
Michelle Kraft
Snezana Lebinac
Loren Hackett
Theresa Kline
Neil Nero
LaDonna Pierce
DeAnna Camara
Mary Pat Harnegie
Mary Schleicher
Shelby Stuart
Olivia Davis
Shelley Ivary
Ethan Haas

James S. Wu
Michelle D. Inkster

Contents of Volume I

Contents of Volume II

Contributors

Armen Aboulian Department of Colon and Rectal Surgery, Kaiser Permanente Woodland Hills Medical Center, Woodland Hills, CA, USA

Amelia Agostinelli WOC Nursing Department, Cleveland Clinic, Cleveland, OH, USA

Eberechi S. Agwa Hematology & Medical Oncology, Cleveland Clinic, Cleveland, OH, USA

Abraham Ahmed Diagnostic Imaging and Interventional Radiology, H. Lee Moffitt Cancer Center & Research Institute, Tampa, FL, USA

Matthew T. Allemang Department of Surgery, Cleveland Clinic, Cleveland, OH, USA

Daniela Allende Pathology & Laboratory Medicine Institute, Cleveland Clinic, Cleveland, OH, USA

Jean H. Ashburn Department of Colon and Rectal Surgery, Atrium Health Wake Forest Baptist, Winston-Salem, NC, USA

H. Nail Aydin Department of Colon and Rectal Surgery, Cleveland Clinic, Cleveland, OH, USA

Joseph T. Azok Radiology & Diagnostic Imaging Institute, Cleveland Clinic, Cleveland, OH, USA

Mark E. Baker Department of Radiology, Cleveland Clinic Lerner College of Medicine, Case Western Reserve University, Cleveland, OH, USA

Joyce M. Balliet Department of Colon and Rectal Surgery, Cleveland Clinic, Cleveland, OH, USA

Hani B. Baradi Mercy Colon and Rectal Surgery, Oklahoma City, OK, USA

David C. Baringer Department of General Surgery, Cleveland Clinic, Cleveland, OH, USA

Ana E. Bennett Pathology & Laboratory Medicine Institute, Cleveland Clinic, Cleveland, OH, USA

Douglas D. Benson Rocky Mountain Colon and Rectal Surgeons, Lone Tree, CO, USA

Ajay Bhardwaj Radiology and Diagnostic Imaging Institute, Cleveland Clinic, Cleveland, OH, USA

Adarsh Bhimraj Department of Infectious Diseases, Cleveland Clinic, Cleveland, OH, USA

Vladimir Bolshinsky Department of Colorectal Surgery, Surgical Health Specialists, Melbourne, Australia

Stephen Brandstetter Department of Colon and Rectal Surgery, Cleveland Clinic Akron General Hospital, Akron, OH, USA

Aaron Brzezinski Department of Gastroenterology, Cleveland Clinic, Cleveland, OH, USA

Sean W. Carlson Department of Radiology, UPMC Children's Hospital of Pittsburgh, Pittsburgh, PA, USA

Christi M. Cavaliere Department of Surgery, Section of Plastic Surgery, Louis Stokes Cleveland VA Medical Center, Cleveland, OH, USA

Sricharan Chalikonda Department of Surgery Allegheny Health Network, Pittsburgh, PA, USA

Michael O. Christian Radiology & Diagnostic Imaging Institute, Cleveland Clinic, Cleveland, OH, USA

James M. Church Department of Colon and Rectal Surgery, Cleveland Clinic, Cleveland, OH, USA

Michael S. Cline Department of Gastroenterology, Cleveland Clinic, Cleveland, OH, USA

Mark A. H. Cohen Radiology & Diagnostic Imaging Institute, Cleveland Clinic, Cleveland, OH, USA

Bradley L. Cole Radiology & Diagnostic Imaging Institute, Cleveland Clinic, Cleveland, OH, USA

Michael W. Cruise Pathology & Laboratory Medicine Institute, Cleveland Clinic, Cleveland, OH, USA

John P. Cullen Department of Colon and Rectal Surgery, Cleveland Clinic, Cleveland, OH, USA

Christopher R. Daigle Department of Surgery, Cleveland Clinic Akron General Hospital, Akron, OH, USA

Amber N. Dalton Dermatology & Plastic Surgery Center, Cleveland Clinic, Cleveland, OH, USA

Robert L. DeBernardo, Jr. Ob/Gyn & Women's Health Institute, Cleveland Clinic, Cleveland, OH, USA

Sandra Dellaportas Department of Internal Medicine, Cleveland Clinic, Cleveland, OH, USA

David W. Dietz Department of Surgery, NYU Langone Medical Center, New York, NY, USA

Lewis A. Diulus III Crystal Plastic Surgeons, Akron, OH, USA

Apollo A. Draco Information Technology Institute, Cleveland Clinic, Cleveland, OH, USA

Richard L. Drake Department of Anatomy, Cleveland Clinic Lerner College of Medicine, Cleveland, OH, USA

John A. Dumot Department of Gastroenterology, University Hospitals of Cleveland, Cleveland, OH, USA

David M. Einstein Radiology & Diagnostic Imaging Institute, Cleveland Clinic, Cleveland, OH, USA

Mohamed I. El Hag Pathology and Laboratory Medicine Institute, Cleveland Clinic, Cleveland, OH, USA

Charis Eng Genomic Medicine Institute and Center for Personalized Genetic Healthcare, Cleveland Clinic, Cleveland, OH, USA

Victor W. Fazio Department of Colon and Rectal Surgery, Cleveland Clinic, Cleveland, OH, USA

Jesus Flores Department of Colon and Rectal Surgery, Cleveland Clinic, Cleveland, OH, USA

Catherine L. Forse Department of Pathology and Laboratory Medicine, Faculty of Medicine, University of Ottawa, Ottawa, ON, Canada

Robert D. Fry Department of Colon and Rectal Surgery, University of Pennsylvania, Philadelphia, PA, USA

Gwendolyn A. Fuller Medical Illustration Team, Enterprise Creative Services, Cleveland Clinic, Cleveland, OH, USA

Clifton G. Fulmer Pathology & Laboratory Medicine Institute, Cleveland Clinic, Cleveland, OH, USA

Thomas E. Garofalo Department of Colon and Rectal Surgery, Cleveland Clinic, Cleveland, OH, USA

Susan L. Gearhart Department of General and Colon & Rectal Surgery, Johns Hopkins Bayview Medical Center, Baltimore, MD, USA

John R. Goldblum Pathology & Laboratory Medicine Institute, Cleveland Clinic, Cleveland, OH, USA

David Hernandez Gonzalo Department of Pathology, Immunology and Laboratory Medicine, University of Florida, Gainesville, FL, USA

Ilyssa O. Gordon Pathology & Laboratory Medicine Institute, Cleveland Clinic, Cleveland, OH, USA

Emre Gorgun Department of Colon and Rectal Surgery, Cleveland Clinic, Cleveland, OH, USA

Ihab S. Haddadin Radiology & Diagnostic Imaging Institute, Cleveland Clinic, Cleveland, OH, USA

Amer A. Hanano Radiology and Diagnostic Imaging Institute, Cleveland Clinic Florida, Weston, FL, USA

James M. Hekman Department of Internal Medicine, Cleveland Clinic, Cleveland, OH, USA

Alexander G. Heriot Department Colorectal Surgery, Peter MacCallum Cancer Centre, Melbourne, Australia

Brian T. Hill Cleveland Clinic Taussig Cancer Institute, Cleveland Clinic, Cleveland, OH, USA

Barbara J. Hocevar Rupert B. Turnbull, Jr., School of WOC Nursing Education, Cleveland Clinic, Cleveland, OH, USA

David A. Horvath Plastic and Cosmetic Surgery, Abbington, PA, USA

Emily Hromi Cleveland Clinic Center for Medical Art and Photography, MI, USA

Emina H. Huang Department of Surgery, University of Texas Southwestern, Dallas, TX, USA

Tracy L. Hull Department of Colon and Rectal Surgery, Cleveland Clinic, Cleveland, OH, USA

Tasadooq Hussain Department of General and Colorectal Surgery, Wrightington Wigan & Leigh Teaching Hospitals NHS Foundation Trust, Manchester, UK

Michelle D. Inkster Department of Gastroenterology, Cleveland Clinic, Cleveland, OH, USA

Katharine L. Jackson Department of Colorectal Surgery, Department of Surgery, Duke University, Durham, NC, USA

Deepa Jagadeesh Cleveland Clinic Taussig Cancer Institute, Cleveland, OH, USA

David G. Jagelman Department of Colon and Rectal Surgery, Cleveland Clinic, Cleveland, OH, USA

Paul C. Janicki Radiology & Diagnostic Imaging Institute, Cleveland Clinic, Cleveland, OH, USA

Sami S. Judeeba Department of Colon and Rectal Surgery, Cleveland Clinic, Cleveland, OH, USA

Leonard A. Kahn Radiology & Diagnostic Imaging Institute, Cleveland Clinic, Cleveland, OH, USA

Hermann Kessler Department of Colon and Rectal Surgery, Cleveland Clinic, Cleveland, OH, USA

Scott E. Kilpatrick Pathology and Laboratory Institute, Cleveland Clinic, Cleveland, OH, USA

Ira J. Kodner Department of Colon and Rectal Surgery, Washington University School of Medicine, St. Louis, MO, USA

Matthew D. Kroh Department of General Surgery, Digestive Diseases Institute, Cleveland Clinic, Cleveland, OH, USA

Kenneth G. Kula Center for Medical Art and Photography, Cleveland Clinic, Cleveland, OH, USA

Keith K. Lai Pathology & Laboratory Medicine Institute, Cleveland Clinic, Cleveland, OH, USA

Irene C. Lalak Department of Dermatology, Cleveland Clinic, Cleveland, OH, USA

James E. Lapinski Pathology & Laboratory Medicine Institute, Cleveland Clinic, Cleveland, OH, USA

Ian C. Lavery Department of Colon and Rectal Surgery, Cleveland Clinic, Cleveland, OH, USA

Brandie Leach Genomic Medicine Institute and Center for Personalized Genetic Healthcare, Cleveland Clinic, Cleveland, OH, USA

Jason E. Leedy Cleveland Plastic Surgery Institute, Mayfield Heights, OH, USA

Jennifer J. Liang Department of Colon and Rectal Surgery, Cleveland Clinic, Cleveland, OH, USA

Susan A. Lintala Department of Gastroenterology, Cleveland Clinic, Cleveland, OH, USA

David Liska Department of Colon and Rectal Surgery, Cleveland Clinic, Cleveland, OH, USA

Careen Y. Lowder Cole Cye Institute, Cleveland Clinic, Cleveland, OH, USA

Sanford S. Luria Glickman Urological & Kidney Institute, Cleveland Clinic, Cleveland, OH, USA

Paresh Mahajan Radiology & Diagnostic Imaging Institute, Cleveland Clinic, Cleveland, OH, USA

Christian G. Massier Department of General Surgery, Cleveland Clinic, Cleveland, OH, USA

Jennifer M. McBride Department of Anatomy, Cleveland Clinic Lerner College of Medicine, Cleveland, OH, USA

Kelsey E. McHugh Department of Laboratory Medicine and Pathology, Mayo Clinic, Phoenix, AZ, USA

Mark J. Melaragno Pathology & Laboratory Medicine Institute, Cleveland Clinic, Cleveland, OH, USA

Amanda C. Mendelsohn Medical Illustration Team, Enterprise Creative Services, Cleveland Clinic, Cleveland, OH, USA

Carla R. Merrick Department of Colon and Rectal Surgery, Cleveland Clinic, Cleveland, OH, USA

Chad M. Michener Ob/Gyn and Women's Health Institute, Cleveland Clinic, Cleveland, OH, USA

Ryan M. Miller Department of Infectious Diseases, Cleveland Clinic, Cleveland, OH, USA

William J. O'Brien Department of Surgery, Cleveland Clinic, Cleveland, OH, USA

Patrick J. O'Keefe Radiology & Diagnostic Imaging Institute, Cleveland Clinic, Cleveland, OH, USA

Charles M. O'Malley, Jr. Radiology & Diagnostic Imaging Institute, Cleveland Clinic, Cleveland, OH, USA

Robert S. O'Shea Department of Gastroenterology and Hepatology, Cleveland Clinic, Cleveland, OH, USA

Rish K. Pai Department of Laboratory Medicine and Pathology, Mayo Clinic, Phoenix, AZ, USA

Joseph A. Pangrace CMI, Medical Illustration Team, Enterprise Creative Services, Cleveland Clinic, Cleveland, OH, USA

Arthur A. Parsee Department of Diagnostic Radiology, H. Lee Moffitt Cancer Center and Research Institute, Tampa, FL, USA

Theodore E. Partridge Department of Surgical Services, South Pointe Hospital, Warrensville Heights, OH, USA

Jessica R. Philpott Department of Gastroenterology, Cleveland Clinic, Cleveland, OH, USA

Melissa Piliang Dermatology & Plastic Surgery Center, Cleveland Clinic, Cleveland, OH, USA

Carolyn L. Power Department of Colon and Rectal Surgery, Cleveland Clinic, Cleveland, OH, USA

Gary W. Procop Pathology & Laboratory Medicine Institute, Cleveland Clinic, Cleveland, OH, USA

Andrei S. Purysko Department of Diagnostic Radiology, Cleveland Clinic, Cleveland, OH, USA

Erick M. Remer Radiology & Diagnostic Imaging Institute, Cleveland Clinic, Cleveland, OH, USA

Feza H. Remzi Inflammatory Bowel Disease Center, NYU Langone Health, New York, NY, USA

Florian Rieder Department of Gastroenterology, Hepatology and Nutrition, Digestive Disease Institute, Cleveland Clinic, Cleveland, OH, USA

Alain G. Rizk Radiology and Diagnostic Imaging Institute, Cleveland Clinic, Cleveland, OH, USA

Scott A. Robertson Pathology & Laboratory Medicine Institute, Cleveland Clinic, Cleveland, OH, USA

Samuel Ruskin Radiology & Diagnostic Imaging Institute, Cleveland Clinic, Cleveland, OH, USA

Chizu Sakai-Imoto WOC Nursing Department, Cleveland Clinic, Cleveland, OH, USA

Janice M. Santisi Digestive Diseases and Surgery Institute, Cleveland Clinic, Cleveland, OH, USA

Erica C. Savage Pathology & Laboratory Medicine Institute, Cleveland Clinic, Cleveland, OH, USA

Thomas K. Schroeder Department of Colon and Rectal Surgery, Cleveland Clinic, Cleveland, OH, USA

Dawn M. Schultz Department of Nursing, Cleveland Clinic, Cleveland, OH, USA

Sebouh Setrakian Pathology & Laboratory Medicine Institute, Cleveland Clinic, Cleveland, OH, USA

Nafis Shafizadeh Department of Pathology, Kaiser Permanente Woodland Hills Medical Center, Woodland Hills, CA, USA

Sherief Shawki Department of Colon and Rectal Surgery, Mayo Clinic Rochester, Rochester, MN, USA

Shu-Jane Shen Radiology and Diagnostic Imaging Institute, Cleveland Clinic, Cleveland, OH, USA

Lena J. Slater-Everhart Department of Surgical Services, South Pointe Hospital, Warrensville Heights, OH, USA

Luca Stocchi Department of Colon and Rectal Surgery, Mayo Clinic, Jacksonville, FL, USA

Todd W. Stultz Radiology & Diagnostic Imaging Institute, Cleveland Clinic, Cleveland, OH, USA

Charles D. Sturgis Hospital Pathology Associates/Allina, Minneapolis, MN, USA

Jacob R. Sweeney Pathology & Laboratory Medicine Institute, Cleveland Clinic, Cleveland, OH, USA

Ursula M. Szmulowicz Department of Colon and Rectal Surgery, Cleveland Clinic, Cleveland, OH, USA

Marisa Tungsiripat Department of Infectious Diseases, Cleveland Clinic, Cleveland, OH, USA

Ralph J. Tuthill Pathology & Laboratory Medicine Institute, Cleveland Clinic, Cleveland, OH, USA

Michael A. Valente Department of Colon and Rectal Surgery, Cleveland Clinic, Cleveland, OH, USA

Ryan D. Ward Radiology & Diagnostic Imaging Institute, Cleveland Clinic, Cleveland, OH, USA

Kenneth D. Webster Department of Obstetrics and Gynecology, Cleveland Clinic, Cleveland, OH, USA

Homer O. Wiland Department of Pathology, OhioHealth Mansfield Hospital, Mansfield, OH, USA

Eric W. Willis Department of Pathology, CORPath, Columbus, OH, USA

Erika B. Woodrum Medical Illustration Team, Enterprise Creative Services, Cleveland Clinic, Cleveland, OH, USA

James S. Wu Department of Colon and Rectal Surgery, Cleveland Clinic, Cleveland, OH, USA

Jing-Jing Yang Departments of Pathology, Medical Diagnostic Laboratories, LLC, Hamilton, NJ, USA

Douglas W. Yoder Department of Surgery, Blanchard Valley Health System, Findlay, OH, USA

Craig D. Zippe Glickman Urological & Kidney Institute, Cleveland Clinic, Cleveland, OH, USA

Gregory Zuccaro, Jr. Department of Gastroenterology, Cleveland Clinic, Cleveland, OH, USA

Massarat Zutshi Department of Colon and Rectal Surgery, Cleveland Clinic, Cleveland, OH, USA

The original version of the book has been revised. A correction to this book can be found at https://doi.org/10.1007/978-3-031-39880-3_236

1 Surgical Diagnosis: Albert A. Berg, MD

Michelle D. Inkster and James S. Wu

Presentation

In 1905, Dr. Albert Berg published a *Manual for Students and Practitioners* entitled *Surgical Diagnosis*.[1] This massive work covered the head and neck, breast, chest, mediastinum, gastrointestinal tract, urinary system, genitalia, and orthopedics in 54 chapters, all written by a single author. Dr. Berg's approach to surgical diagnosis begins with the examiner.

SURGICAL DIAGNOSIS
A MANUAL
FOR STUDENTS AND PRACTITIONERS
BY
ALBERT A. BERG, M.D.
Adjunct Attending Surgeon to the
Mount Sinai Hospital,
New York

PART I.
General Considerations on Diagnosis.
Chapter I.

[1]Berg AA. Surgical Diagnosis. A manual for students and practitioners, Part I., General Considerations on Diagnosis. Lea Brothers & Co., New York and Philadelphia, 1905, Chapter I., pages 17–19.

M. D. Inkster
Department of Gastroenterology, Cleveland Clinic, Cleveland, OH, USA

J. S. Wu (✉)
Department of Colon and Rectal Surgery, Cleveland Clinic, Cleveland, OH, USA

J. S. Wu, M. D. Inkster (eds.), *Cleveland Clinic Colorectal Case Studies*,
https://doi.org/10.1007/978-3-031-39880-3_1

THE EXAMINER—THE TAKING OF THE CLINICAL HISTORY—THE EXAMINATION OF THE PATIENT.

"Success in diagnosis depends upon a careful elicitation of the patient's history and symptoms and upon their logical interpretation. The former demands from the examiner painstaking effort and the sharp use of all his senses; the latter his keenest judgment. Experience trains his discriminating faculties; it teaches him the relative clinical importance of the facts that have been elicited in the anamnesis and examination; it helps him draw conclusions quickly and accurately. The sharper his senses, the better his judgment, and the wider his experience, so much the quicker and so much the more accurate will his diagnosis be. No diagnosis should rest on intuition; it should be the result of a rapid examination, a keen appreciation of the important symptoms, and their significance.

For the beginner in diagnostics, it is essential that the investigation into the history and the examination of the patient be made in a systematic manner. While questioning the patient, the examiner should take note of his general characteristics: the demeanor, the psychical condition (whether hysterical, hypochondriacal, etc.), the accuracy with which statements are made; he should endeavor to dispel fear, or shyness, and to encourage confidence. In eliciting the clinical history, attention should be given to what are apparently minor facts. No point is so small, no symptom so slight, but that it may have quite an important bearing on the diagnosis.

It is to be remembered that the clinical evidences of disease are the most important; the laboratory results aid, elaborate, and substantiate, the bedside findings; they never replace them."

Anatomy-Colon

2

Carolyn L. Power, Jennifer M. McBride, Richard L. Drake, Arthur A. Parsee, and James S. Wu

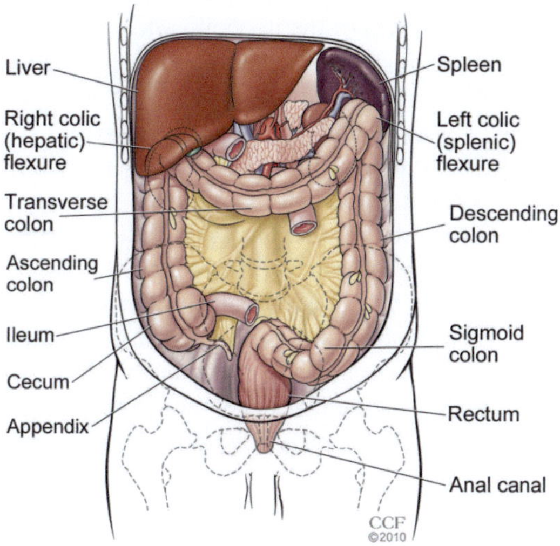

Anatomy-abdomen

C. L. Power · J. S. Wu (✉)
Department of Colon and Rectal Surgery, Cleveland Clinic, Cleveland, OH, USA

J. M. McBride · R. L. Drake
Department of Anatomy, Cleveland Clinic Lerner College of Medicine, Cleveland, OH, USA

A. A. Parsee
Department of Diagnostic Radiology, H. Lee Moffitt Cancer Center and Research Institute, Tampa, FL, USA

J. S. Wu, M. D. Inkster (eds.), *Cleveland Clinic Colorectal Case Studies*,
https://doi.org/10.1007/978-3-031-39880-3_2

Colon Anatomy

The large intestine consists of the cecum, colon, and rectum [1]. The appendix marks the beginning, and the anus marks the end (Fig. 2.1). The cecum is continuous with the small intestine and is typically situated in the right lower quadrant. The appendix is supplied by the appendicular artery. The cecum is the part of the large intestine proximal to the entrance of the terminal ileum into the side of the colon. The posterior aspect of the cecum is variably attached to the retroperitoneum. Proceeding from the cecum superiorly to the right colic or hepatic flexure is the ascending or right colon. The right colon posterior wall is retroperitoneal. The lateral avascular peritoneal attachments of the ascending and descending colons along the right and left paracolic gutters form the "white lines of Toldt." The ascending colon derives its arterial supply from branches of the superior mesenteric artery via the colic branch of the ileocolic artery and the right colic artery. Extending from the hepatic flexure to the left colic or splenic flexure is the intraperitoneal transverse colon, suspended from the posterior abdominal wall by the transverse mesocolon. This structure is supplied primarily by the right and left branches of the middle colic artery from the superior mesenteric artery. The left or descending colon posterior wall is retroperitoneal. Similar to the right colon, there are lateral peritoneal attachments along the left paracolic gutter. The left colon blood supply is from the inferior mesenteric artery.

The sigmoid colon extends from the left colon to the rectum. The sigmoid colon is intraperitoneal and is suspended by a mesentery. It is supplied by multiple sigmoidal arteries derived from the inferior mesenteric artery. The rectum begins where the taenia coli, three longitudinal bands of smooth muscle, disappear. The rectum has lateral curves called the valves of Houston and terminates at the rectal

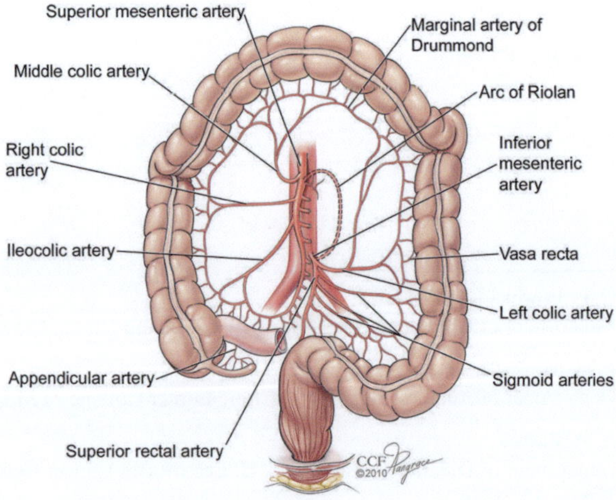

Fig. 2.1 The colon and its arterial supply

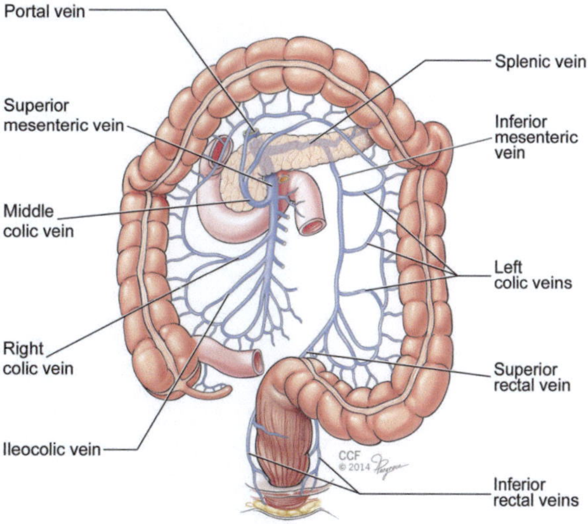

Fig. 2.2 The right and transverse colon venous drainage is by the superior mesenteric vein. Venous drainage of the left colon is by the inferior mesenteric vein. The inferior mesenteric vein joins the splenic vein which then meets the superior mesenteric vein to form the portal vein

ampulla before exiting the pelvis at the anus. The rectum is supplied by the superior rectal artery from the inferior mesenteric artery, the two middle rectal arteries from the internal iliac arteries, and the two inferior rectal arteries from the internal pudendal arteries, branches of the internal iliac arteries.

The large intestine ends at the anus, where the muscular wall of the rectum becomes the internal anal sphincter muscle. The anal canal is supplied by the inferior rectal arteries via the internal pudendal arteries.

The superior and inferior mesenteric circulations communicate by an arterioarterial anastomosis, the marginal artery of Drummond, which runs along the mesenteric edge of the large intestine.

A second arterioarterial collateral, the arc of Riolan, named after the French anatomist Jean Riolan (1580–1657), is an inconstant artery that connects the superior mesenteric artery or one of its branches to the proximal inferior mesenteric artery, classically the middle colic artery to the left colic artery [2].

Right and transverse colon venous drainage is by the superior mesenteric vein. The superior mesenteric vein joins the splenic vein to become the portal vein. The descending colon, sigmoid colon, and proximal rectum are drained by the inferior mesenteric vein. The inferior mesenteric vein joins the splenic vein behind the pancreas (Fig. 2.2).

A radiograph of the colon with air contrast is shown in Fig. 2.3.

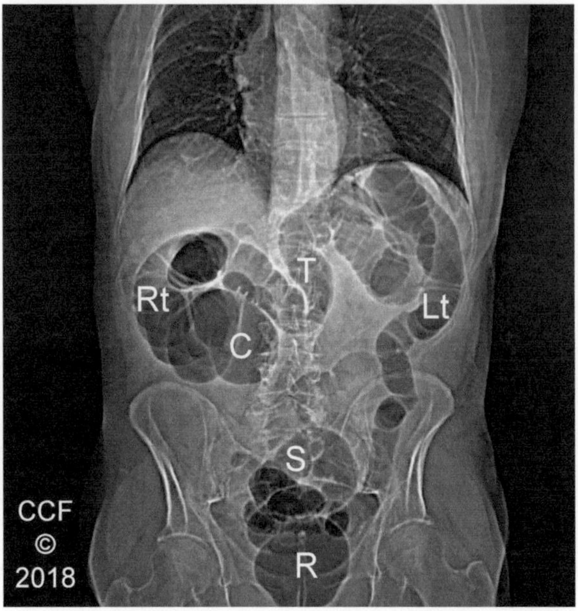

Fig. 2.3 Radiograph of the colon with carbon dioxide insufflation shows the cecum (C), right colon (Rt), transverse colon (T), left colon (Lt), sigmoid colon (S), and rectum (R)

Biographical Note

Hamilton Drummond, MB, BS. Durh, FRCSEd, Major RAMC(T)

Hamilton Drummond graduated, MB, BS, Durham, in 1906 and took the Fellowship of the Royal College of Surgeons of Edinburgh in 1912 [3]. At the outbreak of World War I, he held a commission as a combatant officer in the Northumberland Yeomanry. He was present at the first battle of Ypres and at Neuve Chappelle. In 1917, Captains Fraser and Drummond published their experience with 300 perforating wounds of the abdomen [4]. They found that uncomplicated wounds of the small intestine, which are suitable for suture, recover. Wounds of the colon, however, even when uncomplicated portend a grave prognosis due to infection. He defined the anatomy of the marginal artery that bears his name in 1913 [5].[1] Drummond wrote he found that "by injecting the ileocolic artery at its origin from the superior mesenteric vessel, and with ligatures placed on the right middle and left colic, and the sigmoid branches at points near their origin, that the vessels forming the marginal artery from the cæcum to the middle of the pelvic colon were well filled."

Following ligation of the inferior mesenteric artery, viability of the left colon is preserved by collateral perfusion from the superior mesenteric system through the marginal artery (Fig. 2.4).

[1] Drummond [5]. Permission to republish Figure 4 and the cited excerpt was generously granted by Mr. Craig Myles, under the STM Guidelines, SAGE Ltd. Permissions Team, Ticket numbers RP-5893, August 2, 2021, and RP 6109, September 2, 2021.

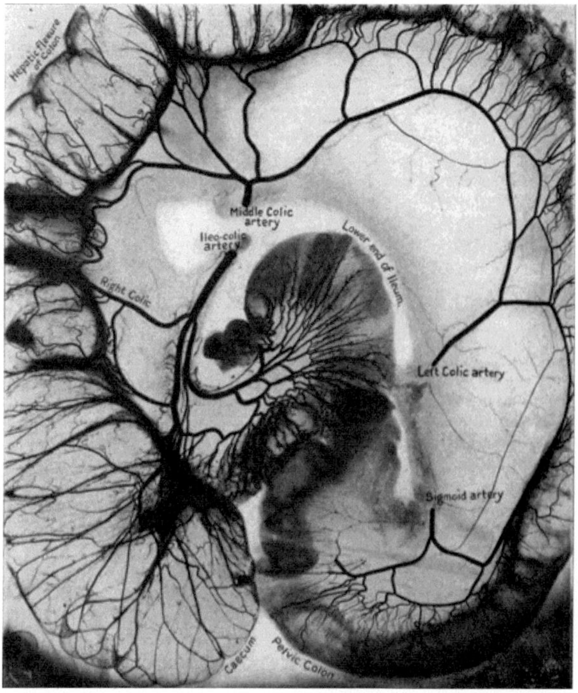

Fig. 2.4 The marginal artery as demonstrated by Drummond in 1913. The whole colon specimen was injected through the ileocolic artery. The injection travels into the pelvic colon area

References

1. Drake RL, Vogl W, Mitchell AWM. 2023. Gray's Anatomy for Students. 5th ed. Philadelphia: Elsevier. https://www.us.elsevierhealth.com/grays-anatomy-for-students-97803239334237.html.
2. Binit S, Mittal MK. Arc of Riolan. Indian J Med Res. 2014;139:965–6.
3. Drummond H. Obituary. Br Med J. 1925;2:181–2.
4. Fraser J, Drummond H. A clinical and experimental study of three hundred perforating wounds of the abdomen. Br Med J. 1917;1:321–30.
5. Drummond H. Some points relating to the surgical anatomy of the arterial supply of the large intestine. Proc R Soc Med. 1914;7:185–93.

Anatomy-Intestinal Mesenteries

3

Carolyn L. Power, Amanda C. Mendelsohn,
Jennifer M. McBride, Richard L. Drake, and James S. Wu

Intestinal Mesenteries

Merriam-Webster's Dictionary defines "mesentery" as follows:

> "One or more vertebrate membranes that consist of a double fold of the peritoneum and invest the intestines and their appendages and connect them with the dorsal wall of the abdominal cavity [1]."

The jejunum, ileum, transverse colon, and sigmoid colon are intraperitoneal structures that are attached to the dorsal abdominal cavity by mesenteries [2]. These mesenteries allow for some movement of the viscera to which they attach. They also provide a route for vessels, nerves, and lymphatics to reach these organs. The cecum is a mobile intraperitoneal structure that normally is not suspended in the peritoneal cavity by a mesentery. The vascular supply to the appendix is encased in the meso-appendix. The transverse mesocolon crosses from the hepatic flexure to the splenic flexure. The sigmoid mesocolon is situated near the bifurcation of the left common iliac artery. The mesentery of the jejunum and the ileum appears in the left upper quadrant just distal to the ligament of Treitz and travels distally toward its

C. L. Power · J. S. Wu (✉)
Department of Colon and Rectal Surgery, Cleveland Clinic, Cleveland, OH, USA

A. C. Mendelsohn
Medical Illustration Team, Enterprise Creative Services, Cleveland Clinic, Cleveland, OH, USA

J. M. McBride · R. L. Drake
Department of Anatomy, Cleveland Clinic Lerner College of Medicine, Cleveland, OH, USA

J. S. Wu, M. D. Inkster (eds.), *Cleveland Clinic Colorectal Case Studies*,
https://doi.org/10.1007/978-3-031-39880-3_3

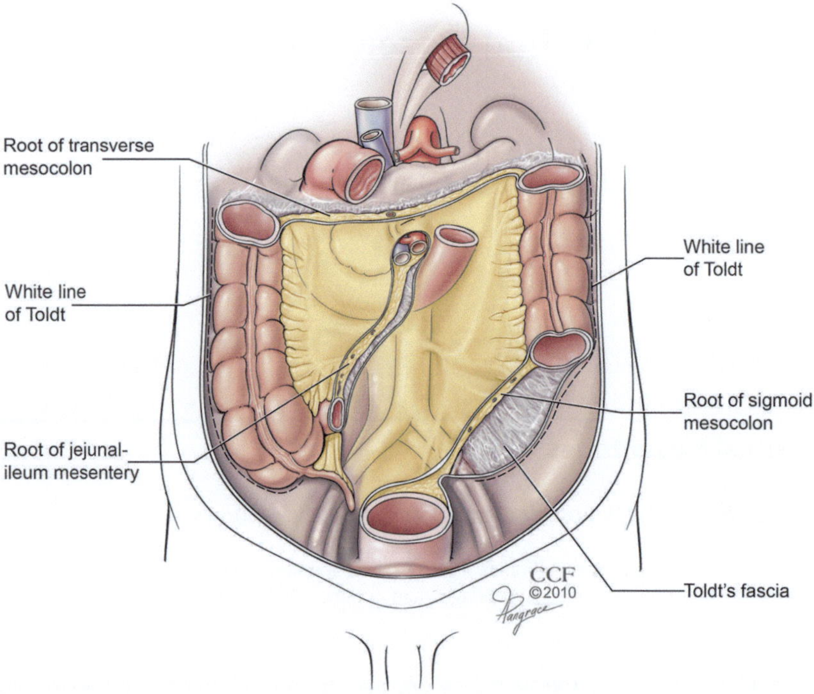

Fig. 3.1 The posterior abdominal wall attachments of the mesenteries to the transverse colon, sigmoid colon, and jejunum/ileum are depicted with the intestine removed. The mesoappendix is seen attached at the appendix. The right and left colons are fixed; they are separated from the posterior abdominal wall by a connective tissue plane (Toldt's fascia)

termination in the right lower quadrant at the ascending colon (Fig. 3.1). The mesenteries of the right and left colon persist into adulthood and remain separated from the posterior abdominal wall by a connective tissue plane formed by fusion of the visceral and parietal peritoneum (Toldt's fascia) [3].

During development, the right colon, the left colon, and their mesenteries become attached to the retroperitoneum; the visceral peritoneum covers the mesentery, but the parietal peritoneum covers the retroperitoneum. This process was illustrated in Toldt's *Atlas of Human Anatomy* (Figs. 3.2 and 3.3) [4, 5].

Anatomischer Atlas Für Studierende und Ärzte unter Mitwirkung von Professor Dr. Allois Dalla Rosa herausgegeben von Dr. Carl Toldt Professor der Anatomie an der Universität Wien	An Atlas of Human Anatomy for Students and Physicians By Carl Toldt, M.D. Professor of Anatomy University of Vienna Assisted by Professor Alois Dalla Rosa, M.D. Translated by M. Eden Paul, M.D., Brux., M.R.C.S., L.R.C.P.

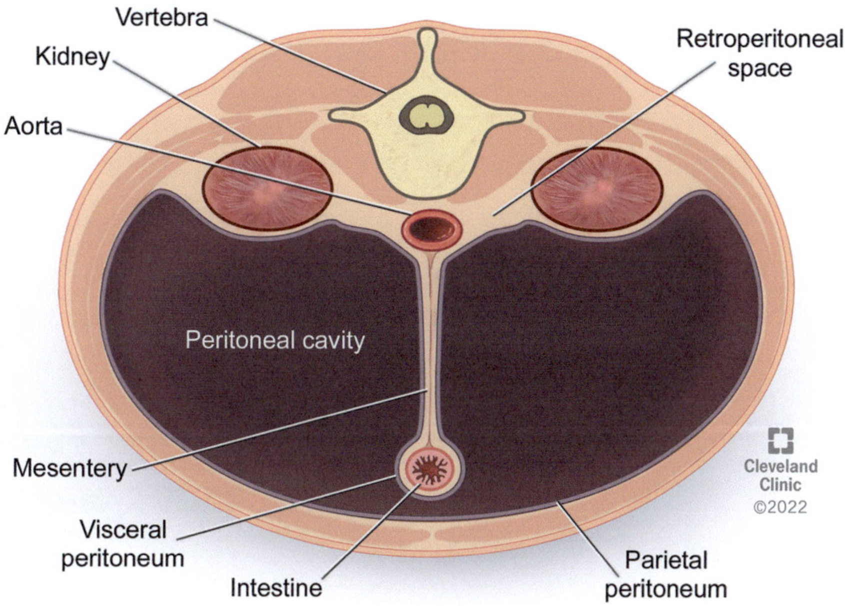

Fig. 3.2 After Toldt (Fig. 657)

Fig 657. Darmstück mit freier, durch eine Tunica serosa geglätteter Oberfläche und freier Beweglichkeit. Verbindung mit der Wand des Eingeweideraumes durch ein freies Gekröse, Mesenterium. Wandteil und Eingeweideteil des Bauchfelles. Schema.

Fig 657.—Portion of intestine, freely mobile, the outer surface having a serous investment (tunica serosa). Connected with the wall of the body-cavity (coelom) by means of a free mesentery. Parietal and visceral layers of the peritoneum. Diagrammatic.

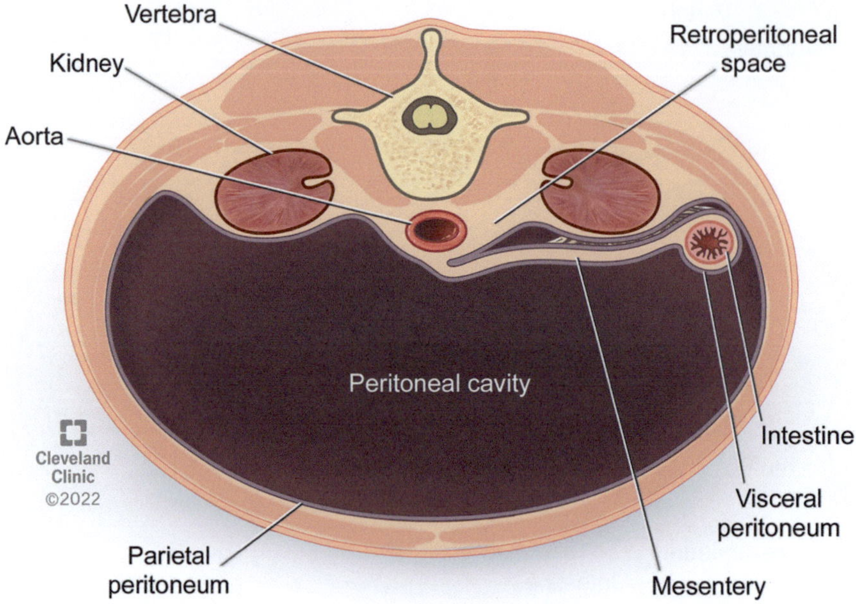

Fig. 3.3 After Toldt (Fig. 658)

Fig. 658. Sekundäre Festheftung eines ursprünglich frei beweglichen Eingeweideteiles (Colon descendens) an der Rumpfwand. Primäres und sekundäres Peritonaeum parietale, Spatium retroperitonaeale, Retroperitonäalraum. Schema.	Fig. 658.—Secondary adhesion to the body-wall of a portion of intestine, originally freely mobile. Primary and secondary parietal peritoneum. Diagrammatic.

References

1. "Mesentery." Merriam-Webster.com Dictionary, Merriam-Webster, https://www.merriam-webster.com/dictionary/mesentery (Accessed 13 June 2022).
2. Drake RL, Vogl W, Mitchell AWM. 2023. Gray's Anatomy for Students. 5th ed., Philadelphia: Elsevier.
3. Culligan K, Coffey JC, Kiran RP, Kalady M, Lavery IC, Remzi FH. The mesocolon: a prospective observational study. Colorectal Dis. 2012;14:421–30.
4. Toldt C, Dalla Rosa A. Splanchnologia. Die Eingeweidelehre. Anatomischer Atlas für Studierende und Ärzte, Achte, Vermehrte und Verbesserte Auflage, vierte Lieferung, Urban & Schwarzenberg, Berlin, 1914;408. Accessed from Archive.org, August 15, 2022.
5. Toldt C, Dalla Rosa A, Paul ME. Splanchnologia Splanchology. In: An Atlas of Human Anatomy for Students and Physicians. New York: Rebman Company; 1904. p. 408. Accessed from Google books, July 1, 2018.

Anatomy-Ileocecal Valve

4

Michelle D. Inkster and James S. Wu

Presentation

Varolius' Valve, Tulp's Valve, Bauhin's Valve, Ileocecal Valve

In their 1932 description of terminal ileitis, Crohn, Ginsburg, and Oppenheimer described the following characteristic physical findings [1]:

> "The characteristic, fully developed hypertrophic process is, as a rule, limited to the distal 25 to 35 cm. (10–14 inches) of the terminal ileum, including the ileal side of Bauhin's valve and terminating rather abruptly at that point."

Before Bauhin, two others described the same structure. In 1573, the Italian anatomist, Costanzo Varoli in his work *Anatomiæ de corporis humani (Anatomy of the Human Body),* stated that he named the *operculum ilii* [2]:

quam ego eiusdem inuentor operculum ilii appello.	It is I who has invented the name of the lid of the ileum.

In 1641, Nicolai Tulp of Amsterdam published *Obersevationes Medicae*, which contained more than 200 systematically organized case histories [3]. In the 1685 edition, Chapter XXI, *Valvula intestinalis*, includes an engraved image labeled *valvula penduli* (pendulum valve) at the junction between the large and the small intestines [4]. In 1605, the Swiss anatomist, Gaspard Bauhin in his *Theatrum Anatomicum,* included Tabula XV (Plate XV) that depicts the *Coli Valvvlam* (colonic valve), a structure located in between the small and large intestines [5, 6].

M. D. Inkster
Department of Gastroenterology, Cleveland Clinic, Cleveland, OH, USA

J. S. Wu (✉)
Department of Colon and Rectal Surgery, Cleveland Clinic, Cleveland, OH, USA

J. S. Wu, M. D. Inkster (eds.), *Cleveland Clinic Colorectal Case Studies*,
https://doi.org/10.1007/978-3-031-39880-3_4

Tabula xv Intestinorum tam tenuium, quam crassorum figorum et ductus, Coli Valvvlam, ani muculos et intestinorum tunicus exprimit.	Plate XV Figures of intestines thin and thick and duct, colonic valve, anal muscle and intestinal tunics are identified.

The common structure to which these three pioneering anatomists referred now is known as the ileocecal valve. The name "valve" given by both Tulp and Bauhin to this structure between the ileum and colon defined its function.

Valvular Action

> "The term "valve" stems from the Latin "valva" meaning leaf or fold, and indicates, by definition, a device for regulating or determining the direction of flow of a liquid, gas, etc., by means of a movable part which opens and closes a passage. From a physiological standpoint, the criterion of a competent valve is unidirectional flow."
> Elliott C. Lasser, Leo G. Rigler, 1954 [7]

In his posthumous papers, published in 1861, John Hunter wrote the following concerning the ileocecal valve [8].

ESSAYS AND OBSERVATIONS
ON
NATURAL HISTORY, ANATOMY,
PHYSIOLOGY, PSYCHOLOGY, AND GEOLOGY
Of the Intestines
By John Hunter, F. R. S.

> "However, this maybe, it is certain that the fæces have not such a quick passage, therefore, must become putrid; which was the cause perhaps of a valve at the termination of the ileum, that these putrid contents might not regurgitate."

In 1950, Fleischner and Bernstein [9] published a comparative roentgen-anatomical study of the ileocecal valve on the basis of normal postmortem specimens and roentgenograms paving the way for the accurate translation of "shadow-pictures" in terms of normal and morbid anatomy. In 1954, Lasser and Rigler [10] demonstrated with barium that the valve can tolerate pressure from the colon side and remain "competent." They also demonstrated that with increasing cecal distension, the valve may become incompetent (Fig. 4.1).

Correlations applicable to clinical practice include:

1. Ileocecal valve competency

   In cases of large bowel obstruction, if the ileocecal valve remains competent, colon ischemia or perforation may ensue as succus entericus and air move antegrade from the small to the large bowel. If the valve becomes incompetent, colonic pressure may decompress into the small intestine.

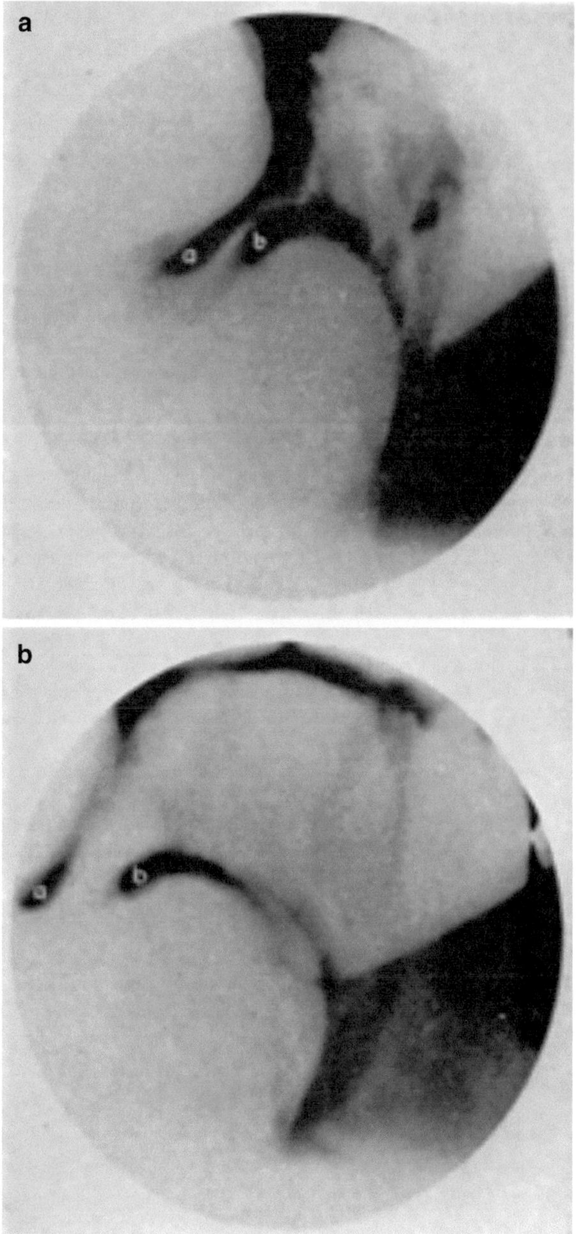

Fig. 4.1 Lasser and Rigler. Ileocecal valve studies with increasing distension of the cecum: (**a**) upper lip, (**b**) lower lip. (**a**) Competent ileocecal valve with the upper and lower lips in approximation; (**b**) The effect of increasing distention of the cecum is here shown. The valve is now incompetent

2. Ileocecal valve hypertrophy

   Hypertrophy of the ileocecal valve may lead to small bowel obstruction attributed to "ileocecal valve syndrome" [11].
3. Ileocecal valve absence [12]

   Surgical removal of the ileocecal valve as part of right colectomy may lead to frequent loose bowel motions.

References

1. Crohn BB, Ginzburg L, Oppenheimer GD. Regional ileitis. A pathologic and clinical entity. J Am Med Assoc. 1932;99:1323–9.
2. Constantii Varolii, Philosophi ac Medici Bononiensis Anatomiæ, sive de Resolvtione Corporis Hvmani ad Cæfarem Mediouillanum libri IIII: a Cortesio IB, ac Mercvriali VC. [Internet]. Francofvrti: Apud Ioannem Wechelum & Petrum Fischerum confortes; 1591; p 70. [cited 2019 Mar 14]. Available from: https://www.google.com/books/edition/Constantii_Varolii_philosophi_ac_medici/u3GiXwAACAAJ?hl=en
3. Koehler PJ. Prevalence of headache in Tulp's *Observationes Medicae* (1641) with a description of cluster headache. Cephalalgia. 1993;13:318–20.
4. Nicolai Tvlpii Amstelredamensis. Obersevationes Medicæ. Amstelædami, apud Henricum Wetstenium, 1585;210–212. Accessed from Google books, March 15, 2020.
5. Bauhin C. Caspari Bauhini, Basileensis: Theatrvm Anatomicum Novis figuris aeneis Illustratum et in lucem emissum opera sumptibus Theodori de Bry p.m. relicta viduae filiorum. Francofurti at [sic] Moenum: Typis M. Beckeri; 1605. Retrieved from: https://archive.org/details/BIUSante_31867/
6. Bauhin C. Caspari Bauhini: Theatrvm anatomicum novis figuris aeneis illustratum et in lucem emissum opera sumptibus Theodori de Bry p.m. relicta viduae filiorum. Francofurti at [sic] Moenum: Typis M. Beckeri. Retrieved from Google books; 1605. p. 116.
7. Lasser EC, Rigler LG. Observations on the structure and function of the ileocecal valve. Radiology. 1954;63:176–83. Permission to republish Figure 1 (A and B) was granted by RNSA, Radiological Society of North America, Order No.: 8001839101; Order date: 08/02/2021
8. Hunter J. Of the Intestines. In: Essays and Observations on Natural History, Anatomy, Physiology, Psychology, and Geology, vol. I. London, John Van Voorst: Paternoster Row; 1861. p. 148–9. Accessed from Google books, September 8, 2022.
9. Fleischner FG, Bernstein C. Roentgen-anatomical studies of the normal ileocecal valve. Radiology. 1950;54:43–58.
10. Lasser EC, Rigler LG. Observations on the structure and function of the ileocecal valve. Radiology. 1954;63:176–83.
11. Nesher E, Schreiber L, Werbin N. Bauhin's ileocecal valve syndrome—A rare cause for small-bowel obstruction: Report of a case. Dis Colon Rectum. 2006;49:527–9.
12. Gazet J-C. The surgical significance of the ileo-caecal junction. Ann R Coll Surg Engl. 1968;43:19–38.

Anatomy-Small Intestine

5

Carolyn L. Power, Jennifer M. McBride, Richard L. Drake, and James S. Wu

Presentation

The small intestine originates at the pylorus of the stomach and terminates at the ileocecal fold, also known as the "bloodless fold of Treves" [1]. Consisting of the duodenum, jejunum, and ileum, this hollow tube narrows in diameter from beginning to end, spanning approximately six to seven meters in length. It is the longest part of the gastrointestinal tract (Fig. 5.1) [2]. The primitive gut tube, from which the gastrointestinal tract is derived, can be divided into three regions: foregut, midgut, and hindgut. The proximal duodenum is a foregut derivative. From the major duodenal papilla, the remainder of the small intestine is derived from the midgut. The first part of the small intestine, the duodenum, is a C-shaped structure approximately 20–25 cm in length between the first and third lumbar vertebrae above the level of the umbilicus. At its origin, the duodenum is attached to the liver by the hepatoduodenal ligament; apart from this, it is a retroperitoneal structure. The duodenum originates at the pylorus of the stomach and ends at the suspensory ligament of the duodenum, a band of smooth muscle extending from the junction of the duodenum and jejunum to the left crus of the diaphragm (a.k.a., the ligament of Treitz). Treitz's ligament is a landmark that identifies the duodenojejunal junction, the site where retroperitoneal duodenum becomes intraperitoneal jejunum. Neighboring structures to the duodenum are the pancreas, gallbladder/biliary tree,

C. L. Power · J. S. Wu (✉)
Department of Colon and Rectal Surgery, Cleveland Clinic, Cleveland, OH, USA

J. M. McBride · R. L. Drake
Department of Anatomy, Cleveland Clinic Lerner College of Medicine, Cleveland, OH, USA

J. S. Wu, M. D. Inkster (eds.), *Cleveland Clinic Colorectal Case Studies*,
https://doi.org/10.1007/978-3-031-39880-3_5

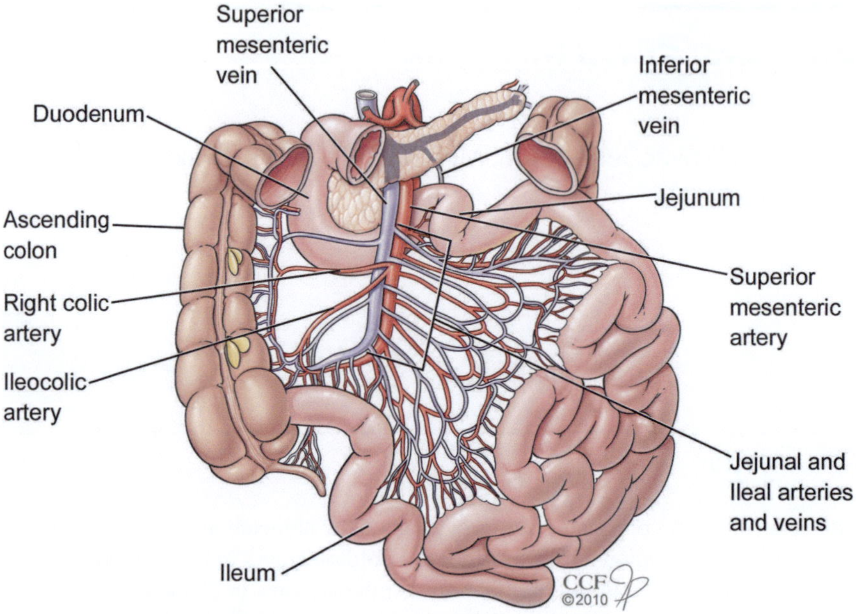

Fig. 5.1 The small intestine consists of duodenum, jejunum, and ileum

gastroduodenal artery, portal vein, superior mesenteric artery/vein, inferior vena cava, aorta, right kidney, and transverse colon.

The remainder of the small intestine is comprised of the jejunum and the ileum, both derivatives of the midgut. The jejunum, which resides mostly in the left upper quadrant of the abdomen, makes up the proximal two-fifths of the remaining small intestine. Compared to the ileum, the jejunum has a larger diameter, a thicker wall, fewer arterial arcades, and longer vasa recta. The remaining three-fifths of the small intestine, which terminates at the ileocecal fold, is made up of the ileum. Mostly occupying the right lower quadrant of the abdomen, the ileum is distinct from the jejunum in that it has thinner walls, a smaller diameter, shorter vasa recta, more arterial arcades, and a greater proportion of mesenteric fat. Being midgut derivatives, the jejunum and ileum receive their entire vascular inflow and output from the superior mesenteric artery and vein via the jejunal arteries, the ileal arteries, and the ileocolic artery. After the superior mesenteric artery gives off its first branch (the inferior pancreaticoduodenal artery), numerous distal branches follow. On the left side, multiple jejunal and ileal branches leave the main artery to supply the jejunum and the ileum. These branches follow a specific pattern. After they branch off the superior mesenteric artery, they travel between two layers of mesentery, anastomosing to form arches (arcades) as they fan out to supply the jejunum and ileum. These arcades increase in frequency distally along the gut, forming both single and double arcades. The straight arteries, or vasa recta, extend from the terminal arcade to provide the final direct vascular supply to the walls of the small intestine. The venous drainage of the jejunum and ileum is via the superior mesenteric vein. The superior mesenteric vein ends behind the neck of the pancreas where it combines with the splenic vein to form the portal vein.

Biographical Notes

Sir Frederick Treves (1853–1923) [3–5]

Frederick Treves attended London Hospital Medical School and during his career was primarily associated with the London Hospital (now known as the Royal London Hospital). He served in South Africa in charge of a Field Hospital during the Second Boer War. Treves was recognized as a highly competent surgeon and a dedicated anatomist, particularly of the abdomen. His Hunterian lectures were based on over 100 dissections he personally performed. His study of anatomy was further developed through his friendship with Joseph Merrick, the "Elephant Man." In 1902, with Lord Lister, he drained an infected appendiceal abscess on King Edward VII on the eve of his coronation, leaving the appendix intact. The ileocecal fold is commonly referred to as the "bloodless fold of Treves."

Václav Treitz (1819–1872) [6–10]

Born in Hostomice, Bohemia, in 1819, Treitz completed his studies in medicine at the Charles-Ferdinand University in Prague. In 1851, Treitz left Prague and was appointed Prosector at the Jagellonian University in Cracow. It was here, in 1853, that he published his paper "Ueber einen neuen Muskel am Duodenum des Menschen, über elastische Sehnen und einige andere anatomische Verhältnisse" ("On a new muscle in the human duodenum, over elastic tendons and some other anatomical relations"). This suspensory muscle, *Musculus suspensorius duodeni*, later became known as the ligament of Treitz. This muscle and its anatomic relationship to neighboring structures as drawn in Treitz's article is shown in Fig. 5.2.

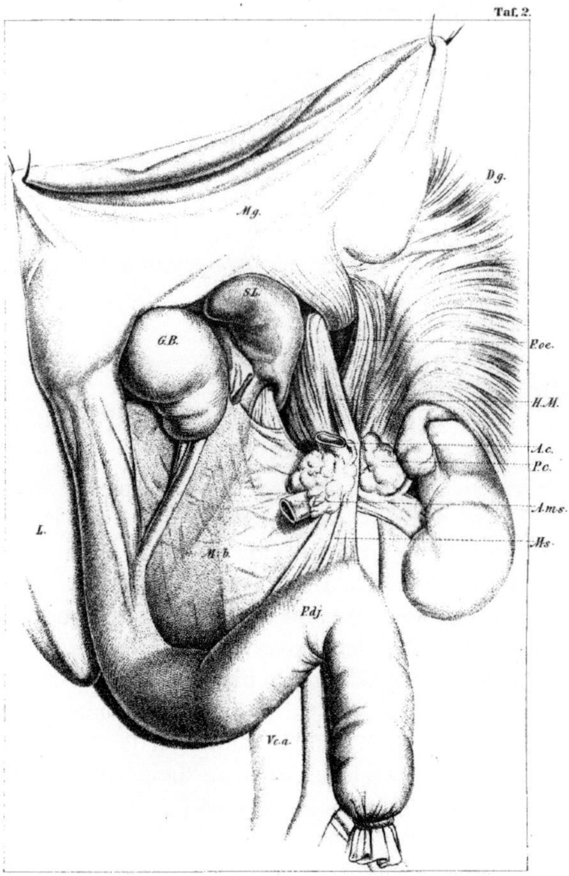

Fig. 5.2 Treitz's illustration of the *Musculus suspensorium duodeni (MS),* eponymously named after him, and its relation to surrounding structures (1853)

Ueber einen neuen Muskel am Duodenum des Menschen, über elastische Sehnen, und einige andere anatomische Verhältnisse
Von Dr. Treitz,
path. Prosector in Krakau
Erklärung der Abbildung
Taf 2.

Die Zeichnung stellt die Anheftung des Zwölffingerdarms durch den M. suspensorious in aufrecter Stellung der Leiche dar. Der Dickdarm, dcr Lccrdarm, dic Gekröse und das Pankreas sind entfernt. — *Dg*. Die untere Fläche des Diaphragma. — *Mg*. Die hintere Fläche des gegen den Thorax geschlagenen Magens. — *L*. Die Leber. — *S. L.* Der Spigel'sche Lappen. — *G. B.* Die Gallenblase mit ihren Gallengängen. — *V. c. a.* Vena cava ascendens. — *A. m. s.* Art. mesenterica sup. — *A. c.* Art. coeliaca. — *P. c.* Plexus coeliacus. — *F. dj.* Flexura duodenojejunalis. — *M. s.* Musculus suspensorius duodeni, dessen Sehne sich mit der Bindegewebshülle der genannten Arterien und Ganglien verwebt, und an welchen die Flexur gleichsam aufgehängt ist. — *H. M.* Der in diesem Falle stark entwickelte Hilfsmuskel. — *Mb*. Die zwischen dem Duodenum, den Arterien, der Vena cava und der Leberpforte ausgespannte Bindegewebsmembran.

Concerning a new muscle in the human duodenum, about elastic tendons, and some other anatomical relations
By Dr. Treitz
path. Prosector in Krakow
Explanation of the figure
Figure 5.2

The drawing represents the attachment of the duodenum though the suspensory muscle in the erect position of the corpse. The large intestine, jejunum, mesentery, and pancreas have been removed. —*Dg*. The under surface of the diaphragm. *Mg*. The posterior surface of the stomach pushed against the thorax. — *L*. The liver. — *S. L.* Spiegel's lobe. — *G. B.* The gallbladder with its bile ducts. — *V. c. a.* Ascending vena cava. — *A. m. s.* Superior mesenteric artery. — A. C. Coeliac artery. — *P. c.* Coeliac plexus. — *F. dj.* Duodenojejunal flexure. — *M. s.* Suspensory muscle of the duodenum, the tendon of which is interwoven with the connective tissue of the arteries and the ganglia mentioned, and on which the flexure as it were, is suspended. *H. M.* The accessory muscle is strongly developed in this case. — *Mb*. The membrane of connective tissue stretched between the duodenum, the arteries, the vena cava and the porta hepatis.

References

1. Haubrich WS. Treves of the fold of Treves. Gastroenterology. 2003;125:676.
2. Drake RL, Vogl W, Mitchell AWM, Gray H. Gray's anatomy for students, 2E. Philadelphia, PA: Churchill Livingstone/Elsevier; 2010.
3. Gibbs DD. Sir Frederick Treves: surgeon, author and medical historian. J Roy Soc Med. 1992;85:565–9.
4. Keith A, Gibbs DD. Treves, Sir Frederick, baronet (1853–1923). In: Oxford Dictionary of National Biography. Oxford: Oxford University Press; 2004. p. 347–9.
5. Treves F. The elephant man and other reminiscences. London: Cassel and Co.; 1923.
6. Ligament of Treitz. Merriam Webster's Medical Dictionary. Merriam-Webster.com/medical/ligament%20of%20Treitz. (Accessed 27 Aug 2016).
7. Treitz V. Ueber einen neuen Muskel am Duodenum des Menschen, über elastische Sehnen, und einige andere anatomische Verhältnisse. Vierteljahrschrift praktische Heilkund. 1853;37:113–44.
8. Fox RS, Fox CG, Graham WP III. Václav Treitz (1819-1872): Czechoslovakian pathoanatomist and patriot. World J Surg. 1985;9:361–6.

9. Costacurta L. Anatomical and functional aspects of the human suspensory muscle of the duodenum. Acta Anat. 1972;82:34–46.
10. Jit I, Grewal SS. The suspensory muscle of the duodenum and its nerve supply. J Anat. 1977;123:397–405.

Anatomy-Rectum

6

James S. Wu, Carolyn L. Power, Richard L. Drake, and Jennifer M. McBride

Presentation

The rectum and anus comprise the end of the gastrointestinal tract. The rectum begins where the taeniae coli of the sigmoid colon disappear and ends at the anus (Fig. 6.1) [1].

The proximal rectum is located within the abdominal cavity. The pelvic rectum is located anterior to the sacrum. The anterior surface of the rectum is variably lined by peritoneum depending on the depth of the *cul de sac* (Fig. 6.2a, b). Anteriorly, the rectum is separated from the urogenital structures by the fascia of Denonvilliers. Posteriorly, the mesorectal fascia abuts the presacral fascia with a connection between the two, the rectosacral fascia (Fig. 6.3).

The pelvic posterior rectal surface resides in the retroperitoneal space anterior to the sacrum. The rectum has lateral curvatures known as the valves of Houston. The length of the rectum is approximately 15–20 cm when measured endoscopically. In the distal rectum, the columnar epithelium of the rectum changes to squamous epithelium of the anal canal with an intervening anal transitional zone. The muscular wall of the rectum differentiates to form the internal anal sphincter muscle. The arterial supply to the rectum is primarily from the inferior mesenteric artery that joins the rectum as the superior rectal artery. Branches of the superior rectal artery perfuse the rectum through a fascia invested mesorectum. As shown in Fig. 6.4, these subdivisions join the right and left branches of the middle rectal arteries (branches of the internal iliac arteries) and the inferior rectal arteries (branches of the internal pudendal arteries).

J. S. Wu (✉) · C. L. Power
Department of Colon and Rectal Surgery, Cleveland Clinic, Cleveland, OH, USA

R. L. Drake · J. M. McBride
Department of Anatomy, Cleveland Clinic Lerner College of Medicine, Cleveland, OH, USA

J. S. Wu, M. D. Inkster (eds.), *Cleveland Clinic Colorectal Case Studies*,
https://doi.org/10.1007/978-3-031-39880-3_6

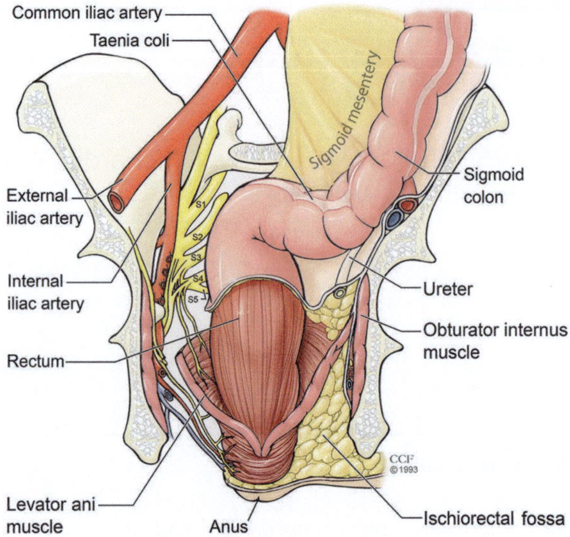

Fig. 6.1 The rectum and its relationship to neighboring structures including the ureter, pelvic floor, and neurovascular structures

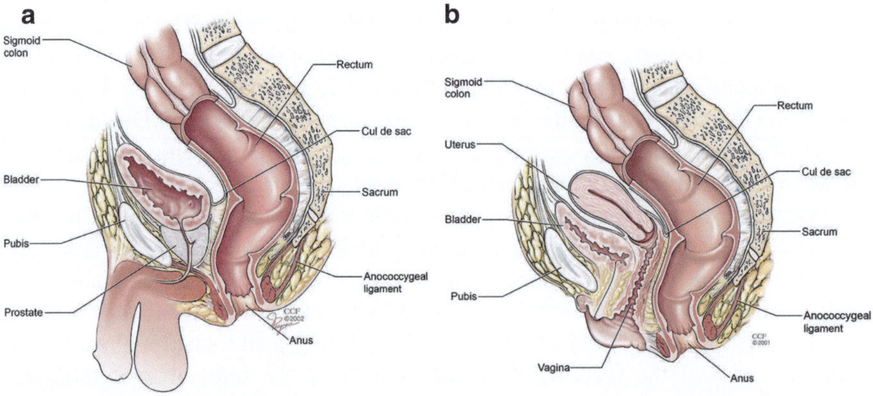

Fig. 6.2 Cross-sections of the rectum. Structures anterior to the rectum include the bladder and prostate in the male (**a**) and the uterus and vagina in the female (**b**)

The rectum has dual venous drainage (Fig. 6.5). The proximal rectum drains to the superior rectal veins which empty into the inferior mesenteric vein (IMV). The IMV joins the splenic vein and becomes part of the portal system. The distal rectum drains through two veins. The middle rectal veins join the internal iliac system leading to the vena cava. The inferior rectal veins also join the iliac system via Alcock's canal.

As shown in Fig. 6.6, anorectal lymphatic drainage is to three major collections of lymph nodes: superior rectal, iliac, and inguinal.

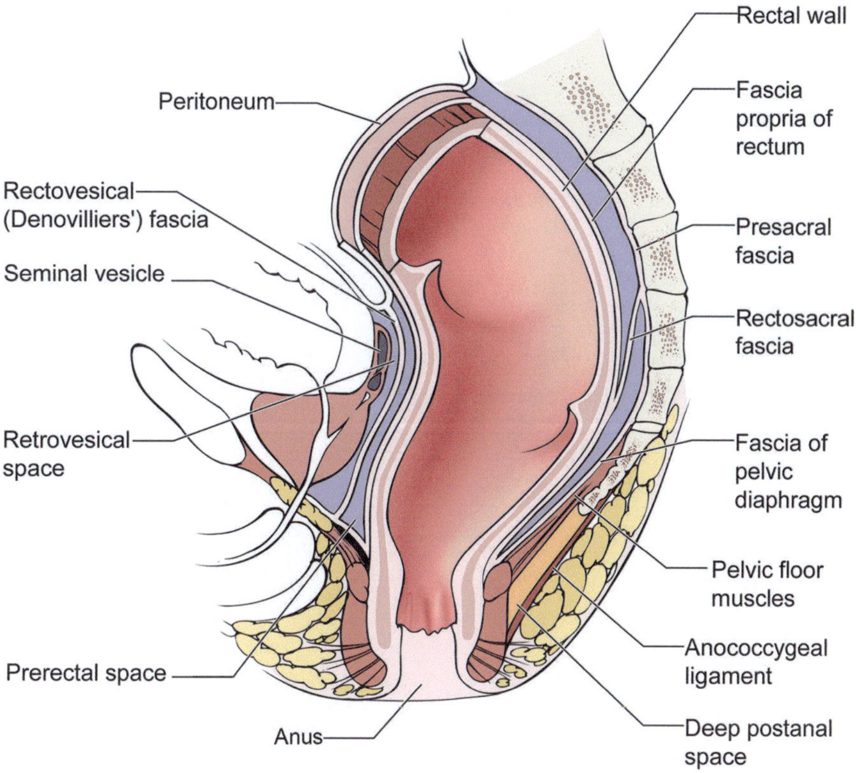

Fig. 6.3 Anteriorly, the rectum is separated from the urogenital structures by Denonvilliers' fascia. Posteriorly, the presacral fascia connects to the mesorectal fascia by the rectosacral fascia. Posteriorly, the anus is attached to the coccyx by the anococcygeal ligament

As shown in Fig. 6.7, the rectum is surrounded by mesorectum encased by fascia. Posterior to the mesorectum is the presacral fascia that covers a plexus of presacral veins. Anteriorly, the mesorectum abuts the fascia of Denonvilliers that separates the rectum from the genitourinary structures. The superior rectal artery enters the rectum posteriorly at the level of the sacral promontory. The middle rectal arteries join the rectum anterolaterally through lateral soft tissue referred to as the lateral stalks or ligaments.

The sympathetic hypogastric nerves associated with male ejaculation can be seen beneath the presacral fascia at the level of the sacral promontory, posterolaterally. The parasympathetic nerves associated with male erection are close to the distal rectum anterolaterally [2].

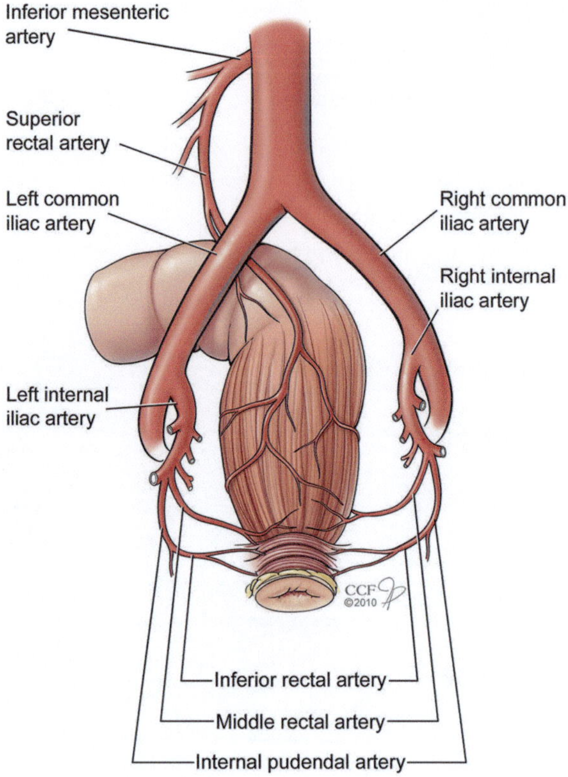

Fig. 6.4 Posterior view of the rectum. The rectum is supplied by three arteries-the superior rectal artery via the inferior mesenteric artery proximally and the middle rectal and inferior rectal arteries distally via the internal iliac artery. The inferior rectal artery travels from the pelvis to the ischiorectal fossa through Alcock's canal becoming the internal pudendal artery supplying blood to the anus

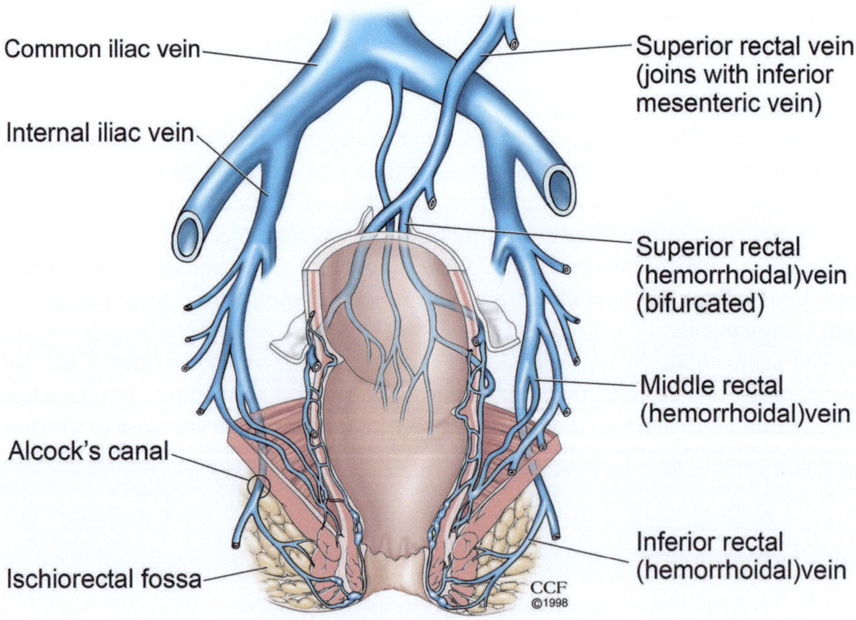

Fig. 6.5 Anterior view of the rectum. Rectal venous drainage from the superior rectal vein is to the portal system via the splenic vein. Venous drainage from the middle and inferior rectal veins is to the systemic circulation

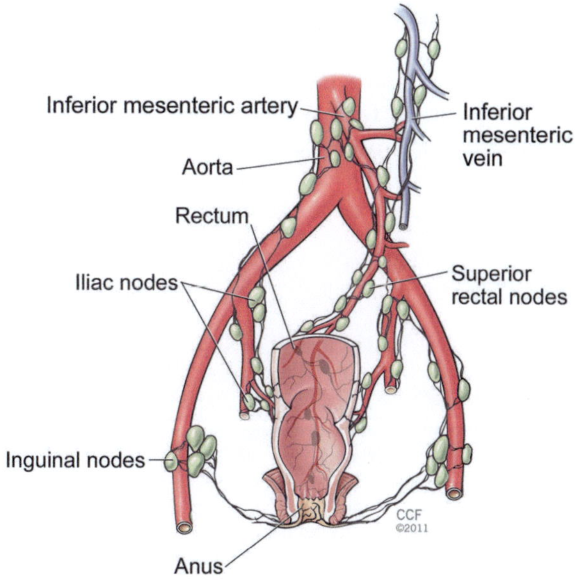

Fig. 6.6 The lymphatic drainage of the anus and rectum is to three major collections of lymph nodes: superior rectal, iliac, and inguinal

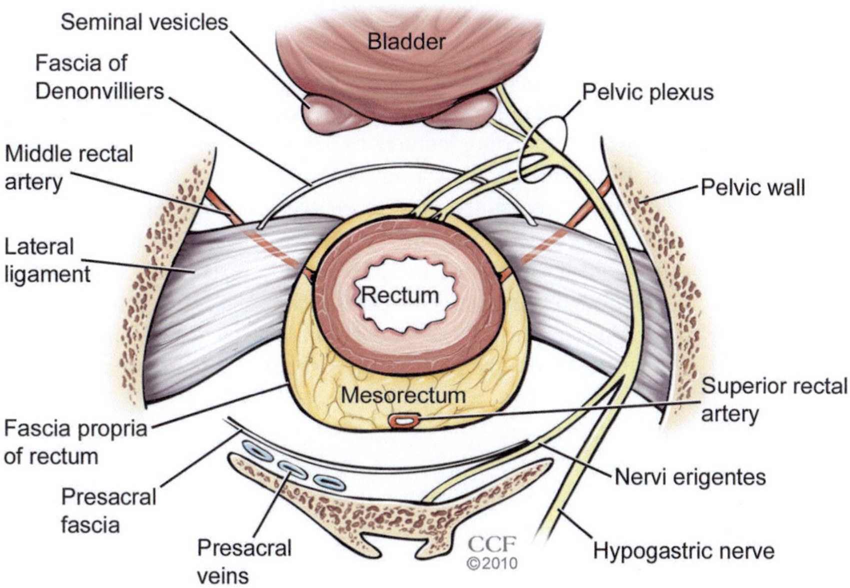

Fig. 6.7 A schematic transverse section showing the relationship of the rectum to surrounding fasciae, blood vessels and nerves at various depths in the male pelvis. Note the lateral position of the pelvic nerve plexus, most of which is embedded in the endopelvic fascia on the pelvic wall (after Church) [3]

Biographical Notes

Charles-Pierre Denonvilliers [4, 5]

Charles-Pierre Denonvilliers (1808–1872) received his medical doctorate in Paris in 1837 and rose to become professor of surgery and anatomy. He provided the first description of the rectoprostatic aponeurosis, now known as Denonvilliers' fascia. The description described in his 1837 thesis reads as follows [6]:

Propositions et observations d'anatomie, de physiologie et de pathologie. Thèse Présentée et soutenue à la Faculté de Médecine de Paris, le 8 août 1837, pour obtenir le grade de Docteur en Médecine Par Charles Denonvilliers, de Paris En arrière de la prostate, entre les vésicules séminales et le rectum, existe un couche membraneuse bien distincte, que j'appelle *prostato-péritonéale*. Voici quelle est sa disposition: Des deux côtés elle se confond avec le tissu cellulaire serré qui entoure les plexus veineux du bas-fond de la vessie; par son bord antérieur, elle se perd sur l'extrémité la plus reculée de la prostate; par son bord postérieur elle adhère à cette portion du péritoine qui descend entre la vessie et le rectum.	Propositions and observations, anatomical, physiological and pathological Thesis Presented to the faculty of Medicine of Paris, August 8, 1837, for the purpose of obtaining the degree of Doctor of Medicine By Charles Denonvilliers, Paris Behind the prostate, between the seminal vesicles and the rectum, there is a distinct membranous layer, which I call *prostato-peritoneal*. This is its position: from the two sides it fuses with the compact cellular tissue which surrounds the venous plexus at the base of the bladder; on the anterior side it runs to the far side of the prostate; on the posterior side it adheres to the part of the peritoneum that descends between the bladder and the rectum [7].

Wilhelm von Waldeyer-Hartz [8]

Wilhelm Waldeyer was born in 1836 in Hehlen, Prussia. He was inspired to study medicine and anatomy after attending lectures by Jakob Henle. He earned the title of medical doctor in 1862. He served as a military surgeon in the Franco-German War of 1870–1871. He subsequently was given the Chair of Anatomy at the University of Strasbourg, Alsace. In 1883, he rose to the prestigious Chair of Anatomy in Berlin where he remained until 1917. He created new terminology including "chromosome" and "neuron." The rectosacral fascia is frequently referred to as Waldeyer's fascia in error. In 1899, Waldeyer published a text of topographical anatomy entitled, "Das Becken" (The Pelvis) [9]. A section on the *Fascia recti* is as follows:

Das Becken Topographisch-Anatomisch Von W. Waldeyer Dr. Med. et Phil. Professor der Medizin und Direktor der Anatomischen Anstalt in Berlin Zwischen Fascia recti und Kreuzbein (Tela adiposa retrorectalis) ist es sehr locker und wenig fetthaltig, so dass man hier von einem retrorectalen (Bindegewebs)-Raume, Spatium retrorectale… sprechen kann. Dieser Raum ist durch Verschiebung des Rectum sehr auszuweiten, und man kann leicht mit den Fingern in ihn eindringen und das Rectum vom Kreuzbeine ablösen. Unten findet dies seine Grenze, indem dort die Fascia recti in die parietale Beckenbodenfascie auf dem Ligamentum anococcygeum übergeht.	The Pelvis Topographic-Anatomic by W. Waldeyer Dr. of Medicine and Philosophy Professor of Medicine and Director of the Anatomic Institute, Berlin Between the rectal fascia and the coccyx (adipose tissues retrorectalis) it is a very loose and a little fatty, so that here one can speak of a retrorectal (connective tissue) space. This space can be expanded by displacement of the rectum; one can easily enter the space with the finger, and the rectum can be peeled off of the coccyx. Beneath this one finds a border where the rectal fascia fuses with the pelvic floor fascia at the anococcygeal ligament.

In 1974, Crapp and Cuthbertson [10] described the rectosacral fascia, a sheet of fascia situated between the periosteum overlying the body of the fourth sacral vertebra and the rectum 3–5 cm above the anorectal junction. The authors concluded that "William Waldeyer described the pelvic fascia but not the rectosacral fascia. The term 'fascia of Waldeyer' is vague and is best avoided."

Benjamin Alcock [11, 12]

Benjamin Alcock was born in 1801 in Kilkenny, Ireland. He studied with Abraham Colles, Professor of Anatomy and Surgery in Dublin University. He received his education at Kilkenny College and Trinity College, Dublin. He became a member of the Royal College of Surgeons in Ireland in 1825. Alcock became the first Professor of anatomy and physiology at Queen's College, Cork. He emigrated to the United States in 1859. Alcock is known for his 1836 anatomic description of a canal leading from the pelvis to the ischiorectal fossa [13].

This canal is part of his detailed description of the anatomic pathway of the internal pudic artery (*internal pudendal artery*), a branch of the anterior division of the internal iliac artery.

> "The first stage of the artery's course, throughout which it is contained in the pelvis, extends from its origin to the lower part of the posterior sacro-sciatic notch, through which it escapes from the cavity…
>
> The third stage of the artery is its longest and most important one; during it the vessel is situate within the skeleton of the pelvis, though not within the pelvis, in the ordinary sense of the phrase, i.e. within its visceral cavity, being excluded therefrom by the structures which form its floor; it lies along the inside of the tuberosity of the ischium and the rami of the ischium and pubis, and its course and relations being different at the posterior and anterior parts of the stage, they may with advantage be considered separately. In the posterior part, or as far forward as the anterior extremity of the tuberosity or the base of the triangular ligament of the perinæum, the artery descends; in the anterior it ascends; in the posterior it is situate in the outer wall of the space which intervenes between the inside of the tuberosity

of the ischium and the rectum—the ischio-rectal space. This space is cuneiform, its base below, toward the surface; its apex above, toward the pelvis; its inner wall is formed by the levator ani and the dense thin expansion by which the muscle is covered externally or inferiorly, its outer by the obturator fascia attached inferiorly to the edge of the great sacro-sciatic ligament and of its falciform process, and by the obturator muscle: the space is occupied by a mass of adipose cellullar structure, traversed by some branches of the pudic vessels and nerves. In a canal in the obturator fascia the artery is contained through the posterior part of the third stage;..."

B. Alcock
Iliac Arteries
The Cyclopadia of Anatomy and Physiology,
1836

In 2011, Colebunders et al. [14] compared Alcock's original description of the pudendal canal with findings from a cadaveric study. The authors concluded: "'Alcock's canal' therefore should be used to describe that the portion of the pudendal nerve within the obturator fascia overlying the obturator internus muscle."

John Houston [15]

John Houston (1802–1845) was born in Ulster, Ireland, and educated in both Dublin and Edinburgh. He was the curator of the museum of the Royal College of Surgeons in Ireland and was elected a member of the Royal Irish Academy in 1829. In his 1830 article "Observations on the mucous membranes of the rectum," he described rectal folds now named after him [16].

> "In the natural state, the tube of the gut does not form, as is usually conceived, one smooth uninterrupted passage, devoid of any obstacles that might impede the entrance of bougies: it is, on the contrary, made uneven in several places by certain valvular projections of its internal membrane, which standing across the passage, must frequently render the introduction of such instruments a matter of considerable difficulty.
>
> Three is the average number, though sometimes four, and sometimes only two are present in a marked degree."

According to Ikard, the physiologic function of the valves is unknown [17].

References

1. Drake RL, Vogl W, Mitchell AWM, Gray H. Gray's anatomy for students. Edinburgh: Churchill Livingstone; 2015.
2. Ahuja V. Open surgical techniques in colorectal cancer. In: Gearhart S, Ahuja N, editors. Stephen C. Yang (Series Editor) Early diagnosis and treatment of cancer series, colorectal cancer. Amsterdam: Saunders-Elsevier; 2010. p. 145–65.
3. Church JM, Raudkivi PJ, Hill GL. The surgical anatomy of the rectum — a review with particular relevance to the hazards of rectal mobilisation. Int J Colorectal Dis. 1987;2:158–66.
4. Charran O, Muhleman M, Shoja MM, Tubbs RS, Loukas M. Charles-Pierre Denonvilliers (1808-1872): renowned anatomist, plastic surgeon, and influential member of French society. Clin Anat. 2013;26:788–92.
5. Ophoven AV, Roth S. The anatomy and embryological origins of the fascia of Denonvilliers: a medico-historical debate. J Urol. 1997;157:3–9.
6. Denonvilliers C. Propositions et observations d'anatomie, de physiologie et de pathologie. Thèses, *Présentée et soutenue à la Faculté de Medicine de Paris, le 8 août 1837, pour obténir le grade de Docteur en Médecine;* 1837, —N° 285; Article Troisieme, p. 23.

7. Charran O, Muhleman M, Shoja MM, Tubbs RS, Loukas M. Charles-Pierre Denonvilliers (1808-1872): renowned anatomist, plastic surgeon, and influential member for French Society. Clin Anat. 2013;26:788–92.
8. Winkelmann A. Wilhelm von Waldeyer-Hartz (1836-1921): an anatomist who left his mark. Clin Anat. 2007;20:231–4.
9. Waldeyer W. Das Becken. Topographisch-anastomisch mit besonderer Berücksichtigung der Chirurgie und Gynäkologie. Bonn, Verlag von Friedrich Cohen, 1899; Fascia recti. p. 269.
10. Crapp AR, Cuthbertson AM. William Waldeyer and the retrosacral fascia. Surg Gynecol Obstet. 1974;138:252–6.
11. Oelhafen K, Shayota B, Muhleman M, Klaassen Z, Tubbs RS, Loukas M. Benjamin Alcock (1801-?) and his canal. Clin Anat. 2013;26:662–6.
12. O'Rahilly R. Benjamin Alcock, anatomist. Ir J Med Sci (1926-1967). 1947;22:622–32.
13. Alcock B. Iliac arteries. In: Todd RB, editor. The cyclopædia of anatomy and physiology, vol. II. London: Sherwood, Gilbert, and Piper, Paternoster-Row; 1835-1859. p. 834–5.
14. Colebunders B, Matthew MK, Broerm N, Persing JA, Dellon AL. Benjamin Alcock and the pudendal canal. J Reconstr Microsurg. 2011;27:349–54. This excerpt is generously reused with the generous permission of Mr. Kariym Bryan, Thieme Publishers, permissions@thieme.com, 16 June 2022
15. Creighton C. Houston John (1802–1845), rev. Bevan M. Oxford Dictionary of National Biography. Oxford University Press 2004. http://www.oxforddnb.com/view/article/13874 (Accessed 22 Apr 2016).
16. Houston J. Observations on the mucous membrane of the rectum. Dublin Hosp Rep. 1830;5:158–65. Accessed from Archiv.org Feb 22, 2024.
17. Ikard RW. Spiral rectal valves: anatomy, eponyms, and clinical significance. Clin Anat. 2015;28:436–41.

Anatomy-Anus

7

James S. Wu, Ana E. Bennett, and Michelle D. Inkster

Presentation

In 1880, Herrmann observed that uniformity of opinion regarding the exact structure of the anal mucosa was lacking [1].

Sur la structure et le développement de la muqueuse anale	On the structure and development of the anal mucosa
Par Gustave Herrmann **Préparteur du Cours d'histologie à La Faculté de médicine.** En lisant dans les traités classiques d'anatomie descriptive et d'histologie, et meme dans les articles spéciaux, les descriptions de la région anale, on remarque qu'il existe entre les auteurs des divergences assez considerable,...	**By Gustave Herrmann** **Preparer for the histology course at the Faculty of Medicine.** In reading the classic treatises of descriptive anatomy and histology, and even in special articles regarding descriptions of the anal area, one remarks that, considerable divergences exist between authors,...

Seventy-eight years later, Parks wrote [2]:

> **Modern concepts of the anatomy of the ano-rectal region.**
> **Introduction**
> It is remarkable that the anatomy of the anal canal should be still the subject of discussion. There are several reasons for this. The region is inaccessible in the cadaver because of the surrounding bony structure. Distinction between muscle fibres and connective tissue is often difficult in fixed specimens and it is easy to create artefacts by blunt dissection. Many

J. S. Wu (✉)
Department of Colon and Rectal Surgery, Cleveland Clinic, Cleveland, OH, USA

A. E. Bennett
Pathology & Laboratory Medicine Institute, Cleveland Clinic, Cleveland, OH, USA

M. D. Inkster
Department of Gastroenterology, Cleveland Clinic, Cleveland, OH, USA

J. S. Wu, M. D. Inkster (eds.), *Cleveland Clinic Colorectal Case Studies*,
https://doi.org/10.1007/978-3-031-39880-3_7

of the complicated arrangements described in anatomical and surgical journals may well be due to excessive zeal in this respect.

A. G. Parks, M.D., M.Ch., F.R.C.S.
Senior Surgical Registrar
Guy's Hospital

Anal Integuments

It was the opinion of Herrmann and Desfosses that the distal rectal lining and the external skin were connected by a transition derived from the embryonic cloaca in the region of the columns of Morgagni [3].

G. Herrmann et L. Desfosses. Sur la muqueuse de la région cloacale du rectum, 1880.	**G. Herrmann et L. Desfosses. On the mucosa of the cloacal region of the rectum, 1880.**
La muqueuse de l'extrémité inférieure du rectum ne se continue pas directement avec le tégument externe. Il existe à ce niveau une zone circulaire, haute de 0^{m}, 006 à 0^{m}, 012, répondant aux sailles musculaires de Morgagni, et qui représente une partie persistante du cloaque de l'embryon. Cette *région cloacale* est revêtue par une muqueuse spéciale qui se trouve nettement limitée du còté du rectum et se continue au contraire avec la peau par une transition sensible.	The lining of the lower end of the rectum is not continued directly with the external integument. There is at this level a circular zone, height 0^{m},006 to, 0^{m},012, corresponding to protruding muscularis of Morgagni, which represents a persistent part of the embryonic cloaca. This *cloacal region* is covered with a special mucosa that is clearly limited on the rectum side and which continues, on the contrary, to the skin by a sensitive transition.

Anal Embryology [4, 5]

The hindgut (endoderm) differentiates into the distal one-third of the transverse colon, the descending and sigmoid colon, rectum and the proximal anal canal. The distal segment of the hindgut fuses with the proctodeum (surface ectoderm). The intervening segment is the cloacal region (Latin for "sewer") also known as the anal transitional zone (ATZ) that is 6–12 mm in length. The presence of a cloacagenic membranous zone interposed between rectal and anal mucosa was restated by Grinvalsky and Helwig in 1956 [6].

> "There exists at the level corresponding to the columns of Morgagni, a circular zone measuring between 0.6 to 1.2 cm. that represents a persistent remnant of the cloaca of the embryo. This cloacal region is covered with a special mucosa that is found limiting the rectum and joining below with skin by a sharp transition."
>
> H.T. Grinvalsky and E.B. Helwig
> The Armed Forces Institute of Pathology
> Washington, DC

In 1978, Fenger stated that the "anal canal extends from the upper to the lower border of the internal sphincter." [7, 8]. He divided the canal histologically into three zones according to the epithelial lining. The epithelium is colorectal type in the upper part and squamous in the lower part. The anal transitional zone (ATZ) is

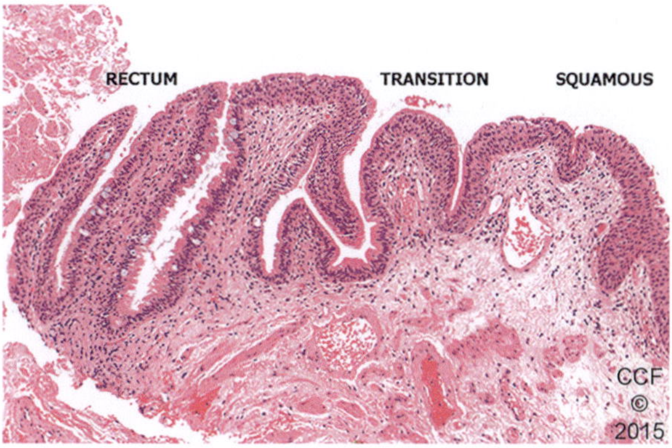

Fig. 7.1 Anal canal anatomy. Rectal (columnar) and squamous linings flank transitional zone epithelium (Courtesy Ana E. Bennett, MD, Cleveland Clinic, Department of Anatomic Pathology)

the zone interposed between uninterrupted colorectal type mucosa above and uninterrupted squamous epithelium below, irrespective of the type of epithelium present in the zone itself.

Histologic section of these three zones in continuity is demonstrated in Fig. 7.1. Proximally, the anal transitional zone joins columnar epithelium of the rectum at the anorectal line (also referred to as Herrmann's line). Concerning this anatomy, Tanaka et al. write [9]:

> "We separated the surgical anal canal into three zones: the upper zone (between the anorectal ring and the anorectal line), the middle zone (between the anorectal line and the dentate line; the part of the anal columns and sinuses), and the lower zone (between the dentate line, and the anal verge).
>
> We recognized that the anal transitional zone was identical to the middle zone, and the suprazonal line and Hermann's line seemed to be identical to the anorectal line, differing from it only in definition."
>
> E. Tanaka, T. Noguchi, K. Nagai,
> Y. Akashi, K. Kawahara, T. Shimada
> Departments of Surgery and Gastrointestinal Surgery, Faculty of Medicine
> Oita University
> Oita, Japan

Distally, the anal transitional zone joins the squamous epithelium at the dentate (pectinate) line. Using high-definition flexible endoscopy, Tanaka and colleagues studied the morphology of the anal canal with focused attention on the epithelium between the anorectal line and the dentate line (Fig. 7.2). Using retroflexion and rectal insufflation, the authors showed that it is easy to see the anorectal line, the dentate line, and the intervening epithelium containing anal columns and sinuses. Furthermore, using electron microscopy, Tanaka and co-workers showed that the columns are composed of stratified squamous epithelium while the sinuses are stratified columnar epithelium.

In our own endoscopy unit, we (MDI/JSW) were able to see team Tanaka's landmarks easily (Figs. 7.3a–f).

The epithelium distal to the dentate (pectinate) line is stratified squamous without keratinization or appendages such as hair or pigment. In 1896, Stroud described certain characteristics to a region that he named the pecten [10].

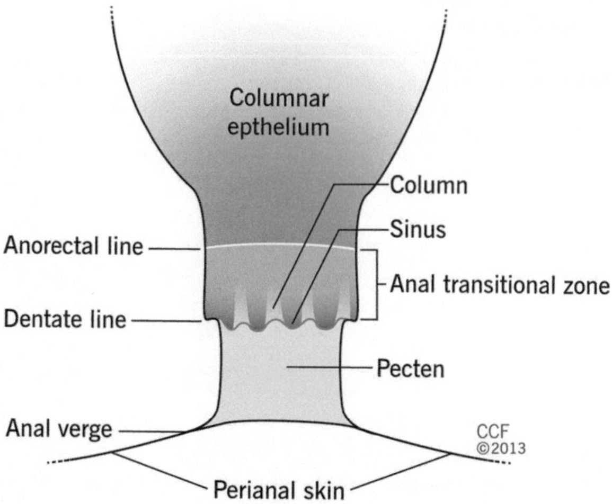

Fig. 7.2 Cross-sectional depiction of the anal canal epithelium. The anal transitional zone is located between the anorectal line and the dentate line flanked proximally by columnar epithelium and distally by the pecten. Proximal to the dentate line are the columns and sinuses of Morgagni. Distal to the pecten is the perianal skin (a.k.a, anal margin). The border between the pecten and the perianal skin is the anal verge (after Tanaka)

"*Characters of the Pecten.* - The pecten is distinguished by the following features:

1. It is bounded caudad (ectad) by the line of junction of the ectal and ental sphincters (Hilton's white line) and cephalad by the linea dentata.
2. It has a smooth, even texture and a glossy, shiny appearance. The color is intermediate between those of the mucosa and skin.
3. It has few or no openings of sweat glands.
4. It is moderately vascular.
5. It is covered by stratified epithelium which is richly supplied with nerve endings.
6. The cephalic dentations vary in size from two to twelve millimetres wide and three to nine millimeters long; and in appearance from broad, truncated, round, or pyramidal to slender, columnar. Sometimes they represent a slender neck and are expanded cephalad to a more or less bulb-like extremity. It is probable that in some cases these develop into papillae."

Bert B. Stroud, D.Sci
Instructor in Physiology, Vertebrate Zoology, and Neurology,
Cornell University,
Ithaca, N.Y.

In 1956, Morgan and Thompson referred to the pecten as the thin anal canal skin [11].

"This anal canal skin, of parchment colour, is delicate, smooth, thin and shiny. There are no hair follicles, sweat or mucous glands, and it passes imperceptibly into the loose, thicker and pigmented corrugated true *skin of the anus* with its hair follicles and glands.

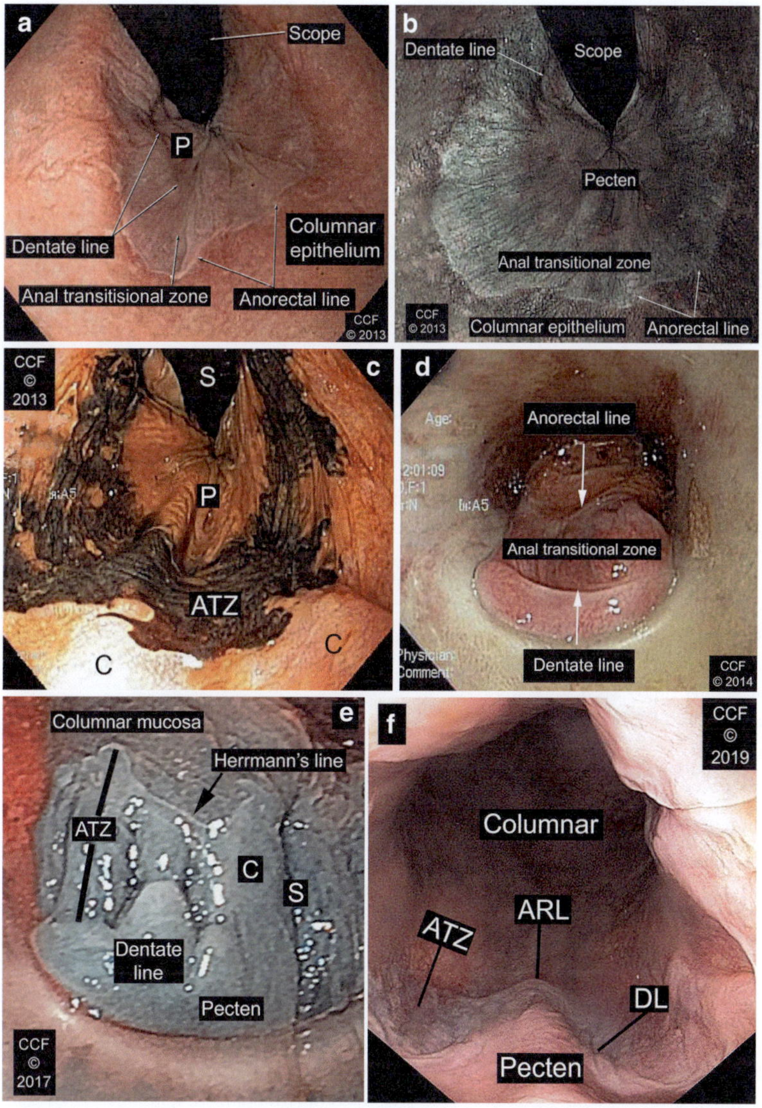

Fig. 7.3 (**a**) Retroflexion in the insufflated rectum with white light shows the dentate line, the ATZ, and the anorectal line. The epithelium between the dentate line and the anorectal line corresponds to the anal transitional zone defined by Fenger. (**b**) Narrow band imaging (same patient as Fig. 7.3a) shows enhancement of the differences between the columnar epithelium, the ATZ and the pecten. (**c**) Retroflex view of the rectum (same patient as in Fig. 7.3a) following treatment with Lugol's iodine shows that the ATZ picks up the iodine while the pecten (P) and the columnar epithelium (C) do not. The scope is identified by the letter S. (**d**) On magnified anoscopy, the anal transitional zone is flanked proximally by columnar epithelium. Nonkeratinized, nonhair-bearing squamous epithelium (pecten) is seen distal to the dentate line. (**e**) When nondistended, the columns (C) and sinuses (S) of Morgagni are apparent in the anal transition zone. The "toothlike" character of the dentate line is apparent in this image. The alternative name for distal border of the ATZ is the pectinate line. Pecten is a genus of scallops; the pectinate line sometimes appears scalloped. (**f**) This *en face* endoscopic white light view of the anoderm shows the ATZ with its distinct borders, the anorectal line (ARL) proximally and the dentate line (DL) distally. The columnar mucosa is proximal to the ATZ while the pecten is distal

Just below the dentate line the anal canal skin is most firmly attached to the deeper structures—Hilton's white line. The zone between the dentate line and the adherent anal canal skin was described by Stroud (1896) as the pecten (Lat. a comb)."

C. Nauton Morgan, M.S., F.R.C.S.
Henry R. Thompson, F.R.C.S.
Consultant Surgeons, St. Mark's Hospital

Hilton's White Line

In Lecture XII of his 1879 course of lectures, *On Rest and Pain*, Hilton described a white line [12].

"That white line corresponds exactly with the linear interval between the external and the internal sphincter muscle. It is an important landmark, exact and truthful, so that it can be relied upon."

John Hilton, F.R.S, F.R.C.S.
Surgeon Extraordinary to her Majesty the Queen,
Consulting Surgeon to Guy's Hospital

Subsequent reports have questioned the identity of this anatomic landmark.

"Below the anal inter-muscular septum, true skin is encountered and cutaneous glandular elements are present. It is at this site that Hilton's white line occurs, but this much described line is only rarely seen."

C. Naunton Morgan, M.B., F.R.C.S.
Senior Assistant Surgeon,
St. Mark's Hospital, 1936 [13]

In 1938, Buie dissected Hilton's definition of the white line and came to the following conclusion:

"Perusal of the foregoing statement reveals the error in Hilton's conception of the problem. His record of the anatomic characteristics of the anus is entirely correct except in one particular, which in itself is truly remarkable, and had he not stated that his white line 'shows the juncture of the skin and the mucous membrane' and that it 'corresponds exactly with the linear interval between the external and external sphincter muscle,' there would have been no evidence of this confusion. It is doubtful if there are instances wherein the white line of Hilton can be seen in the walls of the normal undissected anus. As an anatomic landmark this line is discernable in the undissected specimen only on palpation."

Louis A. Buie, A.B., M.D., F.A.C.S.
Professor of Proctology.
The Mayo Foundation for Medical Education and Research, 1938 [14]

In 1954, Ewing opined,

"The term Hilton's line is so ill-understood and so variously interpreted that it would be wise to discontinue its use altogether".

M. R. Ewing, F.R.C.S.
Department of Surgery, Postgraduate School of Medicine of London, 1954 [15]

A clear description of the most distal region of the anus as seen on external examination was provided by Hirschman in 1937 [16].

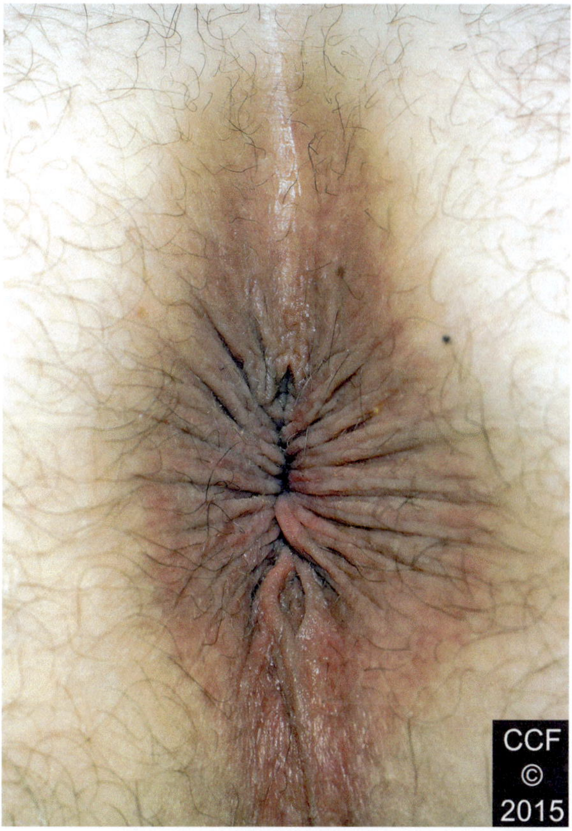

Fig. 7.4 The pigmented circumanal skin with ridges causes by contraction of the underlying corrugator cutis muscle. Note that the anal outlet is a slit not a circle

> "The anus is an oval aperture, longitudinal when in repose, situated at a point equidistant from the tuberosities of the ischii, and about one inch anterior to the tip of the coccyx…The anus is surrounded by integument which is slightly darker than the surrounding skin. The skin around the anus is arranged in radiating folds caused by the contraction of the *corrugator cutis ani* muscle. The circumanal integument contains sweat glands, sebaceous glands, and hair follicles. The circumference of the anal orifice varies from an inch to an inch and three quarters, but it may be dilated to a circumference five to six times greater."
>
> Louis J. Hirschman, M.D., F.A.C.S.
> Consulting Proctologist
> Detroit City Receiving Hospital,
> Detroit

Discovery of the corrugator ani muscle is attributed to George Ellis, Emeritus Professor of Anatomy, University College, London [17]. (Fig. 7.4)

Jabbour and Wilson define the anal verge as follows: "The anal verge, or inferior margin of the anal canal, is the junction of nonkeratinized squamous epithelium of the anal canal with hair-bearing, keratinized, perianal skin." [18] The American Cancer Society states that [19]:

> "At the anal verge, the squamous cells of the lower anal canal merge with the skin just outside the anus. This skin around the anal verge (called the *perianal skin* or the *anal margin*) is also made up of squamous cells,

> but it also contains sweat glands and hair follicles, where are not found in the lining of the lower anal canal."

Cancers of the anal region often are divided into two groups, each with different treatments.

Anal Musculature

Shank et al. [20] define the junction between the anus and the rectum as the anorectal ring.

> "The anorectal ring is defined as the junction where the anal canal meets the rectum. This junction corresponds to the proximal level of the pelvic diaphragm, that is, the levator ani muscle or the muscular floor of the pelvis."
>
> Brenda Shank, M.D., Ph.D., F.A.C.R.
> Clinical Professor
> University of California
> San Francisco, California
> Warren E. Enker, M.D.
> Professor of Surgery
> Albert Einstein College of Medicine
> New York, New York
> Marshall S. Flam, M.D., F.A.C.P.
> Associate Clinical Professor
> University of California,
> San Francisco, California

The muscularis of the rectal wall distally forms the internal sphincter muscle that provides resting sphincter tone under autonomic control. The internal sphincter muscle is surrounded by the somatically innervated external sphincter muscle that joins with the levator ani muscle of the pelvic floor. The intersphincteric groove and the proximal border of the levator muscles are often palpable.

Anal Lymphovascular Supply

The lymphovascular routes to and from the anus vary because of disparate embryologic origins. Above the pectinate line, the arterial supply to the anus is via the superior rectal (hemorrhoidal) artery. Below the pectinate line, the anus is supplied by the middle rectal (hemorrhoidal) artery via the internal iliac artery and by the inferior rectal (hemorrhoidal) artery via the pudendal artery. Venous drainage above the pectinate line is to the portal system via the superior rectal vein. The middle and inferior rectal veins drain into the internal iliac and pudendal veins. Lymphatic drainage of the anus varies according to location. Proximal to the dentate (pectinate) line the lymphatic drainage follows the superior rectal artery to the inferior mesenteric artery or laterally along the middle rectal artery to the iliac nodes. Distal to the dentate line, lymphatics drain to the pudendal and inguinal nodes.

Innervation

The action of the internal sphincter muscle is involuntary. Under sympathetic control, it maintains tonic contraction. Parasympathetic input leads to internal sphincter relaxation. The external anal sphincter is somatically innervated and under voluntary control. The lower part of the anal canal being of ectodermal origin is extremely sensitive to pain.

Anal Glands

Anal glands are intramuscular structures that secrete into the anal canal at the level of the dentate (pectinate)line. McColl credits the first reference to anal glands to Swiss physiologist Albrecht von Haller in 1781 and the suggestion that fistula-in-ano may be caused by infected anal glands to Chiari in 1878. [21, 22] In their 1880 paper on the cloacal region of the rectum, Herrmann and Desfosses [3], describe these glands as follows:

ANATOMIE GÉNÉRALE.—	GENERAL ANATOMY.—
Sur la muqueuse de la région cloacale du rectum. Note de MM. G. Herrmann et L. Desfosses	Concerning the mucosa of the cloacal region of the rectum. Note by Mr. G. Herrmann and Mr. L. Desfosses
Cette region présente de petites glandes en grappe vers la partie moyenne, quelque glandes en tubes simples,... un ou plusieurs conduits, tapissés par le même épithélium et assez semblables à des tubes glandulaires. Ces conduits suivent un trajet sinueux dans les cloisons de tissu cellulaire qui séparent les faisceaux musculaires et traversent ainsi le sphincter dans toute son épaisseur; arrivés dans le tissu conjonctif interposé entre ce muscle et la couche longitudinale,…	This region presents with small glands grouped near the middle, several in simple tubes… one or several ducts, lined by the same epithelium and quite similar to the glandular tubes. These ducts follow a tortuous trajectory in the partitions of tissue that separate the muscle bundles and cross the sphincter entirely, arriving in the conjoined tissue interposed between the muscle and the longitudinal layer, …
Au point de vue chirurgical, ces long conduits tortueux, coiffés à leur extrémité par de petits follicules clos, présentent un certain intérêt, eu égard notamment au rôle qu'ils peuvent jouer dans la production des fistules compliquées qu'on rencontre si fréquemment dans cette région.	From the surgical standpoint, these long tortuous ducts, capped at their ends by small closed follicles, present a certain interest notably with regard to the role they play in the production of complex fistulae so frequently encountered in this region.

Figure 7.6 illustrates the relationships between the anal musculature, epithelial lining and blood supply. The palpable anal canal extends from the anorectal ring at the level of the levators ani to the lower border of the internal anal sphincter muscle at the intersphincteric groove.

In 1920, Hill lamented the lack of familiarity of some physicians with anorectal diseases and their routine omission on anorectal examination [23].

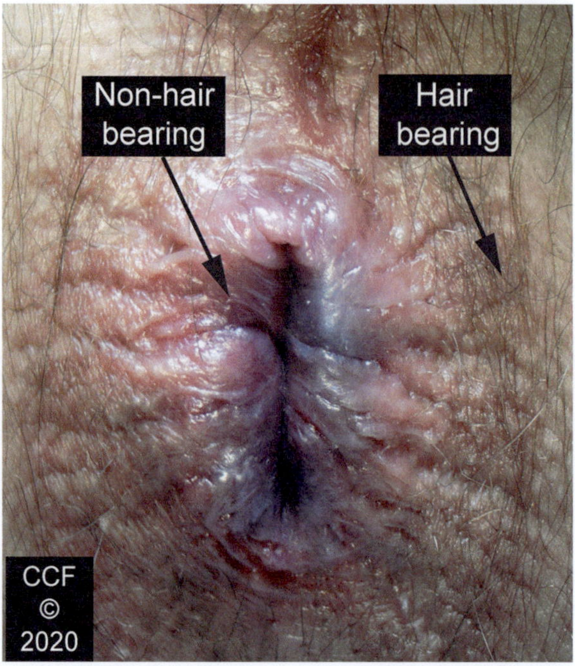

Fig. 7.5 The anal verge is the border between the perianal skin (keratinized squamous epithelium with appendages such as hair) and the distal border of the pecten (nonkeratinized squamous epithelium without appendages)

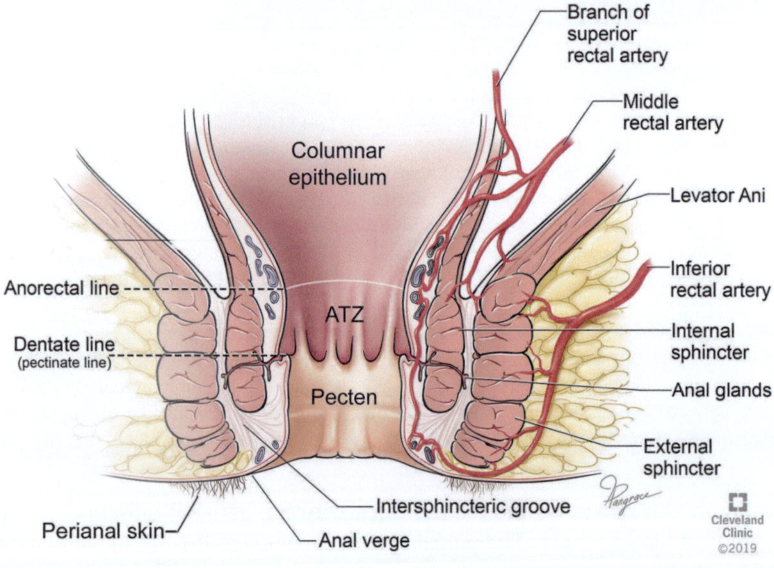

Fig. 7.6 Cross-section of the anus showing the musculature, vascular supply, and epithelia. The mucosal lining is divided into three zones: upper (colorectal), middle (transitional) and lower (squamous). The anal verge is the junction between the nonkeratinized squamous epithelium (pecten) and the keratinized hair-bearing perianal skin (anal margin). Within the anal transitional zone are the columns and sinuses of Morgagni. Anal glands open into the anal canal at the dentate line. The blood supply of the anus is from the superior, middle, and inferior rectal (hemorrhoidal arteries)

Methods of Examination in
Diseases of the Rectum and
Sigmoid Colon
T. Chittenden Hill, Ph.B., M.D.
Instructor in Proctology,
Harvard Graduate School of Medicine;
Surgeon to the Rectal Department
of Boston Dispensary

"The great majority of general practitioners have been afforded opportunities of clinical instruction in nearly every department of medicine and surgery with the notable exception of that large class of diseases common to the anus, rectum, and pelvic colon. It is not remarkable, therefore, that many otherwise skillful practitioners imagine considerable difficulties are associated with the diagnosis of these cases, and that, consequently, the treatment adopted by them is, as a rule, almost entirely perfunctory, haphazard, and unsatisfactory. From personal experience in post-graduate teaching, I have come to the conclusion that most mistakes are due to the practitioner's failure to make a routine examination of his rectal patients, rather than to his lack of knowledge".

Biographical Note

Giovanni Battista Morgagni (1682–1771) is considered the founder of modern pathological anatomy [24]. He studied medicine in Bologna. He was a Prosector in Anatomy to Valsalva and subsequently succeeded him as Demonstrator in Anatomy. His most famous work published in 1761 is De Sedibus, et Causis Morborum per Anatomen Indagatis (The Seats and Causes of Diseases Investigated by anatomy). Zampieri et al. [25] in their etymological autopsy of Morgagni's title write that Morgagni's anatomopathologic approach to medicine was revolutionary in his time because he demonstrated that, "postmortem dissections could be useful to understand pathophysiologic mechanisms and clinical symptoms in the living."

References

1. Herrmann G. Sur la structure et le développement de la muqueuse anale. J Anat Physiol. 1880;16:434–72.
2. Parks AG. Modern concepts of the anatomy of the ano-rectal region. Postgrad Med. 1958;34:360–6.
3. Herrmann G, Desfosses L. Sur la muqueuse de la région cloacale du rectum. C R Hebd Seances Acad Sci. 1880;90:1301–2.
4. Sadler TW. Langman's Medical Embryology. 11th ed. Philadelphia, PA: Wolters Kluwer Health |Lippencott Williams & Wilkins; 2010. p. 230–1.
5. Dudek RW, Fix JD. Embryology. 4th ed. Baltimore, MD: Wolters Kluwer Health|Lippincott, Williams & Wilkins; 2008. p. 119–21.
6. Grinvalsky HT, Helwig EB. Carcinoma of the anorectal junction. I. Histological considerations. Cancer. 1956;9:480–8. This excerpt is reused with the generous permission of John Wiley and Sons, CCC |RightsLink®, License 5165520024935, License date Oct 10, 2021

7. Fenger C. The anal transitional zone. A method for macroscopic demonstration. Acta Path Microbial Scand Sect A. 1978;86:225–30.
8. Fenger C. The anal transitional zone. Acta Path Microbiol Immunol Scand Section A. 1987;suppl 289(95):1–42.
9. Tanaka E, Noguchi T, Nagai K, Akashi Y, Kawahara K, Shimada T. Morphology of the epithelium of the lower rectum and the anal canal in the adult human. Med Mol Morphol. 2012;45:72–9. The excerpt was reproduced with the generous permission of Springer Nature, CCC|RightsLink®, License number 5142220550768, License Date Sep 04, 2021
10. Stroud BB. On the anatomy of the anus. Ann Surg. 1896;24:1–15.
11. Morgan CN, Thompson HR. Surgical anatomy of the anal canal with special reference to the surgical importance of the internal sphincter and conjoint longitudinal muscle. Ann R Coll Surg Engl. 1956;19:88–114. Permission to reuse this excerpt was granted by the Royal College of Surgeons of England, CCC | Marketplace, Order License ID 1249664-1, Order date 20-Jul-2022
12. Hilton J. On rest and pain. Lecture 12. In: Jacobson WHA, editor. 2nd ed. New York: William Wood & Co., 1879. p. 166. Books.Google.com (Accessed 25 Dec 2019).
13. Morgan CN. The surgical anatomy of the anal canal and rectum. Postgrad Med J. 1936;12:287–300.
14. Buie LA. Anatomic aspects. In: Practical proctology. Philadelphia, WB Saunders Company; 1938. p. 51.
15. Ewing MR. The white line of Hilton. Proc R Soc Med. 1954;47:525–30.
16. Hirschman LJ. Synopsis of ano-rectal diseases. St. Louis, MO: The CV Mosby Co.; 1937. p. 17.
17. George Viner Ellis, FRCS. Br Med J 1900;1(2053):1132.
18. Jabbour SK, Frassica D. Anal cancer. In: Haffty BG, Wilson LD, editors. Handbook of Radiation Oncology: Basic Priniciples and Clinic Protocols. Jones and Bartlett Publishers, LLC, Sudbury, Massachusetts, 2009. p. 518.
19. American Cancer Society. What is anal cancer? https://www.cancer.org/cancer/anal-cancer/about/what-is-anal-cancer.html (Accessed 8 Feb 2020).
20. Shank B, Enker WE, Flam MS. Gross and microscopic anatomy. In: Kufe DW, Pollack RE, Weichselbaum RR, et al., editors. Holland-Frei cancer medicine. 6th ed. Hamilton, ON: BC Decker; 2003. NCBI Bookshelf ID: NBK_{13638}.
21. McColl I. The comparative anatomy and pathology of anal glands. Arris and Gale lecture delivered at the Royal College of Surgeons of England on 25th February 1965. Ann R Coll Surg Engl. 1967;40:36–67.
22. Chiari H. Ueber die analen Divertikel der Rectumsschleimhaut und ihre Beziehung zu den Analfisteln. Medizinische Jahrbücher Wien. 1878;8:419–27.
23. Hill TC. Methods of examination in diseases of the rectum and sigmoid colon. Am J Surg. 1920;34:17–20.
24. Adams EW. Founders of modern medicine.-II. Giovanni Battista Morgagni (A.D. 1682-1771). Med Lib Hist J. 1903;1:270–7.
25. Zampieri F, Zanatta A, Thiene G. An etymological "autopsy" of Morgagni's title: *De sedibus et causis morborum per anatomen indagatis* (1761). Hum Pathol. 2014;45:12–6.

Anatomy-Ischiorectal Fossa

8

James S. Wu

Presentation

In 1867, Gray published *Anatomy, Descriptive and Surgical* [1].

Henry Gray, F.R.S.,
Lecturer on Anatomy at Saint-George's Hospital Medical School.
THE DRAWINGS
by
H. V. Carter, M.D.,
Late Demonstrator of Anatomy at St. George's Hospital.
THE DISSECTIONS
Jointly by the author and Dr. Carter.

Surgical Anatomy of the Perineum and
Ischio-Rectal Region.

"The Ischiorectal region corresponds to the portion of the outlet of the pelvis situated immediately behind the perineum: it contains the termination of the rectum. A deep fossa, filled with fat, is seen on either side of the intestine, between it and the tuberosity of the ischium: this is called the *ischiol-rectal fossa*.

The *superficial fascia* is exposed on the removal of the skin: It is very thick, areolar in texture, and contains much fat in its meshes. In it are found ramifying two or three cutaneous branches of the small sciatic nerve; these in turn round the inferior border of the Gluteus maximus, and are distributed to the integument in this region.

The *External sphincter* is a thin flat plane of muscular fibers, elliptical in shape, and intimately adherent to the integument surrounding the margin of the anus. It measures about three or four inches in length, from its anterior to its posterior extremity, being about an inch in breadth, opposite the anus. It arises from the tip of the coccyx, by a narrow tendinous

J. S. Wu (✉)
Department of Colon and Rectal Surgery, Cleveland Clinic, Cleveland, OH, USA

J. S. Wu, M. D. Inkster (eds.), *Cleveland Clinic Colorectal Case Studies*,
https://doi.org/10.1007/978-3-031-39880-3_8

band, and from the superficial fascia in front of that bone; and is inserted into the tendinous center of the perineum, joining with the Transversus perinei, and the other muscles inserted into this part.

Relations. By its *superficial surface*, with the integument; by its *deep surface,* it is in contact with the Internal sphincter; and is separated from the Levator ani by loose areolar tissue.

The *Ischiorectal Fossa* is situated between the end of the rectum and the tuberosity of the ischium on each side. It is triangular in shape, its base directed to the surface is formed by the integument of the ischiorectal region; its *apex,* directed upward, corresponds to the point of division of the obturator fascia, and the thin membrane given off from it, which covers the outer surface of the Levator ani (ischiorectal fascia). Its dimensions are about an inch in breadth, at the base, and about two inches in depth, being deeper behind than in front. It is bounded, *internally*, by the Sphincter ani, Levator ani, and Coccygeus muscles; *externally,* by the tuberosity of the ischium, and the obturator fascia, which covers the inner surface of the Obturator internus muscle; *in front*, it is limited by the line of junction of the superficial and deep perineal fascia; and *behind*, by the margin of the Gluteus maximus, and the great sacro-sciatic ligament. This space is filled with a large mass of adipose substance, which explains the frequency with which abscesses in the neighborhood of the rectum burrow to a considerable depth."

Coronal and axial views of the ischiorectal fossa are shown in Figs. 8.1 and 8.2.

A summary of ischiorectal fossa boundaries and content is shown in Table 8.1 [2].

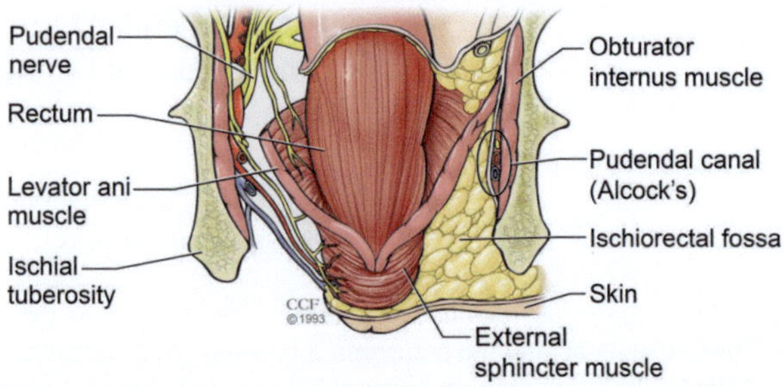

Fig. 8.1 Ischiorectal fossa, coronal view

Table 8.1 Ischiorectal fossa boundaries and content

Ischiorectal fossa boundaries and content
Inferior: skin
Superior: levator ani
Medial: external anal sphincter, levator ani
Lateral: ischial tuberosity, obturator internus muscle
Anterior: superficial transverse perineal muscle
Posterior: gluteus maximus muscle
Contents: fat, Alcock's (pudendal) canal, internal pudendal artery/vein/nerve; inferior rectal artery/vein/nerve

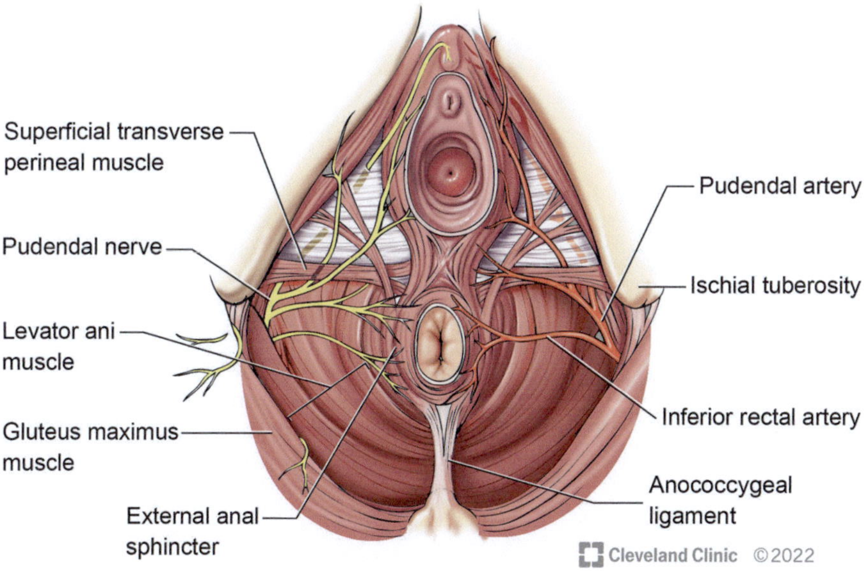

Fig. 8.2 Ischiorectal fossa, axial view

References

1. Gray H. Anatomy, Descriptive and Surgical. The drawings by H. V. Carter, M.D., Second American, from the revised and enlarged London edition, three hundred and ninety-five engravings on wood. Philadelphia, PA: Henry C. Lea, 1867. pp. 775–777. Accessed from Google Books, 14 July 2022.
2. Morgan CN. The surgical anatomy of the ischiorectal space. Proc R Soc Med. 1949;42:189–200.

9 Anatomy-Intestinal Lymphatics

James S. Wu

J. S. Wu (✉)
Department of Colon and Rectal Surgery, Cleveland Clinic, Cleveland, OH, USA

J. S. Wu, M. D. Inkster (eds.), *Cleveland Clinic Colorectal Case Studies*,
https://doi.org/10.1007/978-3-031-39880-3_9

Intestinal Lymphatics

DR. MED. J. Sobotta [1]
ehemals o. ö Professor der Anatomie und Direktor des Anatomischen Instituts in Bonn
Herausgegeben und bearbeitet von
PROF. DR. MED. ET PHIL. H. Becher
Director der Anatomischen Instituts
der Universität Münster i. W.
Das Lymphgefäßsystem,
vasa lymphacea.
Das Lymphgefäßsystem, *vasa lymphacea*, umfaßt die Lymphgefäße und die Lymphknoten (sog. Lymphdrüsen), *lymphonodi* [lymphoglandulae]. Die Lymphgefäße stellen einen Bestandteil des Gefäßsystems dar, und zwar einen (mit blinden Enden beginnenden) Anhang der Venen. Denn die großen Lymphgefäßstämme münden in die vena subclavia sinistra bzw. dextra ein. Die Lymphgefäße enthalten kein Blut, sondern, wie ihr Name sagt, Lymphe. Der Flüssigkeitsstrom in ihnen ist zentripetal gerichtet.

Die Wurzeln der **Lymphgefäße**, *vasa lymphacea*, sind blind; es handelt sich um mikroskopisch kleine, den Blutkapillaren ... ähnliche, aber etwas unregelmäßiger gestaltete, blind in den Organen und Geweben beginnende Lymphkapillaren. Aus diesen gehen kleine, engkalibrige, ihrem Aussehen und ihrem Baue nach den Venen sehr ähnliche, reich mit Klappen ausgestattete vasa lymphacea hervor,...

Die Lymphgefäße des Dünndarms führen den besondern Namen Chylusgefäße; ihr Inhalt — zur Zeit der Verdauung milchweiß — wird auch als chylus bezeichnet. Daher auch der Name: cisterna chyli....
Die Lymphknoten,
Lymphonodi.

Die Lymphknoten (-Drüsen), *lymphonodi* [lymphoglandulae] sind in die Lymphbahn eingeschaltete Filterorgane der Lymphe. Sie werden von der Lymphe durchströmt.

Mit ihnen verwandt sind die Lymphonoduli der Wand mancher Eingeweide wie besonders des Darmes....

Die grossen Lymphgefäßstämme.

1. Der *ductus thoracicus*... ist das mächtigste Lymphgefäß des gesamten Körpers; es sammelt alle Lymphe, außer der aus dem Gebiete des ductus lymphaceus dexter.... Er entsteht in der Höhe des 2. Lendenwirbels aus der Vereinigung der beiden trunci lumbales und des truncus intestinalis in Gestalt einer länglichen Erweiterung des Stammes, *cysterna chyli.*

b. *truncus intestinalis*, der unpaare Lymphgefäßstamm, welcher die Lymphe der Baucheingeweide, namentlich des Darmkanals ableitet.

Lymphknoten des kleinen Beckenraums.

1. *lymphonodi ilici interni*, zahlreiche, neben größeren auch kleinere Lymphknoten; sie liegen teils an der Seitenwand des kleinen Beckens, längs der vasa ilica interna und ihre Äste, teils in der unmittelbaren Umgebung der Beckenorgane....

3. *Lymphonodi anorectales*, klein, aber zahlreicher als die vorigen, seitlich und ventral an der Wand des Mastdarms gelegen (besonders seines kaudalen Abschnittes); nehmen Lymphe vom Mastdarm auf,...

Lymphknoten der Bauchhöhle.

6. *lymphonodi mesosteniales*; sie stellen die größste Ansammlung von Lymphknoten im menschlichen Körper dar; ihre Zahl beträgt 100 bis 150 (und selbst mehr); sie liegen im Dünndarmgekröse so, daß sie mehrere Reihen bilden, von denen die dem Darm zunächst gelegene von den kleinsten Knoten gebildet wird, während an der Gekrösewurzel die größten Lymphknoten gefunden werden. Ihre von der Darmwand kommenden Wurzeln werden als Chylusgefäße... bezeichnet; die vasa efferentia der größten Knoten der radix mesostenii bilden zuzammen mit den obigen (1–5) den ductus intestinalis.

7. *lymphonodi mesocolici*, meist kleiner und stets viel weniger zahlreich als die vorigen, sammeln die Lymphe vom Dickdarm; ihre Anordnung entbehrt der Regelmäßigkeit der Gruppe 6.

DR. Med. J. Sobotta
Formerly Professor of Anatomy and Director of the Anatomical Institute in
Bonn
Issued and edited by
Professor. DR. MED. and PHIL. H. Becher
Director of the Institute of Anatomy
Münster University
The Lymphatic System,
vasa lymphacea.
The lymphatic system, *vasa lymphacea*, includes the lymph vessels and the lymph nodes (so-called lymph glands), *lymphonodi* [lymphoglandulae]. The lymphatic vessels are part of the vascular system, and namely (beginning with blind ends) attachment to the veins. Then the large lymphatic vessel trunks flow into the left subclavian vein, or right respectively. The lymph vessels do not contain blood, but as their name states, lymph. The liquid flow in them is centripetal.

The roots of the **lymph vessels**, *vasa lymphacea*, are blind; concerned with at the small microscopic level, similar to blood capillaries, although somewhat irregularly shaped, lymph capillaries that begin blindly in the organs and tissue. From these emerge vasa lymphacea small, narrow-caliber, similar in appearance and structure to veins, with abundant valves.

The lymphatic vessels of the small intestine follow the particularly named chyle vessels; their content—milk white at the time of digestion—will also be known as chylus. Therefore, also, the name: cisterna chyli.
The lymph nodes,
Lymphnodi.

The lymph nodes (−glands), *lymphonodi* [lymphoglandulae] are connected to the lymph ducts and are organ filters of lymph. Lymph flows through them.

With them are related the lymph nodes of the walls of many gut organs particularly the intestines.

The large lymphatic trunks.

1. The *ductus thoracicus* is the largest lymph vessel of the entire body. It collects all of the lymph, except from the territory of the ductus lymphaceus dexter. It arises high in the second lumbar vertebrae from the union of the two trunci lumbales and from the truncus intestinalis in the shape of a long extension of the *cisterna chyli.*

b. truncus intestinalis, the unpaired lymphatic trunks, that drain the lymph of the abdomen, namely the intestines.

Lymph nodes of the lesser pelvic area.

1. lymphnodi ilici interni, numerous, adjacent to large as well as small lymph nodes; they lie partly in the side walls of the lesser pelvis, along the vasa ilica interna and their branches, the part in the immediate surroundings of the pelvic organs....

3. *Lymphnodi anorectalies*, small, but more numerous than the preceding ones, located laterally and ventrally on the wall of the rectum (particularly its caudal section); carrying lymph from the rectum upward,...

Lymph nodes of the abdominal cavity.

6. *Lymphonodi mesosteniales;* the largest concentration of lymph nodes in the human body are found here; they number 100 to 150 (and even more); they lie in the small intestinal mesentery in such a way that they make up several rows, from which small nodes are developed, while in the root of the mesentery the largest lymph nodes will be found. Their roots arising from the intestinal wall, are called chylous vessels; the *vasa efferentia* of the largest nodes of the radix mesostenii join together with the above (1–5), the ductus intestinalis.

7. *lymphonodi mesocolici*, mostly smaller and always much less numerous as the preceding, collect lymph from the large intestine; their arrangement lacks the regularity of Group 6.

Hamilton summarizes intestinal lymphatic pathways as follows [2]:

"*Superior and Inferior Mesenteric Pathways*

The superior and inferior mesenteric nodes adjoin the origin of the corresponding arteries from the aorta, and they are the terminal nodes of the lymph pathway draining the intestine from the duodenojejunal flexure to the anorectal junction.

Lymph vessels from the jejunum and ileum pass through the mesentery and a large number (100–150) of *mesenteric lymph nodes*. From the terminal ileum, appendix and caecum several lymph vessels proceed to a chain of mesenteric nodes accompanying the ileocolic artery, and finally reach the main superior mesenteric nodes. The lymphatic vessels from the ascending and transverse colon drain to the superior mesenteric nodes, following the branches of the superior mesenteric artery and vein. The efferent vessels from the superior mesenteric nodes join with those from the coeliac nodes to form the *common intestinal lymph trunk*, the largest tributary of the cisterna chyli.

From the splenic flexure to the anorectal junction the lymphatic pathways follow the inferior mesenteric vein and its tributaries. The lymphatics draining the rectum accompany the superior rectal vessels, passing first through the pararectal lymph nodes, and then ascending to join the inferior mesenteric pathway. Vessels from the lower part of the rectum also pass to the internal iliac nodes. The lymph vessels draining the terminal part of the anus go to the proximal superficial inguinal nodes, while those of the rest of the anal canal cross the ischiorectal fossa with the inferior rectal vessels, and then accompany the internal pudendal vessels to reach the internal iliac nodes…."

References

1. Sobotta J, Becher H. Das Lymphgefäßsytem. Atlas der Deskriptiven Anatomie des Menschen. 3. Teil. 15th Edition 1957 ©Urban & Schwarzenberg, München, 1957. pp 354–370. Non-exclusive rights to print and reproduce the citation about Lymphknoten was generously granted by Dr. Cathrin Korz, Lizenzen | Foreign Rights, Elsevier, 13 Sep 2021.
2. Hamilton WJ, editor. Textbook of human anatomy. 2nd ed. St. Louis, MO: CV Mosby Co; 1976. p. 287–8. No objection to reuse of this excerpt was generously granted by Ms. Alice Essenpreis, Rights and Permissions, Springer Nature, on August 10, 2021.

10 Embryology-Intestinal Rotation

Ursula M. Szmulowicz, Carolyn L. Power, Richard L. Drake, and James S. Wu

Intestinal Embryology [1, 2]

The embryologic gut is established by the end of the first trimester. During the second trimester, lengthening and epithelial plus glandular development of the intestine occur. After birth, germinal centers of the gut immune system appear once the infant is exposed to bacteria.

During the 4th week, the gut tube develops into three regions: the foregut, midgut, and hindgut. During the 6th to 8th weeks of gestation, the primitive intestine becomes completely occluded by epithelium, after which it progressively recanalizes. The intestinal epithelium begins to differentiate in the 9th week of gestation. The primitive intestine initially is closely apposed to the dorsal abdominal wall by the mesoderm. By the 5th week of gestation, the mesoderm of the peritoneum forms a thin, two-layered dorsal mesentery in the midline that envelops the gut tube from the abdominal esophagus to the cloaca, suspending it within the peritoneal cavity.

The foregut gives rise to the pharynx, esophagus, stomach, and proximal duodenum. The junction of the fore- and midgut is located just inferior to the ampulla of Vater, the opening of the common bile duct. The straight duodenum develops a C-shape as it pivots to the right, following the rotation of the stomach. These rotations establish the fourth segment of the duodenum in the left upper quadrant. The midgut extends from the duodenum inferior to the opening of the common bile duct to the distal third of the transverse colon. Until approximately the 10th week of gestation, the midgut remains attached to the yolk sac via the narrow vitelline, or omphalomesenteric, duct.

U. M. Szmulowicz · C. L. Power · J. S. Wu (✉)
Department of Colon and Rectal Surgery, Cleveland Clinic, Cleveland, OH, USA

R. L. Drake
Department of Anatomy, Cleveland Clinic Lerner College of Medicine, Cleveland, OH, USA

J. S. Wu, M. D. Inkster (eds.), *Cleveland Clinic Colorectal Case Studies*,
https://doi.org/10.1007/978-3-031-39880-3_10

During the 5th and 6th weeks of gestation, the midgut—particularly the future ileum—rapidly lengthens. Once it exceeds the capacity of the small peritoneal cavity in the 6th week of gestation, the primary intestinal loop begins a physiologic herniation through the umbilicus. While herniated, between the 6th and 8th weeks of gestation, the primary intestinal loop performs a 90° counterclockwise rotation, as viewed from a ventral to dorsal perspective, around an axis composed of the superior mesenteric artery. Two additional 90° counterclockwise rotations transpire at the 9th and 12th weeks of gestation, for a total of 270°. During this process, the cranial limb of the herniated primary intestinal loop—the future small intestine—persists in lengthening and forming loops. In contrast, in the 6th week, the caudal limb changes only by forming a cecal bud, an antimesenteric protuberance that becomes the cecum. The return of the herniated intestine into the abdominal cavity commences in the 10th week of gestation, ending in the 13th week. The series of rotations leaves the proximal jejunum—the first part to re-enter the abdomen—on the left. Initially, the cecal bud—the final segment to return to the abdomen—lies in the right upper quadrant but then travels to the right iliac fossa as the dorsal mesentery suspending the ascending colon shortens and then obliterates. During its descent, the cecal bud gives rise to the appendix. The dorsal mesenteries of the ascending colon and the descending colon recede; the posterior walls of the ascending colon and descending colon become retroperitoneal structures. The mesenteries of the transverse colon and of the sigmoid colon persist; these structures remain intraperitoneal.

The midgut rotates 270° around the axis of the superior mesenteric artery (SMA). The rotation of the midgut is illustrated in Figs. 10.1, 10.2, and 10.3.

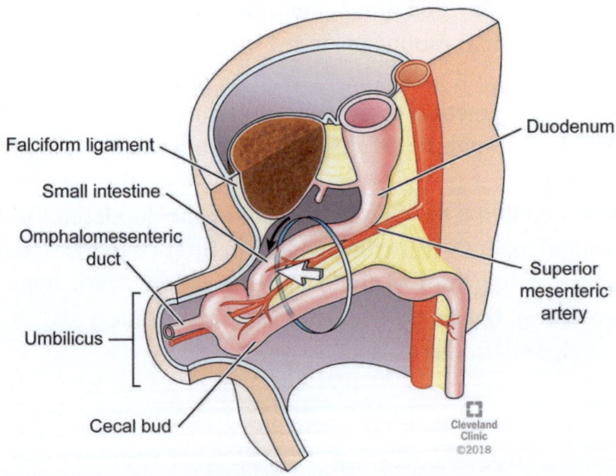

Fig. 10.1 The midgut rotates counterclockwise (black arrow) around the axis of the SMA. The position of the midgut (white arrow) after the first 90° rotation is shown

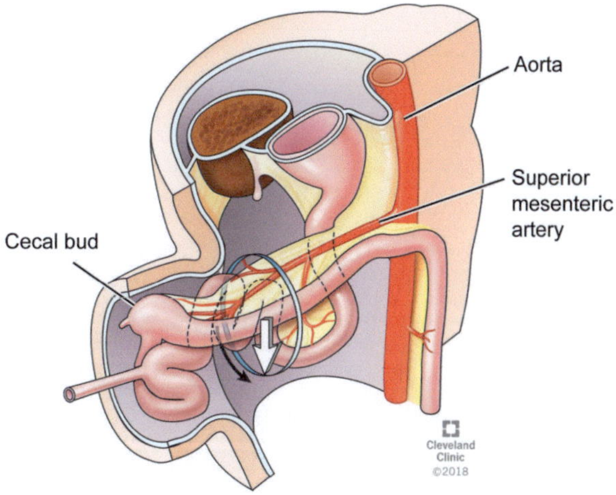

Fig. 10.2 This figure shows the position of the midgut (white arrow) after an additional 90° of rotation (black arrow)

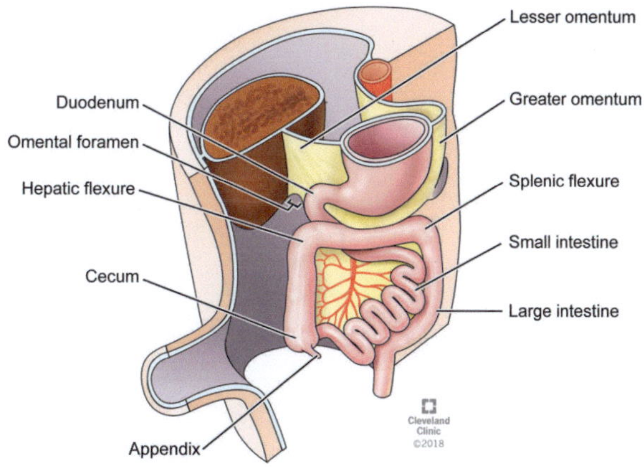

Fig. 10.3 After 270° of rotation, the midgut reaches its final position. The cecum is located in the right lower quadrant. The duodenum is retroperitoneal. The small intestine travels from the left upper quadrant to the right lower quadrant

References

1. Drake RL, Vogl AW, Mitchell AWM. Gray's anatomy for students. Edinburgh: Churchill Livingstone; 2015.
2. Moore KL, Dalley AF. Brief review of the embryological rotation of the midgut. In: Clinically oriented anatomy. 5th ed. Philadelphia, PA: Lippincott Williams & Wilkins; 2006. p. 268–9.

Embryology-Anorectal

11

James S. Wu, Ursula M. Szmulowicz, and Richard L. Drake

Anal Embryology

The hindgut (endoderm) differentiates into the distal one-third of the transverse colon, the descending and sigmoid colon, the rectum, and the proximal anal canal. The cloaca is formed by the allantois anteriorly and the distal hindgut posteriorly (Fig. 11.1a) [1–3]. The boundary between the endoderm and ectoderm is the cloacal membrane [4]. The cloaca then is bisected by the urorectal septum, creating the rectum and anal canal posteriorly and the urogenital sinus anteriorly (Fig. 11.1b). The proctodeum (anal pit) is an indentation of the surface ectoderm located inferior to the posterior cloacal membrane (the anal membrane), resulting from the proliferation of the surrounding mesenchyme. Rupture of the anal membrane creates the anal opening, while the breakdown of the cloacal membrane anteriorly results in an opening for the urogenital structures (Fig. 11.1c).

The former site of the anal membrane is the pectinate (dentate) line. Superior to the dentate line is the 6–12 mm anal transitional zone. Superior to the anal transitional zone is the rectal intestinal lining. Because of its hindgut origin, the rostral anal canal is supplied mainly by the superior rectal artery via the inferior mesenteric artery. Because of its proctodeal origin, the caudal anal canal is supplied by the inferior rectal artery via the internal pudendal artery [3].

J. S. Wu (✉) · U. M. Szmulowicz
Department of Colon and Rectal Surgery, Cleveland Clinic, Cleveland, OH, USA

R. L. Drake
Department of Anatomy, Cleveland Clinic Lerner College of Medicine, Cleveland, OH, USA

J. S. Wu, M. D. Inkster (eds.), *Cleveland Clinic Colorectal Case Studies*,
https://doi.org/10.1007/978-3-031-39880-3_11

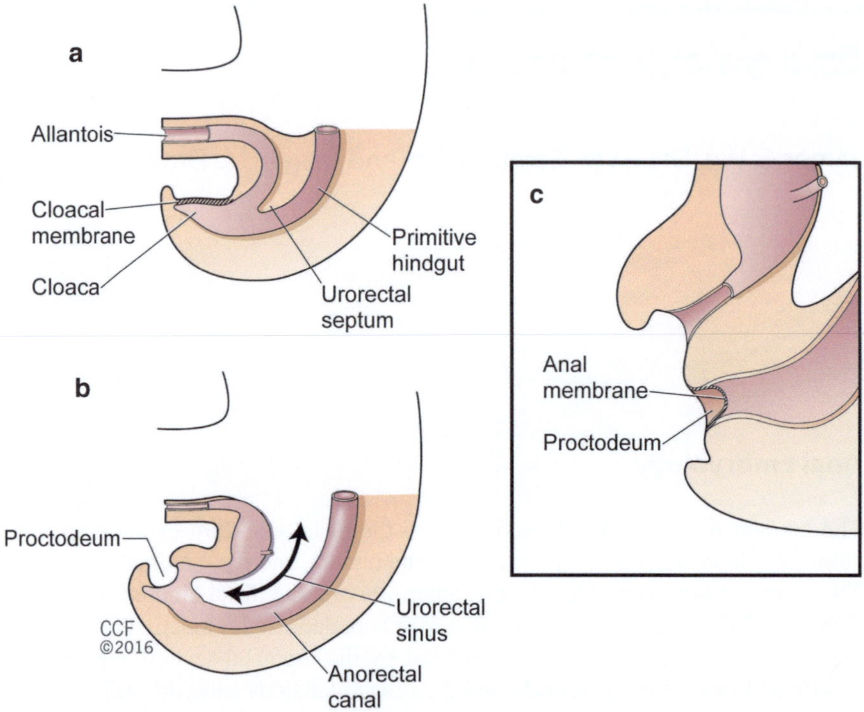

Fig. 11.1 Embryology of the anorectum. (**a**) The primitive hindgut and the allantois terminate as the cloaca. The cloaca is bisected by the urorectal septum [5]. The cloacal membrane is the boundary between the cloaca and the surface ectoderm; (**b**) The urorectal septum separates the gut and urogynecologic structures. The proctodeum (anal pit) is an indentation of the surface ectoderm located inferior to the anal membrane; (**c**) Rupture of the anal membrane creates the anal opening

Comments

Differences in anal embryologic origin lead to different routes for lymphatic drainage and cancer metastases [6]. In his 1961 description of the embryology and anatomy of the anal canal and rectum, Hollingshead stated:

> "Lymphatics: The lymphatic drainage follows four routes, to reach three sets of nodes. The lymphatics of the rectum and anal canal above the pectinate or mucocutaneous line follow the blood vessels: Thus there is the well-known and very important drainage upward along the superior rectal vessels to the inferior mesenteric nodes; and there are two lateral drainages to internal iliac (hypogastric) nodes, one above the levator ani, along the middle rectal vessels, and the second below the levator ani, along the inferior rectal and pudendal vessels. Finally, the lymphatics originating below the mucocutaneous line join perianal lymphatics and drain with these into superficial inguinal nodes."

References

1. "Cloaca." M*erriam-webster.com Dictionary,* Merriam-Webster, https://www.merriam-webster.com/dictionary/cloaca. Accessed 14 June 2021.
2. Dudek RW, Fix JD. Embryology. 4th ed. Baltimore, MD: Wolters Kluwer|Lippincott, Williams & Wilkins; 2008. p. 119–21.
3. Sadler TW. Langman's Medical Embryology. 11th ed. Baltimore, MD: Wolters Kluwer|Lippincott, Williams & Wilkins; 2010. p. 230–1.
4. Hasan RM. Chapter 1: Anatomy of the anal region. In: Hasan R, Mahdi B, editors. New concepts in the management of septic perianal conditions. Elsevier: Amsterdam; 2018. p. 1–8.
5. Moore KL, Persaud TVN. The Developing Human, Clinically Oriented Embryology. 8th ed. Philadelphia, PA: Saunders Elsevier; 2008. p. 236–8.
6. Hollingshead WH. Embryology and anatomy of the anal canal and rectum. Dis Colon Rectum. 1962;5:18–22. Passage reproduced with permission. Wolters Kluwer Health, Inc., and Copyright Clearance Center. License Number 5120750483568. License Date 2 Aug 2021

Transposition of the Viscera

12

Michelle D. Inkster, Arthur A. Parsee, and James S. Wu

Presentation

Computed tomography (CT) of a patient showed *situs inversus* (Fig. 12.1).

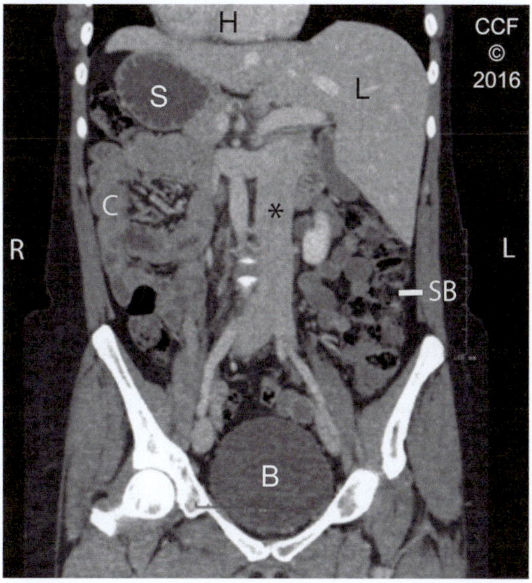

Fig. 12.1 CT of lower chest, abdomen, and pelvis (coronal view) shows *situs inversus*. The heart (H), liver (L), stomach (S), inferior vena cava (asterisk), colon (C), small bowel (SB), and bladder (B) are labeled

M. D. Inkster
Department of Gastroenterology, Cleveland Clinic, Cleveland, OH, USA

A. A. Parsee
Department of Diagnostic Radiology, H. Lee Moffitt Cancer Center and Research Institute, Tampa, FL, USA

J. S. Wu (✉)
Department of Colon and Rectal Surgery, Cleveland Clinic, Cleveland, OH, USA

J. S. Wu, M. D. Inkster (eds.), *Cleveland Clinic Colorectal Case Studies*,
https://doi.org/10.1007/978-3-031-39880-3_12

Comment

In a letter to his uncle, John Hunter, read May 8, 1788, Matthew Baillie gave *An Account of a remarkable Transposition of the Viscera*[1] [1].

Read May 8, 1788

TO JOHN HUNTER, ESQ. F.R.S.

"DEAR SIR,
A VERY singular variety having occurred lately in the
structure of the human body, I beg leave to communi-
cate an account of it by your means to the Royal Society,
if you should think it worthy of their notice. It happens
by a very uncommon concurrence of circumstances, that
while I am naturally led by the ties of affinity to apply to
you upon this occasion, I can gratify my pride by thinking it
is at the same time to the person who is possessed of the first
reputation for his unwearied researches in one of the most ex-
tensive, as well as interesting, parts of the system of nature,
I am, &c.
M. BAILLIE
The person who is the subject of this Paper was a male,
near 40 years of age, somewhat above the middle stature,
and of a clean active shape. He was brought for dissection in
the common way to Windmill-street. Upon opening the
cavity of the thorax and abdomen, the different situation of the
viscera was so striking as immediately to excite the attention of
the pupils who were engaged in dissecting it;…"

Regarding the stomach and the intestines, Baillie records:

> "The stomach was situated on the right side, partly hid by the small lobe of the liver passing to the left, and terminating in the pylorus, rather on the left side of the spine. The duodenum took a most singular course; it first passed to the right-side, behind the small end of the stomach; it then turned upon itself, towards the left side; it afterwards took its proper sweep to the right-side, passing behind the superior mesenteric artery and mesaraica major vein. The mesentery began to be formed on the right-side, instead of the left, as is in ordinary cases. The ileum terminated in the great intestine on the left-side, and there was in it a diverticulum of considerable size, a lusus not unfrequently occurring. The cæcum was situated on the left psoas magnus and iliacus internus muscles. The transverse arch of the colon passed from the left to the right-

[1] For the purposes of clarity, certain letters have been replaced by modern counterparts, e.g., for the word "fhould," the letter "f," used in the original manuscript, has been replaced by the letter "s."

> side of the body, and the sigmoid flexure crossed over the right psoas, to get into the cavity of the pelvis."

Situs inversus (SI), derived from the Latin for "site" and "inverse," refers to the right-to-left mirror image transposition of the viscera. Viscera situated in the usual position is known a *situs solitus*, derived from the Latin for "usual." In 1949, Mayo and Rice [2] reported that during the years 1910 through 1947, of 1,551,047 patients registered at the Mayo Clinic, 76 were found to have SI of both thoracic and abdominal viscera. Seven others showed thoracic transposition only, and four more had transposition of the viscera that was confined to the abdomen. The authors concluded that: "The possibility that situs inversus may be present must always be kept in mind by the physician performing abdominal surgery." In the following Discussion of this paper, Dr. W. J. Potts noted that complete *situs inversus* is a congenital abnormality and cautioned: "It is well to remember that congenital anomalies are frequently multiple." Recognition of SI is an important part of preoperative abdominal operative preparation.

Reference

1. Baillie M. An account of a remarkable transposition of the viscera. Phil Trans Roy Soc Lond. 1788;LXXVIII:350–63. Archiv.org. Accessed 1 Jan 2021
2. Mayo CW, Rice RG. Situs inversus totalis; a statistical review of data on 76 cases with special reference to disease of the biliary tract. Arch Surg 1949;58:724–30

Landmark Nonsurgical Advances (Nineteenth and Twentieth Centuries) 13

James S. Wu and Michelle D. Inkster

Presentation

Advances in surgery are linked closely to discoveries in medicine, anesthesiology, microbiology, blood banking, radiology, endoscopy, genetics, biology, chemistry, and physics [1, 2]. A chronological timeline of major biomedical and basic scientific advances is listed in Table 13.1.

J. S. Wu (✉)
Department of Colon and Rectal Surgery, Cleveland Clinic, Cleveland, OH, USA

M. D. Inkster (✉)
Department of Gastroenterology, Cleveland Clinic, Cleveland, OH, USA

J. S. Wu, M. D. Inkster (eds.), *Cleveland Clinic Colorectal Case Studies*,
https://doi.org/10.1007/978-3-031-39880-3_13

Table 13.1 Chronological timeline of major biomedical and basic science advances

Event	References
1842 C. W. Long describes ether inhalation anesthesia	[3]
1847 J. Y. Simpson describes chloroform inhalation anesthesia	[4]
1895 Wilhelm C. Roentgen announces: "Eine neue Art von Strahlen" (A new kind of ray); awarded the first Nobel prize in physics in 1901	[5, 6]
1880 William Macewen introduces endotracheal intubation	[7]
1899 August Bier describes spinal anesthesia with cocaine	[8]
1900 Karl Landsteiner identifies the four blood groups; awarded the Nobel prize in Physiology or Medicine in 1930.	[9]
1909 S. J. Metzler and John Auer: Continuous respiration without respiratory movements	[10]
1913 Aldred S. Warthin: Heredity with reference to cancer	[11]
1923 A. W. Fischer: Air contrast barium enema	[12]
1929 Alexander Fleming: Penicillin; 1945 Nobel Prize in Physiology or Medicine awarded to Sir Alexander Fleming, Ernst B. Chain, Sir Howard Walter Florey.	[13, 14]
1935 Henry Koenig-Herman W. Rutzen: Ostomy appliance	[15]
1935 Gerhard Domagk: Sulfa drugs. Domagk was awarded the 1939 Nobel prize in Physiology or Medicine.	[16, 17]
1940s World War II American Red Cross establishes a nationwide program for blood collection	[18]
1942 Harold R. Griffith and G. Enid Johnson: Curare in general anesthesia	[19]
1950s Elise Sorensen: Plastic disposable ostomy appliances	[20]
1953 Watson, Crick, Wilkins, Franklin: Double helical structure of DNA 1962 The Nobel Prize in Physiology or Medicine awarded to: Francis H. C. Crick, James D. Watson, and Maurice H. F. Wilkins.	[21–24]
1954 A. C. S. van Heel: Fiberoptics	[25]
1954 S. C. Trulove and L. J. Witts: Therapeutic trial of cortisone in ulcerative colitis	[26]
1961 Hirschowitz: Fiberoptic examination of the stomach and duodenum	[27]
1968 Inkster invents Postive End Expiratory Pressure (P.E.E.P) a.k.a Residual Positive Pressure	[28]
1970s Computed-assisted tomography; the 1979 Nobel Prize in Physiology or Medicine was awarded to Allan M. Cormack and Godfrey N. Hounsfield.	[29]
1976 zur Hausen reports HPV DNA in cervical cancer and warts; awarded the Nobel Prize in Physiology or Medicine in 2008	[30, 31]
Magnetic resonance imaging: Nobel Prizes for nuclear magnetic resonance: 1944 Physics, Isador I. Rabi; 1952—Physics, Felix Bloch and Edward M. Purcell; 1991—Chemistry, Richard R. Ernst; 2002—Chemistry, Kurt Wüthrich.	[32]
1986 Kary B. Mullis—Polymerase chain reaction. Awarded the Nobel Prize in Chemistry in 1993	[33, 34]
1990 Colorectal cancer screening	[35]
1991 Identification of the APC gene	[36, 37]
1991 Identification of germline mismatch repair gene mutations	[38–42]

Biographical Note

Charles Drew (June 3, 1904–April 1, 1950)

Charles Drew received his undergraduate degree from Amherst College and his medical degree from McGill University [43]. He received his surgical training with Dr. Allen O. Whipple at Presbyterian Hospital in New York. As part of his training, Whipple assigned him to the surgical lab of Dr. John Scudder. On November 10, 1942, Scudder and Drew received US patent #2,301,710.

UNITED STATES PATENT OFFICE
2,301,710
APPARATUS FOR PRESERVING BLOOD
John Scudder, New York, N.Y., assignor to
Charles R. Drew, Washington, D.C.

> "This invention relates to the method of and apparatus for preserving blood and more particularly human blood to be used for transfusions.
>
> For a long time in medical and surgical practice it has been customary to inject blood into a patient's veins to take the place of his own which has either been lost or has become altered. Formerly this transfusion of the new blood was done within a few minutes or a few hours after the new blood had been taken from the person giving it. The reason for this prompt transfusion is that blood, when taken from one person soon becomes unfit for injection into another, since it quickly deteriorates unless properly preserved. So long as there is a donor ready to supply blood for injection into a patient or there is time to obtain a donor when needed, there is no special demand for a store or a bank of blood ready to be used. However, it is often the case that blood of the right type is needed immediately in order to save the patient's life. He may be brought into a hospital after losing blood in an accident or he may, being already in a hospital, take a sudden turn for the worse and can be saved only by prompt blood transfusion. In instances such as these it becomes imperative that a supply of typed blood be kept on hand for immediate use.
>
> The larger hospitals have of late years been accustomed to keep a bank or store of blood which has been typed or classified, on hand for emergency use. This has been accomplished by means of refrigeration, keeping the temperature at about four degrees centigrade. By this method human blood can be kept fit for use only a short period of time, after which it is discarded, as it has deteriorated, so much as to be harmful for sick individuals if used.
>
> It is the object of this intervention to preserve blood much longer than was formerly possible."

United States Patent and Trademark Office.

> "The pioneering blood work done by Dr. Drew saved the lives of thousands of allied service men and women during the Second World War. After the war, Dr. Drew became the founding medical director of the Red Cross Blood Bank in the United States and was head of blood collection for the U.S. Army and Navy [44]."

In 1942, the Red Cross announced that it would accept blood from black donors, but would segregate it. Drew objected to this policy. In his 1944 Spingarn Medal acceptance speech, he said:

> "It is fundamentally wrong for any great nation to willfully discriminate against such a large group of its people....One can say quite truthfully that on the battlefields nobody is very interested in where the plasma comes from when they are hurt... [45]."

References

1. Larson MD. History of anesthetic practice. In: Miller RD, editor. *Miller's Anesthesia*, vol. 1. 6th ed. Philadelphia, PA: Elsevier, Churchill Livingstone; 2005. p. 3–52.
2. Wangensteen OH, Wangensteen SD. *The Rise of Surgery. From Empiric Craft to Scientific Discipline.* Minneapolis, MN: The University of Minnesota Press; 1981. 3rd printing

3. Long CW. An account of the first use of sulphuric ether by inhalation as an anæsthetic in surgical operations. South Med Surg J. 1849;5:705–13.
4. Simpson JY. A new anæsthetic agent, more efficient than sulphuric ether. Lancet. 1847;50(1264):549–50.
5. Röntgen W. Eine neue Art von Strahlen. Würzburg, Verlag und Druck der Stahlel'schen K. Hof- und Universitäts-Buch und Kunsthandlung, Ende 1895. Accessed from the Harvard Library Viewer, iiif.lib.harvard.edu, September 11, 2022.1901-The first Nobel prize in physics.
6. Wilhelm Conrad Röntgen — Facts. NobelPrize.org. Nobel prize Outreach AB 2022. Sat 10 Sep 2022. https://www.nobelprize.ora/prizes/physics/1901/rontgen/facts/
7. Macewen W. Clinical observations on the introduction of tracheal tubes by the mouth instead of performing tracheotomy or laryngotomy. Br Med J. 1880;2:163–5.
8. Bier A. Versuche über Cocainisiring des Rückenmarkes. Deutsch Zeitschr Chir. 1899;51:361–9.
9. Landsteiner K. Über agglutinationserscheinungen normalen menschlichen Blutes. Wien Klin Wochenschr. 1901;14:1132–4; Karl Landsteiner - Biographical. nobelprize.org/prizes/medicine/1930/landsteiner/biographical/
10. Meltzer SJ, Auer J. Continuous respiration without respiratory movements. J Exp Med. 1909;11:622–5.
11. Warthin AS. Heredity with reference to carcinoma as shown by the study of the cases examined in the pathological laboratory of the University of Michigan, 1895-1913. Arch Intern Med. 1913;12:546–55.
12. Fischer AW. Über eine neue Röntgenologische Untersuchungsmethode des Dickdarms: Komination von Kontrasteinlauf und Luftaufblähung Klin Wochenschr. 1923;2:1595–8.
13. Fleming A. On a remarkable bacteriolytic element found in tissues and secretions. Proc R Soc B. 1922;93:306–17.
14. The Nobel Prize in Physiology or Medicine in 1945. NobelPrize.org. Nobel Prize Outreach AB 2022. Sat. 10 Sep 2022. https://www.nobelprize.org/prizes/medicine/1945/summary/.
15. Personal communication from Mr. Earl Rutzen, age 81, son of Mr. Herman W. Rutzen, September 10, 2009.
16. Domagk G. Ein Beitrag zur Chemotherapie der bakteriellen Infektionen. Dtsch Med Wochenschr. 1935;61:250–3. 1939 Nobel prize in Physiology or Medicine
17. The Nobel Prize in Physiology or Medicine 1939. NobelPrize.org. Nobel Prize Outreach AB 2022. Sun 11 Sep 2022. https://www.nobelprize.org/prizes/medicine/1939/summary/.
18. Diamond LK. History of blood banking in the United States. J Am Med Assoc. 1965;193:40–4.
19. Griffith HR, Johnson GE. The use of curare in general anesthesia. Anesthesiology. 1942;3:418–20.
20. Coloplast Company. Helios. 40th Anniversary Article. 13.8.1997 Revised, pages 2–3; Coloplast Company. How Coloplast brought a radical change to ostomy care 40 years ago. Humlebæk, September 1997.
21. Watson JD, Crick FHC. Molecular structure of nucleic acids. A structure for deoxyribose nucleic acid. Nature. 1953;171:737–8.
22. The Nobel Prize in Physiology or Medicine 1962. NobelPrize.org. Nobel Prize Outreach AB 2022. Sun 11 Sep 2022. https://www.nobelprize.org/prizes/medicine/1939/summary/.
23. Wilkins MHF, Stokes AR, Wilson HR. Molecular structure of deoxypentose nucleic acids. Nature. 1953;171:738–40.
24. Franklin RE, Gosling RG. Molecular configuration in sodium thymonucleate. Nature. 1953;171:740–1.
25. Van Heel ACS. A new method of transporting optical images without aberrations. Nature. 1954;173:39.
26. Truelove SC, Witts LJ. Cortisone in ulcerative colitis. Preliminary report on a therapeutic trial. Br Med J. 1954;2:375–8.
27. Hirschowitz BI. Endoscopic examination of stomach and duodenal cap with the fiberscope. Lancet. 1961;1:1074–8.

28. Bray RJ. Dr. John Scott Inkster-Obituary. Association of Paediatric Anaesthetists of Great Britain and Ireland. https://web.archive.org/web/20161021073133/http://www.apagbi.org.uk/about-us/membership/obituaries/dr-johnscott-inkster. Accessed February 6, 2024; ii. Craft A. John Scott Inkster. BMJ 2011;343;d7517.
29. The Nobel Prize in Physiology or Medicine 1979. NobelPrize.org. Nobel Prize Outreach AB 2022. Sun 11 Sep 2022. https://www.nobelprize.org/prizes/medicine/1979/summary/.
30. zur Hausen H. Condyloma acuminata and human genital cancer. Cancer Res. 1976;36:794.
31. The Nobel Prize in Physiology or Medicine 2008. NobelPrize.org. Nobel Prize Outreach AB 2022. Sun 11 Sep 2022. https://www.nobelprize.org/prizes/medicine/1979/summary/.
32. Nobel prizes for nuclear magnetic resonance: 1944-Nobel prize for Physics Isador I. Rabi; 1952-Nobel prize for Physics: Felix Bloch and Edward M. Purcell; 1991-Nobel prize for Chemistry-Richard R. Ernst; 2002-Nobel prize for Chemistry: Kurt Wüthrich. Nobel Prize. www.nobelprize.org
33. Mullis K, Faloona F, Scharf S, Saiki R, Horn G, Erlich H. Specific enzymatic amplification of DNA in vitro: the polymerase chain reaction. Cold Spring Harbor Symp Quant Biol. 1986;51:263–73.
34. The Nobel Prize in chemistry 1993. NobelPrize.org. Nobel Prize Outreach AB 2022. Sun 11 Sep 2022. https://www.nobelprize.org/prizes/chemistry/1983/summary/.
35. Winawer SJ. The history of colorectal cancer screening. Digest Dis Sci. 2015;60:596–608.
36. Herrera L, Kakati S, Gibas L, Pietrzak E, Sandberg AA. Brief clinical report: Gardner syndrome in a man with an interstitial deletion of 5q. Am J Med Genet. 1986;25:473–6.
37. Groden J, Thliveris A, Samowitz W, Carlson M, Gelbert L, Albertsen H, et al. Identification and characterization of the familial adenomatous polyposis coli gene. Cell. 1991;66:589–600.
38. Fishel R, Lescoe MK, Rao MRS, Copeland NG, Jenkins NA, Garber J, et al. The human mutator gene homolog *MSH2* and its association with hereditary nonpolyposis colon cancer. Cell. 1993;75:1027–38.
39. Leach FS, Nicolaides NC, Papadopoulos N, Liu B, Jen J, Parsons R, et al. Mutations of a *mutS* homolog in hereditary nonpolyposis colorectal cancer. Cell. 1993;75:1215–25.
40. Nicolaides NC, Papadopoulos N, Liu B, Wei Y-F, Carter KC, Ruben SM, et al. Mutations of two *PMS* homologues in hereditary nonpolyposis colon cancer. Nature. 1994;371:75–80.
41. Bronner CE, Baker SM, Morrison PT, Warren G, Smith LG, Lescoe MK, et al. Mutation in the DNA mismatch repair gene homologue *hMLH1* is associated with hereditary non-polyposis colon cancer. Nature. 1994;368:258–61.
42. Papadopoulos N, Nicolaides NC, Wei Y-F, Ruben SM, Carter KC, Rosen CA, et al. Mutation of a *mutL* homolog in hereditary colon cancer. Science. 1994;263:1625–9.
43. Charles Richard Drew "Father of the Blood Bank," June 3, 1904-April 1, 1950. The American Chemical Society; https://www.acs.org/education/whatischemistry/african-americans-in-science/charlesrichard-drew.html. accessed April 2, 2023.
44. USPTO. Patent for preserving blood issued November 10, 1942. Washingtonian's invention made blood bank possible. November 9, 2001 Press Release # 01-52. Contact Brigid Quinn, brigid.quinn@uspto.gov.(Accessed 21 Apr 2018).
45. The Charles R. Drew Papers. Becoming "the Father of the Blood Bank," 1938-1941. Profiles in Science. NIH/National Library of Medicine. http://profiles.nim.nih.gov/ps/retrieve/Narrative/BG/p-nid/336 (Accessed 6 Apr 2019).

Surgeons and the Nobel Prize

14

Emina H. Huang

Introduction

In the history of the Nobel Prize, several have been given to surgeons. The majority of the awards have been associated with technical innovations; but sprinkled among them are those that would influence a field and change disease management. Common to these investigators have been qualities of curiosity, commitment, determination, passion, and grit [1, 2].

Surgeon Nobel Laureates

1. **Theodor Kocher**: In 1909, this Swiss surgeon became the first surgeon to be awarded the Nobel Prize. While we all know of the eponymously named clamps and mobilization of the duodenum, he received his Nobel Prize for other work. He was trained by contemporaneous mentors including Lister in Edinburgh, Pasteur in Paris, and Billroth in Vienna who gave him his appreciation of bacteria and wound care. However, it was the local absence of iodine in the water and consequent goiter that affected children resulting in airway compression that evolved into his understanding of thyroid surgery. Kocher's thyroidectomy surgery was so thorough that in a few cases his patients developed myxedema, with its classic cretin appearance. These keen observations and understanding of thyroid physiology led the Nobel committee to award Kocher the Prize in Physiology or Medicine [3].
2. **Allvar Gullstrand**: This Swedish ophthalmologist was granted the Nobel Prize in 1911 for seminal work in visual optics addressing astigmatism, cataracts, and, most importantly, the slit lamp [4].

E. H. Huang (✉)
Department of Surgery, University of Texas Southwestern, Dallas, TX, USA

J. S. Wu, M. D. Inkster (eds.), *Cleveland Clinic Colorectal Case Studies*,
https://doi.org/10.1007/978-3-031-39880-3_14

3. **Alexis Carrel:** This French surgeon was awarded the Nobel Prize in Physiology or Medicine in 1912 for suturing techniques for vascular anastomoses. He also is recognized for developing the pump for organ preservation in transplantation. The stabbing death of French president Marie François Sadi Carnot, where the portal vein was severed and could not be successfully repaired, led Carrel to develop the technique of triangulation for the repair of blood vessels. It is reported that he learned from an embroideress. His techniques are used widely to this day [5].
4. **Róbert Bárány**: This Austro-Hungarian surgeon is credited with understanding the physiology of the inner ear. Though he began his career as a neurosurgeon, approximately 1 year into his training, he progressed to a post at the Otological Clinic at the University of Vienna. He advanced understanding of the vestibular apparatus. In particular, he observed that cold and warm irrigation maneuvers resulted in opposing directions of nystagmus due to influences on the semicircular canals. Sadly, when awarded the prize in 1914, he was a Russian prisoner of war. He had been pressed into service in WWI as a surgeon for the German-Austrian alliance to care for otolaryngologic injuries. His talent was recognized by his Russian captors, and he was forced to care for them as well. His release was requested by the Prince of Sweden. He received the Nobel Prize in 1916 [6].
5. **Frederick Banting**: Likely the most famous and one of the most influential surgeons to win a Nobel Prize was Dr. Banting. After serving in France during WWI, he returned to Canada initially to become an orthopedic surgeon. However, the death of a childhood friend from diabetes led Banting to study this disease. Banting worked with physiologist, Professor John J. R. Macleod, at the University of Toronto and with a student, Charles Best. Best and Banting tied off the pancreatic ducts in dogs and injected an extract harvested from the pancreas into a dog whose pancreas had been removed. The recipient dog recovered immediately. The Nobel Prize in Physiology or Medicine 1923 was awarded jointly to Banting and Macleod "for the discovery of insulin." Recognizing that the Nobel committee did not give Best the credit that he deserved, Banting shared his prize money with him [7].
6. **Walter Hess**: An ophthalmologist by training, after WWI, Hess studied physiology. He was intrigued by the association of physiology with the brain and conducted specific experiments to correlate electrical stimulation of the midbrain to autonomic functions such as pupillary dilation, salivation, and bowel movements using cats as his subjects. He was credited with "discovery of the functional organization of the diencephalon as a coordinator of activities of the internal organs." He received the Nobel Prize in Physiology or Medicine in 1949 [8].
7. **Werner Forssmann**: Dr. Forssmann was a physician from Germany who shared the 1956 Nobel Prize in Physiology or Medicine for developing a procedure for cardiac catheterization by advancing a catheter into his own heart. His technique revolutionized both the diagnosis and the management of cardiac disease [9].
8. **Charles Huggins**: Huggins, born Canadian, did his general surgery training at the University of Michigan. Working on prostate cancer, he recognized the hormonal influences of androgen depletion, castration, and estrogen

supplementation on decreasing prostate cancer progression. He was awarded the Nobel Prize in 1966 [10].

9. **Joseph Murray**: Dr. Murray was trained as a plastic surgeon. His interest in transplantation stemmed from experience in World War II where he reconstructed disfigured hands and faces. With burn patients, he recognized that rejection of skin allografts was not as rapid as would be expected; thus, he reasoned that renal allografts were feasible. He was the first to perform a successful human kidney transplant between identical twins. The procedure took place at the Peter Bent Brigham Hospital in 1954. A healthy kidney from one twin was donated to the other twin who had chronic nephritis. The twin then lived for 8 years. He performed the first allograft transplantation in 1959, followed by the first cadaveric renal transplantation in 1962. He received the Nobel Prize in Physiology or Medicine in 1990. [11].

   Shinya Yamanaka: This physician is included here to remind us that sometimes surgery as a career may not be the path forward but may deliver insights into key problems needing to be solved. Although Dr. Yamanaka began a career in orthopedic surgery, he changed his career direction to basic science in order to find the causes and mechanisms of disease. He obtained a PhD in Pharmacology and learned how to design and conduct experiments. At the Nara Institute for Science and Technology, he began the work that would eventually result in his 2012 Nobel Prize which he shared with John Gurdon [5]. They recognized the potential for cellular reprogramming of mature, adult mouse fibroblasts to cells that were pluripotent, or "induced pluripotent stem cells," that were able to generate all of the three germ layer lineages that would eventually be differentiated into terminal cells phenotypically resembling epithelial cells and mesenchyme. Such technology therefore would obviate the need for use of controversial embryonic stem cells. Furthermore, the approach and techniques he developed would then pave the way for individualized reprogramming of cells and tissues both for examination of disease processes and as potential avatars to test therapies [12].

Innovation: Impact and Influence

Each of these innovators was driven by curiosity, a compelling problem, and grit. In order to participate in new areas of research, the colorectal surgeon will need to understand and incorporate into their armamentarium the following:

1. Technology: as the world advances in technology so are there innovations in colorectal surgical science, both at the bench and at the bedside. Here, as a culture, we need to embrace technology, test the technology to develop evidence-based strategies, and then implement those aspects that are both compelling and cost-effective.
2. Gene Editing: With greater comprehension of our genetics, and the influences of the microenvironment on our genes, gene editing with tools such as

CRISPR-Cas9 will transform both single nucleotide and polygenic diseases. The power of these technologies may someday obviate the scalpel as prevention in contexts as simple as colonoscopy and may eventually overtake the need for surgical resection. However, for now, understanding the magnitude of these technologies and seeing a future where their importance is valued for the context of disease is paramount.
3. Stem Cells and regeneration: In colorectal surgery we are always anticipating the next procedure, balancing risk vs. benefit. We are always asking about regeneration of the gut, the skin, the anastomosis, the vessels and nerves and more. Here, stem cell-based technologies both for the epithelia and for the mesenchyme will provide other tools, potentially with roles in transplantation, cancer, and short gut syndrome.
4. Big data: with the advent of the Human Genome project and increased understanding of the intricacies of human genetics both in disease and in health, our ability to manipulate and integrate these data with reference to surgical diseases will provide insights into prevention, biomarkers and cure.
5. Computational biology: Integrating data from all of these data will be increasingly complex. Systems biology approaches to reduce the data to patterns that are comprehensible and facilitate implementation will be of increasing importance.

Challenges

Practical issues abound when we consider where the next generation of colorectal surgeon-scientists will emerge. Equally important are the issues surrounding initiation of careers in surgical science with expansion into areas such as healthcare delivery, molecular epidemiology, healthcare economics, informatics, and bioinformatics. Here more senior surgeons must encourage junior trainees and faculty to be free enough to consider the "right" questions to ask. Such opportunities require insight and sufficient time to reflect on those questions which merit further investigation. Basic questions may not have simple answers. The pedagogy and apprenticeship style that has been the culture of surgical training for decades to centuries may not be the best for producing surgeon scientists and innovators.

While the challenges of funding abound for surgeon scientists, there has never been a more important time for scientists to come to the helm of the clinician to join forces in a synergistic manner to solve some of the most difficult problems. The NIH recognizes the need for more physician scientists, and so too do the most revered institutions in our country.

So, then it falls to the mid-career and senior members of our society to create an environment that nurtures the young and gently nudges them to secure their right to change the field. As coaches, mentors, and especially as sponsors, mid-career and senior colorectal surgeon scientists need to foster such niches and relationships, allowing these young investigators to critically reflect on those most pressing issues with new tools enabled by advances in technology [13].

References

1. Cosimi AB. Surgeons and the Nobel prize. Arch Surg. 2006;141:340–8.
2. Schlich T. Nobel prizes for surgeons: In recognition of the surgical healing strategy. Int J Surg. 2007;5:129–33.
3. The Nobel Prize in Physiology or Medicine 1909 was awarded to Emil Theodor Kocher "for his work on the physiology, pathology and surgery of the thyroid gland." The Nobel Prize in Physiology or Medicine 1909. NobelPrize.org. Nobel Prize Outreach AB 2023. Mon. 6 Feb 2023. https://www.nobelprize.org/prizes/medicine/1909/summary/.
4. The Nobel Prize in Physiology or Medicine 1911 was awarded to Allvar Gullstrand "for his work on the dioptrics of the eye." The Nobel Prize in Physiology or Medicine 1911. NobelPrize.org. Nobel Prize Outreach AB 2023. Mon. 6 Feb 2023. https://www.nobelprize.org/prizes/medicine/1911/summary/.
5. The Nobel Prize in Physiology or Medicine 1912 was awarded to Alexis Carrel "in recognition of his work on vascular suture and the transplantation of blood vessels and organs." The Nobel Prize in Physiology or Medicine 1912. NobelPrize.org. Nobel Prize Outreach AB 2023. Mon. 6 Feb 2023. https://www.nobelprize.org/prizes/medicine/1912/summary/.
6. The Nobel Prize in Physiology or Medicine 1914 was awarded to Robert Bárány "for his work on the physiology and pathology of the vestibular apparatus." The Nobel Prize in Physiology or Medicine 1914. NobelPrize.org. Nobel Prize Outreach AB 2023. Mon. 6 Feb 2023. https://www.nobelprize.org/prizes/medicine/1914/summary/.
7. The Nobel Prize in Physiology or Medicine 1923 was awarded jointly to Frederick Grant Banting and John James Rickard Macleod "for the discovery of insulin." The Nobel Prize in Physiology or Medicine 1923. NobelPrize.org. Nobel Prize Outreach AB 2023. Mon. 6 Feb 2023. https://www.nobelprize.org/prizes/medicine/1923/summary/.
8. The Nobel Prize in Physiology or Medicine 1949 was awarded to Rudolf Hess "for his discovery of the functional organization of the interbrain as a coordinator of the activities of the internal organs." The Nobel Prize in Physiology or Medicine 1949. NobelPrize.org. Nobel Prize Outreach AB 2023. Mon. 6 Feb 2023. https://www.nobelprize.org/prizes/medicine/1949/summary/.
9. The Nobel Prize in Physiology or Medicine 1956 was awarded jointly to André Frédéric Cournand, Werner Forssmann and Dickinson W. Richards "for their discoveries concerning heart catheterization and pathological changes in the circulatory system." The Nobel Prize in Physiology or Medicine 1956. NobelPrize.org. Nobel Prize Outreach AB 2023. Mon. 6 Feb 2023. https://www.nobelprize.org/prizes/medicine/1956/summary/.
10. The Nobel Prize in Physiology or Medicine 1966 was divided equally between Peyton Rous "for his discovery of tumour-inducing viruses" and Charles Brenton Huggins "for his discoveries concerning hormonal treatment of prostatic cancer." The Nobel Prize in Physiology or Medicine 1966. NobelPrize.org. Nobel Prize Outreach AB 2023. Mon. 6 Feb 2023. https://www.nobelprize.org/prizes/medicine/1966/summary/.
11. The Nobel Prize in Physiology or Medicine 1990 was awarded jointly to Joseph E. Murray and E. Donnall Thomas "for their discoveries concerning organ and cell transplantation in the treatment of human disease." The Nobel Prize in Physiology or Medicine 1990. NobelPrize.org. Nobel Prize Outreach AB 2023. Mon. 6 Feb 2023. https://www.nobelprize.org/prizes/medicine/1990/summary/.
12. The Nobel Prize in Physiology or Medicine 2012 was awarded jointly to Sir John B. Gurdon and Shinya Yamanaka "for the discovery that mature cells can be reprogrammed to become pluripotent." The Nobel Prize in Physiology or Medicine 2012. NobelPrize.org. Nobel Prize Outreach AB 2023. Mon. 6 Feb 2023. https://www.nobelprize.org/prizes/medicine/2012/summary/.
13. Keswani SG, Moles CM, Morowitz M, Zeh H, Kuo JS, Levine MH, et al. The future of basic science in academic surgery: identifying barriers to success for surgeon-scientists. Ann Surg. 2017;265:1053–9.

Handwashing

15

James S. Wu

Alexander Gordon

Alexander Gordon (1752–1799), an obstetrician, published a treatise on the epidemic puerperal fever that occurred in Aberdeen in 1789. He recognized the contagious nature of the disease and advocated good hygiene as a preventative measure [1, 2].

> A Treatise on the Epidemic Puerperal Fever of Aberdeen
> Alexander Gordon, 1795
> "Chap. IV.
> CAUSE OF THE DISEASE [3].
> Various causes have been assigned by writers for the production of the Puerperal Fever.
>
> That the cause of this disease was a specific contagion, or infection, I have unquestionable proof.
>
> In short, I had evident proofs of its infectious nature, and that the infection was as readily communicated as that of the small-pox, or measles, and operated more speedily than any other infection, with which I am acquainted.
>
> With respect to the physical qualities of the infection, I have not been able to make any discovery; but I had evident proofs that every person, who had been with a patient in the Puerperal Fever, became charged with an atmosphere of infection, which was communicated to every pregnant woman, who happened to come within its sphere.
>
> The midwife, who delivered No. I. in the table, carried the infection to No. 2, the next woman whom she delivered. The physician, who attended No. I and 2, carried the infection to No. 5 and 6, who were delivered by him, and to many

J. S. Wu (✉)
Department of Colon and Rectal Surgery, Cleveland Clinic, Cleveland, OH, USA

J. S. Wu, M. D. Inkster (eds.), *Cleveland Clinic Colorectal Case Studies*,
https://doi.org/10.1007/978-3-031-39880-3_15

others. The midwife, who delivered No. 3, carried the infection to No. 4; from No. 24 to No. 25, 26, and successively, to every woman whom she delivered. The same thing is true of many others, too tedious to be enumerated.

It is a disagreeable declaration for me to mention, that I myself was the means of carrying the infection to a great number of women. But happily, before I knew that the disease was infectious, I had discovered a remedy which would certainly cure it, if early applied. This discovery was a consolation, which, in a great measure, compensated for the uneasiness which the knowledge of the above-mentioned fact would have otherwise occasioned.

CHAP. VII.
PREVENTION OF THE DISEASE [4].
The patient's apparel and bed-clothes ought, either to be burnt, or thoroughly purified; and the nurses and physicians, who have attended patients affected with the Puerperal Fever, ought carefully to wash themselves, and to get their apparel properly fumigated, before it be put on again [5]."

15.1 Ignaz Philip Semmelweis

The practice of cleaning the hands, clothing, and instruments with disinfectant to limit the transmission of disease from physician to patient was championed by Ignaz Philipp Semmelweis (1818–1865). Semmelweis began his obstetric practice at the Viennese Maternity Hospital in 1846. He recorded his recollections of his experiences there in 1861 [6, 7]. At that time, the maternity ward consisted of a private ward for women who could pay for their care and two gratis clinics. The first gratis clinic was staffed by male obstetricians in training. In the second gratis clinic, female midwives were trained [8]. He noted that between 1841 and 1846, the mortality in the first clinic was three times that of the second clinic (Table 15.1).

The difference between the two gratis clinics was that in the obstetrician trainee clinic, corpses were dissected to correlate clinical and autopsy findings [10].

Table 15.1 Mortality rate in the gratis obstetrics clinics at the Viennese maternity hospital 1841–1846 [9]

First clinic			Second clinic		
Births	Deaths	Mortality (%)	Births	Deaths	Mortality
20,042	1989	9.92	17,791	691	3.38

Semmelweis concluded that this practice was directly responsible for maternal death by childbirth fever.

Die Ätiologie, der Begriff und die Prophylaxis des Kindbettfiebers [11]. Ignaz Philipp Semmelweis, 1861	The Etiology, Concept, and Prophylaxis of Childbed Fever [12]. Ignaz Semmelweis, 1861 (Translated and Edited, with an Introduction by K. Codell Carter)
Am 20. März 1847 übernahm ich zum zweiten Male die Stelle eines wirklichen Assistenten der ersten Gebärklinik, machte früh Morgens meine gynaecologischen Studien in der Todtenkammer, ging dann auf das Kreissezimmer, um sämmtliche auf dem Kreissezimmer befindliche Kreissende, wie es meine und meiner Vorfahren Pflicht war, zu untersuchen, damit ich dann dem die Morgenvisite haltenden Professor über jede einzelne Kreissende einen Bericht erstatten konnte. Dadurch habe ich meinen mit Cadavertheilen verunreinigten Finger mit den Genitalien so vieler Kreissenden in Berührung gebracht, und die Folge war, dass im April von 312 Entbundenen 57, also $18._{26}$ Percent, gestorben. Im Mai sind von 294 Entbundenen 36 gestorben, also $12._{24}$ Percent. Mitte Mai beiläufig war es, ohne mich jedoch des Tages zu entsinnen, wo ich die Chlorwaschungen einführte. Es waren mithin nicht die Beleidigungen der Genitalien durch das rohere Untersuchen der Studirenden, eine an und für sich schon irrige Voraussetzung, welche die grössere Sterblichkeit an der ersten Gebärklinik hervorgebracht, sondern das in Berührungbringen der Genitalien mit Cadavertheilen mittelst des untersuchenden Fingers war es, was die grössere Sterblichkeit an der ersten Gebärklinik hervorbrachte.	On 20 March 1847, I reassumed the position of assistant in the first clinic. Early that morning, I conducted my gynecological studies in the morgue. I then went to the labor room and began to examine all the patients, as my predecessors and I were obliged to do, so that I could report on each patient during the professor's morning rounds. My hands, contaminated by cadaverous particles, were thereby brought into contact with the genitals of so many women in labor that in April, from 312 deliveries, there were 57 deaths (18.26 percent). In May, from 294 deliveries there were 36 deaths (12.24 percent). In the middle of May, without noting the exact day, I instituted chlorine washings. Thus, the great mortality in the first clinic was not caused by injuries in rough examinations—a completely false assumption—but by contaminated fingers that contacted the genitals of the patients.

To combat this iatrogenic cause of mortality, Semmelweis introduced washing with chlorine solutions. The benefit was striking.

Im Jahre 1848, wo das ganze Jahr hindurch die Chlorwaschungen emsig geübt wurden, starben von 3556 Wöchnerinnen 45, $1._{27}$ Percent. An der zweiten Abtheilung starben im Jahre 1848 von 3219 Entbundenen 43, d. i. $1._{33}$ Percent [13].	In 1848, chlorine washings were instituted throughout the year, and of 3,556 patients, 45 died (1.27 percent). In the second clinic in the year 1848, of 3,219 patients, 43 died (1.33 percent) [14].

Semmelweis' method of disinfection targeted not only the hands, but also instruments, bed-clothing, sponges, and bathing bowls among other things.

Die Nothwendigkeit, die Hand zu desinficiren, wird daher immer bleiben, und um dieses Ziel vollkommen zu erreichen, ist es nöthig, die Hand, bevor ein zersetzter Stoff berührt wird, gut zu beöhlen, damit der zersetzte Stoff nicht in die Poren der Hand eindringen könne; nach einer solchen Beschäftigung muss die Hand mit Seife gewaschen, und dann der Einwirkung eines chemischen Agens ausgesetzt werden, welches geeignet ist, den nicht entfernten zersetzten Stoff zu zerstören; wir bedienen uns des Chlorkalkes, und waschen uns so lange, bis die Hand schlüpfrig wird. Eine so behandelte Hand ist vollkommen desinficirt. Träger der zersetzten Stoffe ist übrigens nicht blos der untersuchende Finger, sondern alle Gegenstände, welche mit zersetzten Stoffen verunreinigt sind, und mit den Genitalien der Individuen in Berührung kommen; diese Gegenstände müssen daher vor ihrer Inberührungbringung mit den Genitalien desinficirt, oder ausser Verwendung gesetzt werden, hieher gehören Instrumente, Bettwäsche, Schwämme, Leibschüsseln etc. etc. [15]	In order to disinfect the hands completely, it is necessary to oil them before they are contaminated so that the decaying matter cannot penetrate the pores. Thereafter the hands must be washed with soap and then exposed to the operation of a chemical agent to destroy the decaying matter. I employ chloride of lime and wash as long as it is necessary to make the hands slippery. Hands treated in this way are completely disinfected. Decaying matter is carried not only by the examining finger but also by everything contaminated that can come into contact with the genitals. These items must, therefore, either be disinfected or no longer used [16].

Reflecting back on the consequences of his own practice before his introduction of washing, Semmelweis confesses:

Consequent meiner Ueberzeugung muss ich hier das Bekenntniss ablegen, dass nur Gott die Anzahl derjenigen kennt, welche wegen mir frühzeitig ins Grab gestiegen [17].	In consequence of my conviction I must affirm that only God knows the number of patients who went prematurely to their graves because of me [18].

15.2 Comment

In 2019, at all Cleveland Clinic Hospitals, a computer screen admonishes the person signing on to "Wash Hands." This practice, now accepted as normal and expected, is rooted in the work of both Drs. Gordon and Semmelweis. Both reports are remarkable not only for their descriptions of caregiver to patient transmission of infectious disease in childbed fever (puerperal fever) and their recommendations for remediation of the problem, but also notably for their brutally honest public testaments of their own culpability in causation.

References

1. Gordon A. A treatise on the epidemic puerperal fever of Aberdeen. London: G.G. and J. Robinson; 1795. Accessed from Internet Archive, archive.org, September 12, 2022
2. Gould IM. Alexander Gordon, puerperal sepsis, and modern theories of infection control—Semmelweis in perspective. Lancet Infect Dis. 2010;10:275–8.

3. Gordon A. A treatise on the epidemic puerperal fever of Aberdeen. London: C.G. and J. Robinson; 1795. p. 62–5. Accessed from Internet Archive, archive.org, September 12, 2022
4. Gordon A. A treatise on the epidemic puerperal fever of Aberdeen. London: C.G. and J. Robinson; 1795. p. 96–9. Accessed from Internet Archive, archive.org, September 12, 2022
5. The font used by Dr. Gordon's publisher was changed to a modern font. For example, the letter f in the word nurfe was changed to s making the word nurse.
6. Semmelweiss IP. Die Aetiologie, der Begriff und die Prophylaxis des Kindbettfiebers. C.A. Hartleben's Verlage-Expedition, Pest. Wien and Leipzig, 1861. Deutchestextarchiv.de. Accessed October 24, 2019.
7. Semmelweiss I. *The Etiology, Concept, and Prophylaxis of Childbed Fever*. Translated by K. C. Carter. © 1983 by the board of Regents of the University of Wisconsin System. All rights reserved. Excerpts from this work were reprinted by permission of Ms. Anne T. McKenna, Rights & Permissions Manager | The University of Wisconsin Press, 13 Sep 2021.
8. Semmelweiss I. *The Etiology, Concept, and Prophylaxis of Childbed Fever*. Translated by K. C. Carter. Reprinted by permission of the University of Wisconsin Press. © 1983 by the board of Regents of the University of Wisconsin System. All rights reserved, pp. 17, 63.
9. Semmelweiss I. The Etiology, Concept, and Prophylaxis of Childbed Fever. Translated by K. C. Carter. Reprinted by permission of the University of Wisconsin Press. © 1983 by the board of Regents of the University of Wisconsin System. All rights reserved, p. 64.
10. Semmelweiss I. *The Etiology, Concept, and Prophylaxis of Childbed Fever*. Translated by K. C. Carter. Reprinted by permission of the University of Wisconsin Press. © 1983 by the board of Regents of the University of Wisconsin System. All rights reserved, p. 102.
11. Semmelweiss IP. Die Ätiologie, der Begriff und die Prophylaxe der Kindbettfiebers. C.A. Hartleben's Verlage-Expedition, Pest. Wien and Leipzig, 1861; pp. 72–73. Deutchestextarchiv.de.
12. Semmelweiss I. T*he Etiology, Concept, and Prophylaxis of Childbed Fever*. Translated by K. C. Carter. Reprinted by permission of the University of Wisconsin Press. © 1983 by the board of Regents of the University of Wisconsin System. All rights reserved, pp. 102–103.
13. Semmelweiss IP. Die Ätiologie, der Begriff und die Prophylaxe der Kindbettfiebers. C.A. Hartleben's Verlage-Expedition, Pest. Wien and Leipzig, 1861; p. 56. Deutchestextarchiv.de.
14. Semmelweiss I. *The Etiology, Concept, and Prophylaxis of Childbed Fever*. Translated by K. C. Carter. Reprinted by permission of the University of Wisconsin Press. © 1983 by the board of Regents of the University of Wisconsin System. All rights reserved, p. 89.
15. Semmelweiss, IP. Die Ätiologie, der Begriff und die Prophylaxe der Kindbettfiebers. C.A. Hartleben's Verlage-Expedition, Pest. Wien and Leipzig, 1861; p. 269. Deutchestextarchiv.de.
16. Semmelweiss I. *The Etiology, Concept, and Prophylaxis of Childbed Fever*. Translated by K. C. Carter. Reprinted by permission of the University of Wisconsin Press. © 1983 by the board of Regents of the University of Wisconsin System. All rights reserved, p. 165.
17. Semmelweiss IP. Die Ätiologie, der Begriff und die Prophylaxe der Kindbettfiebers. C.A. Hartleben's Verlage-Expedition, Pest. Wien and Leipzig, 1861; p. 65. Deutchestextarchiv.de.
18. Semmelweiss I. *The Etiology, Concept, and Prophylaxis of Childbed Fever*. Translated by K. C. Carter. Reprinted by permission of the University of Wisconsin Press. © 1983 by the board of Regents of the University of Wisconsin System. All rights reserved, p. 98.

Forgive and Remember: Charles L. Bosk

16

James S. Wu

Presentation

In his work, *Forgive and Remember, Managing Medical Failure,* Dr. Charles Bosk's dedication reads as follows [1]:

> "To the memory of my
> mother and father,
> whose norms I cherish,
> whose quasi-norms I
> miss"

In Chap. 2, Dr. Bosk defines errors, normative, and quasi-normative.

Normative Errors

> "A normative error occurs when a surgeon has, in the eyes of others, failed to discharge his role obligations conscientiously. Technical and judgmental errors are errors in a role; normative errors signal error in assuming a role."

J. S. Wu (✉)
Department of Colon and Rectal Surgery, Cleveland Clinic, Cleveland, OH, USA

J. S. Wu, M. D. Inkster (eds.), *Cleveland Clinic Colorectal Case Studies*,
https://doi.org/10.1007/978-3-031-39880-3_16

Quasi-normative Errors

> "Normative errors are breaches of standards of performance that all attendings share: quasi-normative errors are eccentric and attending-specific. Each attending has certain protocols that he and he alone follows. A subordinate who does not follow these rules mocks his superordinate's authority; his behavior is a claim that his judgment is as adequate as his superior's; and even though in no absolute sense can one claim that a mistake has been made, a subordinate who makes a quasi-normative error risks his reputation as a trustworthy recruit."

Dr. Robert E. Condon in his 2007 editorial opinion, "Forgive and remember revisited," wrote:

> "In 1979, the sociologist, Dr. Charles L. Bosk, published the results of an important study in a major teaching hospital of behavior by surgical residents and attendings. The focus of Bosk's inquiry was the identification and management of error. His epitome of the manner in which surgical error is managed became the title of his book, *Forgive and Remember*. Errors are forgiven if they are remembered and not repeated.
>
> Many directors of surgical residencies were so impressed with the insights Bosk had provided that, in the 1980's they enthusiastically recommended *Forgive and Remember* to their colleagues and to their residents. Some, including myself, bought copies of the book to present to their residents to help guide them in successful behavior during the residency.
>
> *Forgive and Remember* should be read, in my view, by every surgical resident and attending surgeon."[1] [2].

References

1. Bosk CL. Forgive and remember: managing medical failure. Chicago and London, Paperback edition: The University of Chicago Press; 1981. pages 51, 61. These excerpts are reproduced with the generous permission from The University of Chicago Press, CCC|Marketplace™, order License 1143990-1, Order Date 28-Aug-2021
2. Condon RE. Editorial opinion. Forgive and remember revisited. Am J Surg. 2007;194:1–2. These excerpts are reproduced with the generous permission from Elsevier, CCC|RightsLink®, License Number 5222430616492, License date Jan 05, 2022

[1] On the first day of my surgical internship at the Jewish Hospital of St. Louis in 1986, I received a copy of this work from my program Director, Dr. Kenneth J. Bennett.

Evolution of Colorectal Cancer Staging

17

James S. Wu, Shu-Jane Shen, and Amer A. Hanano

Colorectal Cancer staging

> "The classification of cancer by anatomic disease extent, i.e., stage, is the major determinant of appropriate treatment and prognosis."
>
> Union for International Cancer Control [1]

Guided by the critical review of staging systems published in 1983 by Dr. Lewis D. Zinkin, this chapter describes colorectal cancer staging systems reported since the 1920s [2].

1926 Lockhart-Mummery [3]

Perineal excision of rectal cancer

In 1926, Lockhart-Mummery described an A, B, and C staging system for rectal cancer based on 200 cases treated by perineal excision. In this operation, a permanent colostomy is created either before or at the time of resection of the entire rectum. Lockhart-Mummery's description of the operation is as follows:

J. S. Wu (✉)
Department of Colon and Rectal Surgery, Cleveland Clinic, Cleveland, OH, USA

S.-J. Shen
Radiology and Diagnostic Imaging Institute, Cleveland Clinic, Cleveland, OH, USA

A. A. Hanano
Radiology and Diagnostic Imaging Institute, Cleveland Clinic Florida, Weston, FL, USA

J. S. Wu, M. D. Inkster (eds.), *Cleveland Clinic Colorectal Case Studies*,
https://doi.org/10.1007/978-3-031-39880-3_17

Two Hundred Cases of Cancer of the Rectum
Treated by Perineal Excision.
By J. P. Lockhart-Mummery, London

"The patient is placed in the semi-prone position, head down, and if a male a catheter is tied into the bladder. The anus is first closed with a purse-string suture passed subcutaneously with a curved needle, and an incision is made from the base of the sacrum, passing around the anus and about 1 in. from it. The coccyx is removed by dissection, and the deep fascia divided transversely just in front of the sacrum. Both levatores ani muscles are divided close to the pelvic wall with scissors, and the rectum is then dissected off the vagina in the female, or from the urethra and prostate in the male, until the peritoneum is reached. The peritoneum is opened, and as much bowel drawn down as possible. The mesorectum is clamped off as far back as can be managed and divided. The clamps are tied off, and, after dividing the peritoneal coat of the pelvic colon and stripping it back for a short distance, the bowel is crushed and divided with a cautery. The stump is ligatured and turned in with a purse-string suture, and the wound in the peritoneum closed with catgut stitches. The wound itself is closed without drainage in most cases. In a few a small rubber wick is inserted. The wound is not dressed for 48 h, and then the blades of a pair of dressing forceps are introduced between two of the stitches, and any accumulated fluid allowed to escape. If the wound remains quite clean, it is allowed to heal by first intention; but if the accumulation of serum continues, a stitch is removed, a small piece of drainage tube is introduced, and the cavity kept irrigated with weak Dakin or Milton solution. The patient is allowed out of bed on the fourteenth day, and is generally able to return home in from 3 weeks to a month."

Cancer survival was based on the following system.

"A: very favorable cases where the growth was small and had not apparently invaded the muscular coat, and no glands were involved.
B: medium cases where there was involvement of the muscular coat, but where the growth was not unduly fixed and there was no extensive involvement of glands.
C: very bad cases, where the growth was large and fixed, or where there was evidence of extensive involvement of glands. These were borderline cases with a bad prognosis."

The survival of patients operated on with greater than 5 years of followup is shown in Table 17.1.

Table 17.1 Perineal excision in cancer of the rectum: 5-year survival (Lockhart-Mummery)

Stage	Number of cases	Percentage cure
A	30	73.7
B	43	44.1
C	9	44.4

1929 Dukes Classification

In 1929, Dukes made the following observations concerning the spread of cancer of the rectum through continuity of tissue.

The Spread of Cancer of the Rectum Through
Continuity of Tissue
By Cutherbert Dukes
Director of the Research Laboratory at St. Mark's Hospital

> "Cancer of the rectum commences as a proliferation of the columnar epithelium of the mucous membrane, and in its earliest stages takes the form of a mass of atypical epithelium growing in the mucous membrane and protruding to a greater or less extent into the lumen of the bowel. Thus, whether the malignant process begins in a previously level portion of mucous membrane, in a small patch of epithelial hyperplasia, or in a papilloma or adenoma, its first general architecture is that of a protruding epithelial mass. The amount of surface proliferation varies greatly in different cases and is dependent chiefly on the degree of deep infiltration of the rectal wall, which, as will be shown later, leads to a complete transformation in the general contour of the growth. Meanwhile the surface growth enlarges by marginal increase, which tends to be greater in the transverse than in the longitudinal axis of the rectum, and its depth increases by infiltration of the rectal wall. The characteristic features of this deep infiltration are that the growth is more extensive in the submucosa than in the mucous membrane, resulting in an undermining of the mucous membrane at the edge, and that infiltration through the muscular coat takes place by root-like projections which push their way between the segments of the circular muscle [4]."

Dukes proposed a modification of the A, B, C classification suggested by Lockhart-Mummery.

1932 Dukes Classification [5]

The Classification of Cancer of
the Rectum
Cuthbert E. Dukes.
Pathologist to St. Mark's Hospital, London

> "The following classification of cancer of the rectum is of interest in relation to the general pathology of malignant disease and has proved of value in the prognosis of rectal cancer.
>
> *A cases* are those in which the carcinoma is limited to the wall of the rectum, there being no extension into the extrarectal tissues and no metastases in lymph nodes, *B cases* those in which the carcinoma has spread by direct continuity to the extrarectal tissues but has not yet invaded the regional lymph nodes, and *C cases* those in which metastases are present in the regional lymph nodes."

This 1932 classification is recognized as the "Dukes classification" (Fig. 17.1).

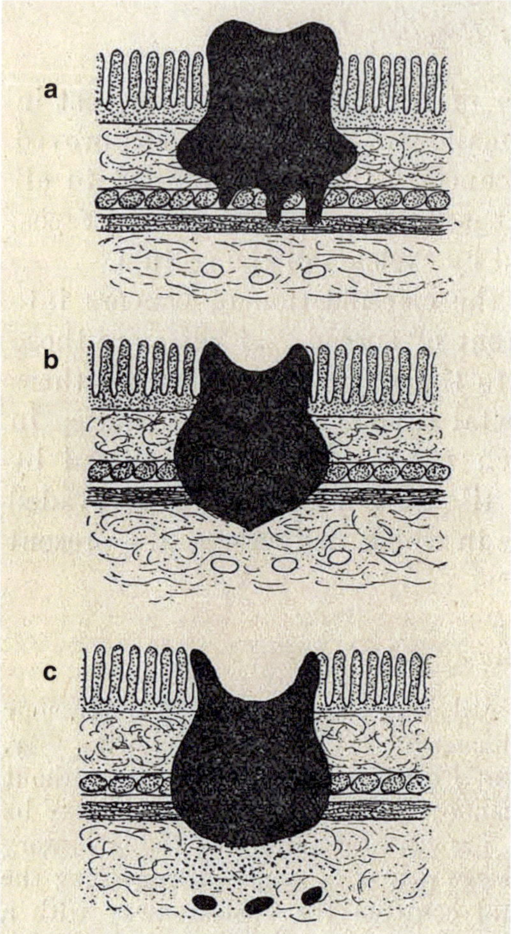

Fig. 17.1 The 1932 Dukes classification of rectal cancer [6]. (**a**) Growth limited to wall of rectum. (**b**) Extension of growth to extra rectal tissues but no metastases in regional lymph nodes. (**c**) Metastasis in regional lymph nodes. Reproduced from Dukes' 1932 article with the generous permission of J. Wiley & Sons - Books, CCC|Marketplace, Order License ID 1449522-1, Order Date 12-Feb-2024

1935 Gabriel, Dukes and Bussey [7]

Gabriel, Dukes, and Bussey performed a 5-year follow-up analysis of 94 cases of rectal cancer treated by perineal excision. Based on classification, the survival was as follows: A (24 cases, 91%), B (36 cases, 64%), and C (34 cases, 16%). The authors found by meticulous dissection of operative specimens that:

> "As a rule the regional glands are the first to be affected by metastases in cancer of the rectum. Lymphatic spread then proceeds from below upwards along the chain of glands accompanying the superior hæmorrhoidal artery. Irregular or interrupted spread is very uncommon. Lateral or downward lymphatic spread is only found in a late stage of the disease when the hæmorrhoidal lymphatics are blocked by metastases."

1967 Turnbull, Kyle, Watson, and Spratt

Turnbull, Kyle, Watson, and Spratt divided adenocarcinoma of the colon into four clinicopathologic stages [8]: The authors added Stage D to account for distant metastatic disease and seeding of tumor, irremovable because of parietal invasion and adjacent organ invasion.

"Stage A—Tumor confined to the colon and its coats
Stage B—Tumor extension into pericolic fat
Stage C—Tumor metastasis to regional mesenteric lymph nodes, but no evidence of distant spread
Stage D—Tumor metastasis to liver, lung, bone, seeding of tumor, irremovable because of parietal invasion; adjacent organ invasion."

Tumor, Node, Metastasis (TNM)

The TNM classification of solid tumors was introduced by Dr. Pierre Denoix in 1946 [9]. TNM is maintained by the Union for International Cancer Control (UICC) and is used by the American Joint Commission on Cancer (AJCC). Each individual aspect of TNM is termed as a category: T—Primary tumor, N—Regional Lymph Nodes, M—Metastases [10]. Definition of TNM categories continues to evolve.

The relation of TNM tumor categories, the 1932 Dukes classification, and Turnbull's Stage D to key anatomic structures are illustrated in Fig. 17.2. The

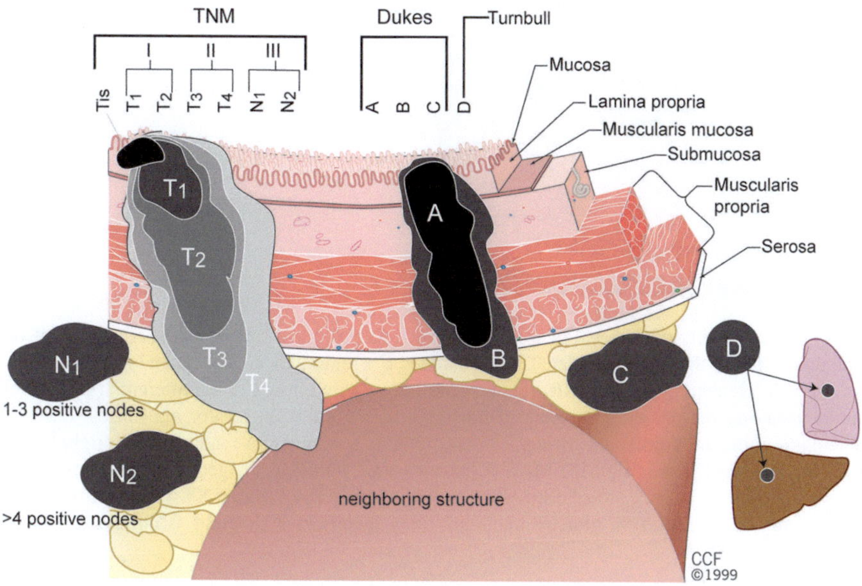

Fig. 17.2 The relation of key anatomic structures to TNM categories for colon and rectal cancer, the 1932 Dukes A, B, C classification for rectal cancer, and Turnbull's stage D (distant metastases) are shown. The Roman numerals I, II, and III refer to TNM stages

primary tumor and regional lymph node categories of low rectal cancers guide therapy. Magnetic resonance imaging (MRI) examples of T3, T4, and node positive rectal cancers are shown in Fig. 17.3a–c.

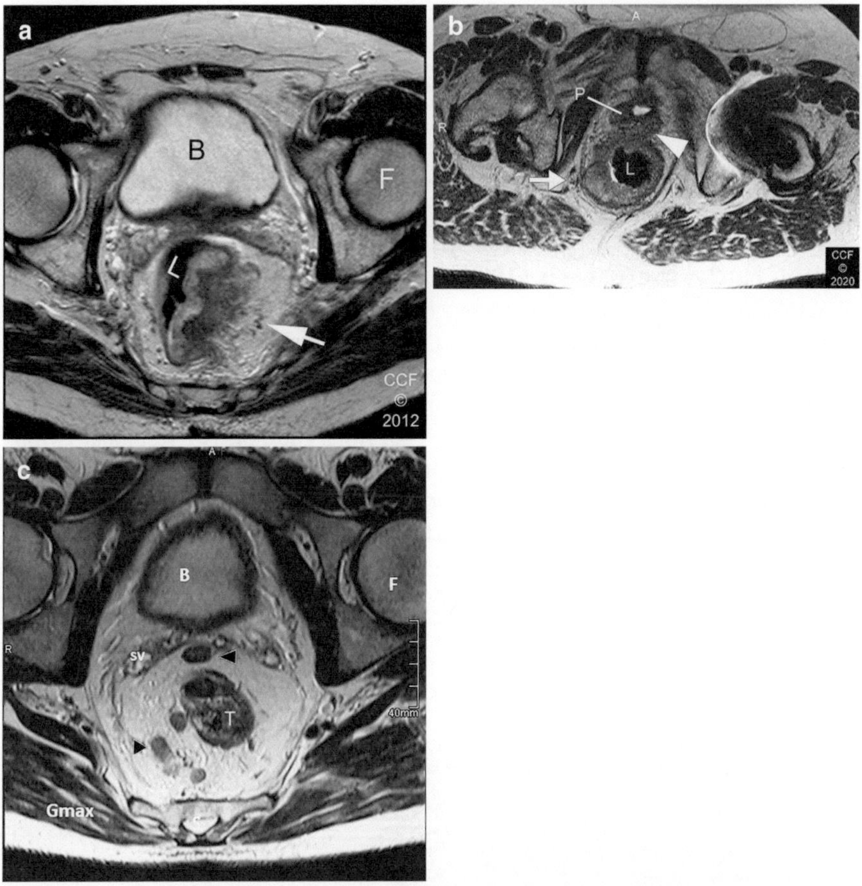

Fig. 17.3 (**a**) MRI, axial view. T2 weighted image. Rectal mass (arrow) with serosal extension and infiltration of the mesorectal fat. T3. B = bladder, F = femoral head, L = rectal lumen (courtesy of Amer A. Hanano, MD). (**b**) MRI, axial view, T2 weighted image. Circumferential low rectal tumor invading the posterior prostate gland (arrowhead) and right levator ani muscle (arrow). There is significant luminal narrowing. T4. P = prostate, L = lumen, A = anterior, R = right (courtesy of Shu-Jane Shen, MD). (**c**) MRI, Axial view, T2 weighted imaged. Multiple mesorectal lymph nodes are seen; two are labelled with arrowheads. N2. B = bladder, SV = seminal vesical, F = Femoral head, Gmax = gluteus maximus; A = anterior, R = right (Courtesy of Amer A. Hanano, MD)

References

1. Union for International Cancer Control. What is the TNM cancer staging system? UICC.org. Accessed 1 Jan 2017.
2. Zinkin LD. A critical review of the classifications and staging of colorectal cancer. Dis Colon Rectum. 1983;26:37–43.
3. Lockhart-Mummery JP. Two hundred cases of cancer of the rectum treated by perineal excision. Br J Surg. 1926;14:110–24. These excerpts were reproduced with permission from Oxford University Press, CCC | RightsLink®, License Number 5165310180241 License date Oct 10, 2021
4. Dukes CE. The spread of cancer of the rectum. Br J Surg. 1929;17:643–8. This excerpt is reused with permission of John Wiley & Sons, CCC|Marketplace™, Order License number ID 1146297-1, Order date 08-Sep-2021
5. Dukes CE. The classification of cancer of the rectum. J Pathol Bacteriol. 1932;35:323–32. This excerpt was reproduced with the generous permission of John Wiley & Sons – Books, CCC|Marketplace™, Order Number: 1146026, Order Date: 07 Sep 2021
6. Dukes CE. The classification of cancer of the rectum. J Pathol Bacteriol. 1932;35:323–32.
7. Gabriel WB, Dukes C, Bussey HJR. Lymphatic spread in cancer of the rectum. Br J Surg. 1935;23:395–413. This excerpt is reused with permission of John Wiley & Sons, LTD, CCC|Marketplace™, Order License ID 1146489-1, Order Date 09 Sep 2021
8. Turnbull RB Jr, Kyle K, Watson FR, Spratt J. Cancer of the colon: the influence of the *No-Touch Isolation* technic on survival rates. Ann Surg. 1967;166:420–7. This excerpt was reused with the generous permission of Wolters Kluwer Health, Inc, CCC | RightsLink® License Number 5165320727430, License date Oct 10, 2021
9. Denoix PF. Enquête permanent dans les centres anticancéreaux. Bull Inst Nat Hyg. 1946;1:70–5.
10. Brierley JD, Gospodarowicz MK, Wittekind C, editors. TNM classification of malignant tumours. 8th ed. Wiley-Blackwell: Chichester, West Sussex, UK; 2017.

Enterorrhaphy

18

James S. Wu

Presentation

Antoine Lembert (1826)

In 1826, Lembert published a treatise entitled *L'énterorraphie* in which he described suture closure of intestinal wounds in the canine model [1].

J. S. Wu (✉)
Department of Colon and Rectal Surgery, Cleveland Clinic, Cleveland, OH, USA

J. S. Wu, M. D. Inkster (eds.), *Cleveland Clinic Colorectal Case Studies*,
https://doi.org/10.1007/978-3-031-39880-3_18

MÉMOIRE
sur l'énteroraphie
avec la description d'un procédé nouveau pour pratiquer cette opération chirurgicale;
par A. Lembert
Chirurgien des Hopitaux Civils de Paris
1826

On a reconnu de tous temps la gravité des solutions de continuité du canal intestinal, et la nécessité de prévenir les épanchemens toujours funestes qui en sont la conséquence presque infaillible. Le danger de ces épanchemens est d'autant plus à redouter que, quel que soit le sens dans lequel l'intestin est divisé, la plaie est toujours élargie par la contraction des fibres circulaires ou longitudinales.

Procédé nouveau.

Le chirurgien ayant la main droite armée d'une aiguille simple, dans laquelle on a engagé un fil de lin ou de matière animale...porte l'index de la main gauche dans la cavité de l'intestin, de manière à soutenir les bords saignans avec la pulpe de ce doigt; tandis que les autre doigts servent à les fixer. On opérera plus facilement si l'on fait tendre les bords de la plaie par un aide. L'aiguille pénétre à 2 lignes [2] environ du bord saignant droit, dans la cavité de l'intestin, ou bien sa pointe glisse entre les tuniques musculeuse et muqueuse, suivant que l'intestin est plus ou moin épais. Lorque cette première ponction est faite, on dirige en haut et à gauche la pointe qui avait primitivement regardé en bas et à gauche, on la fait ressortir à une ligne environ du bord saignant, en sorte que le fil embrasse en dehors de ce bord une ligne à peu près des parois de l'intestin. Ce premier point passé, on dirige la même aiguille vers le bord opposé, on la fair pénétrer à une ligne de ce second bord saignant, et changeant sa direction comme ci-dessus, on la fait ressortir à deux lignes de distance, en sorte que le même fil pénétre deux fois dans les parois de l'intestin, et deux fois en sort.

Cette opération est si simple sur les chiens; que j'en ai vu plusieurs manger, digérer et rendre leur excrémens dès le surlendemain de l'entéroraphie.

Enfin, quoiqu'on ne puisse pas conclure directement du chien à l'homme; je pense que ce procédé présente assez d'avantages pour qu'on doive le tenter dans tous les cas où les solutions de continuité des intestins exposent à des épanchemens, ou à des anus contre nature,...

MEMOIR
On enterorrhaphy
with the description of a new procedure for performing this surgical operation;
by A. Lembert
Surgeon of the Civil Hospitals of Paris
1826

The seriousness of solutions for securing continuity of the intestinal canal has always been recognized because of the need to prevent leaks that are always fatal and that almost always occur.

These leaks are especially feared because whatever direction the intestine is divided, the wound is always enlarged by the contraction of the circular or longitudinal fibers.

New procedure.

The surgeon with the right hand armed with a simple needle, in which a thread of linen or animal has been engaged…positions the index finger of the left hand in the intestinal lumen, so as to support the bleeding edges with the pulp of this finger; while the other fingers are used to stabilize them. Operating is helped by stretching the edges of the wound. The needle enters approximately 2 lignes from the right bleeding edge, into the intestine cavity, or else its point slides between the muscular and mucous layers, depending on whether the intestine is more or less thick. When this first puncture is made, we direct to the surface and to the left point which had originally looked inward and on the left, we bring it out one ligne adjacent to the bleeding edge so that the thread embraces the intestinal wall.

Having completed this first bite, we repeat the maneuver on the opposite side of the wound passing the needle one ligne from the bleeding edge and then changing its direction as above. Thus, there are two separate bites; the same thread penetrates twice into the walls of the intestine and twice leaves.

When done on dogs, this operation is so straightforward, that I have seen many eating and passing bowel movements 2 days after surgery.

In the final analysis, although one cannot extend these conclusions directly from dog to man, I think this procedure has enough advantages that it should be tried on all cases of restoration of intestinal continuity that are at risk for either leak or which otherwise might require an intestinal stoma.

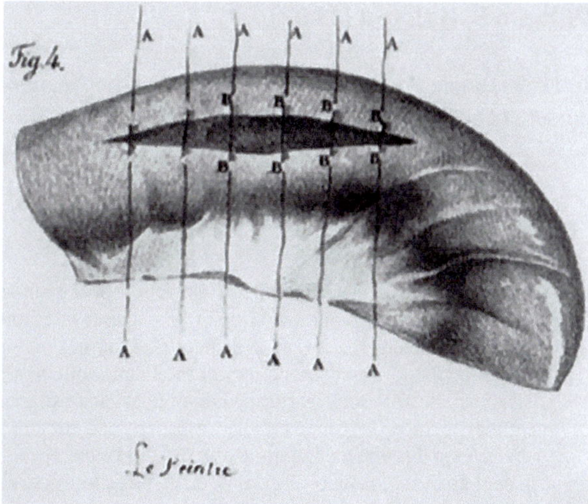

Fig. 18.1 Lembert, *L'énteroraphie* (Fig. 4.). Stitch placement for closure of a longitudinal enterotomy [1]

Lembert's illustration of the suture placement for closure of a longitudinal intestinal wound is shown in Fig. 18.1 (Lembert's Fig. 4).

Samuel D. Gross (1843)

In 1843, Gross published *An Experimental and Critical Inquiry into the Nature and Treatment of Wounds of the Intestines,* work done in the canine model [3]. Gross found that suture closure of intestinal wounds was successful if stitches were introduced through the "cellulo-fibrous lamella," a structure located between the mucous and muscular tunics.

> "EXPERIMENT VIII.—Wound one inch long—continued suture introduced between the mucous and muscular tunics—the animal killed on the fifteen day.
>
> Wishing to ascertain whether the edges of the wound could not be more perfectly approximated by carrying the needle between the muscular and villous tunics, or, in other words, through the cellulo-fibrous lamella,…I instituted this and the following experiments.
>
> Drawing a loop of the ileum from the abdomen of an old tarrier, I made a longitudinal incision, one inch in length, along its convex surface, not far from the cœcum, and sewed it up by carrying the needle, as just intimated, between the villous and muscular tunics. As had been anticipated, my expectations were not disappointed. The operation, without being more painful or protracted than when executed in the ordinary manner, had the effect of bringing the surfaces of the incision into the most perfect apposition. No severe indisposition followed, and the animal was permitted to live until the fifteenth day, when he was killed and his body carefully inspected. The continuity of the villous surfaces was re-established…. The continuity of the serous lips of the wound was unusually perfect."

Gross concludes:

> "The most important circumstances to be observed in making this suture in wounds of the bowels are, to carry the needle through the cellulo-fibrous lamella, and to place the stitches sufficiently near each other to prevent the escape of fæcal and other matters."

William S. Halsted (1887)

In 1887, Halsted reported the results of an experimental investigation done of suture closure of intestinal wounds in the canine model [4].

Circular Suture of the Intestine—An Experimental Study
William S. Halsted, M.D.,
of New York

"In the hope that an experimental investigation of the subject of intestinal suture might contribute somewhat to our knowledge of the causes of failure as well as of the conditions of success of enterorrhaphy, I have undertaken during the past winter a series of experiments in the Pathological Laboratory of the Johns Hopkins University, in Baltimore.

The experiments were performed upon dogs, anæsthetized usually with morphine and ether; they include sixty-nine circular resections and circular sutures of the small intestine.

In looking through the literature of intestinal suture I cannot find that any one has called sufficient attention, from a surgical point of view, to the structure of the different coats of the intestine, particularly to their physical properties.

Between the submucosa and glands of Lieberkühn—in other words, between it and the lumen of the intestine—practically nothing intervenes; and, literally, nothing but the two layers of muscularis mucosae and fibrosa mucosae respectively. It is an easy matter to isolate the submucosa. The outer muscular coats strip from it readily, and the mucous membrane can be rapidly scraped off with a knife. Thus obtained, the submucosa is found to be an exceedingly tough fibrous membrane. It is air-tight and watertight, and is the 'skin' in which sausage meat is stuffed. It is, moreover, the coat of the intestine from which 'catgut' is made.

A needle, on being pushed vertically through the wall of the intestine, meets with considerable resistance when it reaches the submucosa; and still greater resistance is encountered if it be attempted to pass the needle horizontally through its meshes. A delicate thread of this tissue is very much stronger and better able to hold a stitch than is a coarse shred of the entire thickness of the muscular and serous coats. Upon the discovery of the latter fact, at which I was, perhaps, as much surprised as most surgeons will be at the statement of it, it naturally occurred to me that it would, if feasible, be well to include a portion of the submucosa in the suture. Before attempting this, however, I wished to test the merits of a suture which included nothing but the serosa and muscularis, and I, therefore performed the following experiment:

EXPERIMENT A.—Small young dog. Operated on January 18, 1887. Circular resection of intestine. Two rows of interrupted stitches pass as deep as but not including any portion of submucosa-suture of muscular coat. The stitches tore out badly….

January 23. Dog found dead. *Autopsy*: Suppurative peritonitis; sutures had given away completely.

The Experiments of mine to which I particularly wish to invite attention are those of Group II.

Group II. Plain-quilt submucosa stitches (Fig. 18.2).

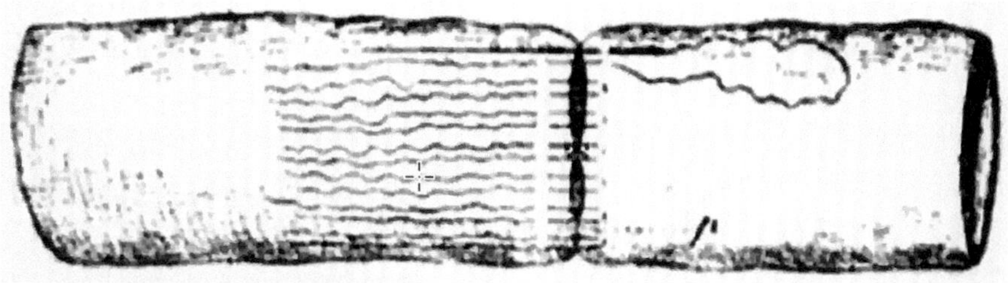

Fig. 18.2 Halsted. Plain-quilt postsection stitches introduced [5]

EXPERIMENT 13.—Small shaggy black dog. Operation February 14, 1887. Circular resection and circular suture. One complete row (eighteen stitches) of plain-quilt stitches.

February 15. Dog is quiet—still affected by morphine.

16th. Dog is very playful.

March 10. Perfectly well. Killed. *Autopsy*: Circular suture perfectly healed.

Experiment 15.—Large, brown and white bitch. Operation March 3, 1887. Circular resection and circular suture. One complete row of plain-quilt, postsection stitches.

March 14. Dog has made an uninterrupted recovery. Given to janitor for a pet.

June 1. Dog perfectly well.

Although there were but 15 experiments in this group, they included 18 circular sutures of the intestine, all of which were successful.

Summary

Each stitch should include a bit of submucosa. A thread of this coat is much stronger than a shred of the entire thickness of the serosa and muscularis. It is not difficult to familiarize one's self with the resistance furnished by the submucosa, and it is quite as easy to include a bit of this coat in each stitch as to suture the serosa and muscularis alone."

Comment

Each of these three investigators identifies an anatomic layer in the intestine that has strength to successfully heal intestinal wounds closed with suture. For Lembert, it is located "lentre les tuniques musculeuse et muqueuse (between the muscularis and the mucosa). For Gross, it is the "cellulo-fibrous lamella" located between the muscular and villous tunics. For Halsted, it is the submucosa. The submucosa is located

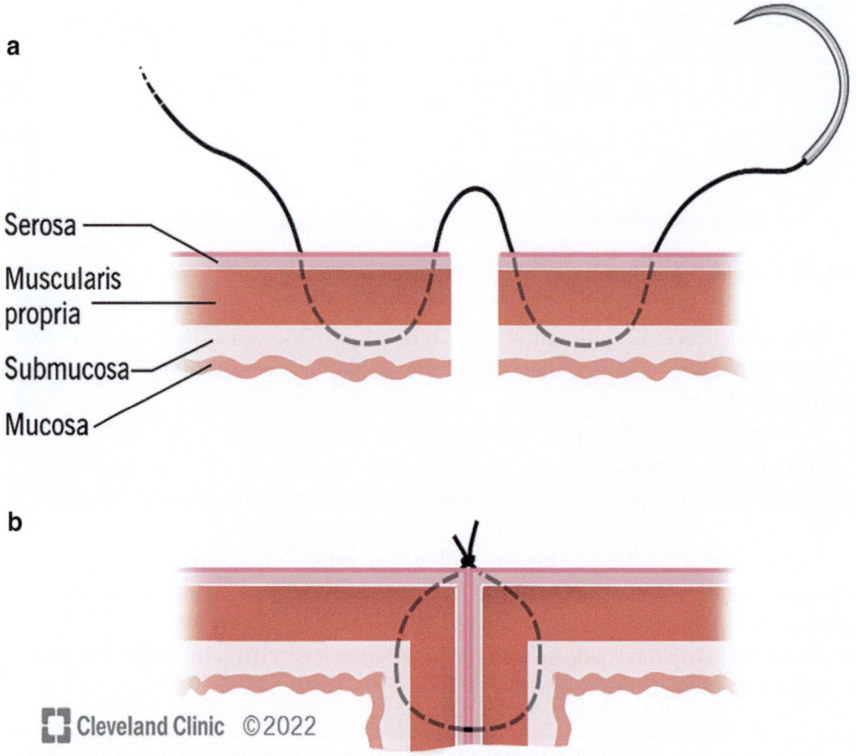

Fig. 18.3 Lembert's suture illustrated (after DeCosta, 1903). The suture on each side of the anastomosis picks up the submucosa because it is strong and will hold suture. When tied, the edges of the intestine are inverted

between mucosa and the muscularis. The submucosal substance that provides fibrous toughness is collagen [6, 7]. This concept was illustrated and described in minute detail by Da Costa in 1903 (Fig. 18.3) [8].

> "*Lembert's suture* was introduced in 1823. Lembert used it on animals but never on man. It is inserted at right angles to the wound. It goes down to, but not through, the mucous membrane. It is formed by picking up a fold of the intestine (one-twelfth to one-eighth of an inch wide) one-eighth of an inch from the edge on one side of the wound, passing the needle through, picking up a fold on the opposite side of the wound, and passing the needle through. On tying the threads the serous membrane is inverted and peritoneum is brought into contact with peritoneum. For many years it was taught that this suture should include only the serous coat, but Halsted in 1887, showed that it must include the tough submucous coat. The submucous coat is strong, and will hold a suture. The other coats are thin, tear easily, and will not hold a suture."

John Chalmers Da Costa
Modern Surgery
Jefferson Medical College
Philadelphia

De Costa included an illustration showing the passage of thread for Lembert's suture (Fig. 18.3).

References

1. Lembert A. Mémoire sur l'entéroraphie avec la description d'un procédé nouveau pour pratiquer cette opération chirurgicale. Répertoire général D'anatomie et de Physiologie Pathologiques, Chez Boiste, Fils Ainé, Libraire, Rue de Sorbonne, N°. 12 Paris, 1826;2:100–107. Accessed from Google Books May 27, 2020.
2. Ligne is defined by the Merriam-Webster Dictionary as: a French unit for watch movements equal to 0.0888 inches. "Ligne." Merriam-Webster.com Dictionary, Merrian-Webster, https://www.meriam-webster.com/dictionary/ligne (Accessed 25 May 2020).
3. Gross SD. *An experimental and critical inquiry into the nature and treatment of wounds of the intestines.* Prentice and Weissinger, Louisville [Ky.], 1843. Accessed from the NIH U.S. National Library of Medicine Digital Collections. http://resource.nlm.nih.gov/65571 1820R.
4. Halsted WS. Circular suture of the intestine—an experimental study. Am J Med Sci. 1887;94:436–61. Accessed from Google Books May 27, 2020.
5. Halsted WS. Circular suture of the intestine—an experimental study. Am J Med Sci. 1887;94:454. Accessed from Google Books May 27, 2020
6. Shi L, Ronfard V. Biochemical and biomechanical characterization of porcine small intestinal submucosa (SIS): a mini review. Int J Burn Trauma. 2013;3:173–9.
7. Lin H-K, Godiwalla SY, Palmer B, Frimberger D, Yang Q, Madihally SV, Fung K-M, Kropp BP. Understanding roles of porcine small intestinal submucosa in urinary bladder regeneration: Identification of variable regenerative characteristics of small intestinal submucosa. Tiss Eng Part B Rev. 2014;20:73–83.
8. Da Costa JC. Modern surgery – Chapter 27. Diseases and Injuries of the Abdomen – Surgery of the Stomach and Intestine (1903). In: Modern Surgery, 4th edition. By John Chalmers Da Costa. Paper 19, pp. 781–3. https://jdc.jefferson.edu/dacosta_modernsurgery/19.

Intestinal Anastomoses

19

Joseph A. Pangrace and James S. Wu

Presentation

Intestinal anastomoses may be stapled or sewn. Successful anastomotic construction depends upon:

1. Viable intestine with adequate blood supply,
2. Intestinal approximation without tension,
3. Airtight and watertight seal.

Intestinal anastomoses commonly used in clinical practice are depicted.

Colocolostomy

Figures 19.1a–d show steps in the creation of a sutured end-to-end, single-layer colon-to-colon anastomosis.

J. A. Pangrace
CMI, Medical Illustration Team, Enterprise Creative Services, Cleveland Clinic, Cleveland, OH, USA

J. S. Wu (✉)
Department of Colon and Rectal Surgery, Cleveland Clinic, Cleveland, OH, USA

J. S. Wu, M. D. Inkster (eds.), *Cleveland Clinic Colorectal Case Studies*,
https://doi.org/10.1007/978-3-031-39880-3_19

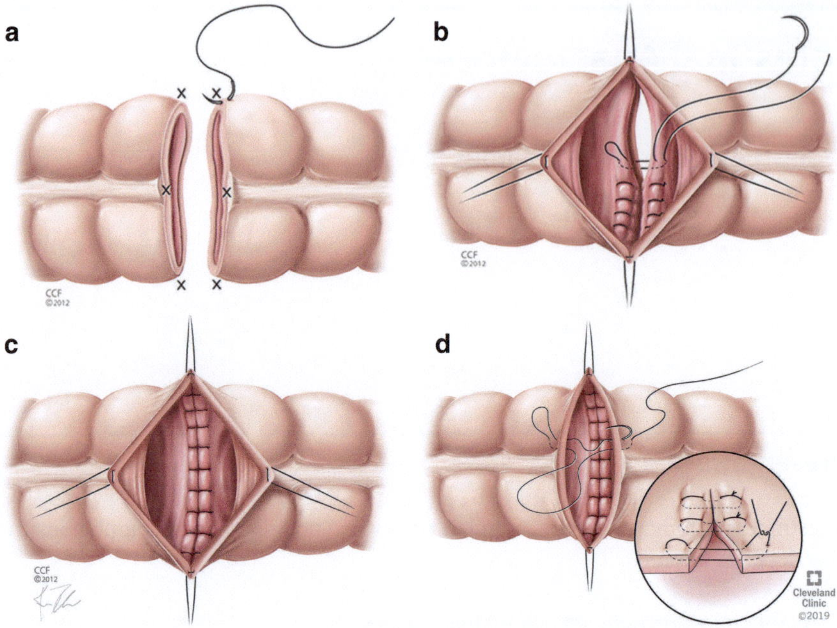

Fig. 19.1 (**a**) Sutures are placed to align the edges of the intestinal segments; (**b**) The back wall is closed by interrupted vertical mattress sutures [1]. For the back row, the knots are sewn on the inside surface of the bowel; (**c**) The completed back wall; (**d**) For the front row, the knots are tied on the outside surface of the bowel. The inset shows details of suture placement (full thickness-full thickness-mucosa-mucosa). The full thickness bites are placed about 1 cm from the cut edge of the colon

Enteroenterostomy

Steps in the creation of a sutured, end-to-end, single-layer enteroenterostomy are shown in Fig. 19.2.

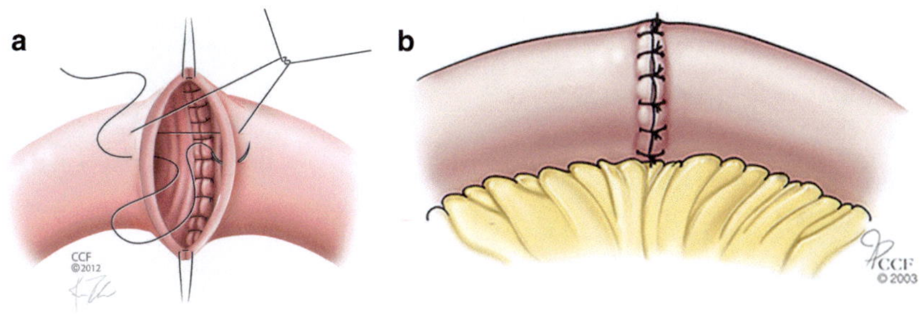

Fig. 19.2 (**a**) End-to-end enterostomy. Similar to colocolostomy, the anastomosis is sewn following the placement of aligning sutures. The bites include the full thickness of the intestinal wall; (**b**) Completed end-to-end sewn anastomosis

End-to-End Anastomosis (Stapled) [2, 3]

Anastomosis of two segments of small intestine using gastrointestinal anastomosis (GIA) and linear stapling devices is shown in Figs. 19.3a–c.

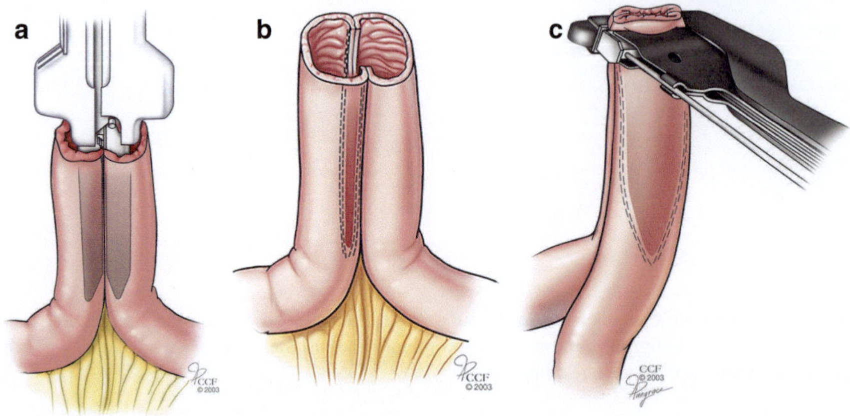

Fig. 19.3 (**a**, **b**) The two ends of the intestine are aligned. The anastomosis is created by connecting the antimesenteric sides of the bowel with a gastrointestinal anastomosis (GIA) device. Care is taken to avoid incorporation of the mesentery in the staple line; (**c**) the enterostomy is closed with a linear stapler

Ileocolic Anastomosis

End of small intestine to side of large intestine, stapled anastomosis is illustrated in Fig. 19.4.

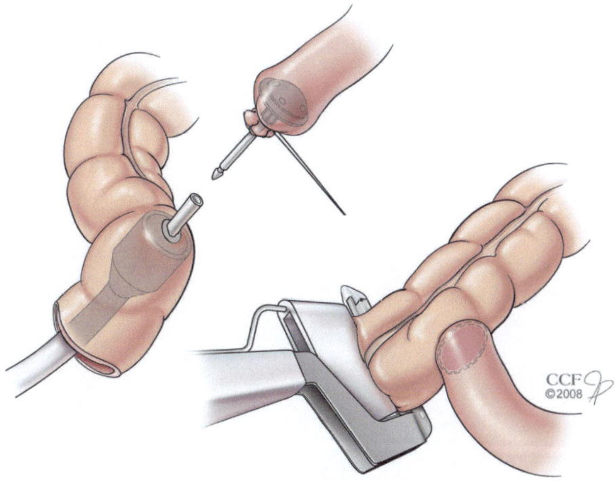

Fig. 19.4 The anvil of an end-to-end anastomosis (EEA) stapler is secured to the end of the ileum. The gun is inserted into the colon lumen, a distance of about 8 cm. The post with a spike is advanced through the side of the colon in between the taenia coli. In this case, an end of ileum-to-side of transverse colon anastomosis is created following right colectomy. The colostomy is closed using a linear stapling device

Colorectal Anastomosis (End-to-End Single Stapled) [4]

End-to-end colorectal single stapled anatomosis using a circular stapling instrument is shown in Fig. 19.5.

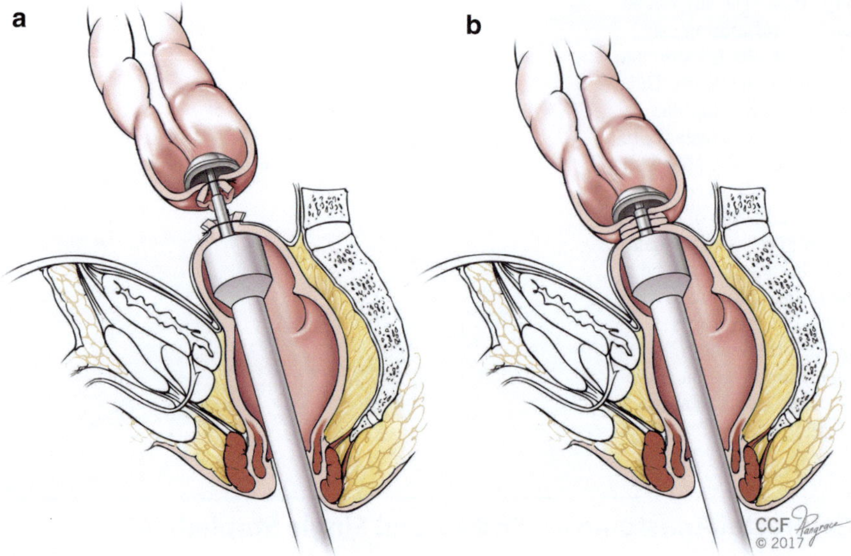

Fig. 19.5 The colon is anastomosed to the rectum. This example illustrates a single-stapled technique where both the anvil and the stapling gun are secured to the intestine with purse-string sutures. (**a**) The anvil is secured to the colon and the stapling gun is secured to the rectum with purse string sutures; (**b**) The stapler is closed and fired, creating the colon-to-rectum anastomosis

Ileorectal Anastomosis (End-to-End Sewn)

Sutured ileorectal anastomosis with a "Cheatle" slit, to increase the diameter of the small intestinal lumen, is shown in Fig. 19.6.

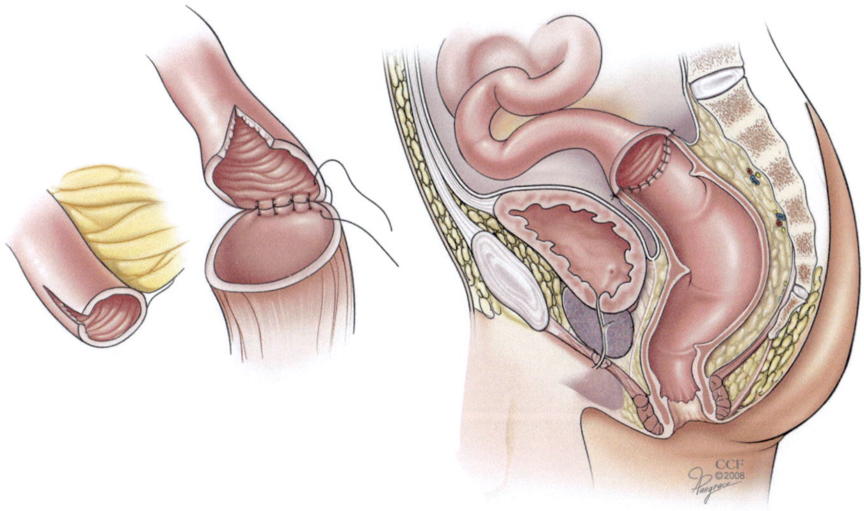

Fig. 19.6 The end of the ileum is sewn to the proximal rectum [5]: Left. A "Cheatle" slit [6] has been made in the terminal ileum to increase the small intestine's luminal diameter. A sutured anastomosis is made. Mattress sutures usually are preferred; Right. Completed sewn ileorectal anastomosis

Colorectal Anastomosis (Double-Stapled)

Anastomosis of the colon to the distal rectum by the double-stapled technique is shown in Fig. 19.7.

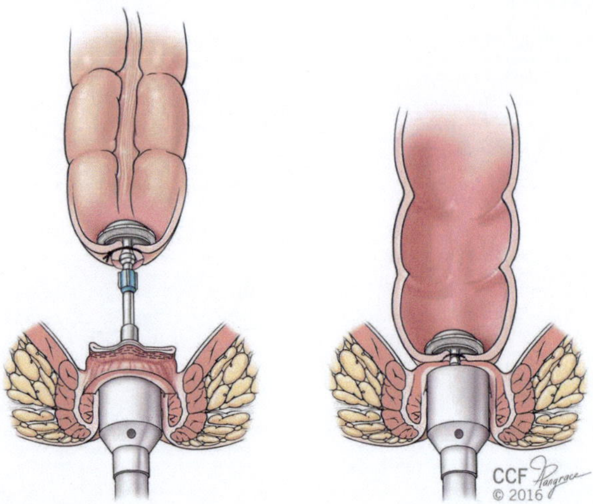

Fig. 19.7 Double-stapled colorectal anastomosis: Left. The distal rectum is closed with a staple line after division. The spike of a circular stapling device is passed through the rectal stump and connected to the anvil part of the stapling gun that has been secured to the colon by a purse-string suture; Right. The stapling gun and anvil have been brought into close apposition in preparation for firing to make the anastomosis. The term double-stapled means that the circular staple line crosses the rectal stump staple line

Coloanal Anastomosis

Anastomosis of the anus to the colon in three configurations (straight, "J"-pouch, and coloplasty) is shown in Figs. 19.8, 19.9, and 19.10.

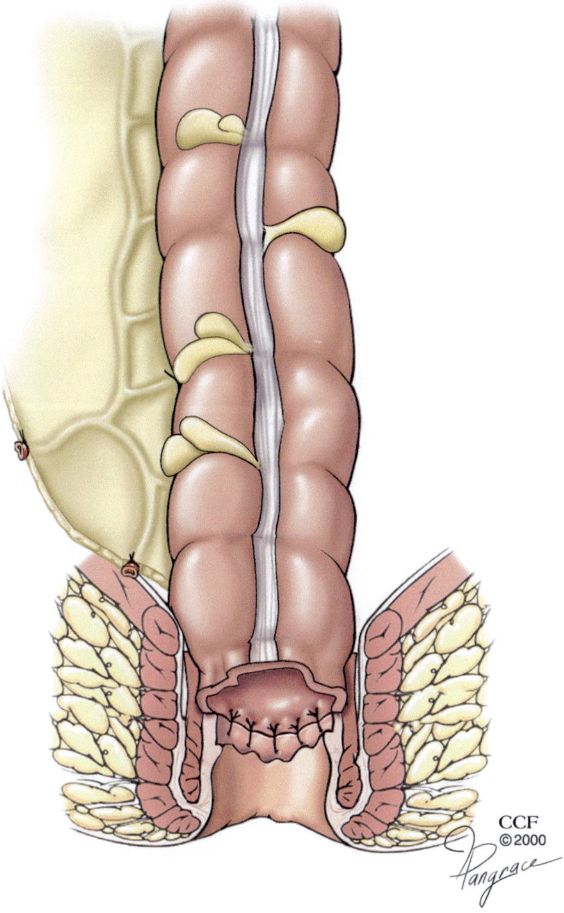

Fig. 19.8 Straight coloanal anastomosis [7]. The end of the colon is anastomosed to the dentate line using sutures

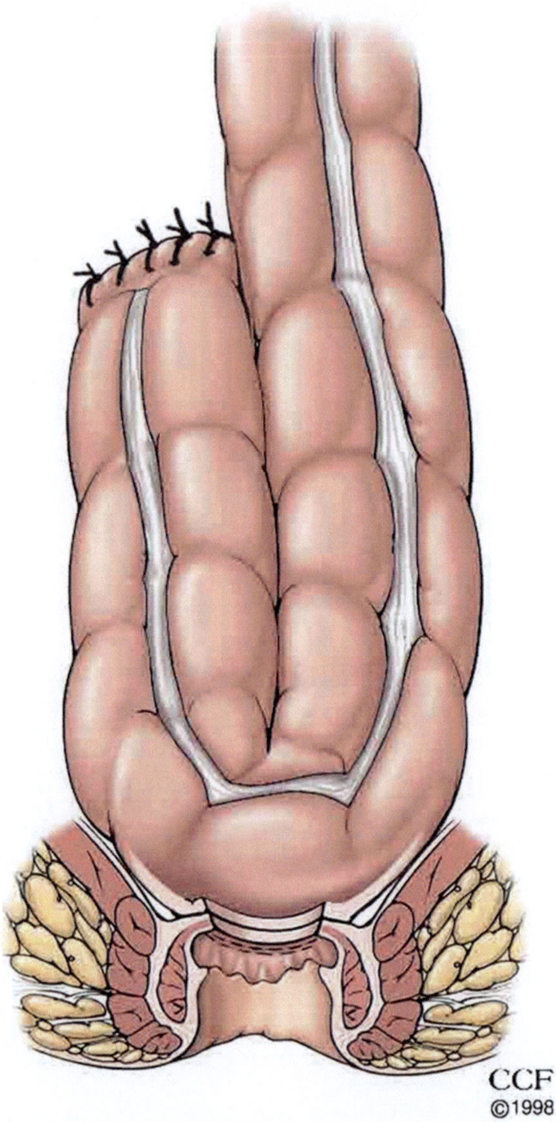

Fig. 19.9 Colonic "J" pouch [8, 9]. The end of the colon is bent in a "J" configuration. The length of the limbs is 5 cm. The opposing walls of the colon are connected with a gastrointestinal anastomosis (GIA) stapler. The tip of the "J" is closed with a linear stapler or, as in this case, with sutures. The pouch anal anastomosis is created by stapled or sewn techniques. In this illustration, the colorectal anastomosis is stapled

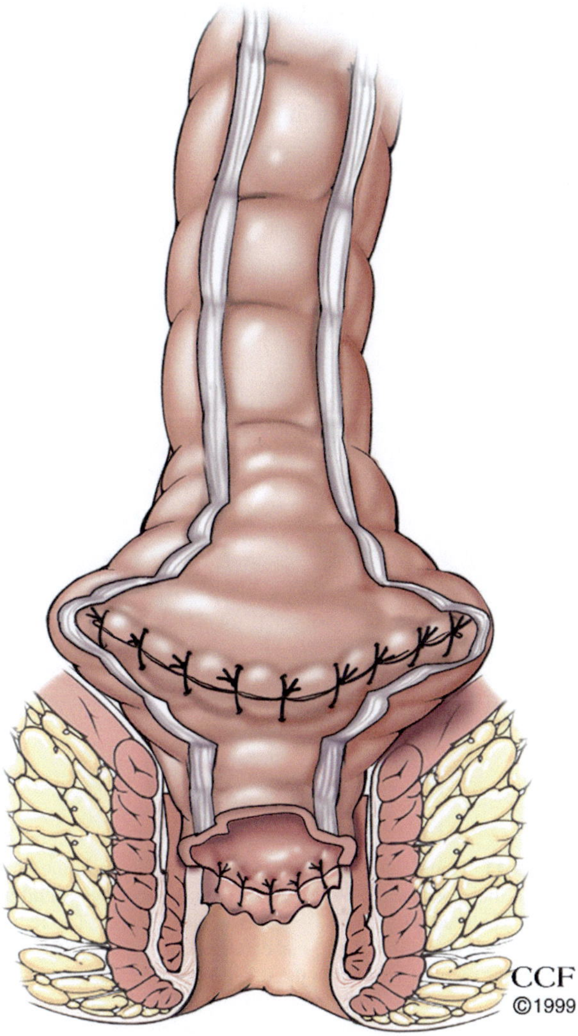

Fig. 19.10 Coloplasty [10, 11]. A longitudinal anti-mesenteric 10-cm incision is made 6 cm proximal to the end of the colon. The colostomy is closed transversely. In this illustration, the coloplasty and the anastomosis to the anus are sewn

Ileal "J"-Pouch-Rectal Anastomosis, Double-Stapled [12]

Figure 19.11 shows the creation of an ileal "J"-pouch that is anastomosed to the rectum by the double-stapling technique.

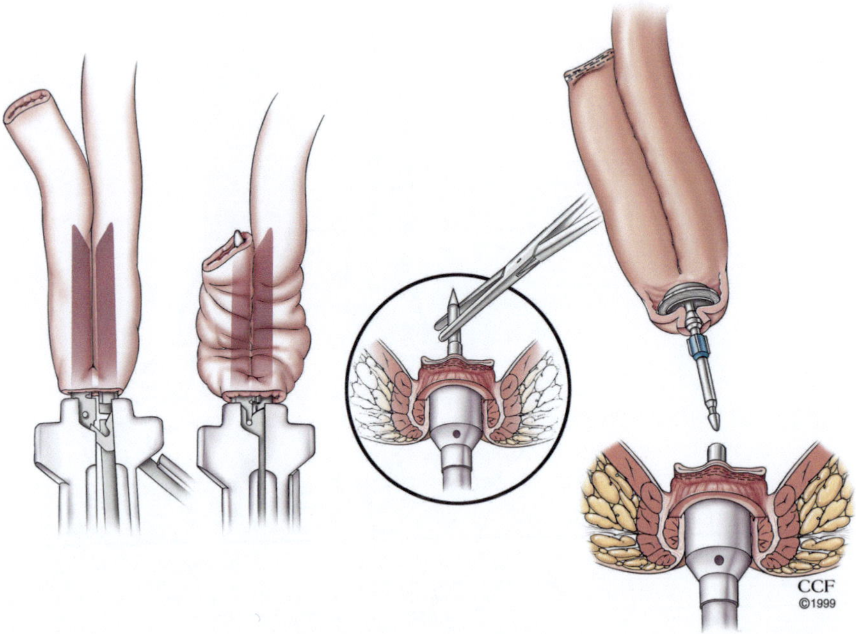

Fig. 19.11 Double-stapled Ileal J-pouch to rectal anastomosis. Left: The common wall between the two limbs of ileum (20 cm each) is connected using several passes of a GIA stapler. The tip of the "J" is closed with a linear stapling device; Center: The rectal stump has been stapled closed. The spike of the stapling gun has been passed through the rectal stump. Preferentially, the spike pierces the rectum posterior to the staple line to decrease the chance of injury to structures anterior to the rectum during anastomosis creation; Right: The ileal pouch-anal anastomosis is created using an end-of-rectum-to-pouch double-stapled anastomosis

Ileal Pouch-Anal Anastomosis (Hand Sewn, "S"-Pouch) [13]

Figure 19.12 shows sequential steps in the creation of an ileal "S"-pouch that is sutured to the anus after mucosectomy.

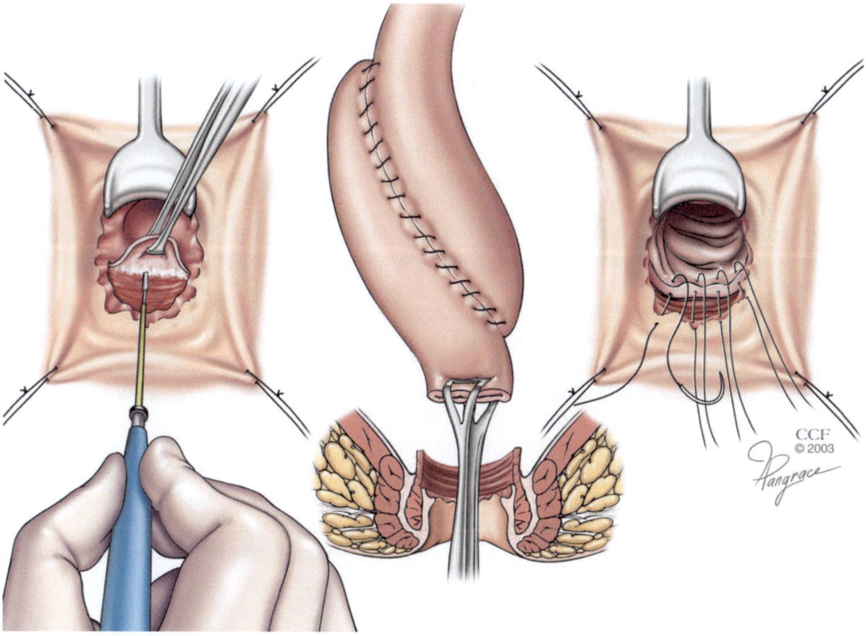

Fig. 19.12 Mucosectomy with sutured ileal pouch-anal anastomosis. Left: In this illustration, the epithelium of the anorectum is removed by mucosectomy. The anal orifice is opened with a retractor. The anus is effaced with traction sutures. Center: The distal end of an ileal three-limbed "S" pouch is positioned above the anoderm, in this case, with Babcock forceps; Right; In this illustration, an anastomosis between the ileal pouch and the anus is created with sutures

References

1. Gambee LP. A single-layer open intestinal anastomosis applicable to the small as well as the large intestine. West J Surg Obstet Gynecol. 1951;59:1–5.
2. Ravitch MM, Rivarola A. Enteroanastomosis with an automatic instrument. Surgery. 1966;59:270–7.
3. Steichen FM, Ravitch MM. Mechanical sutures in surgery. Br J Surg. 1973;60:191–7.
4. Ravitch MM, Steichen FM. A stapling instrument for end-to-end inverting anastomoses in the gastrointestinal tract. Ann Surg. 1979;189:791–7.
5. Fazio W, Turnbull RB Jr, Goldsmith MG. Ileorectal anastomosis: a safe surgical technique. Dis Colon Rectum. 1975;18:107–14.
6. Cheatle GL. A method of uniting the divided intestine. Lancet. 1897;i:1403–4.
7. Steinhagen RM, Weakley FL. Anastomosis to the rectum: operative experience. Dis Colon Rectum. 1985;28:105–9.
8. Lazorthes F, Fages P, Chiotasso P, Lemozy J, Bloom E. Resection of the rectum with construction of a colonic reservoir and colo-anal anastomosis for carcinoma of the rectum. Br J Surg. 1986;73:136–8.
9. Parc R, Tiret E, Frileux P, Moszkowski E, Loygue J. Resection and colo-anal anastomosis with colonic reservoir for rectal carcinoma. Br J Surg. 1986;73:139–41.
10. Z'graggen K, Mauer CA, Mettler D, Stoupis C, Wildi S, Büchler MW. A novel colon pouch and its comparison with a straight coloanal and colon J-pouch — anal anastomosis: preliminary results in pigs. Surgery. 1999;125:105–12.
11. Fazio VW, Mantyh CR, Hull TL. Colonic "coloplasty": novel technique to enhance low colorectal or coloanal anastomosis. Dis Colon Rectum. 2000;43:1448–50.
12. Utsunomiya J, Iwama T, Imajo M, Matsuo S, Sawai S, Yaegashi K, et al. Total colectomy, mucosal proctectomy, and ileoanal anastomosis. Dis Colon Rectum. 1980;23:459–66.
13. Parks AG, Nicholls RJ. Proctocolectomy without ileostomy for ulcerative colitis. Br Med J. 1978;2:85–8.

20 Eponymous Instruments

James S. Wu

Presentation

A surgical instrument often is associated with the name of its creator. The following lists some named surgical instruments commonly used in the colorectal surgical tray at the Cleveland Clinic.

Allis Forceps [1]

Description: Tissue holding forceps
Designer: Oscar Huntington Allis (1836–1921)
Orthopedic surgeon
Presbyterian Hospital
Philadelphia, Pennsylvania

Adson Forceps [2]

Description: Tissue holding forceps
Designer: Alfred Washington Adson (1887–1951)
Neurosurgeon
Mayo Clinic
Rochester, Minnesota

J. S. Wu (✉)
Department of Colon and Rectal Surgery, Cleveland Clinic, Cleveland, OH, USA

J. S. Wu, M. D. Inkster (eds.), *Cleveland Clinic Colorectal Case Studies*,
https://doi.org/10.1007/978-3-031-39880-3_20

Babcock Forceps [3]

Description: Tissue holding forceps
Designer: William W. Babcock (1872–1963)
Surgeon
Temple College
Philadelphia, Pennsylvania

Balfour Self-retaining Abdominal Retractor [4]

Description: Abdominal retractor
Designer: Donald C. Balfour (1882–1963)
Mayo Clinic
Rochester, Minnesota

Barron Hemorrhoid Ligator [5]

Description: Hemorrhoid rubber band ligator
Designer: James Barron (–1996)
Surgeon
Henry Ford Hospital
Detroit, Michigan

Blake Drain [6]

Description: Wound drain catheter
Designers: Larry W. Blake, Ervin R. Harvel, Duane R. Mason, George M. Wright

Bonney Tissue Forceps [7]

Description: Tissue forceps
Designer: William F. V. Bonney (1872–1953)
Gynecologist
England

Bookwalter Retractor [8]

Description: Table mounted self-retaining retractor
Designer: John Bookwalter
Surgeon

Brinkerhoff Speculum [9]

Description: Anoscope
Designer: William C. Brinkerhoff
Surgeon
Chicago, Illinois

Bovie Electrocautery Device [10]

Description: Electrocautery device
Designer: William T. Bovie (1882–1958)
Biophysicist
Harvard University
Boston, Massachusetts

Crile Forceps [11]

Description: Hemostatic clamp
Designer: George W. Crile (1864–1943)
Surgeon
Cleveland Clinic Foundation
Cleveland, Ohio

Deaver Retractor [12]

Description: Abdominal viscera retractor
Designer: John B. Deaver (1885–1931)
Surgeon
University of Pennsylvania
German Hospital
Philadelphia, Pennsylvania

Fansler Anoscope [13]

Description: Operating anoscope
Designer: Walter A. Fansler
Surgeon
University of Minnesota
Minneapolis, Minnesota

Gelpi Retractor [14]

Description: Self-retaining perineal retractor
Designer: Maurice J. Gelpi (1883–1939)
Charity Hospital
New Orleans, Louisiana

Halsted-Rubber Operating Gloves [15]

Description: Rubber Operating Gloves
Designer: William S. Halsted (1852–1922)
Surgeon
Johns Hopkins Hospital
Baltimore, Maryland

Hegar Uterine Dilators [16]

Description: Cylindrical dilators
Ernst L. A. Hegar (1830–1914)
Gynecologist
University of Freiburg
Freiburg, Germany

Hill Anal Retractor [17]

Description: anal retractor
Designer: T. Chittenden Hill
Harvard Graduate School of Medicine
Boston, Massachusetts

Hirschman Anoscope [18, 19]

Description: Anoscope
Designer: Louis J. Hirschman (1878–1965)
Surgeon
Detroit College of Medicine and Surgery
Detroit, Michigan

Jackson-Pratt Drain [20]

Description: Closed suction drain
Designers: Frederick E. Jackson and Richard A. Pratt, III
Naval Hospital
Camp Pendleton, California

Lahey Forceps [21]

Description: Tissue forceps
Designer: Frank H. Lahey (1880–1953)
Surgeon
Lahey Clinic
Boston, Massachusetts

Langenbeck Retractors [22]

Description: tissue retractor
Designer: Bernhard von Langenbeck (1810–1887)
Surgeon
Charité Hospital
Berlin, Germany

Lister Bandage Scissors [23]

Description: Bandage scissors
Designer: Joseph Lister (1827–1912)
Surgeon
Royal Infirmary
Glasgow, Scotland

Kelly Clamp [24]

Description: Curved hemostatic clamp
Designer: Howard A. Kelly (1858–1943)
Gynecology specialist
Johns Hopkins Hospital
Baltimore, Maryland

Kocher Forceps [25]

Description: Hemostatic forceps
Designer: Emil T. Kocher (1841–1917)
Surgeon
Berne University
Bern, Switzerland

Mayo Scissors, Stand, Retractor

Descriptions: scissors, stand, retractors
Designers: William J. Mayo (1861–1939) and Charles H. Mayo (1865–1939)
Surgeons
Mayo Clinic
Rochester, Minnesota

Metzenbaum Scissors [26, 27]

Description: Dissecting scissors
Designer: Myron F. Metzenbaum (1876–1944)
Ear, nose and throat specialist
Mt. Sinai Hospital
Cleveland, Ohio

Mikulicz Pad [28, 29]

Description: Laparotomy sponge
Designer: Jan Mikulicz-Radecki (Johann Freiherr von Mikulicz-Radecki) (1850–1905)
Surgeon
Breslau

Moynihan Intestinal Occlusion Clamp [30, 31]

Description: Intestinal occlusion clamp
Designer: Berkeley George Andrew Moynihan (1865–1936)
Surgeon
University of Leeds
United Kingdom

Ochsner Clamp [11, 32]

Description: tissue clamp
Designer: Alton Ochsner (1896–1981)
Surgeon
Tulane University
Ochsner Clinic,
New Orleans, LA

Péan Clamp (Pince hémostatique de Péan) [33]

Description: hemostat
Designer: Jules-Émile Péan (1830–1898)
Surgeon: Hospitals of Paris
Paris, France

Penrose Drain [34]

Description: surgical drain
Designer: Charles Bingham Penrose (1862–1825)
Gynecologist
Gynecean Hospital
Philadelphia, Pennsylvania

Richardson Retractor [35]

Description: abdominal wall retractor
Designer: Maurice Howe Richardson (1851–1912)
Surgeon
Massachusetts General Hospital
Boston, Massachusetts

Senn Retractor [36]

Description: double ended tissue retractor
Designer: Nicholas Senn (1844–1908)
Surgeon
Rush College of Medicine
Chicago, Ill

St Mark's Pelvic Retractor [37]

Description: deep pelvic retractor
Design: attributed to Oswald Vaughan Lloyd-Davies (1905–1987)
St. Mark's Hospital
London, England

Weitlaner Retractor [38]

Description: self-retaining retractor
Designer: Franz Weitlaner (1872–1944)
Surgeon
Ottenthal, Austria

Wood's Lamp [39]

Description: Optical filter glass that suppresses visible light while transmitting the ultraviolet
Designer: Robert W. Wood (1868–1955)
Physicist
Johns Hopkins University
Baltimore, Maryland

Yankauer Suction Tip [40]

Description: suction tip
Designer: Sidney Yankauer (1872–1932)
Otolaryngologist
Mt. Sinai Hospital
New York, New York

Crile clamps used in the U.S. Army surgical tray are shown in Fig. 20.1.

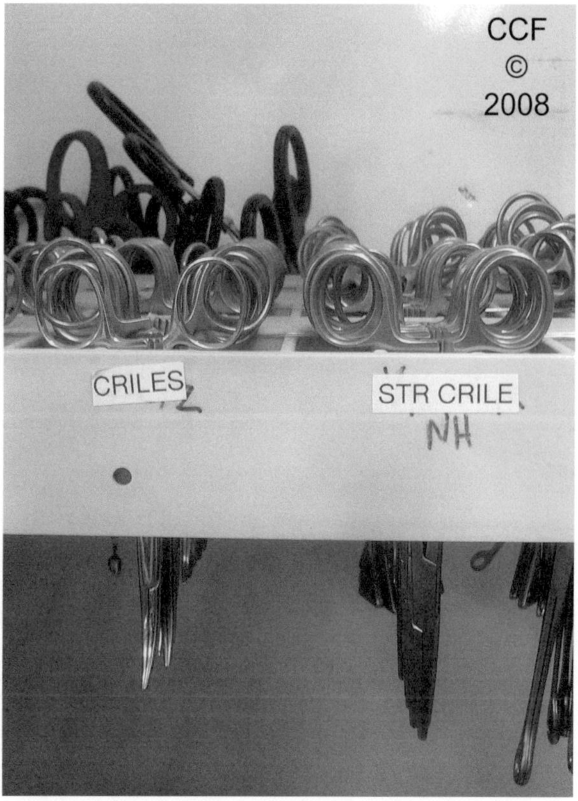

Fig. 20.1 Curved and straight Crile clamps included in the United States Army surgical kit, Iraq, 2008

The Mikulicz Pad

The most ubiquitous of surgical tools is the laparotomy sponge, a.k.a., the Mikulicz pad. Mikulicz's description of this device was in 1887 when abdominal surgery was in its infancy. In order to mitigate against sepsis after pelvic surgery, multiple drains wrapped in large gauze sheet were placed in the "todter Räume (dead space)" of the pelvis and brought out of the anterior abdominal wall wound [41, 42],

Ueber die Ausschaltung todter Räume aus der Peritonealhöhle, mit besonderer Rücksicht auf die Exstirpation der aus der Becken ausgehenden Geschwülste.

Von

Prof. J. Mikulicz

in Krakau

(Mit einem Holzschnitt.)

M. H.! Die Furcht vor Eröffnung der Bauchhöhle im Sinne der vorantiseptischen Zeit gehört zum Glück schon der Geschichte an. Wenn wir heut zu Tage das Bauchfell in was immer für einer Absicht blosslegen, so darf daraus allein für den Operirten keine grössere Gefahr erwachsen, als aus der Verwundung anderer, ausserhalb der Bauchhöhle gelegenen Theile. Die Sicherheit, mit welcher die moderne Operationstechnik der Infection des entblössten Peritoneums vorzubeugen vermag, hat einen so hohen Grad erreicht, dass sich in kürzester Zeit die Abdominalchirurgie auf alle dem chirurgischen Messer zugänglichen Bauchorgane ausdehnen konnte.

Trotz alledem können sich bei Bauchoperationen auch heute noch Complicationen ergeben, welche den exactesten antiseptischen Massregeln trotzen und häufig eine septische Peritonitis zur Folge haben. Ich meine hier nicht jene Fälle, in welchen der verletze Darm oder Magen seinen Inhalt in die Bauchhöhle ergiesst oder etwa eine vereiterte und geborstene Ovarialcyste das Peritoneum direct inficirt: es handelt sich vielmehr um Fälle, in welchen eine directe Infection dieser Art ausgeschlossen ist und die Infectionskeime trotz Antisepsis von aussen hinzukommen. Dahin gehören insbesondere jene Laparotomieen, welche zum Zwecke der Entfernung von umfänglichen, im kleinen Becken festgewachsenen oder subserös im Becken entwickelten Geschwülsten unternommen werden. Namentlich sind es aber derartig situirte Uterusmyome, deren Extirpation mit der Gefahr einer septischen Infection verbunden ist.

Die Gefahr wird in diesen Fällen dadurch bedingt, dass nach der Entfernung des Tumors in der Tiefe des Beckens eine umfängliche Wundhöhle zurückbleibt, welche sich schwer aseptisch erhalten lässt.

I habe mich nun,… bemüht, die Jodoformgaze zur Ausschaltung der todten Räume in einer Weise zu verwenden, welche alle Vortheile, der antiseptischen Tamponnade sichern, aber zugleich den Eigenthümlichkeiten der Peritonealhöhle Rechnung tragen sollte. Insbesondere war ich darauf bedacht, die Schwierigkeiten beim nachträglichen Herausziehen der Gaze zu beseitigen und das Verfahren auch für jene schweren Fälle anwendbar zu machen, in welchen sich für die Wunde im Beckenraum kein Peritonealüberzug gewinnen lässt, der todte Raum also unmittelbar mit der Bauchhöhle communicirt.

On the elimination of dead spaces from the peritoneal cavity, with special reference to the extirpation of tumors arising from the pelvis.

By

Prof. J. Mikulicz

at Crakow

(with one woodcut)

Sirs! Fortunately, the fear of opening the abdominal cavity in the sense of the pre-antiseptic era is already history. If today we expose the peritoneum, for whatever purpose, this alone poses no greater danger for the person who is operated on than from injuring other parts outside the abdominal cavity. The degree of certainty with which modern surgical techniques are able to prevent infection of the exposed peritoneum has reached such a high level that abdominal surgery has been able to extend to all abdominal organs accessible to the surgical knife in a very short time.

In spite of all this, complications still can occur in abdominal operations today, which defy the most exacting antiseptic measures and often result in septic peritonitis. Here, I don't mean those cases in which the injured intestine or stomach spills its contents into the abdominal cavity, or a suppurated and ruptured ovarian cyst directly infects the peritoneum; Rather, we are dealing with cases in which a direct infection of this kind is excluded and the infectious germs come from outside in despite antisepsis. This includes, in particular, those laparotomies which are undertaken for the purpose of removing extensive tumors that have become firmly attached subserosally to the small pelvis. In particular, however, it is uterine fibroids situated in this way that extirpation is associated with the danger of septic infection. The danger in these cases is due to the fact that after the removal of the tumor in the depth of the pelvis a large wound cavity remains which is difficult to preserve aseptically.

I have now tried to use the iodoform gauze to eliminate the dead spaces in a way that should ensure all the advantages of aniseptic tamponade, but at the same time take into account the peculiarities of the peritoneal cavity. In particular, I was intent on eliminating the difficulty of subsequent gauze removal and on making the procedure applicable also for those severe cases in which no peritoneal covering can be obtained for the wound in the pelvic area, i.e. the dead space communicates directly with the abdominal cavity.

Mein Verfahren ist folgendes: Ich nehme ein einfaches Stück 20proc. Jodoformgaze im Umfange eines grösseren Taschentuches. In die Mitte desselben wird ein starker langer aseptischer Seidenfaden festgenäht. Das Ganze wird noch vor der Operation, bei welcher man auf eine Complication in der Beckenhöhle rechnet, in 5 proc. Carbolsäure gelegt. Ist der intraabdominelle Theil der Operation vollendet, so drückt man das Stück Jodoformgaze gut aus und legt es in Form eines Tabaksbeutels zusammen, so dass der Seidenfaden nach innen zu liegen kommt und mit seinem freien Ende beim Halse des Beutels hinaushängt; sein unteres befestiges Ende entspricht dem tiefsten Punkte des Beutels. Nun versenkt man den Beutel mittelst einer geraden oder noch besser gekrümmten Zange bis an den tiefsten Punkt des kleinen Beckens. Ist dies geschehen, so füllt man den im Becken liegenden Theil des Beutels mit 2—5 langen Streifen von Jodoformgaze locker aus, so dass seine Wandungen überall der Wundfläche gut anliegen. Der im Grunde des Beutels befestige Faden dient zum nachträglichen Herausziehen desselben; dem Zuge des Fadens folgt zuerst der tiefste Punkt des Beutels, und indem sich dieser nach oben einstülpt, löst er sich in schonender Weise von der anliegenden Wundfläche.

Derselbe erfüllt einen vierfachen Zweck:

1. Er dient als blutstillender Tampon, was bei ausdehnten, nicht anders zu stillenden Flächblutungen in der Beckenhöhle von grossem Werthe sein kann.
2. Er drainirt die Wundhöhle im Becken in einfacher und vollkommener Weise durch Capillarwirkung;….
3. Der Tampon von Jodoformgaze erhält die Wundhöhle aseptisch und sichert das Peritoneum vor dieser Infectionsquelle.
4. Das beschriebene Vefahren lässt sich in jedem Falle anwenden, unabhängig davon, ob es gelingt, aus der Kapsel oder dem Peritonealüberzug des Tumors einen Sack zu bilden oder nicht.

My procedure is this: I take a plain piece of 20%. Iodoform gauze the size of a large handkerchief. A strong, long, aseptic silk thread is sewn into the middle of it. Prior to operations in which a complication in the pelvic cavity is expected, the whole is soaked 5% carbolic acid. When the intra-abdominal part of the operation is completed, the piece of iodoform gauze is squeezed out well and folded up in the shape of a tobacco-pouch, so that the silk thread hangs out with its free end at the neck of the pouch; its lower fixed end corresponds to the lowest point of the bag. Now the bag is lowered to the lowest point of the pelvis using straight or, even better, curved forceps. After this is done, the pouch is loosely filled with 2–5 long strips of iodoform gauze so that its walls are in good contact with the wound surface. The thread fastened at the bottom of the bag serves to subsequently pull it out; the deepest point of the bag follows the pull of the thread, and as this invaginates upward, it gently detaches itself from the adjacent wound surface.

The above device serves a fourfold purpose:

1. It serves as a hemostatic tampon, which can be of great value in the case of extensive surface bleeding in the pelvic cavity that cannot be stopped in any other way.
2. It drains the wound cavity in the pelvis in a simple and perfect way by capillary action;...
3. The iodoform gauze tampon keeps the wound cavity aseptic and protects the peritoneum from this source of infection.
4. The method described can be used in any case, whether or not a sac can be formed from the capsule or peritoneal lining of the tumor.

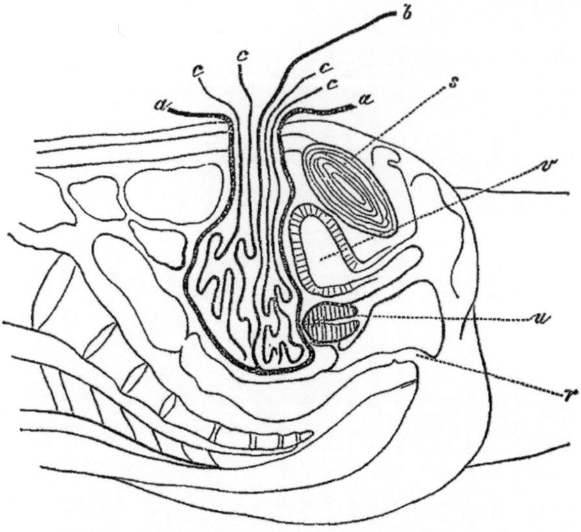

s Symphyse. v Blase. u Uterusstumpf. r Mastdarm. aa Beutel von Jodoformgaze. b Seidenfaden. ccc Gazestreifen.

Fig. 20.2 Mikulicz. Ueber die Ausschaltung todter Räume aus der Peritonealhöhle, mit besonderer Rücksicht auf die Exstirpation der aus der Beckenhöhe ausgehenden Geschwülste, Holzschnitt (On the elimination of dead spaces from the peritoneal cavity, with special reference to the extirpation of tumors arising from the level of the pelvis, woodcut). [s Symphysis. v bladder. u Uterus stump. r rectum. aa pouch of iodoform gauze. b. silk thread. ccc gauze Strips]

Mikulicz illustrated the main features of the bouquet of iodoform gauze drains surrounded by a tobacco pouch-shaped handkerchief-sized gauze sponge in the following woodcut (Fig. 20.2).

Mikulicz's handkerchief-sized iodoform gauze pouch lives on with us in our daily work as our laparotomy sponge, a.k.a., Mikulicz's pad. The silk thread originally placed in the center of the sponge has been moved to the corner.

Biographical Note

Johann von Mikulicz-Radecki (1850–1905)Mikulicz published broadly on subjects that included infection, endoscopy, orthopedics, head and neck, chest, urology, gynecology, and gastrointestinal surgery [43–46]. His obituary was written by his friend, colleague, and student, Ernst Ferdinand Sauerbruch [47].

Johannes v. Mikulicz †. Der deutsche Chirurg Johannes v. Mikulicz ist gestorben.	**Johannes v. Mikulicz †.** The German surgeon, Johnnes v. Mikulicz has died.
Am 14. Juni 1905, mittags, beschloss er sein arbeitsreiches, und wie er in letzer Stunde selbst sagte, glückliches Leben, im rüstigsten Mannesalter, auf der Höhe seines Schaffens. Mit ihm verlieren wir einen der grössten Chirurgen der Jetztzeit, vielleicht einen der grössten überhaupt. Sein Name wird sich anreihen an die unserer Besten.	On June 14, 1905, at noon, he ended his busy life, and as he himself said in the last hour, happy life, in sprightly manhood, at the height of his creativity. With him we are losing one of the greatest surgeons of our time, perhaps one of the greatest ever. His name will join those of our best.
Sein Tod kam nicht unvorbereitet. Etwa 3 Wochen vor Weihnachten diagnostizierte er zuerst bei sich selbst einen inoperablen Tumor, einen Befund, den er mit Rücksicht auf seine Familie bis nach Weihnachten verheimlichte. Dann begab er sich zu seinem Freunde Eiselsberg, der ihn in Gemeinschaft mit Naunyn untersuchte und dringend zur Probelaparotomie riet, welche am 7. Januar in Breslau vorgenommen wurde. Die Hilfe kam zu spät. Es handelte sich um einen jener ungünstigen Fälle von Karzinom der hinteren Magenwand, die ohne Beschwerden zu machen rapid wachsen, auf das Pankreas übergreifen und sehr bald eine Radikaloperation ausschliessen. Von dem Eingriff erholte er sich wider Erwarten schnell und konnte bereits 14 Tage später Breslau verlassen, um sich in Abbazzia, das er gleich seinem grossen Lehrer Billroth über alles liebte, zu erholen. Es war ihm auch vergönnt, wie er und wir hofften, Kräftigung zu finden; uns allen jedenfalls schien es so; denn seine unvergleichliche Energie befähigte ihn trotz seines schwer kranken Zustandes, dessen er sich wohl mehr, als man annahm, bewusst war, am 15. Februar die Leitung der gesamten Klinik noch einmal zu übernehmen. Er hielt Kolleg, er opierierte und arbeitete wie früher. Sein schlechtes Aussehen machte uns bedenklich, als wir mit den Studenten unseren Meister mit der frohen Hoffnung empfingen, ihn dauernd wieder erhalten zu haben. Aber seine Frische und Lebendigkeit im Kolleg und bei einer grösseren Reihe schwieriger Operationen, vor allem aber die Leitung des Operationskursus für Militärärzte warf unsere Bedenken hinsichtlich seines Zustandes wieder über den Haufen. Ende März ging er wie alljährlich nach dem Süden; es sollte seine letzte Reise sein. Ostern bekam er in Meran eine schwere Magenblutung, welcher er fast erlegen wäre. Es drängte ihn nach Hause und er traf am 12. Mai wieder in Breslau ein. Sein Haus hat er seitdem nicht mehr verlassen, bis ihn der Tod von seinen Qualen erlöste. Er ist wie ein Held gestorben; dem Tod, an den er seit Monaten selbst immer dachte, und der in der letzen Woche sich ihm in einer der schrecklichsten Formen — unter dem Bilde der Inanition — näherte, hat er mit Mannesmut ins Auge geschaut; ruhig, gefasst, ohne Furcht und Grauen.	He was not unprepared for his death. About 3 weeks before Christmas he first diagnosed himself with an inoperable tumor, a finding which he kept secret until after Christmas out of consideration for his family. Then he went to his friend Eiselsberg, who examined him together with Naunyn and urgently recommended a probe laparotomy, which was performed in Breslau on January 7th. The help came too late. It was one of those unfavorable cases of carcinoma of the posterior wall of the stomach, which grows rapidly without causing symptoms, spreads to the pancreas, and very soon precludes radical surgery. Contrary to expectations, he recovered quickly from the operation and was able to leave Breslau just 14 days later to recover in Abbazzia, which, like his great teacher Billroth, he loved more than anything. He was also granted, as he and we hoped, to find strength; at least it seemed so to all of us; for his incomparable energy enabled him, in spite of his gravely ill condition, of which he was probably more aware than was assumed, to take over the management of the entire clinic once more on February 15th. He gave lectures, operated, and worked as before. His bad appearance gave us cause for concern when we and the students received our master with the happy hope of having received him again permanently. But his freshness and liveliness at lectures and in a larger series of difficult operations, but above all in conducting the surgical course for military doctors, overturned our concerns about his condition again. At the end of March he went south, as he did every year; it was to be his last journey. At Easter he got a severe stomach hemorrhage in Meran, from which he almost succumbed. He felt compelled to go home and returned to Breslau on May 12th. After that he did not leave his house until death relieved him of his torment. He died like a hero; Death, which he himself had been thinking about for months, and which in the last week had approached him in one of the most terrible forms—under the image of inanition—he faced with manly courage; calm, composed, without fear and horror.
Das ist in kurzen Zügen seine Leidensgeschichte. Eine furchtbare Tragik: Der Mann, der wohl am erfolgreichsten das Magenkarzinom operiert hat, dem viele eine Verlängerung ihres Lebens, manche sogar Heilung verdanken, ist ein Opfer dieses Feindes geworden, der schleichend und hinterrücks ihn überfiel. Grosse Männer haben grosse Schicksale! Die Natur, die in seltener Verschwendung ihn mit dem besten, was sie hat, ausstattete, hat gewissermassen in diesem furchtbaren Tode all das zurückgefordert, was sie der Menschheit in ihm gab — und doch nicht alles. Was er wirkte, was er schuf, das liess er uns zurück als ein köstliches Erbe, das wir dankend aus seinen Händen entgegennehmen, das wir verwahren und vergrössern wollen, so weit es in unseren Kräften steht."	That, in a nutshell, is his story of sadness. A terrible tragedy: the man who probably operated the most successfully on the stomach cancer, to which many owe an extension of their lives, some even healing, became a victim of this enemy, who insidiously attacked him from behind. Great men have great destinies! Nature, which in rare extravagance endowed him with the best that she has, has to a certain extent reclaimed in this terrible death everything that she gave to mankind in him - and yet not everything. What he did, what he created, he left behind for us as a precious legacy, which we gratefully accept from his hands, which we want to preserve and enhance as far as we can.

(continued)

v. Mikulicz ist am 16. Mai 1850 zu Czernowicz geboren, wo sein Vater als Architekt tätig war. Er stammte väterlicherseits aus einer littauischen, mütterlicherseits, aus der preussischen Adelsfamilie v. Damnitz. v. Mikulicz genoss eine strenge Erziehung und als er, der erst orientalische Sprachen studieren sollte, sich der Medizin zuwandte, hatte er ¼ Jahr lang mit dem Groll seines Vaters zu kämpfen, der ihm Anfangs alle Hilfsmittel entzogen hatte. Er studierte in Wien zurzeit der zweiten Blüte dieser Fakultät; Hyrtl, Brücke, Rokitansky, Hebra, Dumreicher und vor allem Billroth waren seine Lehre. Im April 1875 trat er als Operationszögling nach Abschluss seines Staatsexamens in die Billrothsche Klinik ein. Nach 3 Wochen bedeutete ihm sein Lehrer, dass er für die Chirurgie wohl nicht geeignet sei, behielt ihn aber auf v. Miklulicz' Bitte noch bei sich; 1878 wurde er Assistent, 1880 habilitierte er sich als Privatdozent für Chirurgie und verheiratete sich noch im Dezember desselben Jahres. Seine treue Lebensgefährtin hatte er schon lange vorher durch gemeinsame musikalische Beziehungen kennen gelernt. Er musste damasl aus der Klinik austreten und übernahm die Leitung der chirurgischen Abteilung an der allgemeinen Poliklinik in Wien. Im Oktober 1882 wurde er als ordentlicher Professor der Chirurgie nach Krakau berufen. v. Mikulicz war der polnischen Sprache nicht mächtig, deshalb wurde ihm erlaubt, bis zur Erlernung derselben seine Vorlesungen in Deutsch zu halten. Die chirurgische Klinik in Krakau war sehr ärmlich und unmodern eingerichtet. — Hörsaal, Operationssaal, Verbandszimmer, Poliklinik, alles ein Raum — und so nahm er 1887 mit Freuden den Ruf nach Königsberg an. Im Februar 1890 wurde er zum Geheimen Medizinalrat ernannt und kurz darauf nach Breslau berufen; die neue Klinik war für die damalige Zeit ein ausgezeichnetes modernes Institut, dem v. Mikluicz später noch einen grossen, nach seinen eigenen Angaben errichteten Operationssaal anfügte. Hier in Breslau hat er bis zuletz gewirkt. Einen an ihn ergangenen Ruf nach Strassburg und Wien lehnte er ab.	v. Mikulicz was born on May 16, 1850 in Czernowicz, where his father worked as an architect. On his father's side he came from a Lithuanian, on his mother's side, from the Prussian noble family v. Damnitz. v. Mikulicz enjoyed a strict upbringing and when he, who was first supposed to study oriental languages, turned to medicine, he had to fight for a quarter of a year with the resentment of his father, who had initially deprived him of all resources. He studied in Vienna at the time when this faculty was in its second bloom; Hyrtl, Brücke, Rokitansky, Hebra, Dumreicher and above all Billroth were his teachers. In April 1875, after completing his state examination, he entered the Billrothsche Klinik as a surgical trainee. After 3 weeks his teacher informed him that he was probably not suitable for surgery, but, at v. Mikulicz's request, kept him on; In 1878 he became an assistant, in 1880 he became as a lecturer in surgery and married in December of the same year. He had met his true life partner long before that through mutual musical relationships. At that time he had to leave the clinic and took over the management of the surgical department at the general polyclinic in Vienna. In October 1882 he was appointed regular professor of surgery in Kraków. v. Mikulicz did not speak Polish, so he was allowed to give his lectures in German until he learned it. The surgical clinic in Kraków was very poor and unmodern. — Lecture hall, operating room, dressing room, polyclinic, all in one room — and so in 1887 he happily accepted the call to Konigsberg. In February 1890 he was appointed Privy Medical Counselor and shortly thereafter appointed to Breslau; the new clinic was an excellent modern institute for the time, to which v. Mikulicz later added a large operating theater built according to his own specifications. Here in Breslau he worked to the end. He declined calls to Strasburg and Vienna.
Zwei Züge machen vielleicht das Hauptwesen seines Charakters aus, seine Energie und Strenge gegen sich selbst und seine Herzensgüte. Hervorragende Leistungen können nur von selten energischen Naturen verrichtet werden, die ganz im Dienst einer Idee aufgehen und sich selbst vergessen. v. Mikulicz war ein glänzendes Beispiel dafür; von früh bis spät ununterbrochen tätig, mit derselben Frische und Gründlichkeit am frühen Morgen, wie am späten Abend. Müdigkeit kannte er bei der Arbeit nicht, und was sich an Widerstand ihm entgegensetzte, überwand er mit zähem eisernen Willen. Er wollte und er konnte, und er wollte viel! Wir alle, seine Schüler, haben davon die besten Beweise; wurde er am Abend eines mühevollen Tages noch zu einem Fall gerufen, bei dem wir ihn brauchten, so war er stets bereit; und gerade in solchen Augenblicken haben wir nie ein hartes Wort von ihm gehört. Ob reich, ob arm, hoch oder niedrig, wo seine Hilfe nötig war gab er sie gern und ohne Zögern. Die bei seiner Arbeitsüberlastung notwendige Erholung suchte er ausser in den Ferien hier and da auf Reisen, welche er vornehmen musste; und andererseits wiederum kam es ihm in solchen Fällen nicht darauf an, mehrere Nachtruhen bei der Reise zu opfern, um seine klinische Tätigkeit nicht mehr, als unbedingt nötig war, einzuschränken. Neben seiner aufreibenden praktisch chirurgischen Tätigkeit fand v. Mikulicz noch Zeit zu wissenschaftlichen Arbeiten. Wie wenig andere hat er auf fast allen Gebieten der Chirurgie Hervorragendes geleistet, ja auf verschiedenen hat er grundlegende Arbeiten geschaffen.	Two traits perhaps make up the essence of his character, his energy and strictness towards himself, and his goodness of heart. Outstanding achievements can only be achieved by rare energetic natures, who are completely devoted to an idea and forget themselves. v. Mikulicz was a shining example of this; active uninterruptedly from dawn to dusk, with the same freshness and thoroughness early in the morning as late in the evening. He was never tired at work, and whatever resistance he encountered, he overcame with a tenacious iron will. He wanted and he could, and he wanted a lot! All of us, his disciples, have the best evidence of this; if, in the evening of a arduous day, he was called to a case where we needed him, he was always ready; and it was precisely at such moments that we never heard a harsh word from him. Whether rich or poor, high or low, where his help was needed, he gave it willingly and without hesitation. Apart from the holidays, he sought the rest he needed from his excessive workload here and there on trips, which he had to undertake; and, on the other hand, in such cases it did not matter to him to sacrifice several nights' rest during the journey, in order not to limit his clinical work more than was absolutely necessary. In addition to his grueling practical surgical work, v. Mikulicz still found time for scientific work. Like few others, he has achieved excellent results in almost all areas of surgery, indeed he has created foundational works in various areas.

Neben seiner eigenen wissenschaftlichen Tätigkeit, gab er uns, seinen Schülern, die fruchtbarste Anregung zu neuen Arbeiten. Er stellte uns die verschiedenartigsten Aufgaben, liess uns bei der Ausführung volle Freiheit, war aber stets bereit, uns mit seinem Rat zu unterstützen. Er hielt es für seine Pflicht, neben seiner Lehrtätigkeit den Studenten gegenüber, seine Assistenten und Volontäre zu exakten und wissenschaftlichen Arbeiten anzuregen und ihnen zu zeigen, wie fast jeder einzelne entsprechend seiner persönlichen Begabung und seinem Fleisse Anteil nehmen könne an dem langsamen Aufbau der Wissenschaft.	In addition to his own scientific work, he gave us, his students, the most fruitful inspiration for new work. He set us the most diverse tasks, gave us complete freedom in the execution, but was always ready to support us with his advice. In addition to his teaching activities, he considered it his duty to encourage his assistants and trainees to carry out precise and scientific work and to show them how almost every single one according to their personal talent and diligence, could take part in the slow development of science.
Er war nicht bestrebt, den Studenten von Stufe zu Stufe systematisch weiter zu unterrichten, ihm eine Fülle von Kenntnissen mitzugeben, und aus ihm einen gelehrten Mann zu machen. Im Gegenteil, er bemühte sich, seine Schüler chirurgisch denken und ärztlich empfinden zu lehren. Das war sein Hauptziel. Sie sollten sehen und fühlen lernen und sich dabei stets bewusst sein, dass ihre vornehmste Aufgabe sei, den kranken Menschen zu helfen.	He did not strive to teach students systematically, step to step, to give him a wealth of knowledge and to make a learned man out of him. On the contrary, he endeavored to teach his students to think surgically and to feel medically. That was his main goal. They should learn to see and feel and always be aware that their most important task is to help the sick.
Die Studenten verehrten, ja sie liebten ihn. Besonders kam das zum Ausdruck, als er am 15. Februar nach seiner Erholung zum ersten Mal wieder die Klinik betrat. Er wurde mit Begeisterung empfangen, glaubten doch alle, ihr verehrter Lehrer sei genesen aus den Süden zurückgekehrt. Er stand, gerührt von ihrer Anhänglichkeit, tränenden Auges vor ihnen und gab den Studenten und uns allen in einer längeren Rede vielleicht das Beste, was er je geschrieben oder gesprochen hat. Es waren Worte, die sich ein jeder von uns tief ins Herz geschrieben hat, Worte, die ihn uns so recht als grossen Arzt zeigten, und uns immer wieder daran erinnerten, dass die grösste und vornehmste Aufgabe sei, zu helfen —	The students adored, even loved, him. This was particularly evident when he entered the clinic for the first time on February 15 after his recovery. He was received with enthusiasm, as everyone believed that their dear teacher had returned from the south recovered. He stood before them, touched by their devotion, with tears in his eyes, and in a lengthy speech gave the students and all of us perhaps the best thing he has ever written or spoken. They were words that each of us wrote deep in our hearts, words that really showed us how great a physician he was and reminded us again and again that the greatest and most important task is to help —
Die besten Attribute des Chirurgen "tuto et cito" passen auf ihn in vollstem Masse. Trotz der Schnelligkeit, mit der er operierte, litt die Sicherheit niemals. Die grösste Sauberkeit, exaktes Operieren und eine unbedingte Nahtsichterheit betrachtete er stets als die wichtigsten Voraussetzungen eines guten Erfolges. Den schwierigsten Situationen war er stets gewachsen, und je grösser die Gefahr, je ernster die Komplikationen, um so grösser war seine Ruhe."	The best attributes of the surgeon "tuto et cito" [safely and quickly] suit him to in the fullest measure. Despite the speed with which he operated, safety never suffered. He always regarded the greatest cleanliness, precise operation and an unconditional stitch security as the most important prerequisites for good success. He was always able to cope with the most difficult situations, and the greater the danger, the more serious the complications, the greater was his calm."
Breslau, 20. VI. 1905. Sauerbruch	Breslau, June 20 1905. Sauerbruch

References

1. Yap LH, Ahmad T. Allis forceps: notes on the inventor. J Plast Reconstruct Aesthet Surg. 2001;54:561.
2. Ailawadi G, Nagji AS, Jones DR. The legends behind cardiothoracic surgical instruments. Ann Thorac Surg. 2010;89:1693–700.
3. William Wayne Babcock. Whonamedit? www.whonamedit.com. Accessed 12 Nov 2019.
4. Corman ML. Donald Church Balfour 1882-1963. Dis Colon Rectum. 1984;27:559–62.
5. Barron J. Office ligation treatment of hemorrhoids. Dis Colon Rectum. 1963;6:109–13.
6. Blake LW, Harvel ER, Mason DR, Wright GM. United States Patent 4,398,910, Aug. 16, 1983.
7. Berkeley C, Bonney V. A Text-book of Gynæcological Surgery. New York: Funk and Wagnalls Company; 1911. p. 9. Accessed from Google Books, 6 July 2021
8. Barr J, Brayman KL. Development and evolution of self-retaining retractors in surgery: the example of the Bookwalter retractor. J Am Coll Surg. 2015;221:628–34.
9. Brinkerhoff WC. Diseases of the Rectum: Their Consequences and Non-surgical Treatment. Chicago, IL: Orban Publishing Co.; 1907. between pages 106–107. Google books-accessed 26 Dec 2019
10. Carter PL. The life and legacy of William T. Bovie. Am J Surg. 2013;205:488–91.
11. Crile GW, Associates. The thyroid gland. In: Rowland AF, editor. Philadelphia, PA: W. B. Saunders Company, 1923. p. 206. Google books Accessed 26 Nov 2019.
12. Newhook TE, Yeo CJ, Maxwell PJ IV. John Blair Deaver, M.D., and his marvelous retractor. Am Surg. 2012;78:155–6.
13. Fansler WA. Special problems in the proctoscopic examination of the geriatric patient. J Am Geriatr Soc. 1962;10:567–70.
14. Gelpi MJ. A new self-retaining perineal retractor. New Orleans Med Surg J. 1913;66:182–3.
15. Lathan RS. Caroline Hampton Halsted: the first to use rubber gloves in the operating room. Proc (Bayl Univ Med Cent). 2010;23:389–392.
16. Hegar A, Kaltenbach R. Die Operative Gynäkologie. Stuttgart: Verlag von Ferdinand Enke; 1881. p. 87–9. Google books Accessed 25 Nov 2019.
17. Hill TC. A manual of proctology. Philadelphia, PA: Lea & Febiger; 1923. p. 24.
18. Hirschman LJ. Handbook of diseases of the rectum. 2nd ed. CV Mosby Company: St. Louis, MO; 1914. p. 54.
19. Cirocco WC. The Louis J. Hirschman Lineage (Hirschman to Nigro): The rise of a Society and the Fall of a University Department of Colon and Rectal Surgery (Part 1). Dis Colon Rectum 2024;67:7–12.
20. Jackson FE, Pratt RA III. Technical report: a silicone rubber suction drain for drainage of subdural hematomas. Surgery. 1971;70:578–9.
21. Maingot R, Frank H. Lahey-the man, the surgeon and the teacher. Lahey Clin Bull. 1963;13:80–90.
22. Platt WB. Baron von Langenbeck, Surgeon-General of the German Army, Professor of surgery in the University of Berlin. Bull John Hopkins Hosp. 1894;40:62–4.
23. Parks PJ. Giants of Science – Joseph Lister. Farmington Hills, MI: Blackbirch Press; 2005.
24. Haubrich WS. Kelly of the Kelly clamp. Gastroenterology. 2007;132:10.
25. Theodor Kocher-biographical-Nobel Prize. https://www.nobel prize.org. Accessed 24 Nov 2019.
26. Metzenbaum, Myron, MD. Encyclopedia of Cleveland History; www.Case.edu. Accessed 12 Jan 2019.
27. Myron Firth Metzenbaum. Whonamedit.com. Accessed 11 Nov 2019.
28. Mikulicz J. Ueber die Ausschaltung todter Räume aus der Peritonealhöhle, mit besonderer Rücksicht auf die Exstirpation der aus der Beckenhöhe ausgehenden Geschwülste. Arch kiln Chir. 1887;34:635–57.
29. Zajaczkowski T. Johann Anton von Mikulicz-Radecki (1850-1905)—a pioneer of gastroscopy and modern surgery: his credit to urology. World J Urol. 2008;26:75–86.

30. Moynihan's intestinal clamp forceps. Science Museum Group Collection. https://collection.sciencemuseumgroup.org.uk/objects/co168504/moynihans-intestinal-clamp-forceps-intestinal-forceps. Accessed 24 Nov 2019.
31. Bateman D. Berkeley Moynihan: Surgeon. London: MacMillian, & Co. LTD; 1941.
32. Ventura HO. Alton Ochsner, MD: Physician. Ochsner J. 2002;4:48–52.
33. Péan J. Obituary. Lancet. 1898;i:389.
34. Abramson DJ. Charles Bingham Penrose and the Penrose drain. Surg Gynecol Obstet. 1976;143:285–6.
35. Fitz RH. Memorials to Maurice Howe Richardson, MD. Boston Med Surg J. 1912;167:903–11.
36. Meals CG, Meals RA. A history of surgery in the instrument tray: eponymous tools used in hand surgery. J Hand Surg. 2007;32A:942–53.
37. de Jong GM, Clark SK. The St. Mark's retractor. Br J Surg. 2019;106:1818.
38. Sharma A, Swan KG. Franz Weitlaner: the great spreader of surgery. J Trauma Inj Infect Crit Care. 2009;67:1431–4.
39. Dieke GH. Robert Williams Wood, 1868–1955. A Biographical Memoir. National Academy of Sciences. Washington, D.C., Copyright 1993.
40. Yankauer Sidney MD. Death of fellows of the academy. Bull N Y Acad Med. 1932;8:591.
41. Mikulcz J. Ueber die Ausschaltung todter Räume aus der Peritonealhöhle, mit besonderer Rücksicht auf die Exstirpation der aus der Beckenhöhe ausgehenden Geschwülste. Arch Klin Chir. 1887;34:635–57.
42. Whonamedit? – A dictionary of medical eponyms. Jan Mikulicz-Radecki, Mikulicz's pad. whonamedit.com. Accessed 6 Oct 2022.
43. Olch PD. Johann von Mikulicz-Radecki. Ann Surg. 1960;152:923–6.
44. Zajaczkowski T. Johann Anton von Mikulicz-Radecki (1850-1895)—a pioneer of gastroscopy and modern surgery: his credit to urology. World J Surg. 2008;26:75–86.
45. Gorecki P, Gorecki W. Jan Mikulicz-Radecki (1850-1905) – The creator of modern European surgery. Dig Surg. 2002;19:313–20.
46. Kuczkowski J, Stankiewicz C, Kopacz A, Narozny W, Mikaszewski B, Drucis K. Jan-Mikulicz-Radecki (1850–1905): pioneer of endoscopy and surgery of the sinuses, throat, and digestive tract. World J Surg. 2004;28:1063–7.
47. Sauerbruch EF. Johann v. Mikulicz. Muench Med Wochenshr. 1905;52:1297–300.

Colon Evaluation-Historical Overview 21

Michelle D. Inkster, Gwendolyn A. Fuller, and James S. Wu

Radiological Studies

At Röntgen Haus in Würzburg, Germany, a few words memorialize the discovery of X-rays [1].

IN DIESEM HAUSE ENTDECKTE W. C. RÖNTGEN IM JAHRE 1895 DIE NACH IHM BENNANTEN STRAHLEN	IN THIS HOUSE IN 1895, W. C. RÖNTGEN DICOVERED THE RAYS THAT ARE NAMED AFTER HIM

An article commemorating Röntgen published by the American Physical Society in 2001 reads:

> Roentgen was awarded the first Nobel Prize in physics in 1901 for his discovery. When asked what his thoughts were at the moment of discovery, he replied, true to form, "I didn't think, I investigated." Today, Roentgen is widely recognized as a brilliant experimentalist who never sought honors or financial profits for his research. He rejected a title that would

M. D. Inkster
Department of Gastroenterology, Cleveland Clinic, Cleveland, OH, USA

G. A. Fuller
Medical Illustration Team, Enterprise Creative Services, Cleveland Clinic, Cleveland, OH, USA

J. S. Wu (✉)
Department of Colon and Rectal Surgery, Cleveland Clinic, Cleveland, OH, USA

J. S. Wu, M. D. Inkster (eds.), *Cleveland Clinic Colorectal Case Studies*,
https://doi.org/10.1007/978-3-031-39880-3_21

have given him entry into the German nobility, and donated his Nobel Prize money to his university. While he accepted the honorary degree of doctor of medicine offered to him by his own university, he never took out any patents on X-rays, to ensure that the world could freely benefit from his work [2].

Radiologic

In 1904, Schüle noted that prior to the advent of X-rays, Wachsmuth intubated the colon with a flexible tube [3, 4],

Ueber die Sondierung und Radiographie des Dickdarms. Von Prof. Schüle Aus dem ev. Diakonissenhaus zu Freiburg Seit längeren Jahren bis auf die heutige Zeit haben sich Forscher mit dem Problem der Dickdarmsondierung beschäftigt. 1862 behauptete Wachsmuth, dass es „unter günstigen Umständen" gelinge, den Dickdarm bis zur Valv. Bauhini zu passieren und ein Rohr von 166—196 cm einzuführen.	Concerning the probing and radiography of the colon. By Prof. Schüle From the evangelical Deaconess house in Freiburg For many years up to the present day, researchers have been involved with the problem of colonic probing. In 1862, Wachsmuth asserted that "under favorable circumstances," he succeeded in passing a tube through the colon up the valve of Bauhini, a distance of 166–196 cm.

Wachsmuths described the examination and nonoperative management of a patient with "Meteorismus," who presented on March 2, 1861.

Ileus und Enterotomie. Von Prof Adolph Wachsmuth in Dorpat Ein Fall, nicht operirt, mit günstigem Ausgang. Bauch ist hart und stark aufgetrieben.... Druck auf die Bauchdecken in dem Kranken schmerzhaft, namentlich nach vorausgegangenem Druck sieht man sehr deutlich durch die Bauchdecken peristaltische Bewegung des Darms in Gestalt wurmförmiger Bewegungen. Percussion hell tympanitisch,...	Ileus and Enterotomy By Prof. Adolph Wachsmuth Dorpat A case, treated without surgery with a successful outcome. The belly is hard and markedly distended..... Pressure on the surface of the abdomen is painful. After the aforementioned pressure, one can see clearly through the abdominal wall, the peristaltic movement of the intestine with wormlike movements. Percussion is brightly tympanitic....

On March 6, the patient's situation had not improved.

Leib mehr aufgetrieben... In der Frühe Erbrechen von gelblich Grüner Flüssigkeit von fäculentem Geruch.	The body was more distended. The early vomit was yellow green liquid that had a feculent order.

At noon of that day, Wachmuth inserted an elastic sound with a remarkable result.

Um 12 Uhr gelang es das elastische Rohr... mehr als 5 Fuss... hoch hinaufzuführen. Nach 1 Stunde wurden mit dem Wasser wieder einige bröcklige Fäcalmassen entleert. Um 5 Uhr Allgemeinbefinden etwas besser, die Kolikschmerzen haben nachgelassen, Leib weinger aufgetrieben als früher. Am 19. März wurde der Kranke geheilt entlassen.	At noon, an elastic tube was successfully advanced 5 ft. After 1 h, with water irrigation, a chunky stool was emptied. At 5 o'clock, he was generally better, the colicky pain was gone, and his body was less distended than previously. On March 19, the patient was discharged, healed.

Schüle follows with his own studies in which he instilled Bismuth Subn. oil into the large intestine and then documented its structure using X-rays [3].

Die Radiogramme..., auf welche ich hiermit verweise, zeigen mit aller wünchenswerten Deutlichkeit, dass ein Einlauf von 300—400 ccm Oel, appliziert in Knieellenbogenlage mittelst des Hegar'schen Trichters, sehr wohl die Ileocöcalgegend erreichen kann.	The radiograms..., to which I refer, indicate with desired clarity, that the introduction of 300—400 ccm of oil, applied in the knee-elbow position using Hegar-type funnel, can reach the ileocecal region very well.

In 1911, Haenisch [5] described narrowing of the colon seen on contrast enema and the application of the technique for the early diagnosis of colon cancer.

Die Röentgenuntersuchung bei Verengungen des Dickdarms. Röntgenologische Frühdiagnose des Dickdarmkarzinoms Von Dr. G. Fedor Haenisch, Spezialarzt für Röntgenologie in Hamburg	The radiologic investigation of colonic narrowing, radiologic early diagnosis of colon cancer By Dr. G. Fedor Haenisch, Special physician for radiology, Hamburg

In 1925, Fischer described double contrast enema using Barium and air [6]. This method proved particularly useful for the early diagnosis of cancer and was utilized extensively until, gradually, it was replaced by colonoscopy.

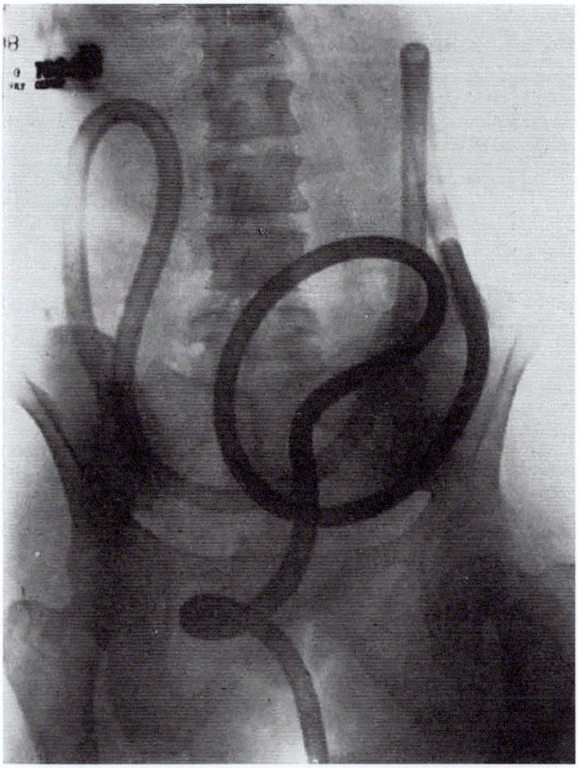

Fig. 21.1 Hoff's retrograde intubation of the colon demonstrates redundant areas. A loop is seen in the sigmoid colon. The mid-transverse colon dips into the pelvis. While the left and right colons are fixed to the posterior wall of the abdominal cavity, the sigmoid and transverse colon are suspended on a mesentery and, therefore, are mobile. This image was reproduced with permission from the American Roentgen Ray Society, Invoice #572, Date 8/9/2021

Über eine neue Röntgenologische Untersuchungsmethode des Dickdarms: Kombination von Kontrasteinlauf und Luft- aufblähung Von Privatdozent Dr. A. W. Fischer Assistant der Chirurgischen Universitätsklinik Frankfurt *Die soeben geschilderte „kombinierte Methode" ist meiner Ansicht nach eine wichtige Ergänzung der bisher gebräuchlichen Verfahren. Sie ist technisch ohne besondere Zusatzapparatur leicht mit jedem Instrumentarium durchzuführen und dürfte besonders berufen sein, uns in der Frühdiagnose des Dickdarmkrebses weiter zu bringen.*	On a new Röntgenologic method of investigating the large intestine: combination of contast instillation and air insufflation By Private lecturer Dr. A. W Fischer Assistant at the Surgical University Clinic, Frankfurt *The "combination method" described above is in my opinion an important addition to procedures used previously.* *Technically, additional special equipment is not needed to perform the procedure which is easily carried out with existing instruments.* *In particular, the method could improve the early diagnosis of colon cancer.*

In 1928, Hoff described retrograde intubation of the cecum using a flexible tube guided by plain radiographs. He documented problems with retrograde colorectal intubation subsequently seen at colonoscopy (Fig. 21.1) [7].

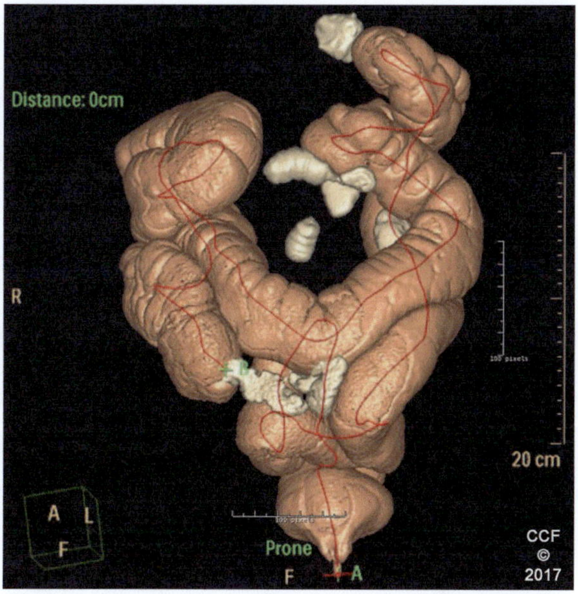

Fig. 21.2 Computed tomographic reconstruction of the large intestine. Optical colonoscopy was incomplete. This examination shows a markedly redundant colon. The tortuous path of the colon is marked with a red line

CT Colonography

In 1994, Vining and colleagues introduced virtual colonoscopy [8, 9]. The term CT colonography was introduced by Johnson et al. in 1998 [10]. CT colonography creates multiple images of the interior of the colon and can detect polyps. Virtual colonoscopy is an accepted method for follow-up after an optical colonoscopy where the procedure cannot be completed or who have contraindications for optical colonoscopy (Fig. 21.2).

Endoscopic Evaluation

Endoscopic evaluation of the large intestine has involved both straight and fiberoptic instruments.

Hippocrates (460–380 BC) [11] used a speculum to remove condyloma from "higher up the anus." In 1806, Bozzini [12, 13] invented a paraffin lamp, named the "Lichtleiter" (guiding light) to illuminate inner parts of the body.

Lichtleiter, eine Erfindung zur Anschauung innerer Theile und Krankheiten, nebst der Abbildung von Dr. Bozzini, Arzt zu Frankfuht a. Mayn	LICHTLEITER, An Invention To visualize the Inner Parts of the Body And their Diseases, With Illustrations by By Dr. Bozzini, Physician, Frankfurt am Main

In 1865, Desormeaux [14] described endoscopy for the diagnosis and treatment of diseases of the urethra and the bladder. He made the first practical cystoscope.

De l'endoscope et de ses applications au diagnostic et au traitement des affections de l'urèthre et de la vessie. Leçons faite a l'Hopital Necker par A.J. Desormeaux Chirurgien de l'Hopital Necker PRÉFACE Nosquoque oculos eruditos habemus (*Cic., Parad. v.*) Un des progrès les plus caractéristiques de l'art médical à notre époque consiste dans la recherche de tous les procédés d'exploration directe des organs…	The endoscope and its applications for the diagnosis and treatment of afflictions of the urethra and the bladder. Lessons learned at Necker Hospital by A.J. Desormeaux Surgeon, Necker Hospital PREFACE Even we have learned eyes (*Cicero, Paradoxa, V*) [15] The most characteristic progress of the medical arts in our epoque is found in research of all procedures that directly explore the organs….

In 1895, Kelly [16] developed a method to examine the rectum by using a speculum and reflected light with the patient in the knee-breast position. The light source was reflected into the viewing area using a head-mirror.

In 1957, Curtiss, Hirschowitz, and Peters at the University of Michigan described a "long fiberscope for internal medical examinations" [17]. In his historical perspective on Dr. Hirschowitz, Burki recounts [18],

> "By early 1957, the first fibre-optic gastroscope was complete. It was almost one metre long and included a lens, a prism, and a tungsten filament bulb (later models transmitted light along a second fibre-optic cable). Hirschowitz tested it on himself. "I looked at this rather thick, forbidding but flexible rod, took the instrument and my courage in both hands, and swallowed it over the protest of my unanaesthetised pharynx and my vomiting centre."

In 1963, Turell introduced the flexible fiber optic coloscope based on the principles of fiber optic examination of the stomach [19].

In a landmark achievement, Provenzale, Camerada, and Revignis in 1966 described *La coloscopia totale trans-anale* [20] (Fig. 21.3).

La coloscopia totale trans-anale mediante una metodica originale (osservazioni preliminari) L. Provenzale - P. Camerada - A. Revignas Instituto di clinica chirurgica generale e terapia chirurgica dell'Universita' di Cagliari Instituto di clinica medica generale e terapia medica dell'Universita' di Cagliari "Esso termina distalmente con un'ansa, in cui si fa passare un secundo tubo, il quale, ripiegato in doppio, viene ad avere i due estremi liberi che fuoriescono dall'ano."	Total trans-anal colonoscopy by an original method (preliminary observations) L. Provenzale, P. Camerada, A. Revignas Institute for general clinical surgery and therapeutic surgery, the University of Cagliari Institute for general clinical medicine and therapeutic medicine, the University of Cagliari "It ends distally with a loop in which a second tube is passed which, folded in double, has the two free ends that protrude from the anus."

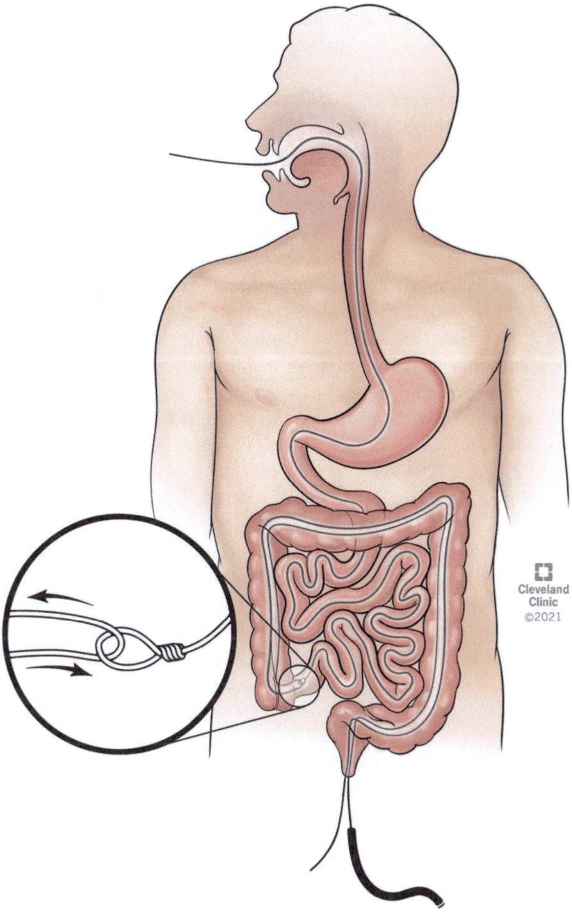

Fig. 21.3 Rappresentazione schematica dello speciale sondino del tipo (end-to-end) ideato per far progredire nel colon in senso antiperistaltico strumenti e dispositivi vari introdotti per via trans-anale (Schematic representations of a special type of probe (end-to-end) designed to advance various instruments and devices introduced transanally into the colon in an antiperistaltic direction)

Schematic representation of the special sound of the (end-end) type intended to advance in the colon in the antiperistaltic sense and introduce various instruments transanally (after Provenzale et al. [20]).

In 1967, Overholt and Pollard reported on the usefulness of a flexible sigmoidoscope equipped with channels for aspiration and instillation of water or air [21]. In 1975, Overholt, in a review, stated that colonoscopy "offers the single most far reaching advance for the diagnosis and treatment of diseases of the colon that has been offered in the last decade" [22]. 1979, Shinya and Wolff reported their analysis of 7000 polyps endoscopically removed and concluded with the following recommendation:

> "A vigorous program for detection and endoscopic removal of colorectal polyps is recommended as a means of reducing the incidence of colorectal cancer [23]."

References

1. Röntgenhaus, 8 Röntgenring, Würzburg, Germany.
2. November 8, 1895: Roentgen's discovery of X-rays. APS News 2001;10(10). Accessed 22 March 2020.
3. Schüle S. Ueber die Sondierung und Radiographie des Dickdarms. Archiv Verdauungskrank 1904;10:111–8.
4. Wachsmuth A. Ileus und Enterostomie. Virch Arch. 1862;23:118–48.
5. Haenisch GF. Die Röntgenuntersuchung bei Verengungen des Dickdarms, Röntgenologische Frühdiagnose des Dickdarmkarzinoms. Muench Med Wochenschr 1911; No. 45, 7. November, 58 Jahrgang:2375–2381. Accessed from Internet Archive, archive.org, September 13, 2022.
6. Fischer AW. Über eine neue Röntgenologische Untersuchungsmethode des Dickdarms. Komination von Kontrasteinlauf und Luftaufblähung. Klin Wochenschr. 1923;2:1595–8.
7. Hoff HC. Retrograde intubation of the cecum. Am J Roent Rad Ther. 1928;20:226–32.
8. Vining DJ, Gelfand DW, Bechtold RE, Scharling ES, Grishaw EK, Shifrin RY. Technical feasibility of colon imaging with helical CT and virtual reality (abstract). Am J Roentgenol. 1994;162(suppl):104.
9. Vining D. Virtual endoscopy: is it reality? Radiology. 1996;200:30–1.
10. Johnson CD, Hara AK, Reed JE. Virtual endoscopy; what's in a name? Am J Roentgenol. 1998;171:1201–2.
11. Hippocrates. On Hemorrhoids – part 5. Translated by Francis Adams. Provided by The Internet Classics Archive. Available online at http://classic.mit.edu//Hippocrates/hemmor.html.
12. Bozzini. Lichtleiter, eine Erfindung zur Anschauung innerer Theile und Krankheiten nebst der Abbildung. J Pract Arzneykunde Wundarzneykunst. 1806;24:107–24.
13. Bush RB, Leonhardt H, Bush IM, Landes RR. Dr. Bozzini's Lichtleiter. A translation of his original article (1806). Urology. 1974;111:119–23.
14. Desormeaux AJ. De L'Endoscope et de ses applications au diagnostic et au traitement des affections de l'urèthre et de la vessie. Leçons faite a l'Hopital Necker. Paris, J. - B. Baillière et fils; 1865.
15. Galinsky K. The age of augustus. Cambridge: Cambridge University Press; 2005. p. 291.
16. Kelly HA. A new method of examination and treatment of diseases of the rectum and sigmoid flexure. Ann Surg. 1895;21:468–78.
17. Curtiss LE, Hirschowitz B, Peters CW. FC63 a long fiberscope for internal medical examinations. J Opt Soc Am. 1957;47:117.
18. Burki TK. In focus|Historical perspective. Let there be light. Lancet Gastroenterol Hepatol 2018;3:151. This excerpt is reproduced with the generous permission of Elsevier and Copyright Clearance Center, License Number 5325800387040, License date Jun 11, 2022.
19. Turell R. Fiber optic coloscope and sigmoidoscope. Am J Surg. 1963;103:133–6.
20. Provenzale L, Camerada P, Revignas A. La coloscopia totale trans-anale mediante una metodica originale. Rass Med Sarda. 1966;69:149–60.
21. Overholt BF, Pollard MH. Cancer of the colon and rectum. Current procedures for detection and diagnosis. Cancer. 1967;20:445–50.
22. Overholt BF. Colonoscopy. A review. Gastroenterology. 1975;68:1308–20.
23. Shinya H, Wolf WI. Morphology, anatomic distribution and cancer potential of colonic polyps. Ann Surg. 1979;190:679–83.

Colonoscopy-Normal Landmarks

22

James S. Wu and Michelle D. Inkster

Colonoscopy Landmarks

Cecum

The appendiceal orifice is located at the proximal end of the colon within the cecum.

Variations of the appearance of the cecum and the appendiceal orifice are shown in Fig. 22.1.

Two appearances of the terminal ileum are shown in Fig. 22.2.

Two views of the hepatic flexure are shown in Fig. 22.3.

The transverse colonic lumen looks triangular (Fig. 22.4).

The spleen can be seen through the colon wall at the splenic flexure (Fig. 22.5).

In the rectum, three valves of Houston are seen as shown in Fig. 22.6.

On retroflexion in the rectum, the anal transitional zone situated between the rectal columnar mucosa and the anal canal pecten is seen (Figs. 22.7, 22.8, and 22.9).

Inspection of the anal orifice shows raised ridges of skin arranged in a radial pattern caused by contraction of the underlying corrugator cutis ani muscle (Fig. 22.10).

J. S. Wu (✉)
Department of Colon and Rectal Surgery, Cleveland Clinic, Cleveland, OH, USA

M. D. Inkster
Department of Gastroenterology, Cleveland Clinic, Cleveland, OH, USA
e-mail: inkstem@ccf.org

J. S. Wu, M. D. Inkster (eds.), *Cleveland Clinic Colorectal Case Studies*,
https://doi.org/10.1007/978-3-031-39880-3_22

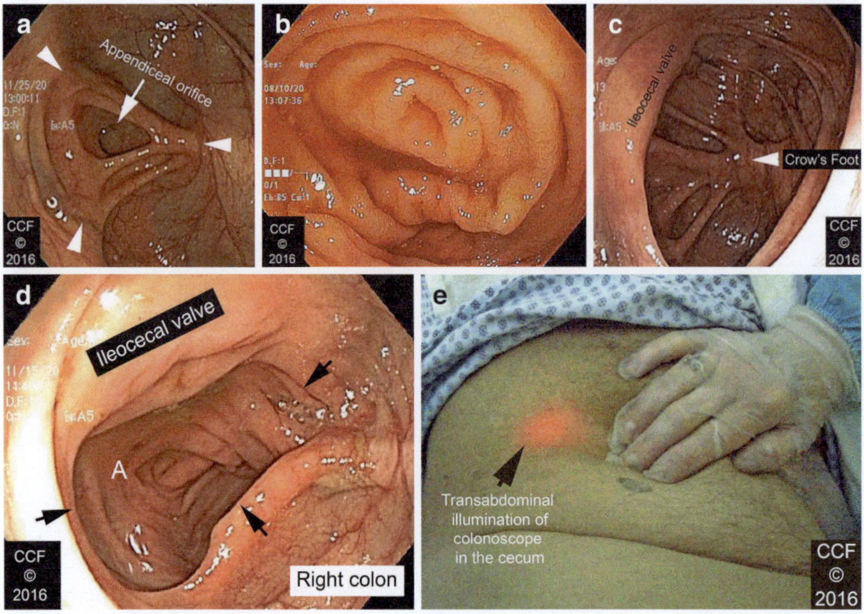

Fig. 22.1 (**a**) The appendiceal orifice is seen at base of the cecum (arrow). Three arrowheads point to the three taenia coli which converge on the base of the cecum; (**b**) The appendiceal orifice has taken on the appearance of a target with concentric rings; (**c**) At the cecum, the muscular bands sometimes take on the appearance of a webbed avian foot (e.g., Crow's foot); (**d**) The lips of the ileocecal valve and the appendiceal orifice (A) are marked. The cecum is the part of the colon that is proximal to the ileocecal valve. The border between the right colon and the cecum in this picture is identified by the black arrows; (**e**) When the cecum is reached, the light of the instrument sometimes can be seen through the abdominal wall of the patient in the right lower quadrant

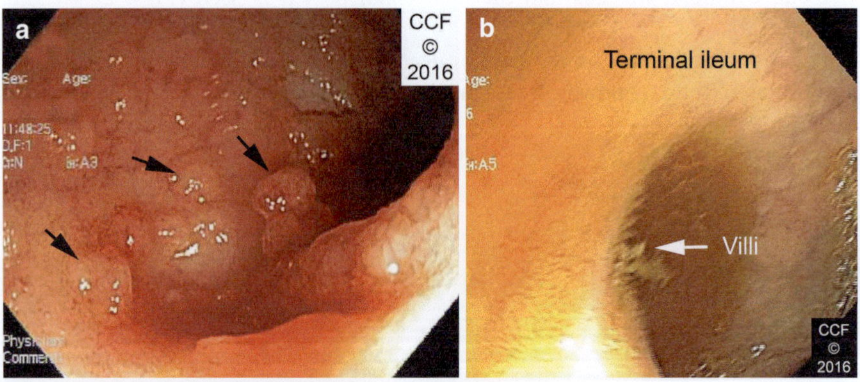

Fig. 22.2 (**a**) Intubation of the terminal ileum shows prominent lymphoid tissue (Peyer's Patches) [arrows]; (**b**) Intubation of the terminal ileum shows villi

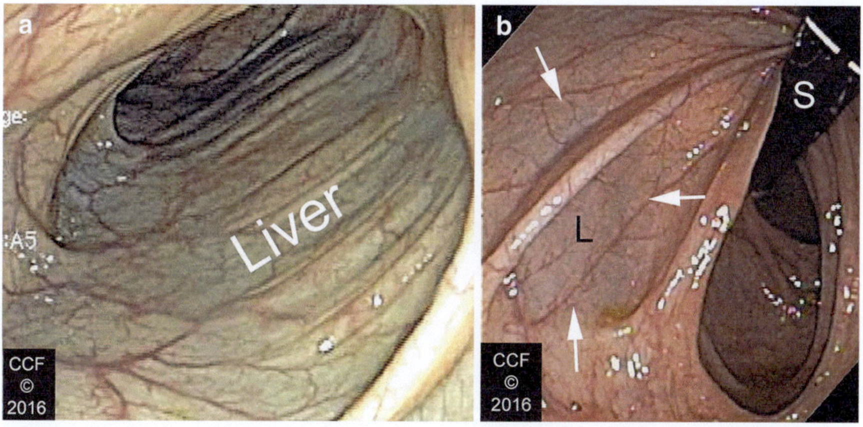

Fig. 22.3 (**a**) The liver is seen through the colon wall at the hepatic flexure; (**b**) The liver (L) and hepatic flexure are seen (arrows) on retroflexed view of the scope (S) from the cecum

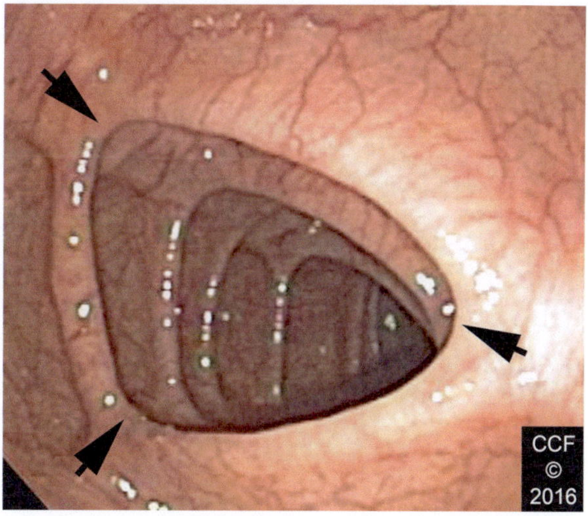

Fig. 22.4 The transverse colon shows a characteristic triangular shape. The three angles (arrows) correspond to the location of the taenia coli (*taenia mesocolica*, *taenia omentalis*, and *taenia libera*)

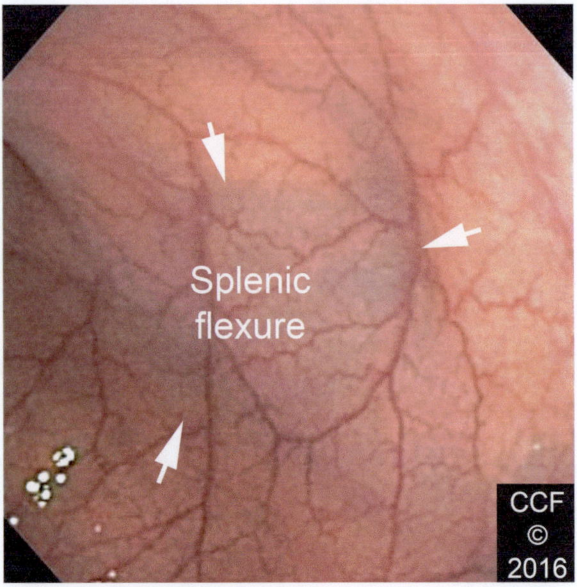

Fig. 22.5 The neighboring spleen is seen through the wall of the colon at the splenic flexure (arrows)

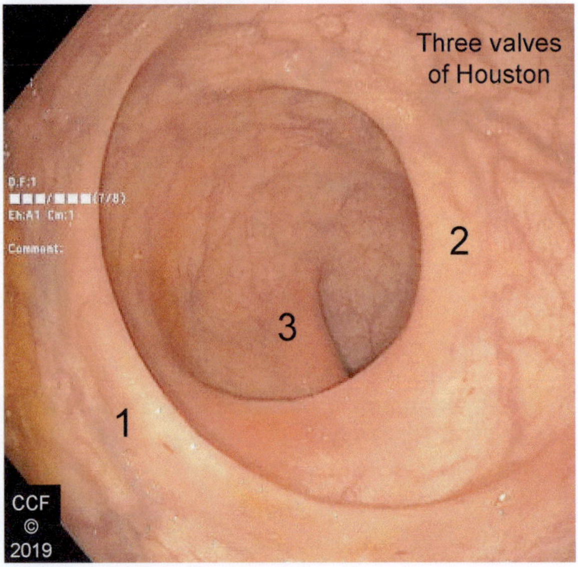

Fig. 22.6 The three valves of Houston (numbered 1, 2, and 3) are seen on antegrade view from the distal rectum

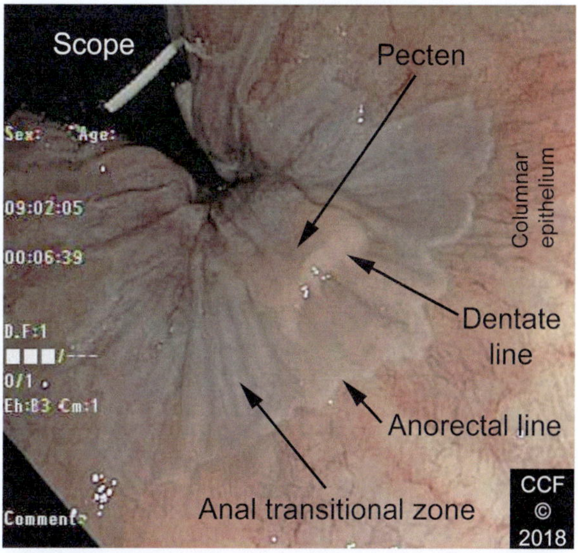

Fig. 22.7 Retroflexed view of the rectum. The anal transitional zone (ATZ) is situated between the pecten and the columnar epithelium of the rectum. The proximal border of the ATZ is the anorectal line; the distal border is the dentate line, also known as the pectinate line

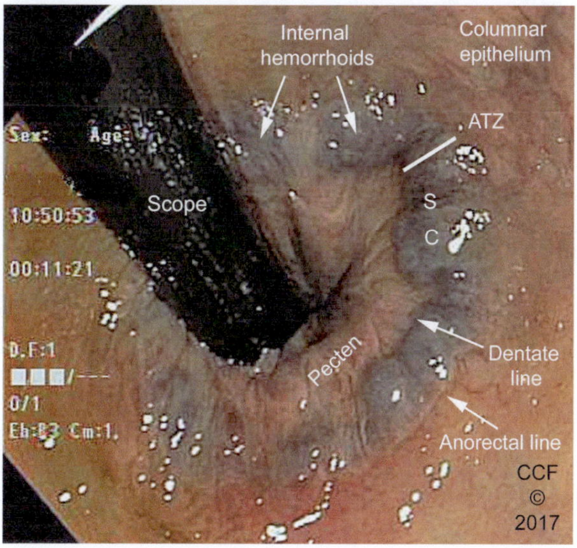

Fig. 22.8 Retroflexed view of the distal rectum shows the anorectal line, anal transitional zone (ATZ), dentate line, pecten, columns/sinuses (C/S) of Morgagni, and the internal hemorrhoids

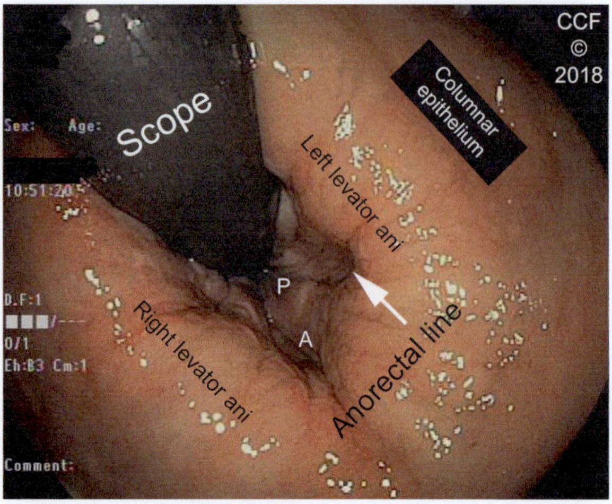

Fig. 22.9 Retroflexed view of the distal rectum shows the pecten (P), the anal transitional zone (A), the anorectal line, the columnar epithelium and the contour of the right and left levator ani muscles. The endoscope is labeled "Scope". When the patient is lying on their left side, water will gravitate to the dependent side and identify which side is "left"

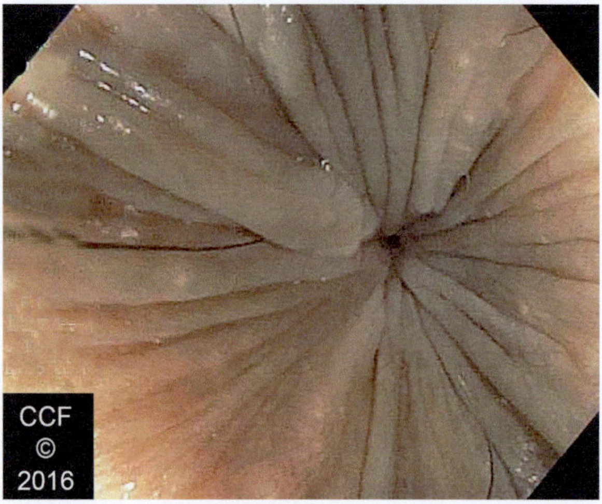

Fig. 22.10 Gray and Lewis define the corrugator cutis anis muscle as follows: "The Corrugator Cutis Ani.—Around the anus is a thin stratum of involuntary muscular fiber, which radiates from the orifice. *Medially* the fibers fade off into the subcutaneous tissue, while *laterally*, they blend with the true skin. By contraction it raises the skin into ridges around the margin of the anus" [1]

Reference

1. Gray H, Lewis WH. The Corrugator Cutis Ani. In: Anatomy of the human body. 20th ed. Philadelphia: Lea & Febiger; 1918. p. 425.

Colonoscopy-Abnormal Findings

23

Susan A. Lintala, Michael S. Cline, Homer O. Wiland, Ilyssa O. Gordon, Clifton G. Fulmer, James E. Lapinski, Mohamed I. El Hag, John R. Goldblum, John A. Dumot, Tracy L. Hull, Michelle D. Inkster, and James S. Wu

Presentation

Abnormalities encountered during routine colonoscopy are seen in perianal structures, the anus, the large intestine, and the distal small intestine. Images of some of these seen at routine colonoscopy are shown.

Figure 23.1 shows buttock ringworm, a skin infection caused by a fungus.

Figure 23.2 shows buttock psoriasis, a scaly rash of autoimmune origin.

Figure 23.3 shows gluteal cleft cutaneous neurofibromas, nerve associated tumors.

Figure 23.4 shows an example of vitiligo, a condition where skin pigmentation is lost.

The patient in Fig. 23.5 treated anal pain with a heating pad resulting in regional *erythema ab igne*.

Figure 23.6a and b were taken at the time of colonoscopy for a patient thought to have rectal bleeding. Separation of the buttocks showed a source other than the anus.

Figure 23.7 shows a raised cutaneous lesion between the anus and the vagina. Biopsy showed high-grade squamous intraepithelial lesion (HSIL).

S. A. Lintala · M. S. Cline · M. D. Inkster
Department of Gastroenterology, Cleveland Clinic, Cleveland, OH, USA

J. A. Dumot
Department of Gastroenterology, University Hospitals of Cleveland, Cleveland, OH, USA

H. O. Wiland
Department of Pathology, OhioHealth Mansfield Hospital, Mansfield, OH, USA

I. O. Gordon · C. G. Fulmer · J. E. Lapinski · J. R. Goldblum
Pathology & Laboratory Medicine Institute, Cleveland Clinic, Cleveland, OH, USA

M. I. El Hag
Pathology and Laboratory Medicine Institute, Cleveland Clinic, Cleveland, OH, USA

T. L. Hull · J. S. Wu (✉)
Department of Colon and Rectal Surgery, Cleveland Clinic, Cleveland, OH, USA

J. S. Wu, M. D. Inkster (eds.), *Cleveland Clinic Colorectal Case Studies*, https://doi.org/10.1007/978-3-031-39880-3_23

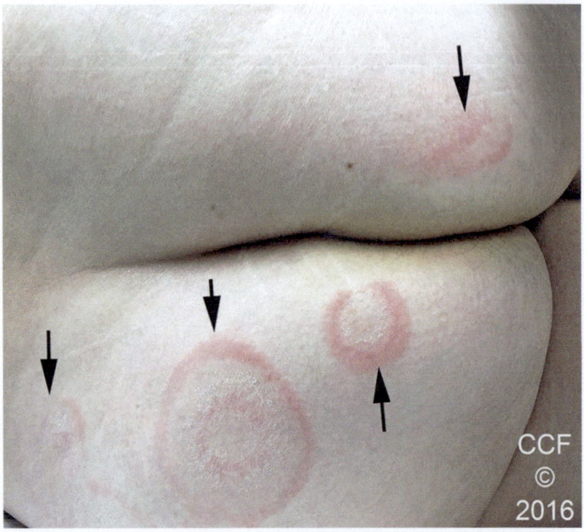

Fig. 23.1 Ringworm (arrows) seen on the buttocks (Diagnosis, courtesy of Ms. Susan A. Lintala)

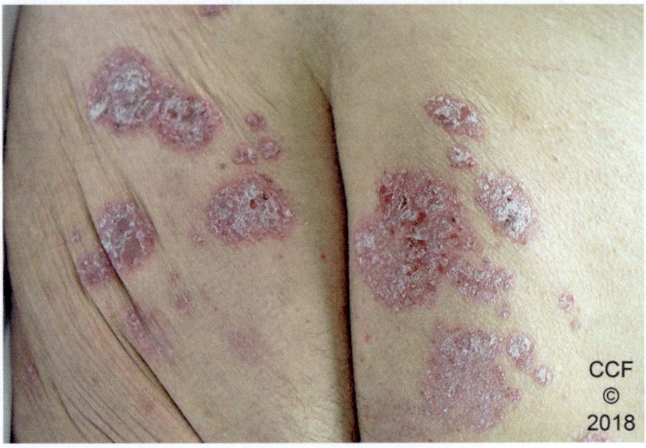

Fig. 23.2 Psoriasis, an itchy, scaly rash of autoimmune origin seen on the buttocks

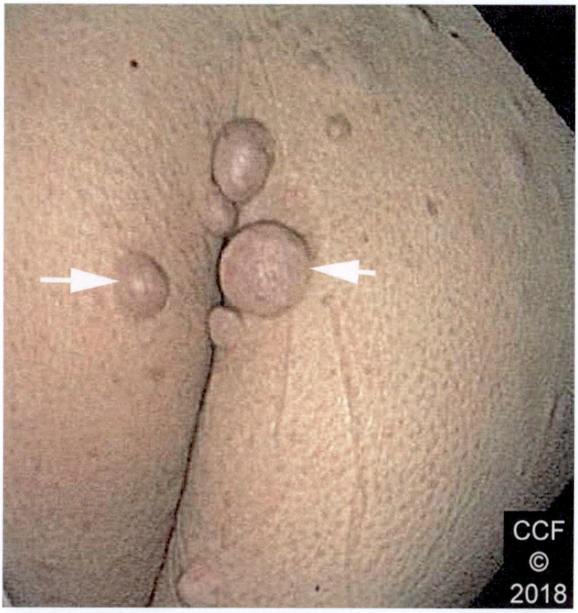

Fig. 23.3 Neurofibromatosis (arrows) located adjacent to the gluteal cleft

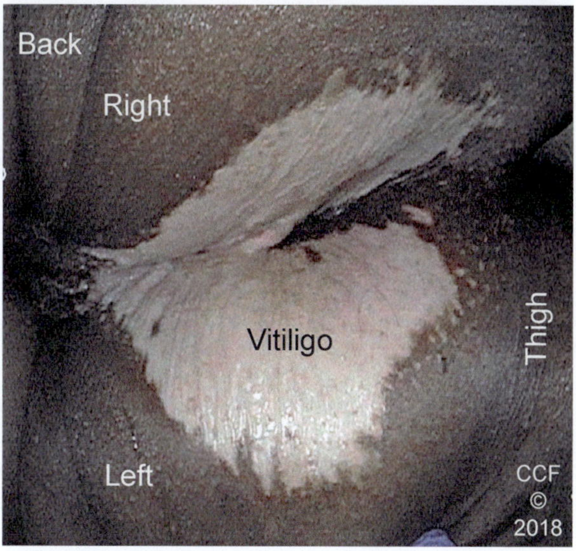

Fig. 23.4 Vitiligo involving the skin on the right and left sides of the buttocks. The back and left thigh are marked

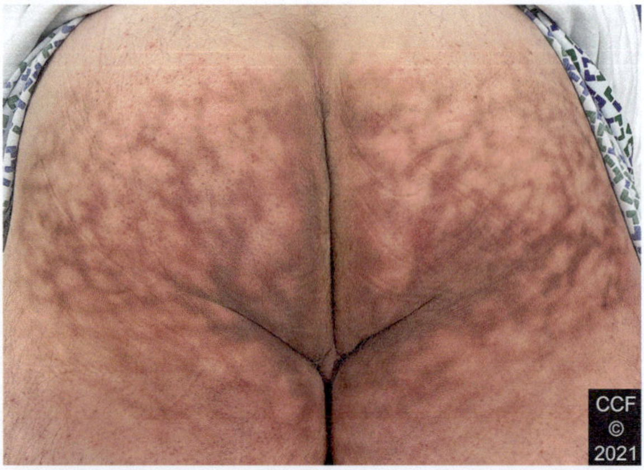

Fig. 23.5 *Erythema ab igne* (redness caused by fire) is an asymptomatic skin condition characterized by reticulated hyperpigmentation of the skin. In this case, the cause was repeated exposure to heat from a heating pad [1, 2]

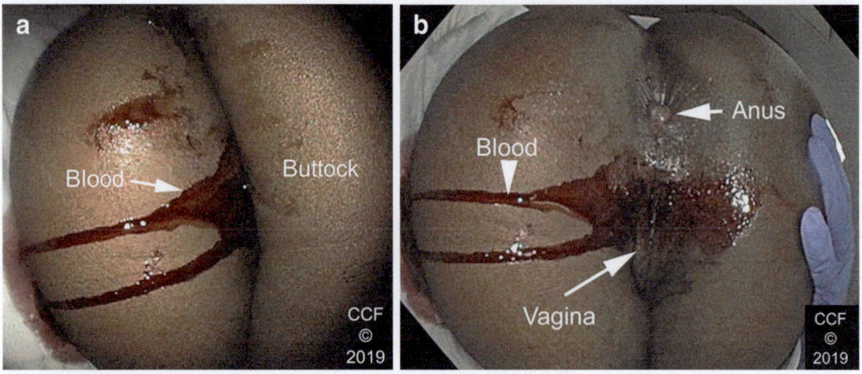

Fig. 23.6 Colonoscopy ordered for hemorrhage: (**a**) Blood is seen emanating from between the closed buttocks; (**b**) Buttock separation showed that the blood originated from the vagina not the anus

Figure 23.8 shows a large circumferential lesion centered around the anus. Biopsies showed HSIL.

Seen in Fig. 23.9 are three prolapsed internal hemorrhoids which are arranged “classically” in the left lateral, right posterior, and right anterior positions. Note that there are three radial lines that lead from the periphery to the center of the anal opening. Figure 23.10 shows rectal prolapse or “true procidentia” in which lines are arranged in circumferential rings.

Figure 23.11a shows prolapsed external hemorrhoids posteriorly and prolapse of the vagina anteriorly. A small bowel follow-through (Fig. 23.11b), done for the same patient, showed an enterocele.

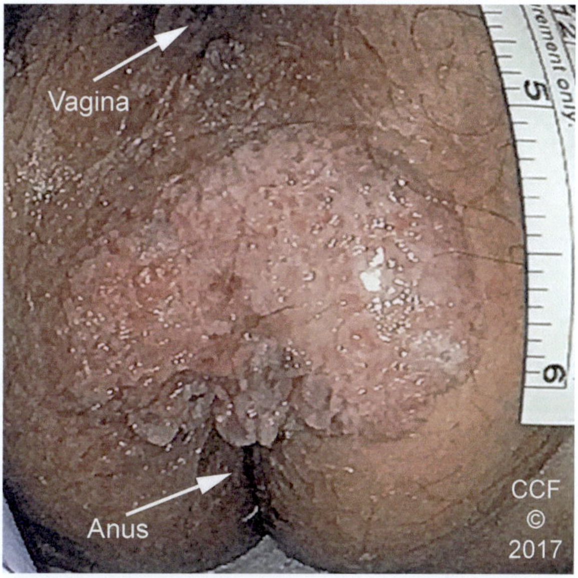

Fig. 23.7 Perineal high-grade squamous intraepithelial lesion (HSIL)

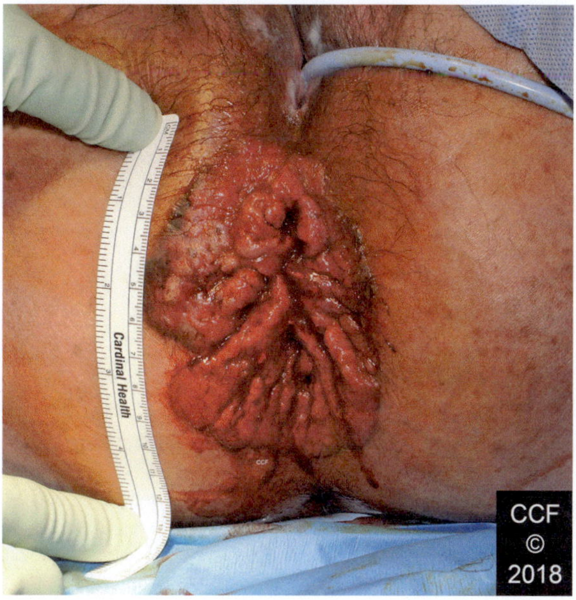

Fig. 23.8 Circumferential involvement of the perianal skin by HSIL. The lesion extended into the anal canal

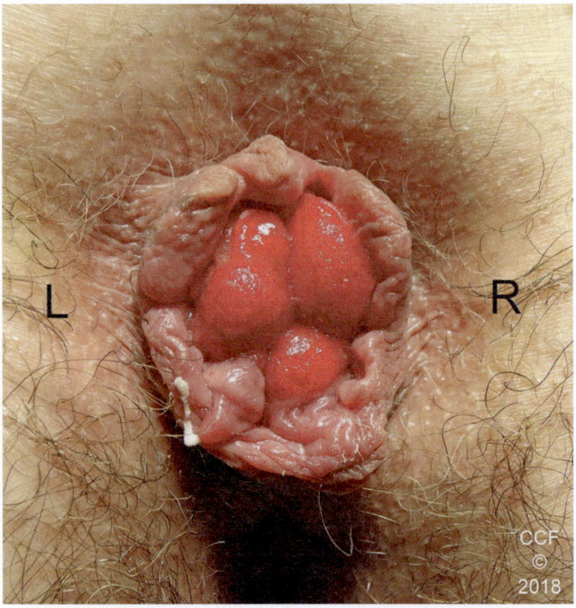

Fig. 23.9 Three prolapsed hemorrhoids, right posterior, right anterior and left lateral

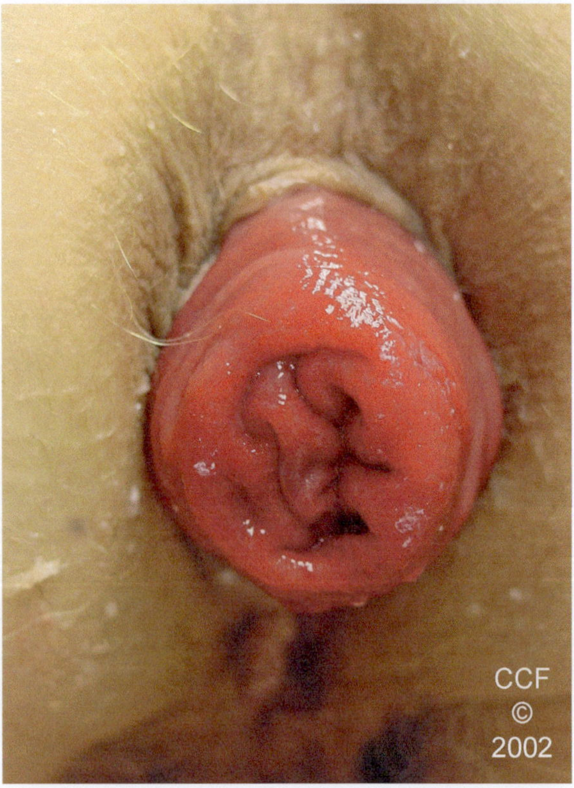

Fig. 23.10 Rectal prolapse (true procidentia). The entire distal rectum has everted

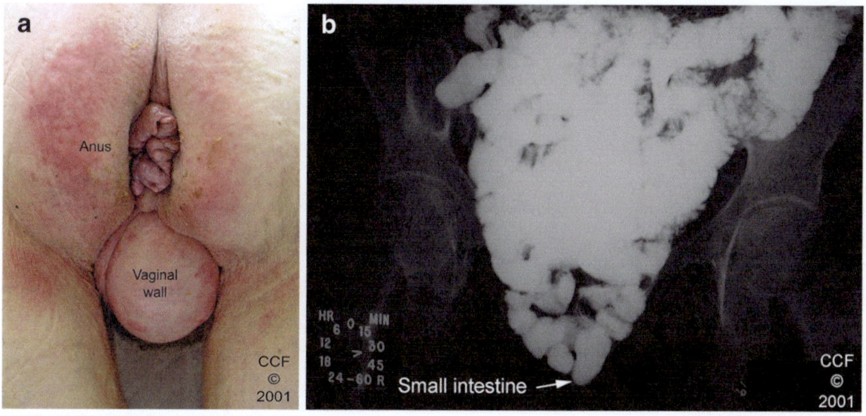

Fig. 23.11 (**a**) The anus shows prominent external hemorrhoids. Anteriorly, prolapse of the vaginal wall is seen. (**b**) Small bowel contrast study for the patient in (**a**) shows an enterocele

Figure 23.12 shows prolapse of the cervix and vagina. The anus is seen on the left side of the image.

Figure 23.13 shows an acute tear in the anoderm (anal fissure).

Retroflexed views of the anorectum with white light (Fig. 23.14a) and narrow band imaging (Fig. 23.14b) show a raised left-sided lesion. Biopsy showed HSIL.

Retroflexed view of the anorectum (Fig. 23.15a) shows an ulcer. Biopsy (Fig. 23.15b) showed squamous cell carcinoma.

Figure 23.16 shows rectal varices in a patient who has end-stage liver disease with portal hypertension.

Figure 23.17 shows proctosigmoiditis.

Seen in Fig. 23.18a is a near-obstructing rectal cancer. A colonic stent was placed to avoid emergency colostomy (Fig. 23.18b).

Figure 23.19 shows diverticulosis.

Figure 23.20 shows purulent discharge from a diverticulum thought to be the source of the patient's diverticulitis.

Figure 23.21 shows a uretero-colonic anastomosis.

Figure 23.22a shows a smooth yellow tumor; indentation of the tumor (Fig. 23.22b) was interpreted as a "pillow sign." Biopsy showed benign lipoma.

Figure 23.23 shows a colonic adenoma that was removed by snare polypectomy.

Figure 23.24a shows melanosis coli involving a colonic diverticulum. Figure 23.24b shows an adenomatous polyp surrounded by melanotic mucosa. Figure 23.24c shows a right colectomy specimen with predominantly melanotic mucosa. The adenomatous polyp and the terminal ileum do not pick up the pigment. Histology shows pigment in the lamina propria (Fig. 23.24d).

Colonoscopy (Fig. 23.25) showed yellow plaques (pseudomembranes) associated with *Clostridioides difficile* infection.

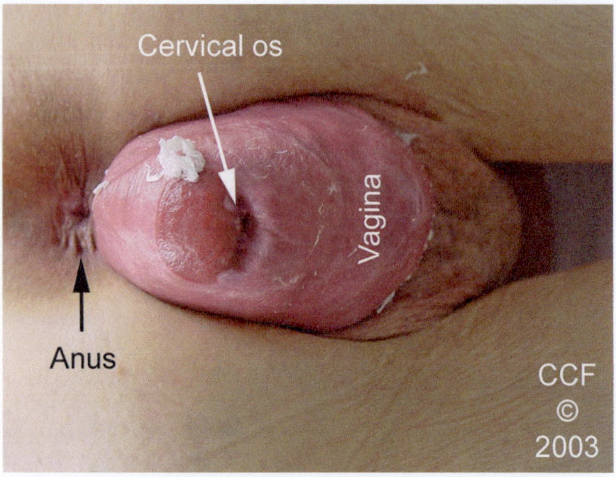

Fig. 23.12 Prolapse of the cervix and the vagina. Note the anus posterior to the prolapsus

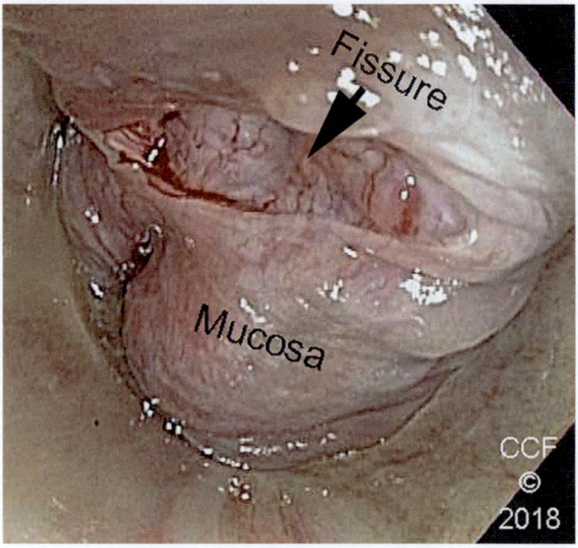

Fig. 23.13 A split in the mucosal surface of the anoderm (stratified squamous) resulted in an acute anal fissure (arrow)

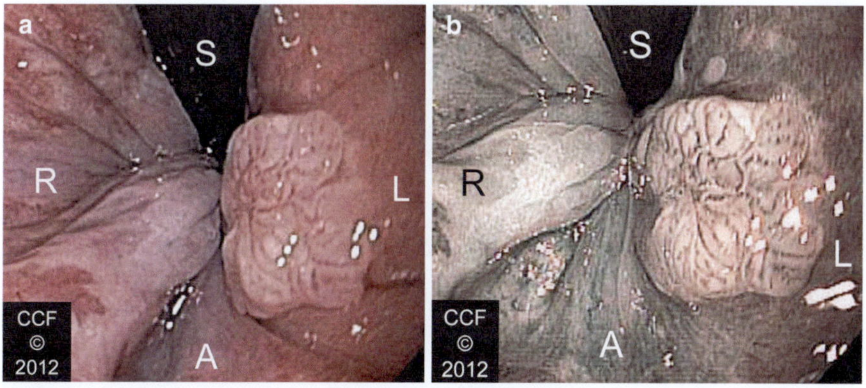

Fig. 23.14 (**a**) A high-grade anal squamous intraepithelial lesion (HSIL) seen at colonoscopy on the left with retroflexion and white light; (**b**) the same lesion seen with narrow band imaging (NBI); S = scope, R = right, A = anterior, L = left [3]. The blood vessels appear red with white light and black with NBI

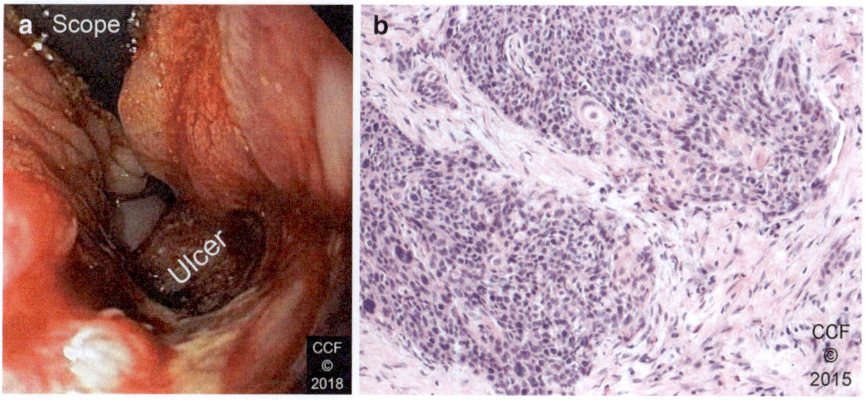

Fig. 23.15 (**a**) A retroflexed view of the anorectum showed an ulcer; (**b**) Biopsies were taken from the edge of the ulcer seen in **a**. Histopathology showed squamous cell carcinoma (Courtesy of John R. Goldblum, MD)

Figure 23.26 shows mucosal implants at the mucocutaneous border of this patient's colostomy.

Retroflexion in a continent ileostomy shows the "nipple valve" (Fig. 23.27).

Figures 23.28a and b show the endoscopic appearance of an end-to-side ileocolic anastomosis.

Figure 23.29 shows the endoscopic view of a colonic J-pouch.

Figure 23.30 shows the endoscopic appearance of an ileal J-pouch.

Figure 23.31 shows terminal ileitis.

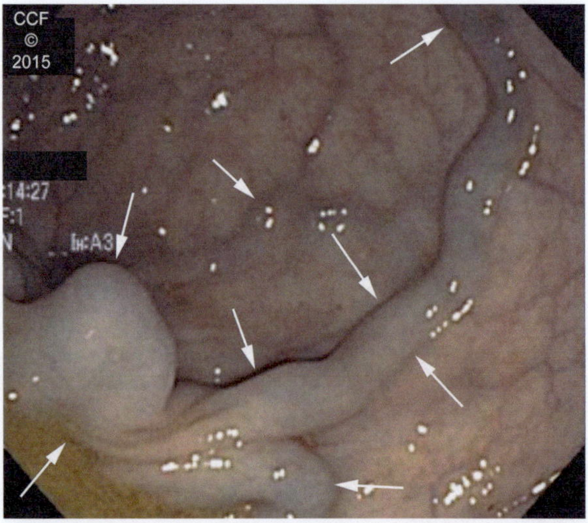

Fig. 23.16 Rectal varices seen at preorthotopic liver transplant colonoscopy in a patient with cirrhosis and portal hypertension. The varices (arrows) are distended and under pressure

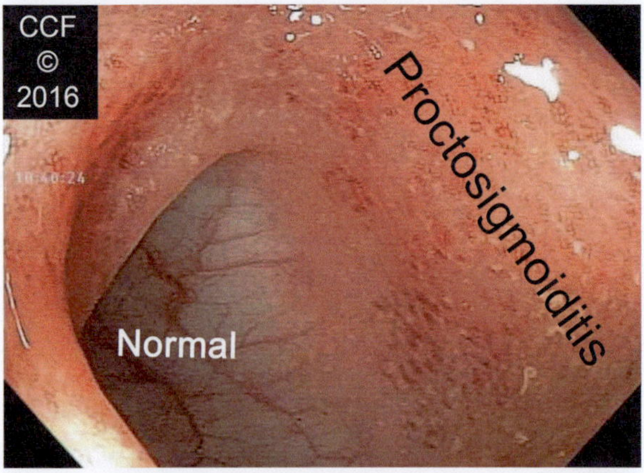

Fig. 23.17 Proctosigmoiditis. Note the sharp division between inflamed (distal) and normal (proximal) mucosa

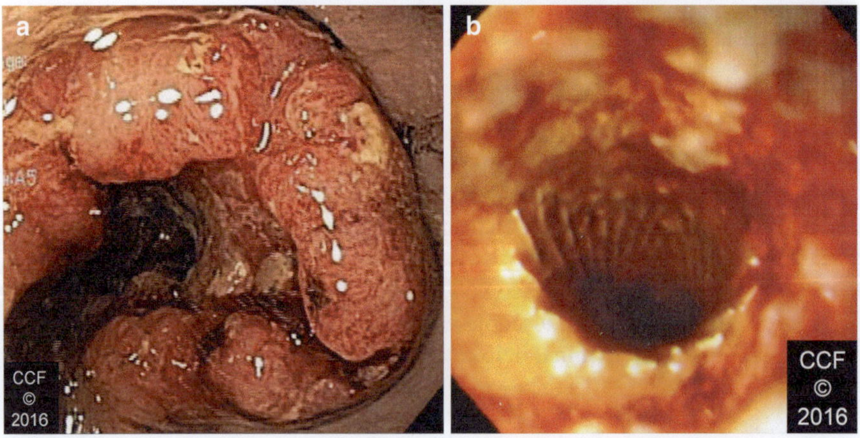

Fig. 23.18 (**a**) Near obstructing rectal cancer. (**b**) The rectal cancer seen in (**a**) after stent placement (Photo, courtesy of John A. Dumot, DO)

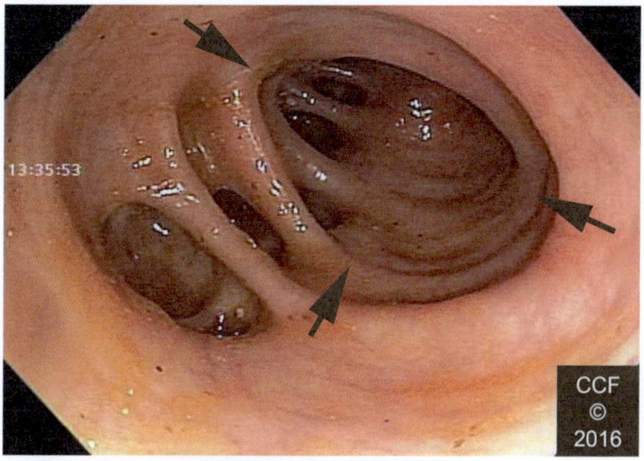

Fig. 23.19 Sigmoid colon diverticulosis. Note the triangular shape of the colonic lumen. The taenia coli are located at the corners of the triangle (arrows). The diverticula appear in between the taenia

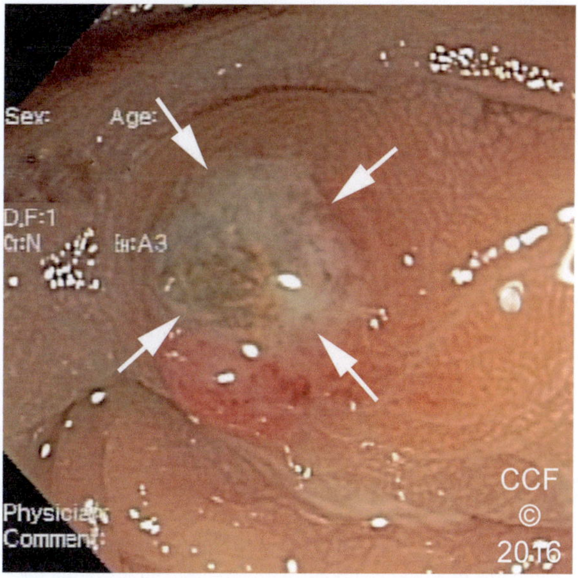

Fig. 23.20 Pus (arrows) is seen emanating from a diverticulum in a patient with acute diverticulitis (Photo, courtesy of Michael S. Cline, DO)

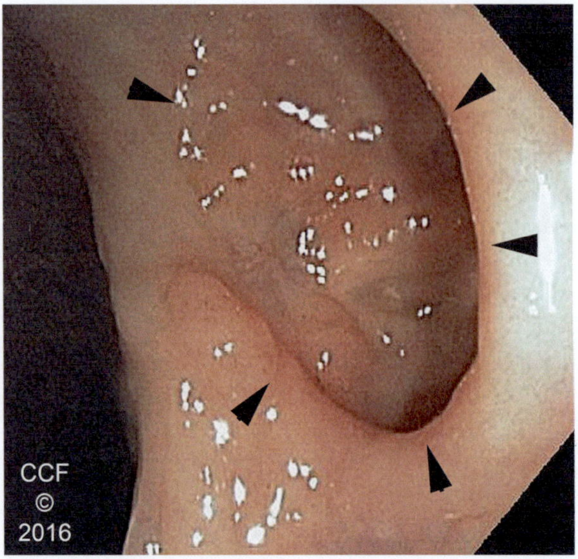

Fig. 23.21 Reconstruction by uretero-sigmoid anastomosis (arrowheads) following cystectomy

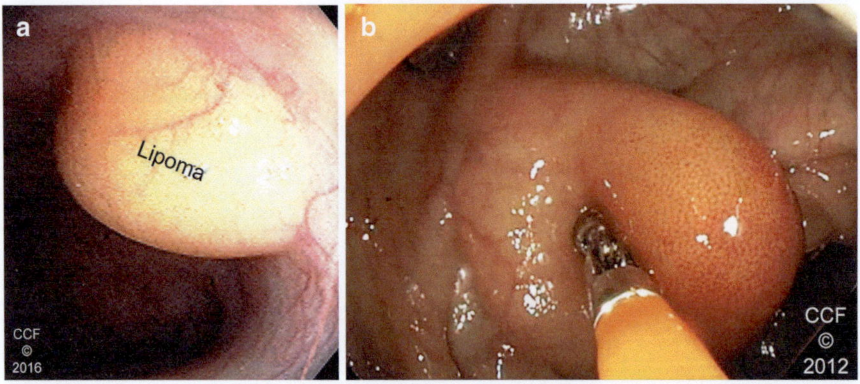

Fig. 23.22 (**a**) Colonic lipoma, a yellow, benign, fatty tumor, located in the submucosa; (**b**) Indentation of a colonic lipoma with forceps demonstrating the "pillow sign"

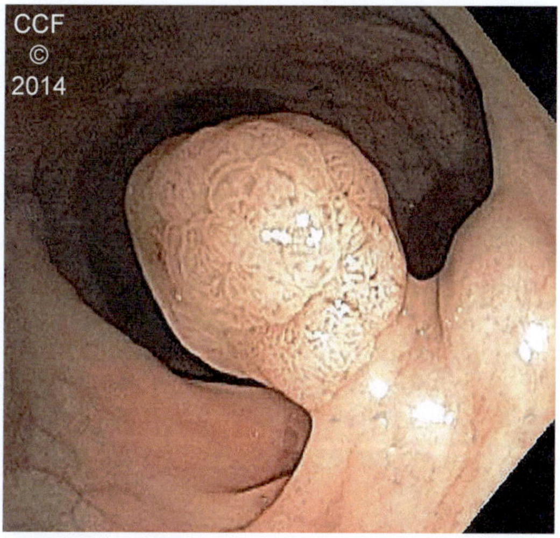

Fig. 23.23 Colon polyp. The polyp was removed endoscopically. Pathology showed that it was a tubular adenoma

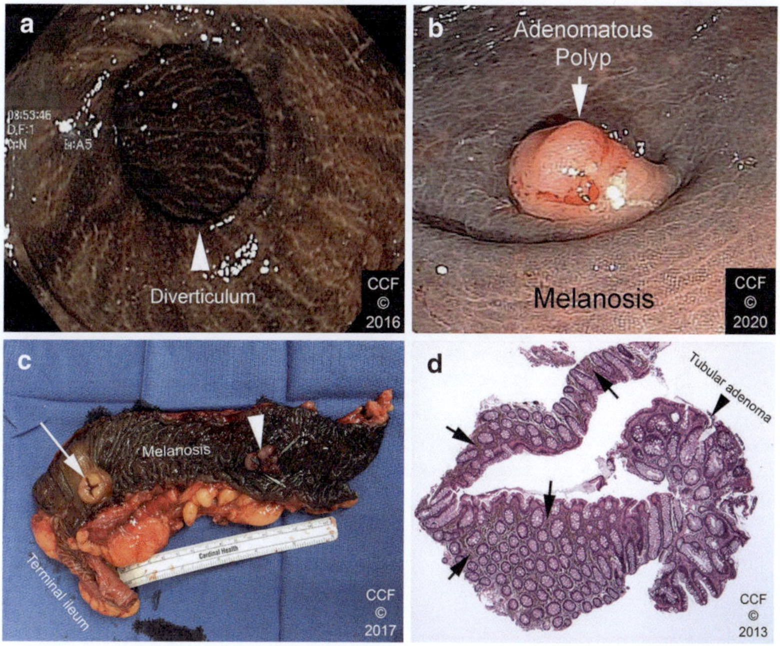

Fig. 23.24 (**a**) Melanosis coli seen in a diverticulum and surrounding colonic mucosa during colonoscopy. This change is seen after chronic anthraquinone laxative use; (**b**) A cecal adenoma (raised white lesion) is seen. Pronounced melanosis, seen in the surrounding colonic mucosa, facilitated detection of the polyp which was not pigmented; (**c**) Right colectomy specimen. An adenomatous polyp (arrowhead, clips), the ileocecal valve (arrow), and the opened terminal ileum (lower left) do not show melanosis. In the surrounding colonic mucosa, melanosis is prominent; (**d**) Low power view of a polypectomy specimen shows areas of adenomatous change (right, arrowhead) characterized by a hyperchromatic surface appearance. The associated colonic mucosa is remarkable for readily conspicuous pigment (melanosis) within the lamina propria (arrows) [H–E, original magnification ×40] (Courtesy of Homer O. Wiland, MD)

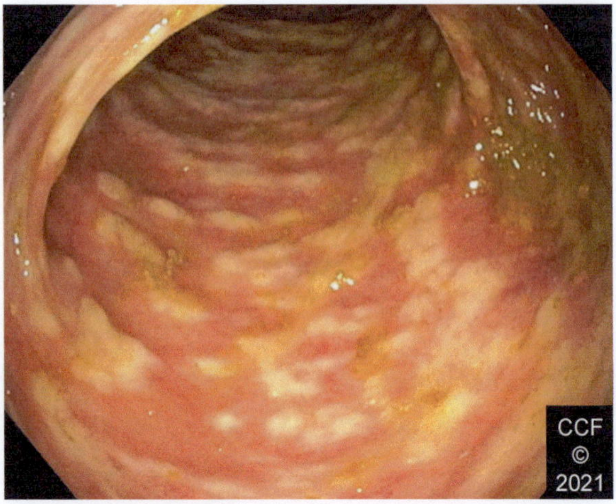

Fig. 23.25 A patient who had received antibiotics to treat urinary tract infections presented with diarrhea. Colonoscopy showed diffuse yellow plaques (pseudomembranes). A test for *C. difficile* was positive

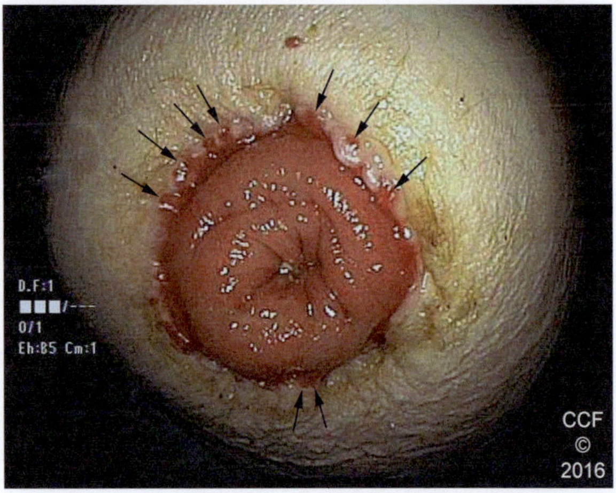

Fig. 23.26 End colostomy. Circumferential mucocutaneous implants are seen (arrows). This phenomenon is associated with stoma maturation by sutures that have traveled through the full thickness of the intestine and the full-thickness of the skin

Fig. 23.27 Continent ileostomy (Kock pouch). An ileoscope has been introduced into the pouch. Upon retroflexion, the nipple valve and the ileoscope are seen

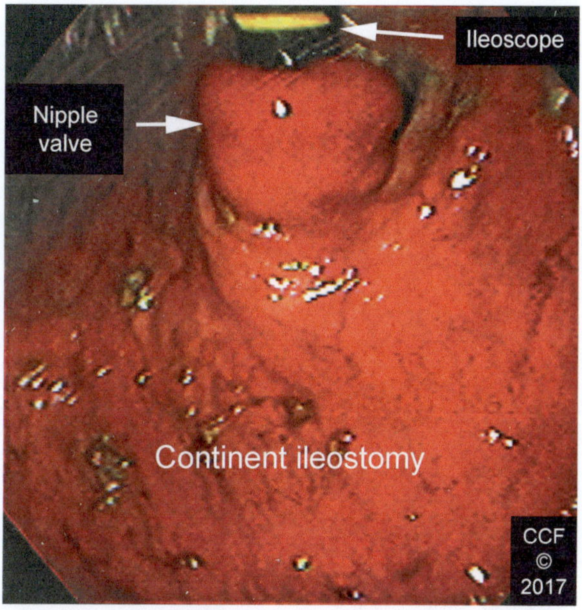

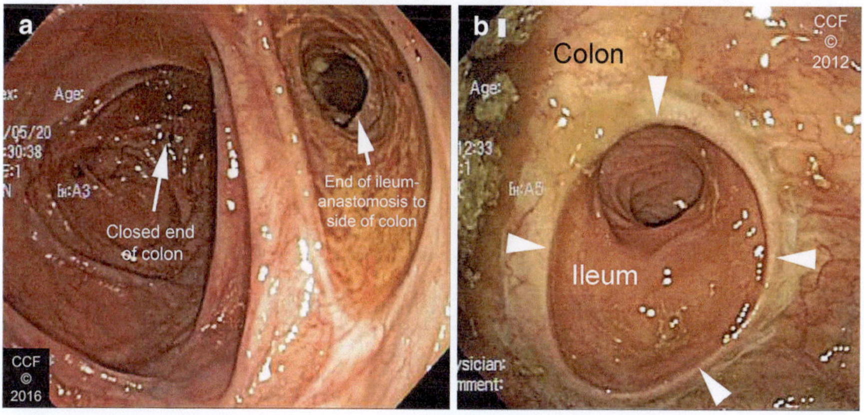

Fig. 23.28 Ileocolic anastomosis, end-to-side: (**a**) The end of the ileum was anastomosed to the side of the colon using a circular stapling device; (**b**) The circular character of this anastomotic scar (arrowheads) show that this structure is man-made

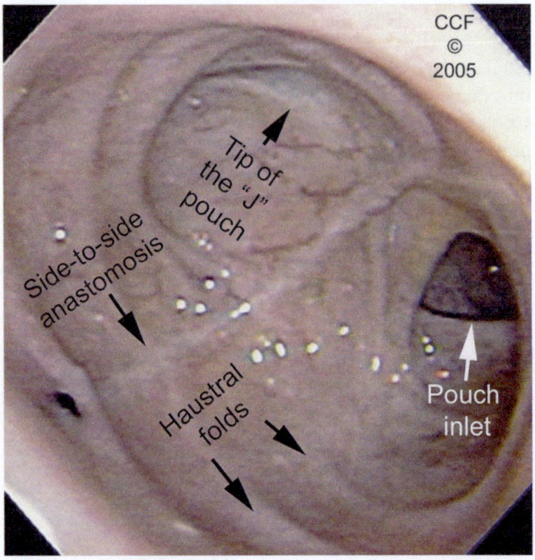

Fig. 23.29 Colonic J-pouch reconstruction after rectal cancer surgery. The tip of the J-pouch is closed. The pouch inlet is widely patent. The side-to-side anastomosis and the colonic haustral folds are identified with arrows

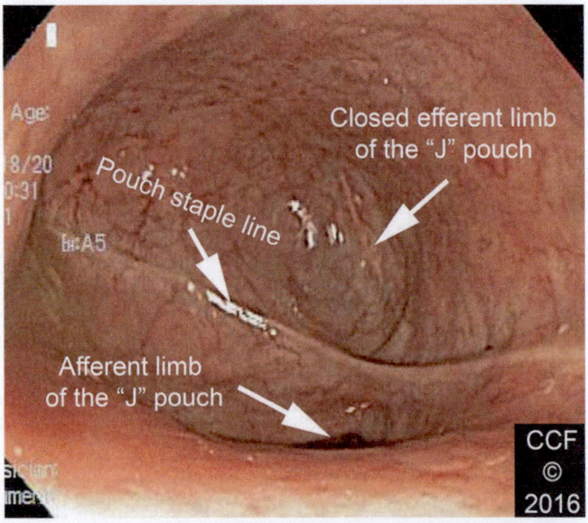

Fig. 23.30 Ileal J-pouch for restorative proctocolectomy. The pouch staple line, entry into the afferent limb and the closed efferent limb are labeled. The pouch mucosa looks mildly inflamed

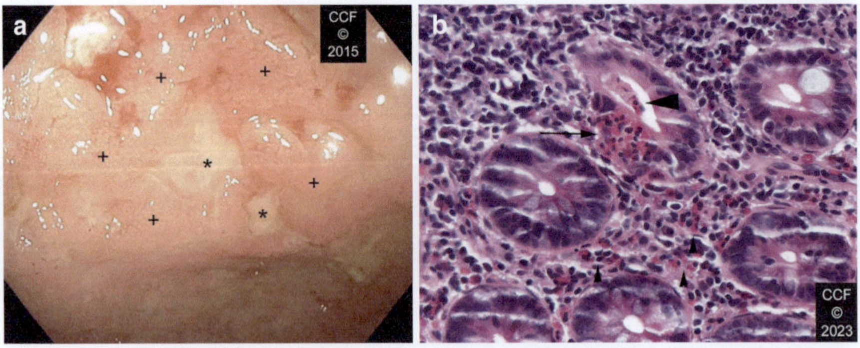

Fig. 23.31 Terminal ileitis. Intubation of the terminal shows inflamed mucosa (+) and ulcers (asterisks) (**a**). Biopsies showed ileal eosinophilia, 40x arrows, (**b**) (Courtesy Ilyssa O. Gordon, MD, PhD)

Uncommon Colonoscopy Observations

Colonic Lymphangioma

The colonic polyp shown in Fig. 23.32a was removed endoscopically. Pathology showed lymphangioma (Fig. 23.32b and c).

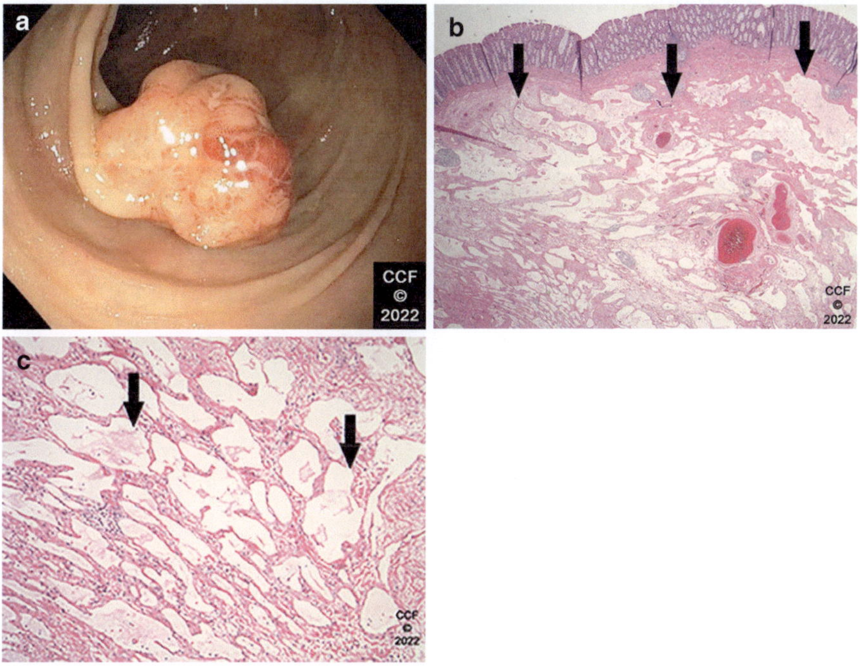

Fig. 23.32 (**a**) Semipedunculated colon polyp removed endoscopically; (**b**) H & E-stained tissue sections show a well-circumscribed submucosal proliferation of anastomosing thin-walled lymphatic spaces that contain serous fluid (low power view) [arrows]; (**c**) Dilated lymphatic channels are lined by uniform cuboidal to flattened endothelial cells that lack any degree of cytologic atypic (high power view) [arrows]. The pathologic diagnosis was lymphangioma (Courtesy of Clifton G. Fulmer, MD)

Comment

Rectal lymphangioma was described by Chisholm and Hillkowitz in 1932 [4]. Colonic lymphangioma, previously thought to be rare, has been found with increased frequency because of endoscopy [5, 6].

Colonic Pyogenic Granuloma

The colonic polyp seen in Fig. 23.33a was removed endoscopically. Pathology showed pyogenic granuloma (Fig. 23.33b).

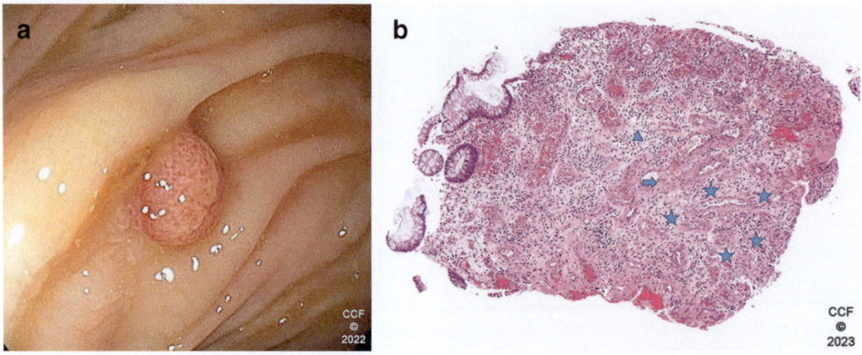

Fig. 23.33 A gay male with a history of anemia underwent colonoscopy (**a**) A 2-mm sessile polyp in the sigmoid colon was removed with forceps; (**b**) Pathology returned the diagnosis of pyogenic granuloma. This image shows a lobular arrangement of capillaries (stars) in an edematous and inflamed stroma (arrowhead). Notice the larger feeder vessel (arrow) in the center of the lesion (Courtesy of Mohamed I. El Hag, MD)

Comment

Pyogenic granuloma (PG), also known as lobular capillary hemangioma, is a benign vascular tumor. As of 2012, Val-Bernal et al. [7] found only eight reported cases of pyogenic granuloma of the large bowel in adults. Endoscopically, lesions are bright red, may bleed profusely when traumatized, and may be a cause of anemia [8]. PG may be misdiagnosed as malignancy, including Kaposi's sarcoma [9]. In this case, immunohistochemistry with antibodies against human herpesvirus-8 was negative.

Colonic Ganglioneuroma

Figure 23.34a shows a small colonic polyp that was removed. Pathology (Fig. 23.34b, c) showed colonic ganglioneuroma.

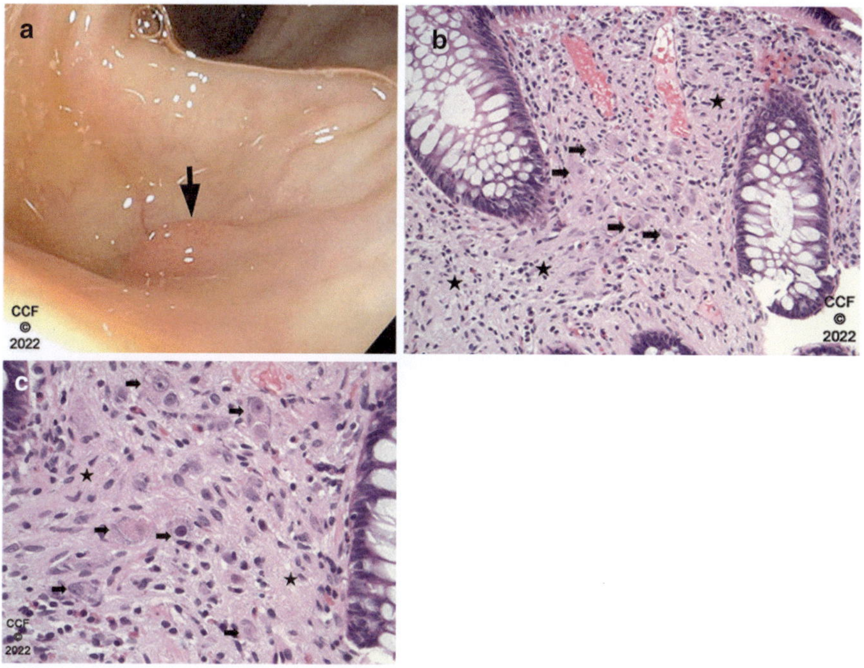

Fig. 23.34 (**a**) A sessile polyp was removed at colonoscopy (arrow); Histopathology (**b** ×200, **c** ×400) showed a spindle cell (Schwannian) stroma (marked with stars). Interspersed ganglion cells are labeled with arrows (Courtesy of James E. Lapinski, MD)

Comment

Colonic ganglioneuromas (GN) are rare neuroectodermal tumors. Histologically colonic GN are characterized by ganglion cells, nerve fibers, and cells of the enteric nervous system [10]. Single lesions are usually an isolated finding, not associated with any genetic syndrome [11]. Certain subtypes may be associated with familial adenomatous polyposis, Cowden's disease, tuberous sclerosis, juvenile polyposis, von Recklinghausen's disease, and multiple endocrine neoplasia type IIb [12–14].

Two More…

Figure 23.35 shows a large pill and undissolved time release medication spheres. Figure 23.36 shows what appears to be an ingested mosquito.

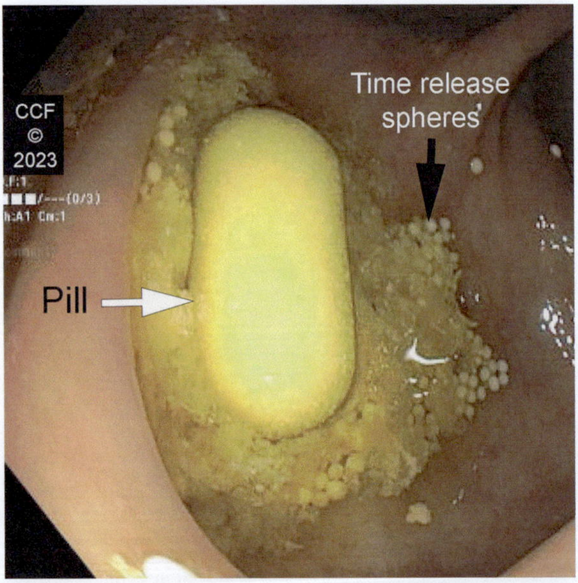

Fig. 23.35 Large pill (white arrow) and undissolved time release medication spheres (black arrow)

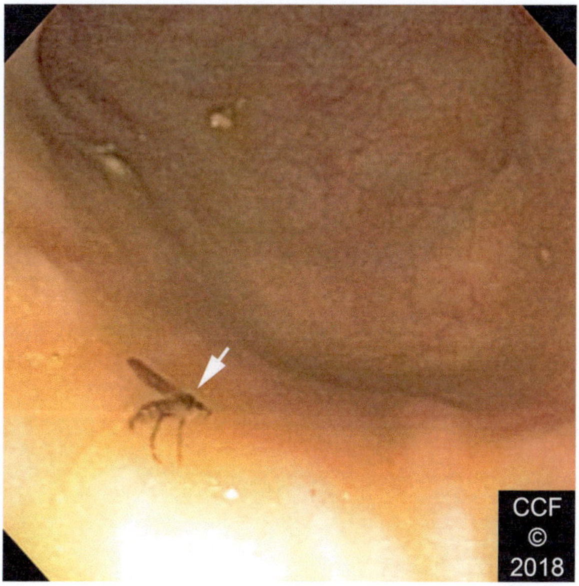

Fig. 23.36 Mosquito. There once was an old woman who… (photo, courtesy of Tracy L. Hull, MD)

References

1. Smith T III, Nambudiri VE. Erythema ab igne. Cleve Clin J Med. 2018;85:96–7.
2. Aria AB, Chen L, Silapunt S. Erythema ab igne from heating pad use: A report of three clinical cases and a differential diagnosis. Cureus. 2018;10(5):e2635. https://doi.org/10.7759/cureus.2635.
3. Inkster MD, Wiland HO, Wu JS. Detection of anal dysplasia is enhanced by narrow band imaging and acetic acid. Colorectal Dis. 2015;18:O17–21.
4. Chisholm AJ, Hillkowitz P. Lymphangioma of the rectum. Am J Surg. 1932;17:281–2.
5. Kim KM, Choi KY, Lee A, Kim BK. Lymphangioma of large intestine: report of ten cases with endoscopic and pathologic correlation. Gastrointest Endosc. 2000;52:255–9.
6. Matsuda T, Matsutani T, Tsuchiya Y, Okihama Y, Egami K, Yoshioka M, et al. A clinical evaluation of lymphangioma of the large intestine. A case presentation of lymphangioma of the descending colon and a review of 279 Japanese cases. J Nippon Med Sch. 2001;68:262–5.
7. Val-Bernal JF, Mayorga M, García-Somacarrera E. Pyogenic granuloma of the large intestine: Case report and review of reported cases in the adult. Pathol Res Pract. 2012;208:687–90.
8. Meyer-Herbon P, Brugnolaro C, Frei R, Sulz MC. Pyogenic granuloma of the descending colon: A rare cause of lower gastrointestinal bleeding. ACG Case Rep J. 2015;2:74–5.

9. Meeks MW, Kamal UM, Hammami MB, Taylor JR, Omran ML, Chen Y, et al. Gastrointestinal pyogenic granuloma (lobular capillary hemangioma): an underrecognized entity causing iron deficiency anemia. Case Rep Gastrointest Med. 2016;2016:8. Article ID 4398401.
10. Mendez IM, Pereda T, Rodriquez FJ, Funez R, Sanchez A. Solitary colonic polypoid ganglioneuroma. Diagnostic Pathol. 2008;3:20.
11. Nehme C, Ghazaleh S, Patel D, Hasan S, Nawras A. Incidental ascending colon ganglioneuroma in the setting of hematochezia. Cureus. 2020;12:e9447.
12. Abraham G, Prakash SR. Solitary colonic ganglioneuroma: A rare incidental finding of hematochezia. Case Rep Gastrointest Med 2015, Article ID 794985.
13. Baiomi A, Abbas H, Niazi M, Remotti H, Daniel M, Balar B. Colonic ganglioneuroma: A rare lesion with extremely different presentations and outcomes in two patients. Gastroenterol Res. 2021;14:194–8.
14. Ofori E, Ona M, Ramai D, Huang T, Xiao P, Reddy M. Colonic ganglioneuroma: A rare finding during colorectal cancer screening. Case Rep Gastroenterol. 2017;11:434–9.

Position for Prone Cases; Operative Field Preparation and Draping

24

Lena J. Slater-Everhart, Theodore E. Partridge, and James S. Wu

Presentation

A Wilson spinal frame™ is useful for performing anorectal operations (Figs. 24.1 and 24.2) [1]. The frame maintains patients in a stable, adjustable, flexed position with excellent access to the anus and distal rectum. The prone position provides the surgeon the benefit of a surgical assistant located directly across the table. The genitalia are free from pressure.

After the patient is positioned, the buttocks are separated with tape to expose the anal orifice (Fig. 24.3).

L. J. Slater-Everhart · T. E. Partridge
Department of Surgical Services, South Pointe Hospital, Warrensville Heights, OH, USA

J. S. Wu (✉)
Department of Colon and Rectal Surgery, Cleveland Clinic, Cleveland, OH, USA

J. S. Wu, M. D. Inkster (eds.), *Cleveland Clinic Colorectal Case Studies*,
https://doi.org/10.1007/978-3-031-39880-3_24

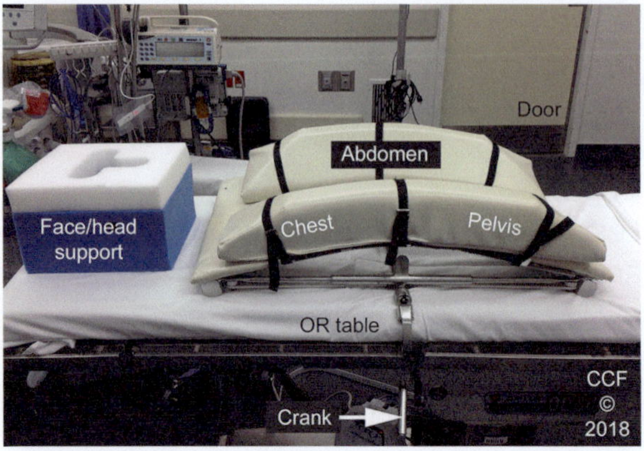

Fig. 24.1 Wilson spinal frame™. The face rest is located on the left of the photograph. The crank (arrow) allows for adjustment of lordosis. The space in between the two lateral ridges supports the chest, abdomen, and pelvis

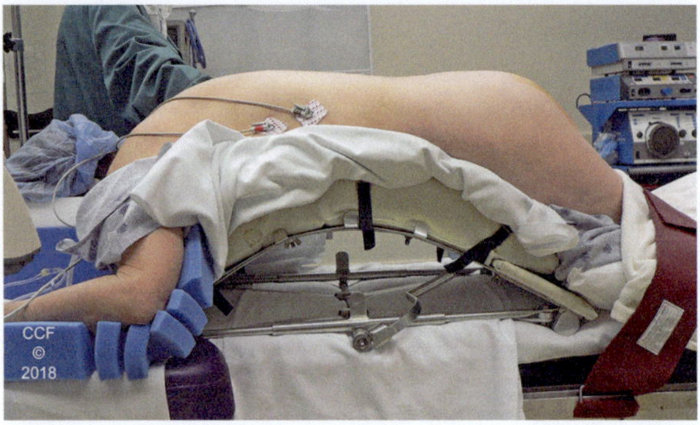

Fig. 24.2 Wilson spinal frame™: A patient is positioned on the table in the prone position in preparation for anorectal surgery

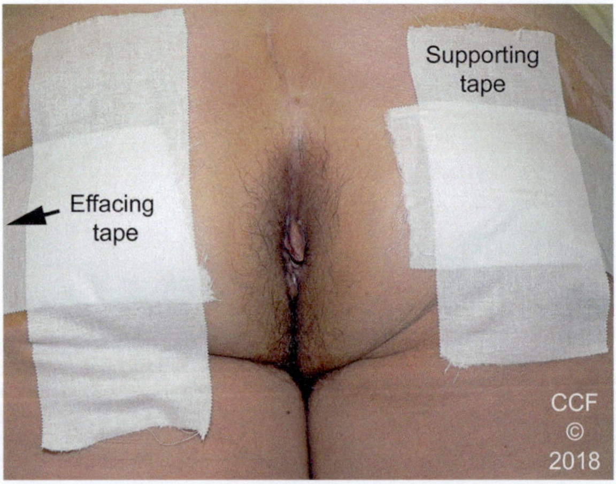

Fig. 24.3 The buttocks are separated with wide tape. The effacing tape is secured to the operating table. The effacing tape has been reinforced with two additional pieces placed orthogonally

Operative Field Preparation and Draping

The operative field is prepared, in this example, with Povidone-iodine solution (Fig. 24.4).

The surgical site is draped with sterile towels as demonstrated in (Figs. 24.5, 24.6, 24.7, 24.8, and 24.9).

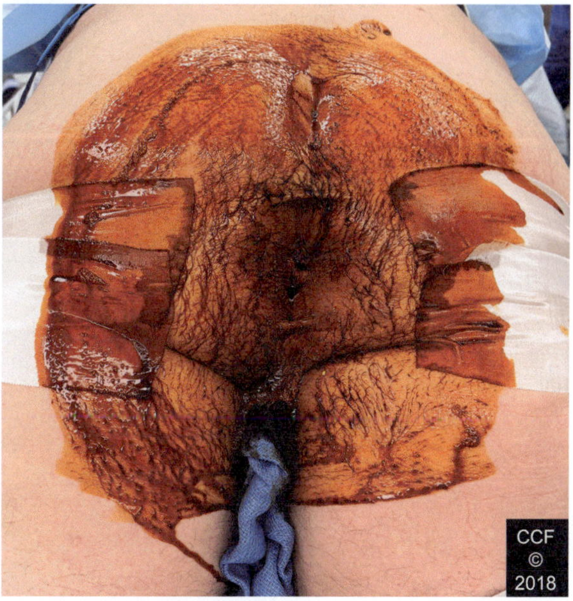

Fig. 24.4 The anus and perianal skin are prepared with Povidone-iodine solution. A sterile towel is placed between the legs

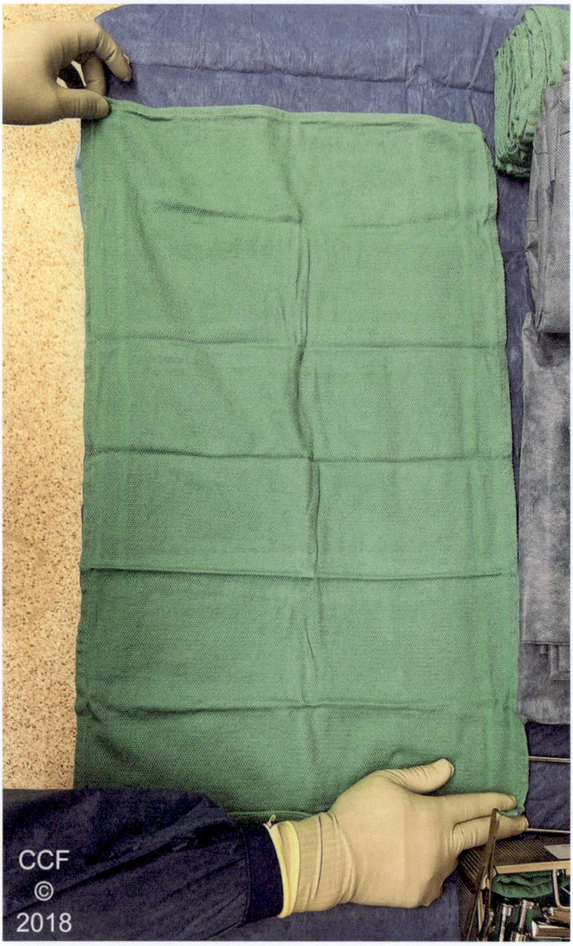

Fig. 24.5 Draping towels are grasped at opposite corners

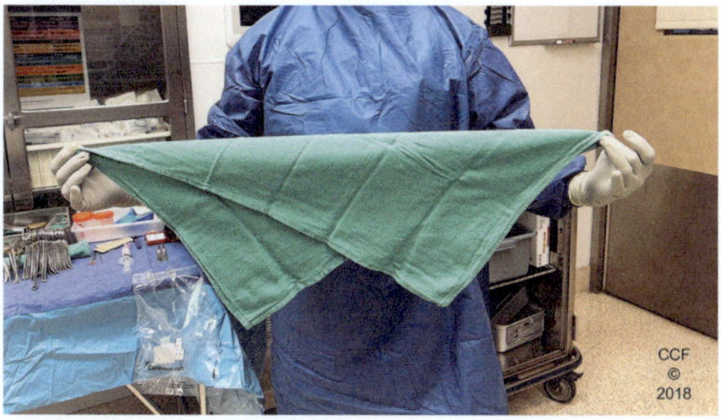

Fig. 24.6 Each towel is folded as shown

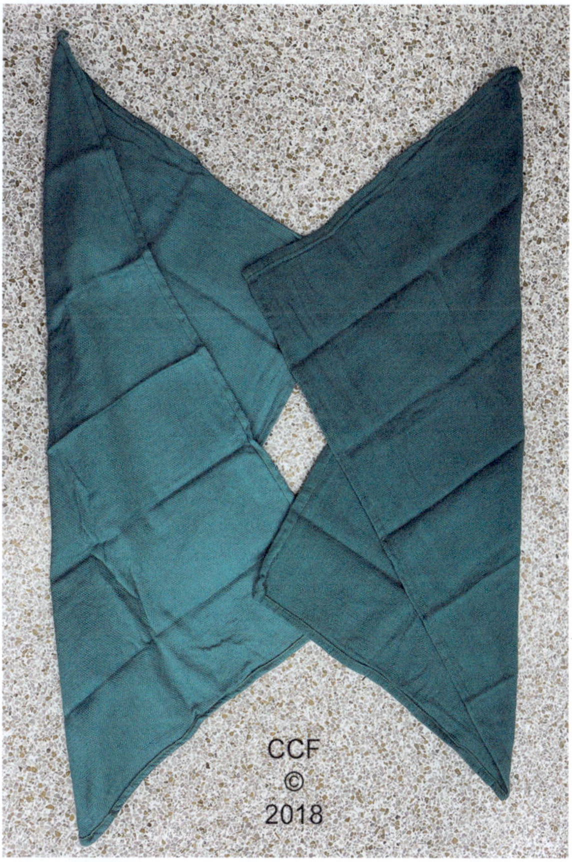

Fig. 24.7 Two towels are positioned with a central opening for the operative field

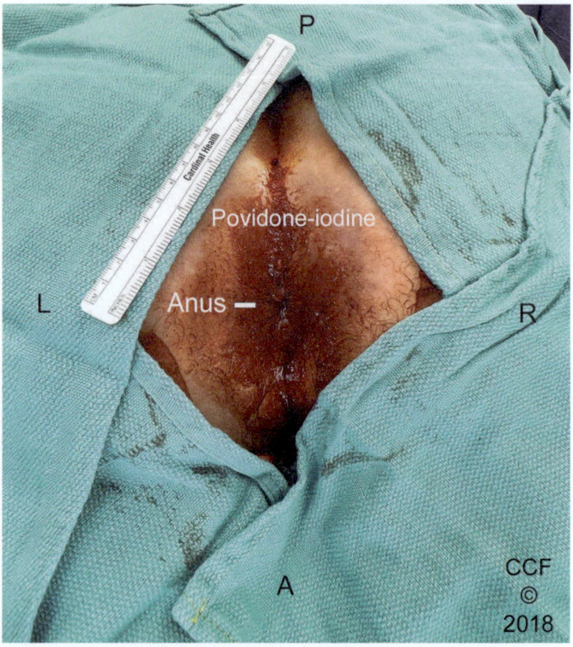

Fig. 24.8 Two folded towels are positioned around the operative field. R = right, L = left, A = anterior, P = posterior

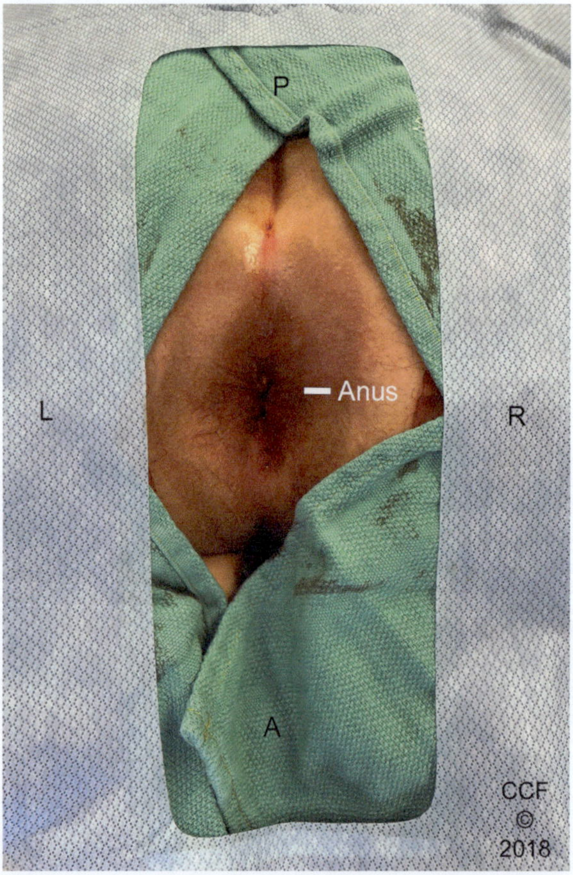

Fig. 24.9 Surgical drapes area placed over the towels. R = right, L = left, A = anterior, P = posterior

Reference

1. Anderton JM. The prone position for the surgical patient: A historical review of the principles and hazards. Br J Anaesth. 1991;67:452–63.

25 Gluteal Cleft Abscess

James S. Wu

Presentation

A patient presented with fever and pain localized to the gluteal cleft.

The gluteal cleft skin was red, painful, firm, and swollen (Fig. 25.1).

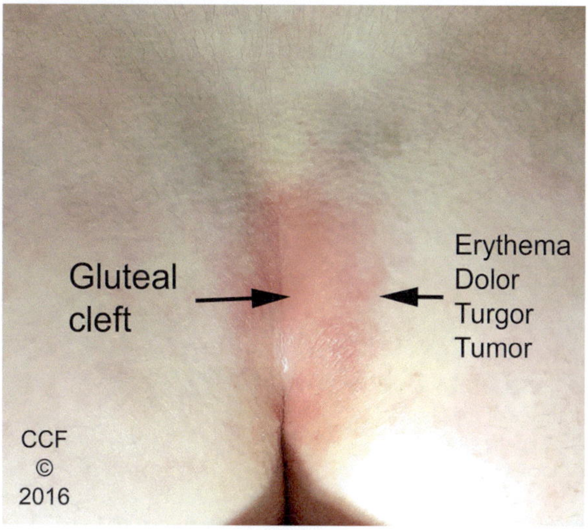

Fig. 25.1 A pointing abscess in the gluteal cleft

J. S. Wu (✉)
Department of Colon and Rectal Surgery, Cleveland Clinic, Cleveland, OH, USA

J. S. Wu, M. D. Inkster (eds.), *Cleveland Clinic Colorectal Case Studies*,
https://doi.org/10.1007/978-3-031-39880-3_25

Management

The patient underwent immediate incision and drainage of the gluteal cleft abscess (Figs. 25.2 and 25.3).

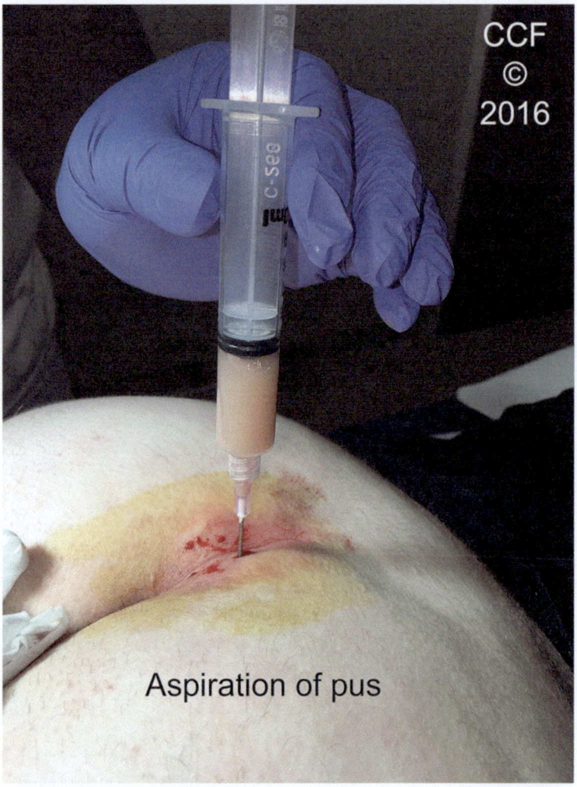

Fig. 25.2 After sterile preparation with an iodinated skin solution and administration of local anesthesia, the abscess was located by aspiration with an 18 Gauge needle

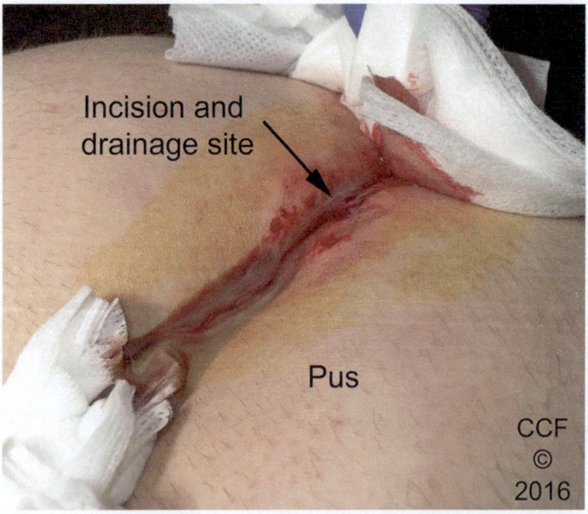

Fig. 25.3 Incision and drainage of the abscess allowed the egress of a large amount of pus

Comment

Classic signs of inflammation are calor (warmth), dolor (pain), tumor (swelling), and rubor (redness). In his text, *De Medicina*, Celsus described the association of three of these features with suppuration.

De Medicina [1]	**MEDICINE** [2]
Quibus sine febre aliqua [ex] parte dolor aut prurigo cum rubore et calore est, ibi aliquid suppurat. Aulus Cornelius Celsus (c. 25 BC–c. 50 AD)	To whom there is pain in some part without fever, or itching, with redness and with heat, there some (thing) suppurates. Aurelius Cornelius Celsus (c. 25 BC–c. 50 AD)

Gluteal cleft abscesses are associated with ingrown subcutaneous hairs.[1] Incision facilitates abscess drainage. Hair, if not removed, can lead to chronic draining sinuses.

References

1. Aulus Cornelius Celsus. De Medicina. PHI Latin Texts; https://latin.packhum.org; 2.7.22.3-5. Accessed 15 Oct 2019.
2. Celsus AC, Underwood JW. The eight books of medicine of Aurelius Cornelius Celsus, with a literal and interlineal translation on the principles of the Hamiltonian System, Vol 1. London, printed for the author, 1830, p. 110. Accessed from Archiv.org. 7 Feb 2023.

[1] See cases of pilonidal disease in this work.

26 Pilonidal Sinus-Unroofing

James S. Wu

Presentation

A young male complained of drainage from the region of the gluteal cleft (Fig. 26.1).

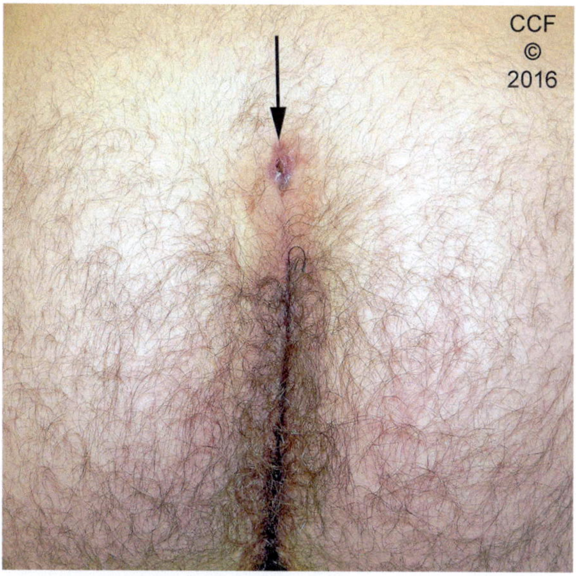

Fig. 26.1 Draining sinus (arrow) in the gluteal cleft in a hirsute young male

J. S. Wu (✉)
Department of Colon and Rectal Surgery, Cleveland Clinic, Cleveland, OH, USA

J. S. Wu, M. D. Inkster (eds.), *Cleveland Clinic Colorectal Case Studies*,
https://doi.org/10.1007/978-3-031-39880-3_26

Management

At surgery, hair in the area of the gluteal cleft was removed with clippers (Fig. 26.2). The exposed gluteal cleft revealed multiple sinus openings (Fig. 26.3). Hair fibers were seen within these sinuses (Fig. 26.4).

A probe was passed into a sinus tract that lay beneath all of the midline pits (Fig. 26.5).

The skin overlying the pilonidal sinus was unroofed. Within the sinus were multiple hair fibers (Fig. 26.6).

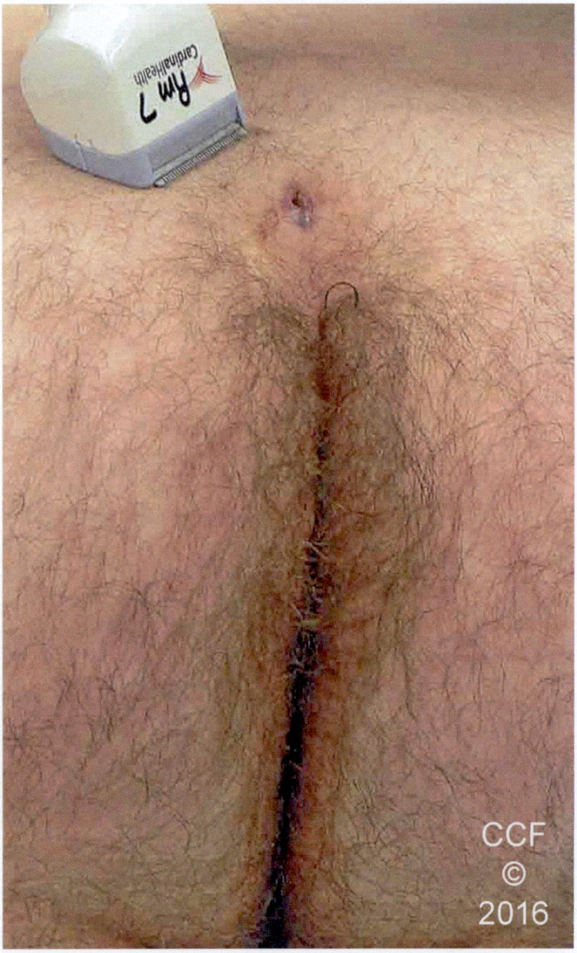

Fig. 26.2 The gluteal cleft is shaved

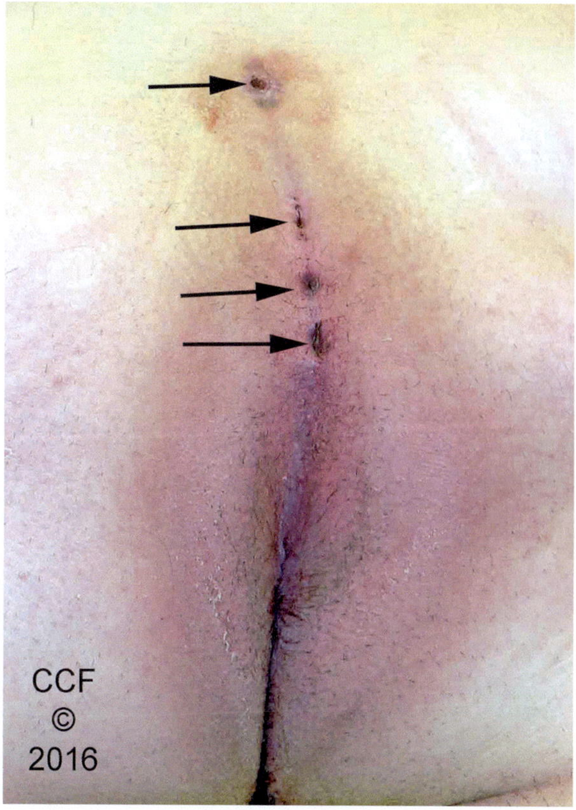

Fig. 26.3 Multiple midline pits are seen in the gluteal cleft (arrows)

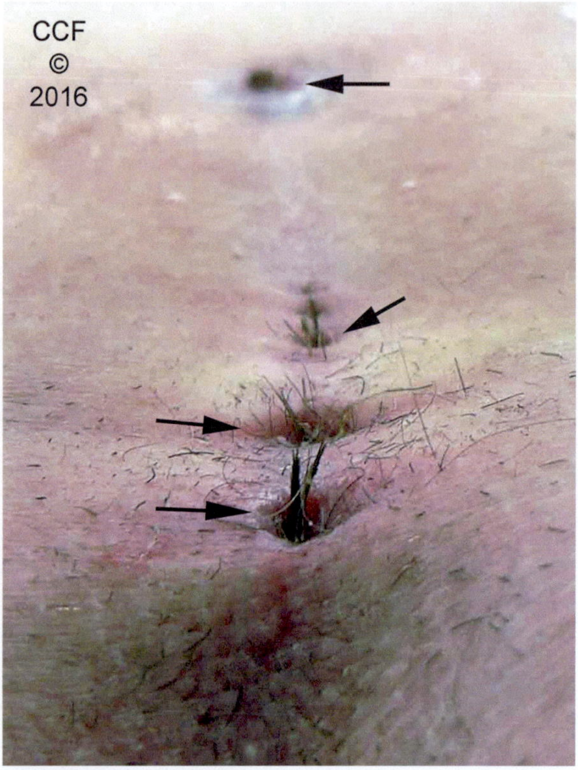

Fig. 26.4 Shows a close-up of the hair fibers within the lower three midline pits (arrows)

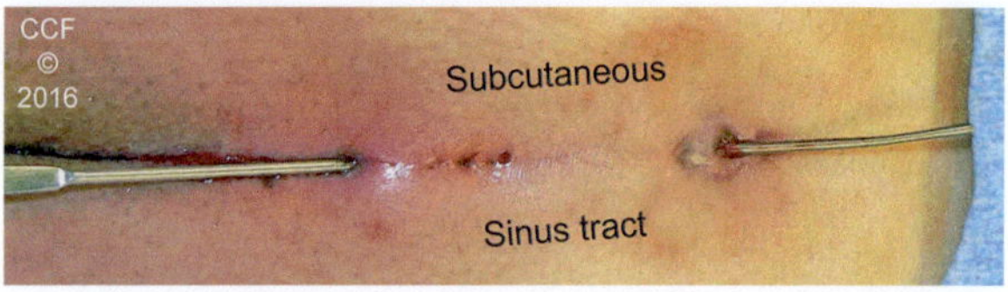

Fig. 26.5 A probe defines a subcutaneous sinus tract beneath all midline pits

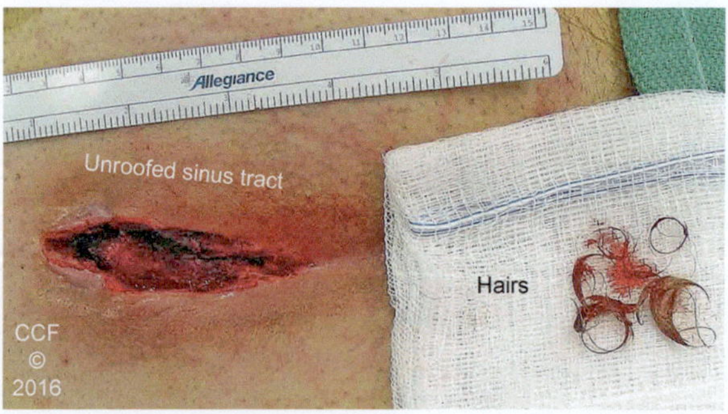

Fig. 26.6 Wound after unroofing of the sinus tract. A nest of hair was found within the sinus tract. The wound was curetted and allowed to heal by secondary intention

Comment

In 1847, Anderson described: Hair extracted from an ulcer [1].

> "Dear Sir,—I take the liberty to send you a short account of the following case, which I am vain enough to think may be interesting to you.
>
> Last year I was called upon by Capt. ———, who stated that his son had a troublesome sore on his back.
>
> About a week after this conversation he called on me with the young man…I found, upon examination, a *fistula* opening near the os coccygis,…I then made an opening into a cavity,…
>
> About three weeks after I made the opening, while at work upon it I drew out a black substance, in a loop form, as large round, when straight, as a large-sized rye straw, and very offensive. I found it was hair, very fine, closely matted, and about two inches in length. When it dried, the next day, I examined it again, and found it soft and fine, the color a dark brown. The discharge stopped, the wound healed rapidly, and he was entirely well in three weeks from the time he lost his hair."

In 1880, Hodges coined the term pilo-nidal, "pilus" meaning hair and "nidus" meaning nest [2]. Pilonidal disease occurs when hairs, trapped beneath the sacrococcygeal skin, create an abscess that may rupture leaving a chronically draining sinus. The condition is seen most commonly in young adults. Anatomic features that predispose to the development of pilonidal disease include a deep natal cleft, a hirsute body habitus, obesity, moisture, bacteria, and midline depressions or "pits" that trap hairs. In 1944, Buie [3] coined the term, "Jeep disease" to describe pilonidal disease associated with mechanized warfare and stated: "It was feared that riding on jeeps, trucks and tanks would play havoc even with the innocent sacrococcygeal dimple." Pilonidal abscesses present as a painful fluctuant swelling in the sacrococcygeal area. The abscess is drained. Hair and necrotic debris are removed, and the wound is allowed to heal by secondary intention. Care is taken to prevent the reintroduction of hair into the wound during healing. If the abscess bursts spontaneously, a draining pilonidal sinus results. Many surgical procedures have been used to treat pilonidal disease [4]. Unroofing/curettage and healing by secondary intention, as used in this case, removes the causative in-grown hair. The advantage of this approach is that it is easy to perform. The disadvantage is that prolonged convalescence may be needed for complete wound closure. Skin openings off the midline almost always connect to a midline pit (Figs. 26.7 and 26.8).

The sinus tract was unroofed, and the hair within the sinus tract was removed. Healing occurred by secondary intention.

Figures 26.9 and 26.10 show a two limbed pilonidal sinus before unroofing and after healing by secondary attention.

Unfortunately, impaired wound healing and recurrence impairs the success of all operations for pilonidal disease (Fig. 26.11). The hope of success is weighed against the possibility of failure in offering a particular operation. More complex operations may be associated with larger complications. Persistent or recurrent pilonidal disease impairs quality of life and carries long-term risks for osteomyelitis and squamous cell carcinoma [5].

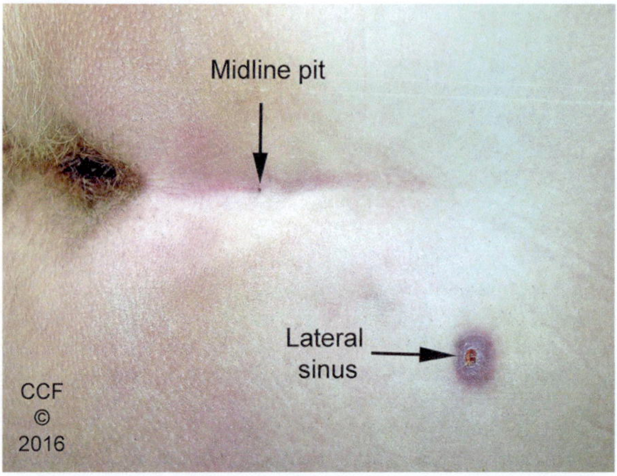

Fig. 26.7 A draining buttock sinus is seen (arrow). In the midline, there is a minute midline pit (arrow)

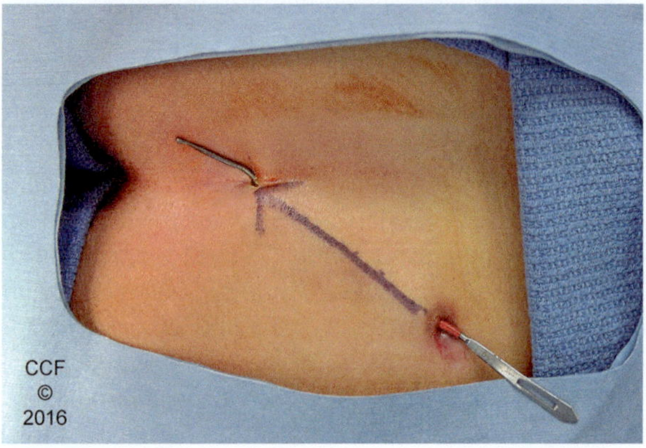

Fig. 26.8 A probe passes from the buttock draining sinus directly to the midline pit

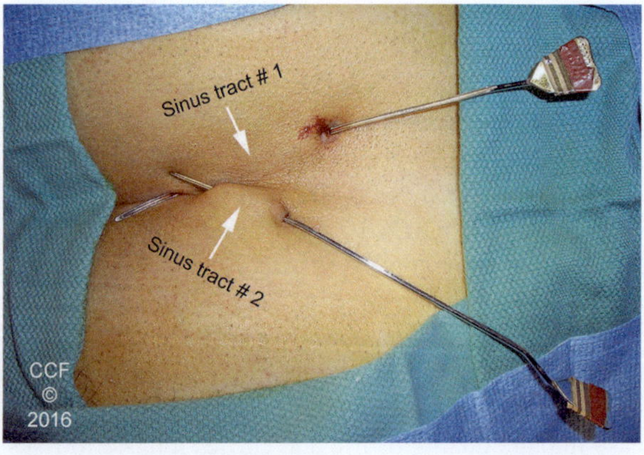

Fig. 26.9 Two draining sinuses connect to midline gluteal cleft pits

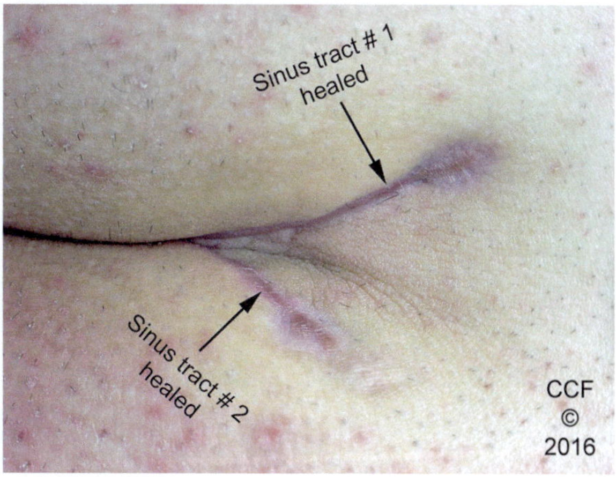

Fig. 26.10 Wound appearance after healing by secondary intention

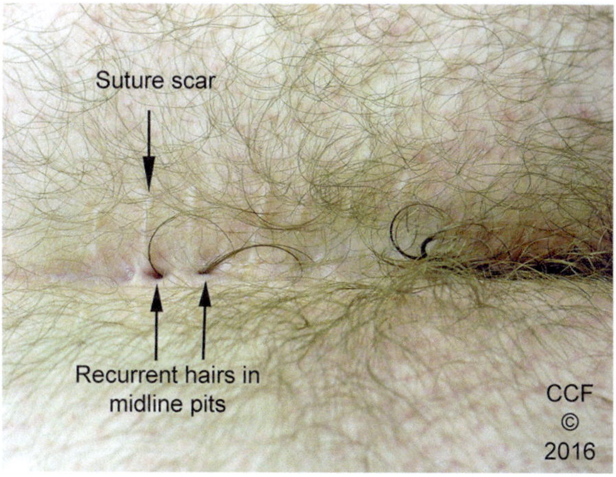

Fig. 26.11 Recurrent pilonidal sinus after excision and primary closure. Hair protruding from a midline pit and scars associated with wound closure sutures are highlighted by arrows

References

1. Anderson AW. Hair extracted from an ulcer. Boston Med Surg J. 1847;36:74.
2. Hodges RM. Pilo-nidal sinus. Boston Med Surg J. 1880;103:485–6.
3. Buie LA. Jeep disease (pilonidal disease of mechanized warfare). South Med J. 1944;37:103–9.
4. Hull TL, Wu J. Pilonidal disease. Surg Clin N Am. 2002;82:1169–85.
5. de Bree E, Zoetmulder FA, Christodoulakis M, Aleman BM, Tsiftsis DD. Treatment of malignancy arising in pilonidal disease. Ann Surg Oncol. 2001;8:60–4.

Pilonidal Disease-Limberg Flap

27

Carolyn L. Power, Emre Gorgun, and James S. Wu

Presentation

A 23-year-old male patient presented with pilonidal disease exacerbated by an acute abscess (Fig. 27.1).

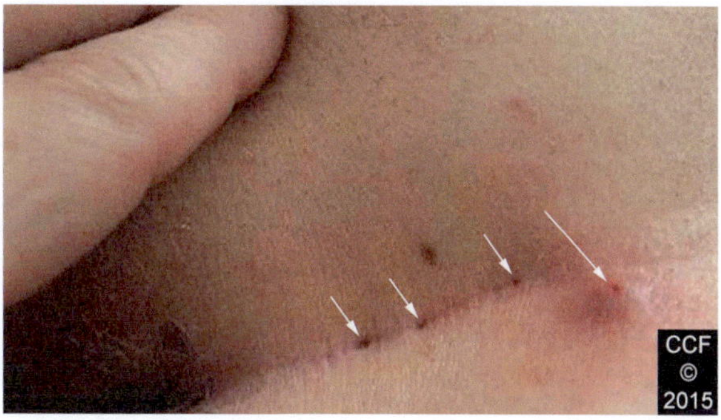

Fig. 27.1 Pilonidal disease. Three pits are located in the midline (short arrows). One (off the midline) pit is acutely infected (long arrow)

C. L. Power · E. Gorgun · J. S. Wu (✉)
Department of Colon and Rectal Surgery, Cleveland Clinic, Cleveland, OH, USA

J. S. Wu, M. D. Inkster (eds.), *Cleveland Clinic Colorectal Case Studies*,
https://doi.org/10.1007/978-3-031-39880-3_27

Management

Operative management involved excision of the pilonidal disease within a rhomboid-shaped skin island (Fig. 27.2) [1–5]. Fig. 27.3 shows injection of the pilonidal sinus with methyene blue to identify subcutaneous sinus tracts.

The operative strategy of pilonidal excision and flap reconstruction is illustrated in Fig. 27.4.

The surgical incision is marked with numbers and letters that show the beginning (top) and end-positions (bottom) of the flap.

Figure 27.5 shows the operative field following excision of the diamond-shaped skin containing the pilonidal disease.

Figure 27.6 shows the rhomboid flap that has been mobilized off of the gluteus maximus muscle.

In Fig. 27.7, the rhomboid flap is rotated to cover the site where the pilonidal disease has been excised.

Figure 27.8 shows the flap sewn into position.

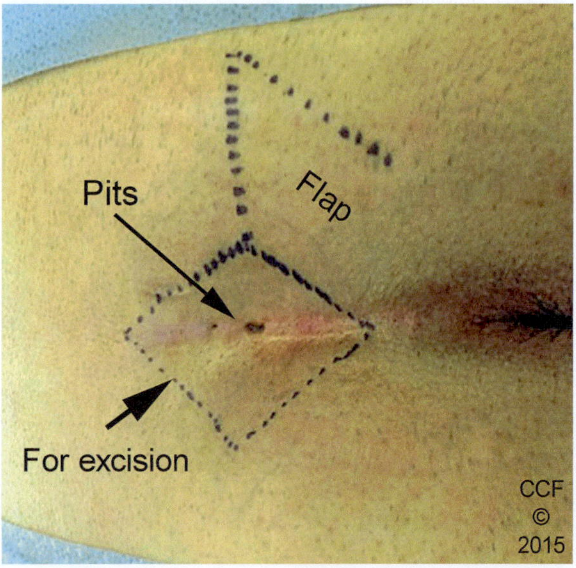

Fig. 27.2 A diamond-shaped island of skin surrounds the pilonidal disease. An adjacent rhomboid-shaped reconstruction flap is defined. Methylene blue injection defines subcutaneous pilonidal tracts (Fig. 27.3)

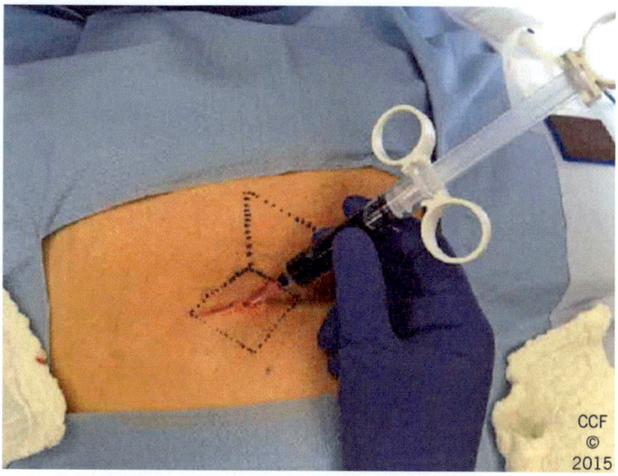

Fig. 27.3 Subcutaneous methylene blue injection identifies subcutaneous sinus tracts

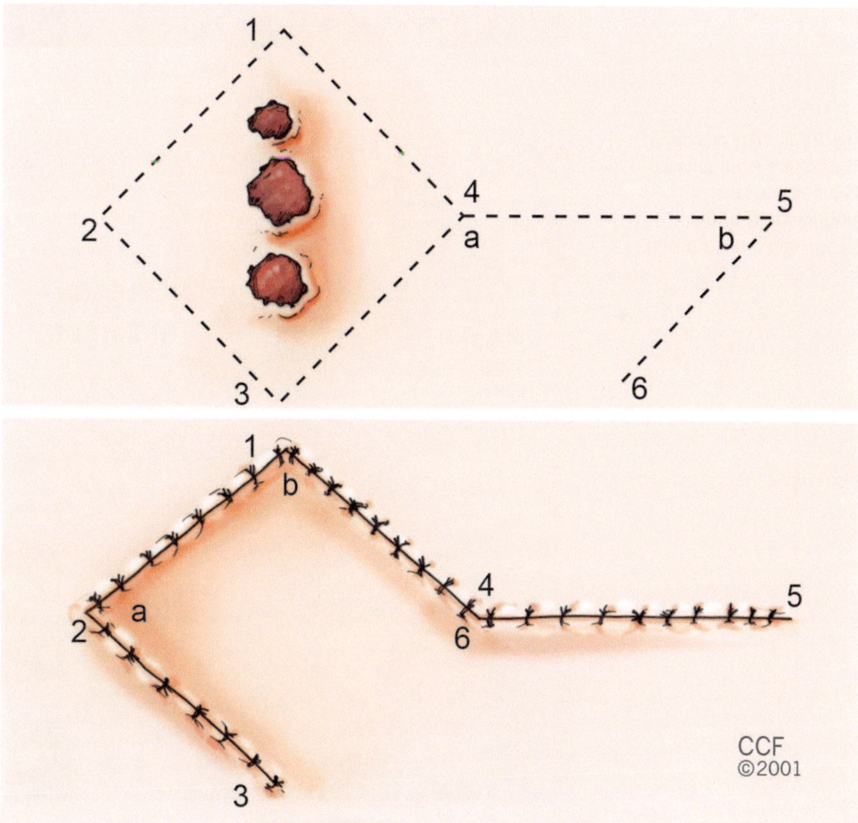

Fig. 27.4 Limberg flap reconstruction after excision of pilonidal disease

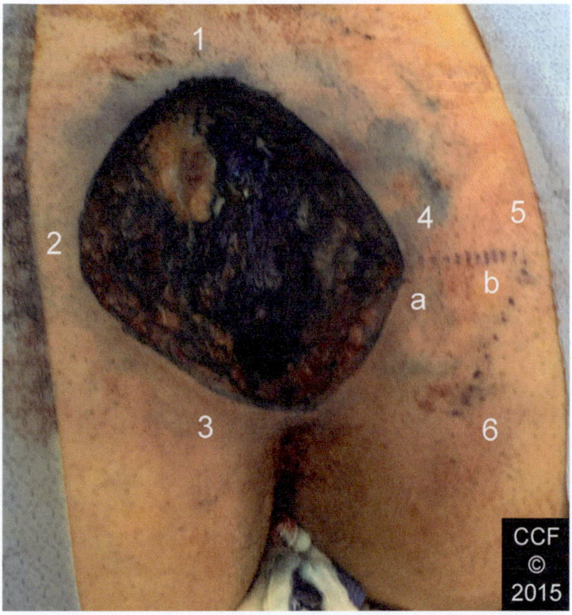

Fig. 27.5 Operative layout for flap reconstruction of defect left after excision of pilonidal disease. The pilonidal anatomy was defined by methylene blue by injecting the sinus tracts

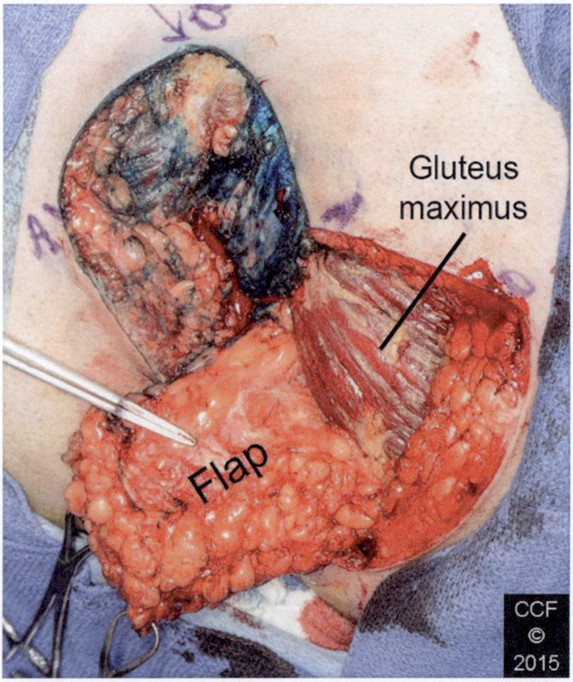

Fig. 27.6 The pilonidal disease has been excised. The flap has been mobilized off of the gluteus maximus muscle

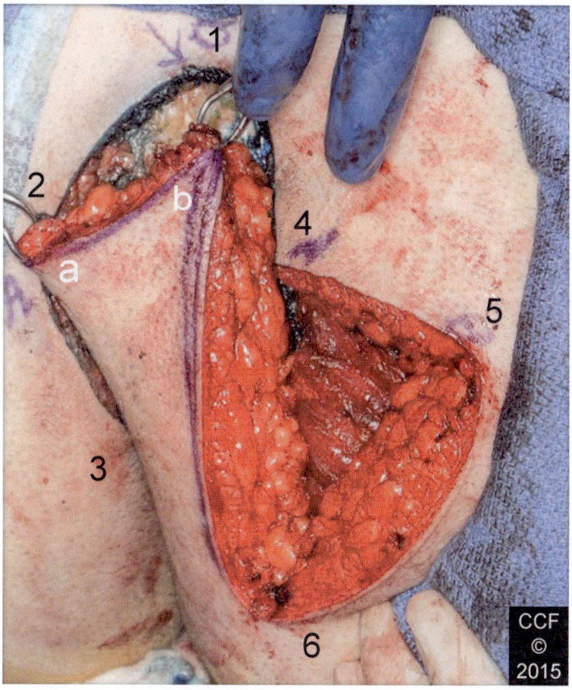

Fig. 27.7 The flap is rotated to cover the site of pilonidal disease excision

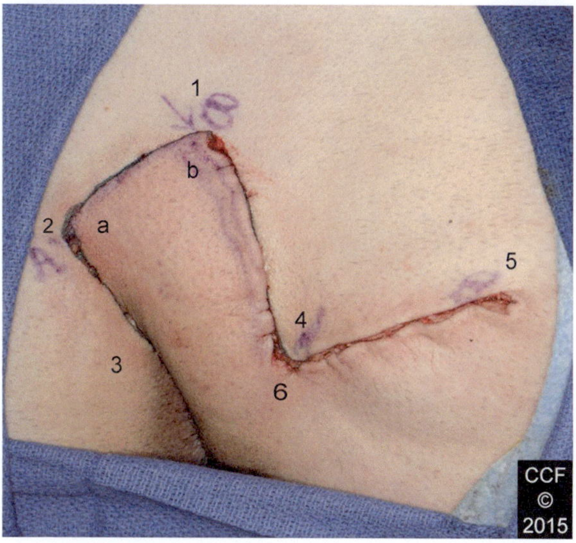

Fig. 27.8 The rhomboid flap rotated and sewn into position

Comment

Flap procedures offer several advantages:

1. wide removal of all sinus tracts and infected tissue,
2. tension-free closure using healthy tissue,
3. elimination of the gluteal cleft.

In Limberg's procedure, the sinus or sinuses are excised down to the presacral fascia using a rhombic incision. The rhomboid-shaped flap is made of skin, fat, and fascia. The flap with fascia is stripped off of the gluteus muscle, rotated, and then secured. Similar to other flap procedures, the rhomboid flap procedure permits wide excision and primary closure with well-vascularized tissue. The patient described in this case had an uneventful recovery.

References

1. Limberg AA. Ch 3: Design of local flaps. In: Gibson T, editor. Modern Trends in Plastic Surgery. vol. 2. London: Butterworth & Co.; 1966. p. 38–61.
2. Gwynn BR. Use of the rhomboid flap in pilonidal sinus. Ann R Coll Surg Eng. 1986;68:40–1.
3. Erdem E, Sungurtekin U, Neşşar M. Are postoperative drains necessary with the Limberg flap for treatment of pilonidal sinus? Dis Colon Rectum. 1998;41:1427–31.
4. Milito G, Cortese F, Casciani CU. Rhomboid flap procedure for pilonidal sinus: results from 67 cases. Int J Colorect Dis. 1998;13:113–5.
5. Chasmar LR. The versatile rhomboid (Limberg) flap. Can J Plast Surg. 2007;15:67–71.

28 Gluteal Cleft and Perianal Herpes Simplex

Christi M. Cavaliere, Amber N. Dalton, Melissa Piliang, and James S. Wu

Presentation

A patient who 1 year earlier had received a kidney transplant developed gluteal cleft ulcers (Fig. 28.1).

C. M. Cavaliere
Department of Surgery, Section of Plastic Surgery, Louis Stokes Cleveland VA Medical Center , Cleveland, OH, USA

A. N. Dalton
Dermatology & Plastic Surgery Center, Cleveland Clinic, Cleveland, OH, USA

M. Piliang
Dermatology & Plastic Surgery Center, Cleveland Clinic, Cleveland, OH, USA

J. S. Wu (✉)
Department of Colon and Rectal Surgery, Cleveland Clinic, Cleveland, OH, USA

J. S. Wu, M. D. Inkster (eds.), *Cleveland Clinic Colorectal Case Studies*,
https://doi.org/10.1007/978-3-031-39880-3_28

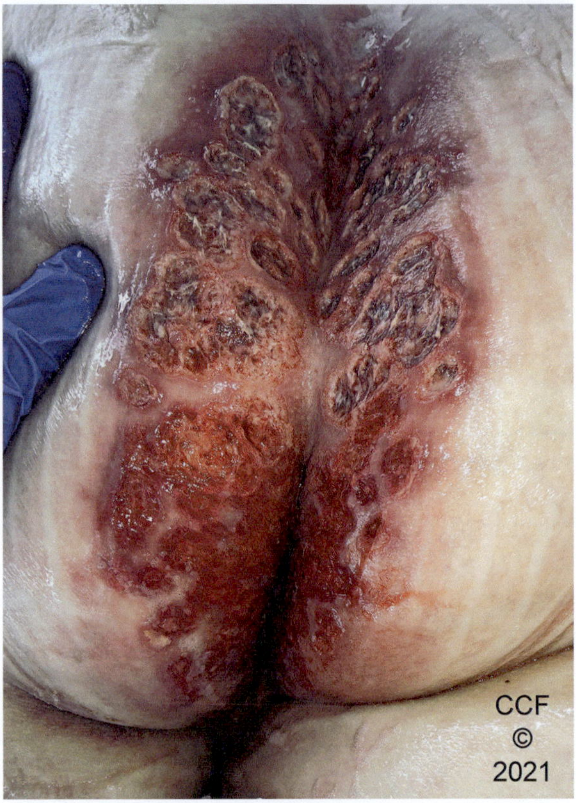

Fig. 28.1 Multiple gluteal cleft ulcerations

Management

Biopsies were taken (Fig. 28.2).

A wound culture was positive for herpes simplex virus. Molecular detection was positive for herpes simplex virus type 2. The patient was treated with intravenous and oral antiviral medication active against herpes simplex and local wound care. Skin ulcerations steadily improved on this regimen.

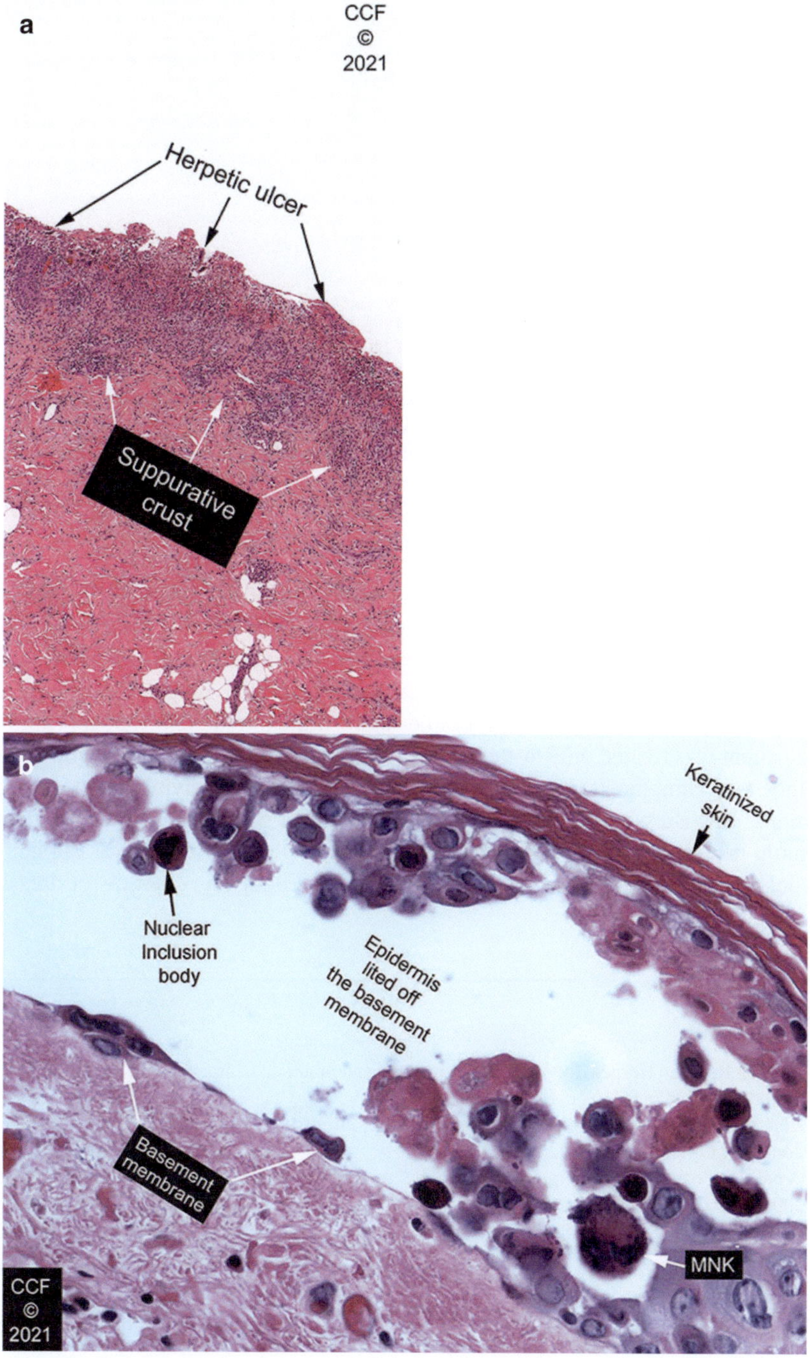

Fig. 28.2 (**a**) Herpetic ulcer ×5.5 magnification. This image shows an ulcer with a suppurative crust (arrow); (**b**) herpetic ulcer, ×40 magnification. This image shows herpetic changes: keratinized skin lifted off of the basement membrane, multinucleated keratinocytes (MNK), and a nuclear inclusion body

Comment

In 1713, Boulton described *herpes simplex*[1] [1].

Richard Boulton,
Late of Brazen-Nose College in Oxford
A System of Rational and Practical Chirurgery.
CHAP. XIV.
Of an Herpes.

> "Herpes is so called, a *serpendo*, from its creeping and spreading Quality.
>
> There are three Sorts of it, which take their Difference from the Temper of the Humour that Occasions them. The first is Herpes *simplex*, proceding from a cholerick Humour.
>
> A simple *Herpes* is a Pustle, with a sharp Head of a yellowish inflamed Colour; Matter soon appears in the top of it, though the basis is inflamed; but when the Matter is discharged they presently heal, the Inflammation going off. They often appear in single in the Face and other Parts;.... They are caused by the Grossness of that Serum which ought to go off by Transpiration; which making an Obstruction in the Glands of the Cutis, and being strongly impregnated with Choler, produces this Tumour."

Patients are at risk for both opportunistic infection and squamous cell carcinoma after renal transplantation [2, 3]. Tissue biopsy was, therefore, necessary to confirm a diagnosis for this ulcerated lesion. For patient comfort, thorough examination and punch biopsies were performed under general anesthesia. Biopsies demonstrated herpes infection; therefore, medical rather than surgical treatment was appropriate. The patient was treated with systemic acyclovir and valacyclovir. Local wound care included washing the area gently with soap and water and applying a non-adherent dressing. The dressing included a layer of fine mesh gauze impregnated with 3% bismuth tribromophenate in petrolatum. Additional petroleum jelly was applied as needed to prevent adherence to the wound surface. Finally, an outer cover dressing was applied.

References

1. Boulton R. Of an Herpes. In: A system of rational and practical Chirurgery. W. Taylor, W. Innys, London, 1713, Ch. XIV, pp. 87–88.
2. Hörl MP, Schmitz M, Ivens K, Grabensee B. Oppportunistic infections after renal transplantation. Curr Opinon Urol. 2002;12:115–23.
3. Penn I. Post-transplant malignancy. The role of immunosuppression. Drug Safety. 2000;23:101–13.

[1] For ease of readability, the letter "f," as in "fo called," has been changed to "s," and reads "so called."

Perianal Hidradenitis Suppurativa

29

Scott E. Kilpatrick, Carla R. Merrick, and James S. Wu

Presentation A

A 50-year-old female presented with multiple perianal draining sinuses which had been present for years. Some of the sinuses closed spontaneously only to be replaced by new abscesses that either drained spontaneously or required surgical incision. The appearance of the perianal skin at presentation is shown in Fig. 29.1a.

S. E. Kilpatrick
Pathology and Laboratory Institute, Cleveland Clinic, Cleveland, OH, USA

C. R. Merrick · J. S. Wu (✉)
Department of Colon and Rectal Surgery, Cleveland Clinic, Cleveland, OH, USA

J. S. Wu, M. D. Inkster (eds.), *Cleveland Clinic Colorectal Case Studies*,
https://doi.org/10.1007/978-3-031-39880-3_29

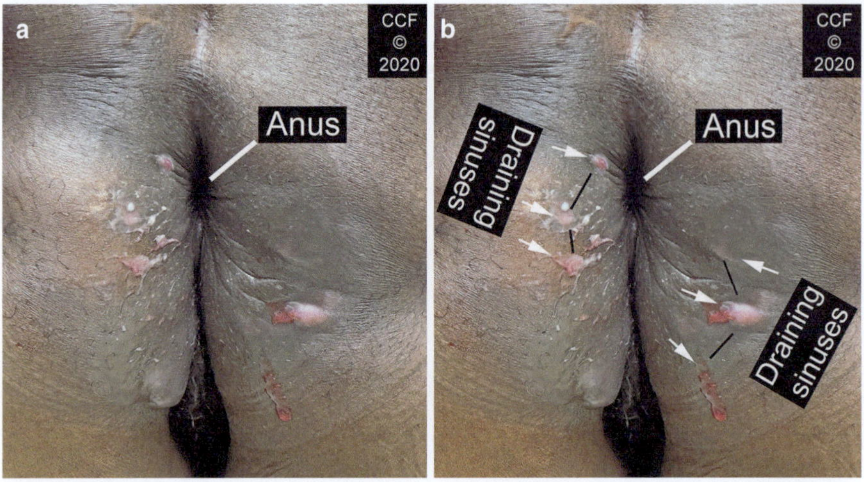

Fig. 29.1 The appearance of the perianal skin in a patient with a history of multiple draining sinuses: (**a**) Anus labeled (white line); (**b**) Three draining sinuses are seen on the perianal skin on each side of the anus (white arrows). The draining sinuses were shown to be connected subcutaneously by sinus tracts (black lines)

Management

A course of oral antibiotics had no benefit. Examination under anesthesia was done. Interrogation of the draining sinuses with probe showed that they were connected by subcutaneous tracts (black lines), as shown in Fig. 29.1b. A connection of these sinus tracts to the anal canal was not demonstrated.

The sinus tracts were unroofed and curetted (Fig. 29.2). Pathologic examination of the curettage showed granulation tissue without evidence of malignancy. The wounds were allowed to heal by secondary intention. The appearance of the skin one month after surgery is shown in Fig. 29.3. Drainage had stopped. The skin was dry.

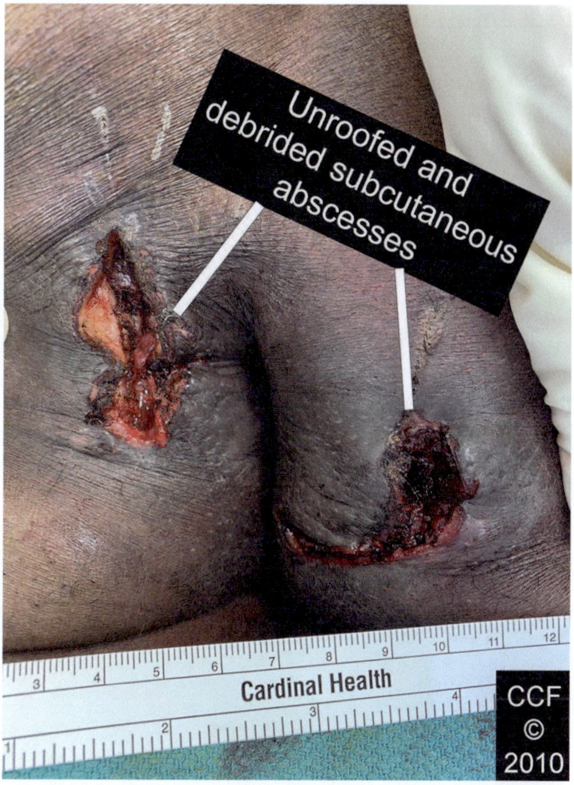

Fig. 29.2 The subcutaneous abscess cavities after unroofing

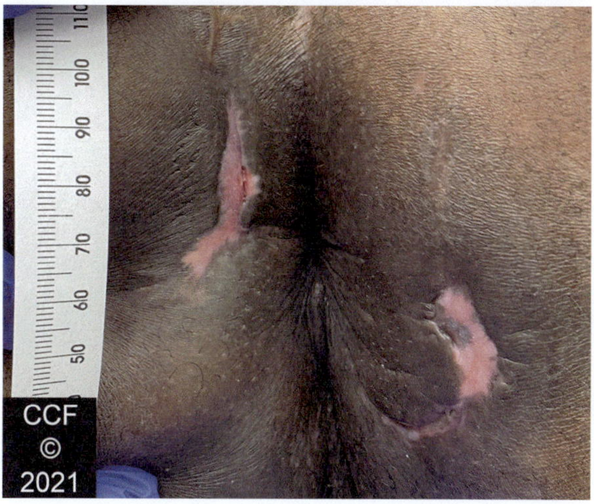

Fig. 29.3 Wound healing 4 weeks after surgery

Presentation B

A 72-year-old debilitated man presented with multiple draining buttock sinus tracts. Four years earlier, he developed multiple abscesses that were drained by local incision. The appearance of the buttocks at presentation is shown in Figs. 29.4a, b.

Management

At surgery, a fistulous connection to the anus was not identified. Subcutaneous sinus cavities and tracts were defined using probes and clamps as shown in Fig. 29.5. All were all unroofed and debrided. The appearance of the buttocks after sinus tract unroofing and debridement is shown in Figs. 29.6a, b.

The pathologic diagnosis was hidradenitis suppurativa (HS) (Figs. 29.7a, b).

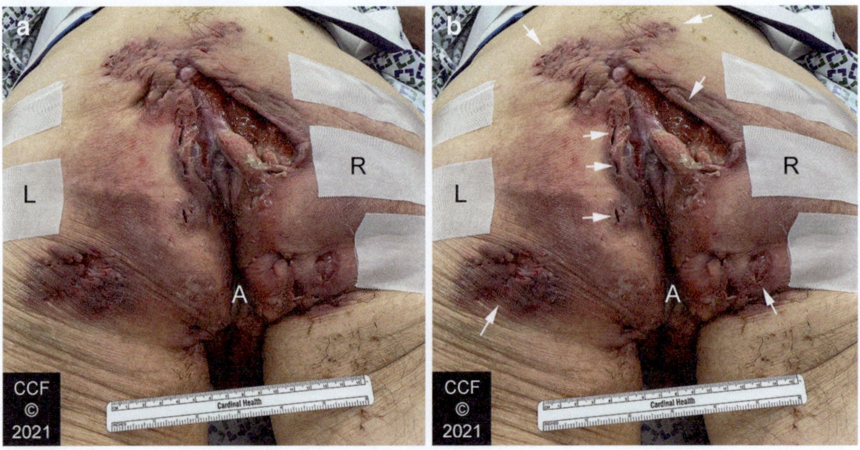

Fig. 29.4 (**a**) Perianal and buttock appearance at presentation. The anus (A) is labeled; (**b**) Cutaneous sites leading to subcutaneous sinuses and cavities are marked with arrows

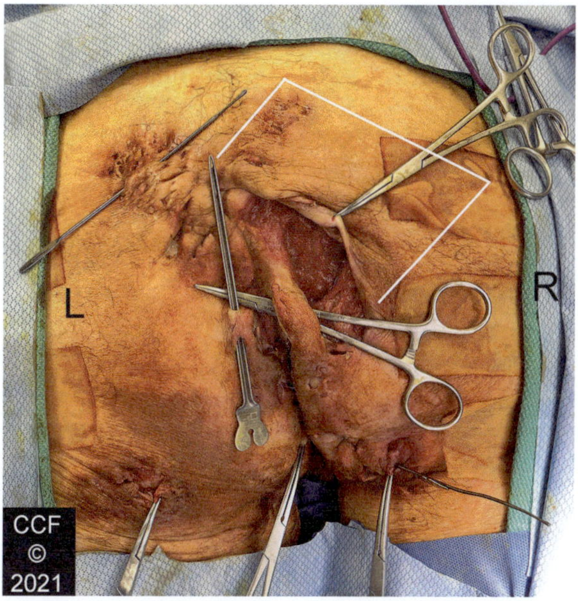

Fig. 29.5 Identification of sinus tracts and cavities with clamps and probes. The white lines mark the borders of a large subcutaneous cavity covered by an unattached skin flap

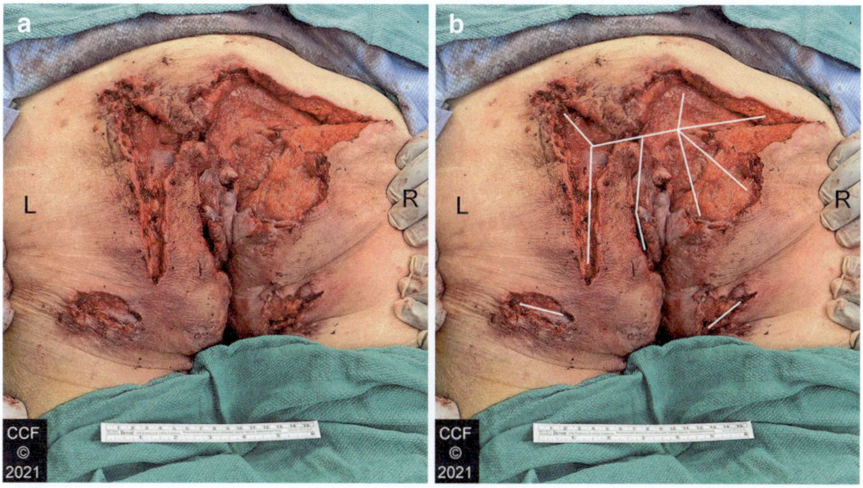

Fig. 29.6 (**a**) The appearance of the buttocks and perianal skin following unroofing and debridement of sinus tracts and cavities; (**b**) The sinus tracts and cavities posterior to the anus all were interconnected as illustrated by the white lines. The right and left and right posterior thigh sites were not connected to other sites

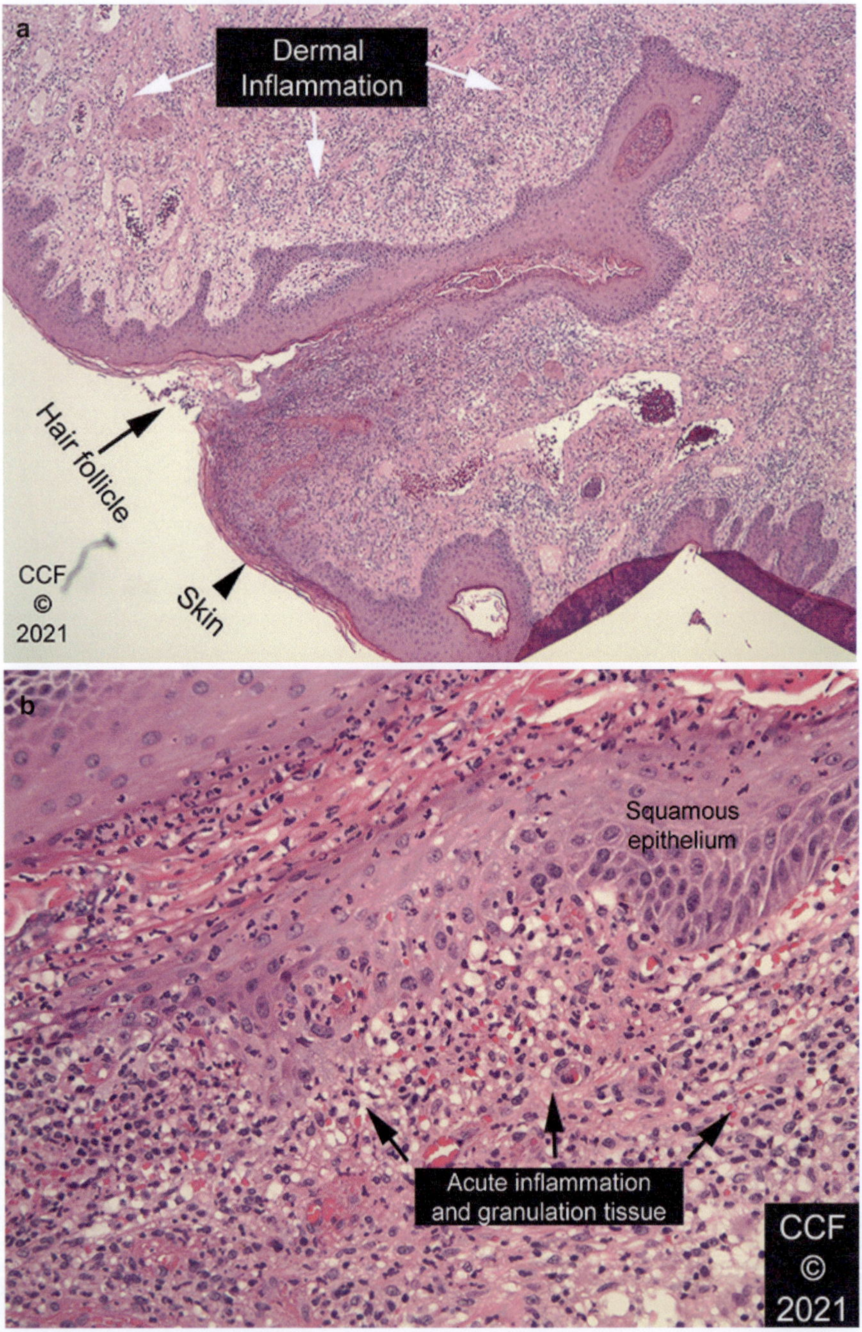

Fig. 29.7 Hidradenitis suppurativa. (**a**) Low power view shows a hair follicle with adjacent dermal inflammation (arrows); (**b**) High power view shows acute inflammation and granulation tissue (arrows)

Comment

In 1833, Velpeau described four phlegmonous or inflammatory conditions of the arm pit: "*Phlegmons superficiels ou tubériformes, phlegmons érysipélateux, phlegmons ganglionnaires, Inflammation profonde* (*superficial or tuberiform phlegmons, erysipelatous phlegmons, lymph node phlegmons, deep inflammation*)" [1]. In 1864, Verneuil published a memoir entitled, *De l'hidrosadénite phlegmoneuse et des abcès sudoripares* [2].

De l'hidrosadénite phlegmoneuse et des abcès sudoripares, Par M. le Dr. Verneuil.	Hidradenitis phlegmonosa and sweat abscesses, By M. le Dr. Verneuil.
Il y a dix années en environ, pour la première fois, j'ai cherché à fixer l'attention sur les affections chirurgicales des glandes sudoripares; j'ai décrit à cette époque, et d'après l'examen cadavérique, une variété d'abcès sous-cutanés qui me semblaient avoir pour origine l'inflammation de ces glandes.	For the first time, about 10 years ago, I tried to focus attention on surgical conditions of the sweat glands; at that time based on cadaveric examination, I described a variety of subcutaneous abscesses which appeared to me to be caused by inflammation of these glands.
Étiologie.—L'hidrosadénite phlegmoneuse est rarement idiopathique, elle reconnaît presque toujours des causes locales ou générales.	Etiology.—Phlegmonous hidradenitis rarely is idiopathic. Almost always, local or general causes are recognized.
Il en résulte que l'hidrosadénite est toujours sous-cutanée à son début, et qu'elle progresse de dedans en dehors, caractère important qui la distingue du furoncle, de l'ecthyma et de certaines dermites pustuleuses qui apparaissent de prime abord à la surface et n'envahissent les couches profondes du derme que consécutivement.	The result is that hidradenitis is always subcutaneous at its start, and it progresses from the inside out. This is an important characteristic that distinguishes it from certain pus forming dermatidities that, at first glance, appear at the surface and then consecutively invade the deep layers of the dermis.

Hidradenitis suppurativa (HS) is also known as eponymously as Verneuil's disease [3]. The Cleveland Clinic defines HS as follows: [4]

> "Hidradenitis suppurativa is a chronic inflammatory skin disease involving the hair follicles and sweat glands. Also known as acne inversa, this condition usually begins with the appearance of pimple-like bumps on the skin. Without treatment, there bumps can worsen, grow deep into the skin and turn into painful hard lumps or pockets of pus (boils). The pockets often break open. After they heal, thick scars often form.
>
> Hidradenitis suppurativa typically affects areas of the body where skin touches skin. These areas may include the underarms, buttocks, breasts, and groin (genitals and around the anus), and the inner thigh".

Hurley notes that HS abscesses may be single, multiple, or diffuse [5]. Multiple interconnected tracts between abscesses may occur. Squamous cell carcinoma is a rare complication [6]. Management options include medication, laser, drainage, excision, and deroofing [7].

In presentation A, bilateral perianal subcutaneous sinus tracts each with three external connections to the perianal skin were detected. On each side, only one opening was actively draining. Examination with a probe under anesthesia demonstrated the underlying subcutaneous sinus tracts. The sinus tracts were completely unroofed with electrocautery, curetted, and allowed to heal by secondary intention as described by van der Zee [8]. The unroofing procedure proved to be effective, minimally invasive, and tissue sparing. In presentation B, multiple interconnected subcutaneous sinus tracts and cavities crossing both buttocks plus additional separated lesions were found at examination under anesthesia. All tracts and cavities were unroofed. The extensive wounds were allowed to heal by secondary intention with the aid of a negative pressure dressing. In both cases, anal fistulous disease was excluded.

References

1. Velpeau. Des maladies propres a l'aisselle et des opérations qui s'y pratiquent. Dictionnaire de Médecine ou répertoire général des sciences médicales, vol. II. 2nd ed. Paris: Béchet jeune; 1833. p. 91–109.
2. Verneuil A. De l'hidrosadénite phlegmoneuse et des abcès sudoripares. Arch Gén Méd (Paris). 1864;115:537–57.
3. Ben Dhaou B, Boussema F, Aydi Z, Baili L, Rokbani L. Hidradenitis suppurative (Verneuil's disease). J Saudi Soc Derm Derm Surg. 2013;17:1–5.
4. Hidradenitis suppurativa. My.clevelandclinic.org (Accessed 14 Sept 2022).
5. Hurley HJ. Axillary hyperhidrosis, apocrine bromhidrosis, hidradenitis suppurativa, and familial benign pemphigus: Surgical approach. In: Roenigk RK, Roenigk Jr HH, editors. Roenigk and Roenigk's Dermatologic Surgery: Principles and Practice. 2nd ed. New York: Marcel Dekker; 1996. p. 623–45.
6. Anderson MJ Jr, Dockerty MB. Perianal hidradenitis suppurativa. A clinical and pathologic study. Dis Colon Rectum. 1958;1:23–31.
7. Sabat R, Jemec GBE, Matusiak L, Kimball AB, Prens E, Wolk K. Hidradenitis suppurativa. Nat Rev Dis Primers. 2020;6:18.
8. van der Zee HH, Prens EP, Boer J. Deroofing: a tissue-saving surgical technique for the treatment of mild to moderate hidradenitis suppurativa lesions. J Am Acad Dermatol. 2010;63:475–80.

Perianal Hidradenoma Papilliferum

30

Ursula M. Szmulowicz, Eric W. Willis, and James S. Wu

Presentation

A 39-year-old woman presented with pain from a blue-colored perianal mass that had been present for years but now was getting larger (Fig. 30.1). An excisional biopsy was done. The cyst was removed intact and submitted to pathology (Fig. 30.2).

The histopathology is shown in Fig. 30.3a, b.

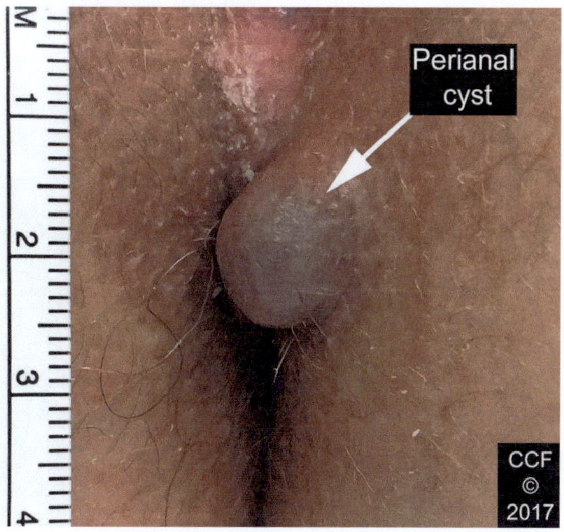

Fig. 30.1 Examination shows a left-anterior blue-colored perianal cyst

U. M. Szmulowicz · J. S. Wu (✉)
Department of Colon and Rectal Surgery, Cleveland Clinic, Cleveland, OH, USA

E. W. Willis
Department of Pathology, CORPath, Columbus, OH, USA

J. S. Wu, M. D. Inkster (eds.), *Cleveland Clinic Colorectal Case Studies*,
https://doi.org/10.1007/978-3-031-39880-3_30

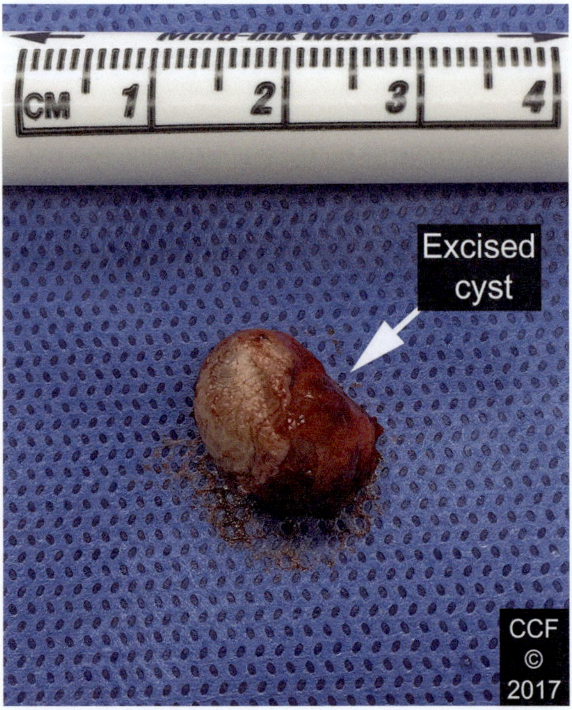

Fig. 30.2 Excised perianal cyst

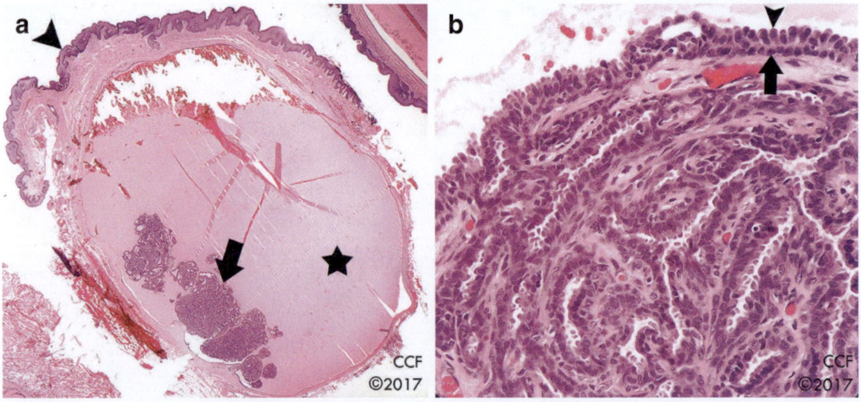

Fig. 30.3 (**a**) On low power, sections demonstrate an unremarkable epidermis (arrowhead) with a subcutaneous cystic lesion containing eosinophilic proteinaceous material (star). A mural nodule with papillary architecture is present (arrow); (**b**) on high magnification, the papillary fronds are lined by two cell layers: an eosinophilic luminal layer with apocrine snouts (arrowhead) and an abluminal myoepithelial layer (arrow)

Comment

The pathology was consistent with a hidradenoma papilliferum, a benign tumor that originates from the apocrine sweat glands [1, 2]. The first case report is attributed to Werth who, in 1878, described the anatomy of a cyst excised from the vulva of a 21-year-old woman [3]. These tumors mainly arise in the anogenital region of middle-aged women [4]. Usually, these lesions are asymptomatic with only a lump noticed by the patient [4]. Symptoms, when present, are nonspecific: bleeding, pruritus ani, drainage, and pain. Most lesions measure less than 1 cm. Rare cases of the malignant transformation of hidradenoma papilliferum have been reported [5]. Excision is both diagnostic and therapeutic.

References

1. Daniel F, Mahmoudi A, de Parades V, Fléjou J-F, Atienza P. An uncommon perianal nodule: Hidradenoma papilliferum. Gastroenterol Clin Biol. 2007;31:166–8.
2. Meeker JH, Neubecker RD, Helwig EB. Hidradenoma papilliferum. Am J Clin Pathol. 1962;37:182–95.
3. Werth R. Zur Anatomie der Cysten der Vulva. Centralblatt Gynäkol. 1878;22:513–6.
4. Handa Y, Yamanaka N, Inagaki H, Tomita Y. Large ulcerated perianal hidradenoma papilliferum in a young female. Dermatol Surg. 2003;29:790–2.
5. Rosmaninho ADN, de Almeida MTDP, Costa V, Sanches MMV, Lopes C, Meirinhos MMSG. Ectopic hidradenoma papilliferum. Dermatol Res Pract. 2010:709371. https://doi.org/10.1155/2010/709371.

31 Perianal Epidermal Inclusion Cyst

Catherine L. Forse, Erika B. Woodrum, and James S. Wu

Presentation

A 60-year-old male presented with a firm perianal mass (Fig. 31.1).

C. L. Forse
Department of Pathology and Laboratory Medicine, Faculty of Medicine, University of Ottawa, Ottawa, ON, Canada

E. B. Woodrum
Medical Illustration Team, Enterprise Creative Services, Cleveland Clinic, Cleveland, OH, USA

J. S. Wu (✉)
Department of Colon and Rectal Surgery, Cleveland Clinic, Cleveland, OH, USA

J. S. Wu, M. D. Inkster (eds.), *Cleveland Clinic Colorectal Case Studies*,
https://doi.org/10.1007/978-3-031-39880-3_31

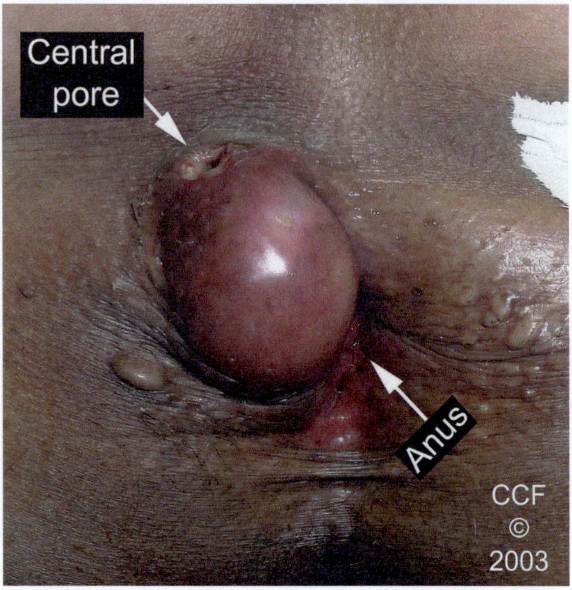

Fig. 31.1 A perianal cyst with a "central pore" was seen

Management

Surgical excision was done (Fig. 31.2).

Pathology showed epidermal inclusion cyst.

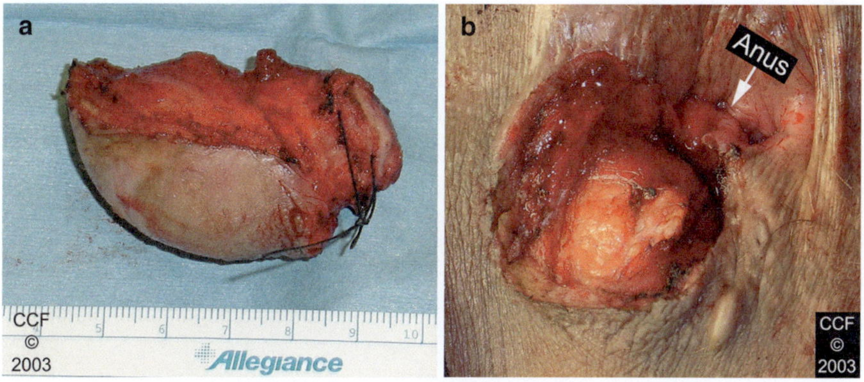

Fig. 31.2 (**a**) The perianal mass, completely excised. The specimen was oriented with a stitch; (**b**) The surgical site after excision

Comment

An epidermal inclusion cyst is derived from the epithelial lining of a hair follicle in which the epidermis invaginates into the dermis resulting in a keratin-filled epidermal lined cyst. A central pore and cheesy, foul smelling discharge is diagnostic (Fig. 31.3) [1].

Histologically, epidermal inclusion cysts show keratinized stratified squamous epithelium with keratin debris within the cyst. An example of the histology observed from a submucosal gluteal cyst is shown in Fig. 31.4.

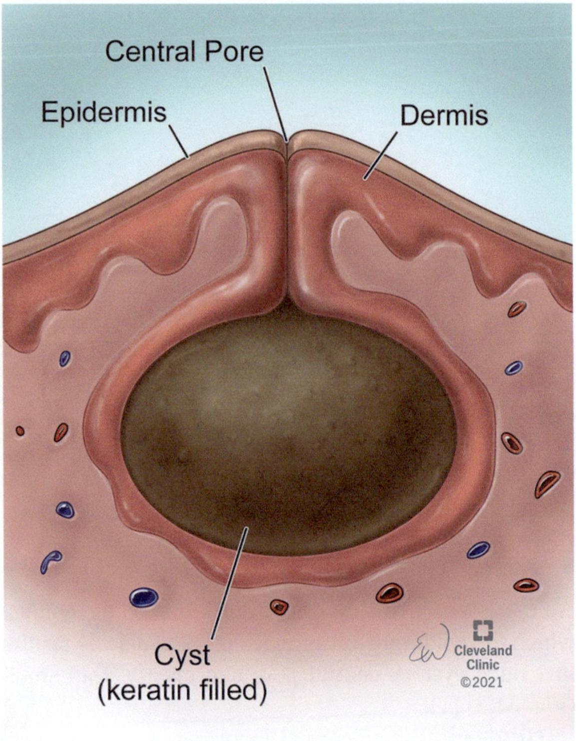

Fig. 31.3 Illustration depicting an epidermal inclusion cyst. Epidermis invaginates into dermis leading to a keratin-filled, epidermal-lined cyst (after Marks and Lookingbill)

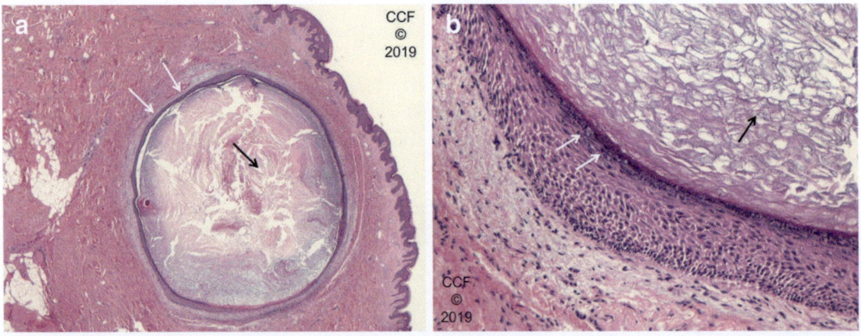

Fig. 31.4 (**a**) Submucosal gluteal cyst lined by keratinized stratified squamous epithelium (white arrows), consistent with an epidermal inclusion cyst. Note the laminated keratin/keratin debris within the cyst lumen (black arrow). H&E, ×20 magnification; (**b**) Keratinized stratified squamous epithelial lining of an epidermal inclusion cyst. Note the granular layer (white arrows) and the intraluminal keratin debris (black arrow). H&E, ×200 magnification

Reference

1. Marks JG Jr, Miller JJ. Ch 7: Dermal and subcutaneous growths. In: Lookingbill and Marks' Principles of Dermatology. 6th ed. Philadelphia, PA: Elsevier; 2019. p. 75–94.

Perianal Basal Cell Carcinoma

32

James S. Wu, Homer O. Wiland, and Eric W. Willis

Presentation

An 82-year-old female presented with a perianal mass (Fig. 32.1). The mass was located peripheral to the anal verge, was mobile, and was not fixed to underlying structures. Its diameter was 1.5 cm. Biopsy showed basal cell carcinoma.

Management

Local excision with a two-centimeter margin of skin and subcutaneous fat was done (Fig. 32.2). Final pathology showed basal cell carcinoma with nodular and morpheaform types (Fig. 32.3). Margins were negative for neoplasia.

Comment

Basal cell carcinoma is the most common skin cancer. Basal cell carcinoma in non-UV-exposed areas such as the anogenital region is considered a dermatological rarity [1]. It rarely metastasizes. Treatment of anal margin basal cell cancer by wide local excision with a negative margin is adequate therapy [2]. Flap reconstruction of large surgical defects has been reported [3].

J. S. Wu (✉)
Department of Colon and Rectal Surgery, Cleveland Clinic, Cleveland, OH, USA

H. O. Wiland
Department of Pathology, OhioHealth Mansfield Hospital, Mansfield, OH, USA

E. W. Willis
Department of Pathology, CORPath, Columbus, OH, USA

J. S. Wu, M. D. Inkster (eds.), *Cleveland Clinic Colorectal Case Studies*,
https://doi.org/10.1007/978-3-031-39880-3_32

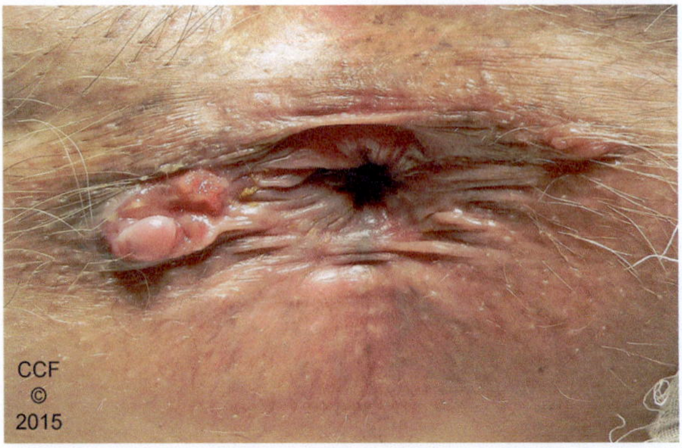

Fig. 32.1 Right lateral perianal mass

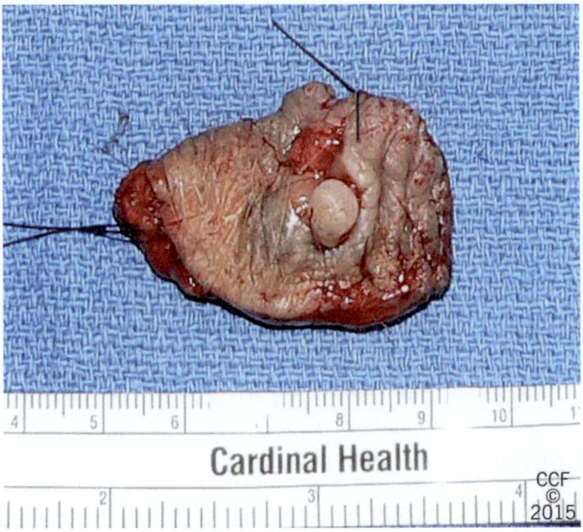

Fig. 32.2 Anal margin basal cell carcinoma completely excised with negative margins. The long stitch is lateral. The short stitch is posterior

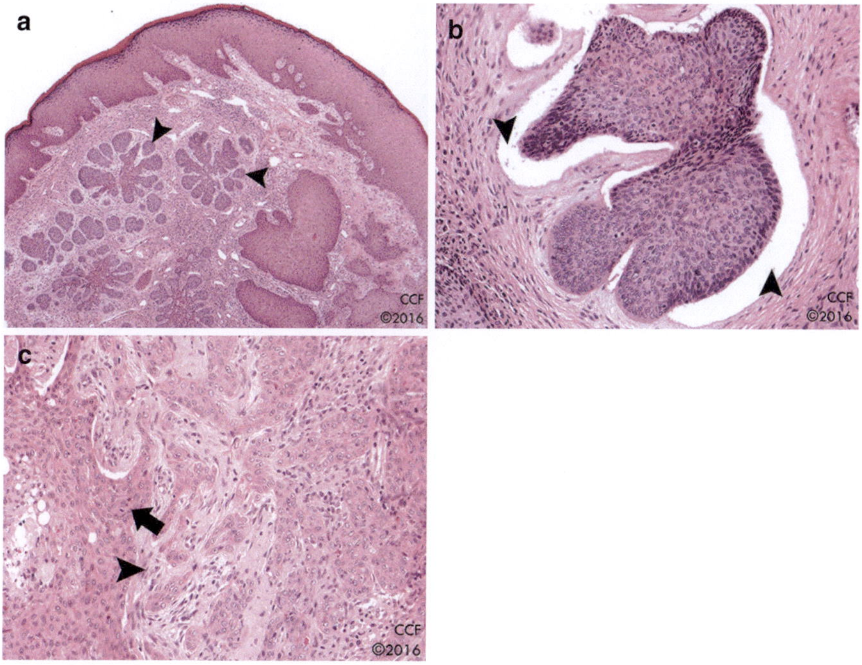

Fig. 32.3 (**a**) Low power view shows anal squamous mucosa undermined by nodules (arrowheads) of cuboidal blue squamous cells (H–E, original magnification ×40); (**b**) The nodules show typical features of basal cell carcinoma, including cellular palisading at the periphery of cell nests and retraction artifact (arrowheads) between the nests and surrounding stroma (H–E, original magnification ×400); (**c**) Areas of the tumor showed features of a morpheaform basal cell carcinoma, characterized by thin strands of basaloid cells (arrow) infiltrating a dense sclerotic stroma (arrowhead) (H–E, original magnification ×400)

References

1. Kreuter A, Bechara FG, Stücker M, Brockmeyer NH, Altmeyer P, Wieland U. Perianal basal cell carcinoma-unusual localization of a frequent tumor. J Dtsch Derm Gesell. 2012;10:59–61.
2. Berking C, Hauschild A, Kölbl O, Mast G, Gutzmer R. Basal cell carcinoma—Treatments for the commonest skin cancer. Dtsch Arztebl Int. 2014;111:389–95.
3. Ruiz-de-Erenchun R, Rodriguez N, Hernández JL, García-Tutor E. Reconstruction of a perianal defect after basal cell carcinoma using bilateral V-Y advancement fasciocutaneous flaps. Plast Reconstr Surg. 2003;111:1360–2.

Perianal Extramammary Paget's Disease 33

Sandra Dellaportas, Irene C. Lalak, David A. Horvath, Ralph J. Tuthill, Eric W. Willis, Michelle D. Inkster, and James S. Wu

Presentation

A 71-year-old white female presented with a pruritic perianal rash that had been present for more than a year (Fig. 33.1).

Treatment with topical medications did not improve her symptoms. Biopsy showed single atypical cells and nests (arrowheads) infiltrating in the epidermis (Fig. 33.2a). Extension of atypical cells into the dermis was not identified. Immunohistochemical stains were performed to evaluate the atypical cells within the epidermis. The cells were negative with antibodies to S-100 protein and melan-A, excluding melanoma. The atypical cells in question were positive (brown staining) with antibodies to carcinoembryonic antigen, cytokeratin AE 1/3, and cytokeratin CAM 5.2 (Fig. 33.2b). The pathologic interpretation was extramammary Paget's disease (EMPD).

S. Dellaportas
Department of Internal Medicine, Cleveland Clinic, Cleveland, OH, USA

I. C. Lalak
Department of Dermatology, Cleveland Clinic, Cleveland, OH, USA

D. A. Horvath
Plastic and Cosmetic Surgery, Abbington, PA, USA

R. J. Tuthill ·
Pathology & Laboratory Medicine Institute, Cleveland Clinic, Cleveland, OH, USA

E. W. Willis
Department of Pathology, CORPath, Columbus, OH, USA

M. D. Inkster
Department of Gastroenterology, Cleveland Clinic, Cleveland, OH, USA

J. S. Wu (✉)
Department of Colon and Rectal Surgery, Cleveland Clinic, Cleveland, OH, USA

J. S. Wu, M. D. Inkster (eds.), *Cleveland Clinic Colorectal Case Studies*,
https://doi.org/10.1007/978-3-031-39880-3_33

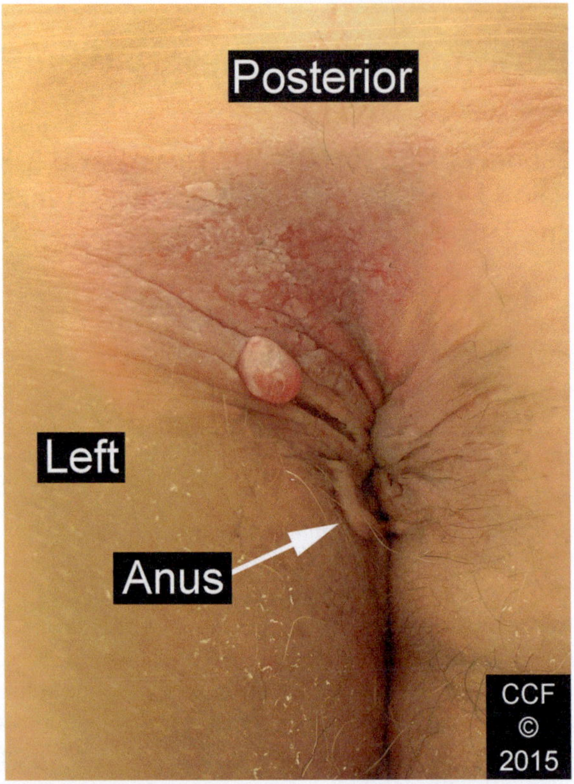

Fig. 33.1 Left posterior perianal skin rash. The anus is identified by an arrow

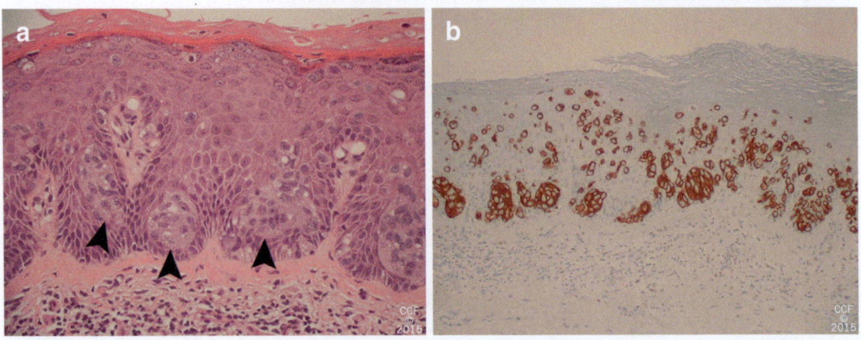

Fig. 33.2 Biopsy of perianal skin rash; (**a**) Biopsy showed single atypical cells and nests (arrowheads) infiltrating in the epidermis; (**b**) The atypical cells in question were positive (brown staining) with antibodies to carcinoembryonic antigen, cytokeratin AE 1/3 and cytokeratin CAM 5.2

Management

Following the pathologic diagnosis of extramammary Paget's disease, the histologic extent of disease was defined by perianal mapping biopsies (Fig. 33.3). Full-thickness wide excision of diseased skin was done (Figs. 33.4a, b). Margins were tumor free. Immediate perianal reconstruction was accomplished by split-thickness skin grafting (Fig. 33.5). Healing occurred without stricture (Fig. 33.6). Surveillance biopsies of the anoderm proximal to the skin graft were negative for Paget's disease 49 months after excision.

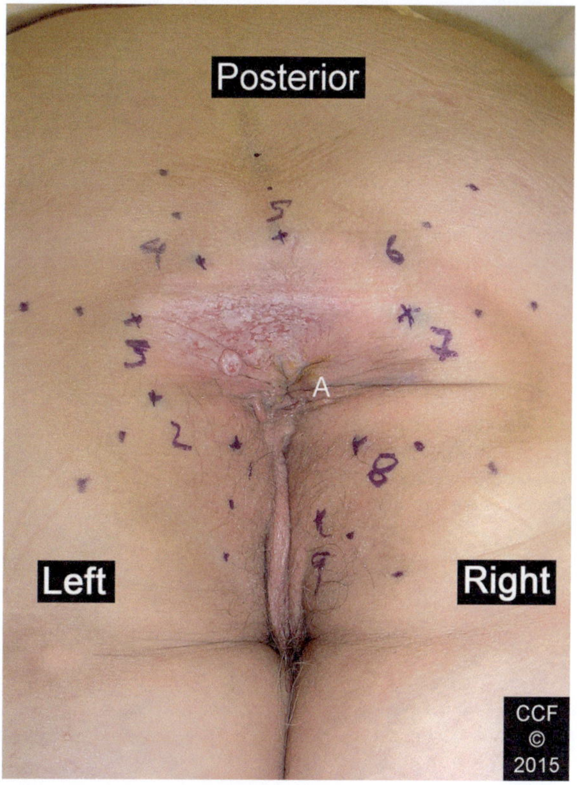

Fig. 33.3 Perianal mapping biopsies. Circumferential blind biopsies were taken from the anus (A) and at progressively greater distances from the peripheral border of the lesion. Biopsy sites were individually identified with a number and an indelible mark

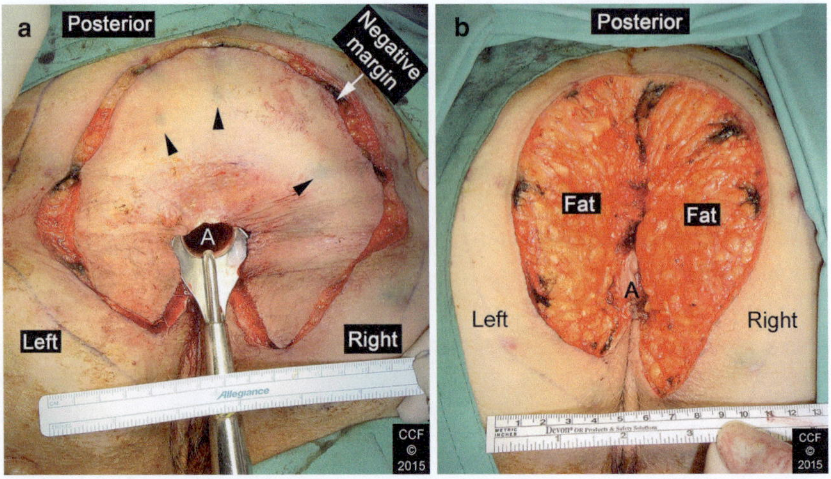

Fig. 33.4 (**a**) A circumferential full-thickness incision was made in histologically negative skin (arrow). Tattoo sites from mapping procedures in which the biopsy site was involved with disease are marked with arrowheads. A lighted Hill anoscope has been placed in the anus (A); (**b**) Full-thickness excision of the perianal skin involved with Paget's disease leaves behind exposed fat. The anus is marked (A)

Fig. 33.5 The perianal fat is covered with a split-thickness skin graft. The graft surrounds the left, posterior, and right borders of the anus (A)

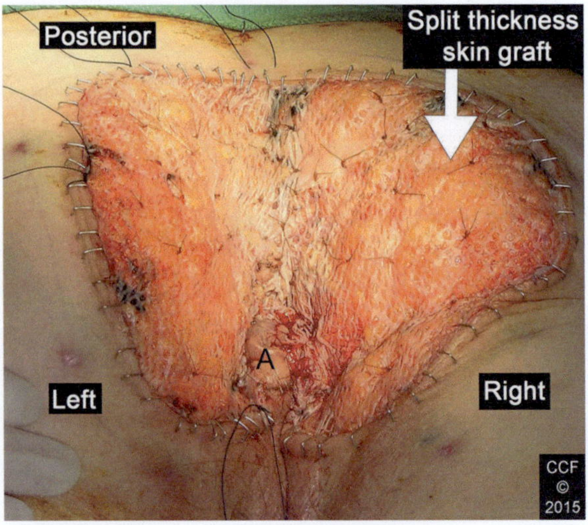

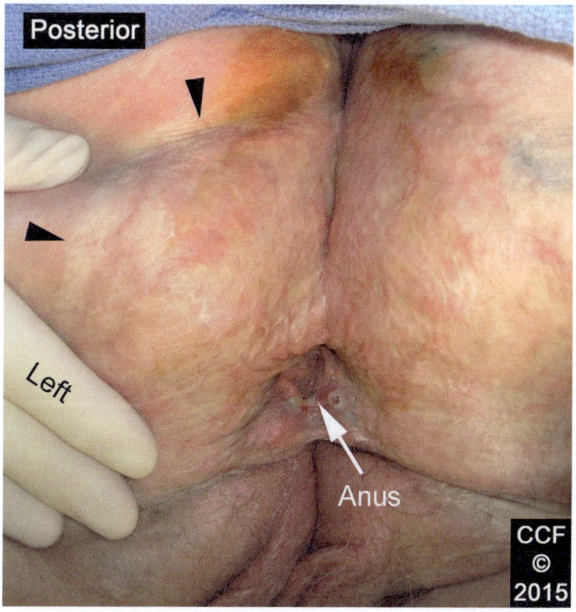

Fig. 33.6 The postoperative appearance of the skin-grafted surgical site 49 months after surgery. Arrowheads identify the border between the native skin and the skin graft. Anal canal biopsies were negative for Paget's disease

Comment

Perianal EMPD is uncommon. In this case, because a perianal rash did not resolve with common topical treatments, biopsy was done to look for uncommon diagnoses. Prior to surgery, circumferential mapping biopsies were done, not once but three times in order to reach skin histologically uninvolved by disease and to determine the margins required for complete surgical removal [1]. Grossly, the rash appeared localized to a small area of skin to the left and posterior to the anus. Mapping, however, showed extensive bilateral involvement. Preoperative colonoscopy was done to exclude colon cancer. Full-thickness wide excision with skin grafting removed the disease and provided an acceptable cosmetic and functional result [2]. Final pathology showed no evidence of invasion and clear margins. The operation chosen in this case worked particularly well because the disease did not extend into the anal canal. Had extensive anoderm excision been required, the operation likely would have been complicated by stricture formation.

References

1. Beck DE, Fazio VW. Perianal Paget's disease. Dis Colon Rectum. 1987;30:263–6.
2. Lam DTY, Batista O, Weiss EG, Nogueras JJ, Wexner SD. Staged excision and split-thickness skin graft for circumferential perianal Paget's disease. Dis Colon Rectum. 2001;44:868–70.

Perianal Extramammary Paget's Disease with Rectal Adenocarcinoma

34

Armen Aboulian and Nafis Shafizadeh

Presentation

A 71-year-old male presented with perianal irritation, pruritus, and discharge. Examination revealed a 10 cm flat perianal mass with numerous fine nodules (Fig. 34.1). Biopsy showed perianal mucinous adenocarcinoma with signet ring cell features and overlying Paget's disease (Fig. 34.2). Staging PET scan demonstrated intense PET activity in the perianal area in addition to the right inguinal lymph node (Fig. 34.3).

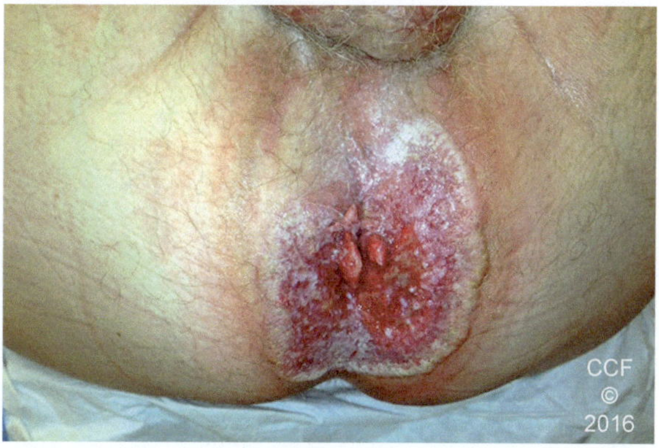

Fig. 34.1 A pruritic perianal lesion

A. Aboulian (✉)
Department of Colon and Rectal Surgery, Kaiser Permanente Woodland Hills Medical Center, Woodland Hills, CA, USA

N. Shafizadeh
Department of Pathology, Kaiser Permanente Woodland Hills Medical Center, Woodland Hills, CA, USA

J. S. Wu, M. D. Inkster (eds.), *Cleveland Clinic Colorectal Case Studies*,
https://doi.org/10.1007/978-3-031-39880-3_34

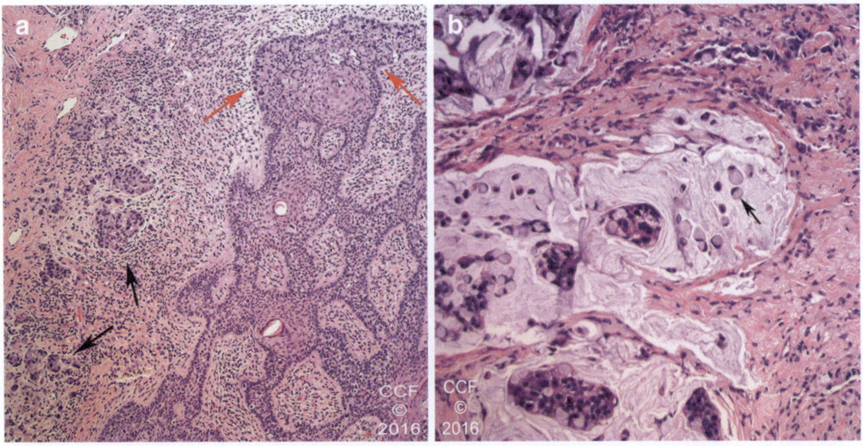

Fig. 34.2 (**a**) Invasive poorly-differentiated signet ring cell carcinoma is seen invading the dermal collagen of the perianal tissue (black arrows). Signet ring cells are also seen infiltrating the overlying epidermis (Paget's disease, red arrows); (**b**) Note the cells lying in pools of mucin that contain abundant intracytoplasmic mucin compressing an eccentric nucleus (signet ring cells; black arrow)

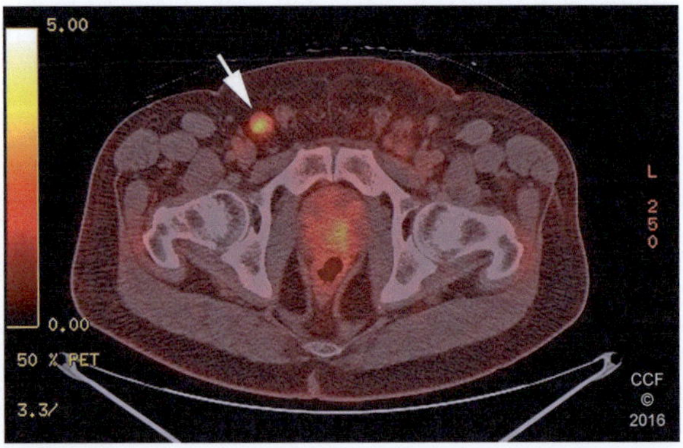

Fig. 34.3 PET scan shows activity in the right inguinal lymph node suspicious for metastatic disease

Management

Following neoadjuvant chemoradiation therapy (Fig. 34.4), abdominoperineal resection with wide excision of the perianal skin was done. The perineal defect was closed with a transrectus abdominal musculocutaneous (TRAM) flap (Fig. 34.5). Unilateral inguinal lymph node biopsy was positive for metastatic carcinoma.

The postoperative recovery was unremarkable. Two years after surgery, pulmonary and mediastinal metastases appeared. Perianal Paget's disease is uncommon. Synchronous visceral malignancy may be seen [1]. In this case, perineal wound construction was accomplished by rectus abdominis flap [2].

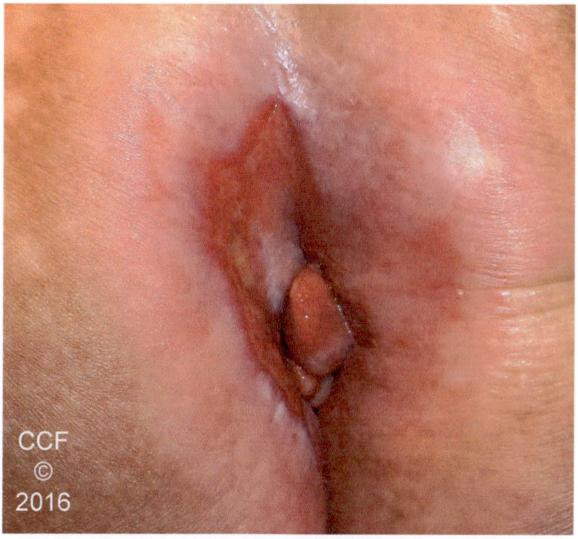

Fig. 34.4 The appearance of the perianal skin after chemoradiation therapy

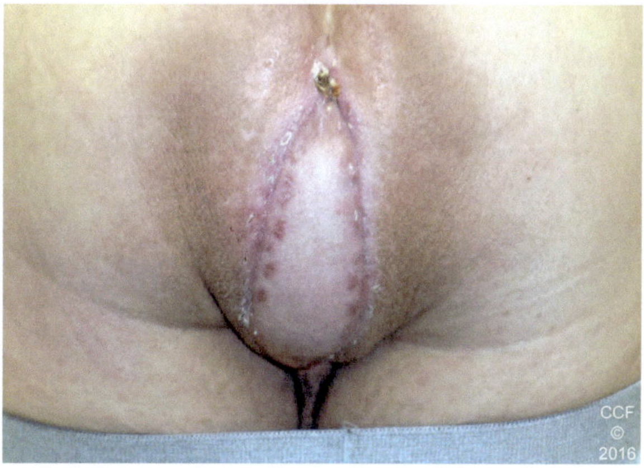

Fig. 34.5 Rectus abdominis muscle (TRAM) myocutaneous flap closure of the perineal defect following APR with wide excision of the perianal skin

References

1. Goldblum JR, Hart WR. Perianal Paget's disease: a histologic and immunohistochemical study of 11 cases with and without associated rectal adenocarcinoma. Am J Surg Pathol. 1998;22:170–9.
2. Nisar PJ, Scott HJ. Myocutaneous flap reconstruction of the pelvis after abdominoperineal excision. Color Dis. 2009;11:806–16.

Perial Extramammary Paget's Disease-Discussion

35

James S. Wu

Presentation

Intraepithelial adenocarcinoma was observed in the breast by Sir James Paget in 1874 [1].

> "I believe it has not yet been published that certain chronic affections of the skin of the nipple and areola are very often succeeded by the formation of scirrhous cancer in the mammary gland. I have seen about fifteen cases in which this has happened, and the events were in all of them so similar that one description may suffice.
>
> The patients were all women, various in age from 40 to 60 or more years, having in common nothing remarkable but their disease. In all of them the disease began as an eruption on the nipple and areola. In the majority it had the appearance of a florid, intensely red, raw surface, very finely granular, as if nearly the whole thickness of the epidermis were removed; like the surface of very acute diffuse eczema, or like that of an acute balanitis. From such a surface, on the whole or greater part of the nipple and areola, there was always copious, clear, yellowish, viscid exudation. The sensations were commonly tingling, itching, and burning, but the malady was never attended by disturbance of the general health."
>
> Sir James Paget, Bart., FRS

In 1893, Darier and Couillaud described a case of Paget's disease of the perineal-anal and scrotal region [2]. The authors credit Wickham with the first description.

J. S. Wu (✉)
Department of Colon and Rectal Surgery, Cleveland Clinic, Cleveland, OH, USA

J. S. Wu, M. D. Inkster (eds.), *Cleveland Clinic Colorectal Case Studies*,
https://doi.org/10.1007/978-3-031-39880-3_35

Sur un cas de maladie de Paget de la région périnéo-anale et scrotale.
Par MM. J. Darier et P. Couillaud

Le malade que nous avons l'honneur de vous présenter occupe á la salle Saint-Louis, le lit n° 20, il est âgé de 72 ans et porteur d'une lésion durant depuis une quinzaine d'années et présentant les caractères cliniques de la maladie de Paget. L'examen histologique fait par l'un de nous confirme ce diagnostic.

C'est en réalité le second cas publié de cette affection ainsi localisée. Le premier cas est de Radcliffe Crocker et est rapporté dans la thèse de M. Wickham, mais le dermatologiste anglais, après examen histologique conclut négativement, tandis que M. Wickham, par l'examen histologique de la même lésion conclut affirmativement.

On a case of Paget's Disease of the perineal-anal and scrotal region
By MM. J. Darier and P. Couillaud

The illness that we have the honor of presenting to you occupied bed no. 20 in the Hospital of St. Louis. He was 72 years old and bore a lesion for 15 years that had clinical features of Paget's disease. Histologic examination by one of us confirmed the diagnosis.

In reality, this is the second published case of this condition. The first is a case of Radcliffe Crocker reported in the thesis of Mr. Wickham. The English dermatologist, after histologic examination, concluded negatively, while the histological examination of Mr. Wickham of the same lesion arrived at an affirmative conclusion.

Shepherd et al.[1] summarize extramammary Paget's disease (EMPD) as follows:

> "EMPD is a rare condition that poses difficulties of diagnosis and management. Suspicious skin lesions not responding to topical therapy after four to six weeks should be biopsied to exclude EMPD. There is an associated malignancy in 20% to 30% of cases and a detailed investigation of the patient should be carried out at presentation to exclude invasive disease. Surgery remains the mainstay of treatment for EMPD but carries a 40% local recurrence rate."

Biographical Note

OBITUARY [4]
Sir James Paget, Bart., F. R. C. S.Eng., F.R.S.,
Sergeant-Surgeon to Her Majesty the Queen, and Consulting Surgeon to St. Bartholomew's Hospital

> "He was born at Great Yarmouth in 1814 and was one of seventeen children, of whom eight died in infancy or childhood. His father was a brewer and shipowner of Yarmouth;….
>
> He was apprenticed in 1830 to Mr. Charles Costerton, a St. Bartholomew's man in busy practice in Yarmouth. His first eight of surgery was on February 17th, 1830, and he never again saw a similar case—a double amputation, thigh and arm, for gunshot wounds. It may console present students to know that he fainted at the operation. The routine work of his apprenticeship was less exciting. He was in the surgery from 9 till 1 daily, and again in the afternoon; he dispensed and sent out the medicines, rolled the pills, kept the books, made out the accounts, bandaged and dressed and treated such patients as came to the surgery, and bled many of them especially on market days, and at the spring and fall of the year.
>
> Of his first year at St. Bartholomew's Hospital it is enough to say that he was left without such help and teaching as are now given to students. He worked hard in the dissecting

[1] Shepherd et al. [3]. Permission to reproduce this excerpt was generously provided by Blackwell Publishing LTD, CCC|Marketplace™, Order License ID 1139327-1, Order date August 09, 2021.

rooms, with the aid of Stanley's *Anatomy, the Dublin Dissector*, and a translation of Cloquet's *Anatomy*, which last book he so valued that once, when a fire broke out in the house next to his lodgings, he seized Cloquet as the one thing that must at all risks be saved.

He taught himself German, and read Hildebrandt and Müller with a dictionary; and Marshall Hall asked him to call on him and to translate to him what Müller had just published about reflex action. This year in the dissecting rooms, he made his discovery of the *trichina spiralis*; and at the end of the year he swept the board of all four prizes-medicine, surgery, chemistry, and botany.

On May 13th, 1836, he passed at the College of Surgeons. His examiners were Sir Astley Cooper and Mr. Anthony White of Westminster Hospital. He was asked the branches of the fifth nerve, and gave them a minute account of the otic ganglion which was at that time a structure hardly known at the College.

In 1839 he caught typhus fever, and nearly died of it; this same year he was appointed Demonstrator of Morbid Anatomy at St. Bartholomew's Hospital, and in 1841 he became Surgeon to the Finsbury Dispensary.

With this appointment as Demonstrator of Morbid Anatomy Paget's career as a teacher began. His demonstrations drew crowded classes, for hitherto scientific pathology had hardly ever been taught in British schools, and few if any teachers, excepting Lawrence, knew how to make the subject interesting to the student. So well did Paget succeed that his pupils begged the authorities that he should be made a lecturer rather than a mere demonstrator, and the request was granted.

In 1842 Paget, working at first with Stanley, undertook one of his great feats, the preparation of the *Descriptive Catalogue of the Pathological Specimens contained in the Museum of the Royal College of Surgeons of England.* He set up a model of catalogue literature which is all but universally adopted at the present day, and which by its nature cannot be improved upon. He knew his work and his heart was in it,... To him searching through hundreds of pages of manuscript in order to find a single reference was no drudgery, and when he found it he almost made merry, like a keen sportsman who has made a good shot.

On February 24th, 1847, two years before he had finished the College Catalogue, he was appointed Assistant Surgeon to St. Bartholomew's Hospital. He was already a Fellow of the College for four years, having been made an Honorary Fellow in 1843, when the higher diploma was instituted.

It was not till July, 1861, that Paget was elected full Surgeon to St. Bartholomew's Hospital. ...during his many years as assistant, and almost to the end as senior surgeon, he taught surgery as a science rather than as an art in a manner which has never been surpassed. The mantle of John Hunter had indeed fallen upon Paget."

References

1. Paget J. On disease of the mammary areola preceding cancer of the mammary gland, vol. 10. London: St. Bartholomew's Hospital Reports, St. Bartholomew's Hospital; 1874. p. 87–9.
2. Darier J, Couillaud P. Sur un cas de maladie de Paget de la région périnéo-anale et scrotale. Bull Soc Française Dermatol Syphil. 1893;4:25–31.
3. Shepherd V, Davidson EJ, Davies-Humphreys J. Extramammary Paget's disease. Br J Obstet Gynecol. 2005;112:273–9.
4. Obituary. Sir James Paget. Br Med J. 1900;1:49–54.

36 Perivulvar and Perianal Warts-Ablation

Robert L. DeBernardo, Jr and James S. Wu

Presentation

A female presented with vulvar, vaginal, and perianal condyloma acuminata (Fig. 36.1).

R. L. DeBernardo, Jr
Ob/Gyn & Women's Health Institute, Cleveland Clinic, Cleveland, OH, USA

J. S. Wu (✉)
Department of Colon and Rectal Surgery, Cleveland Clinic, Cleveland, OH, USA

J. S. Wu, M. D. Inkster (eds.), *Cleveland Clinic Colorectal Case Studies*,
https://doi.org/10.1007/978-3-031-39880-3_36

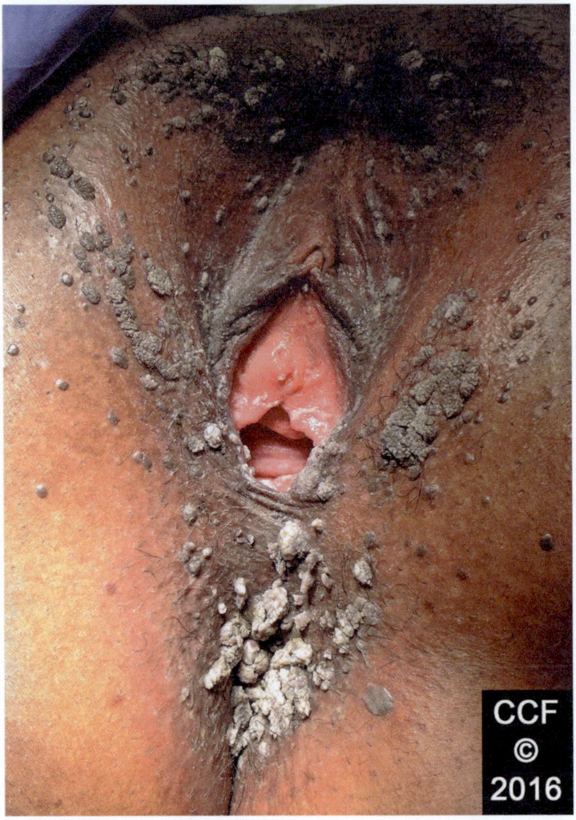

Fig. 36.1 Perianal anal and perivulvar warts

Management

The vulvar warts were ablated with the CO_2 laser (Figs. 36.2 and 36.3). The perianal warts were ablated with electrocautery (Fig. 36.3).

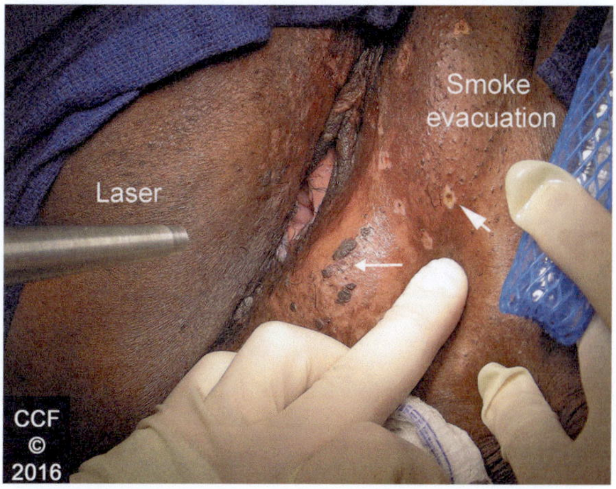

Fig. 36.2 CO_2 laser poised to ablate perivulvar condyloma acuminata (long arrow). The short arrow points to an ablated wart. Smoke is evacuated

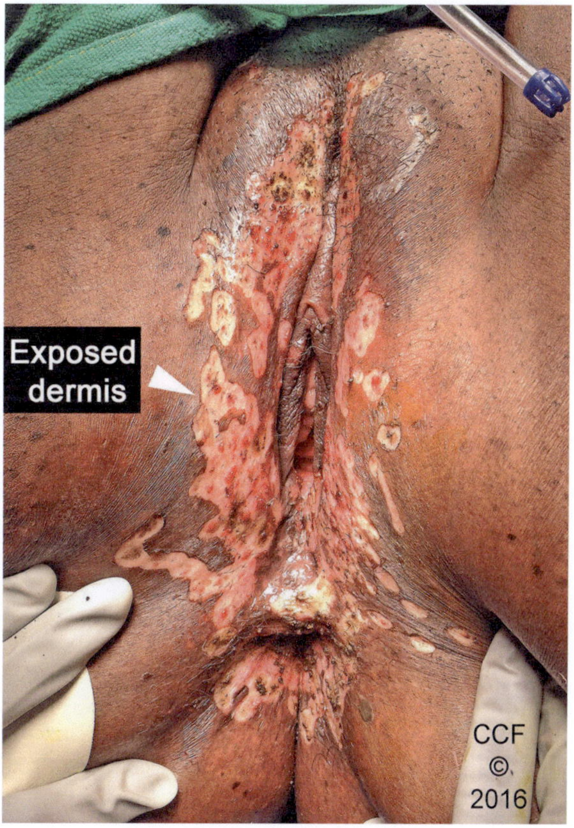

Fig. 36.3 Perivulvar warts were ablated with a CO_2 laser; perianal warts were ablated with electrocautery. The postablation appearance of the perivulvar and perianal skin is shown. The desiccated lesions have been scraped away leaving exposed dermis

Comment

Condyloma acuminata are human papillomavirus-associated lesions that affect the epidermis. Lesion ablation is superficial. In this case, two techniques, carbon dioxide laser and electrocautery, were used with similar results. When performed correctly, the desiccated condyloma can be debrided with a gauze sponge leaving exposed dermis. Skin regeneration usually occurs with minimal scarring [1, 2].

References

1. Padilla-Ailhaud A. Carbon dioxide laser vaporization of condyloma acuminata. J Low Genit Tract Dis. 2006;10:238–41.
2. Yanofsky VR, Patel RV, Goldenberg G, Genital warts. A comprehensive review. J Clin Aesthet Dermatol. 2012;5:25–36.

Perianal Condyloma Acuminata-Excision with V–Y Advancement Flap Reconstruction

37

James S. Wu, Homer O. Wiland, and Eric W. Willis

Presentation

A 25-year-old male presented with confluent condyloma acuminata involving the perianal skin (Fig. 37.1). Biopsies confirmed the diagnosis (Fig. 37.2).

J. S. Wu (✉)
Department of Colon and Rectal Surgery, Cleveland Clinic, Cleveland, OH, USA

H. O. Wiland
Department of Pathology, OhioHealth Mansfield Hospital, Mansfield, OH, USA

E. W. Willis
Department of Pathology, CORPath, Columbus, OH, USA

J. S. Wu, M. D. Inkster (eds.), *Cleveland Clinic Colorectal Case Studies*,
https://doi.org/10.1007/978-3-031-39880-3_37

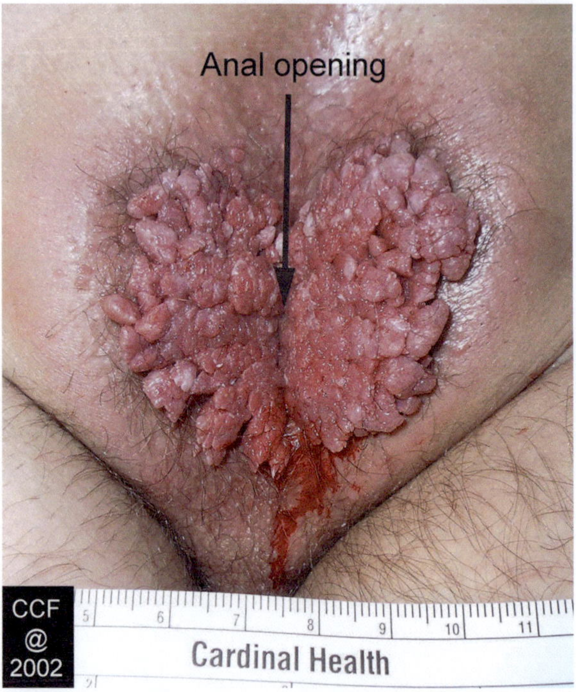

Fig. 37.1 Confluent perianal condyloma acuminata. The arrow points to the location of the anal opening

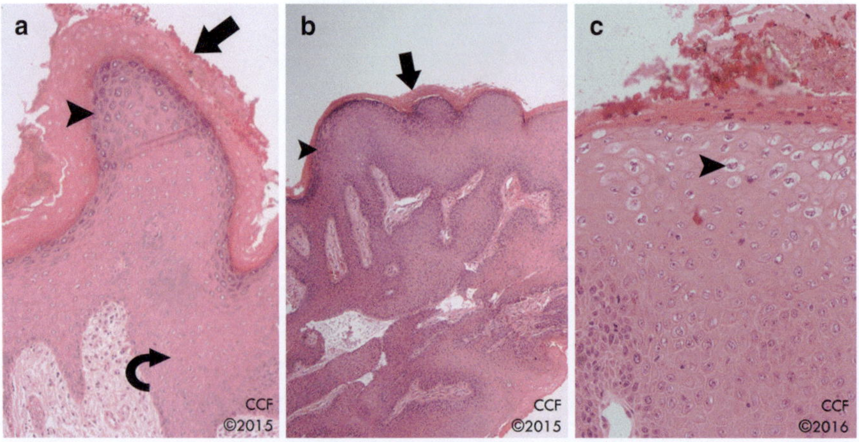

Fig. 37.2 (**a**, **b**) Low power views of the perianal condyloma show a papillary squamous proliferation with associated hyperkeratosis (arrow), hypergranulosis (arrowhead), and acanthosis (curved arrow) (H–E, original magnification ×40; H–E, original magnification ×100). (**c**) Focally, the keratinocytes are remarkable for koilocytic change (arrowhead) (H–E, original magnification ×200)

Management

The condyloma with the underlying skin was completely excised. The perianal defect was closed by bilateral V–Y advancement flaps. The concept of this reconstruction is illustrated in Fig. 37.3 [1, 2].

In this case, first, the condyloma and the underlying skin were excised (Fig. 37.4).

The surgical wound involves the perianal area. The epithelial lining of the anal canal was not removed (Fig. 37.5).

Following condyloma excision, a "V"-shaped incision is made laterally creating a triangular-shaped flap (Fig. 37.6).

The skin flaps are advanced medially toward the anal orifice (Fig. 37.7).

Each flap is well perfused from the subcutaneous fat which remains attached to its site of origin with its blood supply.

The flaps are sewn in place at the anal orifice. On each side, the closure looks like the letter "Y" (Fig. 37.8). The proximal anastomosis is to the anoderm distal to the end of the internal sphincter.

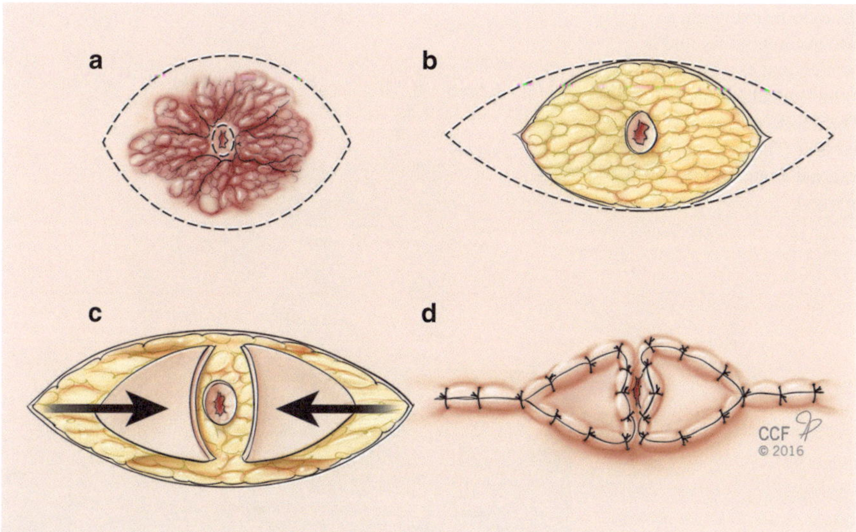

Fig. 37.3 (**a**) For circumferential perianal condyloma, the external condyloma are completely excised (outer dotted line). The anal canal epithelium is left in place (inner dotted line); (**b**) The subcutaneous fat beneath the excised condyloma is seen. The epithelial lining at the anal canal, left in place, is visible. The dotted lines show where bilateral, full-thickness, "V"-shaped incisions are made; (**c**) The triangular-shaped flaps are moved medially toward the anus (arrows); (**d**) The flaps are secured in place with interrupted suture. The final shape of each flap looks like the letter, "Y"

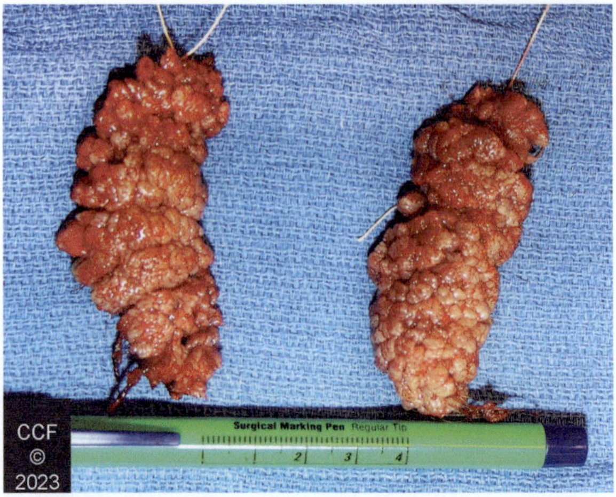

Fig. 37.4 Two excised masses of condyloma acuminata, one from the left and one from the right are shown

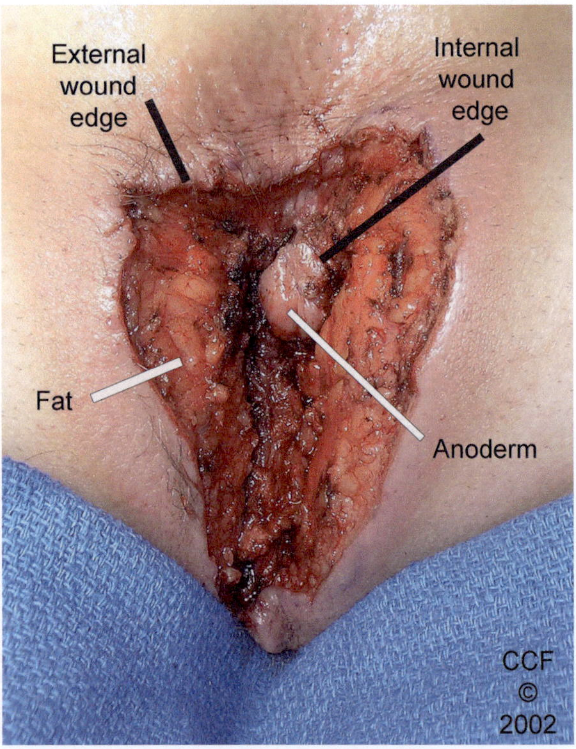

Fig. 37.5 Following condyloma excision, a circumferential wound is created that extends down to the subcutaneous fat. The anoderm was not excised. The external and internal wound edges are marked

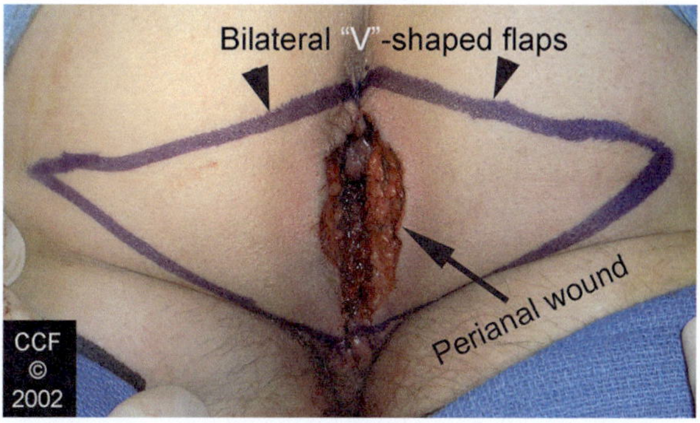

Fig. 37.6 Following excision of the condyloma, triangular-shaped skin flaps are created from the lateral edges of the perianal wound with a "V"-shaped incision

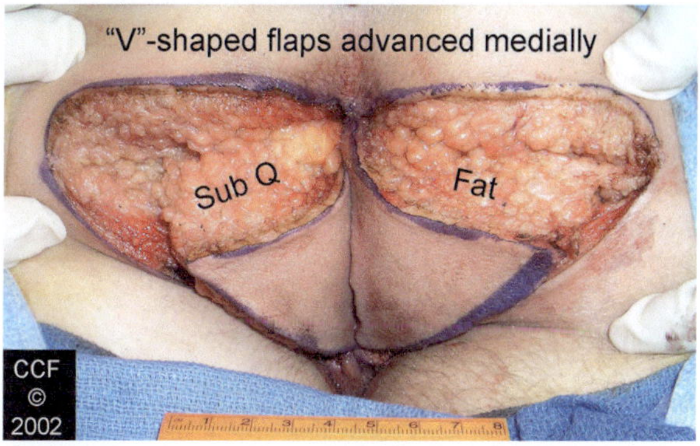

Fig. 37.7 The "V"-shaped flaps have been moved medially toward the anus

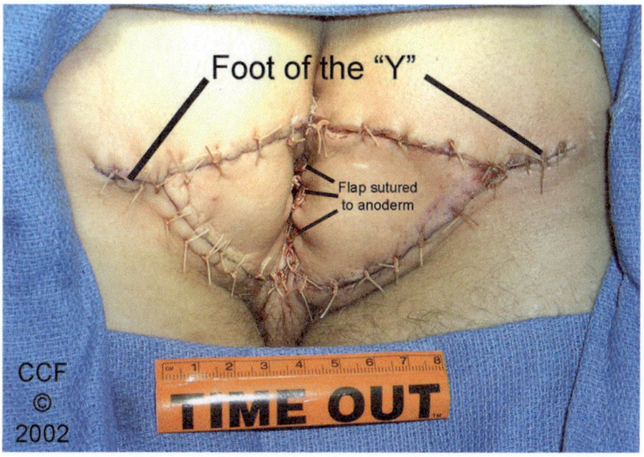

Fig. 37.8 The surgical site appearance at the end of the case. The foot of the "Y" on each side is marked with a line

Comment

Excision of condyloma with the underlying skin leaves a large wound. Reconstruction by advancement flaps avoids large open perianal wounds and permits relatively rapid healing with minimal scarring. In this approach, the squamous epithelium

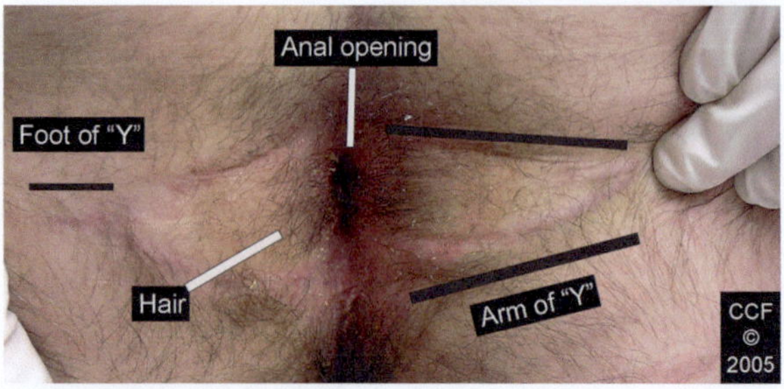

Fig. 37.9 The postoperative appearance of bilateral V–Y advancement flap reconstruction following circumferential condyloma acuminata excision is shown

lining the anal canal defined by the internal anal sphincter is not removed. If the anal canal lining is removed, anal stricture likely will occur. The postoperative appearance of the bilateral V–Y flaps is shown in Fig. 37.9.

The foot and arm of the letter "Y" are indicated by black lines. The anal opening is patent. The hair bearing perinal skin of the flaps has moved closer to the anal opening.

References

1. Kiran RP, Kalavagunta S, Berube M, Brown W, Richi AA, Dudrick SJ. Bilateral V-Y advancement flaps for the management of extensive defects of the perianal skin. Am Surg. 2006;72:631–2.
2. Uribe N, Millan M, Flores J, Asencio F, Díaz F, Ruiz Del Castillo J. Excision and V-Y plasty reconstruction for giant condyloma acuminatum. Tech Coloproctol. 2004;8:99–101.

Perianal (Anal Margin) Squamous Cell Carcinoma-Local Excision

38

James S. Wu, Homer O. Wiland, and Eric W. Willis

Presentation

A 51-year-old HIV-positive homosexual male presented with a 4.5 cm × 2.5 cm perianal mass (Fig. 38.1). A biopsy was taken that showed squamous cell carcinoma (Fig. 38.2).

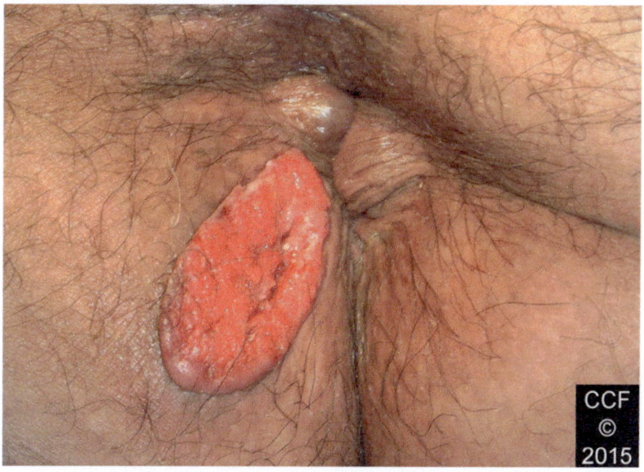

Fig. 38.1 Perianal mass in an HIV-positive homosexual male

J. S. Wu (✉)
Department of Colon and Rectal Surgery, Cleveland Clinic, Cleveland, OH, USA

H. O. Wiland
Department of Pathology, OhioHealth Mansfield Hospital, Mansfield, OH, USA

E. W. Willis
Department of Pathology, CORPath, Columbus, OH, USA

J. S. Wu, M. D. Inkster (eds.), *Cleveland Clinic Colorectal Case Studies*,
https://doi.org/10.1007/978-3-031-39880-3_38

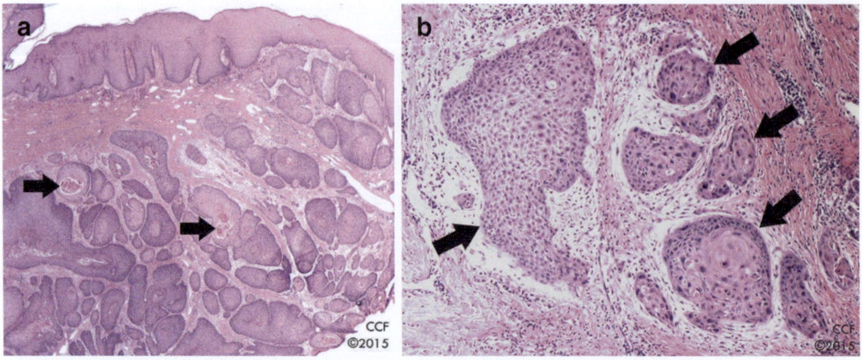

Fig. 38.2 (**a**) Biopsy of the perianal mass shows an invasive squamous carcinoma with irregular nests of squamous cells invading deep into the underlying stroma. Keratin pearls are identified by arrows (H–E, original magnification ×20). (**b**) Arrows highlight invasive nests of squamous cells with irregular, jagged contours, set within a pale-staining, loose desmoplastic stroma. The squamous cells are well-differentiated with abundant glassy, eosinophilic cytoplasm, and intercellular bridges (H–E, original magnification ×100)

Management

Adenopathy was not detected on examination of the inguinal lymph nodes. Examination of the lesion borders showed that it was entirely located on the hair bearing skin. The tumor was not attached to the anal sphincter. No additional lesions were detected on examination of the anoderm from the verge to the anorectal line. The lesion was removed by wide local excision with >1 cm margin (Figs. 38.3, 38.4, 38.5, and 38.6).

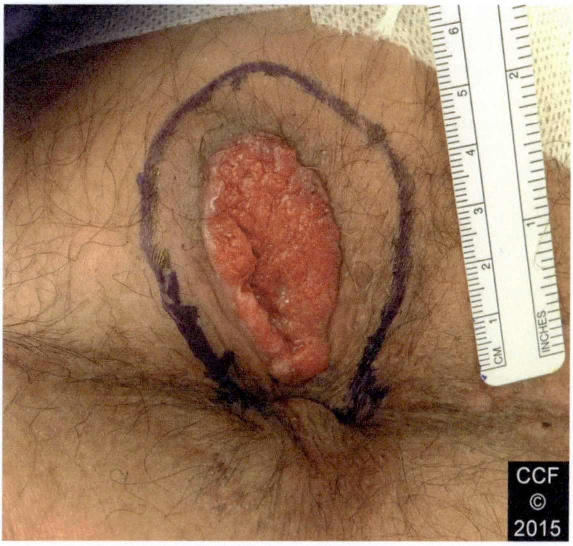

Fig. 38.3 The perianal mass is marked with a 1 cm margin

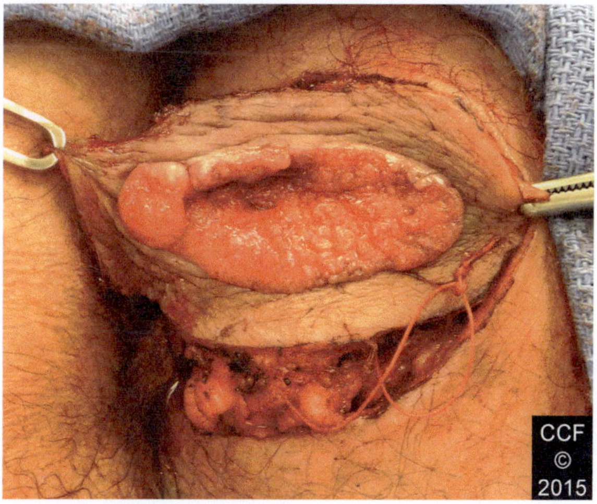

Fig. 38.4 The mobilized lesion with surrounding skin

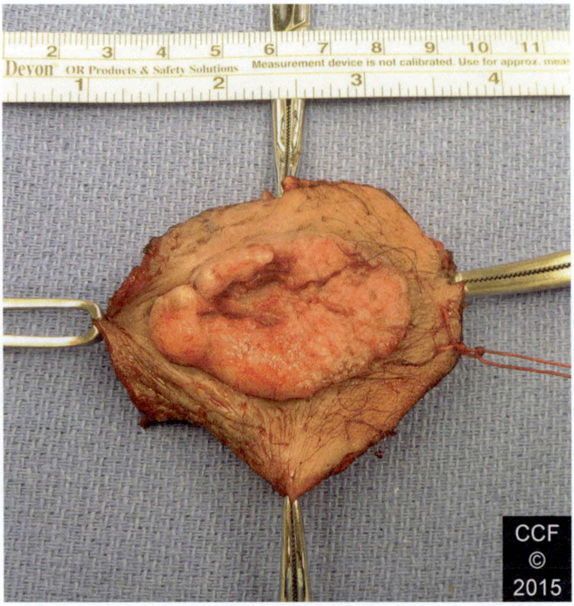

Fig. 38.5 The excised specimen. The lateral margin is identified with a stitch

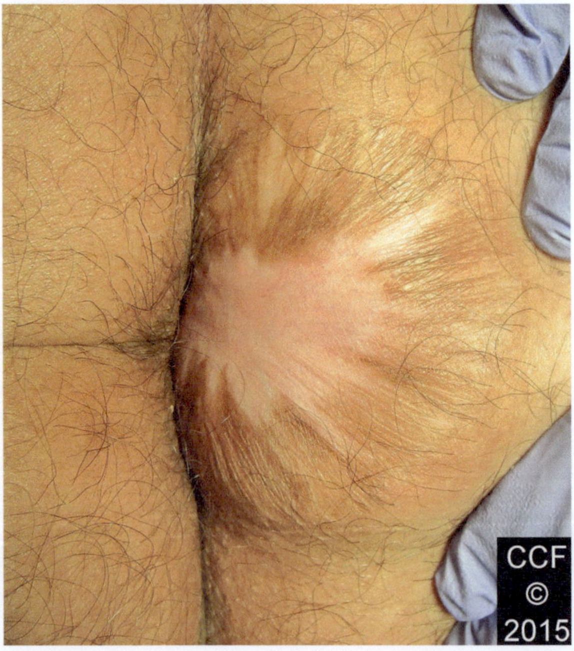

Fig. 38.6 The surgical site following healing by secondary intention

Comment

The behavior and treatment of carcinomas located on the perianal skin (previously referred to as the anal margin) and those in the anal canal are different:

> "ANAL MARGIN CANCER
>
> Carcinoma of the anal margin is anatomically and clinically distinct from tumors in the anal canal. The anal margin begins at the anal verge and includes the perianal tissues surrounding the anal canal. Malignancy in this region is rare, with an incidence estimated at approximately one fifth of that of anal canal cancer. Squamous cell cancers in this region are staged as skin cancers elsewhere in the body and generally have a favorable prognosis. Most tumors of the anal margin are well-differentiated, keratinized variants of squamous cell carcinoma. Visceral metastases are rare and inguinal involvement is also significantly less common than with anal canal malignancies. The optimal management of these tumors depends on their location, extent, and other patient factors, with options including local excision, abdominoperineal resection, and radiotherapy.
>
> Local Excision
>
> If an adequate (i.e., > 1 cm) margin can be obtained around the tumor, local excision of an anal margin cancer generally provides satisfactory local control and overall survival rates."
>
> Ashish K. Chawla and Christopher G. Willett[1]
>
> Massachusetts General Hospital, 2001

> "The proximal region of the anus encompasses true mucosa of three different histologic types: glandular, transitional, and squamous (proximal to distal, respectively). Distally, the squamous mucosa transitions into the perianal skin (true epidermis) at the point that historically has been called the anal verge. Thus, two distinct categories of tumors arise in the anal region. Tumors that develop from mucosa (of any of the three types) are termed anal canal cancers, whereas those that arise within the skin at or distal to the squamous mucocutaneous junction are termed perianal cancers."
>
> American Joint Committee on Cancer[2]
>
> Cancer Staging Handbook, 2010

References

1. Chawla AK, Willett CG. Squamous cell carcinoma of the anal canal and anal margin. Hematol Oncol Clin N Am. 2001;15:321–44.
2. Edge SB, Byrd DR, Compton CC, Fritz AG, Greene FL, Trotti A III, eds. Anus. AJCC cancer staging handbook. 7th ed., Springer, New York: 2010, pp 165–173.

---

[1] Chawla and Willett [1]. This excerpt is reproduced with the generous permission of Elsevier, Inc. All right reserved, CCC|Rightslink®, License number 5146130714609, License date Sep 11, 2021.

[2] Edge et al. [2]. Ch 15 Permission to reuse this excerpt was generously granted by Ms. Sara Martínez, Book Permissions, SpringerNature, 15 Sep 2021.

Perianal (Anal Margin) Squamous Cell Carcinoma-Local Excision with Fasciocutaneous Flap Reconstruction

39

Jason E. Leedy and James S. Wu

Presentation

A 65-year-old male presented with a perianal mass (Fig. 39.1). Biopsy showed squamous cell carcinoma. Mapping biopsies at 1 and 2 cm from the outer edge of the lesion were negative for dysplasia (Fig. 39.2). Colonoscopy was unremarkable. Adenopathy was not detected on inguinal examination. Wide local excision of the cancer with negative margins was done (Fig. 39.3). Final pathology showed squamous cell carcinoma with focal severe Bowenoid dysplasia of the skin. Margins were free of dysplasia.

Figure 39.4 shows the postexcision wound with a plan for gluteal fasciocutaneous flap closure.

The gluteal flap was raised with a lower border located in a skin crease (Fig. 39.5).

The gluteus flap was rotated medially to close the wound without tension (Fig. 39.6).

The flap was sewn into place (Fig. 39.7).

J. E. Leedy
Cleveland Plastic Surgery Institute, Mayfield Heights, OH, USA

J. S. Wu (✉)
Department of Colon and Rectal Surgery, Cleveland Clinic, Cleveland, OH, USA

J. S. Wu, M. D. Inkster (eds.), *Cleveland Clinic Colorectal Case Studies*,
https://doi.org/10.1007/978-3-031-39880-3_39

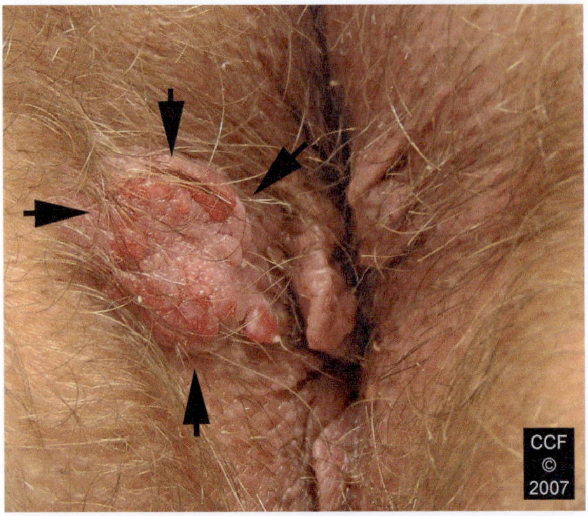

Fig. 39.1 Squamous cell carcinoma. The lesion (arrows) is located entirely on the hair-bearing skin (perianal skin/anal margin)

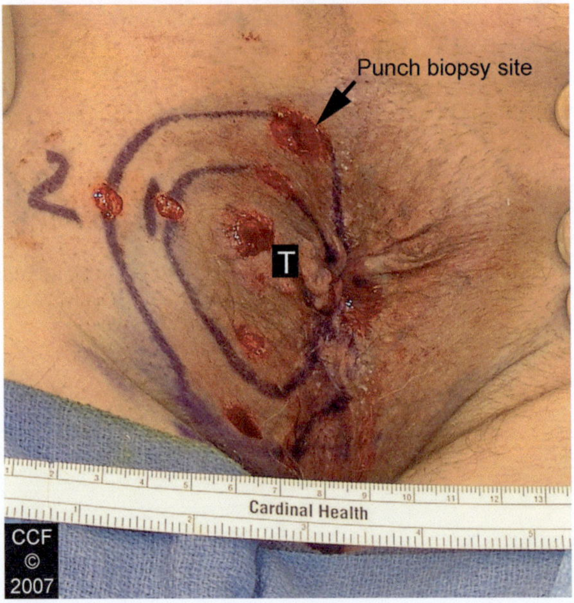

Fig. 39.2 Punch biopsies at 1 and 2 cm from the edge of the lesion (T) were negative for dysplasia

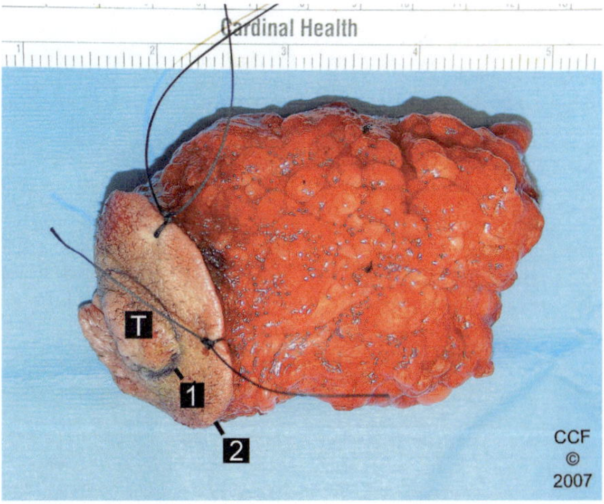

Fig. 39.3 Anal margin squamous cell carcinoma excised with a 2 cm negative margin

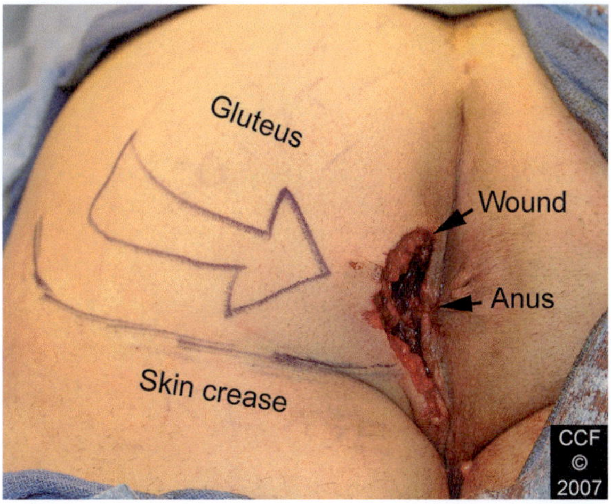

Fig. 39.4 The perianal wound is shown. The outline of a gluteal flap is marked

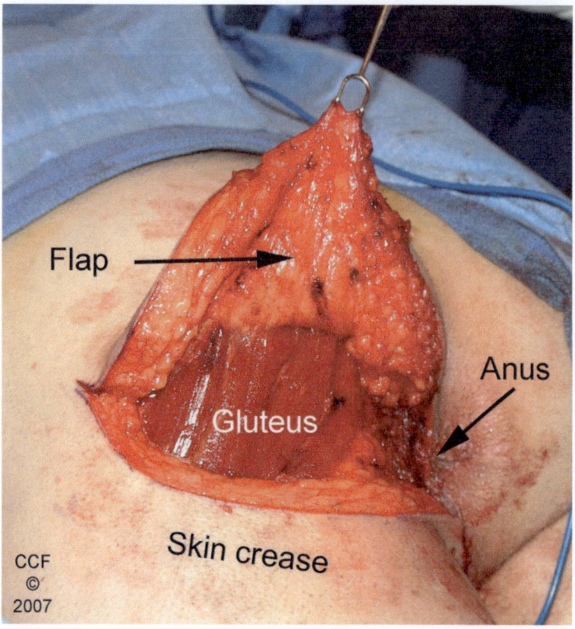

Fig. 39.5 The skin, subcutaneous fat, and fascia are raised off of the gluteus muscle

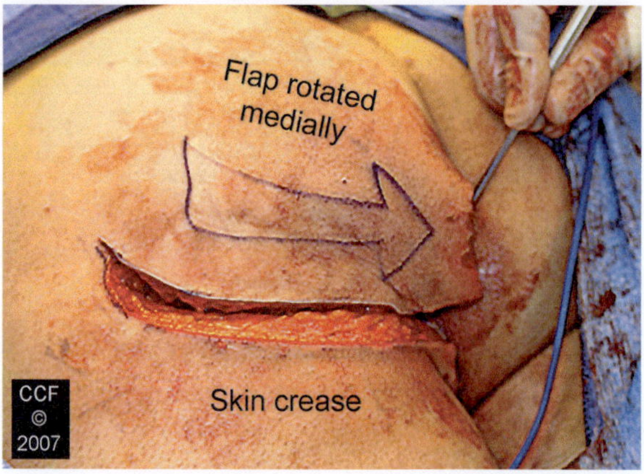

Fig. 39.6 The flap is rotated medially to close the perianal wound without tension

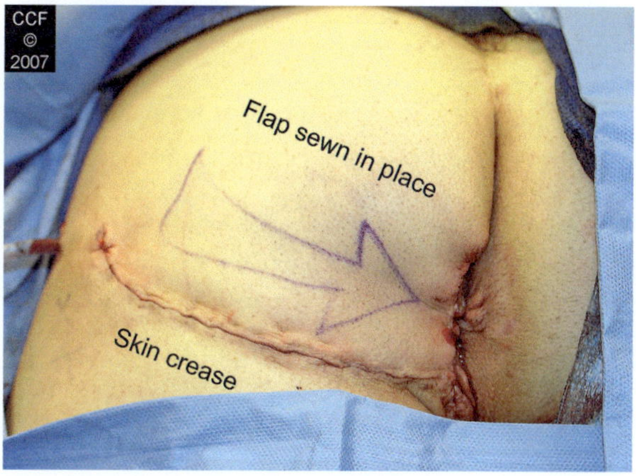

Fig. 39.7 The flap is seen sewn into place. A temporary drain is seen (far left)

Comment

This squamous cell carcinoma is located entirely on the hair-bearing skin. This places it in the perianal skin (anal margin). Treatment was wide local excision with a negative margin [1]. In 1993, Yamamoto described the fasciocutaneous flap in reconstruction of sacral pressure sores [2]. In this case, tensionless wound closure was achieved by a gluteal fasciocutaneous flap [3, 4]. The gluteal fold rotational flap reliably reconstructs pelvic, perineal, perianal, and sacral defects.

References

1. Wietfeldt ED, Thiele J. Malignancies of the anal margin and perianal skin. Clin Colon Rectal Surg. 2009;22:127–36.
2. Yamamoto Y, Ohuro T, Shintomi Y, Sugihara T, Nohira K, Igawa H. Superiority of the fasciocutaneous flap in reconstruction of sacral pressure sores. Ann Plast Surg. 1993;30:116–21.
3. Winterton RIS, Lambe GF, Ekwobi C, Oudit D, Mowatt D, Murphy JV, et al. Gluteal fold flaps for perineal reconstruction. J Plast Reconstr Aesthet Surg. 2013;66:397–405.
4. Wong TC, Ip FK. Comparison of gluteal fasciocutaneous rotational flaps and myocutaneous flaps for the treatment of sacral sores. Int Orthop. 2006;30:64–7.

40 Perianal/Anal Buschke-Loewenstein Tumor

Matthew T. Allemang, Eberechi S. Agwa, Ryan D. Ward, and James S. Wu

Presentation

A 42-year-old female was referred for anal pain and bleeding. Examination of the anal outlet and the perianal skin at presentation is shown in Fig. 40.1.

M. T. Allemang
Department of Surgery, Cleveland Clinic, Cleveland, OH, USA

E. S. Agwa
Department of Hematology & Medical Oncology, Cleveland Clinic, Cleveland, OH, USA

R. D. Ward
Radiology & Diagnostic Imaging Institute, Cleveland Clinic, Cleveland, OH, USA

J. S. Wu (✉)
Department of Colon and Rectal Surgery, Cleveland Clinic, Cleveland, OH, USA

J. S. Wu, M. D. Inkster (eds.), *Cleveland Clinic Colorectal Case Studies*,
https://doi.org/10.1007/978-3-031-39880-3_40

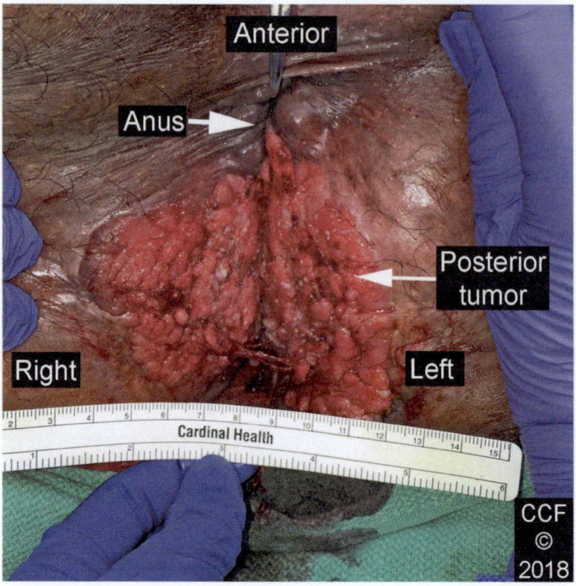

Fig. 40.1 A 10 cm × 8 cm tumor extends from the anal canal posteriorly

Management

At examination under anesthesia, an ulcerated tumor involving the posterior anal canal and the posterior perianal skin was found. Multiple superficial biopsies were taken. Pathology showed high-grade squamous intraepithelial lesion (HSIL). The patient was returned to surgery to obtain additional tissue for pathological examination. At the second examination, samples were obtained circumferentially that contained full-thickness normal skin/anoderm in addition to tumor. Repeat pathology showed anal squamous cell carcinoma (SCC) and anal margin SCC. Gynecologic examination revealed cervical cancer. The patient was referred to Oncology. Magnetic resonance imaging of the pelvis (MRI) showed a mesorectal lymph node in addition to findings in the posterior perianal skin and the cervix (Fig. 40.2). Treatment with combined chemoradiation was initiated.

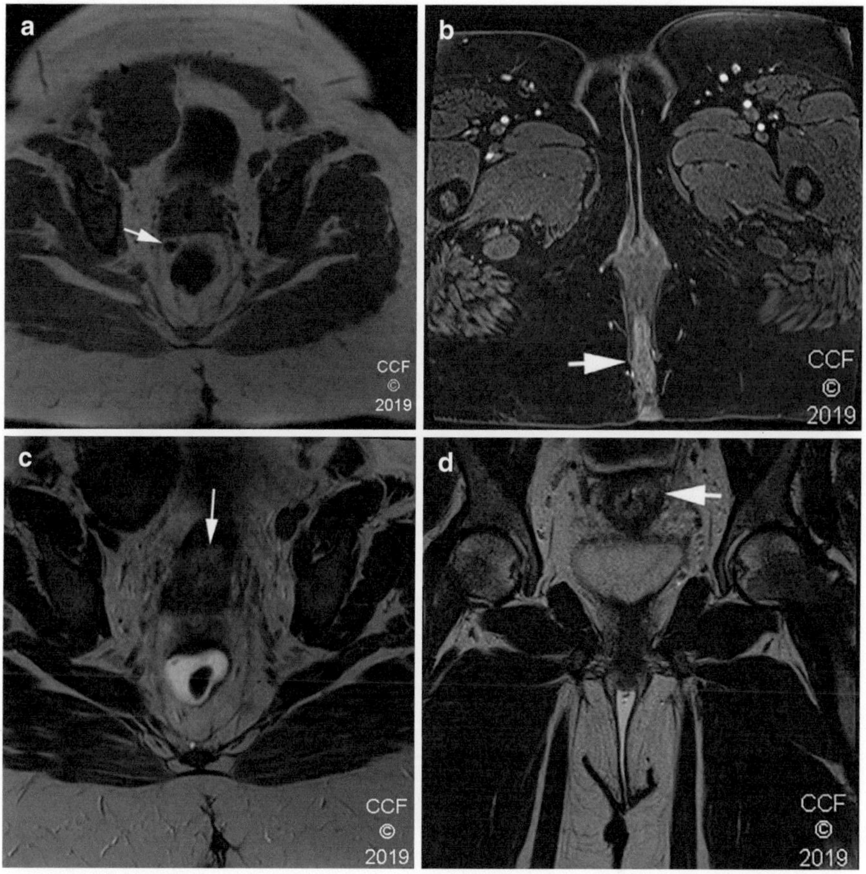

Fig. 40.2 Pelvic MRI (**a**) Right anterior mesorectal lymph node (arrow), T1-weighted in phase image; (**b**) Anal margin cancer (arrow), axial T1-weighted arterial phase post-contrast fat suppressed image; (**c**) Cervical cancer (arrow), axial T2-weighted image; (**d**) Cervical cancer (arrow), coronal T2-weighted image

Comment

This tumor looked malignant. Although multiple superficial biopsies only showed HSIL, additional full-thickness biopsies containing normal-appearing skin/anoderm and tumor were obtained in order to detect invasion below the basement membrane and to make the diagnosis of squamous cell carcinoma. Gynecologic examination, done because of the likelihood of gynecologic HPV coinfection, revealed cervical carcinoma [1]. Initial therapy consisted of combined chemotherapy and radiation.

Buschke and Loewenstein in 1925 reported three patients with "carcinomähnliche (carcinomalike)" condyloma acuminata of the penis.[1]

[1] Buschke and Loewenstein [2]. This excerpt was reproduced with the generous permission of Mr. Dirk Einecke, Springer.de.

ÜBER CARCINOMÄHNLICHE CONDYLOMATA ACUMINATA DES PENIS
Von
Prof. Dr. A. Buschke und
Dr. Ludwig Loewenstein
Aus der Dermatologischen Abteilung des Rudolph-Virchow-Krankenhauses zu Berlin
Genitale: Der distale Teil des Penis ist stark angeschwollen, die Haut darüber ist gerötet und gespannt. Die Vorhaut ist nach rechts verzogen und umschließt die Eichel derartig, daß von ihr nur eine erbsengroße Stelle sichtbar ist, die Erosionen zeigt. Betastung ist sehr schmerzhaft. Aus dem Vorhautsack entleert sich schmierig-eitriges Sekret. Nach *Dorsalinzision.* in örtlicher Betäubung quillt die Glans als ein kleinapfelgroßer, blumenkohlartig zerklüfteter Tumor hervor. Nur ein Teil des rechten oberen Quadranten zeigt normale Beschaffenheit. Der Rest der Eichel ist in den oben erwähnten blumenkohlartigen Tumor verwandelt. Die Geschwulstmasse ist fest in die Glans übergegangen und nicht verschieblich auf der Unterlage. Das Orificium externum ist nicht sichtbar und auch vermittels Sondierung nicht aufzufinden. Probeexcision vom 8. 11. 1924 ergibt nach histolgischer Untersuchung: Condylomata acuminata mit infiltrierendem Wachstum. 8 Tage später Amputatio penis an der Wurzel wegen der schweren Zerstörung des Gliedes und Ausräumen einiger bohnen- bis haselnußgroßer Drüsen aus der Leiste. Histologische Untersuchung der Leistendrüsen: Drüsengewebe: einfache Entzündung.

Dem kontinuierlichen Einwachsen destruierender Neubildungen in die Umgebung schließt sich aber außerdem vielfach eine diskontinuierliche Form des Wachstums an: Durchbrüche in Blut- und Lymphbahnen vermitteln die Geschwulstmetastasen in den regionären Lymphdriisen. *Bei den von uns angeführten Fällen ist nicht eine Metastase nachweisbar gewesen*, auch keine Verschleppung von Tumormaterial in die Lymphdrüsen.

In therapeutischer Hinsicht haben wir es für berechtigt gehalten, da die Versuche einer konservativeren Behandling wohl wegen der schweren anatomischen Veränderungen scheiterten, in einem Teile der Fälle die Amputation des Penis vorzunehmen. In letzer Zeit beginnen wir auch diese Geschwülste — nachdem ihre Gutartigkeit feststeht — versuchsweise mit Röntgenbestrahlung und Radium…zu behandeln, zumal uns letztere Methode bei spitzen Kondylomen schon gute Dienste geleistet hat.

CONCERNING CARCINOMALIKE CONDYLOMATA ACUMINATA OF THE PENIS
By
Prof. Dr. A. Buschke and
Dr. Ludwig Loewenstein
from the Dermatology Department of the Rudolph-Virchow Hospital in Berlin.
Genitals: The distal part of the penis is very swollen, the skin above it is red and and taut. The foreskin is distorted on the right side and encloses the glans in such a way that only one pea-sized spot is visible, showing erosions. Touching is very painful. The foreskin sac empties greasy-purulent secretions. After *dorsal incision,* under local anesthesia, the glans exposes a small apple-sized, cauliflower-like fissured tumor. Only part of the right upper quadrant shows normal texture. The rest of the glans is transformed into the cauliflower tumor mentioned above. The tumor mass has passed firmly into the glans and is not displaceable on the surface. The external orifice is not visible and cannot be found by probing. Trial excision on 8. 11. 1924 provides tissue for histologic examination: Condyloma acuminata with infiltrating growth. Eight days later, amputation of the penis was done due to the severe destruction of the penis; in addition, several hazelnut-sized glands were cleared out of the groin. Histologic examination of the groin nodes: simple inflammation.

The continuous ingrowth of destructive neoplasm into the area is often followed by a discontinuous form of growth: Breakthrough into the blood and lymph channels mediate the tumor metastases into the regional lymphatic glands. In our cases, no metastasis was detectable, nor was any transport of tumor material into the lymphatic glands.

From a therapeutic standpoint, since attempts of a more conservative treatment failed due to the severe anatomical changes, we have considered amputation of the penis justified. Recently, we also have started to treat these tumors – after their benign nature has been determined-experimentally with X-rays and radium…, especially as the latter method has already served us well in acute condylomas.

Buschke and Loewenstein's tumor (BLT) had the following characteristic features: (1) Condylomata acuminata mit infiltrierendem Wachstum (condyloma acuminata with infiltrating growth) (2) *ist nicht eine Metastase nachweisbar gewesen*, auch keine Verschleppung von Tumormaterial in die Lymphdrüsen (no metastases were detected and no transport of any tumor material into the lymphatic glands).

Strictly speaking, the tumor presented in this case differs from that described by Buschke and Loewenstein first because the affected organ is not the penis and second because tumor has progressed to squamous cell carcinoma with metastases. Currently, the moniker BLT has expanded to included giant condyloma acuminata involving the anal canal [3–10]. Malignant transformation of anal "BLT" also is recognized [3, 4, 6, 8, 9].

Assessment includes tests that look for local and distant metastatic spread and that examine secondary organ systems at risk for HPV-related malignancy. Treatment options for BLT include surgery [3], chemoradiation [4, 5], surgery/chemoradiation [6, 7], interferon [8], retinoids/interferon [9], interleukin 2/Cidofovir [10], laser therapy [11], and imiquimod/laser [12].

References

1. Inkster MD, Szmulowicz UM, Wiland HO, Wu JS. Ch 8: Anal condyloma acuminata and anal dysplasia. In: Zutshi M, editor. Anorectal Disease. Springer: New York; 2016. p. 189–209.
2. Buschke A, Loewenstein L. Über carcinomähnliche Condyloma Acuminata des Penis. Klin Wochenschr. 1925;4:1726–8.
3. Balik E, Eren T, Bugra D. A surgical approach to anogenital Buschke Loewenstein tumours (Giant condyloma acuminata). Acta Chir Belg. 2009;109:612–6.
4. Armstrong N, Foley G, Wilson J, Finan P, Sebag-Montefiore D. Successful treatment of a large Buschke-Lowenstein tumour with chemo-radiotherapy. Int J STD AIDS. 2009;20:732–4.
5. Hague W, Kelly E, Dhingra S, Carpenter LS. Successful treatment of recurrent Buschke-Lowenstein tumor by radiation therapy and chemotherapy. Int J Color Dis. 2010;25:539–40.
6. Tytherleigh MG, Birtle AJ, Cohen CE, Glynne-Jones R, Livingstone J, Gilbert J. Combined surgery and chemoradiation as a treatment for Buschke-Löwenstein tumour. Surgeon. 2006;4:378–83.
7. Sobrado CW, Mester M, Nadalin W, Nahas SC, Bocchini SF, Habr-Gama A. Radiation-induced total regression of a highly recurrent perianal condyloma. Dis Colon Rectum. 2000;43:257–60.
8. Geusau A, Heinz-Peer G, Volc-Platzer B, Stingl G, Kirnbauer R. Regression of deeply infiltrating giant condyloma (Buschke-Löwenstein tumor) following long-term intralesional interferon alpha therapy. Arch Dermatol. 2000;136:707–10.
9. Tian YP, Yao L, Malla P, Song Y, Li SS. Successful treatment of giant condyloma acuminatum with combination retinoid and interferon-γ therapy. Int J STD AIDS. 2012;23:445–7.
10. Nambudiri VE, Mutyambizi K, Walls AC, Fisher DC, Bleday R, Saavedra AP. Successful treatment of perianal giant condyloma acuminatum in an immunocompromised host with systemic interleukin 2 and topical cidofovir. JAMA Dermatol. 2013;149:1068–70.
11. Martín JM, Molina I, Monteagudo C, Marti N, López V, Jorda E. Buschke-Lowenstein tumor. J Dermatol Case Rep. 2008;4:60–2.
12. Heinzerling LM, Kempf W, Kamarashev J, Hafner J, Nestle FO. Treatment of verrucous carcinoma with imiquimod and CO_2 laser ablation. Dermatology. 2003;207:119–22.

Anal Adenocarcinoma

41

James S. Wu, Thomas E. Garofalo,
David Hernandez Gonzalo, and Eric W. Willis

Presentation

A 79-year-old female presented with an anal mass (Fig. 41.1). A biopsy was taken (Fig. 41.2). Pelvic magnetic resonance imaging is shown in Fig. 41.3. Colonoscopy revealed normal appearing colorectal mucosa.

J. S. Wu (✉) · T. E. Garofalo
Department of Colon and Rectal Surgery, Cleveland Clinic, Cleveland, OH, USA

D. Hernandez Gonzalo
Department of Pathology, Immunology and Laboratory Medicine, University of Florida, Gainesville, FL, USA

E. W. Willis
Department of Pathology, CORPath, Columbus, OH, USA

J. S. Wu, M. D. Inkster (eds.), *Cleveland Clinic Colorectal Case Studies*,
https://doi.org/10.1007/978-3-031-39880-3_41

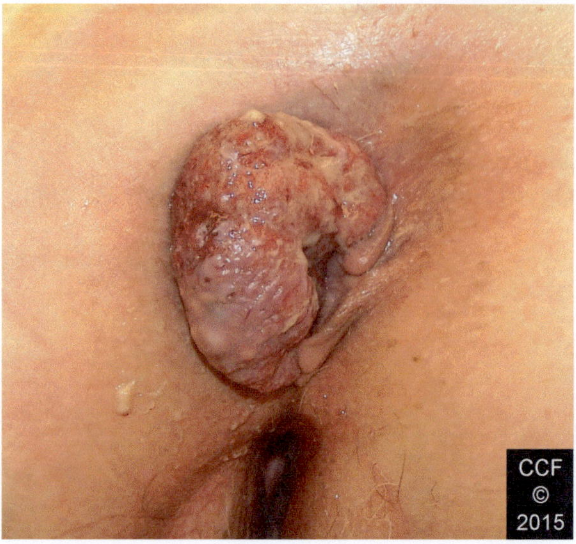

Fig. 41.1 Anal mass

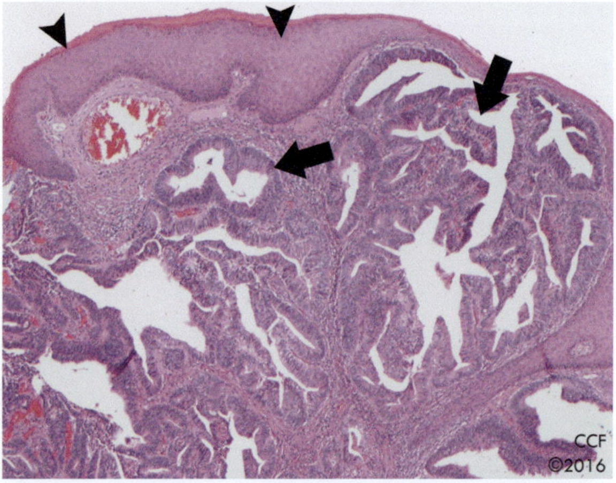

Fig. 41.2 At low power, infiltrating glands (arrows) with overlying uninvolved squamous epithelium (arrowheads) (H&E, original magnification ×50)

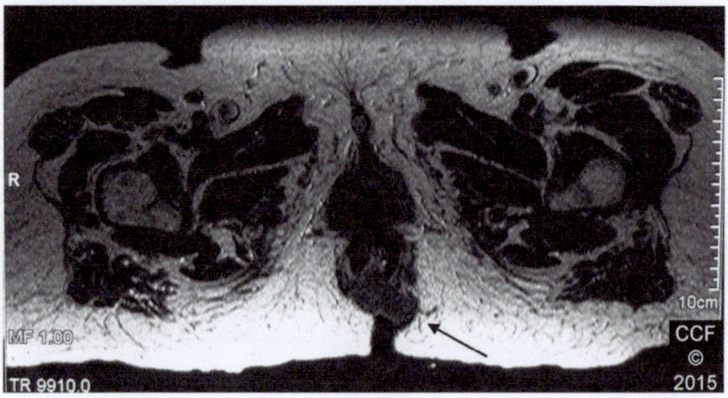

Fig. 41.3 MRI revealed an anal mass with a large exophytic/pedunculated component involving the posterior anal sphincter (arrow). Intrapelvic extension, osseous extension, lymphadenopathy, or metastatic disease in the pelvis was not seen

Management

Biopsy showed adenocarcinoma. MRI showed that the tumor was located primarily on the anal margin but involved the distal anal sphincter. The patient declined abdominoperineal resection or chemoradiation. The tumor was removed by local excision with a 1 cm margin (Fig. 41.4). The anal sphincter was partially removed. The wound healed by secondary intention. Pathology of the resected specimen showed adenocarcinoma (Fig. 41.5). All margins were tumor free.

In this case, local excision was done because the patient refused more aggressive measures. Follow-up 3.5 years after surgery revealed no evidence of recurrent carcinoma.

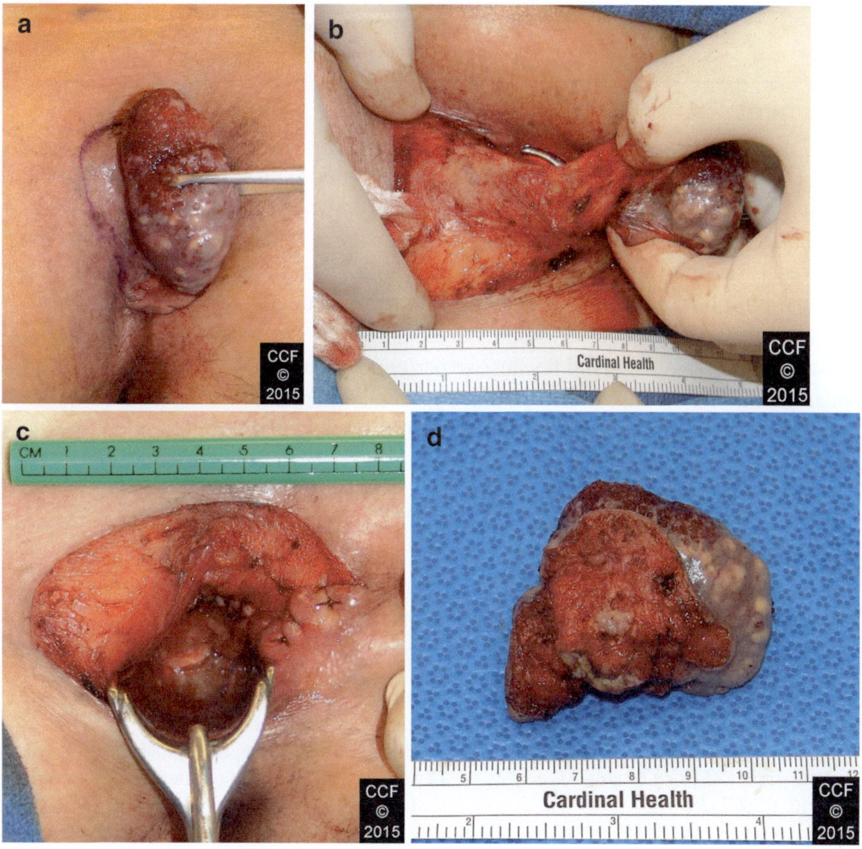

Fig. 41.4 (**a**) A 1 cm margin is drawn around the tumor; (**b**) tumor removal by local excision; (**c**) the tumor bed following excision; (**d**) the excised specimen

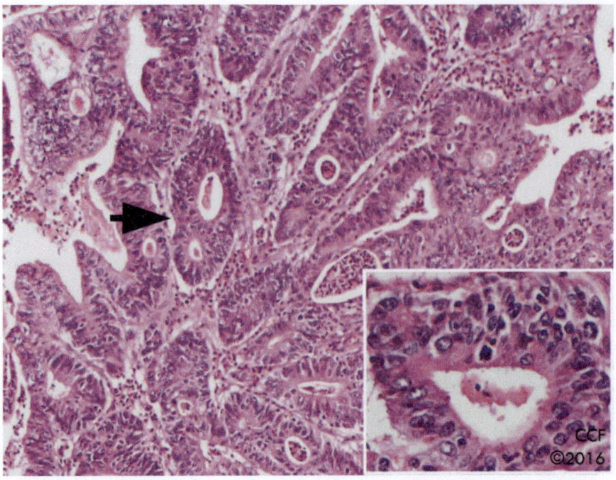

Fig. 41.5 Tumor histopathology shows adenocarcinoma. High-power view showing back-to-back glands (arrow) with dirty necrosis (inset) (H&E, original magnification ×20, ×50)

Comment

In 1937, Manning described a patient who presented with a painful anal mass [1]. The tumor was removed by local excision. Pathology, unexpectedly, showed adenocarcinoma, not squamous cell carcinoma. The patient subsequently developed local recurrence of anal adenocarcinoma with inguinal metastases. Metastases to the inquinal lymphatics attest to the anal origin of this adenocarcinoma. The origin of anal adenocarcinoma includes anal fistulae, anal ducts, or anal glands [2–4]. Optimal management is controversial because experience is limited. Distinction of anal adenocarcinoma from anal involvement by rectal adenocarcinoma also is needed. Treatment options include abdominoperineal excision, chemoradiation therapy, and local excision.

References

1. Manning VR. Adenocarcinoma of the anus. Trans Am Proctol Soc. 1937;38:70–4.
2. Close AS, Schwab RL. A history of the anal ducts and anal-duct carcinoma. Report of a case. Cancer. 1955;8:979–85.
3. Chang GJ, Gonzalez RJ, Skibber JM, Eng C, Das P, Rodriguez-Bigas MA. A twenty-year experience with adenocarcinoma of the anal canal. Dis Colon Rectum. 2009;52:1375–80.
4. Belkacémi Y, Rouanet P, Jafari M. Primary adenocarcinoma of the anal canal. In: Belkacémi Y, Mirimanoff RO, Ozsahin M, editors. Management of Rare Adult tumours. Paris: Springer; 2010. p. 167–73.

Anal Melanoma (Amelanotic)-Local Excision

42

James S. Wu, Homer O. Wiland, and Eric W. Willis

A 73-year-old male was referred for management of a firm anal mass (Fig. 42.1). The mass was removed by excisional biopsy with a 1 cm margin (Fig. 42.2). Histopathology is shown in Fig. 42.3.

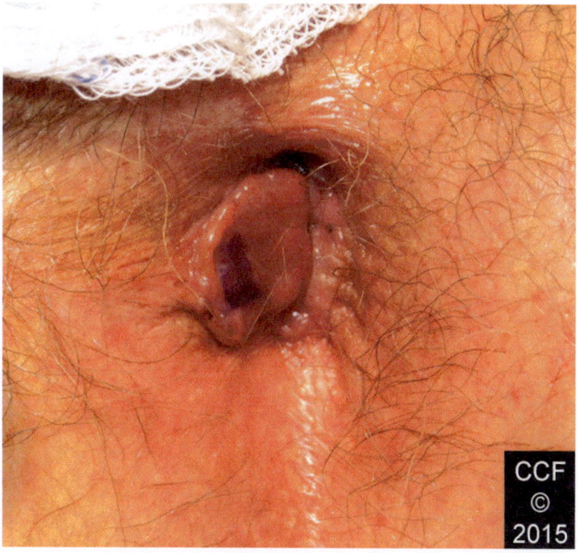

Fig. 42.1 Right lateral perianal mass. Its most distal border is located at the anal verge. The mass has been marked with purple ink

J. S. Wu (✉)
Department of Colon and Rectal Surgery, Cleveland Clinic, Cleveland, OH, USA

H. O. Wiland
Department of Pathology, OhioHealth Mansfield Hospital, Mansfield, OH, USA

E. W. Willis
Department of Pathology, CORPath, Columbus, OH, USA

J. S. Wu, M. D. Inkster (eds.), *Cleveland Clinic Colorectal Case Studies*,
https://doi.org/10.1007/978-3-031-39880-3_42

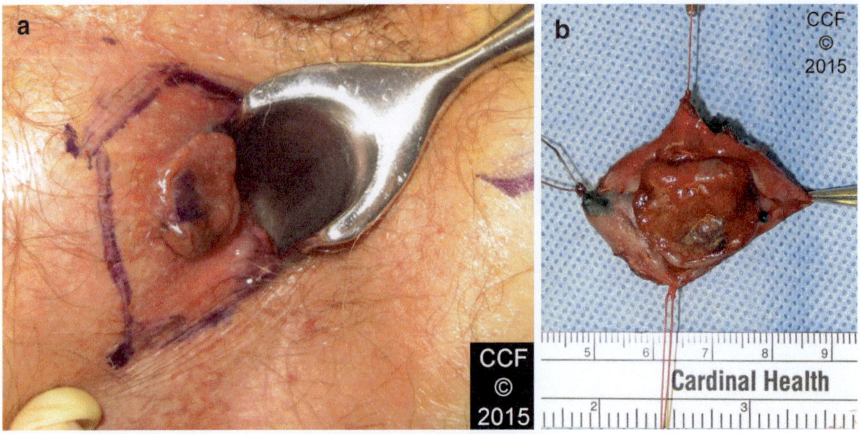

Fig. 42.2 (**a**) Perianal mass with circumferential 1 cm margins marked in ink; (**b**) excised specimen oriented with sutures of different length and color

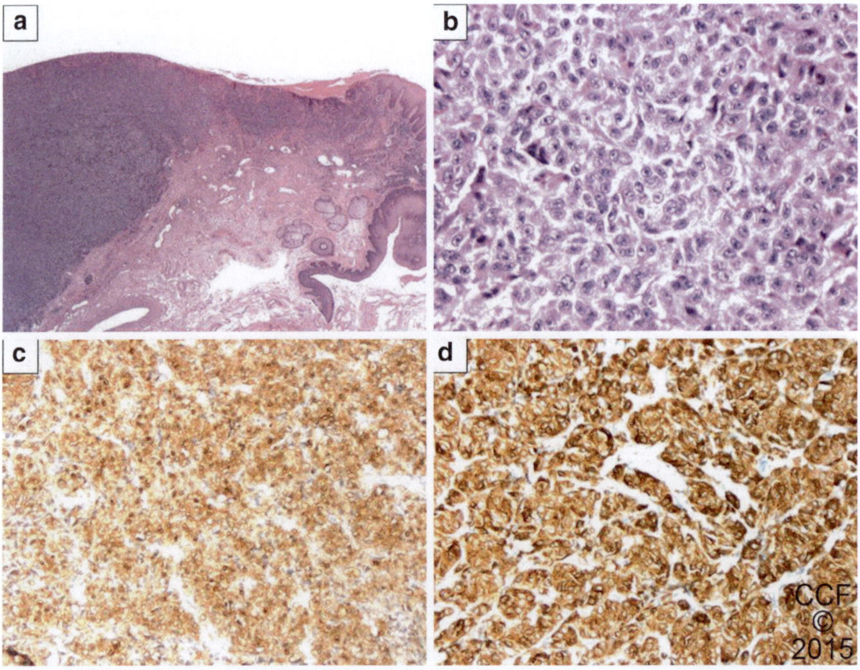

Fig. 42.3 Amelanotic melanoma. The perianal skin is remarkable for a nodular mass which extends into the deep dermis with overlying epidermal ulceration (**a**; H–E original magnification ×20). On high power, the malignant cells appear epithelioid to spindled in shape and have prominent macronucleoli (**b**; H–E original magnification ×400). The cells stain strongly and diffusely with immunohistochemical stains for S100 (**c**) and Melan-A (**d**) (original magnifications ×200)

Comment

The word melanoma is derived from the Greeks words "melas" (dark) and "oma" (tumor) [1]. The descriptive catalogue of the pathological specimens contained in the museum of the Royal College of Surgeons of England, Volume I, General Pathology, contains a section entitled *f. The Melanotic Variety of the Medullary Tumour or Soft Cancer* [2].

[Melanoma; Melanosis; True Melanosis]

> "All the specimens of melanotic disease in the Museum appear to be examples, either of tumours which, in addition to the general characteristics of medullary disease, present more or less of blackness from the deposit of colouring matter, like black pigment, in their substance; or of deposits of black colouring matter in the organs of persons in whom such tumours existed. The specimens in the following group are arranged according to the degrees in which the medullary substance which forms the basis of the tumour is blackened by the melanotic matter; so that they show several stages of transition from the pale nearly colourless tumour, through such as are, in deepening shades, mottled with grey, brown, or black, to those in which an intense blackness pervades the whole mass.
> 282. Sections of a tumour removed from behind the angle of a jaw. It is of an oval shape, smooth on its outer surface, and invested by a thin but dense and tough capsule. It measures nearly 3 inches in its chief diameter, and its interior is arranged in many lobes. Half of it is composed of a uniform pale, close textured, medullary substance. The other half, separated from the preceding by a definite line similar to others by which the tumour is partitioned into lobes, is composed of the same pale substance, mottled, in various and mingling shades grey and black, by melanotic matter."
> *Hunterian*

An account of the case was published by Sir Everard Home in his "Observations on Cancer." London, 1805. 8ve. P. 48, Case VIII [3].

> "A gentleman, about 35 years of age, had a tumour formed behind the angle of the lower jaw, which was considered as an enlarged lymphatic gland. This increased so much in size as to induce him to have it removed. Three years later, a second tumour was observed in nearly the same situation: this was slow in its increase, but gradually enlarged to the size of a pullet's egg. It was insensible to the touch, and gave neither pain nor uneasiness. While it was it this state he went to Vauxhall; and being engaged in a drunken squabble, received a violent blow with a stick upon the tumour. The blow produced no injury to the skin, but the tumour very rapidly increased, and in a few weeks had doubled its original size. It was removed by Mr. Hunter, and afterward examined. On making a section of it, the original tumour was white in its substance, and of an uniform texture; the part formed since the accident was spongy and soft, of a dark black appearance, resembling what is commonly termed a cancerous fungous excrescence; and an exact line, the whole breadth of the tumour, separated the two appearances."

In 1806, Laennec described black tumors of the lung as "melanoses" [4, 5].

Extrait du Mémoire de M. Laennec, sur les mélanôses	*Extracts of a memoire of M. Laennec, on melanoses*
M. *Laennec* a décrit sous ce nom dérivé du mot μξλοα, noir qui indique le caractère le plus saillant de la substance dont il s'agit, une des *matières morbifique visible* qui se rencontrent dans nos organes, et qui, quoique très différentes entre elles, sont ordinairement confondues sous les noms vagues d'obstructions, ou de squirrhes.	M. Laennec used the word melanoses, derived from the word, black, to indicate the most salient characteristic of the substance in question-one of the morbid visible materials that occur in our organs, and which, although very different from each other, are usually confused under the vague names of obstructions or hard cancers.

In 1857, Moore described a case of human melanosis of the anorectum [6].

"Melanosis of the rectum and anus is a circumstance of the greatest rarity, that has not hitherto been noticed by any writer on affections of that part of the body.

In the short abstract which we give of the patient at present in the Middlesex Hospital, whom we had the opportunity of again seeing on the 13th instant, the disease first affected the verge of the anus, was removed nearly two years ago, but has re-appeared higher up in the rectum.

Thomas M——, aged 65, was a patient in this hospital in May, 1855, with disease of the anus for upwards of two years. At this period, he had a black fungoid growth, situated at the right edge of the sphincter ani, in an ulcerated condition, and which bled freely. At this time, the disease did not extend far into the bowel, and it was excised by Mr. Moore on the 11th of May, a large portion of the external sphincter being removed. This was followed by recovery, with perfect control over the bowel. He remained tolerably well for upwards of a year, but began to suffer from a sensation of heat and bearing down in the middle of 1856; and as these symptoms increased, he again became a patient on the 15th of December last, under Mr. Moore's care. The rectum is now affected higher up, with no external manifestation of the disease.

When we last saw him, on the 13th instant, his pallor was extreme, with a slight yellowish tinge about the cheeks;... His debility seems extreme, and there can be no doubt the disease is spreading upwards, and possibly may recur in other parts of the body as well as the rectum."

In 1963, Morson and Volkstädt described the clinical features of 15 cases of malignant melanoma of the anal canal [7]. Bleeding was a common complaint. Misdiagnoses included cancer of the rectum, "piles," and epithelioma. The average survival rate was 15½ months. In 1996, Roumen described 63 cases of anorectal melanoma collected in the Netherlands [8]. Most tumors presented in an advanced stage due to the obscure location and lack of specific symptoms.

Two surgical options for anal melanoma often are considered, abdominoperineal resection (APR) and wide local excision (WLE). Treatment preferences include the following.

> "It is concluded that, in the future, patients presenting with an anorectal melanoma should be treated with a sphincter-saving surgical approach whenever possible."
>
> RMH Roumen, 1996 [9]

"Since the mortality rate is high, wide local excision offers the advantage of avoiding a permanent colostomy and should be considered the procedure of choice when excision is feasible."

Amara Malik, Tracy L. Hull, Crina Floruta, 2004 [10]

"The extent of surgical treatment is not associated with outcome in primary anorectal melanoma. Therefore, LE *(local excision)* of the primary tumor is recommended when technically feasible."

Jen Jen Yeh, Jinru Shia, Wen Jen Hwu,
Klaus J. Busam, Philip B. Paty, Jose G. Guillem,
et al., 2006 [11]

"Here we present a patient who was referred to the surgeon for treatment of hemorrhoids but was diagnosed with anal melanoma.

A wide local excision (WLE) including these lesions was performed with a margin of 2 cm, en bloc with 25% of the circumference of the rectal wall."

M. van't Riet, R. W. M. Giard, J. H. W. de Wilt,
and W. Vles, 2007 [12]

"Both APR (*abdominoperineal resection*) and LE (*local excision*) seem appropriate for anorectal melanoma provided clear margins can be achieved; prognosis is poor regardless of surgical approach."

P. J. Nilsson and B.K. Ragnarsson-Olding, 2010 [13]

"Survival of patients with anal melanoma is similar after local excision or rectal resection irrespective of whether patients have localized or regional stage of disease."

Ravi P. Kiran, Matteo Rottolo,
Naveen Pokola, Victor W. Fazio, 2010 [14]

"This study, the largest to analyze surgical treatment and outcomes for patients with anorectal melanoma in the USA, did not reveal a survival difference comparing TAE *(transanal excision)* and APR (*abdominoperineal resection)*."

Douglas M. Iddings, Ani J. Fleisig, Steven L. Chen, Mark B. Faries, Donald L. Morton, 2010 [15]

"The limited information available in the scientific literature on AM *(anal melanoma)* does not support the use of aggressive surgical procedures such as APR (*abdominoperineal resection*). A WLE (*wide local excision)* with negative margins is associated with equivalent survival."

Ari-Nareg Meguerditchian, Sarkis H. Meterissian,
Kelli Bullard Dunn, 2011 [16]

Biographical Notes

John Hunter, FRS (1728–1793)

AN ADDRESS
ON
THE UNVEILING OF THE STATUE OF
JOHN HUNTER BY PRINCESS CHRISTIAN.

By Sir James Paget, F. R. C. S., D.C.L., LL.D., F.R.S [17].

'It was in the year 1786, one hundred years ago, that John Hunter, after years and years of laborious toil, finished and arranged, the museum which he planted in Leicester Square, and then, for the first time, opened it to the public and his scientific friends; himself the curator, himself the demonstrator, himself the promoter of all the good work to which it could lead.

Becoming an insatiable collector, he at the same time became insatiable in the pursuit of knowledge. And everything that he collected he studied profoundly, till, to be brief, he ended in the completest study of everything living, or that had ever lived, and of all things living in health, or in disease. No man covered a wider range of ground than he did; no man studied with more care. I doubt whether, amongst all, could be found one who studied with more insight into facts, with more ingenuity and experiment, with more capacity of interpreting all he saw, with more caution, with more earnest desire to arrive at the truth, whatever it might be.

...I think, may be told more briefly, and seen more commonly, is that we owe to Hunter the habitual introduction of science into the study of surgery, and into its practice. Before his time, it was thought a decoration, an ornament, for a man if he knew some science; since the time of Hunter, it has been a necessary study for every man who is deemed even competent for practice. Since the time of Hunter, I think one might say the very language of science in relation to surgery has been, for the first time, adopted. Hunter's language was that in which the scientific truths of surgery could always best be expressed.

I know no one whose writings might be more studied for an example how, in the best scientific inquiry, the expressions of certainty are rare. His customary expressions are "I think there is reason to believe," "I am disposed to believe," "There is some evidence for holding," this or that; never such statements as "I am sure," "I have finally settled this." Hunter showed clearly that element of the scientific mind, the element of doubt—doubt repeated and prolonged, doubt justifying continual revision and fresh thought, doubt which, within the proper range of a man's own scientific study, it is better to hold and easier to maintain that complete belief.'

René Théophile Hyacinthe Laennec (1781–1826)

In addition to his description of melanoma, Laennec is credited with coining the word cirrhose (cirrhosis) in his description of liver disease published in the first volume of *De L'ausucultation Médiate* [18, 19].

p. 368	p.368
Le foie, réduit au tiers de son volume ordinaire, se trouvait, pour ainsi dire, caché dans la région qu'il occupe; sa surface externe, légèrement mamelonée et ridée, offrait une teinte grise-jaunâtre; incisé, il paraissait entièrement composé d'une multitude de petits grains de forme ronde ou ovoide, dont la grosseur variait depuis celle d'un grain de millet jusqu'à celle d'un grain de chenevis. Ces grains, faciles à séparer les uns des autres, ne laissaient entre eux presqu'aucun intervalle, dans lequel on pût distinguer encore quelque reste du tissu propre du foie; leur couleur était fauve ou d'un jaune roux, tirant par endroits sur le verdâtre; leur tissu, assez humide, opaque, était flasque au toucher plutôt que mou, et en pressant les grains entre les doigts, on n'en écrasait qu'une petite partie: le reste offrait au tact la sensation d'un morceau de cuir mou (a).	The liver, reduced to a third of its ordinary volume, so to speak, hidden in the region it occupies; its external surface, slightly hilly and wrinkled, had a gray-yellowish tint; incised. It appeared entirely composed of a multitude of small round or ovoid grains, the size of which varied from that of a grain of millet to that of a grain of hemp. These grains, easy to separate from each other, left almost no space between them, in which some remnant of the liver's own tissue could still be distinguished; their color was fawn or a reddish yellow, tending to greenish in places; their tissue, quite moist, opaque, was flaccid to the touch rather than soft, and by pressing the grains between the fingers, only a small part was crushed: the rest gave to the touch the sensation of a piece of leather soft (a).
(a) Cette espèce de production est encore du nombre de celles que l'on confound sous le nom de *squirrhe.* Je crois devoir la désigner sous le nom de *cirrhose*, à cause de sa couleur.	(a) This species of production is also one of those which we confound under the name of *squirrhe*. I think I should call it *cirrhose* (cirrhosis), because of its color. [20]

In addition, Laennec is credited with the invention of the stethoscope as well as authoring an authoritative treatise of the diseases of the chest.

De L'auscultation Médiate,
ou,
Traité du Diagnostic des Maladies
des Poumons et du Coeur,
fondé principalement sur ce nouveau moyen d'exploration
Par R. T. H. Laennec [21],
D. M. P., Médecin de l'Hòpital Necker,
Médecin honoraire des Dispensaires, Membre de la Societé de la Faculté de Médecine de Paris et de plusieurs autres sociétés nationales et étrangères
1819
De L'auscultation
Médiate

8. Je fus consulté, en 1816, pour une jeune personne qui présentait des symptômes généraux de maladie du cœur, et chez laquelle l'application de la main et la percussion donnaient peu de résultat à raison de l'embonpoint.
…je vins à me rappeler un phénomène d'acoustique fort connu: si l'on applique l'oreille à l'extrémité d'une poutre, on entend très distinctement un coup d'épingle donné à l'autre bout. J'imaginai que l'on pouvait peut-être tirer parti, dans le cas don't il s'agissait, de cette propriété des corps. Je pris un cahier de papier, j'en formai un rouleau fortement serré dont j'appliquai une extrémité sur la région précordiale, et posant l'oreille à l'autre bout, je fus aussi supris que satisfait d'entendre les battemens du cœur d'une manière beaucoup plus nette et plus distincte que je ne l'avais jamais fait par l'application immédiate de l'oreille.

9. Je présumai dès-lors que ce moyen pouvait devenir un méthode utile, et applicable non-seulement à l'etude des battemens du cœur, mais encore à celle de tous les mouvemens qui peuvent produire du bruit dans la cavité de la poitrine, et par conséquent à l'exploration de la respiration, de la voix, du râle, et peut-être même de la fluctuation d'un liquide épanché dans les plèvres ou le péricarde.

11. Le premier instrument dont j'aie fait usage était un cylindre ou rouleau de papier de seize linges de diamètre et d'un pied de longueur, formé de trois cahiers de papier battu, fortement serré, maintenu par papier collé, et applani à la lime aux deux extrémités. Quelque serré que soit un semblable rouleau, il reste toujours au centre un conduit de trois à quatre lignes de diamètres, dû à ce que les cahiers qui le composent ne peuvent se rouler complètement sur eux-mêmes. Cette circonstance fortuite m'a, comme on le verra, donné occasion de faire une observation importante: ce conduit est indispensable pour l'exploration de la voix. Un corps tout-à-fait plein est le meilleur instrument dont on puisse se servir pour l'exploration du cœur: il suffirait même pour celles de la respiration et du râle; cependent ces deux derniers phénomènes donnent plus d'intensité de son à l'aide d'un cylindre perforé et évasé à aon extrémité, jusqu'à la profondeur d'environ un pouce et demi, en forme d'enntonnoir.

13. Je me sers, en conséquence, actuellement d'un cylindre de bois percé dans son centre d'un tube de trois lingnes de diamètre et brisé au milieu à l'aide d'une vis, afin de le rendre plus portatif. L'une des pièces est évasée à son extrémité, à une profondeur d'environ un pouce et demi, en forme d'entonnoir. Le cylindre ainsi disposé est l'instrument qui convient pour l'exploration de la respiration et du râle. On le convertit en un simple tube à parois épaisses, pour l'exploration de la voix et des battemens du cœur, en introduisant dans l'entonnoir ou pavillon un *en-bout* de même bois qui le remplit exactement, et qui se fixe à l'aide d'un petit tube de cuivre qui le traverse et entre dans la tubulure du cylindre jusqu'à une certaine profondeur.

Je pense que si l'on veut lui donner un nom, celui qui conviendrait le mieux serait *stéthoscope*.

A Treatise on the Diseases of the Chest and on
Mediate Auscultation
By R. T. H Laennec, M.D.
Regius Professor of Medicine in the College of France,
Clinical Professor to the Faculty of Medicine of Paris,
Physician to Her Royal Highness the Duchess of Berri,
&c., &c, &c.
Translated from the latest French edition, with notes and a sketch of the author's life
By John Forbes, M. D. [22]
Member of the Royal College of Physicians, and Senior Physician to the Chichester Infirmary
On Diseases of the Chest

In 1816, I was consulted by a young woman laboring under general symptoms of diseased heart, and in whose case percussion and the application of the hand were of little avail on account of a great degree of fatness.
…I happened to recollect a simple and well-known fact in acoustics, and fancied, at the same time, that it might be turned to some use on the present occasion. The fact I allude to is the augmented impression of sound when conveyed through certain solid bodies,—as when we hear the scratch of a pin at one end of a piece of wood, on applying our ear to the other. Immediately, on this suggestion, I rolled a quire of paper into a kind of cylinder and applied one end of it to the region of the heart and the other to my ear, and was not little surprised and pleased, to find that I could thereby perceive the action of the heart in a manner much more clear and distinct than I ever have been able to do by the immediate application of the ear. From this moment I imagined that the circumstance might furnish means for enabling us to ascertain the character, not only of the action of the heart, but of every species of sound produced by the motion of all the thoracic viscera, and consequently, for the exploration of the respiration, the voice, *the rattle* or *rhonchus*, and perhaps even the fluctuation of fluid extravasated in the pleura or pericardium.

The first instrument which I used was a cylinder of paper, formed of three quires, compactly rolled together and kept in shape by paste. The longitudinal aperture which is always left in the center of the paper thus rolled, led accidentally in my hands, to an important discovery. This aperture is essential to exploration of the voice. A cylinder without any aperture is best for the exploration of the heart: the same kind of instrument will indeed suffice for the respiration and rattle; but both these are more distinctly perceived by means of a cylinder which is perforated throughout, and excavated into somewhat of a funnel-shape, at one of its extremities, to the depth of an inch and a half.
…I now employ a cylinder of wood, an inch and a half in diameter and a foot long, perforated longitudinally by a bore three lines wide, and hollowed out into a funnel-shape, to the depth of an inch and a half at one of its extremities. It is divided into two portions, partly for the convenience of carriage, and partly to permit its being used of half the usual length. The instrument in this form—that is, with the funnel-shaped extremity,—is used in exploring the respiration and rattle: when applied to the exploration of the heart and the voice, it is converted into a simple tube, with thick sides, by inserting into its excavated extremity a stopper or plug traversed by a small aperture, and accurately adjusted to the excavation. This instrument I have denominated *the Stethoscope*.

Explication des planches [21].
Figure 42.4 [Figure 1]. Le cylindre, réduit au tiers de ses dimensions naturelles.
(a) L'obturateur ou en-bout.
(b) Le corps inférieur de stéthoscope.
(c) Le corps supérieur.
(d) L'extrémité auriculaire ou destinée à être appliquée contre l'oreille.
Figure 42.4 [Figure 2]. Coupe du stéthoscope dans le sens de sa longueur.
(a) L'obturateur ou en-bout.
(b) Point de réunion des deux corps du cylindre.
(c) Le corps supérieur.
Figure 42.4 [Figure 3]. Cette figure représente la même coupe, l'obturateur étant enlevé.
(a) Corps supérieur ou auriculaire.
(b) Corps inférieur ou pectoral.
Figure 42.4 [Figure 4]. L'obturateur ou en-bout.
(c) Le corps de l'obturateur, fait de même bois que le reste du stéthescope.
(d) Petit tube de cuivre qui traverse l'en-bout et sert à le fixer dans le canal du stéthoscope.
Figure 42.4 [Figure 5]. Le corps supérieur du stéthoscope.
(a) Le corps du stéthescope.
(b) Vis an moyen de laquelle il s'articule avec le corps inférieur ou pectoral.
Figure 42.4 [Figure 6]. Diamètre réel du stéthoscope.
(a) Diamètre du canal du stéthoscope.

Explanation of the plates [22].
Figure 42.4 [Fig. 1]. The stethoscope, or cylinder, reduced to one-third its actual dimensions.
(a) The stopper
(b) The lower end
(c) The upper half
(d) The auricular or upper extremity.
Figure 42.4 [Fig. 2]. Longitudinal section of the same.
(a) The stopper
(b) Point of union of the two parts
(c) The upper half
Figure 42.4 [Fig. 3]. The same section with the stopper removed.
Figure 42.4 [Fig. 4]. The stopper
(a) The body of it, formed of the same wood as the rest of the instrument.
(b) Small brass tube traversing the stopper, for fixing it in the tube of the stethoscope.
Figure 42.4 [Fig. 5]. Upper half of the stethoscope.
(a) Body of it
(b) *Pin,* covered with leather or waxed thread, by which the two parts of the instrument are joined together.
Figure 42.4 [Fig. 6]. Actual diameter of the stethoscope.
(a) Diameter of the canal of the stethoscope.

Laennec's treatise included *Planche* Ire (Fig. 42.4) which shows the details of his stethoscope design.

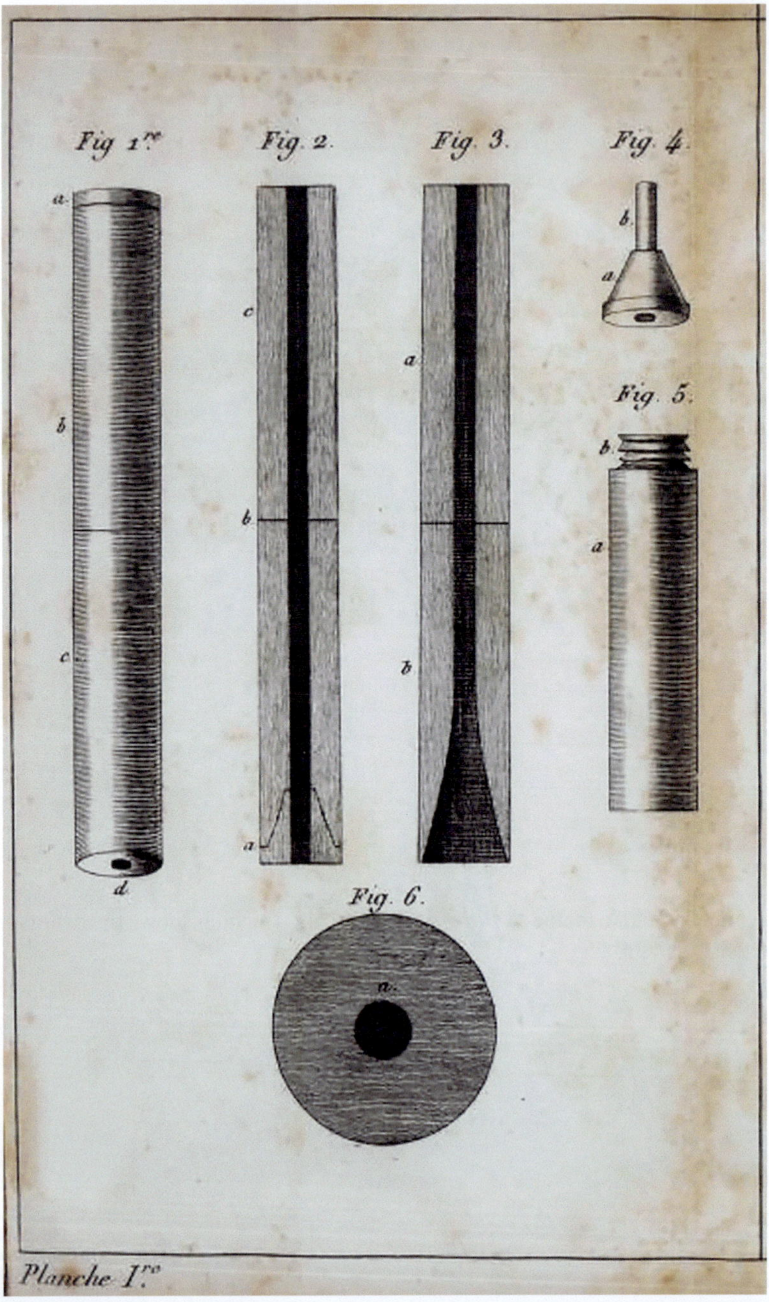

Fig. 42.4 Laennec's stethoscope design. Laennec RTH. De l'auscultation médiate, ou, Traité du diagnostic des maladies des poumons et du coeur, fondé principalement sur ce nouveau moyen d'exploration. Tome premier. A Paris. Chez J.-A. Brosson et J.-S. Chaudé. Libraires rue Pierre-Sarrazin, n°9, 1819. Accessed from Archive.org, March 13, 2022

References

1. Rebecca VW, Sondak VK, Smalley KSM. A brief history of melanoma: From mummies to mutations. Melanoma Res. 2012;22:114–22.
2. The Melanotic variety of the Medullary tumor or Soft Cancer. [Melanoma; Melanosis; True Melanosis]. The Royal College of Surgeons of England, Vol I, General Pathology. In: Descriptive Catalogue of the Pathological Specimens contained in the Museum of the Royal College of Surgeons of England. William Clowes and Sons, London, 1846. pp 128–129. Google Books, Accessed March 20, 2021.
3. Case VIII. In: Home E. Observations on Cancer connected with Histories of the Disease. London: Bulmer and Co. Cleveland Row, St. James's; 1805. p. 48–9. Archive.org, Accessed 16 Aug 2022.
4. Laënnec RTH, Extrait du mémoire de M. Laennec, sur les mélanôses. Bull École Méd (Paris), 1806;1:24–6.
5. Karamanou M, Stratigos AJ, Saridaki Z, Tsoucalas G, Androutsos G. René-Théophile-Hyacinthe Laennec (1781-1826) and the description of metastatic pulmonary melanoma. JBUON. 2015;20:354–6.
6. Moore. Recurrent melanosis of the rectum, after previous removal from the verge of the anus, in a man aged sixty-five. Lancet. 1857;69, Issue 1751:290.
7. Morson BC, Volkstädt H. Malignant melanoma of the anal canal. J Clin Path. 1963;16:126–32.
8. Roumen RM. Anorectal melanoma in The Netherlands: a report of 63 patients. Eur J Surg Oncol. 1996;22:598–601.
9. Roumen RM. Anorectal melanoma in The Netherlands: a report of 63 patients. Eur J Surg Oncol. 1996;22:598–601. The excerpt is reused with the generous permission of Elsevier, CCC I RightsLink™, License Number 5166161341009, License date Oct 11, 2021
10. Malik A, Hull TL, Floruta C. What is the best surgical treatment for anorectal melanoma? Int J Colorectal Dis. 2004;19:121–3. This excerpt is reused with the generous permission of Springer Nature, CCC I RightsLink®, License Number 5166170759872, license date Oct 11, 2021
11. Yeh JJ, Shia J, Hwu WJ, Busam KJ, Paty PB, Guillem JG, et al. The role of abdominoperineal resection as surgical therapy for anorectal melanoma. Ann Surg. 2006;244:1012–7. This excerpt is reused with the generous permission of Wolters Kluew Health, Inc., CCC I RightsLink®, License Number 5166001081845, License date Oct 11, 2021
12. van't Riet M, Giard RWM, de Wilt JHW, Vles W. Melanoma of the anus disguised as hemorrhoids: Surgical management illustrated by a case report. Dig Dis Sci. 2007;52:1745–7. These excerpts are reused with the generous permission of Springer Nature, CCC I RightsLinks®, License Number 5173830398042, License date Oct 21, 2021
13. Nilsson PJ, Ragnarsson-Olding BK. Importance of clear resection margins in anorectal malignant melanoma. Br J Surg. 2010;97:98–103. This excerpt is reused with the generous permission of Oxford University Press, CCC I RightsLink®, License Number 5166421455149, License date Oct 12, 2021
14. Kiran RP, Rottoli M, Pokola N, Fazio VW. Long-term outcomes after local excision and radical surgery for anal melanoma: Data from a population database. Dis Colon Rectum. 2010;53:402–8. This excerpt is reused with the generous permission of Wolters Kluwer Health, Inc., CCC I RightsLink®, License Number 5166080281288, License date Oct 11, 2021
15. Iddings DM, Fleisig AJ, Chen SL, Faries MB, Morton DL. Practice patterns and outcomes for anorectal melanoma in the USA, reviewing three decades of treatment: Is more extensive surgical resection beneficial in all patients? Ann Surg Oncol. 2010;17:40–4. This excerpt is reused with the generous permission of Springer Nature, CCC I RightsLink®, License number 5166091065848, License Date Oct 11, 2021

16. Meguerditchian A-N, Meterissian SH, Dunn KB. Anorectal melanoma: Diagnosis and treatment. Dis Colon Rectum. 2011;54:638–44. The excerpt is reused with the generous permission of Wolters Kluwer Health, Inc., CCC |RightsLink®, License Number 5166081017645; License date Oct 11, 2021
17. Paget J. An address on the unveiling of the statue of John Hunter by Princess Christian. Br Med J. 1886;i:1093–5.
18. Braillon A. Laennec's cirrhosis. Lancet. 2019;393(10167):131–2.
19. Laennec RTH. De L'auscultation Médiate, ou, Traité du Diagnostic des Maladies des Poumons et du Coeur, fondé principalement sur ce nouveau moyen d'exploration. Tome premier. A Paris, Chez J.-A. Brosson et J.-S. Chaudé, Libraires, rue Pierre-Sarrazin, n°9, 1819:368. Accessed from Archive.org, March 13, 2022.
20. The etymology of the word cirrhosis is: "New Latin, from Greek *kirrhos* orange-colored. "Cirrhosis." Merriam-Webster.com Dictionary, Merriam-Webster, https://www.merriamwebster.com/dictionary/cirrhosis. Accessed 7 Jan.2024.
21. Laennec RTH. De l'auscultation médiate, ou, Traité du diagnostic des maladies des poumons et du coeur, fondé principalement sur ce nouveau moyen d'exploration. Tome premier. A Paris, Chez J.-A. Brosson et J.-S. Chaudé, Libraires, rue Pierre-Sarrazin, no9, 1819:7–11, Explication des Planches. Accessed from Archive.org, March 13, 2022.
22. Laennec RTH. A treatise on diseases of the chest and on mediate auscultation. Translated by John Forbes, published by Samuel Wood & Sons, and Collins & Hannay. Philadelphia,—John Grigg, and G. Auner. R. & G. S. Wood, Printers, 1830:4–7, 721. Accessed in Google Books, March 13, 2022.

Presacral Dermoid

43

Carolyn L. Power, Luca Stocchi, Homer O. Wiland, Eric W. Willis, and James S. Wu

Presentation

A 48-year-old woman was referred for evaluation of a rectal mass.

Assessment

A nontender posterior rectal mass close to the tip of the coccyx was palpated on digital examination. Magnetic resonance imaging was done (Fig. 43.1).

C. L. Power · J. S. Wu (✉)
Department of Colon and Rectal Surgery, Cleveland Clinic, Cleveland, OH, USA

L. Stocchi
Department of Colon and Rectal Surgery, Mayo Clinic, Jacksonville, FL, USA

H. O. Wiland
Department of Pathology, OhioHealth Mansfield Hospital, Mansfield, OH, USA

E. W. Willis
Department of Pathology, CORPath, Columbus, OH, USA

J. S. Wu, M. D. Inkster (eds.), *Cleveland Clinic Colorectal Case Studies*,
https://doi.org/10.1007/978-3-031-39880-3_43

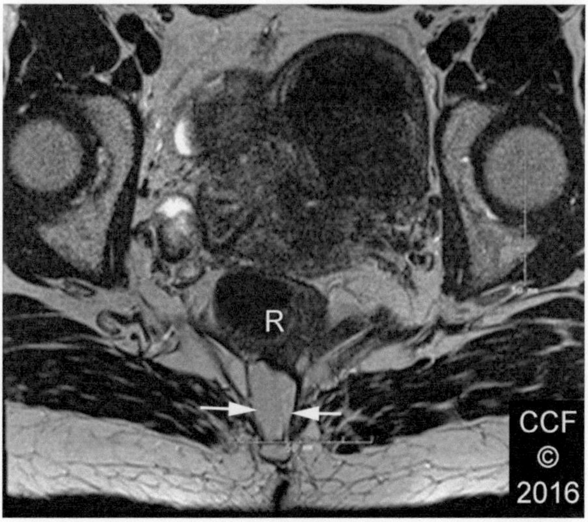

Fig. 43.1 MRI showed a fat-filled retrorectal cystic mass (arrows) abutting the adjacent rectum (R) without notable signs of invasion

Management

En bloc resection of the cyst and coccyx was performed using a posterior approach in the Kraske position. A midline incision was made just caudal to the distal part of the coccyx (Fig. 43.2). The sphincter muscle fibers were close to the distal portion of the cyst (Fig. 43.3). Following circumferential dissection around the cyst, which measured 3–4 cm, the coccyx was dissected and transected off the sacrum. The excised specimen is shown in Fig. 43.4. The sphincter, rectum, and mesorectum were entirely preserved.

The final pathological diagnosis was ruptured dermoid cyst (Fig. 43.5).

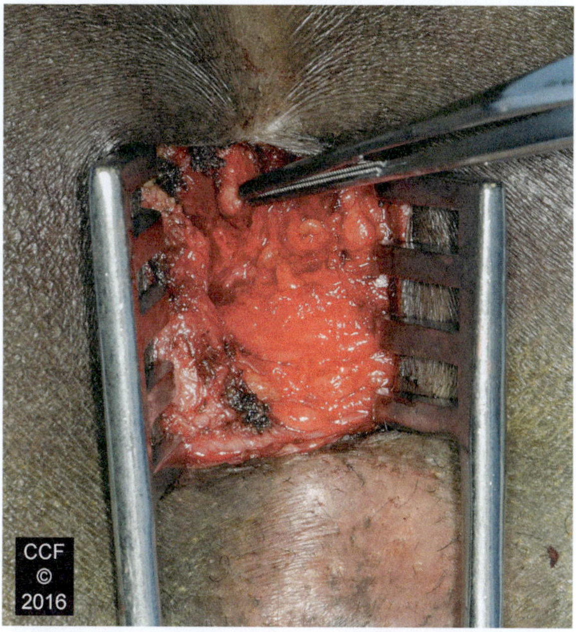

Fig. 43.2 Through a midline incision, the tip of coccyx (forceps) is exposed

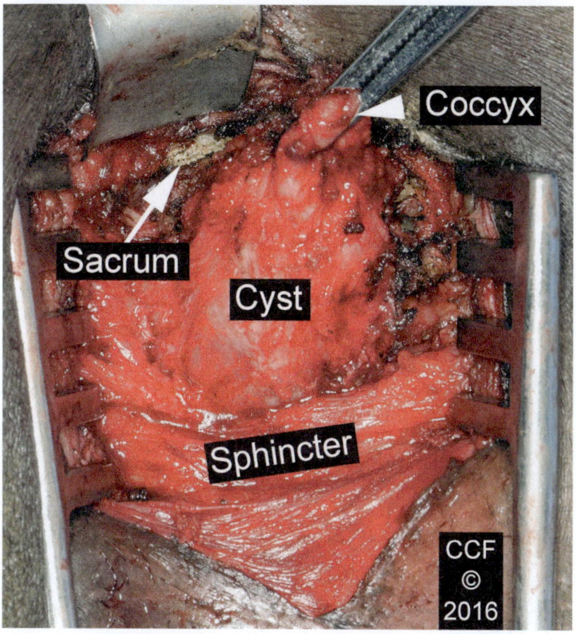

Fig. 43.3 The coccyx (arrow/clamp) has been transected off the sacrum. The presacral cyst has been partially dissected free from the sphincter muscle

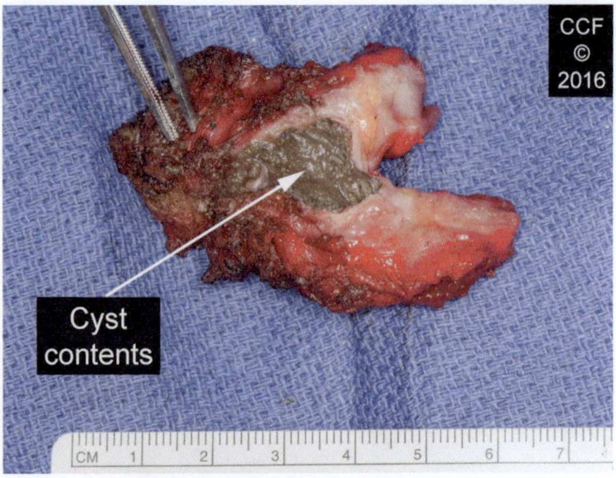

Fig. 43.4 The opened resected specimen. The cyst contents are indicated by the arrow

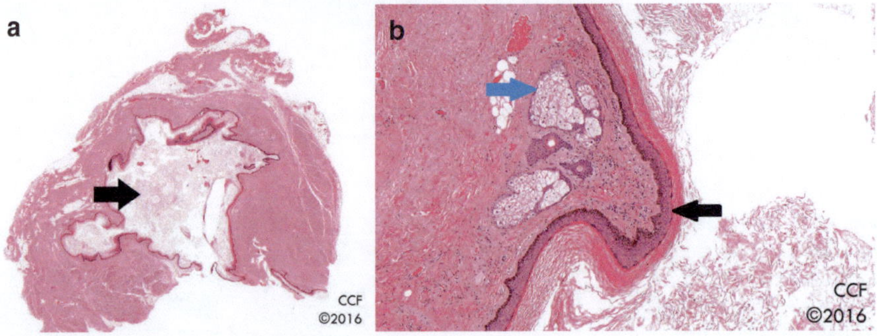

Fig. 43.5 (**a**) Low power view of the retrorectal cyst shows a well-developed cystic space (arrow) set within a muscular wall (H–E, original magnification ×1). (**b**) Higher power view of the cyst lining shows a stratified squamous mucosa with hyperkeratosis and luminal keratin debris. The wall of the cyst shows adnexal structures including sebaceous glands. The findings are those of a dermoid cyst (H–E, original magnification ×40)

Comment

Retrorectal tumors are heterogeneous. Types include congenital, inflammatory, neurogenic, osseous, and other less common variants. Benign and malignant lesions occur both in children and in adults. Complete resection is standard treatment. Surgical approaches are abdominal, perineal, or combined abdominoperineal. The perineal-only approach utilized in this case usually is used for tumors caudal to S4 [1, 2]. The trans-coccygeal approach to the rectum was described by Kraske in 1885 [3]. At the time, it was a revolutionary advance in rectal cancer surgery because it allowed mobilization of the tumor and the tumor-bearing segment of intestine without the benefit of general anesthesia, antibiotics, bowel preparation, or blood transfusion. His technique is still used to gain access to tumors located in the retrorectal space.

Zur Exstirpation hochsitzender Mastdarmkrebse. Von Prof. Dr. P. Kraske [4] In Freiburg Die Operation führte ich an der Leiche in folgender Weise aus: An dem auf der rechten Seite liegenden Cadaver machte ich in der Mittellinie etwa von der Mitte des Kreuzbeins bis zum After einen Schnitt bis auf der Knochen. Darauf löste ich die Glutäälmusculatur an ihrer Insertion von dem untersten Theile des linken Kreuzbeinflügels ab, umschnitt und excidirte das Steissbein und durchtrennte nun den untersten Theil des nach Anspannung des äusseren Wundrandes frei zu Tage tretenden Lig. tuberoso-sacrum und darunter das Lig. spinoso-sacrum dicht an deren Anheftung am Kreuzbein. Schon als ich die Bänder durchschnitten hatte und mir die Weichtheile mit scharfen Wundhaken kräftig nach aussen ziehen liess, war ich überrascht, wie weit ich mit dem Finger von unten und von der Seite her auf der inneren Fläche des Kreuzbeines vordringen und den durch lockeres Zellgewebe angehefteten Mastdarm ablösen konnte.	Concerning extirpation of high sitting rectal cancer by Professor Dr. P. Kraske Freiburg I performed the operation in a cadaver in the following manner. With the cadaver lying on the right side, I made an incision in the midline of the sacrum to the anus down to the bone. Then I raised the gluteus muscle to its insertion of the lowest part of the left sacral wing, cut around and excised the coccyx and then severed the underlying ligamentum tuberosacrum and spinososacrum close to their attachments to the sacrum. When I divided the bands and retracted outward, I was surprised, how wide my finger was able to penetrate from below and sideways the inner surface of the sacrum and could detach the loose connective tissue of the rectum.

Biographical Note [5]

Paul Kraske (1851–1930)

Paul Kraske was born in 1851 in Berg b. Muskau. He received his surgical training with Richard v. Volkmann. At the age of 32, he became Director of the Surgical Clinic in Freiburg. As surgical scientist, he demonstrated the feasibility of the transcoccygeal approach to rectal cancer in cadavers first. As a military surgeon during World War I, he strongly advocated early laparotomy for abdominal trauma. He was beloved by his students as noted by Oehler writing his obituary:

Prof. Paul Kraske Mit seinen vielen Schülern fühlte er sich zeitlebens eng verbunden. Sie sahen in dankbarer Ehrfurcht zu ihm empor und wuβten seinen Rat sehr zu schätzen. Wir, die wir seine Schüler waren, werden uns seiner kraftvollen Persōnlichkeit allezeit dankbar und in Verehrung erinnern. J. Oehler, Hannover, 1930 [6]	**Prof. Paul Kraske** He felt a lifelong link to his many students who appreciated and treasured his advice. We, who were his students, will always remember his powerful personality with gratitude and admiration. J. Oehler, Hannover, 1930

References

1. Messick CA, Hull T, Rosselli G, Kiran RP. Lesions originating within the retrorectal space: A diverse group requiring individualized evaluation and surgery. J Gastrointest Surg. 2013;17:2143–52.
2. Glasgow SC, Dietz DW. Retrorectal tumors. Clin Colon Rectal Surg. 2006;19:61–8.
3. Kraske P, Perry EG, Hinrichs B. A new translation of professor Dr. P. Kraske's Zur Exstirpation Hochsitzender Mastdarmkrebse. 1885. Aust N Z J Surg 1989;59:421–4.
4. Kraske P. Zur Extirpation hochsitzender Mastdarmkrebse. Verhandlung Tagung Deutsch Gesell Chir 1885;14:464–74.
5. Corman ML. Classic articles in colonic and rectal surgery: Paul Kraske, 1851–1930.
6. Oehler J. Prof. Paul Kraske. Zentralbl Chir. 1930;57:1777–8.

44 Thrombosed External Hemorrhoids-Observation

James S. Wu

Presentation

A 64-year-old male had diarrhea due to the "flu." Four days later, he developed severe anal pain and bulging hemorrhoids. Examination beyond inspection was not possible (Fig. 44.1).

J. S. Wu (✉)
Department of Colon and Rectal Surgery, Cleveland Clinic, Cleveland, OH, USA

J. S. Wu, M. D. Inkster (eds.), *Cleveland Clinic Colorectal Case Studies*,
https://doi.org/10.1007/978-3-031-39880-3_44

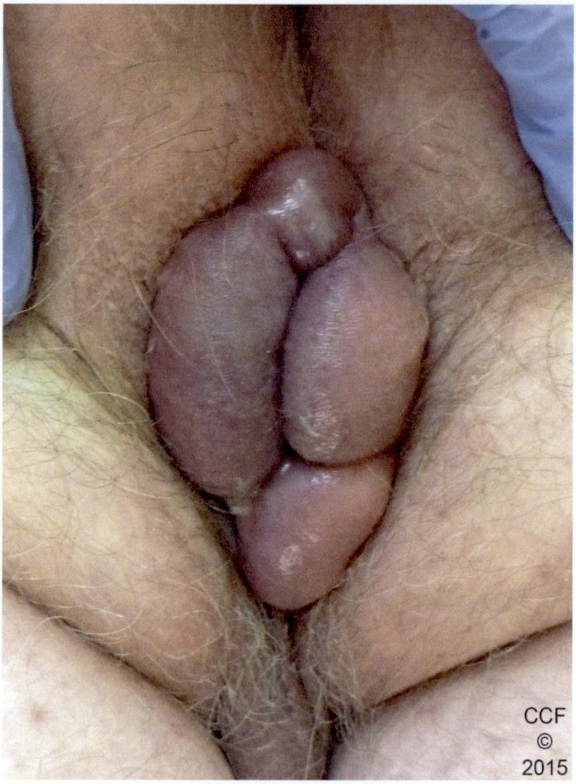

Fig. 44.1 Massive acutely thrombosed external hemorrhoids

Management

Oral analgesics were administered for pain management. The patient was instructed to sit in warm water twice a day and as needed. Topical 2% diltiazem (a calcium channel blocker) ointment was prescribed for application to the perianal skin in the morning, at night, and before bowel movements. Fiber and stool softeners were recommended to avoid constipation or diarrhea. Resolution of pain and thrombosis occurred gradually and steadily over a period of several weeks (Fig. 44.2).

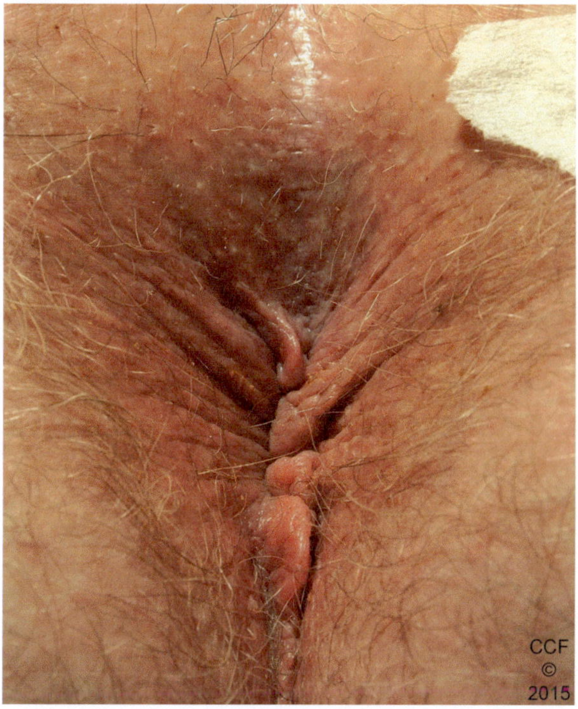

Fig. 44.2 The appearance of the perianal skin 6 weeks after initial presentation

Comment

Because of the extensive nature of the thrombosis and because the skin was viable, nonoperative therapy was chosen. Internal sphincter spasm was treated with heat and a topical smooth muscle relaxant. Topical nitrates and calcium channel blockers decrease internal anal sphincter hypertonicity. The medication is applied several times a day. Application before bowel movements relaxes the sphincter before defecation. Warm sitz baths or tub soaks accomplish the same objective. Fiber is taken to bulk the stool. In this case, resolution of symptoms and thrombosis occurred slowly but steadily without surgery [1–3]. Flexible endoscopy was done in follow-up to exclude a mucosal disorder.

References

1. Perrotti P, Antropoli C, Molino D, De Stefano G, Antropoli M. Conservative treatment of acute thrombosed external hemorrhoids with topical nifedipine. Dis Colon Rectum. 2001;44:405–9.
2. Silverman R, Bendick PJ, Wasvary HJ. A randomized, prospective, double-blind, placebo-controlled trial of the effect of calcium channel blocker ointment on pain after hemorrhoidectomy. Dis Colon Rectum. 2005;48:1913–6.
3. Gebbensleben O, Hilger Y, Rohde H. Do we at all need surgery to treat thrombosed external hemorrhoids? Results of a prospective cohort study. Clin Exp Gastroenterol. 2009;2:69–74.

Thrombosed External Hemorrhoid-Excision

45

James S. Wu and Kenneth G. Kula

Presentation

A 52-year-old man developed a painful anal lump while straining at stool. He was seen a day later. He appeared distressed. He could/would not sit down. Examination showed a tender perianal mass (Fig. 45.1).

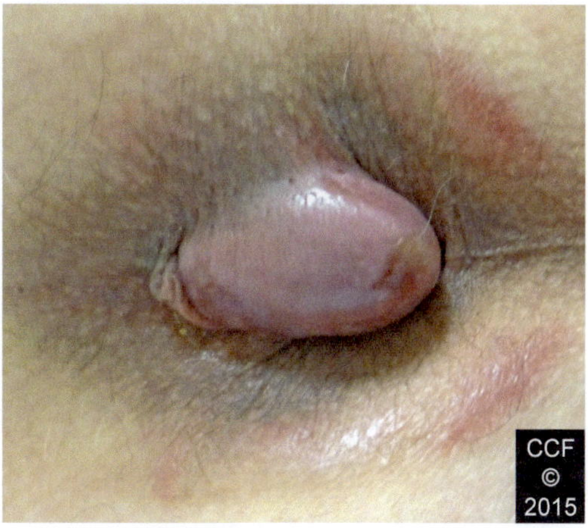

Fig. 45.1 A tender anal mass appeared suddenly after straining at stool

J. S. Wu (✉)
Department of Colon and Rectal Surgery, Cleveland Clinic, Cleveland, OH, USA

K. G. Kula
Center for Medical Art and Photography, Cleveland Clinic, Cleveland, OH, USA

J. S. Wu, M. D. Inkster (eds.), *Cleveland Clinic Colorectal Case Studies*,
https://doi.org/10.1007/978-3-031-39880-3_45

Management

The patient has an acute thrombosed external hemorrhoid. The hemorrhoidal clot was removed under local anesthesia with immediate relief of symptoms. After cleaning the surgical site, the skin overlying the hemorrhoid was injected with a local anesthetic (Fig. 45.2). The skin overlying the thrombosed hemorrhoid was incised exposing the clot (Fig. 45.3). A cruciate incision was used in order to delay skin closure and prevent clot re-accumulation. The clot was mobilized by squeezing the base of the hemorrhoid between the thumb and forefinger. The extracted clot is seen in Fig. 45.4. Figure 45.5 shows the hemorrhoid excision site after clot removal.

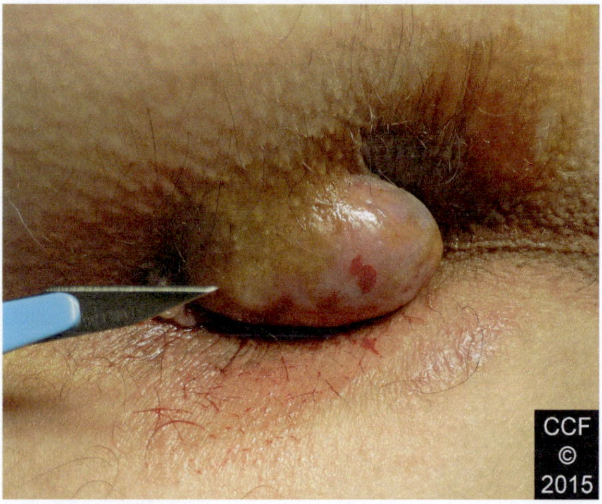

Fig. 45.2 The skin overlying the thrombosed external hemorrhoid has been cleansed and injected with local anesthetic (note red injection sites). A No. 11 blade is at the ready

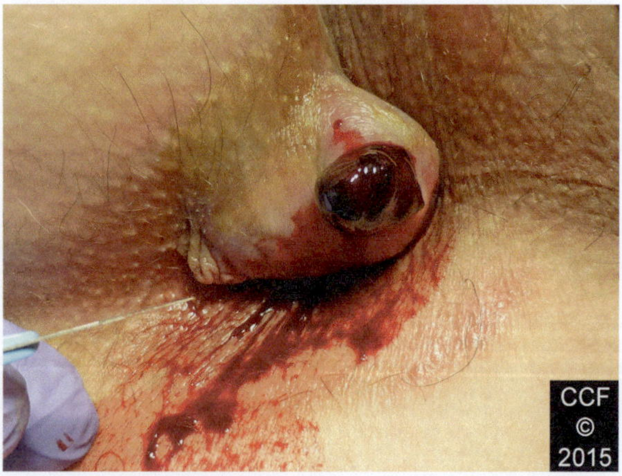

Fig. 45.3 The skin overlying the thrombosis has been incised. The clot bulges at the incision site

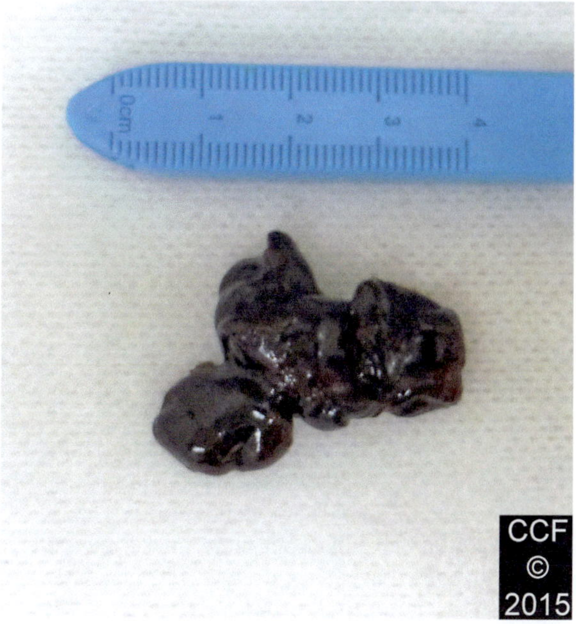

Fig. 45.4 The excised clot

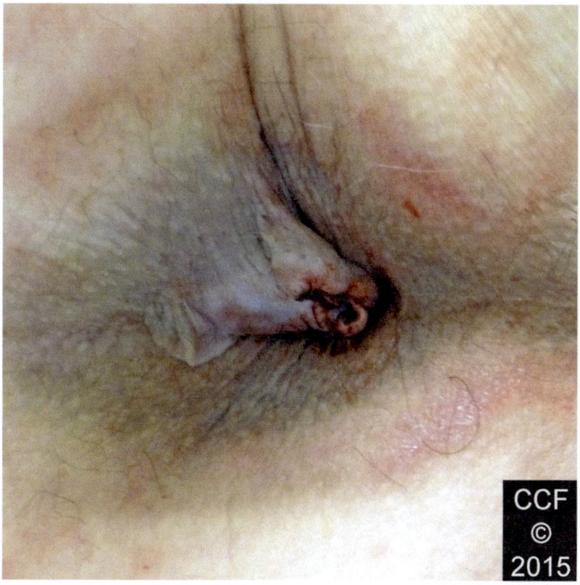

Fig. 45.5 The surgical site following clot removal

Comment

External hemorrhoidal thrombosis presents as an acute painful lump around the anus that cannot be reduced. Management can be by surgical excision or by observation (Fig. 45.6). Indications for surgery include: pain in the acute situation or skin

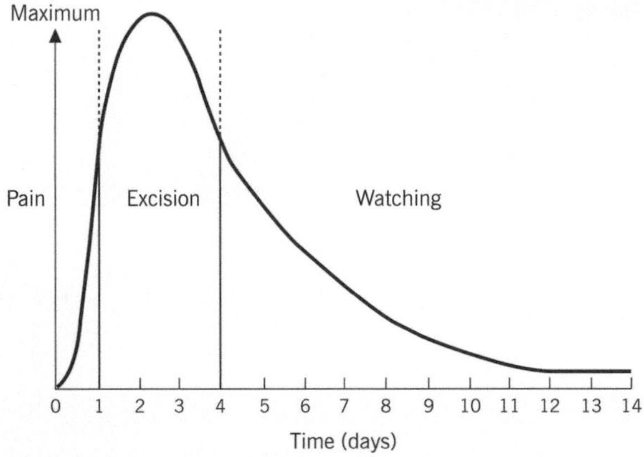

Fig. 45.6 Pain is maximal immediately after the appearance of the thrombosed external hemorrhoid. Surgical excision during this period results in immediate pain relief (graph courtesy of Victor W. Fazio, AO, MS)

perforation. When pain abates, observation is appropriate. Without surgery, most thrombosed hemorrhoids eventually resolve [1].

Increased dietary fiber and fluid intake may alleviate the tendency to strain at stool and help prevent recurrence. Flexible endoscopy is done in follow-up to exclude a rectal mucosal disorder.

Reference

1. Rivadeneira DE, Steele SR, Ternent C, Chalasani S, Buie WD, Rafferty JL, et al. Practice parameters for the management of hemorrhoids (revised 2010). Dis Colon Rectum. 2011;54:1059–64.

46 Hemorrhoid Banding

James S. Wu and Michelle D. Inkster

Presentation

A patient requested treatment of a hemorrhoid that prolapses with straining but can be reduced manually (Fig. 46.1). Office hemorrhoidal elastic band ligation was done (Fig. 46.2). Banding can also be done at the time of flexible endoscopy as shown in Fig. 46.3.

J. S. Wu (✉)
Department of Colon and Rectal Surgery, Cleveland Clinic, Cleveland, OH, USA

M. D. Inkster
Department of Gastroenterology, Cleveland Clinic, Cleveland, OH, USA

J. S. Wu, M. D. Inkster (eds.), *Cleveland Clinic Colorectal Case Studies*,
https://doi.org/10.1007/978-3-031-39880-3_46

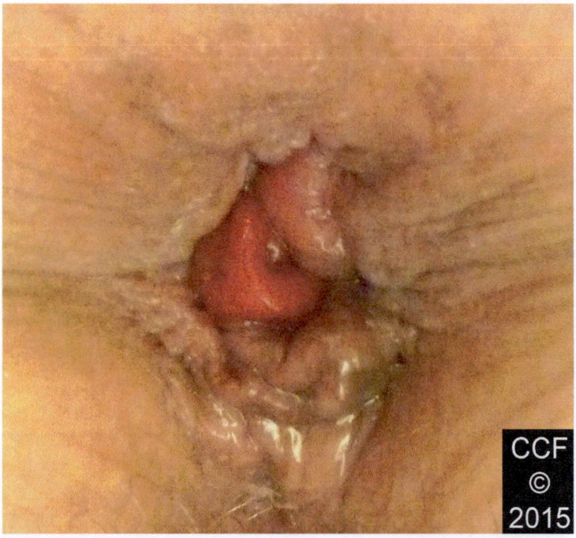

Fig. 46.1 Third-degree prolapsing internal hemorrhoid

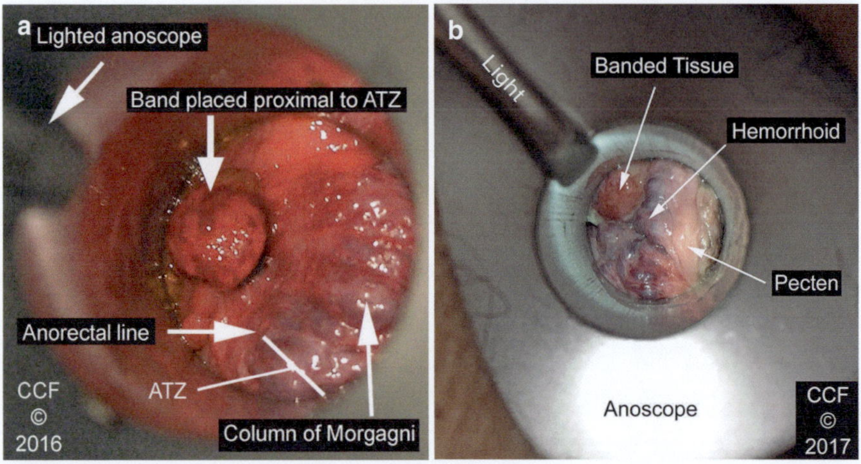

Fig. 46.2 (**a**, **b**) Photographs taken through a lighted beveled anoscope. The band is placed proximal to the sensate anal transitional zone (ATZ) whose borders are the anorectal line (the proximal border of the ATZ) and the dentate line. Within the ATZ are the internal hemorrhoids and the column/sinuses of Morgagni. Distal to the ATZ is the pecten

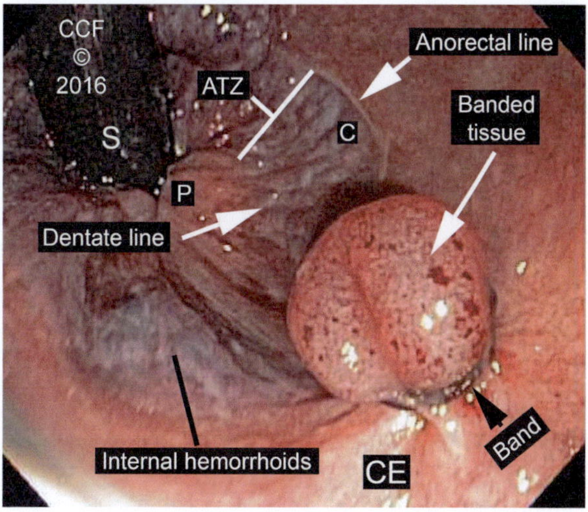

Fig. 46.3 Endoscopic internal hemorrhoidal banding. A band has been placed proximal to the ATZ and the anorectal line. The dentate line, pecten (P), and a column of Morgagni (C) have been labeled. The vascular tissue within the ATZ are the internal hemorrhoids. *CE* columnar epithelium; *S* Scope

Comment [1]

In 400 BC, Hippocrates described hemorrhoids as follows [2]:

On Hemorrhoids

"The disease of the hemorrhoids is formed in this way: if bile or phlegm be determined to the veins in the rectum, it heats the blood in the veins; and these veins becoming heated attract blood from the nearest veins, and being gorged the inside of the gut swells outwardly, and the heads of the veins are raised up, and being at the same time bruised by the faeces passing out, and injured by the blood collected in them, they squirt out blood, most frequently along with the faeces but sometimes without faeces [1]."

In 1937, Louis J. Hirschman, 1912 president of the American Proctologic Society, (subsequently the American Society of Colon and Rectal Surgeons) published *Synopsis of Ano-rectal Diseases*, a concise summary by a master surgeon [3].

Concerning hemorrhoids he opined:

CHAPTER XII
HEMORRHOIDS

> "We see more quack advertising about, more nostrum remedies sold for, more irregular practitioners promising to cure hemorrhoids than any other disease.
>
> There must be several reasons for this, and these reasons are: the lack of instruction to the medical student on the subject of rectal disease, in the first place; the paucity of such instruction when given as an incident in the teaching of general surgery; the repugnance with which the average practitioner approaches a case requiring rectal examination; the cursory character of such examination; the distaste of the average practitioner for local treatment of the anorectal region; the inability to make a correct diagnosis; and the superficial treatment given and the early discharge of the patient by the practitioner, who is anxious to get rid of a case that is unpleasant for him to treat—."

In 1907, W. C. Brinkerhoff in his book entitled *Diseases of the Rectum: Their consequences and non-surgical treatment*, stated concerning the management of hemorrhoids [4]:

> "There is no good reason why, in the treatment of hæmorrhoids, commonly called piles, suffering should be added to suffering in order that suffering may be cured."

In 1958, Blaisdell described an office procedure for the ligation of hemorrhoids [5].

The author remarked that:

> "…application was strictly limited to internal hemorrhoids. Such restriction renders this office technique possible because the area of the internal hemorrhoids is, of course, wholly insensitive."[1]

The technique involved placement of a ligature at the base of the internal hemorrhoid.

Barron noted that Blaisdell's first ligating instruments used silk as the ligation material and that this led to an increased incidence of delayed bleeding. In 1963, Barron introduced:

> "…the use of rubber bands which provide a much longer period of hemostasis by compression which persists until sloughing of the hemorrhoids is complete."

Barron's recommended band placement site is shown in Fig. 46.4 [6]. Specifically, he states that,

"Care must be taken not to include the stratified squamous and transitional epithelium in the ligating bands because they contain sensory nerve fibers."[7]

Modestly, he referred to his technique as a modification of the "Blaisdell method of ligation."

[1] Blaisdell [5]. Reprinted with permission from Mr. Spencer Dimmick, the Journal of the American College of Surgeons, formerly Surgery Gynecology & Obstetrics, August 30, 2021.

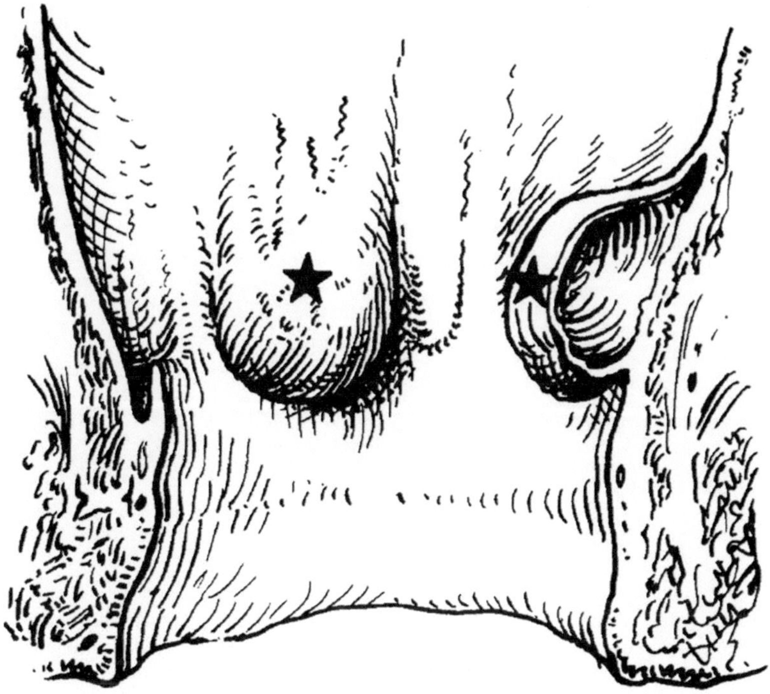

Fig. 46.4 In this drawing, Barron identifies the best site for rubber band placement with stars. Reproduced with permission. James Barron. Office ligation treatment of hemorrhoids. Diseases of the Colon & Rectum; Wolter Kluwer Health, Inc.; License number 5116690798856; License date Jul 26, 2021

Figure 46.5 illustrates the banding technique.

The 2001 American Society of Colon and Rectal Surgeons classification of hemorrhoids is shown in Table 46.1.[2]

The concept behind hemorrhoidal banding is suspension. The procedure works for hemorrhoids that bleed and do not prolapse or bleed and prolapse and can be replaced either spontaneously or by manually back into the anal canal.

[2] Rivadeneira et al. [8]. Permission to reproduce this excerpt was generously provided by Wolters Kluwer Health, Inc., CCC|RightsLink License Number 5124731454040; License date Aug 9, 2021.

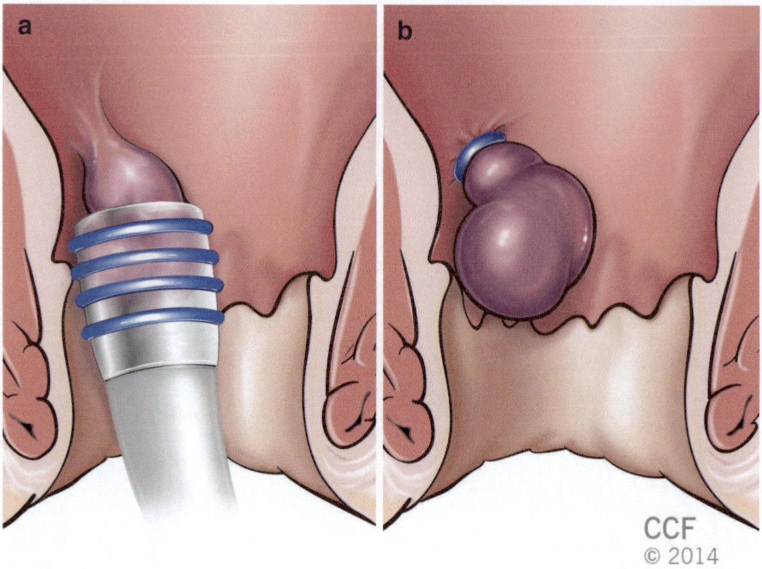

Fig. 46.5 Left upper frame. The tissue to be banded is seen; (**a**) a cylinder with rubber bands stretched over it approaches the tissue to be banded; (**b**) the tissue to be banded is brought into the cylinder; (**c**) the band is released from the cylinder at the base of the tissue to be banded

Table 46.1 Classification of internal hemorrhoids

Grade	Physical findings
I	Prominent hemorrhoidal vessels, no prolapse
II	Prolapse with Valsalva and spontaneous reduction
III	Prolapse with Valsalva requires manual reduction
IV	Chronically prolapsed manual reduction ineffective

There are several complications associated with hemorrhoidal banding. Band placement involving the sensate anoderm may cause immediate pain, sometimes with a vasovagal reaction (bradycardia, arteriolar dilatation) [9]. Immediate band removal reverses the symptoms. Bleeding may occur if a band either falls off or cuts through the banded tissue prematurely. Anal/pelvic floor spasm can lead to urinary retention. A rare but potentially lethal complication of hemorrhoidal banding is perineal sepsis (Fournier's gangrene) [10, 11].

References

1. Holley CJ. History of hemorrhoidal surgery. South Med J. 1946;39:536–41.
2. Hippocrates. On hemorrhoids. Translated by Francis Adams. Internet Classics Archive. http://classics.mit/edu//Hippocrates/hemmor.html (Accessed 25 Oct 2019).
3. Hirschman LJ. Synopsis of ano-rectal diseases. C.V. Mosby: St. Louis, MO; 1937. p. 186.
4. Brinkerhoff WC. Diseases of the Rectum: Their consequences and non-surgical treatment. Chicago, IL: Orban Publishing Co.; 1907. p. 6.
5. Blaisdell PC. Prevention of massive hemorrhage secondary to hemorrhoidectomy. Surg Gynecol Obstet. 1958;106:485–8.
6. Barron J. Office ligation treatment of hemorrhoids. Dis Colon Rectum. 1963;6:109–13.
7. Barron J. Office ligation of internal hemorrhoids. Am J Surg. 1963;105:563–70.
8. Rivadeneira DE, Steele ST, Ternent C, Chalasani S, Buie WD, Rafferty JL. Standards Practice Task Force of the American Society of Colon and Rectal Surgeons. Practice parameters for the management of hemorrhoids (revised 2010). Dis Colon Rectum. 2011;54:1059–64.
9. van Lieshout JJ, Wieling W, Karemaker JM, Eckberg DL. The vasovagal response. Clin Sci. 1991;81:575–86.
10. Bat L, Melzer E, Koler M, Dreznick Z, Shemesh E. Complications of rubber band ligation of symptomatic internal hemorrhoids. Dis Colon Rectum. 1993;36:287–90.
11. McCloud JM, Jameson JS, Scott AND. Life-threatening sepsis following treatment for haemorrhoids: a systematic review. Colorectal Dis. 2006;8:748–55.

Hemorrhoid Sclerosis

47

Stephen Brandstetter and James S. Wu

Presentation

A patient underwent colonoscopy because of anorectal bleeding. Retroflexion showed evidence of recent hemorrhage from the distal anorectum (Fig. 47.1).

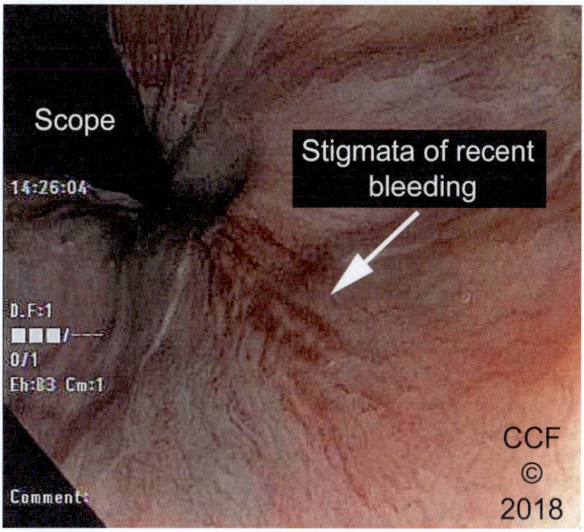

Fig. 47.1 Retroflexed view of the anorectum shows evidence of recent hemorrhage (arrow)

S. Brandstetter
Department of Colon and Rectal Surgery, Cleveland Clinic Akron General Hospital, Akron, OH, USA

J. S. Wu (✉)
Department of Colon and Rectal Surgery, Cleveland Clinic, Cleveland, OH, USA

J. S. Wu, M. D. Inkster (eds.), *Cleveland Clinic Colorectal Case Studies*,
https://doi.org/10.1007/978-3-031-39880-3_47

Management

Injection sclerosis with hypertonic saline was done[1] (Figs. 47.2a–c).

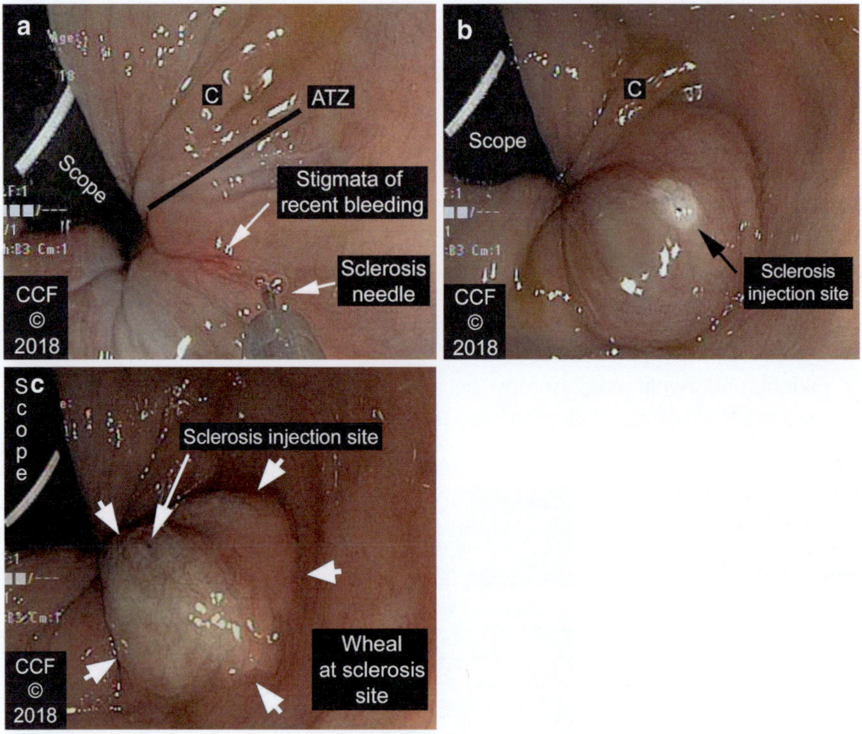

Fig. 47.2 (**a**) A split in the anal transitional zone (ATZ, black line) overlying hemorrhoidal vessels is seen (labeled-stigmata of recent bleeding). A column (C) of Morgagni within the ATZ has been labelled. Endoscopic sclerosis was done using 23% NaCl solution (9 mL) containing 2% Lidocaine (1 mL). Using a retroflexed approach, the sclerosing needle is positioned to inject 1 mL of the sclerosant into the submucosa; (**b**) the sclerosis injection site immediately after needle removal is shown (black arrow). The column (C) of Morgagni shown defines the anatomic location of the anal transitional zone and the underlying hemorrhoids; (**c**) about a minute following submucosal injection of the hypertonic saline, a wheal (short arrows) appears. The mucosal injection site is identified by the long white arrow

[1]The hypertonic saline/lidocaine mixture was made prepared as follows: 23.4% sodium chloride solution (9 mL)-2% Lidocaine (1 mL).

Comment

Sclerosis is defined as an induration or hardening [1]. In 1869, Morgan described treatment of external hemorrhoids by injection of tincture of persulfate of iron [2].

> "Two favourable cases of very large external hæmorrhoids having presented themselves, I used the persulfate injection with much success.
>
> The projecting masses were seized in an ordinary slide forceps and three drops of the persulphate of iron tincture injected into each. Coagulation took placed in a few minutes, and the patient got permanent relief; the tumours becoming dense and full of coagulum were effectually occluded."
>
> John Morgan, 1869

Since then, a variety of agents have been used as sclerosants. Several are shown in Table 47.1.

Sclerosis may be used for small, bleeding internal hemorrhoids with success rates reported in 75% to 89% of patients [9]. Because the risk of bleeding is low, sclerosis may be particularly attractive for patients with bleeding tendencies such as those receiving antiplatelet or anticoagulation therapy. Potential complications include rectal perforation, fistula, hemorrhage, infection, and pain. Sclerosis has been done under direct vision through an anoscope or endoscopically with or without anesthesia. The site of injection varies in the literature. In this case, the procedure was done endoscopically under conscious sedation in an endoscopy suite after mechanical bowel preparation. Retroflexion facilitated visualization of the anal transitional zone (the anatomic location of the hemorrhoids, Fig. 47.2). Injection was done into the apex of the internal hemorrhoid [8]. The addition of a local anesthetic to the hypertonic saline helped prevent pain after the procedure.

Table 47.1 Sclerosants used to treat hemorrhoids

	References
5% Phenol	[3, 4]
5% Quinine and urea hydrochloride	[5]
Alcohol	[6]
Aluminum potassium sulfate	[7]
23.4% Hypertonic saline	[8]

References

1. Sclerosis. The free Dictionary by Farlex; https://www.the freedictionary.com (Accessed 15 Sept 2022).
2. Morgan J. Hospital Reports. Mercer's Hospital. Varicose state of saphena veins, erectile tumour of the forehead, external hæmorrhoids treated successfully by the injection of tincture of persulphate of iron. Medical Press & Circular July 14, 1869. pp. 29–30.
3. Andrews E. The treatment of hemorrhoids by injection. The Medical Record 1879;15:451.
4. Kilbourne NJ. Internal hemorrhoids: comparative value of treatment by operative and by injection methods. Ann Surg. 1934;99:600–8.
5. Terrell EH. Treatment of hemorrhoids by injection. Virginia Med Monthly, April 1926. pp. 13–16.
6. Elsner H. Die nichtoperative Radikalbehandlung der Hämorrhoiden. Klin Wochenschschr. 1931;10:1032–4.
7. Takano M, Iwadare J, Ohba H, Takamura H, Masuda Y, Matsuo K, et al. Sclerosing therapy of internal hemorrhoids with a novel sclerosing agent: Comparison with ligation and excision. Int J Colorectal Dis. 2006;21:44–51.
8. Ponsky JL, Mellinger JD, Simon IB. Endoscopic retrograde hemorrhoidal sclerotherapy using 23.4% saline: a preliminary report. Gastrointest Endosc. 1991;37:155–8.
9. Rivadeneira DE, Steele SR, Ternent C, Chalasani S, Buie WD, Rafferty JL. Practice parameters for the management of hemorrhoids (revised 2010). Dis Colon Rectum. 2011;54:1059–64.

Anal Block

48

James S. Wu

Presentation

In 2004, Nyström et al. [1] described a technique for local block of all terminal nerve branches to the anus. The block was applied to patients undergoing hemorrhoid and anal fistula operations. Local anesthetic is injected into the ischiorectal fat peripheral to the external sphincter in eight directions as shown in Fig. 48.1.

Local anal block targets the terminal nerve branches of the anus. Nyström and coworkers found that their methods could be used as the sole method of anesthesia for proctologic operations. Also in 2004, Ong et al. [2] described a technique for circular stapled hemorrhoidectomy under local anesthesia in which an anesthetic solution is infiltrated into the anal sphincter, levator ani muscles, and the surrounding perianal skin. In 2012, Bansal et al. [3] reported hemorrhoidectomy under local anesthesia administered around the anus skin and into the intersphincteric plane. In 2011, Gorfine et al. [4] reported Bupivicaine extended-release liposome injection for prolonged postsurgical analgesia in patients undergoing hemorrhoidectomy. This formulation demonstrated a statistically significant reduction in pain through 72 h.

J. S. Wu (✉)
Department of Colon and Rectal Surgery, Cleveland Clinic, Cleveland, OH, USA

J. S. Wu, M. D. Inkster (eds.), *Cleveland Clinic Colorectal Case Studies*,
https://doi.org/10.1007/978-3-031-39880-3_48

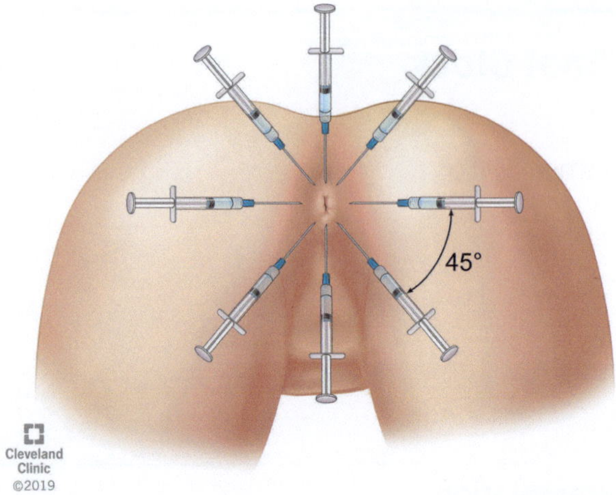

Fig. 48.1 Local anesthetic solution is injected peripheral to the external sphincter into the ischiorectal fat (after Nyström)

References

1. Nyström PO, Derwinger K, Gerjy R. Local perianal block for anal surgery. Tech Coloproctol. 2004;8:23–6.
2. Ong CH, Foo ECB, Keng V. Ambulatory circular stapled haemorrhoidectomy under local anaesthesia versus circular stapled haemorrhoidectomy under regional anaesthesia. ANZ J Surg. 2005;75:184–6.
3. Bansal H, Jenaw RK, Mandia R, Yadav R. How to do open hemorrhoidectomy under local anesthesia and its comparison with spinal anesthesia. Indian J Surg. 2012;74:330–3.
4. Gorfine SR, Onel E, Patou G, Krivokapic ZV. Bupivacaine extended-release liposome injection for prolonged postsurgical analgesia in patients undergoing hemorrhoidectomy: A multicenter, randomized, double-blind, placebo-controlled trial. Dis Colon Rectum. 2011;54:1552–9.

Hemorrhoidectomy

49

James S. Wu

Presentation

A 59-year-old female presented with bright red anorectal bleeding associated with bowel movements. Examination revealed a prolapsed anterior hemorrhoid that could not be reduced (4th degree). Colonoscopy was normal. Hemorrhoidectomy was done (Figs. 49.1a–c). Pathology showed hemorrhoids with adjacent chronic inflammation.

J. S. Wu (✉)
Department of Colon and Rectal Surgery, Cleveland Clinic, Cleveland, OH, USA

J. S. Wu, M. D. Inkster (eds.), *Cleveland Clinic Colorectal Case Studies*,
https://doi.org/10.1007/978-3-031-39880-3_49

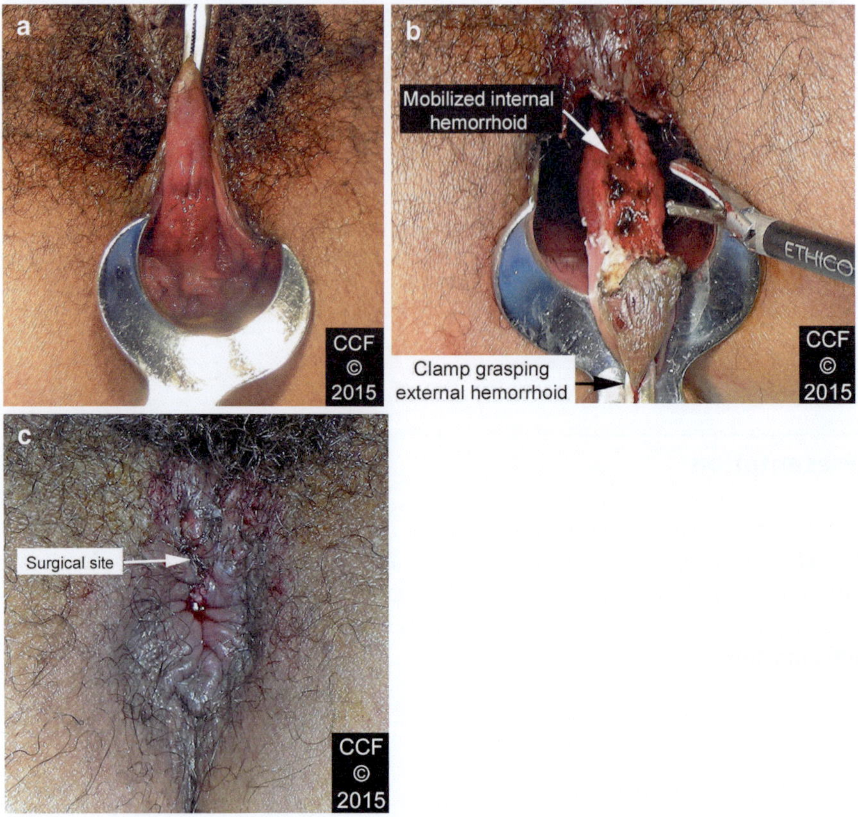

Fig. 49.1 (**a**) The anterior prolapsed hemorrhoid is exposed under traction; (**b**) the hemorrhoid is dissected off of the internal anal sphincter, in this case using the harmonic scalpel [1, 2]; (**c**) the postoperative appearance of the anus after hemorrhoidectomy

Comment

In 1937, Milligan, Morgan, Jones, and Officer described the operative treatment of hemorrhoids.[1] The authors defined three primary hemorrhoids:

> 'It is now possible to consider the blood-vessels concerned in the formation of each of the three primary hæmorrhoids. The blood-vessels supplying both the internal and its corresponding external hæmorrhoid lie in the submucous layer under the fold of pink rectal mucosa forming the "pile pedicle." '

The authors identify three primary pile pedicles. Their operation, illustrated in Fig. 49.2, is described as follows:

[1] Milligan et al. [3]. This excerpt is reproduced with the generous permission of Elsevier Science &Technology journals, CCC|Marketplace®, Order License 1141087-1, Order date 16-Aug-2021.

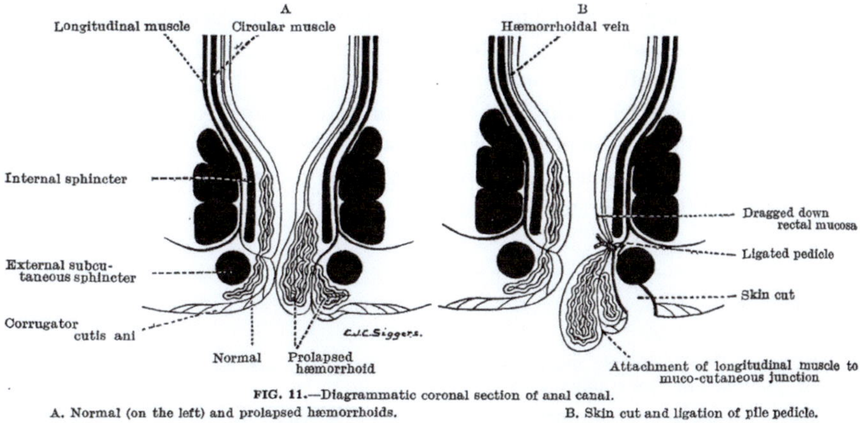

Fig. 49.2 Excisional hemorrhoidectomy as illustrated by Milligan, Morgan, Jones, and Officer, 1937. Reproduced with permission from Elsevier Ltd., CCC|RightsLink®, License number 5136851018331, License date Aug 26, 2021

> 'With the anæsthetized patient in the lithotomy position one or more of the primary hæmorrhoids tend to prolapse. The tag of skin corresponding with the hæmorrhoid showing the greatest tendency to prolapse is grasped with dissecting forceps and drawn laterally, away from the anus. This tension causes the anal mucosa covering the internal hæmorrhoid to appear outside the anal canal. The hæmorrhoid is now grasped and further traction brings into view a longitudinal fold of rectal mucous membrane. This rectal fold is caught with artery forceps—the "pedicle forceps."
>
> With scissors, two cuts are now made in the skin of the anus, one on either side of the skin forceps and extending from the anocutaneous line to the outer border of the distended external hæmorrhoidal plexus. The incisions are made to meet at their outer extremities, thus outlining a V-shaped section of tissue over the external hæmorrhoidal plexus. The incisions are extended through the corrugator cutis ani until the circular band of the subcutaneous external sphincter is laid bare. Starting at the apex of the V the tissues are dissected away from the subcutaneous external sphincter until the inner border is exposed, where the fibers of the longitudinal muscle may be seen.
>
> The dissection having been completed, the entire hæmorrhoid—that is, the internal and external hæmorrhoidal plexuses with their coverings of anal mucosa and skin of anus—swings free on its pedicle. An assistant now exerts traction on both pedicle and skin forceps directly outwards from the anus, while a No. 16 hollow-woven silk ligature is tied very tightly around the pedicle above the pedicle forceps.
>
> The excess tissue distal to the ligature is now excised and the ligatures cut short.'

In 1959, Ferguson and Heaton described closed hemorrhoidectomy [4].Their rationale for wound closure is as follows.

> "Incisions are closed because they heal more dependably, discomfort is lessened, the danger of postoperative bleeding is reduced, postoperative hospital visits are required less frequently, and the healed anal canal has a natural and complete pliability which we believe the open method of hemorrhoidectomy does not provide consistently."

The principles of excisional hemorrhoid surgery remain the same today. The tools used to achieve the dissection have been modified to include instruments that simultaneously cut and coagulate such as the ultrasonically activated scalpel and electrocautery. Key advantages of these techniques are meticulous hemostasis. A common complaint after hemorrhoidectomy is anal pain. In 1953, Eisenhammer identified anal sphincter spasm as the cause of postoperative pain after anal canal surgery [5]. Administration of an anal block prior to hemorrhoid excision plus postoperative warm water soaks and topical medications to relax the internal anal sphincter partially ameliorates this pain.

References

1. McCarus SD. Physiologic mechanism of the ultrasonically activated scalpel. J Am Assoc Gynecol Laparosc. 1996;3:601–8.
2. Khan S, Pawlak SE, Eggenberger JC, Lee CS, Szilagy EJ, Wu JS, Margolin DA. Surgical treatment of hemorrhoids. Prospective, randomized trial comparing closed excisional hemorrhoidectomy and the Harmonic Scalpel® technique of excisional hemorrhoidectomy. Dis Colon Rectum. 2001;44:845–9.
3. Milligan ETC, Morgan CN, Jones LE, Officer R. Surgical anatomy of the anal canal, and the operative treatment of hæmorrhoids. Lancet. 1937;230(5959):1119–24.
4. Ferguson JA, Heaton JR. Closed hemorrhoidectomy. Dis Colon Rectum. 1959;2:176–9.
5. Eisenhammer S. The internal sphincter: its surgical importance. S Afr Med J. 1953;27:266–70.

50 Hemorrhoid-Doppler Arterial Ligation

Massarat Zutshi, Gwendolyn A. Fuller, and James S. Wu

Presentation

Patients usually present with rectal bleeding. The bleeding usually is painless, bright red, and associated with bowel movements. The patient was referred for hemorrhoid-Doppler arterial ligation.

Preoperative Management

Other causes lower gastrointestinal bleeding are eliminated by colonoscopy. Two disposable enemas are given on the morning of the procedure. Oral intake is withheld for 6 h before general anesthesia.

Technique

Surgery is done in the operating room, under general anesthesia in the lithotomy position. Instruments used for the procedure are shown in Fig. 50.1.

An examination is done to evaluate the hemorrhoids. An anal block is administered (e.g., 1% Lidocaine). The lighted Doppler anoscope, lubricated with the ultrasound jelly, is inserted into the anal canal (Fig. 50.2) and positioned with the suture window at the site of a potential Doppler signal (Fig. 50.3).

M. Zutshi · J. S. Wu (✉)
Department of Colon and Rectal Surgery, Cleveland Clinic, Cleveland, OH, USA

G. A. Fuller
Medical Illustration Team, Enterprise Creative Services, Cleveland Clinic, Cleveland, OH, USA

J. S. Wu, M. D. Inkster (eds.), *Cleveland Clinic Colorectal Case Studies*,
https://doi.org/10.1007/978-3-031-39880-3_50

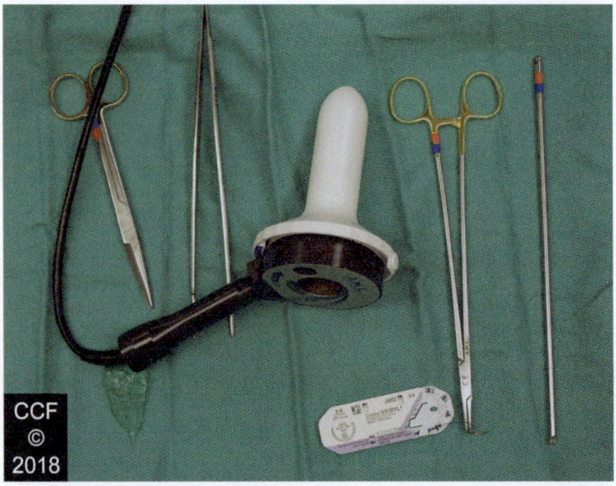

Fig. 50.1 Equipment used for Doppler-guided hemorrhoidal ligation (left to right): long scissors, long non-tooth forceps, lighted anoscope with Doppler attachment, polyglycolic acid absorbable suture, long needle-holder, knot pusher

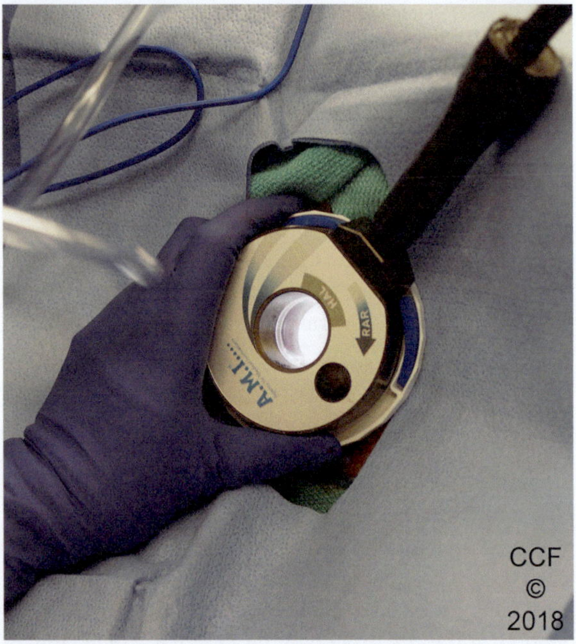

Fig. 50.2 The lighted Doppler anoscope is positioned with the Doppler over the internal hemorrhoids

A prominent Doppler signal is sought (Fig. 50.3) such that the vessel is not deep (7, 8, 9) or too superficial (1, 2, 3).

The hemorrhoidal artery is suture ligated (Fig. 50.4) using two sutures. The first marks the spot, and the next goes deeper to ligate the vessel. The knots are advanced to the mucosa with the aid of a knot pusher (Fig. 50.5). Disappearance of the Doppler sound is evidence of a successful ligation. The device then is rotated to the

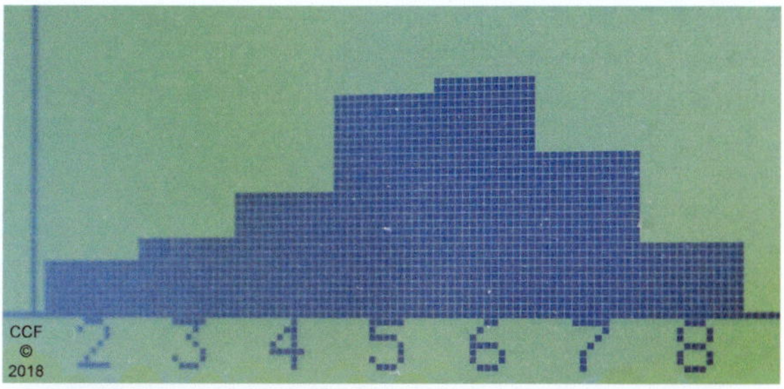

Fig. 50.3 A prominent Doppler signal locates a candidate internal hemorrhoid

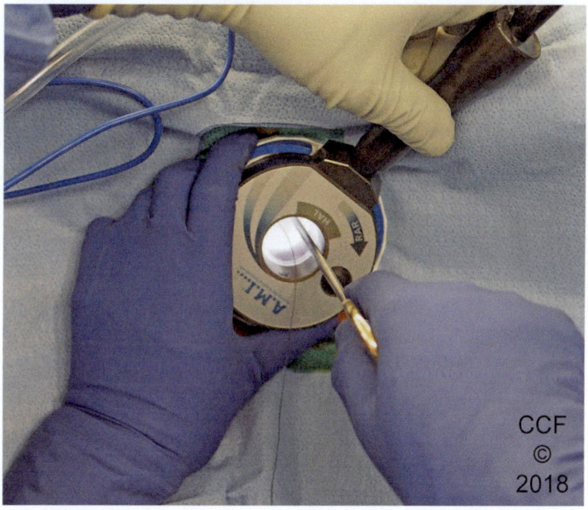

Fig. 50.4 Suture ligation of an internal hemorrhoidal artery selected by the Doppler

next hemorrhoid, and the procedure is repeated. After completing ligations at the entire circumference, the device is pulled out by 1 cm, and a second ring of suture ligations is placed. Typically, 6 to 11 hemorrhoidal vessels are ligated.

After completion of the ligations, the anoscope-Doppler is removed. Anoscopy is done at the end of the procedure to ensure hemostasis.

Mucopexy or rectoanal repair is done using a 2-0 polyglycolic acid suture and is initiated proximal to the area of the hemorrhoid ligation and tied. The same suture is continued as a running suture distally and is concluded just above the dentate line. As the suture is tied, using the index finger, the hemorrhoidal tissue is pushed up. This causes the hemorrhoidal pedicle to be pulled up into the anal canal (Figs. 50.6 and 50.7).

Following the Doppler arterial ligation, the prolapsed hemorrhoids are suspended with stitches (mucopexy, Figs. 50.8a, b). The prolapsed hemorrhoids seen before the procedure in Fig. 50.8a are pulled up after the mucopexy as seen in Fig. 50.8b. A local anal block is added for pain control.

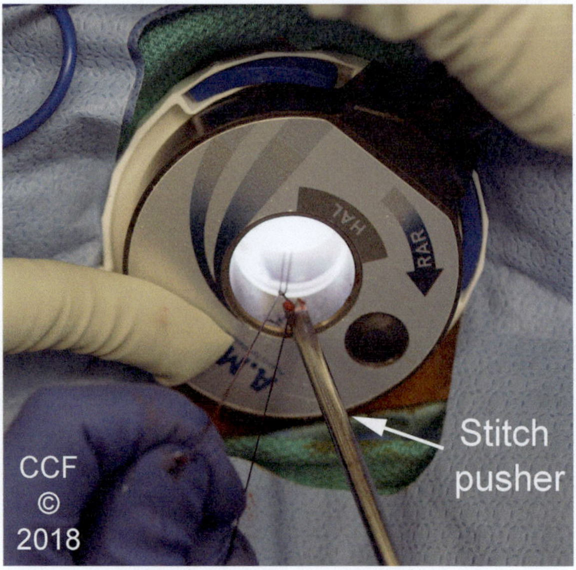

Fig. 50.5 The knot is advanced to the mucosa with the aid of a knot (stitch) pusher

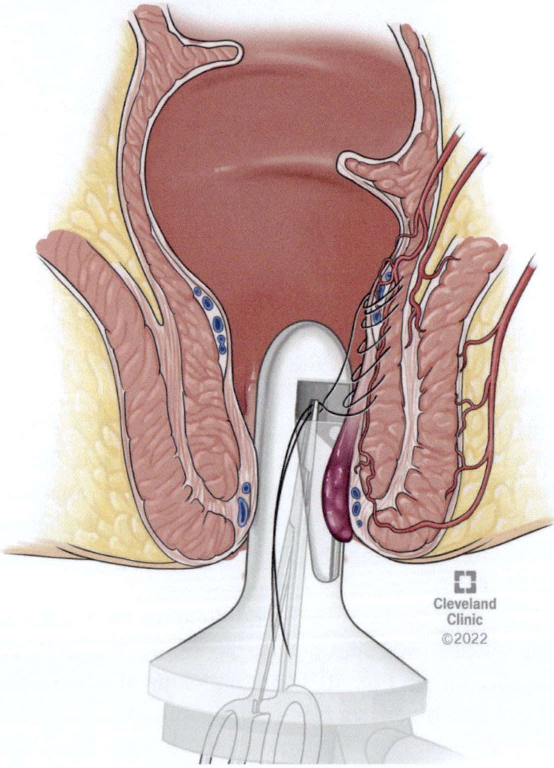

Fig. 50.6 Mucopexy or rectoanal repair done through the window in the proctoscope without the Doppler probe in place. The suture is initiated proximal to the area of ligation and ends above the dentate line

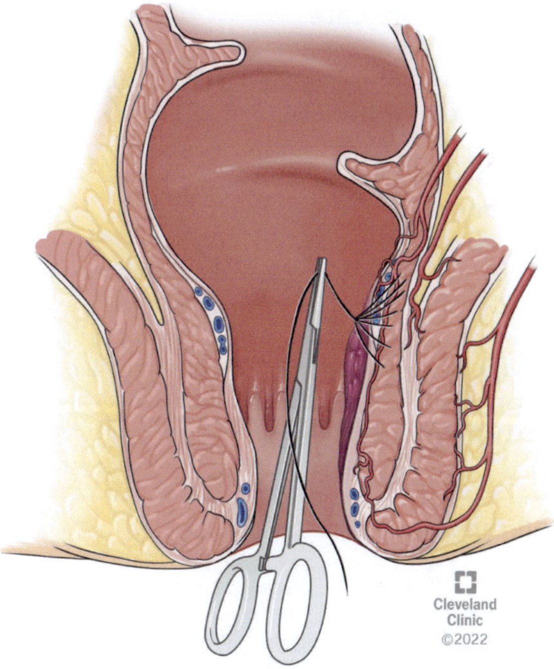

Fig. 50.7 Mucopexy when concluded shows the hemorrhoidal tissue pushed into the anal canal proximally as the suture is tied

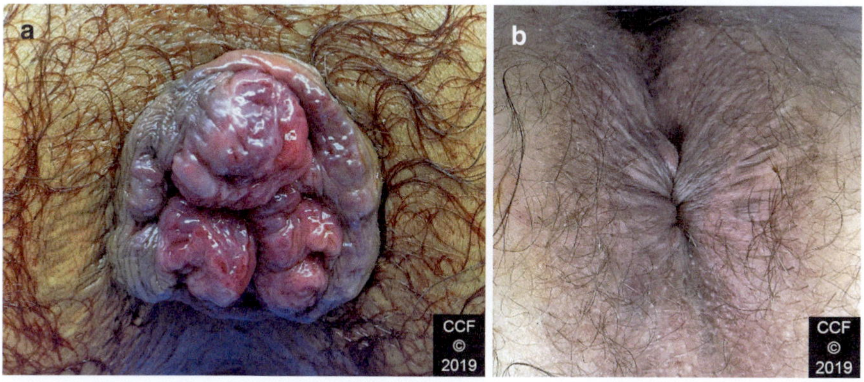

Fig. 50.8 (**a**) Prolapsed hemorrhoids before mucopexy; (**b**) prolapsed hemorrhoids after mucopexy

Postprocedure Care

Stool softeners, fiber, and mineral oil are used to keep stools soft after surgery. Sitz baths are used for cleanliness.

Comment

In 1995, Morinaga et al. [1] described hemorrhoidal artery ligation for internal hemorrhoids with a device called the Moricorn, a cylinder with a Doppler transducer and a window for arterial ligation, as shown in Fig. 50.1. A review of outcomes after 20 years by Figueiredo and Campos found that the Doppler-guided hemorrhoidal dearterialization was especially useful in patients who had undergone previous anal surgery and in those with alterations of fecal continence [2].

References

1. Morinaga K, Hasuda K, Ikeda T. A novel therapy for internal hemorrhoids: Ligation of the hemorrhoidal artery with a newly devised instrument (Moricorn) in conjunction with a Doppler flowmeter. Am J Gastroenterol. 1995;90:610–3.
2. Figueiredo MN, Campos FG. Doppler-guided hemorrhoidal dearterialization/transanal hemorrhoidal dearterialization: Technical evolution and outcomes after 20 years. World J Gastrointest Surg. 2016;8:232–7.

51 Incarcerated Prolapsed Hemorrhoids and Distal Rectum

James S. Wu

Presentation

A 56-year-old male developed severe anal pain when straining at stool. He was seen in the emergency room late at night. Examination showed acutely incarcerated prolapsed hemorrhoids and distal rectum (Fig. 51.1). Attempts at manual reduction caused pain.

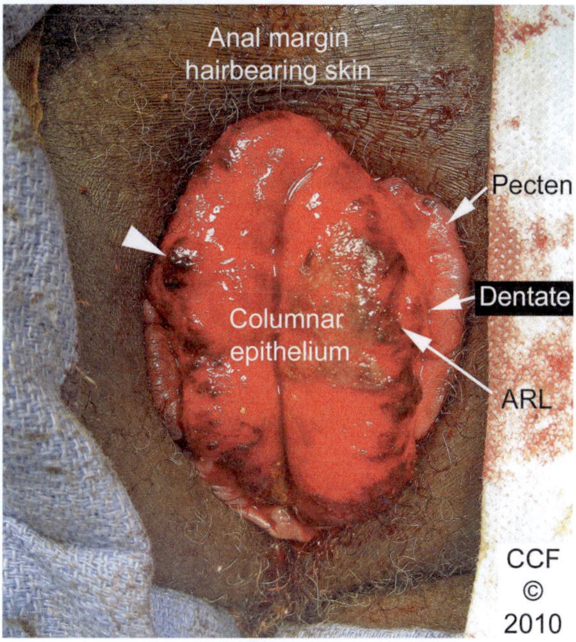

Fig. 51.1 Acutely incarcerated hemorrhoid and distal rectal prolapse. The prolapsus is viable. Anatomic landmarks include the anal margin, anal canal pecten, dentate line, anorectal line, and columnar epithelium. Thrombosis in an internal hemorrhoid is marked with an arrowhead

J. S. Wu (✉)
Department of Colon and Rectal Surgery, Cleveland Clinic, Cleveland, OH, USA

J. S. Wu, M. D. Inkster (eds.), *Cleveland Clinic Colorectal Case Studies*,
https://doi.org/10.1007/978-3-031-39880-3_51

Management

The patient was positioned prone. The buttocks were separated. The prolapsed mucosa was covered with sucrose (table sugar) (Fig. 51.2). After several minutes, the prolapsed hemorrhoids shrank; simultaneously, the sucrose became moist. The prolapsed hemorrhoids then were manually reduced (Fig. 51.3).

A piece of wide tape was placed across the buttocks to prevent re-prolapse, and the patient was admitted to the hospital. The following day, he was brought to surgery electively. Operation was done in the prone position. The prolapse was easily re-exteriorized and then amputated with a circumferential incision (Fig. 51.4).

Following prolapsus amputation, additional sutures were placed to approximate the wound edges (Fig. 51.5).

The final external appearance of the anus after circular hemorrhoidectomy is shown in Fig. 51.6.

The operative specimens are shown in Fig. 51.7.

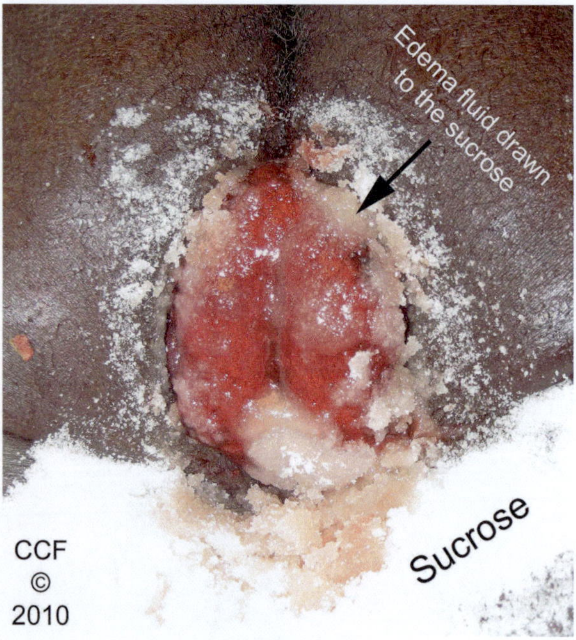

Fig. 51.2 Sucrose in contact with the prolapsed mucosa. The sucrose creates an osmotic gradient that draws edema fluid from the prolapsus and moistens the sugar

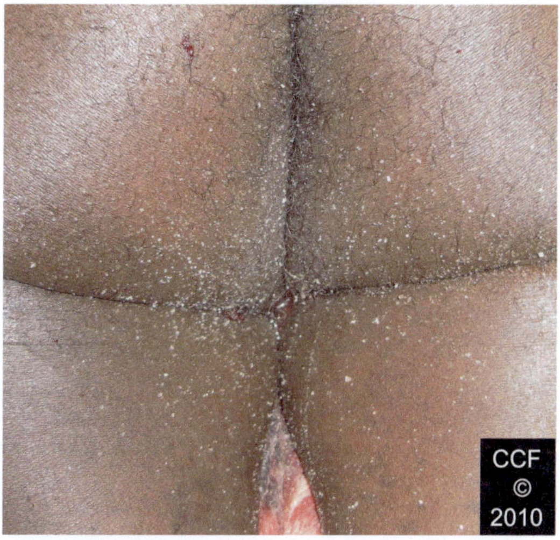

Fig. 51.3 Following treatment with topical sucrose, prolapse reduction was achieved

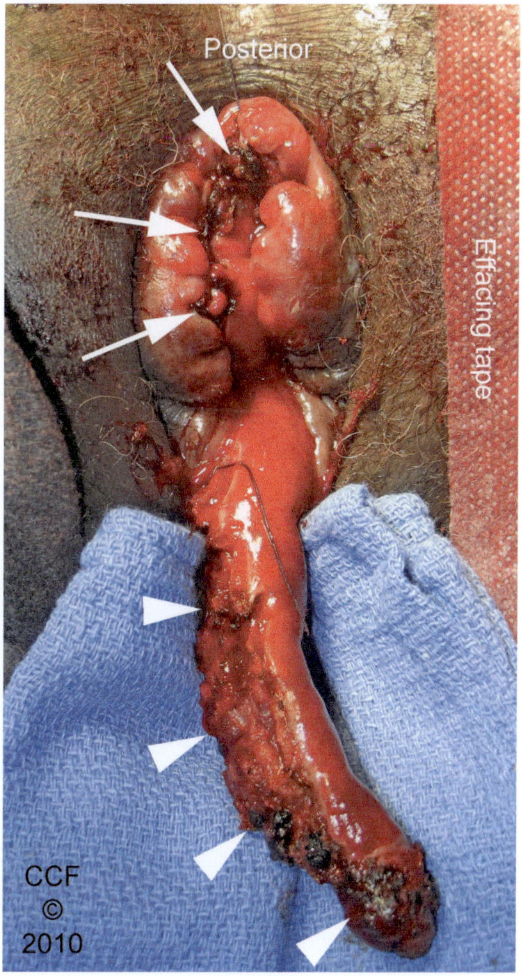

Fig. 51.4 The circumferentially excised prolapsus is indicated with arrowheads. Arrows point to suture approximation of the anoderm to the rectal mucosa

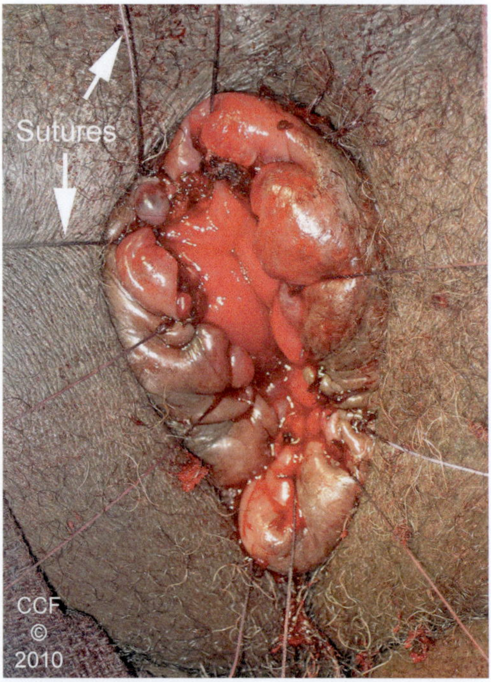

Fig. 51.5 The postamputation wound is approximated with circumferentially placed absorbable suture

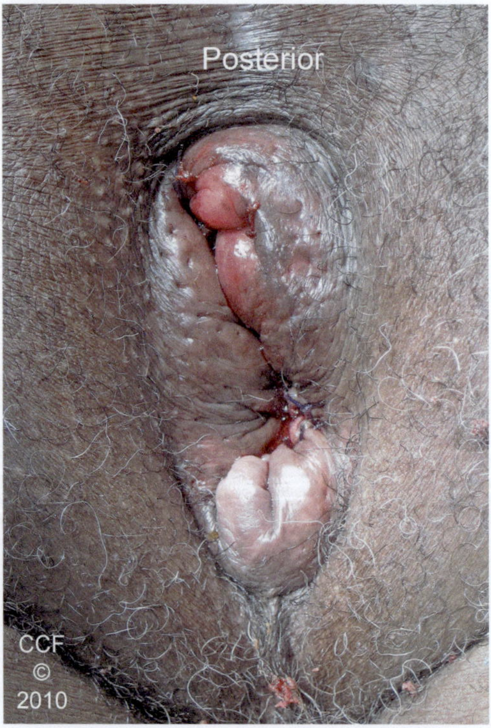

Fig. 51.6 Final appearance of the anus following circumferential amputation of the prolapse

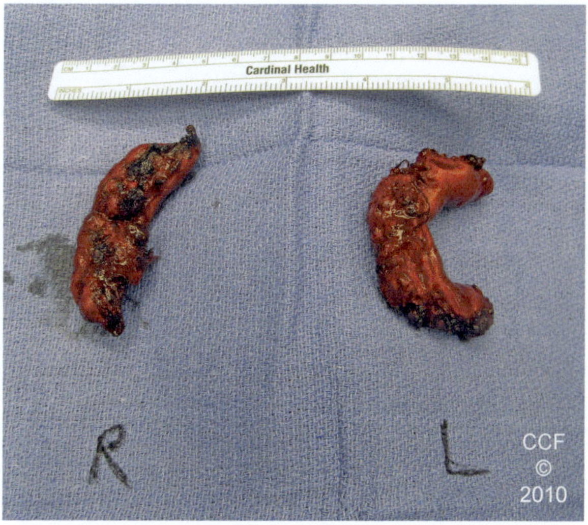

Fig. 51.7 Circumferentially excised hemorrhoid and distal rectum specimens submitted in two pieces, right (R) and left (L)

Comment

In 1991, Meyers and Rothenberger described the role of sugar in the reduction of incarcerated bowel [1]. Sucrose in contact with the prolapsed edematous mucous membrane creates an osmotic gradient that draws water from the mucosa into the sugar. As shown in Fig. 51.2, the sucrose applied to the prolapsus is moistened by the extracted water. Successful prolapse reduction relieved the patient's pain obviating the need for emergency surgery. The following day, the patient was brought to surgery electively. The prolapse was easily re-exteriorized and amputated by a circumferential incision. The principle followed in this operation was similar to trans-anal amputation and colo-anal anastomosis reported by Mikulicz for the treatment of rectal prolapse in 1889 [2].

References

1. Myers JO, Rothenberger DA. Sugar in the reduction of incarcerated prolapsed bowel. Dis Colon Rectum. 1991;34:416–8.
2. Mikulicz J. Zur operativen Behandlung des prolapsus recti et coli invaginati. Arch Klin Chir. 1889;38:74–97.

Squamous Intraepithelial Lesion in an Excised Hemorrhoid

52

James S. Wu, Homer O. Wiland, and Eric W. Willis

Presentation

A 67-year-old female underwent excision of a prolapsed 4th degree hemorrhoid (Figs. 52.1 and 52.2).

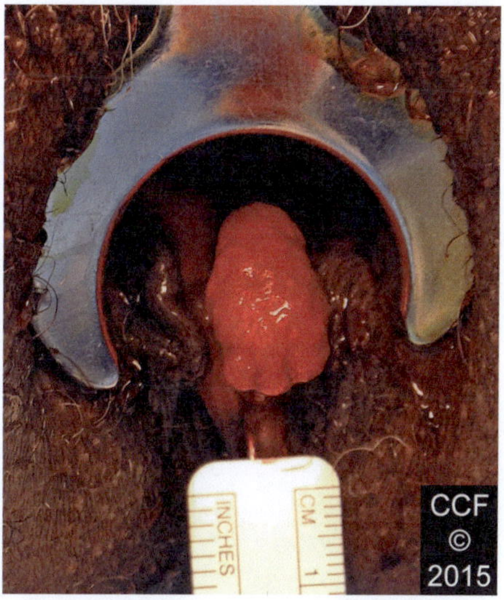

Fig. 52.1 Prolapsing hemorrhoid

J. S. Wu (✉)
Department of Colon and Rectal Surgery, Cleveland Clinic, Cleveland, OH, USA

H. O. Wiland
Department of Pathology, OhioHeatlh Mansfield Hospital, Mansfield, OH, USA

E. W. Willis
Department of Pathology, CORPath, Columbus, OH, USA

J. S. Wu, M. D. Inkster (eds.), *Cleveland Clinic Colorectal Case Studies*,
https://doi.org/10.1007/978-3-031-39880-3_52

Fig. 52.2 Excised hemorrhoid

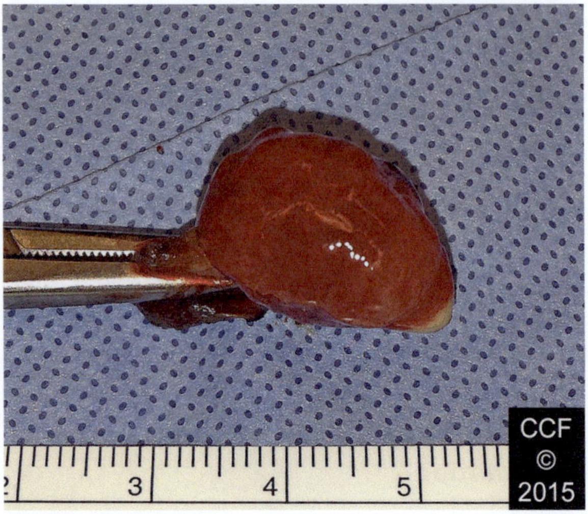

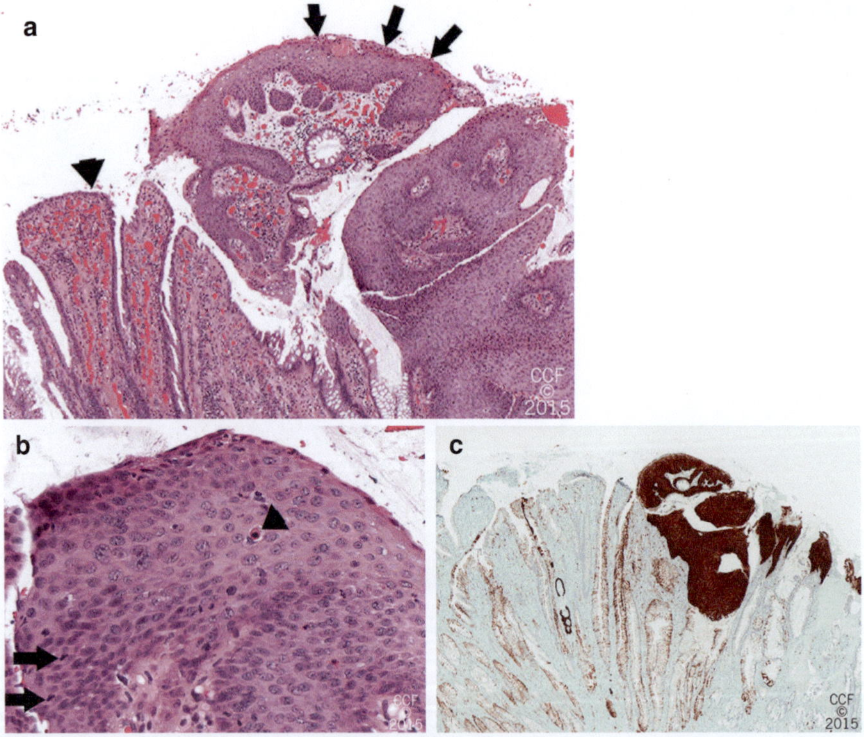

Fig. 52.3 (**a**) Low power view shows benign columnar mucosa (arrow head) and immature-appearing, dysplastic squamous mucosa (arrows) (H–E, original magnification ×40); (**b**) At higher power, there is full thickness nuclear enlargement and hyperchromasia (dark-staining nuclei) as well as increased mitotic activity (arrows). A necrotic, "dyskeratotic keratinocyte" is present (arrowhead) (H–E, original magnification ×200); (**c**) the p16 immunohistochemical stain shows diffuse, dark staining of the dysplastic squamous mucosa, suggesting human papillomavirus (HPV) integration

Histopathology is shown in Fig. 52.3.

Comment

The histopathologic findings are consistent with a high-grade squamous intraepithelial lesion (HSIL). In 1981, Fenger and Nielsen examined material from 306 minor anal surgical specimens [1]. Unexpected dysplastic changes were found in 7 (2.3%). The authors concluded that all surgical specimens from the anal canal should be evaluated histologically so that the diagnosis of anal dysplasia is not missed. Current nomenclature for squamous intraepithelial lesions follows the Lower Anogenital Squamous Terminology (LAST) recommendations [2]. Anal SIL is associated with HPV Infection and with overexpression of the protein p16 [3–5]. In this case, a p16 immunohistochemical stain showed diffuse, dark staining along the areas of squamous mucosa consistent with HSIL. Following surgery, patients are entered into a SIL surveillance program. The presence of anal dysplasia prompts examination of other structures at risk for human papilloma virus infection and SIL, e.g., cervix, vagina, vulva, penis, and oropharynx [6, 7].

References

1. Fenger C, Nielsen VT. Dysplastic changes in the anal canal epithelium in minor surgical specimens. Acta Path Microbiol Scand Sect A. 1981;89:463–5.
2. Darragh TM, Colgan TJ, Cox JT, Heller DS, Henry MR, Luff RD, et al. The lower anogenital squamous terminology standardization project for HPV-associated lesions: Background and consensus recommendations from the College of American Pathologists and the American Society for Colposcopy and Cervical Pathology. Arch Pathol Lab Med. 2012;136:1266–97.
3. Lu DW, El-Mofty SK, Wang HL. Expression of p16, Rb, and p53 proteins in squamous cell carcinomas of the anorectal region harboring human papillomavirus DNA. Mod Pathol. 2003;16:692–9.
4. Walts AE, Lechago J, Bose S. P16 and Ki67 immunostaining is a useful adjunct in the assessment of biopsies for HPV-associated anal intraepithelial neoplasia. Am J Surg Pathol. 2006;30:795–801.
5. Bean SM, Eltoum I, Horton DK, Whitlow L, Chhieng DC. Immunohistochemical expression of p16 and Ki-67 correlates with degree of anal intraepithelial neoplasia. Am J Surg Pathol. 2007;31:555–61.
6. Stanley MA, Winder DM, Sterling JC, Goon PKC. HPV infection, anal intra-epithelial neoplasia (AIN) and anal cancer: current issues. BMC Cancer. 2012;12:398.
7. Chung CH, Bagheri A, D'Souza G. Epidemiology of oral human papillomavirus infection. Oral Oncol. 2014;50:364–9.

Anal Squamous Intraepithelial Lesions

53

Michelle D. Inkster, Charles D. Sturgis, Homer O. Wiland, and James S. Wu

Background

Anal squamous intraepithelial lesions (SIL) are human papillomavirus (HPV)-associated precursors to anal squamous cell carcinoma (SCC) [1]. Increased risk is seen in the presence of immunosuppression, human immunodeficiency virus (HIV) infection, urogynecologic dysplasia, inflammatory bowel disease, and solid organ transplantation [2]. However, anal SIL can occur in anyone. Pathogenesis begins with the introduction of HPV into the basement layer of the squamous epithelium (Fig. 53.1).

Terminology is by the Lower Anogenital Squamous Terminology LAST standardization system [3]. Anal cytology is a method used to screen for anal SIL [4]. Examples of anal cytology, interpreted according to the Bethesda system, are shown in Fig. 53.2 [5].

M. D. Inkster
Department of Gastroenterology, Cleveland Clinic, Cleveland, OH, USA
e-mail: inkstem@ccf.org

C. D. Sturgis
Hospital Pathology Associates/Allina, Minneapolis, MN, USA

H. O. Wiland
Department of Pathology, OhioHealth Mansfield Hospital, Mansfield, OH, USA

J. S. Wu (✉)
Department of Colon and Rectal Surgery, Cleveland Clinic, Cleveland, OH, USA

J. S. Wu, M. D. Inkster (eds.), *Cleveland Clinic Colorectal Case Studies*,
https://doi.org/10.1007/978-3-031-39880-3_53

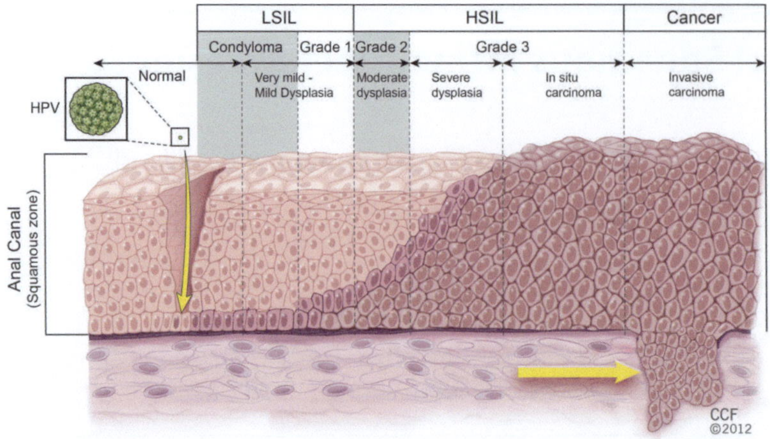

Fig. 53.1 HPV pathogenesis begins with introduction of the virus through a break in the epithelium (vertical arrow) into the basal stem cells of the squamous epithelium. A dysplastic cell population expands from the basal layer to the surface. Extension beneath the basement membrane defines carcinoma (horizontal yellow arrow). Synonymous terms used to describe dysplasia are included

Histopathologic examples of LSIL and HSIL are shown in Fig. 53.3.

Lesion detection is important for management. Methods of SIL detection include physical examination, direction inspection, anal colposcopy [6] aka high-resolution anoscopy (HRA) [7], and anal chromoendoscopy (ACE) [8]. Detection of SIL is facilitated by chromoendoscopy with acetic acid (AA) and narrow band imaging (NBI) in conjunction with rectal insufflation and retroflexion (Fig. 53.4) [9, 10].

The chromoendoscopic appearance of low-grade SIL is shown in Fig. 53.5. A complex high-grade lesion is seen on retroflexion and rectal insufflation with NBI after treatment of the anoderm with 3% acetic acid (Fig. 53.6).

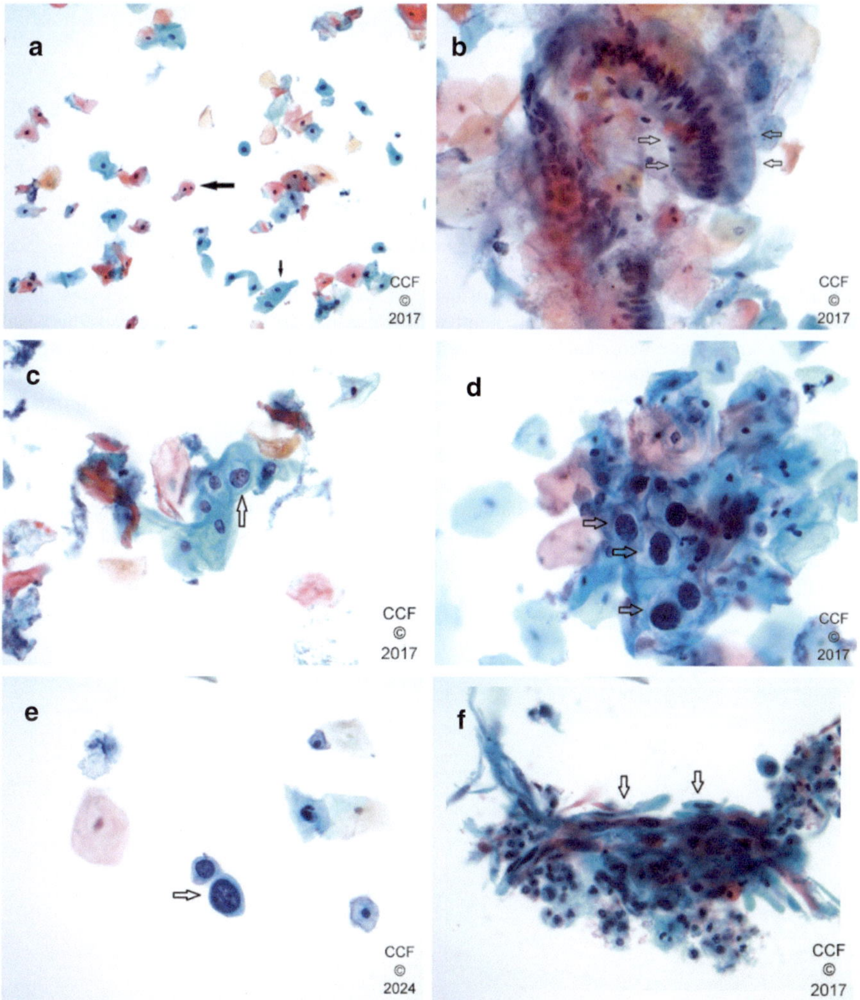

Fig. 53.2 (**a**) Negative for intraepithelial lesion and malignancy (NILM) exfoliative anal cytology, 45 M, admixture of unremarkable nucleated superficial (large arrow) and intermediate (small arrow) squamous epithelial cells, ThinPrep Papanicolaou, ×200. (**b**) Negative for intraepithelial lesion and malignancy (NILM) exfoliative anal cytology with rectal glandular transformation zone component (columnar cells between arrows), 49 M, ThinPrep Papanicolaou, ×400. (**c**) Atypical squamous cells of undetermined significance (ASC-US) exfoliative anal cytology, 44 M, squamous cells with mild nucleomegaly and nuclear hyperchromasia (arrow), ThinPrep Papanicolaou, ×400. (**d**) Low-grade squamous intraepithelial lesion (LSIL) exfoliative anal cytology, 51 M, squamous cells >×3 nuclear enlargement, coarse hyperchromasia, perinuclear halos, and binucleation, (arrows) ThinPrep Papanicolaou, ×400. (**e**) High-grade squamous intraepithelial lesion (HSIL) exfoliative anal cytology, 50 M, dysplastic squamous cells with nucleomegaly, high nuclear/cytoplasmic ratios, and coarsely granular hyperchromasia, (arrow) ThinPrep Papanicolaou, ×400. (**f**) Squamous carcinoma exfoliative anal cytology, 37 M, individual HSIL cells and many associated atypical spindled squamous cells (arrows) with accompanying inflammation and clinging tumor diathesis, ThinPrep Papanicolaou, ×400

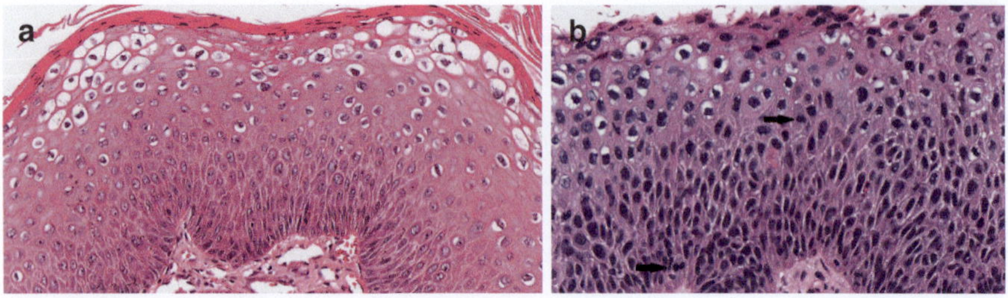

Fig. 53.3 (**a**) LSIL (AIN1). This biopsy of flat anal mucosa shows numerous koilocytes in the superficial layer of the squamous epithelium with overlying parakeratosis. However, the basal layer of the squamous mucosa appears preserved with no evidence of nuclear enlargement or pleomorphism, and mitotic figures are not increased (H–E, original magnification ×100). (**b**) HSIL (AIN2). The squamous mucosa appears abnormal as keratinocytes have enlarged, hyperchromatic, and pleomorphic nuclei filling the basal zone and extending into the middle third of the epithelium. Nuclear to cytoplasmic ratios are markedly increased. The nuclei are extensively crowded; there is overall loss of polarity with irregular nuclear orientations, and mitotic activity is increased at the base and in the middle third of the epithelium (arrows). There is a minimal degree of maturation toward the epithelial surface and scattered superficial koilocytes are seen. Accordingly, the findings are best classified as a high-grade squamous intraepithelial lesion (AIN 2) (H–E, original magnification ×200)

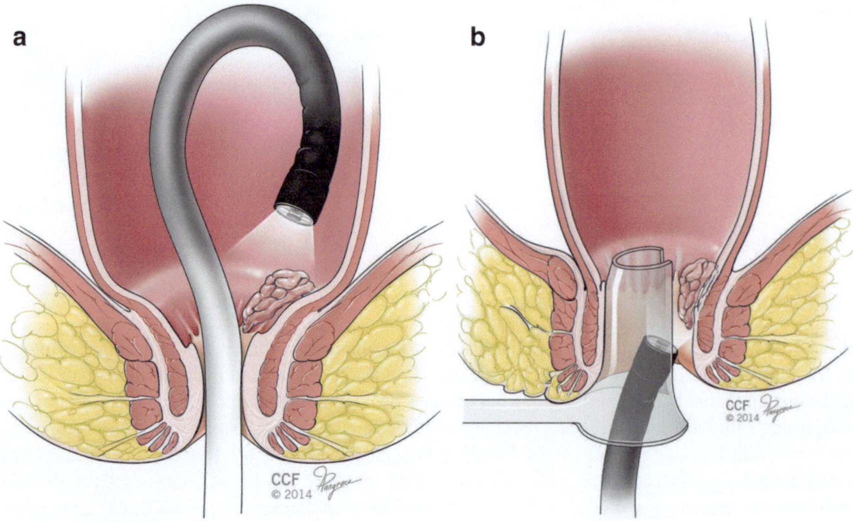

Fig. 53.4 (**a**) Endoscopic view of the anal transitional zone by retroflexion; (**b**) *en face* examination of the anoderm through an anoscope

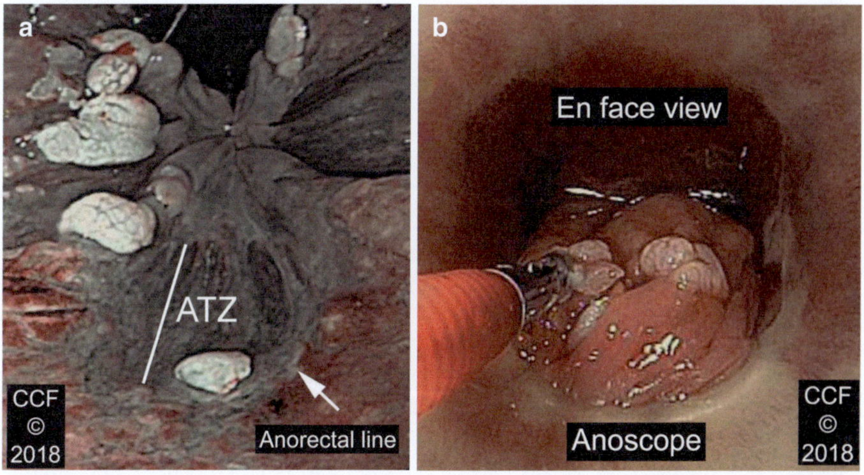

Fig. 53.5 (**a**) Multiple low-grade SIL lesions seen on retroflexion with NBI after anoderm treatment with acetic acid. The ATZ and anorectal line have been labelled; (**b**) biopsy and ablation of lesions with hot forceps through an anoscope (*en face* view)

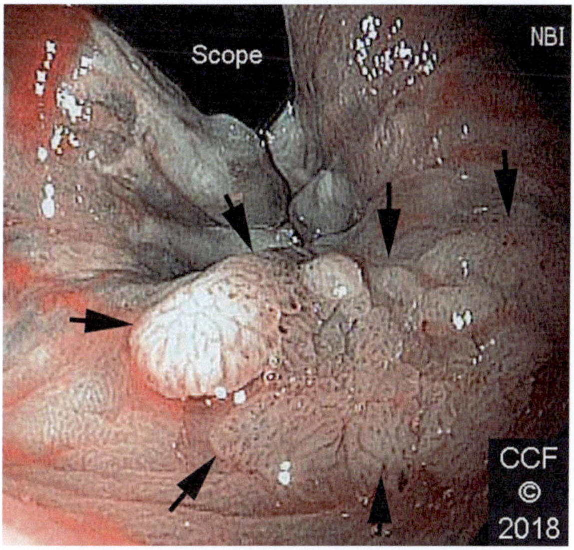

Fig. 53.6 HSIL (outlined with arrows) seen on retroflexion with rectal insufflation with NBI after treatment with acetic acid. The endoscope "scope" is labeled

Screening for Anal Cancer and Anal Dysplasia

While no published guidelines exist regarding general population screening for anal cancer/anal dysplasia, a few organizations have offered recommendations for specific high-risk groups (Table 53.1).

The 2013 primary care guidelines for persons infected with HIV, by the HIV Medicine Association of the Infectious Diseases Society of America recommends that MSM, women with a history of anoreceptive intercourse or abnormal cervical Pap test results, and HIV-infected persons with genital warts should have anal

Table 53.1 Populations recommended for screening for anal dysplasia/anal cancer

Persons who practice anoreceptive intercourse
Persons with genital tract neoplasia
Immunocompromised state
– HIV positivity
– Organ transplantation
– Immunosuppressive medication

Pap tests [11]. In 2015, the American Society for Colposcopy and Cervical Pathology and the Anal Intraepithelial Neoplasia Society together recommended that HIV-infected women and women with lower genital tract neoplasia may be considered for screening anal cytology with triage to treatment if HSIL is diagnosed [12]. The 2024 position of the American Cancer Association on early detection of anal cancer is that some people at increased risk for anal intraepithelial neoplasia might benefit from screening [13]. This group includes MSM, women who have had cervical cancer, vaginal cancer, or vulvar cancer, anyone who is HIV-positive, and anyone who is immunocompromised (such as people who have had received an organ transplantation or who are on long term steroids), anyone with a history of anal warts and women older than 45 years old who are HPV 16 positive.

References

1. Muñoz N, Castellsagué X, Berrington de González A, Gissmann L. Chapter 1: HPV in the etiology of human cancer. Vaccine. 2006;24S3:S3/1-S3/10.
2. Suneson KG, Nørgaard M, Thorlacius-Ussing O, Laurberg S. Immunosuppressive disorders and risk of anal squamous cell carcinoma: a nationwide cohort study in Denmark, 1978–2005. Int J Cancer. 2010;127:675–84.
3. Darragh TM, Colgan TJ, Cox JT, Heller DS, Henry MR, Luff RD, et al. The lower anogenital squamous terminology standardization project for HPV-associated lesions. Arch Pathol Lab Med. 2012;136:1266–97.
4. Bean SM, Chhieng DC. Anal-rectal cytology: A review. Diagn Cytopathol. 2010;38:538–46.
5. Nayar R, Wilbur DC, editors. The Bethesda System for Reporting Cervical Cytology. 3rd ed. New York: Springer-Verlag; 2015.
6. Scholefield JH, Sonnex C, Talbot IC, Palmer JG, Whatrup C, Mindel A, Northover JMA. Anal and cervical intraepithelial neoplasia: possible parallel. Lancet. 1989;ii:765–9.
7. Jay N, Berry JM, Hogeboom CJ, Holly EA, Darragh TM, Palefsky JM. Colposcopic appearance of anal squamous intraepithelial lesions. relationship to histopathology. Dis Colon Rectum. 1997;40:919–28.
8. Oette M, Wieland U, Schünemann M, Haes J, Reuter S, Jensen BEO, et al. Anal chromoendoscopy using gastroenterological videoendoscopes: A new method to perform high-resolution anoscopy for diagnosing intraepithelial neoplasia and anal carcinoma in HIV-infected patients. Z Gastroenterol. 2017;55:23–31.
9. Inkster MD, Wiland HO, Wu JS. Detection of anal dysplasia is enhanced by narrow band imaging and acetic acid. Colorectal Dis. 2015;18:O17–21.
10. Inkster MD, Wu JS. Detection of anal dysplasia by chromoendoscopy with narrow band imaging and acetic acid (NBIA) in 182 patients. Clin Surg. 2017;2:1583.
11. Aberg JA, Gallant JE, Ghanem KG, Emmanuel P, Zingman BS, Horberg MA. Primary care guidelines for the management of persons infected with HIV: 2013 update by the HIV Medicine Association of the Infectious Diseases Society of America. Clin Infect Dis. 2014;58:1–10.
12. Moscicki A-B, Darragh TM, Berry-Lawhorn JM, Roberts JM, Khan MJ, Boardman LA, et al. Screening for anal cancer in women. J Lower Gen Tract Dis. 2015;19:S27–42.
13. American Cancer Society. Can anal cancer be found early? Cancer.org. Accessed 10 Nov 2024.

Anal Squamous Cell Carcinoma

54

James S. Wu and Eric W. Willis

Presentation

A 45-year-old female presented with an anal mass (Fig. 54.1). Biopsy was done (Fig. 54.2).

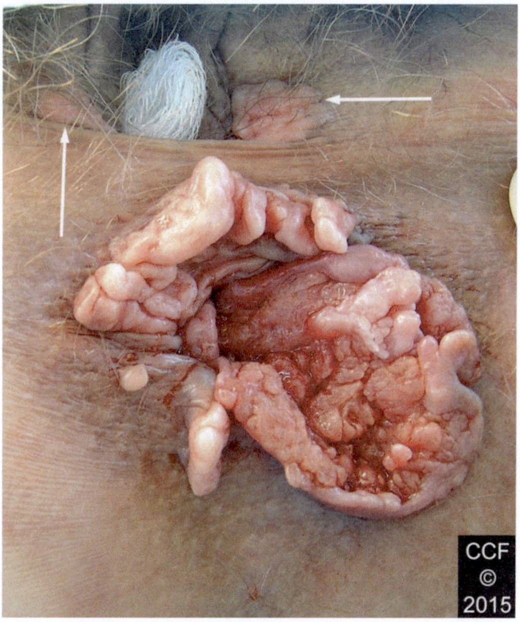

Fig. 54.1 A 3.5 cm × 3.0 cm left posterior two-thirds circumference ulcerated mass involving the anal canal and the anal margin is seen. Arrows point to two vulvar lesions

J. S. Wu (✉)
Department of Colon and Rectal Surgery, Cleveland Clinic, Cleveland, OH, USA

E. W. Willis
Department of Pathology, CORPath, Columbus, OH, USA

J. S. Wu, M. D. Inkster (eds.), *Cleveland Clinic Colorectal Case Studies*,
https://doi.org/10.1007/978-3-031-39880-3_54

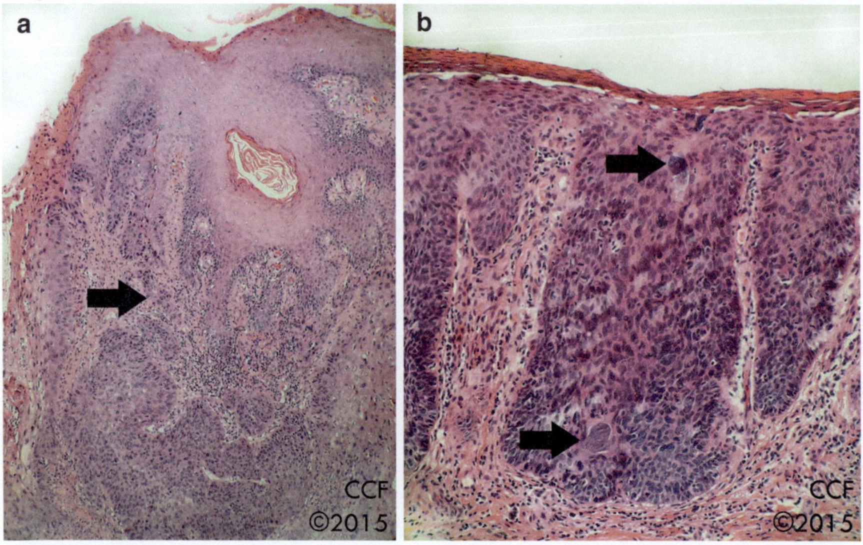

Fig. 54.2 (**a**) This invasive squamous cell carcinoma of the anus shows an irregular dermal-epidermal junction (arrow), invasive nests of carcinoma and single cells (Original magnification, H&E, ×100); (**b**) Vulvar squamous epithelium with marked nuclear atypia (arrows), consistent with high-grade squamous intraepithelial lesion (VIN3). The dermal–epidermal junction is smooth, indicating the noninvasive nature of this lesion (Original magnification, H&E, ×100)

Management

The patient underwent chemoradiation therapy. Follow-up at 1 and 2 years showed scars in the anus and vagina (Fig. 54.3). Biopsies were negative for dysplasia.

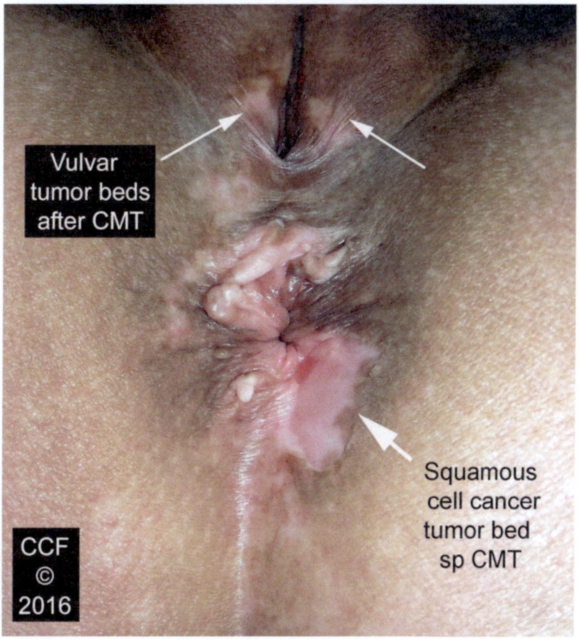

Fig. 54.3 Both the anal squamous cell carcinoma and the vulvar HSIL were eliminated by combined modality therapy (CMT)

Comment

The estimated new cases and deaths from cancer of the anus, anal canal, and anorectum in the United States in 2018 were 8580 with 1160 deaths [1].

Squamous cell carcinomas comprise the majority of cases. Anal squamous cell carcinoma is associated with human papillomavirus (HPV) infection, genital dysplasia, immunosuppression, and smoking.

Treatment of Squamous Cell Carcinoma of the Anus

A full therapeutic circle: from radiotherapy and back again.

Following World War I, radiation was the primary effective treatment for anal cancer. In 1935, Gordon-Watson wrote on the radium treatment of malignant disease of the anus:

> "I can only deal briefly here with squamous cell carcinoma of the anus. Early cases do well with radium and are much less resistant than rectal cases; the rectum with its sphincters can often be preserved intact and no colostomy performed" [2].

Because of complications, radiotherapy was abandoned in favor of radical surgery, namely abdominoperineal resection (APR). Five-year survival in large series for this surgery was between 48% and 71% (Table 54.1) [3–6].

In 1974, Nigro and co-workers described preoperative radiation and chemotherapy prior to APR. [7] The original protocol involved pelvic radiation, 5-Fluorouracil and Mitomycin C followed by APR. Nigro explained his rationale for combined modality therapy, as follows:

> "The anatomic features of the anal canal are such as to promote early spread of malignant cells. The area has both a profuse blood supply and an abundant lymphatic drainage system which leads in all directions. At the same time, there is a serious limitation in the amount of tissue around the anal canal which can be removed.
>
> It appears to us that surgical excision is not likely to be adequate treatment for many patients with cancer of the anal canal. Consequently, we believe the therapeutic approach should be changed to include other treatment modalities. Squamous-cell cancers are known to be sensitive to irradiation. Furthermore, there is evidence that chemotherapy, given simultaneously with irradiation, tends to potentiate its effect."[1]

Because chemoradiation therapy eliminated the tumor in five of the first six patients, Nigro discontinued routine APR. Among 104 anal cancers treated with chemoradiation, no gross tumor remained in 97 patients 6 weeks after treatment [8].

Combined chemoradiation therapy remains the primary mode of treatment for anal squamous carcinoma. Local excision is offered in selected early cases. APR may be offered for salvage [9].

---

[1] Nigro et al. [7]. Permission to reproduce this excerpt was generously provided by Wolters Kluwer Health, Inc., CCC|RightsLink License Number 5124730319376; License date Aug 9, 2021.

Table 54.1 Anal cancer survival following APR

Study	Year	*N*	5-year survival (%)
Hardcastle, Bussey	1968	83	48
Boman	1984	114	71
Frost	1984	109	62
Greenall	1985	103	55

On Anal Squamous Cell Carcinoma and Its Variants

Concerning invasive squamous cell cancer located in the area of the dentate line, Nigro observed in 1984 [10].[2]

> "These cancers, most of which arise in or just below the cloacogenic tissue that lines the part of the canal immediately above the dentate line, are often described as either cloacogenic, transitional, basaloid, epidermoid or squamous cell cancers. The terms, of course, refer to the predominant cell type present in the tumor. All of them are variants of squamous cells and, because their management does not depend upon the cell type, we prefer to call them squamous cell cancer of the anal canal; this simplifies the discussion of therapy."

Biographical Note [11]

Norman D. Nigro (1912–2009)

Norman Nigro was born in Syracuse, New York. He received his medical degree from Syracuse University in 1937. He became a preceptee in surgery in Detroit under Dr. Louis J. Hirschman. He served with the 17th Army General Hospital attached to the 5th Army in Italy during World War II. After the war, he practiced at Wayne State University in Detroit where he remained for his entire career. His report on combined therapy for cancer of the anal canal effectively displaced surgery as the primary treatment modality for anal cancer.

[2] Nigro [10]. Permission to reproduce this excerpt was generously provided by Wolters Kluwer Health, Inc.; CCC|RightsLink License Number 5124720590871; License date Aug 9, 2021.

References

1. Siegel RL, Miller KD, Jemal J. Cancer statistics, 2018. CA Cancer J Clin. 2018;68:7–30.
2. Gordon-Watson C. Discussion on the radium treatment of malignant disease of the rectum and anus. Proc R Soc Med. 1935;28:1251–63.
3. Hardcastle JD, Bussey HJR. Results of surgical treatment of squamous cell carcinoma of the anal canal and anal margin seen at St Mark's Hospital 1928–66. Proc R Soc Med. 1968;61:629–30.
4. Boman BM, Moertel CG, O'Connell MJ, Scott M, Weiland LH, Beart RW, et al. Carcinoma of the anal canal. A clinical and pathologic study of 188 cases. Cancer. 1984;54:114–25.
5. Frost DB, Richards PC, Montague ED, Giacco GG, Martin RG. Epidermoid cancer of the anorectum. Cancer. 1984;53:1285–93.
6. Greenall MJ, Quan SHQ, Urmacher C, DeCosse JJ. Treatment of epidermoid carcinoma of the anal canal. Surg Gynecol Obstet. 1985;161:509–17.
7. Nigro ND, Vaitkevicius VK, Considine B Jr. Combined therapy for cancer of the anal canal: a preliminary report. Dis Colon Rectum. 1974;17:354–6.
8. Nigro ND. Multidisciplinary Management of Cancer of the Anus. World J. Surg 1987;11:446–51.
9. Longo WE, Vernava AM III, Wade TP, Coplin MA, Virgo KS, Johnson FE. Recurrent squamous cell carcinoma of the anal canal: predictors of initial treatment failure and results of salvage therapy. Ann Surg. 1994;220:40–9.
10. Nigro ND. An evaluation of combined therapy for squamous cell cancer of the anal canal. Dis Colon Rectum. 1984;27:763–6.
11. Corman ML. Classic articles in colon and rectal surgery: Norman D. Nigro 1912. Dis Colon Rectum. 1993;36:709–11.

Cloacogenic Polyp

55

Sebouh Setrakian and James S. Wu

Presentation

A polyp in the anal transitional zone was biopsied (Fig. 55.1).

Pathology showed a cloacogenic polyp (Fig. 55.2).

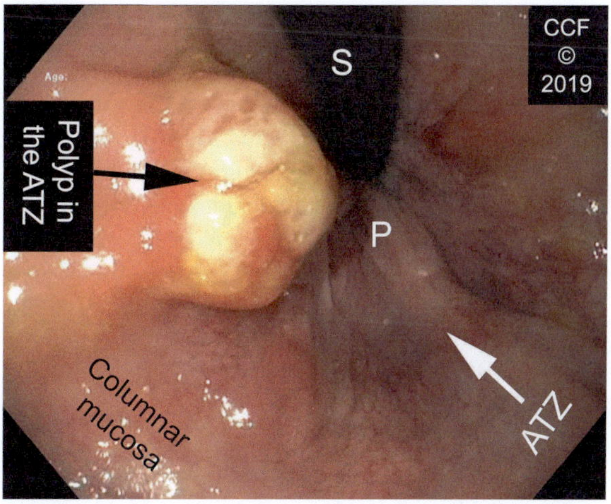

Fig. 55.1 Retroflexed endoscopic view of the distal rectum shows a polyp in the anal transitional zone (ATZ). The endoscope (S), pecten (P), and columnar mucosa are labeled

S. Setrakian
Pathology & Laboratory Medicine Institute, Cleveland Clinic, Cleveland, OH, USA

J. S. Wu (✉)
Department of Colon and Rectal Surgery, Cleveland Clinic, Cleveland, OH, USA

J. S. Wu, M. D. Inkster (eds.), *Cleveland Clinic Colorectal Case Studies*,
https://doi.org/10.1007/978-3-031-39880-3_55

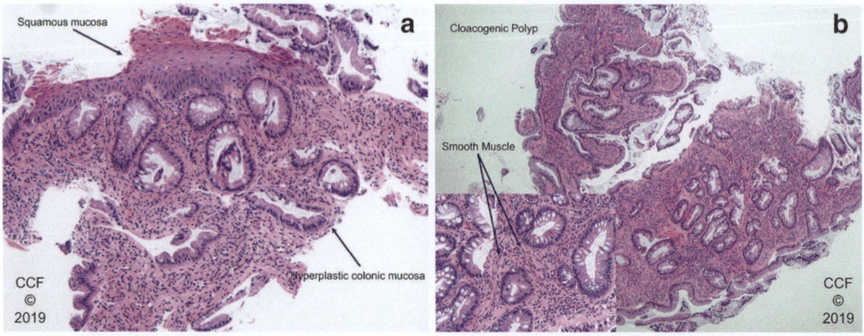

Fig. 55.2 (**a**) Reactive squamous epithelium overlying hyperplastic colorectal glands (H&E, original magnification ×200); (**b**) faint serrated appearance of hyperplastic glands (H&E, original magnification ×20) and fibromuscular proliferation in the lamina propria (Inset, H&E ×400)

Management

The polyp was removed by snare polypectomy.

Comment

Cloacogenic polyps are inflammatory lesions that occur in and around the anal transitional zone. They are considered to be part of the spectrum of mucosal prolapse [1]. They are benign but have features which mimic neoplsia including adenocarcinoma and squamous intraepithelial lesion [2–6].

References

1. Tendler DA, Aboudola S, Zacks JF, O'Brien MJ, Kelly CP. Prolapsing mucosal polyps: An underrecognized form of colonic polyp—a clinic-pathological study of 15 cases. Am J Gastroenterol. 2002;97:370–6.
2. Mathialagan R, Turner MJ, Gorard DA. Inflammatory cloacogenic polyp mimicking anorectal malignancy. Eur J Gastroenterol Hepatol. 2000;12:247–50.
3. Zaman S, Mistry P, Hendrickse C, Bowley DM. Cloacogenic polyps in an adolescent: A rare cause of rectal bleeding. J Pediatr Surg. 2013;48:E5–7.
4. Parfitt JR, Shepherd NA. Polypoid mucosal prolapse complicating low rectal adenomas: beware the inflammatory cloacogenic polyp! Histopathology. 2008;53:91–6.
5. López-Ramos CS, Rodríguez-Gómez S, Bailador-Andrés C, Baizán-García MJ. Inflammatory cloacogenic polyp: A rare cause of lower gastrointestinal bleeding. Rev Esp Enferm Dig (Madrid). 2013;105:240–1.
6. Hanson IM, Armstrong GR. Anal intraepithelial neoplasia in an inflammatory cloacogenic polyp. J Clin Pathol. 1999;52:393–4.

56 Hypertrophied Anal Papilla

Michelle D. Inkster and James S. Wu

Presentation

A 60-year-old patient complained of a prolapsing "hemorrhoid." Examination showed a prolapsed hypertrophied anal papilla (Fig. 56.1).

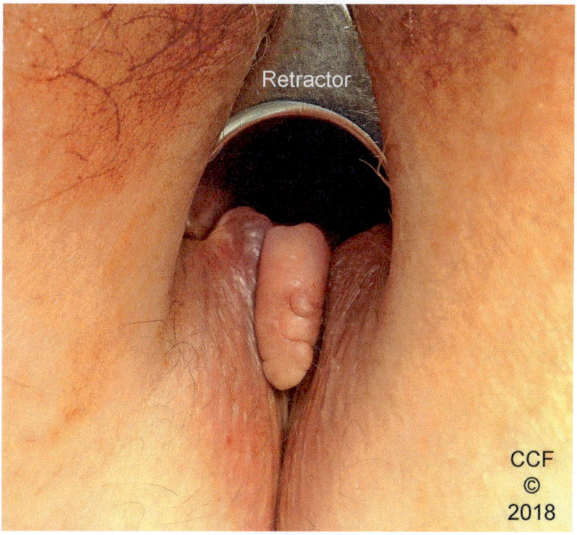

Fig. 56.1 Hypertrophied anal papilla prolapsing from the anus

M. D. Inkster
Department of Gastroenterology, Cleveland Clinic, Cleveland, OH, USA

J. S. Wu (✉)
Department of Colon and Rectal Surgery, Cleveland Clinic, Cleveland, OH, USA

J. S. Wu, M. D. Inkster (eds.), *Cleveland Clinic Colorectal Case Studies*,
https://doi.org/10.1007/978-3-031-39880-3_56

Management

Colonoscopy showed a hypertrophied anal papilla (HAP) but was otherwise normal. Surgical excision was done (Figs. 56.2a–c) .

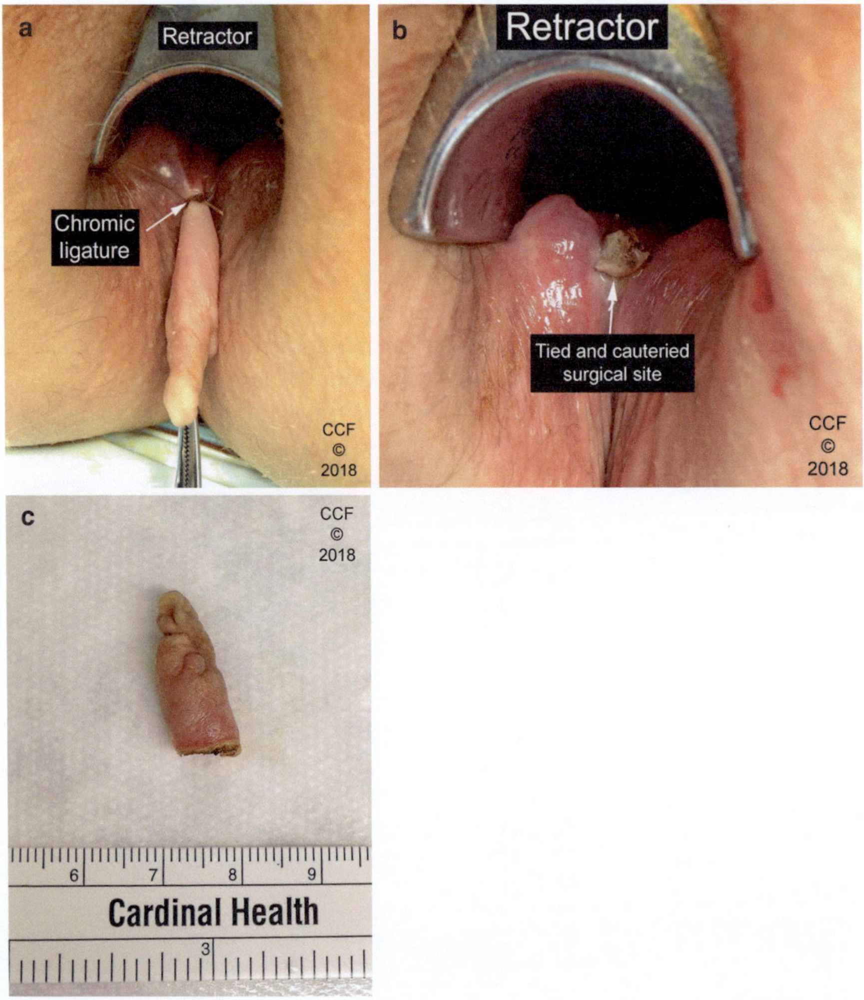

Fig. 56.2 (**a**) The papilla was exposed with an operating anoscope and exteriorized with traction. The base of the papilla was tied with a suture ligature to secure the vascular supply. (**b**) The surgical site following HAP excision. (**c**) The excised anal papilla. Pathology showed squamous epthelium without dysplasia

Comment

Anal papillae arise from the squamous mucosa at the proximal extent of the pecten of Stroud [1] and the distal border of the anal transitional zone [2]. These papillae are prone to hypertrophy. Gant described "Papillitis (hypertrophied anal papillae)" in 1920 [3]:

> "Hypertrophied papillae may persist without manifestations, but when large they incite sphincteralgia, pruritis ani, desire to stool, tickling sensations, slight mucoid discharge, and they intensify constipation by causing sphincterismus.
>
> Hypertrophied papillae are occasionally mistaken for skin tabs, polyps and venereal warts, from which they are distinguished by their reddish base, pointed extremity and hypersensitiveness."

The anatomic appearance of hypertrophied anal papillae was described by Drueck in 1922 [4].

> "The pyramidal teats have a pinkish colored base continuous with the mucous membrane below but a pearl white tip. They are always present although not easily seen except when hypertrophied and elongated, at which time they appear as saw tooth projections with their bases directed upward and inward often associated with inflammation or ulceration of neighboring crypts (cryptitis), and many hang down as slender ribbons, perhaps an inch long, or may be a rounded balllike tumor easily mistaken for a skin tab or polyp or an anal wart."

Hypertrophied anal papillae seen at colonoscopy are shown in Fig. 56.3a, b.

Surgical removal of hypertrophied anal papillae is indicated when symptoms develop.

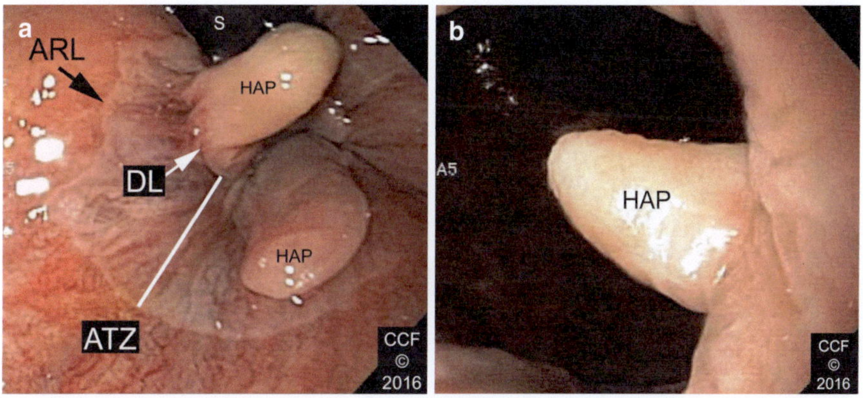

Fig. 56.3 (**a**) Two hypertrophied anal papillae (HAP), seen during colonoscopy on retroflexion, arise from the proximal pecten adjacent to the dentate line (DL) which is also the distal border or the anal transitional zone (ATZ). The proximal border of the ATZ is the anorectal line (ARL). (**b**) One of the HAP when seen *en face* during colonoscopy has a toothlike or "dentate" appearance

References

1. Stroud BB. On the anatomy of the anus. Ann Surg. 1896;24:1–15.
2. Tanaka E, Noguchi T, Nagai K, Akashi Y, Kawahara K, Shimad. Morphology of the epithelium of the lower rectum and the anal canal in the adult human. Med Mol Morphol. 2012;45:72–9.
3. Gant SG. Papillitis (Hypertrophied anal papillae). Am J Surg. 1920;34:25–6. Google books. https://books.google.com. Accessed 29 Dec 2, 2019.
4. Drueck CJ. Hypertrophied anal papillæ (Papillitis). New York Med J Med Rec. 1922;CXVI:448–9. Google Books. http://books.google.com. Accessed 29 Dec 2019

Anal Abscess

57

James S. Wu

Presentation A

A 37-year-old diabetic male was seen in the emergency room with anal pain. A tender, fluctuant, erythematous, and edematous mass was seen in the left perirectal area (Fig. 57.1).

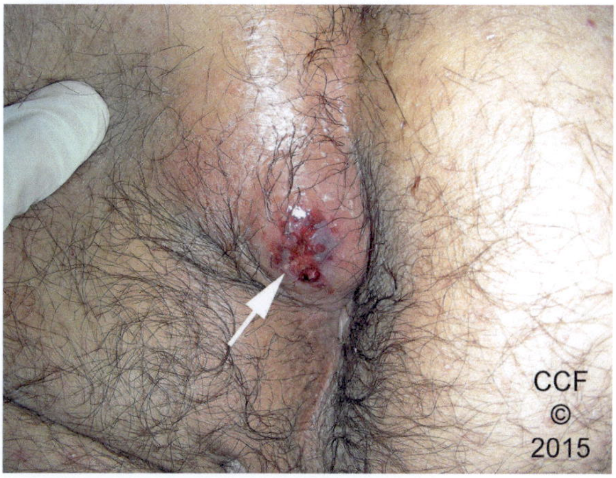

Fig. 57.1 Tender, fluctuant, erythematous, and edematous left perirectal mass (arrow)

J. S. Wu (✉)
Department of Colon and Rectal Surgery, Cleveland Clinic, Cleveland, OH, USA

J. S. Wu, M. D. Inkster (eds.), *Cleveland Clinic Colorectal Case Studies*,
https://doi.org/10.1007/978-3-031-39880-3_57

Management

This patient has a perirectal abscess that was treated by immediate incision and drainage under local anesthesia (Fig. 57.2). Purulent drainage was discharged in abundance. Pain relief soon followed. Because of his history of diabetes, the patient was admitted and received intravenous antibiotics. His recovery was uneventful.

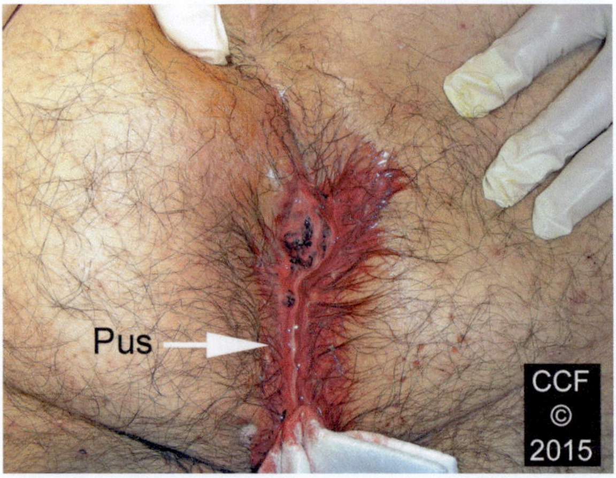

Fig. 57.2 Following administration of a local anesthetic, the abscess was drained through a cruciate incision made in the skin overlying the point of maximum fluctuance

Presentation B

A patient with an acute perianal abscess underwent drainage with a Malecot™ catheter (Figs. 57.3, 57.4, 57.5, and 57.6).

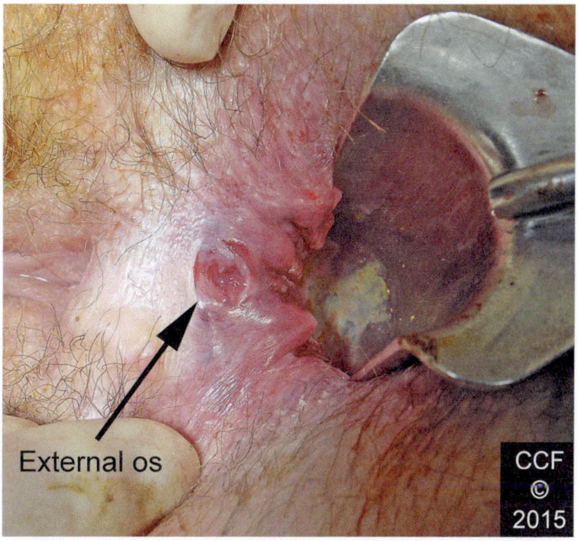

Fig. 57.3 The anus is dilated with an anoscope. The external opening in the skin (external os) of an abscess after incision and drainage is marked with an arrow

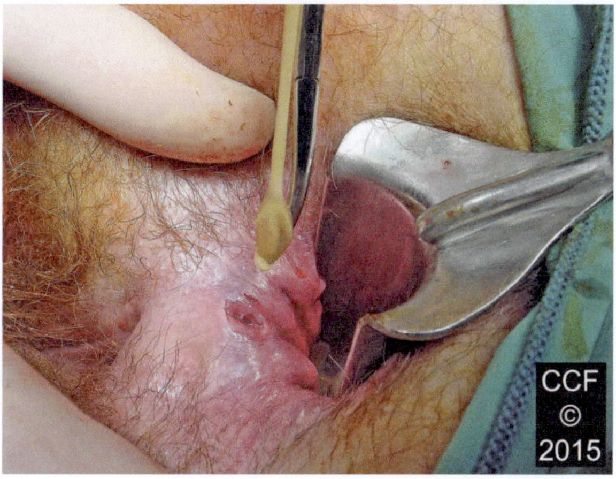

Fig. 57.4 A Malecot™ drain is stretched over a curved hemostat

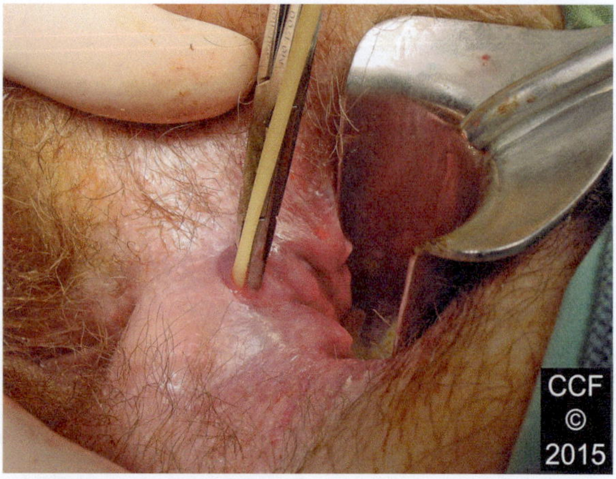

Fig. 57.5 The Malecot™ drain is inserted into the abscess cavity aided by the curved hemostat

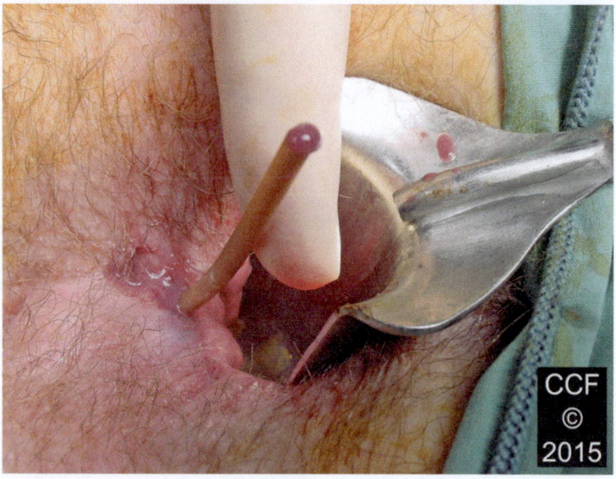

Fig. 57.6 Purulent drainage following drain placement exudes from the catheter tail

Presentation C

A 30-year-old male, BMI 39, presented with anorectal pain of 5 days' duration. He reported chills. He had extreme pain when straining for a bowel movement. Examination showed focal tenderness in the anal canal posteriorly. A CT scan showed a 2.5 × 1.8 cm focal density consistent with a perianal abscess (Fig. 57.7).

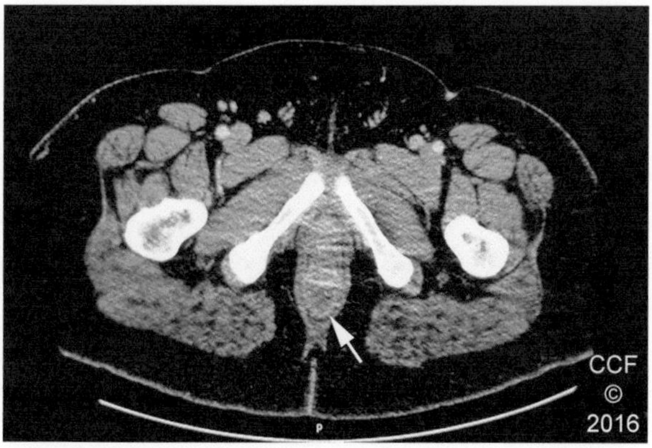

Fig. 57.7 A density posterior to the anus (arrow) is seen on this CT scan

Management

Examination under anesthesia in search of a postanal abscess was done in the prone position. Aspiration with a spinal needle was attempted without success. When pressure was applied to the skin between the anus and coccyx, pus was seen in the anal canal (Fig. 57.8). The posterior internal anal opening was dilated with a curved clamp resulting in brisk drainage of pus into the anal canal (Fig. 57.9). The patient's symptoms resolved following this internal abscess drainage.

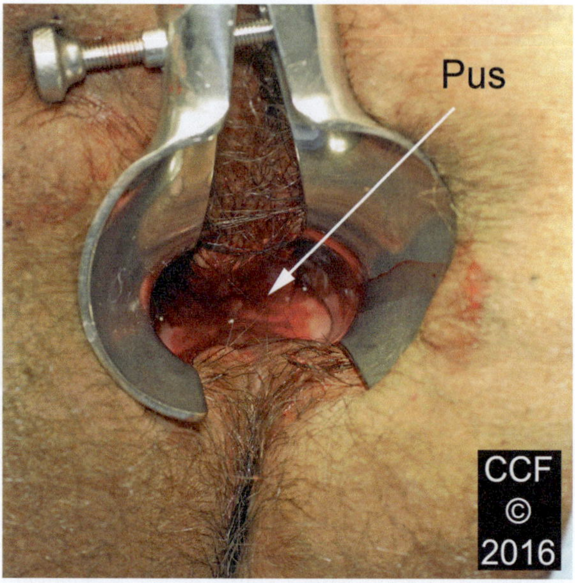

Fig. 57.8 The anal canal was observed while pressure was applied to the space posterior to the anus. Internal drainage of pus was seen.

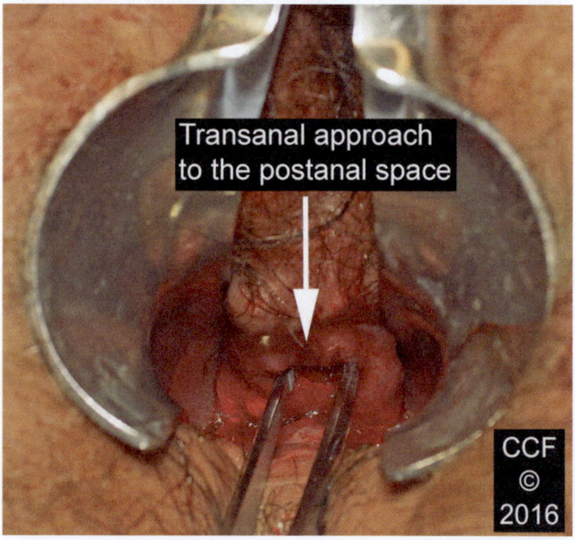

Fig. 57.9 Adequate drainage of the postanal space abscess was achieved by trans-anal dilation of the tract between the anal canal and the abscess cavity (Fig. 57.10)

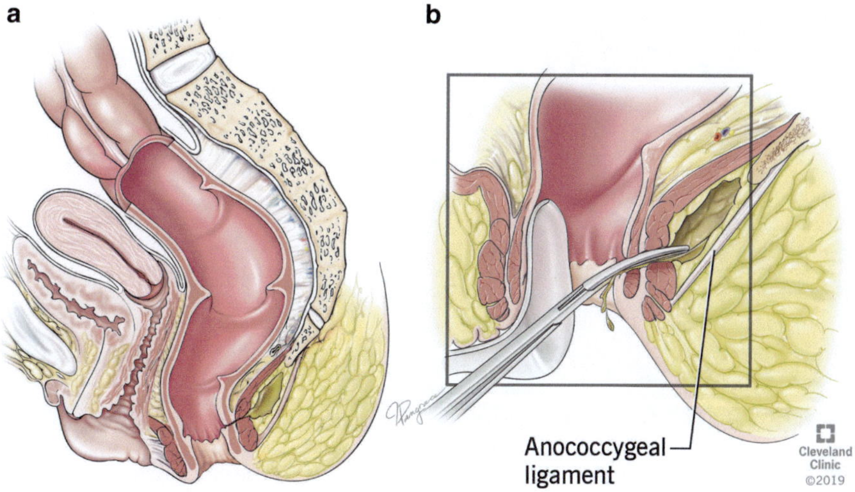

Fig. 57.10 Trans-anal drainage of a posterior midline deep postanal space abscess (Fig. 57.10a). In this case, a curved clamp is passed from the internal opening in the anus into the abscess cavity (Fig. 57.10b). The anococcygeal ligament is labeled

Presentation D

A 33-year-old morbidly obese male was seen in the clinic because of anorectal pain. He could not stay still and moved about restlessly. He was febrile and was unable to sit or to tolerate examination. Broad spectrum intravenous antibiotics were given, and the patient was taken to the operating room for examination under anesthesia. Palpation of the anal canal, perianal skin, buttock, and gluteal cleft did not reveal fluctuance. Anoscopy did not show thrombosis or fissure. Transrectal ultrasound was done (Fig. 57.11a). The abscess was drained using silastic setons, an example of which is shown in Fig. 57.11b.

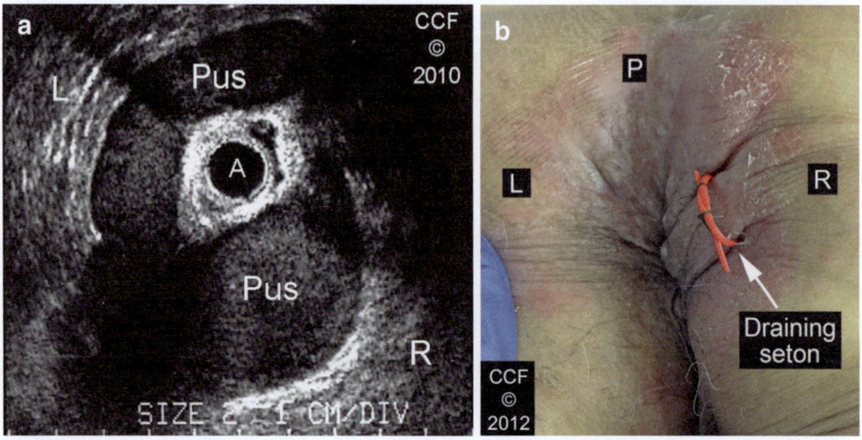

Fig. 57.11 (**a**) Trans-anal ultrasound examination shows a large bilateral collection of fluid in the ischiorectal fossae consistent with a "horseshoe abscess." Incision and drainage with setons was done to allow for egress of suppuration. The anus (A), right (R), left (L), and areas containing pus are labeled. (**b**) Right-sided ischiorectal fossa abscess drained with a silastic vessel loop seton

Discussion

Suppuration within anal "Divertikel" as the cause of anal abscess and fistula was proposed by Chiari in 1878 [1].

Ueber die analen Divertikel der Rectumsschleimhaut und ihre Beziehung zu den Analfisteln. **Von** Dr. Hanns Chiari Assistenten am path.-anat. Institute in Wien Es lässt sich das aber auch unschwer verstehen. Man hat sich nur vorzustellen, dass Fäcalmassen in solchen Divertikeln stagniren, was gewiss leicht geschehen kann, zumal dann, wenn die Divertikel bereits ausserhalb der Sphincteren herausgetreten sind, wobei dann die Rückentleerung von Inhalt aus den Divertikeln in das Darmrohr bedeutend erschwert ist. Die stagnirenden Fäcalmassen regen Ulceration an und so kommt es im Grunde des Divertikels allmälig zu Durchbruch durch die Haut und damit zur Herstellung einer Fistula ani…	**Concerning anal diverticula of the rectal mucosa and their relation to anal fistulae.** **By** Dr. Hanns Chiari Assistant in path.-anat. Institute in Wien It is not difficult to understand. One has only to imagine that fecal masses stagnate in such diverticula which certainly can be done easily, especially if the diverticula are then emerged already outside of the sphincters, in which case the retrograde emptying of the contents from the diverticula into the intestinal tube is made considerably more difficult. The stagnant fecal masses stimulate ulceration, and basically the diverticulum gradually breaks through the skin and thus makes an anal fistula…

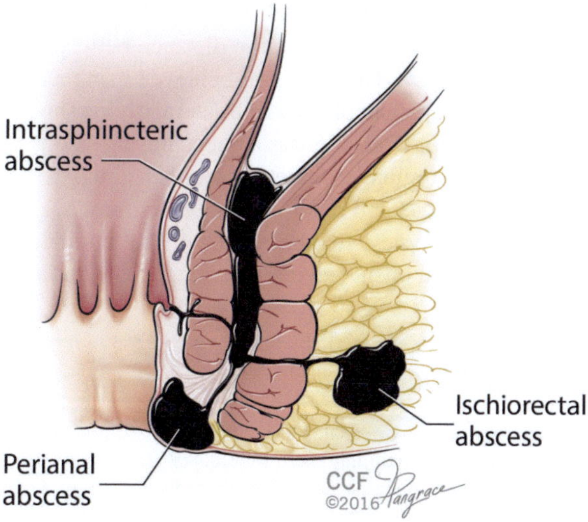

Fig. 57.12 Anal gland abscesses form in the intersphinteric groove. Infections can ascend to the supralevator space, descend to the skin adjacent to the intersphincteric groove or traverse the external sphincter into the ischiorectal fossa

Table 57.1 Boundaries of the ischiorectal fossa

Floor: skin
Superior levator ani
Medial: external anal sphincter
Lateral: ischial tuberosity, obturator internus muscle
Anterior: superficial transverse perineal muscle
Posterior: gluteus maximus muscle

Table 57.2 Common causes of anal pain

Anal fissure
Thrombosed external hemorrhoid
Abscess

The presence of inflammation in the perianal or rectal regions raises the possibility for abscess. Perirectal abscesses arise from the anal glands. According to Parks [2], infection from an anal gland creates an abscess in the space between the internal and external anal sphincter. The abscess can travel in several directions. Downward spread results in a perianal abscess. Spread across the external sphincter results in an abscess in the ischiorectal fossa. An abscess in the intersphincteric space, rarely can ascend into the supralevator space Fig. 57.12. Ischiorectal abscesses occur in the ischiorectal fossa. The boundaries of the ischiorectal fossa are listed in Table 57.1 (see Chap. 8). Anal pain commonly is associated with three causes (Table 57.2)

In these cases, pain was due to an abscess that required drainage [3]. In presentation A, drainage was done percutaneously through a cruciate skin incision. Small abscesses such as this can be drained under local anesthesia in an office setting. Larger abscesses are drained in the operating room. In general, blunt probing of the abscess cavity is not necessary and may lead to bleeding that is difficult to control. In presentation B, drainage was done by placing a Malecot® catheter into the abscess cavity through a small incision. In presentation C, percutaneous drainage was not successful due to a large distance between the skin and the abscess and a small abscess size. Drainage was achieved using a transanal approach. In presentation D, the diagnosis of a large bilateral "horseshoe" abscess was made by transanal ultrasound. Drainage was achieved using setons.

Following drainage, three subsequent outcomes may occur: (1) the drainage wound may close and recurrent abscesses may not ever recur; (2) the wound may close, and an abscess may recur at some future date; and (3) the draining perianal site may remain open, leaving behind an anal fistula.

References

1. Chiari H. Ueber die analen Divertikel der Rectumsschleimhaut und ihre Beziehung zu den Analfisteln. Medizin Jahrbüch. 1878;8:419–27.
2. Parks AG. Pathogenesis and treatment of fistula-in-ano. Br Med J. 1961;i:463–9.
3. Rickard MJFX. Anal abscesses and fistulas. ANZ J Surg. 2005;75:64–72.

Anal Fistula-Introduction

58

James S. Wu and Michelle D. Inkster

Introduction

A fistula is an abnormal connection between two epithelialized surfaces. An anal fistula (fistula-in-ano) is a sinus secondary to a diseased anal gland. Fistula-in-ano is suspected if a persistent sinus remains after drainage of a perirectal abscess. Symptoms include pain, drainage, and chronic inflammation [1].

On fistulae, Hippocrates wrote:

> "But if a fistula be already formed when you undertake the case, take a stalk of fresh garlic, and having laid the man on his back and separated his thighs on both sides, push down the stalk as far as it will go, and thereby measure the depth of the fistula" [2].

With this statement, Hippocrates defined the first principle of anal fistula surgery, namely, definition of fistula anatomy. There are three fistula components: the external opening (external os), the internal opening (internal os), and the tract connecting the two. In 1878, Chiari described the anatomy of anal fistula discovered at autopsy of a 46 year-old man who had died from tuberculosis (Fig. 58.1) [3].

J. S. Wu (✉)
Department of Colon and Rectal Surgery, Cleveland Clinic, Cleveland, OH, USA

M. D. Inkster
Department of Gastroenterology, Cleveland Clinic, Cleveland, OH, USA

J. S. Wu, M. D. Inkster (eds.), *Cleveland Clinic Colorectal Case Studies*,
https://doi.org/10.1007/978-3-031-39880-3_58

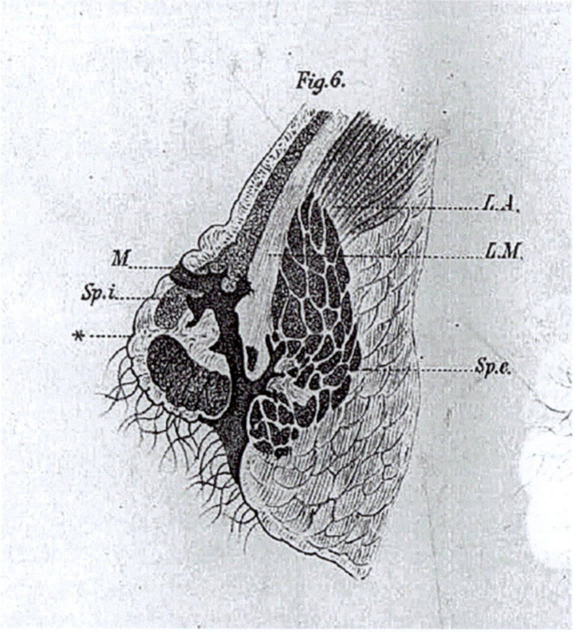

Fig. 58.1 Chiari's drawing of an anal fistula found at the autopsy of a 46-year-old man who had died of tuberculosis, Fig. 6. Zum 7 Falle. Längschnitt durch das rectum in der Mitte der Protuberanz (Fig. 6 Case 7). Longitudinal section through the rectum in the middle of the protuberance. Medially, there is an opening at the lacune of Morgagni (*M*) that passes across the internal anal sphincter (*Sp. i*) across the longitudinal muscle of the rectum (*L.M.*-Längsmusculatur des Rectums) and across the external anal sphincter (*Sp.e.*) to the skin. The levator ani muscle *(L.A.)* is identified proximal to the external sphincter. Two short extensions in the space between the sphincters are seen

Ueber die analen Divertikel der Rectumsschleimhaut und ihre Beziehung zu den Analfisteln Von Dr. Hanns Chiari path.-anat. Institute in Wien	Concerning anal diverticulum of the rectal mucosa and their relation to anal fistulas By Dr. Hanns Chiari Pathologic Anatomy Institute, Vienna
7. Fall. Analportion des Rectums eines 46jährigen an Tuberculose verstorbenen Mannes. » Am vorderen Rande der Analöffnung und von da auf das Perinäum sich erstreckend eine sagittal gestellte, längliche, im ganzen haselnussgrosse Vorwölbung der Haut, an deren vorderem Ende (2 Ctm. von dem Anus entfernt) eine trichterartig eingezogeoe, von narbigem Gewebe begrenzte, hanfkorngrosse Lücke sich findet. Diese Lücke leitet in einen der früher genannten Vorwölbung in der Haut correspondirenden Kanal, der 2·5 Ctm. lang, an der inneren Oberfläche der vorderen Rectumswand genau entsprechend einer Morgagni'schen Lacune ausmündet. Auf diesem Wege durchsetzt der Kanal die unterste Partie des M. sphincter ani int. et ext., so dass von diesen Muskeln auf dem Querschnitte etwas 4 Mm. dicke Antheile nach innen von ihm liegen.	7th case. Anal portion of the rectum of a 46-year-old man who died of tuberculosis. » At the anterior border of the anal opening and from there to the perineum, a sagittally elongated, hazelnut-sized protrusion of the skin, at the anterior end (2 cm. from the anus) a funnel-like reticulated, scarred tissue, hemp grain big gap is found. This gap leads into one of the previously mentioned protrusions in the skin corresponding to a channel, 2–5 cm. long, opening at the inner surface of the anterior rectum wall exactly corresponding to a Morgagni's Lacune. In this way the channel penetrates inwardly the lowest part of the internal and external anal sphincter muscles (on cross-section some 4 mm. thick).

In 1961, Parks wrote: "In fact, a fistula-in-ano is virtually a sinus secondary to a diseased anal gland,…" [4].

In 1976, Parks, Gordon and Hardcastle published their classification of fistula-in-ano (Fig. 58.2) [5]. Fistulas are classified according to their relationship to the anal sphincter. There are four main anatomical types. The external sphincter mass is regarded as the keystone. The terms "trans," "supra," and "extra" refer to it.

An anal fistula may be deemed complex when certain features are present (Table 58.1) [1].

Causes of anal fistula are listed in Table 58.2 [6].

Diagnosis is established by examination, usually under anesthesia, and radiologic studies.

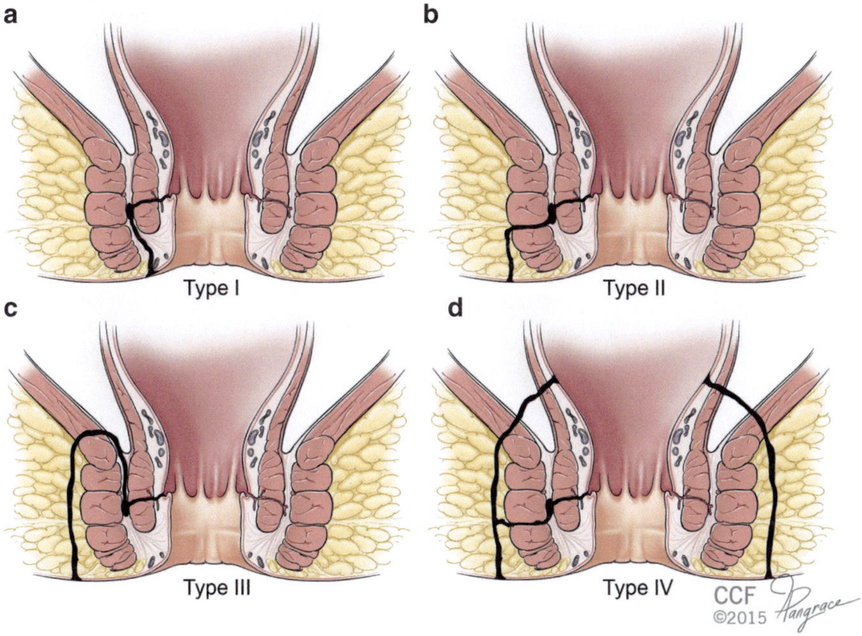

Fig. 58.2 Classification of anal fistula (after Parks, Gordon and Hardcastle): (**a**) intersphincteric, (**b**) transsphincteric, (**c**) suprasphincteric, and (**d**) extrasphincteric

Table 58.1 Features associated with "complex" anal fistulas

Features
Fistula track crosses >30%–50% of the external sphincter (high-transsphincteric, suprasphincteric, and extrasphincteric)
Anterior anal fistula in a female
Multiple fistula tracks are present
Recurrent anal fistula
Preexisting fecal incontinence
Local irradiation
Inflammatory bowel disease
Malignant fistula

Table 58.2 Causes of anal fistula

Causes of anal fistula
Anorectal (cryptoglandular) sepsis
Malignancy
Hidradenitis suppurativa
Tuberculosis
Crohn's disease
Trauma

References

1. Whiteford MH, Kilkenny J, Hyman N, Buie WD, Cohen J, Orsay C, et al. Practice parameters for the treatment of perianal abscess and fistula-in-ano (revised). Dis Colon Rectum. 2005;48:1337–42.
2. Adams F. On fistulae. The genuine works of Hippocrates, translated from the Greek with a preliminary discourse and annotation, Vol II. William Wood and Co., New York, 1886. p. 311. Accessed from Google Books February 20, 2020.
3. Chiari H. Ueber die analen Divertikel Rectumsschleimhaut und ihre Beziehung zu den Analfisteln. Med Jahrbüch. 1878;8:419–27.
4. Parks AG. Pathogenesis and treatment of fistula-in-ano. Br Med J. 1961;i:463–9.
5. Parks AG, Gordon PH, Hardcastle JD. A classification of fistula-in-ano. Br J Surg. 1976;63:1–12.
6. Jacob TJ, Perakath B, Keighley MR. Surgical intervention for anorectal fistula. Cochrane Database Syst Rev. 2010;(5):CD006319.

Anal Fistula-Fistulotomy

59

James S. Wu and Michelle D. Inkster

Presentation

A patient underwent incision and drainage of a left anterolateral perirectal abscess. Six months later, a small amount of drainage soiling the underwear each day was noted. Inspection revealed a sinus tract in the left anterior perianal skin (Fig. 59.1). There was no history of prior anal surgery, inflammatory bowel disease, pelvic irradiation, or fecal incontinence.

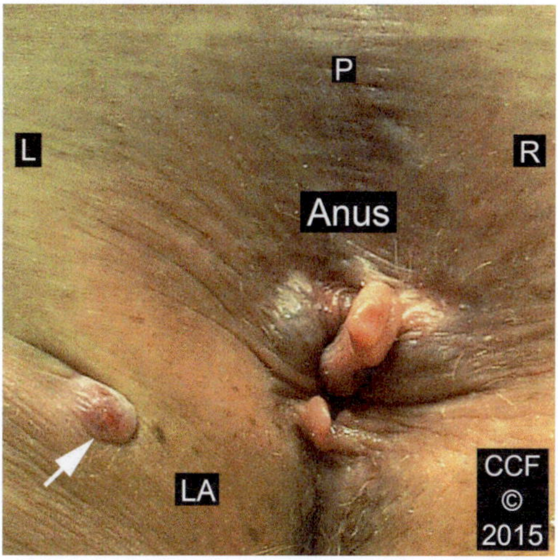

Fig. 59.1 Draining left anterior (LA) perianal skin opening (arrow). The left (L), Right (R), and posterior (P) positions around the anus are labeled

J. S. Wu (✉)
Department of Colon and Rectal Surgery, Cleveland Clinic, Cleveland, OH, USA

M. D. Inkster
Department of Gastroenterology, Cleveland Clinic, Cleveland, OH, USA

J. S. Wu, M. D. Inkster (eds.), *Cleveland Clinic Colorectal Case Studies*,
https://doi.org/10.1007/978-3-031-39880-3_59

Management

At examination under anesthesia, a left anterior external os was seen (Fig. 59.2). A probe was passed from the external os through a fistula tract to an internal os in the anal canal (Fig. 59.3). The fistula tract was divided with electrocautery (Figs. 59.4 and 59.5).

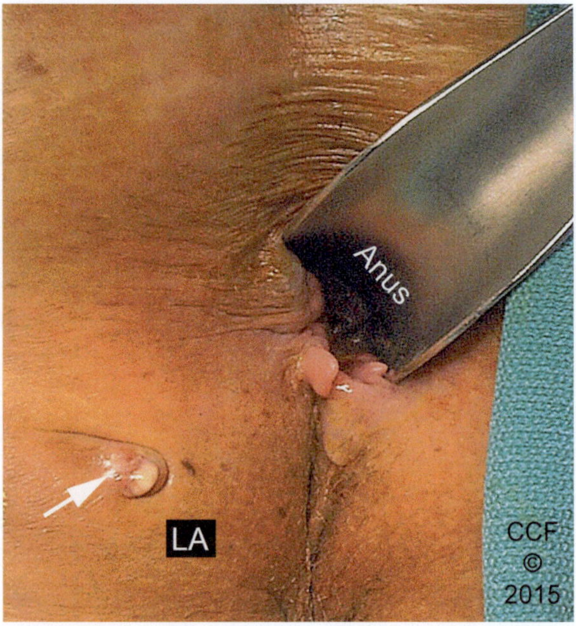

Fig. 59.2 An operating anoscope is positioned in the anal canal. The arrow points to the external os in the left anterior (LA) position

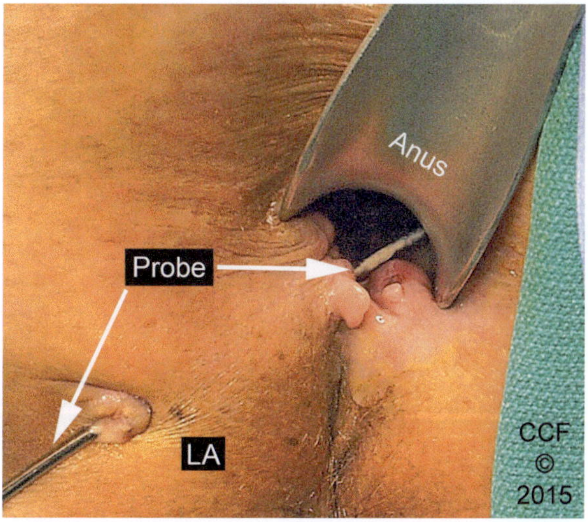

Fig. 59.3 An anal probe inserted into the external os at the perianal skin opening passes directly into the anal canal at the internal os. Left anterior (LA)

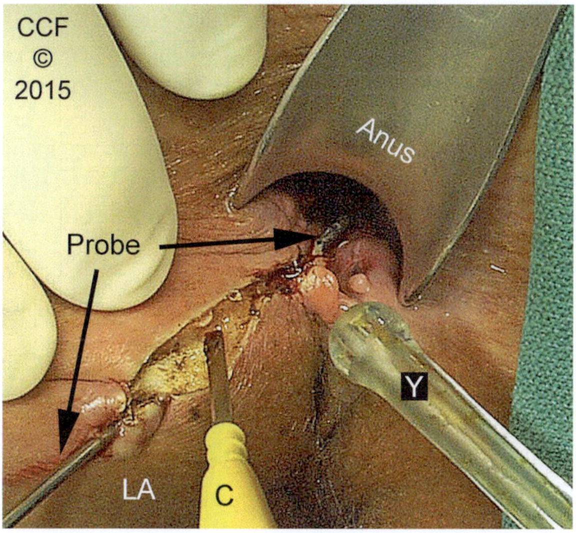

Fig. 59.4 The skin, fat, and muscle overlying the fistula probe were divided using electrocautery (C). Smoke was evacuated using a Yankauer suction catheter (Y). The amount of sphincter muscle divided was estimated to be less than 30%. Left anterior (LA)

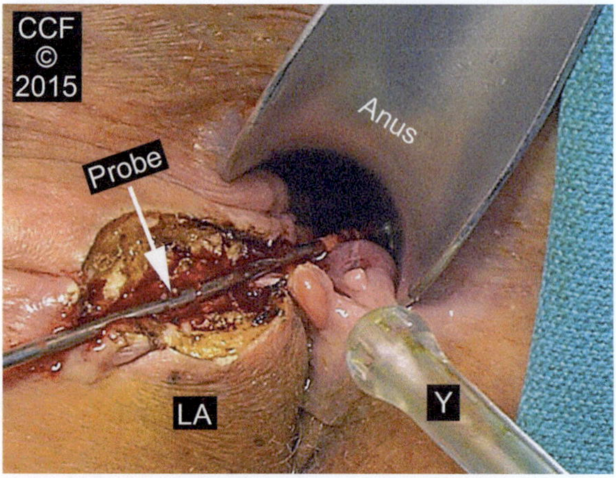

Fig. 59.5 Surgical site after complete fistulotomy. The probe within the tract has been exposed. Left anterior (LA), Yankauer suction (Y)

Comment

A fistula is an abnormal connection between two epithelialized surfaces. The anal fistula in this case was a sinus tract between a diseased anal gland and the skin. Fistula-in-ano is suspected if a persistent cutaneous opening remains after drainage of a perirectal abscess. Symptoms include pain, drainage, and chronic inflammation [1].

This case illustrates the diagnosis and management of a cryptogenic low transsphincteric anal fistula by fistulotomy in which the soft tissue and the skin overlying the fistula tract was unroofed and laid open [2]. Healing occurred by secondary intention.

References

1. Whiteford MH, Kilkenny J, Hyman N, Buie WD, Cohen J, Orsay C, et al. Practice parameters for the treatment of perianal abscess and fistula-in-ano (revised). Dis Colon Rectum. 2005;48:1337–42.
2. Rizzo JA, Naig AL, Johnson EK. Anorectal abscess and fistula-in-ano: evidence-based management. Surg Clin N Am. 2010;90:45–68.

Anal Fistula (Horseshoe)-Hanley's Procedure

60

James S. Wu and Alain G. Rizk

Presentation A

A 36 year-old male presented with a draining right-sided perianal skin opening that had been present for more than five years. Although the site periodically closes, without fail, it resuppurates and redrains. Examination under anesthesia was done.

Management

The appearance of the perianal skin is shown in Fig. 60.1.

J. S. Wu (✉)
Department of Colon and Rectal Surgery, Cleveland Clinic, Cleveland, OH, USA

A. G. Rizk
Radiology and Diagnostic Imaging Institute, Cleveland Clinic, Cleveland, OH, USA

J. S. Wu, M. D. Inkster (eds.), *Cleveland Clinic Colorectal Case Studies*,
https://doi.org/10.1007/978-3-031-39880-3_60

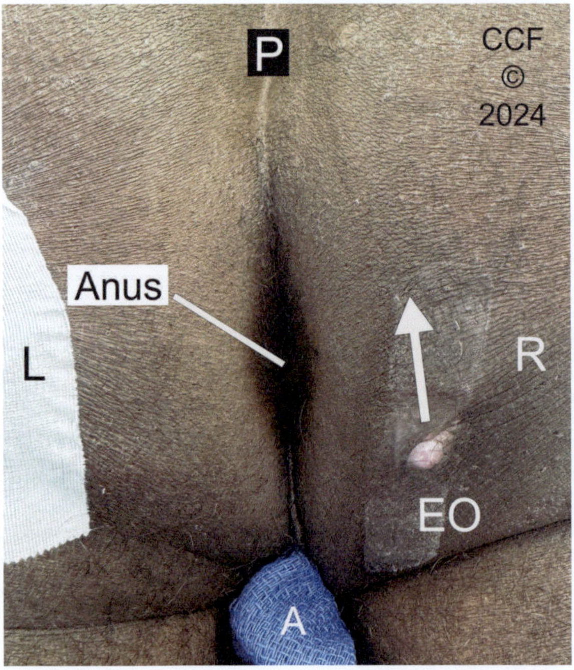

Fig. 60.1 Appearance of the perianal area during examination under anesthesia in the prone jackknife position. The external draining skin opening (external os, EO) is seen in the right anterior position relative to the anus. When the EO was gently probed, a sinus tract was found that moved in a direction lateral and posterior to the anus (arrow). Anterior (A), left (L), posterior (P), right (R)

The finding of a subcutaneous tract moving from the EO in the posterolateral direction suggested the presence of an anal fistula originating from the posterior midline. The anal canal was gently probed with a malleable sterling silver anal probe. An internal opening was found in the posterior midline that connected to a space outside the anal sphincter muscles. The skin and fat overlying the probe was divided; a fistula tract that passed through the anal sphincter muscle was found as shown in Fig. 60.2.

The silver probe with two 0-silk threads attached at the tip was withdrawn. The two attached silk threads were tied around the anal sphincter muscles as cutting setons. A "needle eye" probe was passed easily from the EO through the right "horseshoe" fistula extension to the unroofed posterior perianal space (Fig. 60.3).

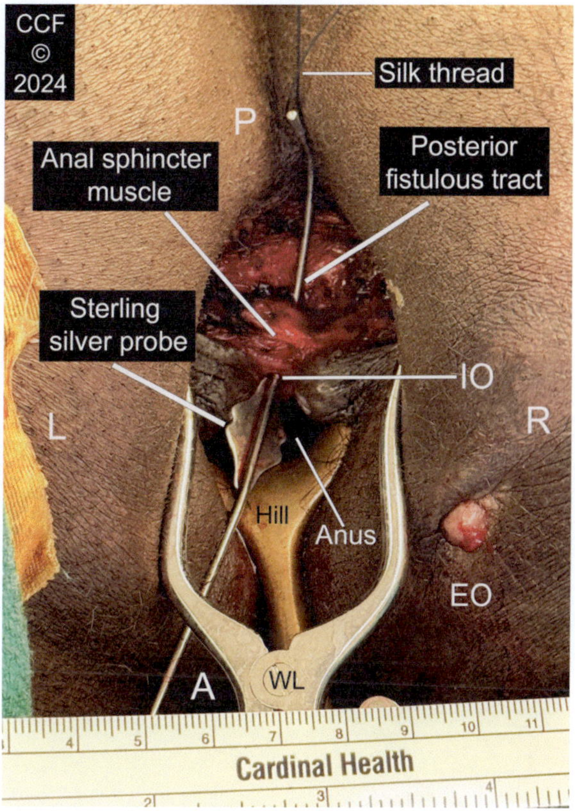

Fig. 60.2 A malleable sterling silver probe passes from the posterior midline of the anal canal (internal os, IO) through the anal sphincter muscle and into a posterior perianal space. The posterior fistulous tract, the external os (EO) and anus are labelled. An 0-silk thread has been attached to the tip of the probe. Anterior (A), left (L), posterior (P), right (R), Hill anoscope (Hill), Weitlaner self-retaining retractor (WL)

Two draining Silastic® setons were drawn through the right lateral extension of the fistula tract (Fig. 60.4).

The ends of the Silastic® draining setons are tied together with silk suture (Fig. 60.5).

The final appearance of the anus after partial posterior fistulotomy. Midline cutting silk setons and right posterolateral draining setons have been placed (Fig. 60.6).

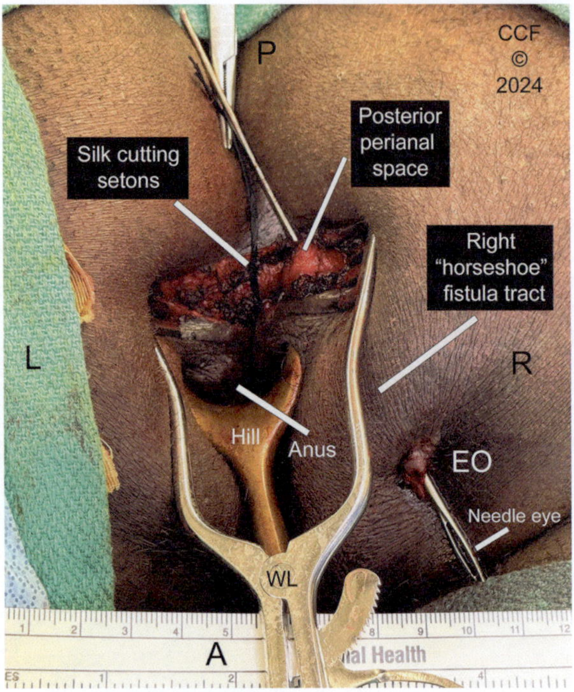

Fig. 60.3 The malleable silver probe with 0-silk ties attached to its tip was withdrawn. Two attached silk threads were tied around the anal sphincter muscle as cutting setons. The tails of the threads (held by a hemostat) were left in place to aid with future cutting seton identification. A probe with a "needle eye" easily traversed the fistula tract from the EO passing through the right "horseshoe" fistula tract to the unroofed posterior perianal space. External os (EO), Hill anoscope (Hill), Weitlaner self-retaining retractor (WL), anterior (A), left (L), posterior (P), right (R)

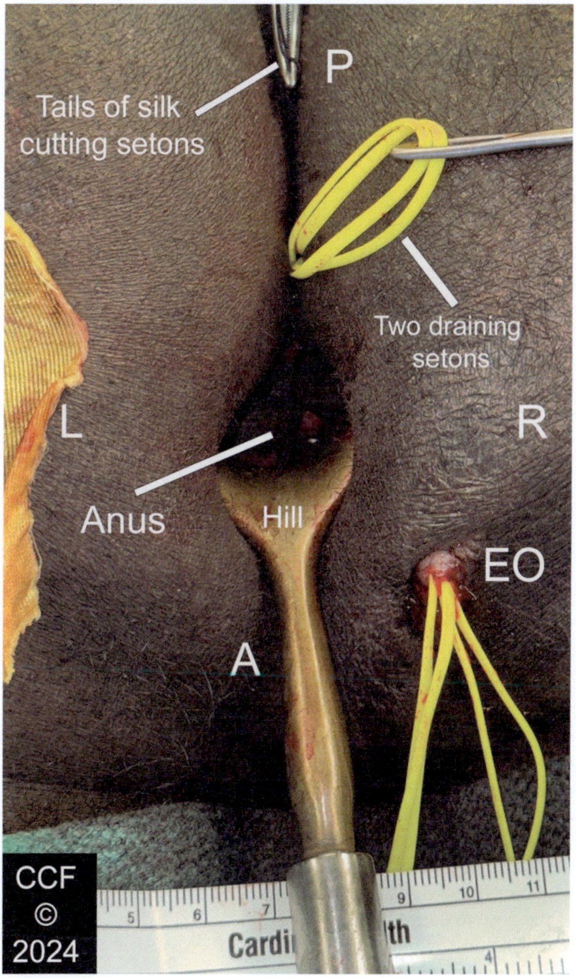

Fig. 60.4 Two Silastic® vessel loops have been drawn through the right-sided "horseshoe" fistula tract to act as draining setons. The tails of the posterior midline cutting setons encircling the anal sphincter muscle are marked with a hemostat. The anus has been labeled. External os (EO), Anterior (A), Left (L), Posterior (P), Right (R), Hill anoscope (Hill)

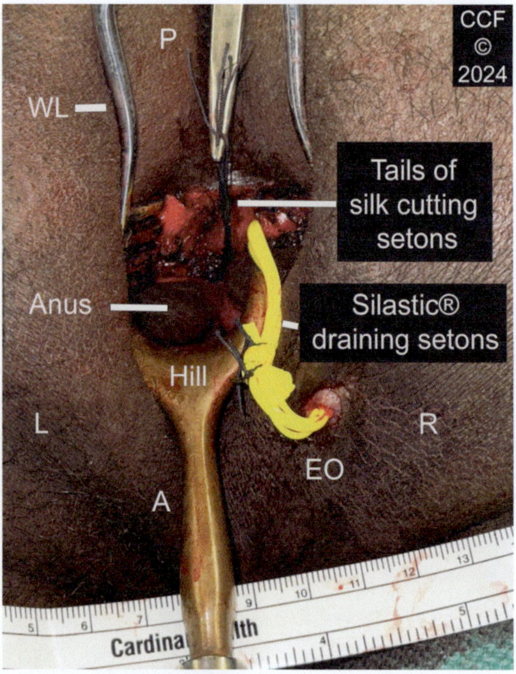

Fig. 60.5 The right lateral "horseshoe" extension of the fistula tract is encircled by Silastic® draining setons. The tails of the cutting setons encircling the sphincter muscle are tagged with a hemostat. The anus is labeled. EO = external os, Hill = Hill anoscope, WL = Weitlaner self retracting retaining retractor, A = anterior, L = left,
P = posterior, R = right

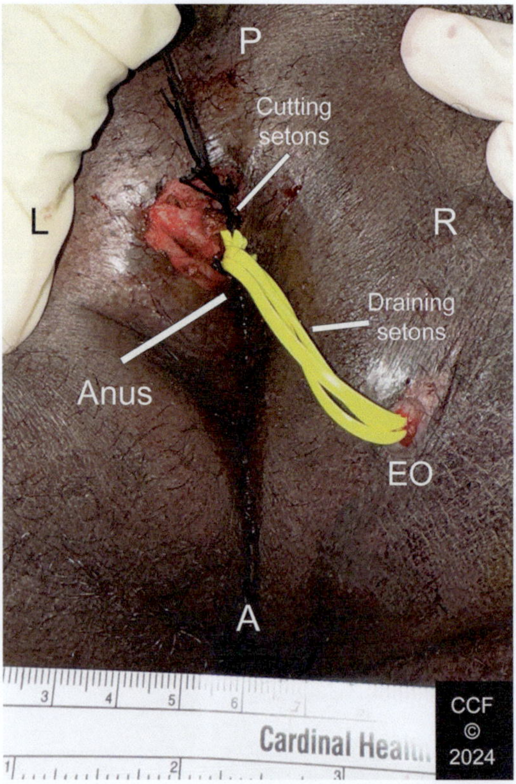

Fig. 60.6 The final appearance of the anus after treatment of a right-sided "horseshoe" anal fistula by partial posterior midline fistulotomy and drainage of the posterolateral fistula tract. The posterior midline silk cutting setons and right posterolateral Silastic® draining setons are shown. The anus and external os (EO) are labeled. Anterior (A); left (L); posterior (P); right (R)

Presentation B

A patient presented for management of recurrent anorectal abscesses for which incision and drainage procedures have been performed over 10 years. The appearance of the perianal area is shown in Fig. 60.7.

A pelvic magnetic resonance imaging (MRI) scan was obtained to define subcutaneous anatomy (Fig. 60.8).

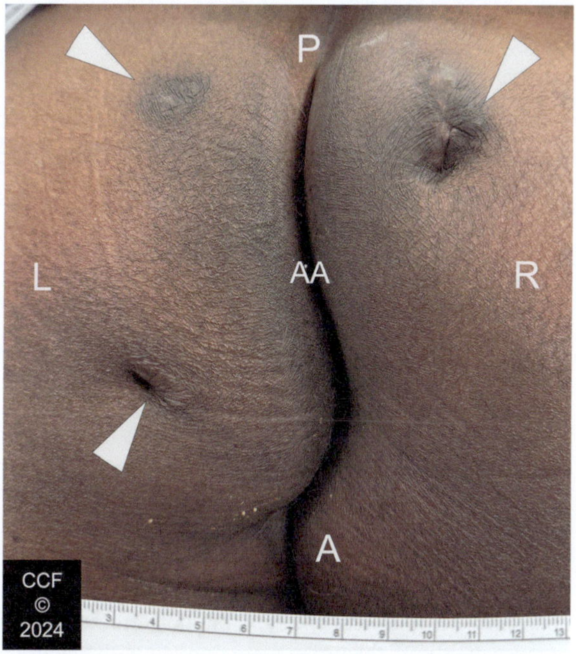

Fig. 60.7 Inspection of the perianal skin shows three surgical scars (arrowheads) in the right posterior, left posterior, and left anterior locations. Anterior (A), left (L), P posterior (P), right (R), anal area (AA)

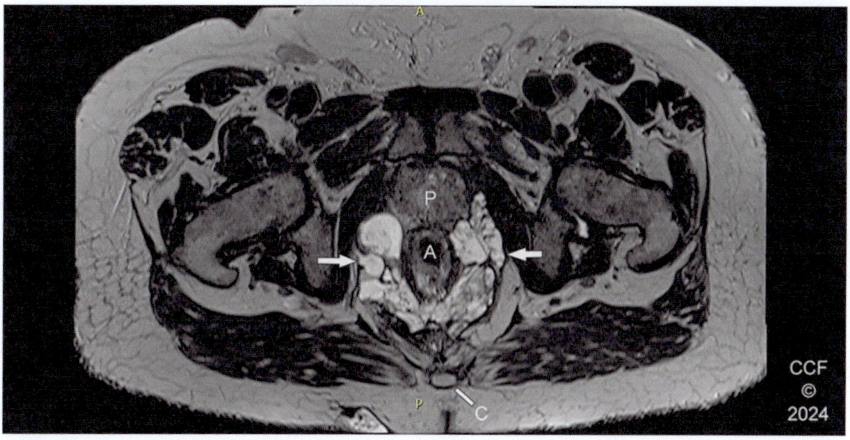

Fig. 60.8 Pelvic MRI, axial view, T2 weighted image, shows a "U" or "horseshoe"-shaped fluid collection (arrows) surrounding the anus (A), outside the external anal sphincter and centered in the ischiorectal fossa.Prostate (P), coccyx (C), anterior (A), posterior (P)

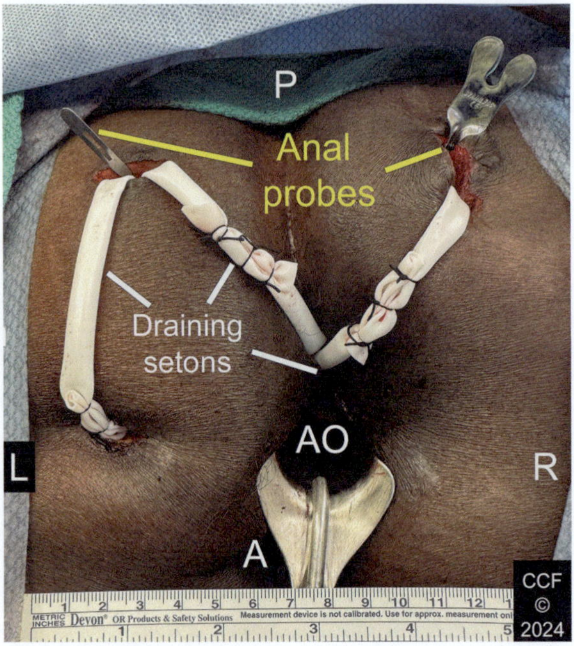

Fig. 60.9 Right and left horseshoe fistulous extensions originating from the posterior midline are encircled by draining 1/4" Penrose drains. Probes have passed from the right posterior and left posterior surgical incisions to the anal canal posterior midline. Anterior (A), left (L), posterior (P), right (R), anal orifice (AO)

Management

Examination under anesthesia in the prone jackknife position was done. During anoscopy, the anal canal was examined with a curved anal probe. An internal opening was found in the posterior midline. The probe entered a sinus tract that traversed the anal sphincter muscles. The skin, fat, posterior anal sphincter muscles, and anal canal mucosa overlying the probe were divided with electrocautery. The skin and fat at the right posterior, left posterior, and left anterior perianal scars were incised. Using probes, the lateral horseshoe fistulous extensions emanating from the posterior midline were defined and encircled with draining 1/4" Penrose draining setons (Fig. 60.9).

Comment

In 2009, Zbar published an article entitled, "David Henry Goodsall: reassessment of the rule" [1]. Zbar attributes to Edwards the original articulation of "the rule" at a meeting of the West London Medico-Chirurgical Society [2].

"*Some of the Rarer Forms of Rectal Fistulæ.*—Mr. Edwards read a paper upon this subject.

After touching upon some of the more frequent errors in diagnosis and operative treatment, the author pointed out that there seemed to be a definite relation between the internal and external orifices of a fistula. For fistulæ having their external orifices situate behind a plane passing transversely through the centre of the anus usually have their internal aperture in the middle line dorsally, while those with their external orifice in front of this plane generally terminate in an internal opening immediately opposite, thus forming a simple, straight complete fistula. The author then spoke of horseshoe fistulæ, which he defined as being a fistula with one or more external orifices on either side of the anus with an internal one in the middle line behind."

F. Swinford Edwards. 1887

Illustration of Goodsall's rule is shown in Fig. 60.10.

The anatomic structure associated with horseshoeing is the posterior subsphincteric space of Courtney.[1]

"Dissection of a series of cadavers has shown a definite, fatty, areolar tract joining the two ischioanal fossae. This tract lies posterior to the anus and between two prolongations of the puborectalis is muscle. The location of this space coincides with the location of posterior horseshoe fistula."

Harold Courtney B.S., M.D., M.Sci. (Med),
Syracuse, New York
1949

The pathogenesis of horseshoe fistulous abscess and a conservative method of its correction was described by Hanley in 1965.[2].

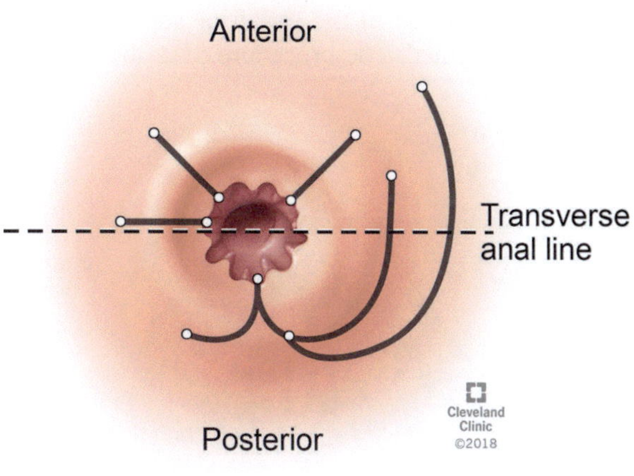

Fig. 60.10 Goodsall's rule illustrated

[1] Courtney [3]. This excerpt is reproduced with the generous permission of Mr. Spencer Dimmick, Journal of the American College of Surgeons, September 1, 2021.

[2] Hanley [4]. Permission to reproduce this excerpt and figures 1, 2, and 3 was generously provided by Wolters Kluwer Health, Inc., CCC|RightsLink, License number 58565620490999, License date Aug 26, 2024; License number Number 5124861267869, License date Aug 9, 2021, and License number 5118590520669, License date Jul 30, 2021 respectively.

Conservative Surgical Correction of Horseshoe Abscess and Fistula
Patrick H. Hanley, M.D.
Department of Colon and Rectal Surgery
Ochsner Clinic and Tulane University School of Medicine
New Orleans, Louisiana

> "Horseshoe fistulous abscess is a suppurative, anorectal clinical entity, originating initially from infected anal glands that connect with an anal crypt usually situated in the posterior midline of the anal canal. These glands penetrate the internal sphincter. At the onset, the abscess may be located between the internal sphincter and longitudinal muscle of the rectum. The pus further dissects through the longitudinal muscle into the superior posterior anal space, passing either superiorly or inferiorly, to the deep profunda of the external sphincter. This phase of suppuration is confined to the postanal space. Since both ischiorectal spaces communicate with the posterior superior anal space above the surface of the superficial external sphincter muscle, the pus will extend in the plane of least resistance into one or both ischiorectal spaces. (Fig 60.11)"

Hanley noted that complete unroofing of horseshoe fistulous tracts is associated with anterior displacement of the lower anal canal, anal deformity, prolonged hospitalization, and some degree of incontinence in the early postoperative period.

Therefore, he described a more conservative surgical procedure that minimizes these disadvantages. An abscess in the deep postanal space will extend into one or both ischiorectal spaces (Fig. 60.11). Hanley's procedure is based on the premise that: "The primary opening is a drainage site that inadequately drains the chronic abscess in the posterior superior anal space, and heals when it is adequately drained. The procedure described provides adequate drainage of the

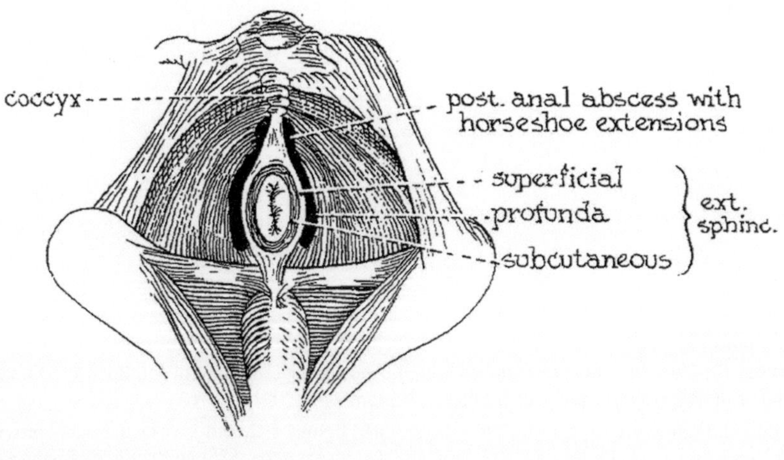

Fig. 60.11 Horseshoe fistula (Hanley). Postanal suppuration extends in a horseshoe fashion, under the puborectalis near the deep external sphincter [4] (Hanley Fig. 2)

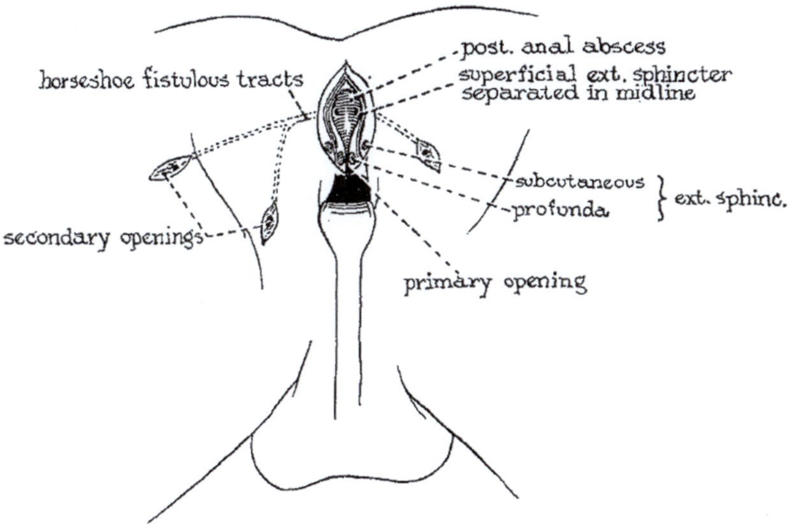

Fig. 60.12 The posterior anal space is unroofed. Lateral tracts are not unroofed. Hanley's procedure [4] (Hanley) (Fig. 3)

postanal space, and the horseshoe abscess fistulous extensions from the postanal space will resolve spontaneously."

In Hanley's procedure, the posterior anal space is unroofed. The lateral tracts are curetted but their lengths are not unroofed (Fig. 60.12).

Two modifications of Hanley's procedure are presented. In Presentation A, the right lateral "horseshoe" anatomy of the fistula was determined at examination under anesthesia by finding that insertion of a probe into the EO tracked in the posterolateral direction. The anal sphincter overlying the fistula tract was not divided; instead it was encircled with a cutting seton. The lateral extension was not curetted; instead, controlled drainage was established with Silastic® (silicone rubber) setons.

In Presentation B, MRI demonstrated the bilateral "horseshoe" fistula anatomy and pointed to the posterior midline as the fistula origin. In this case, the posterior anal sphincter muscles overlying the fistula were divided. Drainage of the lateral extensions again was accomplished with drains.

References

1. Zbar AP. David Henry Goodsall: reassessment of the rule. Tech Coloproctol. 2009;13:185–8.
2. Edwards FS. Some of the rarer forms of rectal fistulae. Lancet. 1887;1:1089–90.
3. Courtney H. The posterior subsphincteric space. Its relation to posterior horseshoe fistula. Surg Gynecol Obstet. 1949;89:222–6.
4. Hanley PH. Conservative surgical correction of horseshoe abscess and fistula. Dis Colon Rectum. 1965;8:364–8.

Anal Fistula-Cutting Seton Placement

61

James S. Wu

Presentation

A 35-year-old female presented with a right anterior fistula-in-ano.

Management

A cutting seton using 0-silk suture was placed (Figs. 61.1, 61.2, 61.3, 61.4, 61.5, and 61.6).

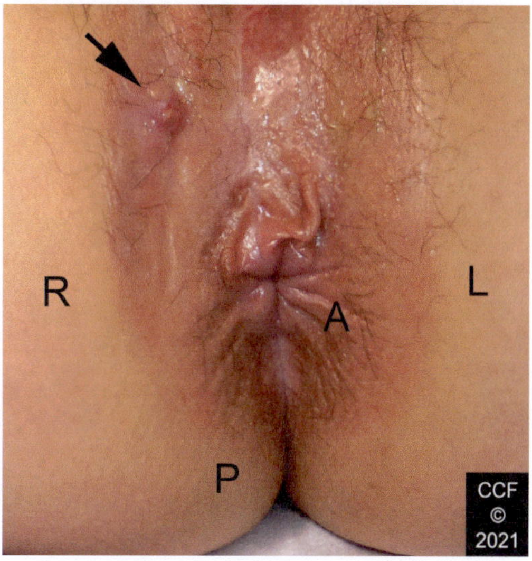

Fig. 61.1 The external os (arrow) is identified in the right anterior position. Right (R), left (L), posterior (P)

J. S. Wu (✉)
Department of Colon and Rectal Surgery, Cleveland Clinic, Cleveland, OH, USA

J. S. Wu, M. D. Inkster (eds.), *Cleveland Clinic Colorectal Case Studies*,
https://doi.org/10.1007/978-3-031-39880-3_61

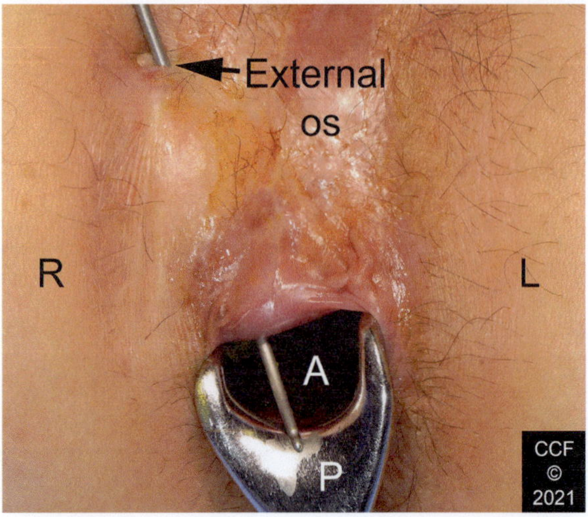

Fig. 61.2 A probe passes radially from the right anterior external os into the anal canal (A) at the dentate line at the dentate line. Right (R), left (L), anus (A), Posterior (P)

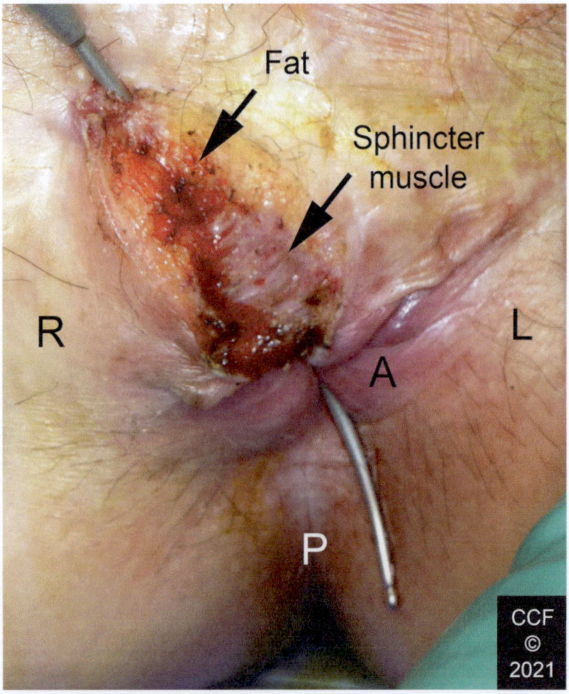

Fig. 61.3 The skin, anoderm, and subcutaneous fat are divided. The probe remains in the fistula tract. The sphincter muscle is left intact Right (R), left (L), anus (A), posterior (P)

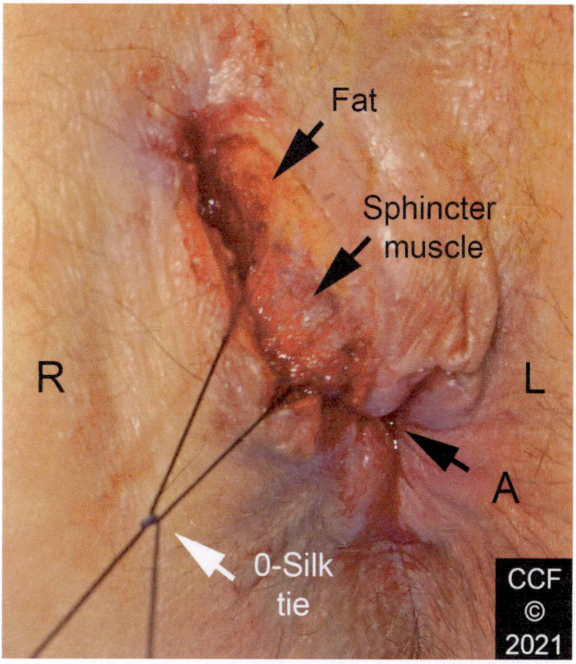

Fig. 61.4 The sphincter muscle involved in the fistula is encircled with a braided 0-silk tie (white arrow). The fat has been divided. The anal orifice (A) is identified by the black arrow. Right (R), left (L)

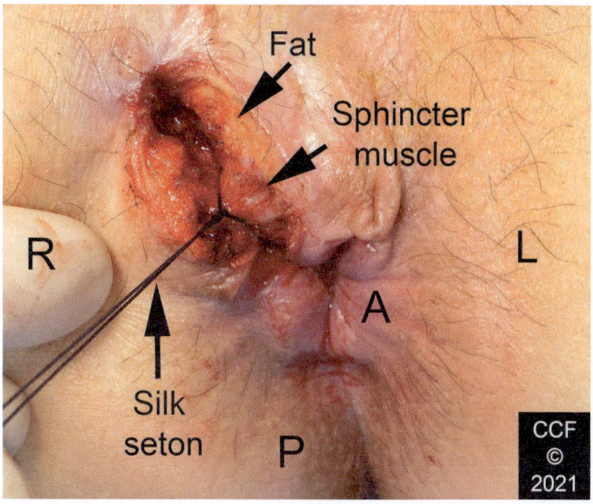

Fig. 61.5 The silk thread (arrow) is tied down around the sphincter muscle snugly. The anal orifice (A) is labelled. Right (R), left (L), posterior (P)

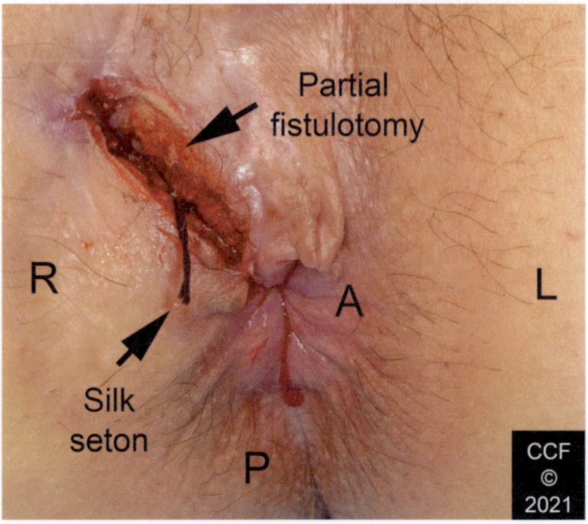

Fig. 61.6 The silk thread encircling the right anterior partial fistulotomy is trimmed leaving behind a tail. Right (R), left (L), anus (A), posterior (P)

Comment

The mechanism of action, technique, indications, contraindications, efficacy, and complications of cutting seton surgery in the management of anal fistulas are the subject of varied opinions. They are relatively easy and inexpensive to place. In general, they are less commonly used for the management of high transphincteric fistulas and anterior fistulas in women [1–3].

> "We report a standardized technique for placement and management of cutting setons in the treatment of transsphincteric fistula-in-ano which permits minimal manipulation and harm to the anal structures."
>
> A non-absorbable, braided thread…is inserted in an olive tip cannula…. After excision of the entire external opening and the extrasphincteric parts of the fistula, this cannula is used to probe for the tract of the fistula…. Once the internal opening of the fistula is identified, the thread is grasped at the tip of the cannula with a pair of forceps and is pulled out of the anus…. The mucosa is incised over the muscular bridge…to ensure that the thread is tied around the "naked" muscle only."
>
> Christian T. Hamel, Walter R. Marti, and
> Daniel Oertli
> General Surgical Service
> University Hospital of Basel, Switzerland
> 2004[1]

[1] Hamel et al. [4]. Permission to reuse this excerpt was generously granted by Springer Nature BV, CCC|Marketplace™, Order License ID 1141081-1; Order date 16, Aug 2021.

"Cutting seton yields fairly good results in regard to cure of fistula, but the risk of anal incontinence, despite its minor degree, seems to be too high to recommend its routine use for all high fistulas. The suprasphincteric fistulas and some extrasphincteric fistulas are difficult to treat otherwise, but especially for high transsphincteric fistulas, other methods of treatment (preferably those in which sphincter division can be avoided and the risk of anal canal deformity and incontinence are minimized) are advocated."[2]

Kari-Pekka J. Hämäläinen, M.D.
and A. Peter Sainio, M.D.
Fourth Department of Surgery
Helsinki University Central Hospital,
Helsinki, Finland,
1997

"Cutting setons have been used for many years to manage complex fistula-in-ano. In this procedure, the seton is secured tightly within the fistula tract, with intentional pressure placed on the tract itself. The theory behind this procedure is similar to regelation, where a frozen object melts under pressure, but then freezes again when the pressure is released. This is a common high-school science project, where a wire or paper clip is placed on an ice cube, and the cube retains its form as the wire advances through. For a cutting seton, the slow division of muscle as the seton becomes more superficial allows buildup of a fibrotic tract, with less muscle separation than if a primary fistulotomy was performed."

Emily J. Bubbers, MD
St. Peter's Hospital
Helena, Montana
Kyle G. Cologne, MD
Division of Colorectal Surgery
Keck School of Medicine,
University of Southern California, Los Angeles
2016[3]

Cutting setons have the advantage that they are inexpensive to use compared to other procedures. Because cutting setons divide muscle, other techniques are often chosen for high fistulae and anterior fistulae in women.

[2] Hämäläinen and Sainio [5]. Permission to reuse this excerpt was generously granted by Wolters Kluwer Health, Inc, CCC | RightLink® 5152490064255, License date Sep 19, 2021.

[3] Bubbers and Cologne [6]. License permission to reuse this excerpt was generously granted by Mr. Kariym Bryan, Thieme Publishers, 21 Sept 2021.

References

1. Graf W, Påhlman L, Ejerblad S. Functional results after seton treatment of high transsphincteric anal fistulas. Eur J Surg. 1995;161:289–91.
2. Saeed El MM. Cutting seton in management of complex perianal fistula – is it a safe procedure? Menoufia Med J. 2018;31:867–70.
3. Savom EP, Bwelle Motto GR, Bang GA, Ekani Boukar MY, Guifo ML, Essomba A. Cutting seton fistulotomy for the management of high anal fistula: Prospective evaluation of clinical results in Yaoundé. Health Sci Dis. 2016;17:14–8.
4. Hamel CT, Marti WR, Oertli D. Simplified placement and management of cutting setons in the treatment of transsphincteric anal fistula: technical note. Int J Colorectal Dis. 2004;19:354–6.
5. Hämäläinen K-PJ, Sainio AP. Cutting seton for anal fistulas: high risk of minor control defects. Dis Colon Rectum. 1997;40:1443–7.
6. Bubbers EJ, Cologne KG. Management of complex anal fistulas. Clin Colon Rectal Surg. 2016;29:43–9.

Anal Fistula-Internal Os Not Identified

62

James S. Wu

Presentation A

A patient presented with a chronic left posterior draining sinus (Fig. 62.1). Examination under anesthesia 2 years earlier had not identified the internal os. Re-examination under anesthesia showed a curved sinus tract between the external os and the anus (posterior midline) (Fig. 62.2).

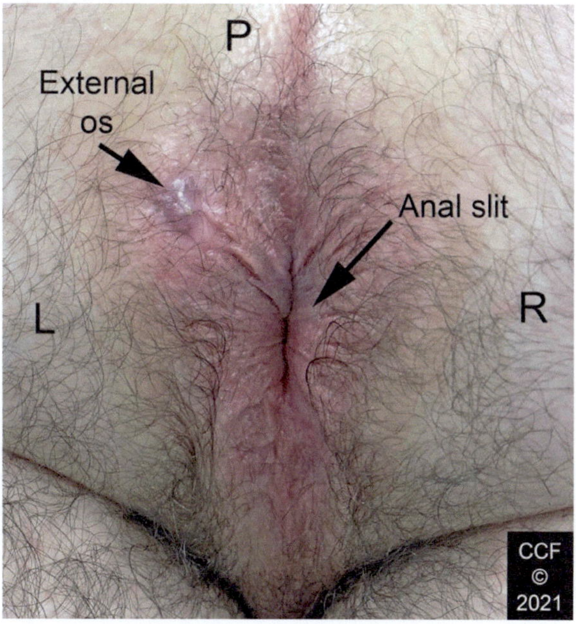

Fig. 62.1 An external os is seen in the left posterior perianal skin. The anal slit is identified. Left (L), posterior (P), right (R)

J. S. Wu (✉)
Department of Colon and Rectal Surgery, Cleveland Clinic, Cleveland, OH, USA

J. S. Wu, M. D. Inkster (eds.), *Cleveland Clinic Colorectal Case Studies*,
https://doi.org/10.1007/978-3-031-39880-3_62

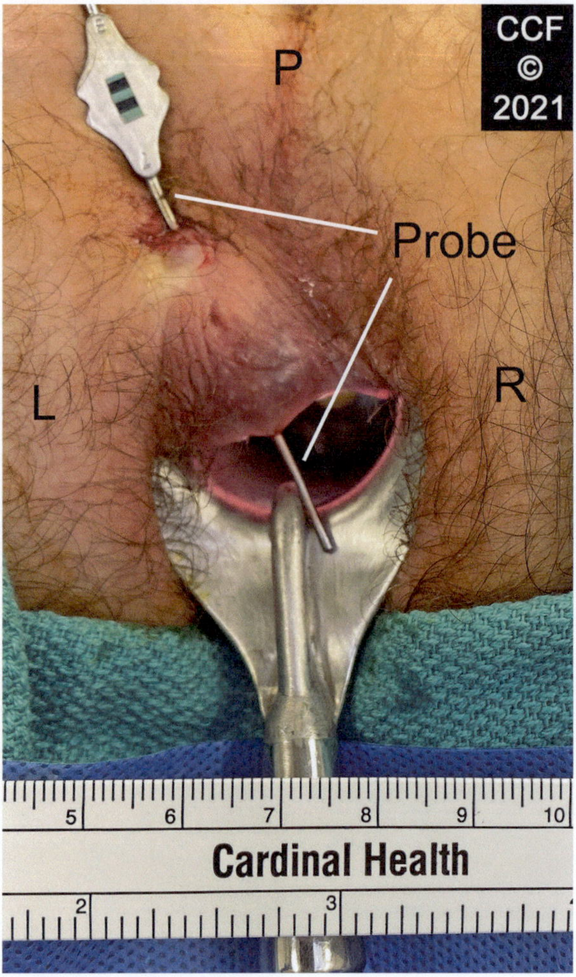

Fig. 62.2 On re-examination, an anal probe passed easily from the left posterior external os into the anal canal at the posterior midline. Left (L), posterior (P), right (R)

Comment

Two years earlier, examination failed to identify the external os, the internal os, and the intervening fistula tract. After several minutes, the procedure was stopped, and the patient went home with the fistula unchanged but not worse. The fistula was easily defined at a subsequent re-examination.

Presentation B

A 50-year-old patient was referred for management of a presumed anal fistula after an initial examination under anesthesia had failed to identify the internal anal opening of the fistulous tract 1 year earlier. The patient complained of discomfort and drainage from the skin opening behind the anus.

Management

Examination under anesthesia was done in the prone position. The external os was probed. The probe passed easily toward the posterior midline but could not be advanced into the anal canal. The skin and the soft tissue overlying the probe were divided (Fig. 62.3). The wound was curetted and allowed to heal by secondary intention. Examination 1 month later showed complete wound healing (Fig. 62.4), and the patient's symptoms had resolved.

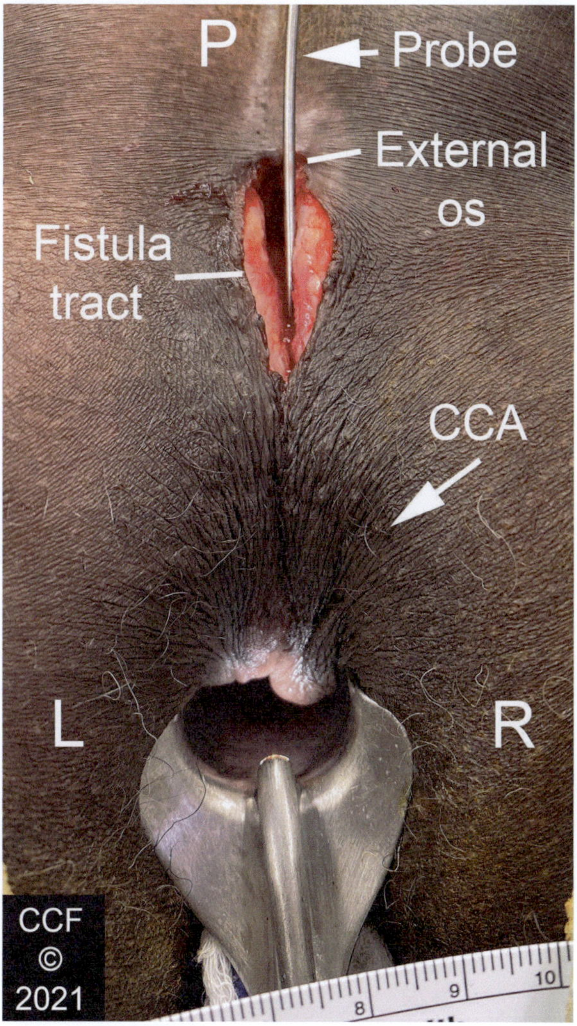

Fig. 62.3 A probe (arrow) passed through an external os (line) and sits in a posterior (P) midline fistulous tract but has not passed into the anal canal. The fistula tract external to the anal sphincter has been unroofed and the wound curetted. Pathologic examination of the curettage specimen did not show dysplasia or malignancy. Corrugator cutis anis (CCA), left (L), right (R)

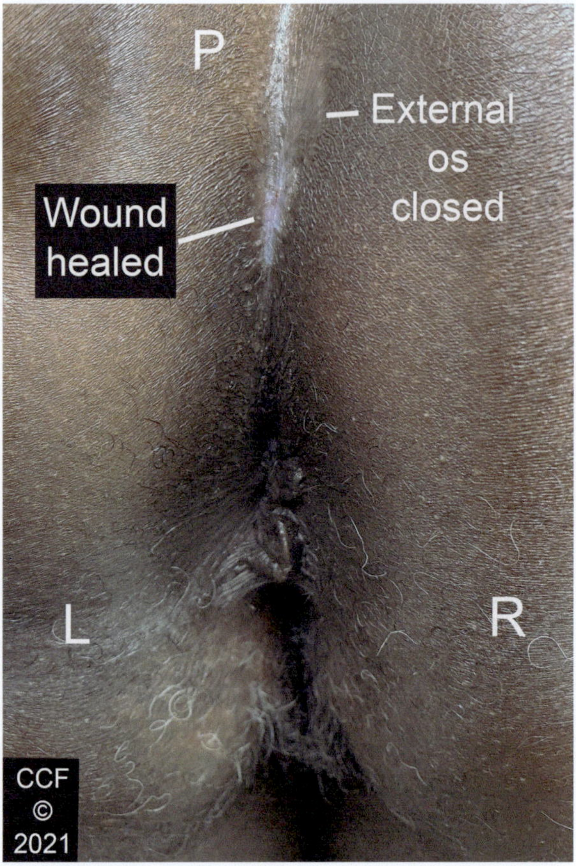

Fig. 62.4 The postoperative appearance of the surgical site. The curetted wound (including the external os site) has healed. The external os is closed. Left (L), posterior (P), right (R)

Comment

In this case, an internal os of a presumed fistula was not defined. It is possible that the internal os was closed or that the drainage site was not due to a fistula at all. Curettage and unroofing of the extra-sphincteric tract with subsequent wound healing by secondary intention led to wound closure.

Anal Fistula-Crohn's Disease 63

James S. Wu

Presentation

A 35-year-old female with a history of ileocolic Crohn's disease presented with anal suppuration and drainage. Anal inspection showed multiple perianal external skin openings as shown in Fig. 63.1.

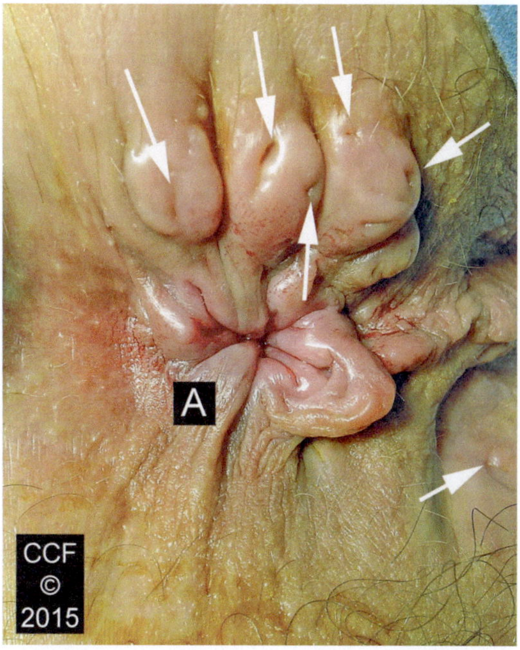

Fig. 63.1 Inspection reveals multiple openings in the perianal skin (arrows). The anus (A) is labelled

J. S. Wu (✉)
Department of Colon and Rectal Surgery, Cleveland Clinic, Cleveland, OH, USA

J. S. Wu, M. D. Inkster (eds.), *Cleveland Clinic Colorectal Case Studies*,
https://doi.org/10.1007/978-3-031-39880-3_63

Management

Examination under anesthesia was done using probes and dilute hydrogen peroxide. The hydrogen peroxide solution forms bubbles when injected into an external os that can be seen at an open internal os. Three anal fistulae were successfully defined as shown in Figs. 63.2a–d.

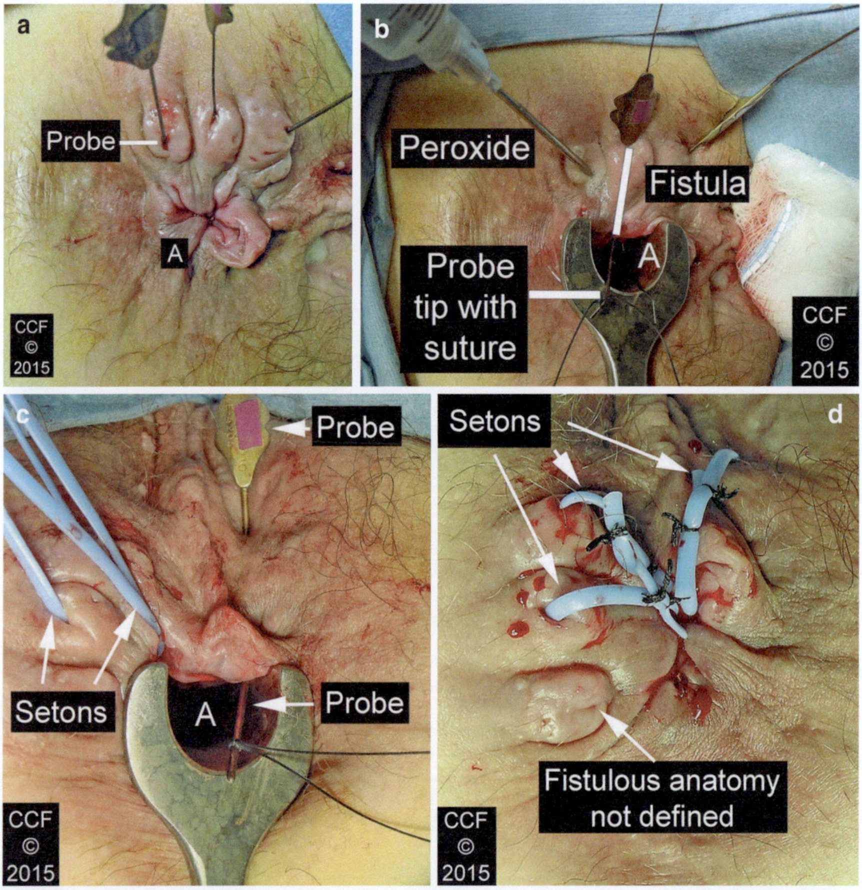

Fig. 63.2 (**a**) Lacrimal duct probes have been inserted into three perianal skin openings. The anus (A) is labelled; (**b**) two anal fistulae have been defined with lacrimal duct probes. A suture has been attached to the tip of a probe that passed through a fistula tract. Half strength peroxide is being injected in the external opening at 11 o'clock; however, a connection to the anal canal was not demonstrated. A= anus; (**c**) two fistula tracts are controlled with vessel loops (arrows). A third fistula tract is defined with a lacrimal duct probe. The silk suture at the end of the probe is used to draw a silastic seton through the fistula tract. A= anus; (**d**) three anal fistulae are encircled with blue silastic draining setons. The anatomy of a additional fistulae were not defined. Hence, no additional intervention was done at this examination

Comment

Following the publication of *Regional Ileitis* in 1932 by Crohn, Ginsburg and Oppenheimer, reports of other clinical patterns of the disease bearing Dr. Crohn's name appeared, among them, perianal abscesses and fistulae [1–5]. Management depends on the complication and its severity. Asymptomatic perianal fistulas may not require surgical treatment. Surgical options include observation, drainage, fistulotomy, and advancement flaps. Fecal diversion and proctectomy may be offered in severe cases [6]. This case demonstrates two methods useful for fistula tract identification. Gentle probing and injection of external skin openings with dilute hydrogen peroxide is done under anesthesia. The anal canal is inspected circumferentially to identify internal openings, commonly originating from the anal glands. In this case, fistulous drainage was controlled with Silastic® (silicon rubber) setons [7]. In the instance where fistula anatomy was not easily defined, probing was stopped in order to avoid creating a false iatrogenic passage.

References

1. Crohn BB, Ginzburg L, Oppenheimer GD. Regional ileitis. JAMA. 1932;99:1323–9.
2. Farmer RG, Hawk WA, Turnbull RB Jr. Clinical patterns in Crohn's disease: a statistical study of 615 cases. Gastroenterology. 1975;68:627–35.
3. Stein BL, Gordon PH. Perianal inflammatory conditions in inflammatory bowel disease. Curr Opin Gen Surg. 1993:141–6.
4. ten Cate Hoedemaker HO. Perianal Crohn's disease. Neth J Med. 1994;45:72–5.
5. Danelli P, Bartolucci C, Sampietro GM, Panizzo V, Sartani A, Maconi G, et al. Surgical options in the treatment of perianal Crohn's disease. Ann Ital Chir. 2003;74:635–40.
6. Williams JG, Hughes LE. Abdominoperineal resection for severe perianal Crohn's disease. Dis Colon Rectum. 1990;33:402–7.
7. Seton; "a skein of cotton or other absorbant material passed below the skin and left with both ends protruding, to promote drainage of fluid or to act as a counterirritant." Apparently from Latin seta "bristle." Definition of SETON by Oxford Dictionary on lexico.com (Accessed 19 June 2021).

Rectovaginal Fistula-Advancement Flap 64

James S. Wu and Mark E. Baker

Presentation

A 46-year-old female with colonic Crohn's disease complained that she was passing stool from her vagina. A vaginogram and examination under anesthesia were done as shown in Figs. 64.1 and 64.2.

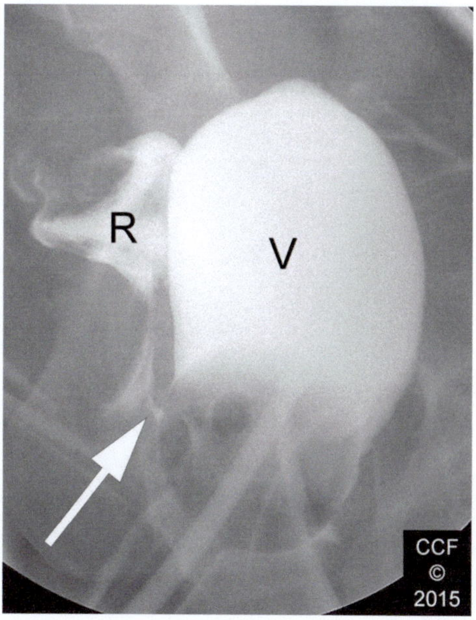

Fig. 64.1 Vaginogram. Water soluble contrast instilled into the vagina (V) through a balloon catheter, extravasates into the rectum (R). A low rectovaginal fistula is seen (arrow)

J. S. Wu (✉)
Department of Colon and Rectal Surgery, Cleveland Clinic, Cleveland, OH, USA

M. E. Baker
Department of Radiology, Cleveland Clinic Lerner College of Medicine, Case Western Reserve University, Cleveland, OH, USA

J. S. Wu, M. D. Inkster (eds.), *Cleveland Clinic Colorectal Case Studies*,
https://doi.org/10.1007/978-3-031-39880-3_64

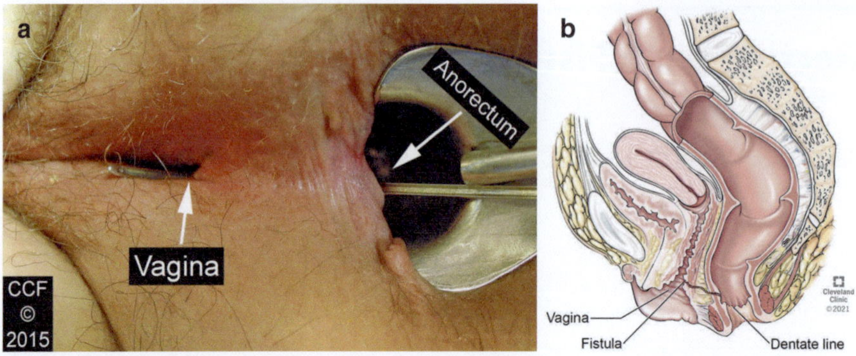

Fig. 64.2 (**a**) Examination of the anal canal under anesthesia. A probe passes from the distal rectum into the vagina; (**b**) illustration showing the path of a fistula from the dentate line of the anorectum to the vagina

Management

The vaginogram and examination demonstrate a low rectovaginal fistula. Advancement flap repair was done (Fig. 64.3a–f). Illustrations showing key steps in the advancement flap repair are shown in Fig. 64.4.

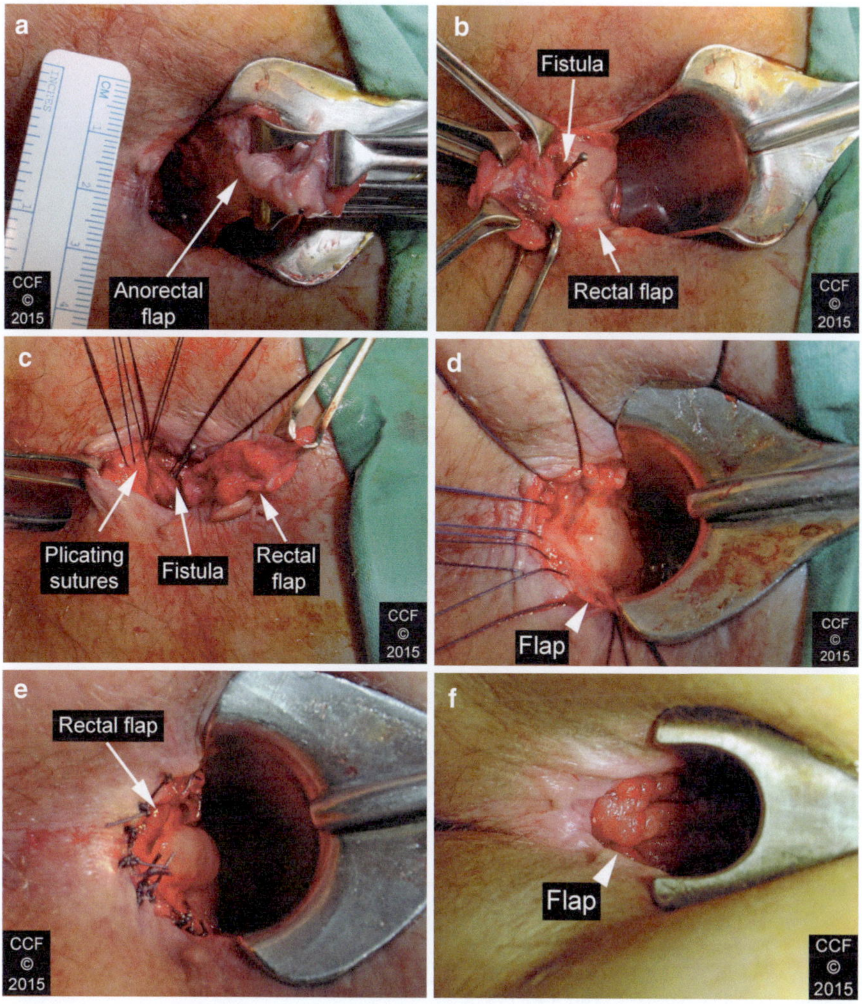

Fig. 64.3 (**a**) An anterior rectal mucosal flap is raised; (**b**) the rectal flap with the fistula (identified by the probe) is displayed; (**c**) the submucosal soft tissue is plicated, covering the fistulous opening; (**d**) the flap is sutured to the skin; (**e**) the completed advancement flap repair; (**f**) the healed advancement flap

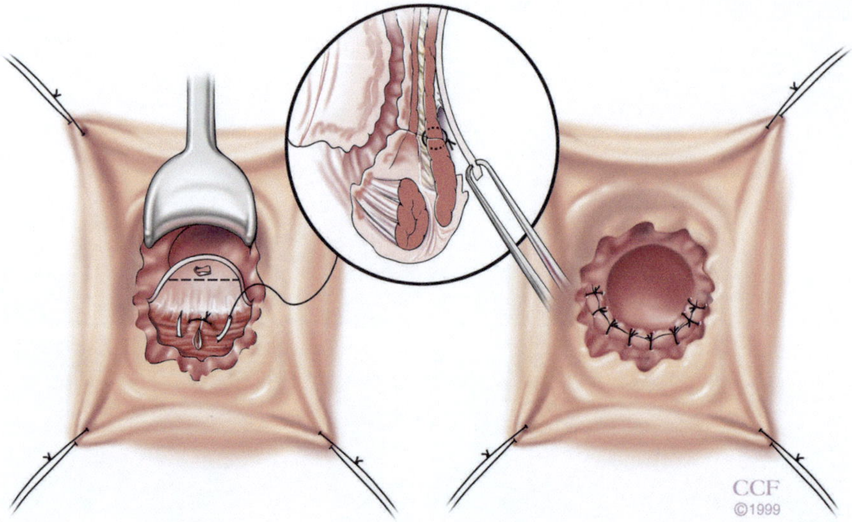

Fig. 64.4 Left. The mucosal flap has been dissected free of the underlying muscularis. The defect in the muscularis is closed with suture; Center. The mucosal flap (held by forceps) is advanced to cover the fistula tract in the muscularis; Right. The advancement flap is sewn in place

Comment

Rectovaginal fistulas can be repaired by mucosal advancement flap. Healing of Crohn's related rectovaginal fistulae after surgical repair ranges from 40% to 60% [1–3].

References

1. Halverson AL, Hull TL, Fazio VW, Church J, Hammel J, Floruta C. Repair of recurrent recto-vaginal fistulas. Surgery. 2001;130:753–8.
2. El-Gazzaz G, Hull T, Mignanelli E, Hammel J, Gurland B, Zutshi M. Analysis of function and predictors of failure in women undergoing repair of Crohn's related rectovaginal fistula. J Gastrointest Surg. 2010;14:824–9.
3. Gaertner WB, Madoff RD, Spencer MP, Mellgren A, Goldberg SM, Lowry AC. Results of combined medical and surgical treatment of recto-vaginal fistula in Crohn's disease. Color Dis. 2011;13:678–83.

Rectovaginal Fistula-Abdominoperineal Pull-Though (Turnbull–Cutait)

65

Tracy L. Hull, Vladimir Bolshinsky, Sherief Shawki, and James S. Wu

Presentation

The patient developed an iatrogenic rectovaginal fistula following a complicated gynecological procedure. At the time of gynecological surgery, a proctotomy was made inadvertently, identified and repaired in layers with interrupted dissolvable sutures. This repair broke down, and the patient developed a distal rectovaginal fistula. Multiple local repairs in the setting of fecal diversion (loop ileostomy) were unsuccessful over a period of 3 years. At examination under anesthesia, a rectovaginal fistula was found (Fig. 65.1).

T. L. Hull · J. S. Wu (✉)
Department of Colon and Rectal Surgery, Cleveland Clinic, Cleveland, OH, USA

V. Bolshinsky
Department of Colorectal Surgery, Surgical Health Specialists, Melbourne, Australia

S. Shawki
Department of Colon and Rectal Surgery, Mayo Clinic Rochester, Rochester, MN, USA

J. S. Wu, M. D. Inkster (eds.), *Cleveland Clinic Colorectal Case Studies*,
https://doi.org/10.1007/978-3-031-39880-3_65

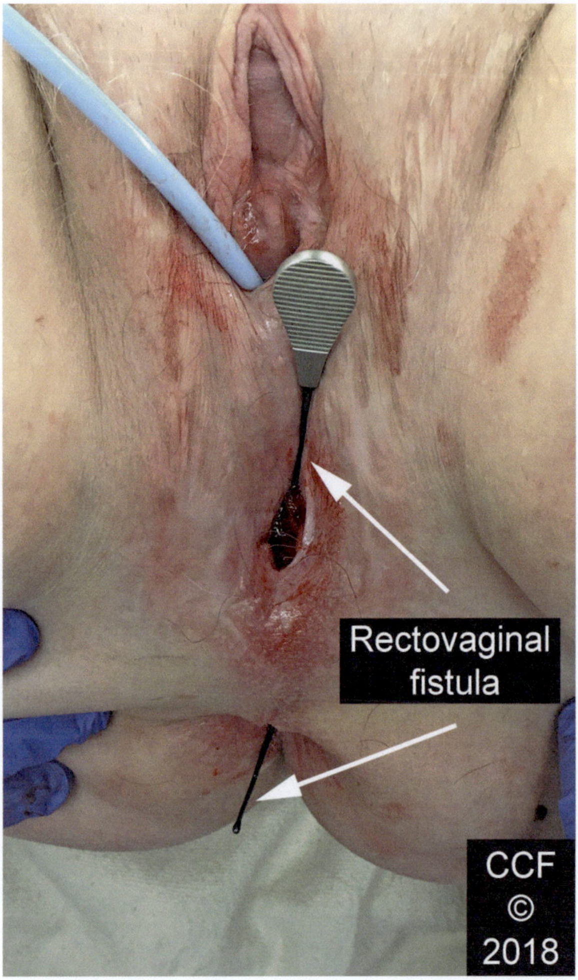

Fig. 65.1 A probe passes from the vagina to the anus (arrows)

Management

Proctectomy and pull-through reconstruction was chosen as the method of repair. The proximal rectum, sigmoid colon, left colon, and splenic flexure were mobilized using an open anterior approach. Mobilization of the distal rectum with simultaneous takedown of the rectovaginal fistula was accomplished by a trans-anal approach (Fig. 65.2). Following low ligation and division of the superior rectal artery close to the rectal wall, the rectum was elevated from the pelvis to facilitate placement of anal canal sutures at the dentate line. The rectum and sigmoid colon then were pulled through the anal canal (Figs. 65.3 and 65.4). The rectosigmoid pull-through

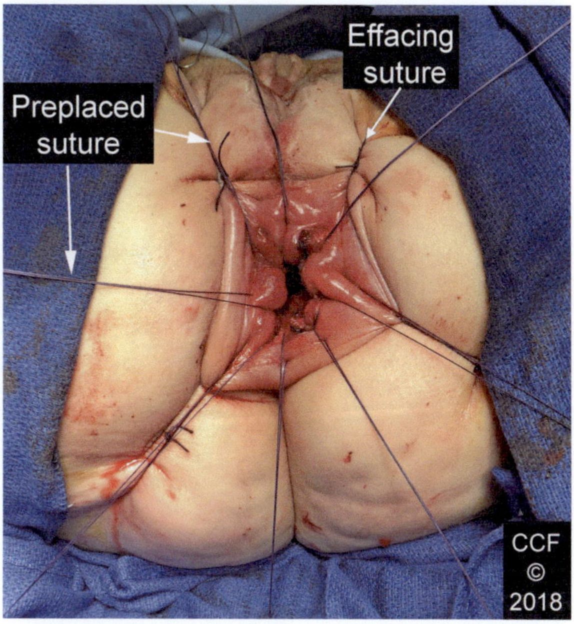

Fig. 65.2 The anus has been effaced with sutures allowing access to the distal rectum for trans-anal mobilization

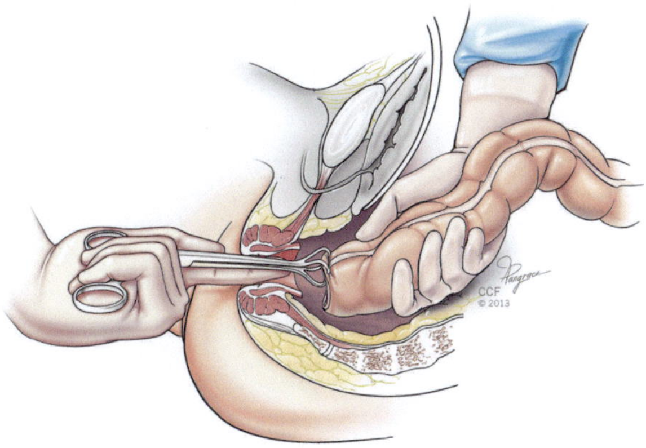

Fig. 65.3 Illustration showing the large intestine prepared for anal pull-through

was partially amputated, and the remaining exteriorized colon was secured outside the anus with a surgical sponge (Fig. 65.5). One week later, the sponge was removed (Fig. 65.6). Excess length of large intestine was amputated and bowel continuity was restored by hand-sewn colo-anal anastomosis (Fig. 65.7).

An illustration of abdominoperineal pull-through for delayed colorectal anastomosis is shown in Fig. 65.8.

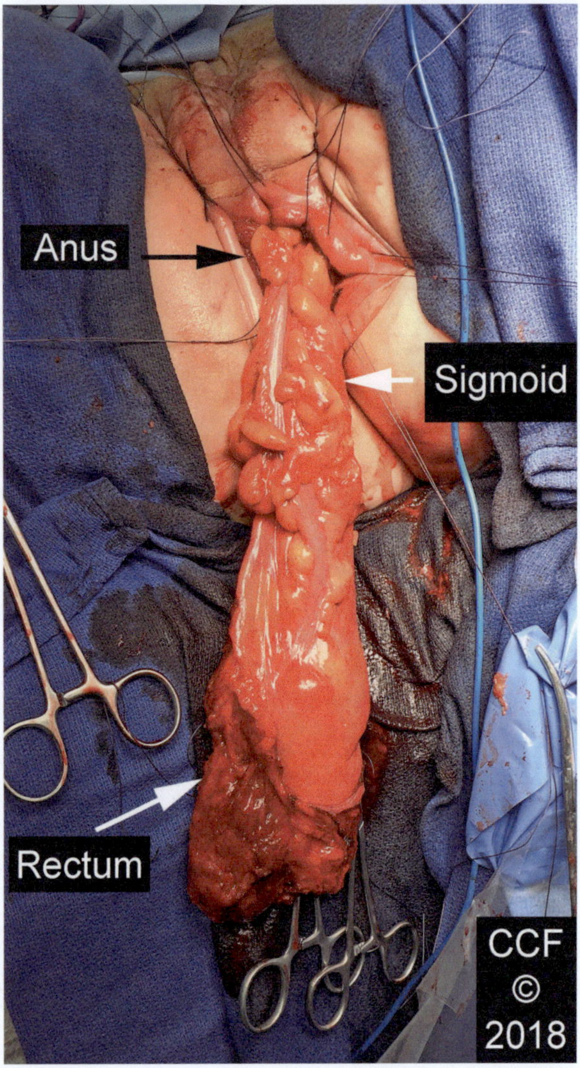

Fig. 65.4 The rectum and sigmoid are exteriorized through the anus

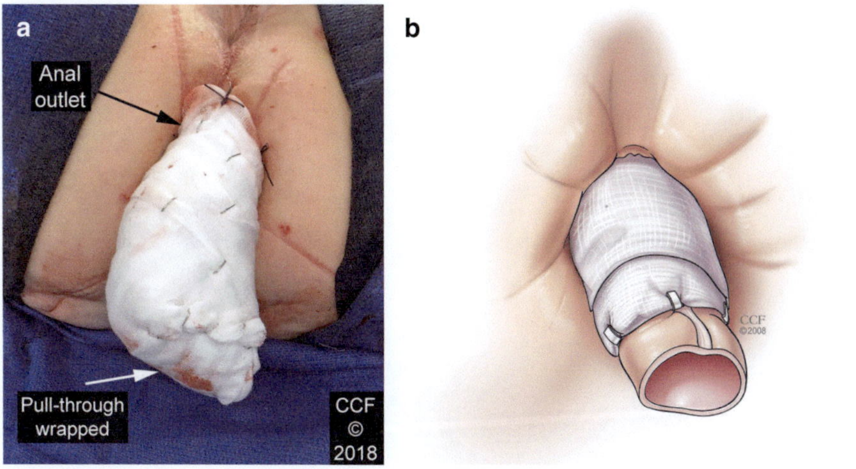

Fig. 65.5 (**a**) The exteriorized colon is secured in place by a surgical sponge. The sponge is attached to the gut by staples; (**b**) illustration showing sponge surrounding exteriorized large intestine

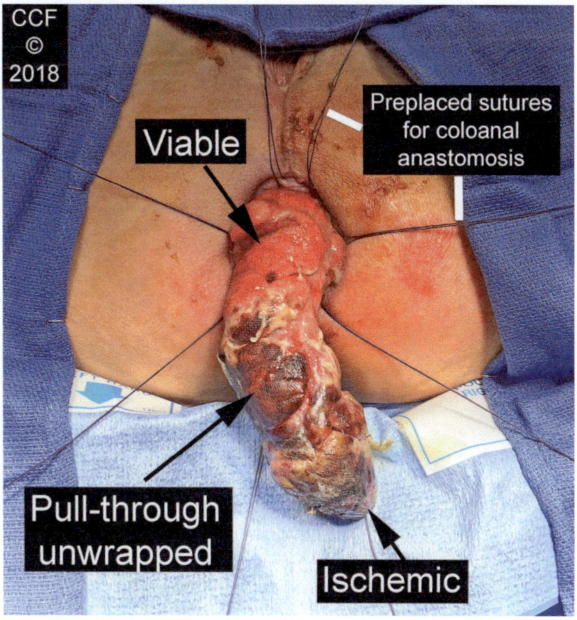

Fig. 65.6 Following removal of the surgical sponge, the exteriorized colon is exposed. Note the demarcation between viable and nonviable intestine. Preplaced sutures (arrows) used for the coloanal anastomosis are positioned circumferentially around the anus

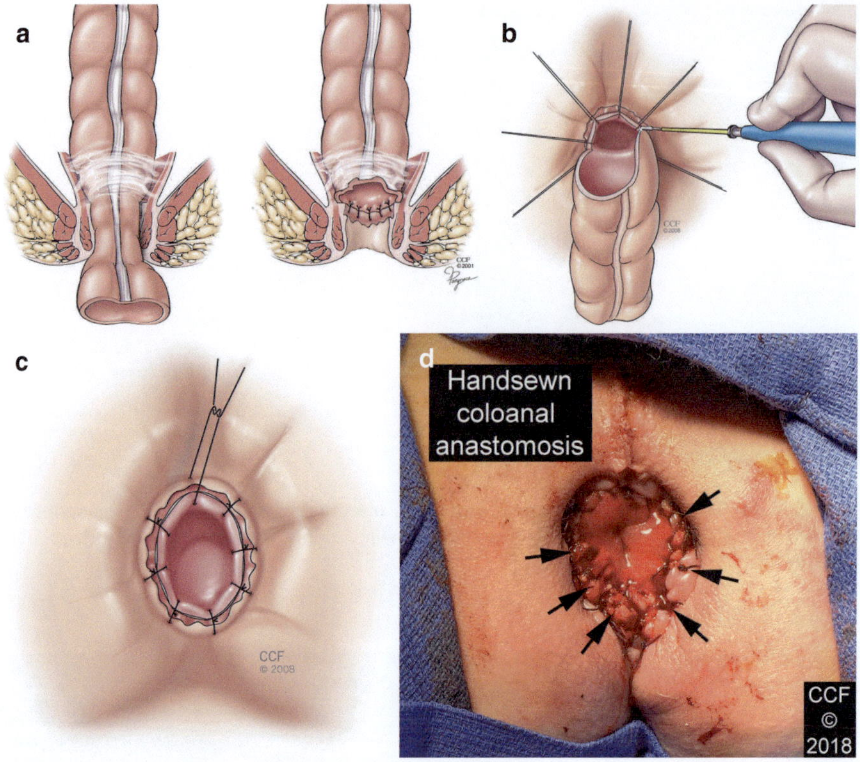

Fig. 65.7 (**a**) Illustration showing adhesions securing the large intestine in place following pull-through and after coloanal anastomosis; (**b**) amputation of redundant colon; (**c**) hand-sewn coloanal anastomosis; (**d**) final appearance after coloanal anastomosis. Arrows point to individual sutures

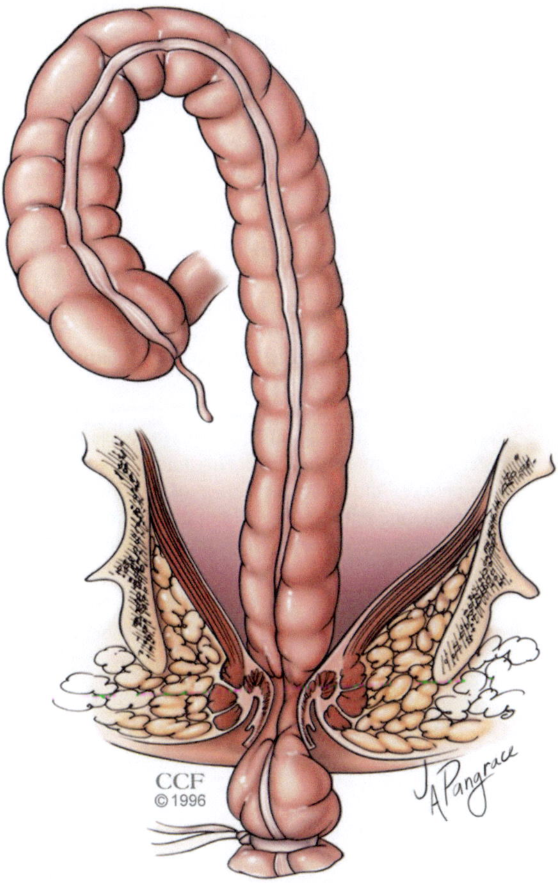

Fig. 65.8 Abdominoperineal pull-through for delayed colorectal anastomosis. Viable colon is pulled through the anal canal and secured in place. Delayed coloanal anastomosis follows

Comment

Abdominoperineal resection with pull-through and delayed reconstruction was described by two groups in 1961 for the surgical management of acquired megacolon of Chaga's disease, Hirschsprung's disease, and rectal cancer (Fig. 65.8).[1, 2] Working separately on both the Northern and the Southern hemispheres of the Americas, the authors faced and overcame the daunting problem of anastomotic failure commonly seen after restitution of bowel continuity following rectosigmoidectomy.

[1]Turnbull and Cuthbertson [1]. Permission to reproduce this excerpt was generously granted by the Cleveland Clinic Foundation; Copyright ©1961 The Cleveland Clinic Foundation. All rights reserved.

[2]Cutait and Figliolini [2]. Permission to reproduce this excerpt was generously granted by Wolters Kluwer Health, Inc., CCC|RightsLink®, License Number 5125190700284, License date Aug 10, 2021.

A New Method of Colorectal Anastomosis in Abdominoperineal Resection

Daher E. Cutait, M.D. and Felipe José Figliolini, M.D.
Department of Surgery, Medical School of the University of São Paulo, São Paulo, Brazil

"Abdominoperineal rectosigmoidectomy is, at present, considered the operative method of choice for treatment of megacolon.

To remedy this condition, removal of the diseased, as well as the dilated portion of colon, with immediate re-establishment of bowel continuity by colorectal anastomosis, seems therefore to be a rational surgical procedure. This is why rectosigmoidectomy has been performed by most experienced surgeons all over the world. Notwithstanding its effectiveness, there are some restrictions owing to the high incidence of post-operative complications, most of which are due to disruption, of varying degrees, of the colorectal anastomosis.

In order to lessen the incidence of disruption and to obviate its harmful effects after abdominoperineal rectosigmoidectomy, we devised and began to perform a new technic of colorectal anastomosis in 1959. This method is based on the principle of "adhesion by contact between the muscular surface of the everted rectum and the serosa surface of the pulled colon, and in the suture of the mucosa coat of the rectum to the mucosa coat of the colon" (primary-secondary colorectal anastomosis). We feel that the gratifying results obtained by this technic justify presentation of this report."

Abdominorectal Pull-through Resection for Cancer and For Hirschsprung's Disease

Rupert B. Turnbull, Jr., M.D., and Alan Cuthbertson, M.D.
Department of General Surgery, Cleveland Clinic Foundation
Cleveland, Ohio

"The complications following conventional pull-through procedures for cancer of the mid-rectum or Hirschsprung's disease are certainly not to be minimized. Ischemic necrosis of the pulled-through segment, and retraction and abscess of the presacral space are the most difficult complication to treat.

We believe that ischemic necrosis, retraction, and presacral infection are due to: (1) the too frequent reliance on the sigmoid colon as the pulled-through segment, (2) insufficient external fixation of the exteriorized colonic segment, and (3) immediate replacement of a colorectal anastomosis into a compartmented pelvic hematoma (as in Swenson's operation). The technic reported here ensures the removal of the sigmoid colon (which occasionally is of doubtful viability after mobilization), adequate and absolute fixation of the exteriorized colonic segment on the perineum, and a safe, delayed colorectal anastomosis after the incubation period of pelvic abscess is past, or the infection, if present, has been controlled.

The delayed anastomosis technic described here was evolved by us in 1952 for adults having small cancers located in the mid-rectum, and in whom a Swenson type of pull-through resection was performed. In 1953, we utilized the same technic in children undergoing resections for Hirschsprung's disease. In September, 1960, in Sao Paolo, Brazil, one of us (R.B.T.) was pleased to note that Dr. Daher E. Cutait had independently utilized the delayed anastomosis in adults who had undergone pull-though resections for the acquired megacolon of Chagas' disease."

Although coloanal anastomosis commonly is achieved by primary anastomosis, pull-through and delayed anastomosis still is useful for reconstruction of complex and septic anorectal conditions [3–8].

References

1. Turnbull RB Jr, Cuthbertson A. Abdominorectal pull-through resection for cancer and for Hirschprung's disease. Delayed posterior colorectal anastomosis. Clev Clin Q. 1961;28:109–15.
2. Cutait DE, Figliolini FJ. A new method of colorectal anastomosis in abdominoperineal resection. Dis Colon Rectum. 1961;4:335–42.
3. Kirwan WO, Turnbull RB. The Turnbull-Cutait pullthrough procedure for certain cancers of the rectum and Hirschprung disease. Int Adv Surg Oncol. 1981;4:173–87.
4. Halverson AL, Hull TL, Fazio VW, Church J, Hammel J, Floruta C. Repair of recurrent rectovaginal fistulas. Surgery. 2001;130:753–8.
5. Lane BR, Stein DE, Remzi FH, Strong SA, Fazio VW, Angemeier KW. Management of radiotherapy induced rectourethral fistula. J Urol. 2006;175:1382–8.
6. Gorgun IE, Milsom JW. Rectal reconstruction using the Turnbull-Cutait abdominoperineal pull-through anastomosis: indications and outcomes. Semin Colon Rectal Surg. 2009;20:73–7.
7. Remzi FH, El Gazzaz G, Kiran RP, Kirat HT, Fazio VW. Outcomes following Turnbull-Cutait abdominoperineal pull-through compared with coloanal anastomosis. Br J Surg. 2009;96:424–9.
8. Rosselli Londono JM, Aytac E, Gorgun E. Turnbull-Cutait abdominoperineal pull-through: a safe approach for recurrent sacrococcygeal teratoma complicated by rectovaginal fistula. Tech Coloproctol. 2014;18:761–3.

References

Anal Fissure-Introduction

66

James S. Wu and Thomas K. Schroeder

Introduction

An anal fissure is a tear of the anoderm. A history of local trauma such as passage of a large stool, diarrhea, sexual penetration, or anal procedure may be present. They are also associated with inflammatory bowel and sexually transmitted diseases. Symptoms include sharp pain accompanied by bright red bleeding per anus during and after defecation. The fissure usually can be seen with gentle separation of the buttocks. Most are located in the midline, posterior, or anterior. The white fibers of the internal sphincter muscle are exposed at the base of the fissure. The edematous skin tag located at the outermost edge of the fissure, also known as the sentinel pile or tag, indicates a chronic condition. The importance of the internal sphincter in fissure pathogenesis was stated by Eisenhammer.

The Surgical Correction of Chronic Internal Anal (Sphincteric) Contracture
Stephen Eisenhammer, B.M. (Edin.), F. R. C. S. (Eng)
Johannesburg, 1951 [1]
THE INTERNAL SPHINCTER

> "The internal sphincter plays a leading role in the normal functioning of the anal canal. It is a pronounced thickening and continuation of the circular muscle coat of the rectum, and is composed of unstriped muscle which exhibits continuous involuntary postural tone. It is about one inch long and two to four mm. thick. The pectinate or dentate line is situated at its half-way point.
>
> The strength of the anal musculature varies considerably. In some subjects, it is only with great difficulty that instrumentation can be performed. In others, the sphincter muscles are atonic and weak. They offer little or no resistance to the examining finger or instrument. On withdrawal, the anal canal gapes before closing slowly and yet perfect continence exists.

J. S. Wu (✉) · T. K. Schroeder
Department of Colon and Rectal Surgery, Cleveland Clinic, Cleveland, OH, USA

J. S. Wu, M. D. Inkster (eds.), *Cleveland Clinic Colorectal Case Studies*,
https://doi.org/10.1007/978-3-031-39880-3_66

> The postural tone of the combined sphincter muscles maintains closure of the anal canal. The internal sphincter co-operates in this action, but functions best with moderate or even low tone.
>
> The internal sphincter absolutely controls the degree of dilatation permissible. This obtains because this muscle is the inner sleeve of the double-lined muscular tube of which the inner involuntary muscle alone is liable to undergo narrowing. Adequate relaxation and full dilatation is the most important function of the internal sphincter. It is the only muscle of the anal group that is liable to undergo spastic or structural narrowing from pathologic stimuli.
>
> Unfortunately, the internal sphincter possesses the inherent character of the involuntary circular muscle of the alimentary tract, viz. liability to spasm. This appears to be greatest at the exit of the tract because of the many abnormal influences to which it is exposed there. The commonest irritating stimuli are those of chronic medicinal purgation, cryptitis, hemorrhoidal congestion, dysenteric and simple proctitis, and sympathetic over-stimulation. The spasm, if persistent, leads to organic structural changes in the muscle which gives rise to permanent contracture. The anal canal is then unable to relax and dilate sufficiently to extrude a full fecal mass. The muscle now impedes evacuation and abnormal straining ensues. In the later stages, the inner lining tissues of the anal canal also appear to lose their elasticity and become rigid allowing a tear or fissure to develop generally at the weak mid-posterior site."

Anal manometry demonstrates anal sphincter hypertonicity and spasm (Fig. 66.1).

Examination with the slightest pressure causes immediate pain. Thorough digital exam without anesthesia is not possible because of pain and internal sphincter spasm. Most acute anal fissures heal spontaneously following correction of the inciting event. Persistent fissures require additional measures. Both medical and surgical therapies are used [2]. Nonoperative treatments are listed in Table 66.1 [3].

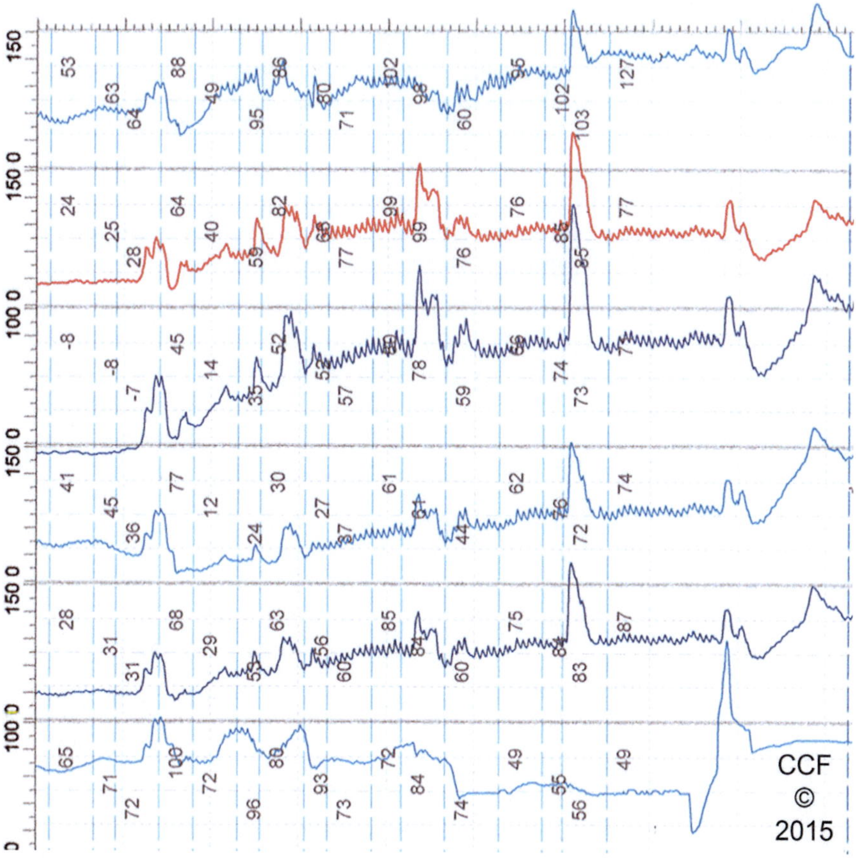

Fig. 66.1 This multichannel anal manometry tracing of a patient with anal fissure shows elevated resting anal sphincter pressures with a "saw tooth" pattern indicative of internal sphincter muscle spasm with rapid increases and decreases in muscle contraction (pressures in mm Hg)

Table 66.1 Nonoperative treatments for anal fissure

Correct inciting stimulus
Warm water baths
Fiber
Topical analgesics
Topical steroids
Topical nitrates
Topical calcium channel blockers
Anal dilation
Botulinum toxin

References

1. Eisenhammer S. The surgical correction of chronic internal anal sphincteric contracture. S Afr Med J. 1951;25:486–9. Permission to reproduce this except was obtained from the South African Medical Association on 2021.08.17, Invoice number 20210817, VAT Number 4600106662
2. Stewart DB, Gaertner W, Glasgow S, Migaly J, Feingold D, Steele SR. Clinical practice guidelines for the management of anal fissures. Dis Colon Rectum. 2017;60:7–14.
3. Nelson RL. Non surgical therapy for anal fissure (Review). Cochrane Database Syst Rev. 2006;(4):CD003431. https://doi.org/10.1002/14651858. CD003431.pub2.

Anal Fissure-Botulinum Toxin and Balloon Dilation

67

James S. Wu and Thomas E. Garofalo

Presentation

A 59-year-old patient presented with chronic anal pain due to anal fissure. Examination revealed anterior and posterior anal fissures. Topical nitrate and calcium channel blocker therapy administered over 2 months were not beneficial. The patient declined lateral anal sphincterotomy, fearing fecal incontinence. Combination anal sphincter balloon dilation and chemodenervation with botulinum toxin injection were done.

Technique

The two procedures were done under general anesthesia in the lithotomy position after sterile skin preparation.

Procedure 1

Anal Sphincter Chemodenervation with Botulinum Toxin

Botulinum toxin (BTX) dissolved in sterile normal saline and injected circumferentially through the prepared perianal skin into the anal sphincter.[1]

[1] In this particular case, 100 units of botulinum toxin dissolved in 10 cc of normal saline was used.

J. S. Wu (✉) · T. E. Garofalo
Department of Colon and Rectal Surgery, Cleveland Clinic, Cleveland, OH, USA

J. S. Wu, M. D. Inkster (eds.), *Cleveland Clinic Colorectal Case Studies*,
https://doi.org/10.1007/978-3-031-39880-3_67

Procedure 2

Anal Sphincter Dilation

An esophageal balloon dilator [1] was placed into the anal canal and inflated (Fig. 67.1).

At 1-month follow-up, both fissures had healed.

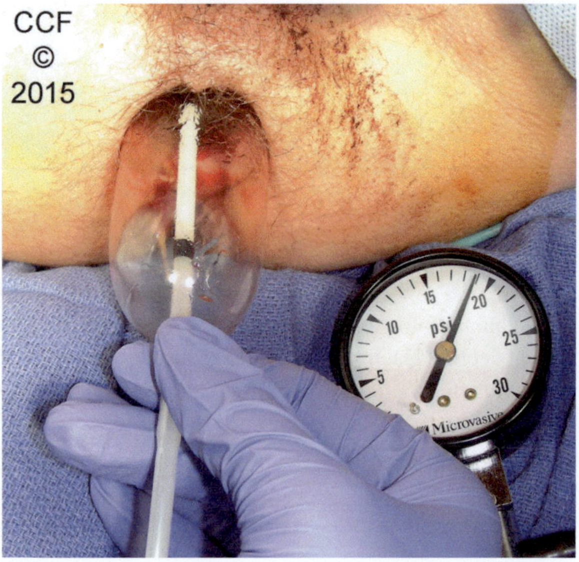

Fig. 67.1 Anal balloon dilation. An esophageal balloon (40 mm diameter) was inserted into the anus and inflated, in this case, to 19 psi for 15 min

Comments

Chemodenervation With BTX

BTX inhibits acetylcholine release into the synaptic gap. In 1993, Jost and Schimrigk described the use of botulinum toxin to treat anal fissure.

Use of Botulinum Toxin in Anal Fissure
Wolfgang H. Jost, M.D., Klaus Schimrigk, M.D.
Hamburg/Saar, Germany

"Important in the origin of a chronic fissure is the vicious circle of inflammation, pain, and sphincter spasm. Medical management can tackle the inflammation and the pain and, hence, the spasm. Anal dilation, like lateral sphincterotomy acts by a direct reduction in anal tone; posterior sphincterotomy by removal of the ulcer and the secondary changes as well as causing a reduction in tone. We investigated a new mode of therapy involving injection of the external anal sphincter with botulinum toxin. This works by causing a temporary paresis of the injected muscle, allowing the ulcer to heal."[2]

While Jost and Schimrigk recommended injection into the external sphincter, injection into the internal anal sphincter also has been reported [3] .

Anal Sphincter Dilation

Stretching of the anal sphincter in the treatment of fissure-in-ano was described by Watts et al. in 1964.

Stretching of Anal sphincters in Treatment of Fissure-in-Ano
J. McK. Watts, F.R.A.C.S.; R. C. Bennett, F.R.C.S., F.R.A.C.S.;
J. C. Goligher, CH.M., F.R.C.S.
General Infirmary at Leeds

"From its inception in 1955 up to the present, it has been the practice of this clinic to employ either simple sphincter stretching or internal sphincterotomy in the treatment of fissure-in-ano. In the earlier years internal sphincterotomy was employed almost exclusively, but since 1960 simple stretching of the anal sphincter has become the routine treatment,...

In all patients the anal sphincters were stretched under general anaesthesia, and in the great majority this was done as an out-patient procedure. Dilatation was usually begun by inserting and gradually opening a bivalve speculum, which permitted careful inspection of the site of the fissure. After withdrawal of the instrument, two and ultimately four fingers were introduced into the anal canal. With both forearms strongly pronated, lateral distraction was exerted on the anal sphincters, at first gently but eventually with considerable force, the total period of the stretch being not less than four minutes." [4]

[2] Jost and Schimrigk [2]. Permission to reuse this excerpt was generously granted by Wolters Kluwer Health, Inc., CCC|RightsLink®; License Number 5125870252529, License date Aug 11, 2021.

In 2005, Renzi et al. described their results of pneumatic balloon dilation to treat chronic anal fissure.

Pneumatic Balloon Dilatation for Chronic Anal Fissure: A Prospective, Clinical, Endosonographic, and Manometric Study
A. Renzi, M.D., L Brusciano, M.D., M. Pescatori, M.D., D. Izzo, M.D., V. Napoletano, M.D., G. Rossetti, M.D., G. del Genio, M.D., A. del Genio, M.D.
Stefano Hospital, Naples, Italy; Second University, Naples, Italy
Villa Flaminia Hospital, Rome

"With the patient lying in the lithotomy position, local anesthesia was performed… in the four perianal quadrants…. A 40-mm diameter and 60-mm mm long anal balloon… was inserted in the anal canal after adequate lubrication and was positioned with 1 cm protruding from the anus. The balloon was rapidly inflated up to a 20 psi pressure (1.4 atm) and maintained *in situ* for 6 minutes."[3]

The authors reported that fissures healed between the third and fifth week in most patients. While the sphincter is stretched, it is not divided.

Comment

Over concerns of incontinence, procedures such as BTX and balloon dilatation now precede lateral internal sphincterotomy in the treatment of anal fissure. The procedures can be done together as in this case or separately. Addition of an anal anesthetic block at the start of the case is done routinely.

[3] Renzi et al. [5]. Permission to reuse this excerpt was generously granted by Wolters Kluwer Health, Inc., CCC|RightsLink®; License Number 5152550951712, Sep 19, 2021.

References

1. Boston Scientific Corporation. Esophageal balloon dilator specifications. Boston Scientific, RIGIFLEX™ II single use achalasia balloon dilator. Boston Scientific Corporation, Marlborough, Massachusetts 01752.
2. Jost WH, Schimrigk K. Use of botulinum toxin in anal fissure. Dis Colon Rectum. 1993;36:974.
3. Brisinda G, Maria G, Bentivoglio AR, Cassetta E, Gui D, Albanese A. A comparison of injections of botulinum toxin and topical nitroglycerin ointment for the treatment of chronic anal fissure. N Engl J Med. 1999;341:65–9.
4. Watts JM, Bennett RC, Goligher JC. Stretching of anal sphincters in treatment of fissure-in-ano. Br Med J. 1964;2:342–3.
5. Renzi A, Brusciano L, Pescatori M, Izzo D, Napoletano V, Rossetti G, et al. Pneumatic balloon dilatation for chronic anal fissure: A prospective, clinical endosonographic, and manometric study. Dis Colon Rectum. 2005;48:121–6.

Anal Fissure-Sphincterotomy

68

James S. Wu

Presentation

A 62-year-old male experienced sharp anal pain and bright red anal bleeding with bowel movement. The pain was spastic and could last for hours once started. Only sitting in a tub of warm water gave relief. Symptoms had been present for 5 years. He had been treated with topical analgesics, steroids, stool softeners, and fiber without benefit. He felt a "hemorrhoid" on the outside of the anus. Examination under anesthesia was done (Fig. 68.1).

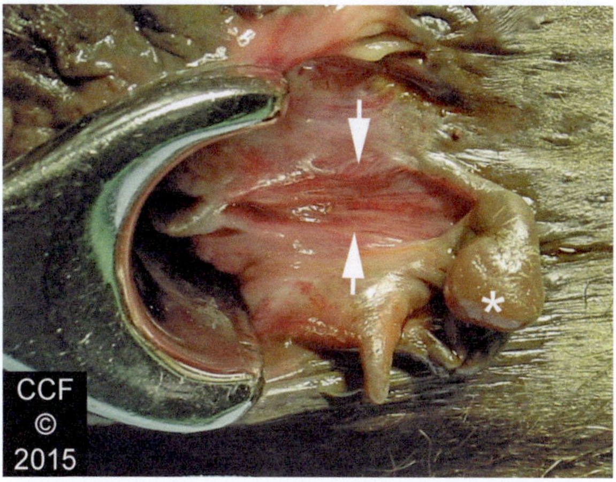

Fig. 68.1 Anal fissure. The split in the distal anoderm (arrows) exposes the underlying internal sphincter. The perianal skin tag (asterisk) is also known as a "sentinel pile"

J. S. Wu (✉)
Department of Colon and Rectal Surgery, Cleveland Clinic, Cleveland, OH, USA

J. S. Wu, M. D. Inkster (eds.), *Cleveland Clinic Colorectal Case Studies*,
https://doi.org/10.1007/978-3-031-39880-3_68

Management

This patient has a chronic anal fissure. Lateral internal sphincterotomy was done by open technique. With an operating anoscope in place, a small incision was made in the lateral intersphincteric groove. The distal internal sphincter muscle was isolated (Fig. 68.2) and then divided under direct vision. The wound was left open.

At follow-up examination, the fissure had healed. The patient did not experience any loss of fecal continence.

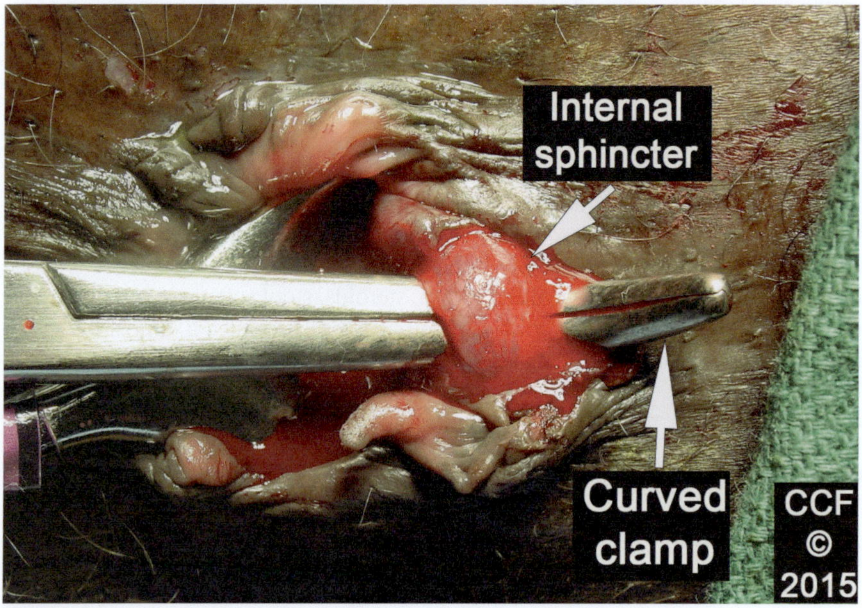

Fig. 68.2 Lateral internal sphincterotomy. The distal aspect of the internal sphincter has been isolated and displayed over a curved clamp prior to division under direct vision

Comment

In 1951, Eisenhammer proposed an operation for the surgical correction of anal fissure.[1]

> "The operation has been adopted for the treatment of the chronic fissure syndrome. It is performed in the consulting-room surgery under local anesthesia.
>
> The patient lies in the left lateral position,…chest supine, the knees well drawn up.
>
> The rectum is now swabbed out with Dettol solution [antiseptic]…. The largest single-ended Sim's speculum which will be admitted is introduced. About 2 c.c. of Novutox [local anesthetic] is then injected submucosally along the left lateral line of the anal canal axis from ¼ inch above the dentate line to the anal verge over the subcutaneous external sphincter. A straight incision is made in this line, parallel with the long axis of the canal. The incision commences a ¼ inch above the dentate line, between two rectal columns and anal papillae, and through the corresponding crypt. The incision is extended outwards to the outer edge of the subcutaneous external sphincter. Digital palpation finds the taut bowstring of the lower border of the internal sphincter, with below it the sulcus of the anal intermuscular septum, separating the internal sphincter from the subcutaneous external sphincter.
>
> The pearly white internal sphincter is now exposed throughout the length of the wound by further knife dissection.
>
> At least four-fifths of the internal sphincter is divided".

In 1953, Eisenhammer identified the left lateral mid-point of the internal sphincter as the site of choice for sphincterotomy.[2]

> "INTERNAL ANAL SPHINCTEROTOMY
> This term has been applied to the operation of linear division of the internal sphincter… The left lateral mid-point is the site of choice,... Posterior incisions may tend to gutter and leave a mucous leak".

Subsequently, lesser degrees of internal sphincter division have been used to decrease the chances of postsphincterotomy fecal incontinence [3].

---

[1] Eisenhammer [1]. Permission to reuse this excerpt was granted by the South African Medical Association, Invoice number 20210921, 2021.09.21.

[2] Eisenhammer [2]. Permission to reuse this excerpt was granted by the South African Medical Association, Invoice number 20210921, 2021.09.21.

References

1. Eisenhammer S. The surgical correction of chronic internal anal (sphincteric) contracture. S Afr Med J. 1951;25:486–9.
2. Eisenhammer S. The internal sphincter: its surgical importance. S Afr Med J. 1953;27:266–70.
3. Perry WB, Dykes SL, Buie WD, Rafferty JF. Practice parameters for the management of anal fissures (3rd Revision). Dis Colon Rectum. 2010;53:1110–5.

Anal Sphincter Repair

69

Ira J. Kodner and James S. Wu

Introduction

Continence is the controlled elimination of the rectal contents at a socially acceptable time and place. Factors affecting anal continence are shown in Table 69.1. Synchronized function of all components results in normal control of defecation [1–4].

Problems with the internal sphincter that may lead to fecal incontinence are listed in Table 69.2. The anterior portion of the anal sphincter mechanism contains

Table 69.1 Factors affecting anal continence

Involuntary anal sphincter-involuntary resting tone
External anal sphincter-voluntary squeeze pressure
Puborectalis muscle
Maintenance of anorectal angle
Adequate rectal capacity
Consistency of stool
Normal anal sensation

Table 69.2 Origins of internal sphincter injury

Cut
•Trauma (including obstetrics)
•Surgery for abscess/fistula (Fournier's gangrene)
•Sphincterotomy for ulcer/fissure
Stretch
•Obstetric
•Extreme sex
•Surgery (keyhole deformity)
•Obstructed defecation leading to descending perineum

I. J. Kodner
Department of Colon and Rectal Surgery, Washington University School of Medicine, St. Louis, MO, USA

J. S. Wu (✉)
Department of Colon and Rectal Surgery, Cleveland Clinic, Cleveland, OH, USA

J. S. Wu, M. D. Inkster (eds.), *Cleveland Clinic Colorectal Case Studies*,
https://doi.org/10.1007/978-3-031-39880-3_69

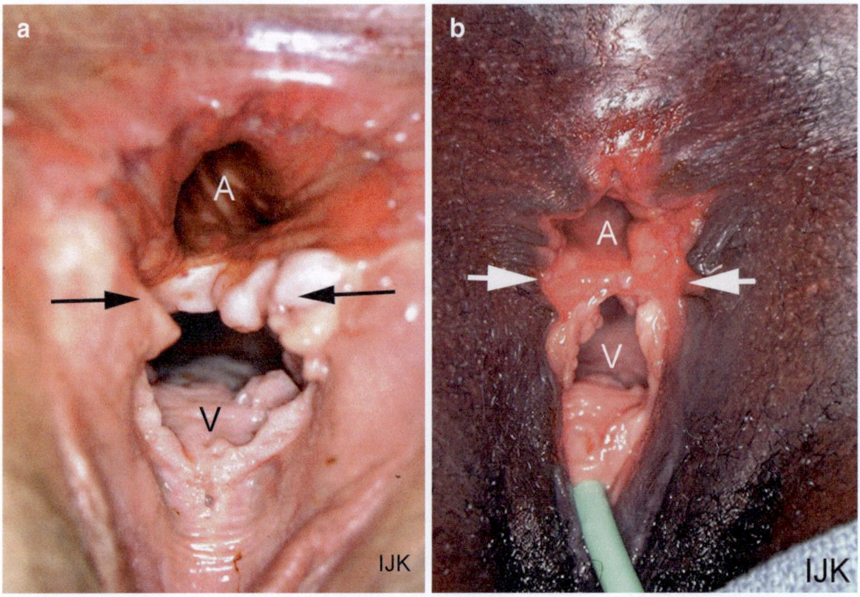

Fig. 69.1 (**a**, **b**) Arrows point to the anterior anal sphincter defect. The anus (A) and vagina (V) are labeled [5]

only one loop of muscle, is shorter than posterior, is weaker than posterior and will cause incontinence if transected. Anal sphincter reconstruction is focused on this part of the sphincter. However, before embarking on surgery, several key questions have to be answered. Is the tissue to be used in the repair normal? Does the sphincter function? Is systemic evaluation necessary to identify inflammatory bowel disease or malignancy? Has the tissue been irradiated?

Common presentations for fecal incontinence secondary to anal sphincter injury include obstetric injuries, Crohn's disease, and fistulotomy damage. Examples of internal sphincter injury in two patients are demonstrated in Fig. 69.1a, b.

Trans-anal ultrasound (TAUS) of an intact internal anal sphincter and an internal sphincter with an anterior defect are shown in Fig. 69.2a, b.

Surgical considerations prior to surgery include the immediate cause of the sphincter injury and possible complicating factors such as previous unsuccessful repairs, age, and systemic disease (Crohn's disease, diabetes, severe irritable bowel syndrome). Special diagnostics include evaluation of sphincter innervation, assessment of the muscle present available for repair, and defecography. It is also important to determine from the outset which patients are not appropriate candidates for anal sphincter repair. For example, if the sphincter is denervated, scarred or there is inadequate sphincter muscle, then other surgical options are considered as shown in Table 69.3. Finally, one must determine what price to pay for continence. In the end, preservation of defecation by the normal route may not be desirable if the post-surgical outcome is a "perineal colostomy."

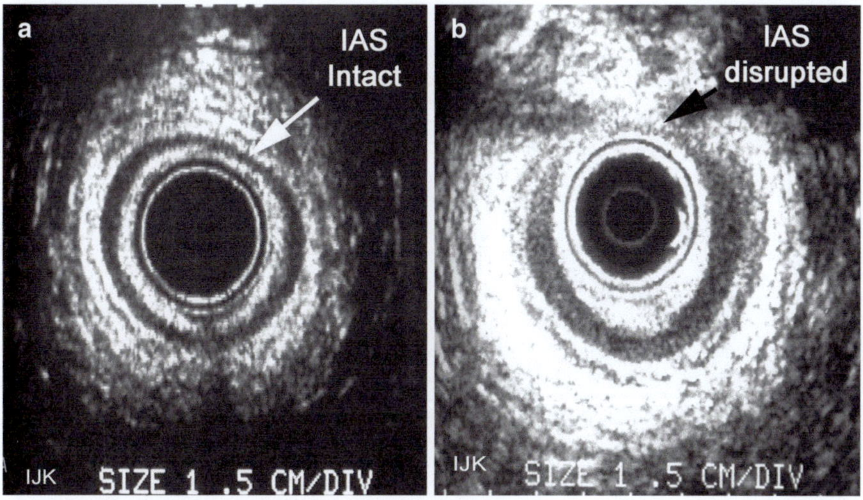

Fig. 69.2 (**a**) Trans-anal ultrasound (TAUS) shows an intact internal anal sphincter (IAS, dark ring); (**b**) TAUS shows disruption of the IAS

Table 69.3 Surgical options other than sphincter repair for fecal incontinence

Anal encirclement (gracilis muscle, synthetic band)
Park's posterior repair (often combined with perineal proctectomy)
Gracilis/gluteus muscle substitution ± electronic stimulator
Artificial anal sphincter
Good colostomy

Once the decision to perform sphincter repair is made, surgical preparation includes complete bowel preparation, constipation, and prophylactic antibiotics. Surgical technique involves spinal or epidural anesthesia, prone/flexed position, anal effacement, and repair with nonabsorbable suture.

Operative Details

As shown in Fig. 69.3, the perianal skin is retracted to provide exposure of the anus. The sphincter is exposed by a curved incision (Fig. 69.4).

The scar at the site of sphincter injury is identified (Fig. 69.5a, b).

Following division of the midline scar, the divided ends are mobilized (Fig. 69.6a, b).

Sphincter repair is completed by suturing the ends of the sphincter together so that the anal lumen is narrower in diameter (Fig. 69.7a, b).

The surgical site closed anterior-to-posterior increases the distance between the anus and vagina (Fig. 69.8a, b).

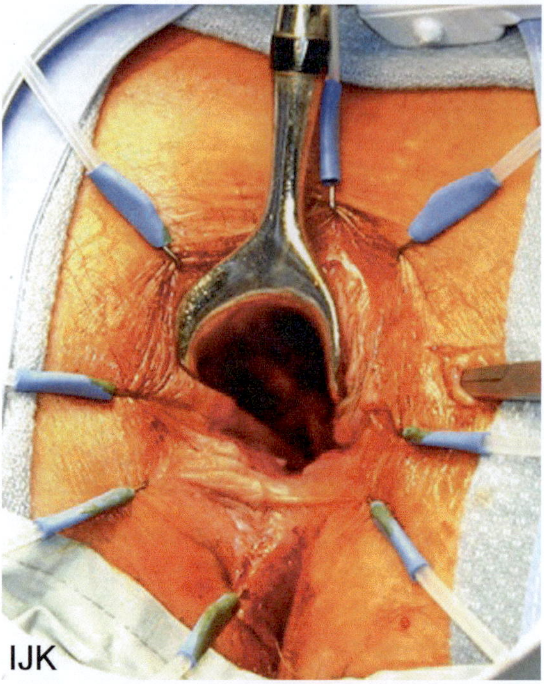

Fig. 69.3 Following preparation of the operative field, the perianal skin is retracted, in this case, using a Lone Star™ retractor

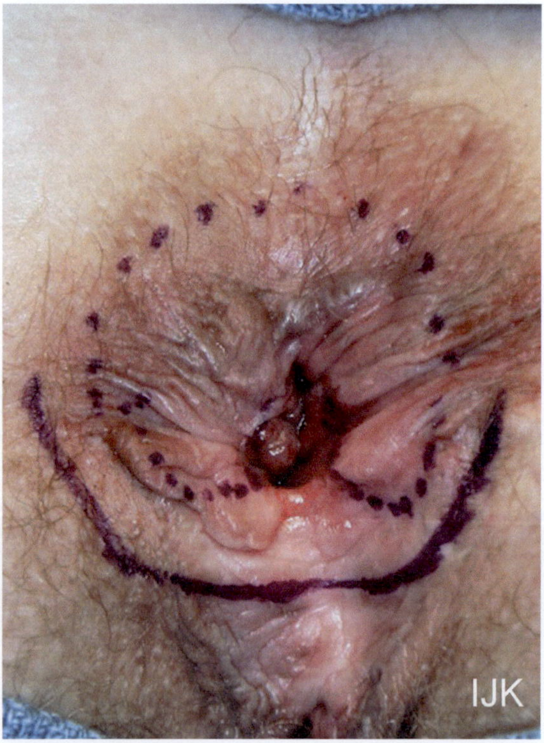

Fig. 69.4 The sphincter is exposed using a curved transverse incision (solid line). The internal anal sphincter is identified by the dotted line

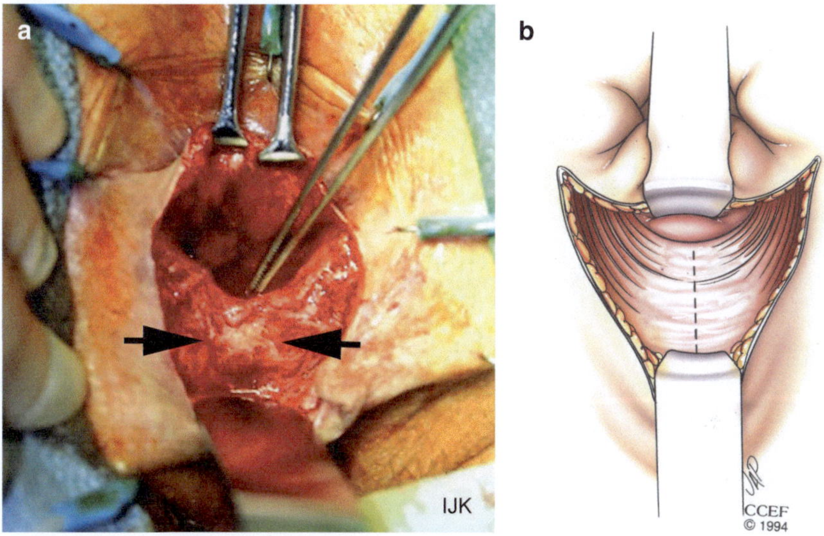

Fig. 69.5 Illustration (**a**) A midline scar (arrows) is demonstrated in this operative photograph; (**b**) the dotted line in this illustration shows the site of midline scar division

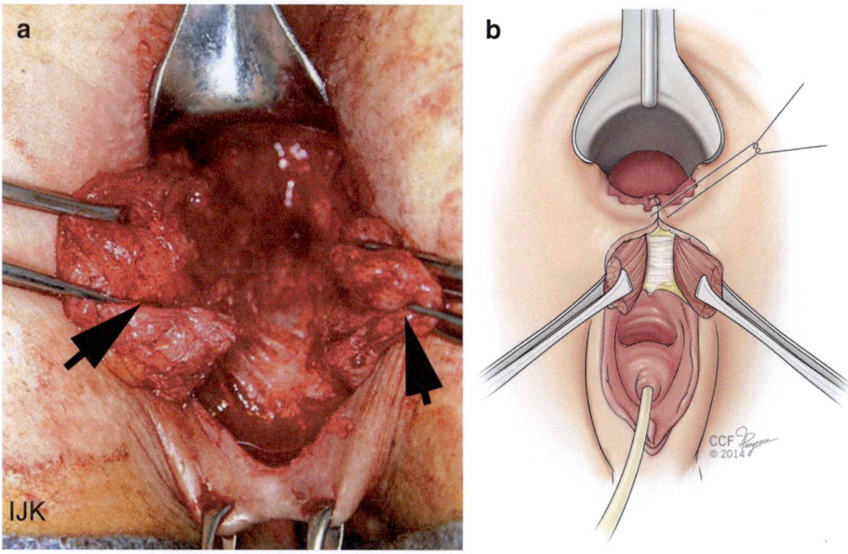

Fig. 69.6 (**a**) The mobilized ends of the anal sphincter (arrows) are displayed with Allis clamps in this operative photograph; (**b**) this illustration shows the mobilized end of the anal sphincter

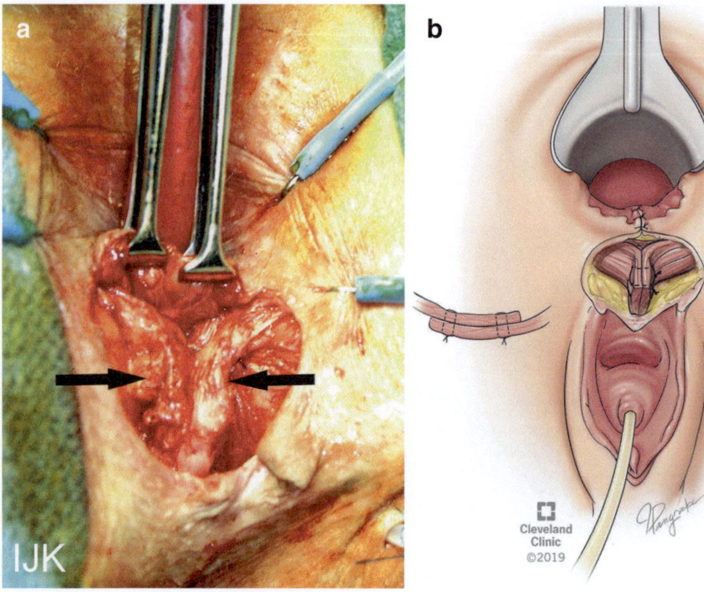

Fig. 69.7 (**a**) The mobilized sphincter has been re-approximated by side-to-side sphincter repair (arrows); (**b**) illustration of side-to-side repair and alternative overlapping sphincter repair

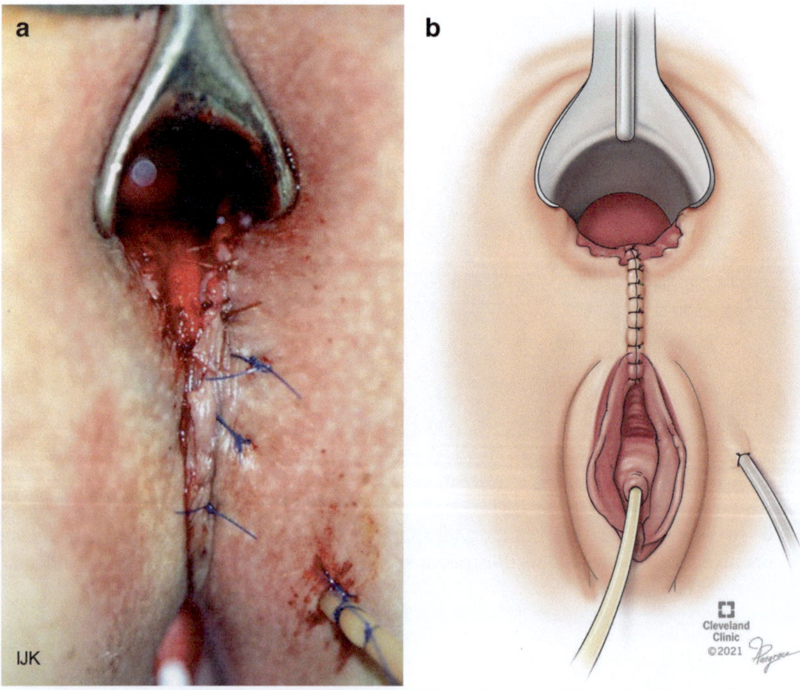

Fig. 69.8 (**a**) Operative photo showing the wound closure and a drain; (**b**) illustration showing closure of the surgical site

In the postoperative period, the patient is constipated, kept *nil* per os for 48 hours and then discharged with a drain in place on oral antibiotics.

Fecal incontinence-summary/advice:

- Know the cause,
- Diagnose and treat systemic disease,
- Verify the presence of muscle and adequacy of nerve function before surgical reconstruction,
- You cannot put a bag on a perineal colostomy.

References

1. Fleshman JW, Dreznik Z, Fry RD, Kodner IJ. Anal sphincter repair for obstetric injury: manometric evaluation of functional results. Dis Colon Rectum. 1991;34:1061–7.
2. Simmang C, Birnbaum EH, Kodner IJ, Fry RD, Fleshman JW. Anal sphincter reconstruction in the elderly: Does advancing age affect outcome? Dis Colon Rectum. 1994;37:1065–9.
3. Tsang CBS, Seow-Choen F. Anal incontinence. In: Holzheimer RG, Mannick JA, editors. Surgical treatment: Evidence-based and problem oriented. Munich: Zuckschwerdt; 2001.
4. Grey BR, Sheldon RR, Telford KJ, Kiff ES. Anterior anal sphincter repair can be of long term benefit: a 12–year case cohort from a single surgeon. BMC Surg. 2007;7:1.
5. Permission to reuse images marked IJK was given exclusively for this work only by Professor Ira J. Kodner.

Rectal Prolapse-Perineal Rectosigmoidectomy

70

Robert D. Fry and James S. Wu

Presentation

An elderly female presented with rectal prolapse (Figs. 70.1a, b).

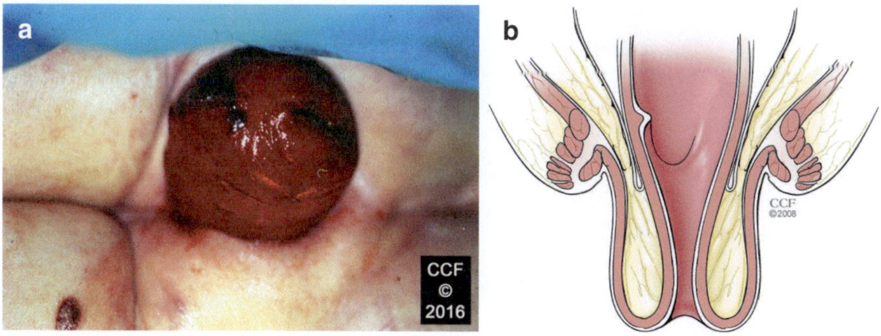

Fig. 70.1 (**a**) Rectal prolapse (procidentia). The whole thickness of the rectum has descended through the anus. Hemorrhagic trauma to the exposed mucosa is apparent. (Photos courtesy of Alan E. Timmcke, M.D.). (**b**) Rectal prolapse, cross-section, illustration

R. D. Fry
Department of Colon and Rectal Surgery, University of Pennsylvania, Philadelphia, PA, USA

J. S. Wu (✉)
Department of Colon and Rectal Surgery, Cleveland Clinic, Cleveland, OH, USA

J. S. Wu, M. D. Inkster (eds.), *Cleveland Clinic Colorectal Case Studies*,
https://doi.org/10.1007/978-3-031-39880-3_70

Management

The patient underwent surgical correction for rectal prolapse by perineal proctectomy with single-stapled colorectal anastomosis as shown in Figs. 70.2, 70.3, 70.4, and 70.5. Figures 70.2a and b show division of the outer wall of the prolapsed rectum.

Figure 70.3 shows the exteriorized rectosigmoid colon after perineal mobilization. As shown in Fig. 70.4, the exteriorized rectum is amputated.

As the redundant rectosigmoid colon is exteriorized, its mesentery is divided.

The colorectal anastomosis can be sewn or stapled. In this case, a single-stapled anastomosis was created as shown in Figs. 70.5a–e.

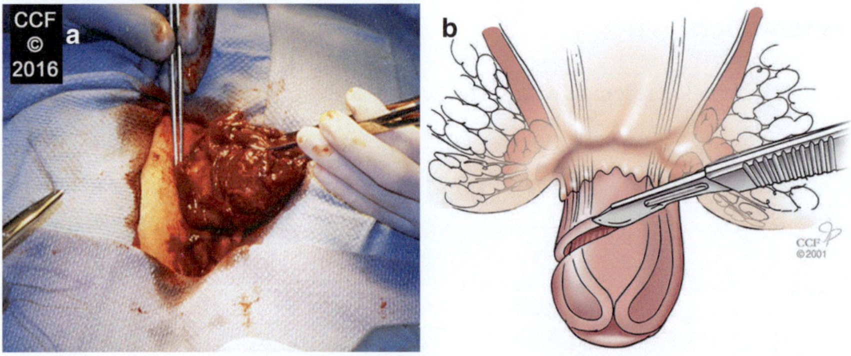

Fig. 70.2 (**a**, **b**) Proctotomy. In the prone position, the outer wall of the prolapsus is divided

Fig. 70.3 The rectosigmoid colon is exteriorized after perineal mobilization

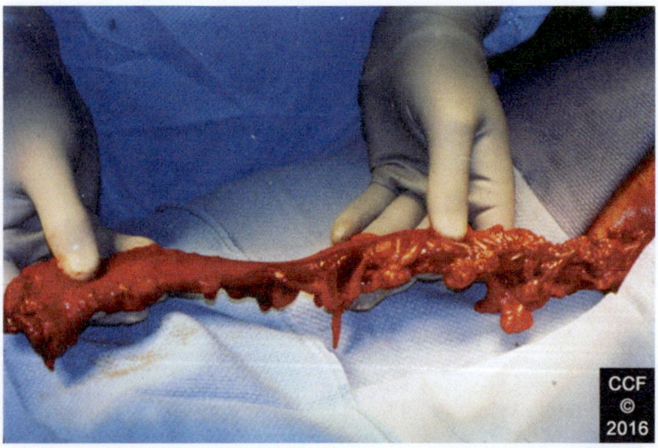

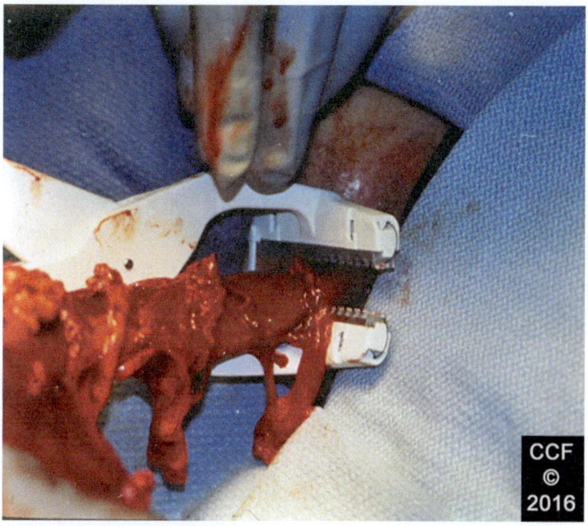

Fig. 70.4 The exteriorized rectosigmoid colon is amputated

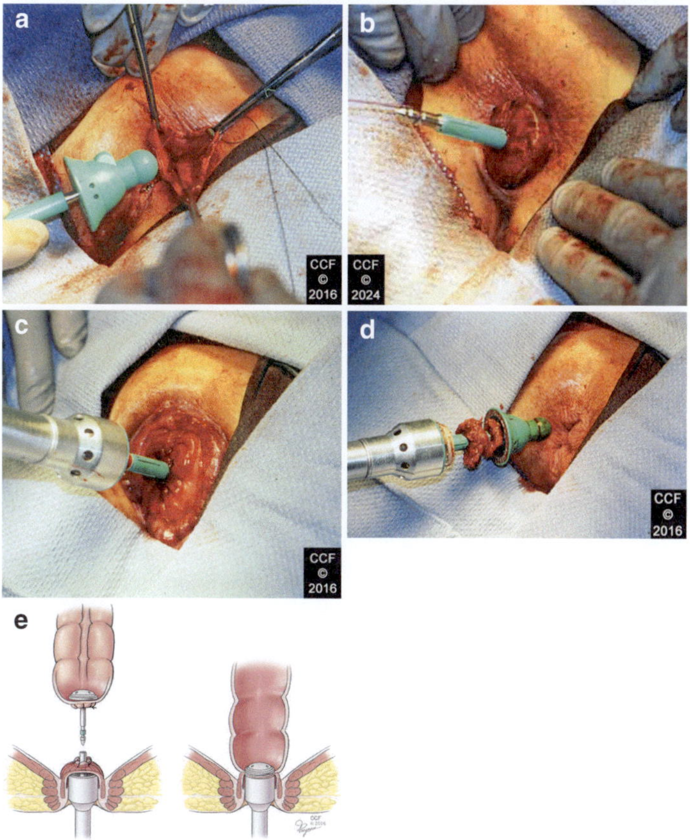

Fig. 70.5 Single-stapled colorectal anastomosis; (**a**) the anvil is inserted into the colon; (**b**) the anvil is secured to the colon with a purse-string suture; (**c**) a second purse-string suture secures the rectum to the stapling gun; (**d**) two intact donuts are obtained after completion of the anastomosis, (**e**) Illustration of the single-stapled end-to-end-colorectal anastomosis

Comments

In 1873, Allingham defined rectal prolapse or procidentia as follows:

> "True procidentia is the descent of the upper part of the rectum, in its whole thickness, or all its coats, through the anus [1]."

The anatomic arrangement of the intestinal layers is shown in Fig. 70.1. The condition tends to occur in the very young and the very old. Factors associated with the development of rectal prolapse include:

1. Low lying cul-de-sac
2. Diastasis of the levator ani muscles
3. Lax lateral ligaments
4. Patulous anus
5. Loose attachment of the rectum to the sacrum.

Although numerous operations have been devised to treat rectal prolapse, none has successfully displaced all others. The prime objective of surgery is the elimination of the prolapse with greatest success and the least morbidity. The choice of the best operation depends on surgeon experience and patient suitability [2]. Full thickness perineal amputation of the rectum was reported in 1882 by Auffret [3].

CLINIQUE CHIRURGICALE Un cas de procidence du gros intestin d'une longueur de 90 centimèters.— Opération par excision. Par M. Auffret professeur à l'école de Brest	SURGERY CLINICS A case of prolapse of the large intestine a length of 90 centimeters.—Operation by excision. By M. Auffret Professor at the School of Brest

In 1889, Mikulicz described his experience of rectal prolapse treatment by transperineal amputation and immediate coloanal anastomosis (Fig. 70.6a and b) [4]. Modestly, he begins by eschewing credit.

Zur operativen Behandlung des Prolapsus recti et coli invaginati Von Dr. Johann Mikulicz Professor der Chirurgie in Königsberg	On the operative management of rectal prolapse and invaginated colon By Dr. Johann Mikulicz Professor of Surgery at Königsberg
M.H.! Die Operation, für welche ich Ihre Aufmerksamkeit in Anspruch nehmen möchte, ist keine neue.	Sirs! The operation, for which I would like to call your attention, is not new.
Nun durchtrennt man 1 bis 2 Ctm. von der Analfalte entfernt schichtweise zunächst das äussere Darmrohr in seinem vorderen Umfange. Man geht Schritt vor Schritt vor, indem man jedes blutende Gefäss fasst und mit feinen Catgut unterbindet. Hat man auf diese Weise die vordere Hälfte des äusseren Darmrohres bis auf die Serosa quer durchtrennt, so kommt die gegenüberliegende Serosa des inneren Darmrohres zum Vorschein, die Peritonealtasche zwischen beiden Darmrohren ist in ihrer ganzen Breite eröffnet. Nun sieht man nach, ob nicht etwa Intestina vorgefallen sind. Sollte ihrer Reposition der contrahirte Sphincter ani widerstehen (bei acuten Vorfällen), so müsste er gespalten werden. Ist die Peritonealtasche leer, so sorgt man sofort für den vollständigen Abschluss der Peritonealhöhle an dieser Stelle. Dies geschieht, indem man durch eine Reihe von Knopfnähten die einander zugekehrten Peritonealflächen der zwei Darmrohre an der Schnittlinie vereinigt.	Now, 1–2 cm from the anal fold, one cuts through the outer intestinal tube in its front circumference in layers. One goes step by step, holding and stopping every bleeding vessel with Catgut. When the anterior half of the outer tube has been severed transversely, except for the serosa, the opposite serosa of the inner intestinal tube is revealed. The peritoneal pocket between the two intestinal tubes is opened in its entire width. Now one sees if or if not any intestine has fallen into the area. Should the contracted anal sphincter resist its reduction (in acute cases), it should be split. If the peritoneal pouch is empty, it is immediately closed at this point. This is done by joining, by suturing the cut edge of the mutually facing peritoneal surface of the two intestinal tubes.
Erst wenn die Peritonealspalte bis in ihre äussersten Winkel exact verschlossen ist, geht man weiter. Man durchschneidet zunächst schichtweise den vorderen Umfang des inneren Darmrohres, indem man auch hier jedes blutende Gefäss fasst. Ist nun auch das innere Darmrohr zur Hälfte durchtrennt, so vereinigt man in der ganzen Schnittlinie beide Darmrohre durch eine Reihe tiefgreifender, alle Schichten fassender Knopfnähte. Die Fadenenden lässt man lang, den sie dienen im weiteren Verlaufe der Operation zum Festhalten des Darmes. Nun durchschneidet man schichtweise den hinteren Abschnitt beider Darmrohre. Zwischen ihnen liegt hier in der Regel kein Peritoneum mehr; sie umschliessen das Mesocolon, dessen zahlreiche Gefässe man am besten sofort mit Catgut unterbindet, da sie sich sonst leicht weit hinauf zurückziehen. Die Blutung in der Darmwand selbst wird am besten auch hier durch die tiefgreifenden Nähte gestillt, welche man der schrittweisen Durchschneidung des Darmes gleich folgen lässt. In dieser Weise vollendet man schrittweise die vollständige Vereinigung beider Darmenden.	When the peritoneum is closed, one goes on. First one slices through the front of the inner intestinal tube in layers, here also securing every bleeding blood vessel. Now, the inner intestinal tube is divided halfway, so the entire incision line of both intestinal tubes is united by a single row of stitches deeply gripping all layers. The ends of the sutures are left long as they serve in the further course of the operation to hold the intestine. Now one cuts through the back section of both intestinal tubes in layers. Between them, as a rule, there is no longer any peritoneum that encloses the mesocolon whose numerous blood vessels are best immediately secured with catgut since they otherwise easily can retract far back above. Bleeding from the intestinal wall itself is also controlled with deep sutures. This is followed immediately by the stepwise division of the intestine. In this manner, one stepwise completes the complete union of both intestinal ends.

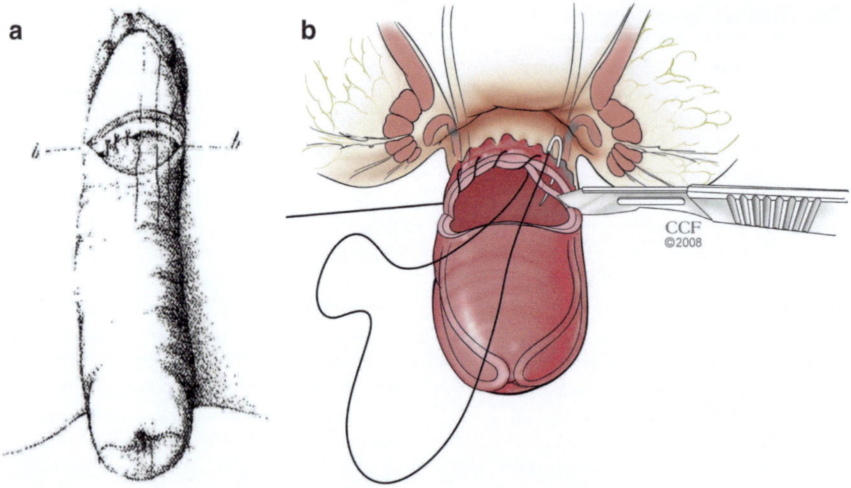

Fig. 70.6 (**a**) Perineal amputation with immediate coloanal anastomosis as drawn by Mikulicz in 1889; (**b**) Contemporary illustration of Mikulicz's operation. The two layers of prolapsed rectum have been divided. Primary coloanal anastomosis is done

In 1920, Miles described his adoption of the Mikulicz operation (Fig. 70.6). This was followed by his description of rectosigmoidectomy in 1933 for the removal of the rectum along with the prolapsed portion of the colon via a perineal approach [5]. In 1958, Gabriel renamed rectosigmoidectomy as the Auffret–Mikulicz–Miles procedure in recognition of their pioneering work [6]. In the 1950s, Altemeier and colleagues advocated perineal rectosigmoidectomy primarily for aged or debilitated persons with rectal prolapse [7].

In 2006, Auguste et al. noted more than 300 different surgical procedures for the treatment of rectal prolapse [8]. Operations for rectal prolapse are divided broadly into two groups: abdominal and perineal. Abdominal operations tend toward lower recurrence rates but require entrance into the abdominal cavity. Perineal procedures are associated with fewer complications, but recurrence rates are higher. Less risky operations are favored in the elderly and those with medical co-morbidities. The choice of operation depends on individual patient characteristics and surgeon experience. Concerning the plurality of operations for rectal prolapse, Lenormant wrote in 1907 [9].

La Colopexie	**Colopexy**
Ch. Lenormant, 1907	Ch. Lenormant, 1907
Le nombre des méthodes et des procédés opératoires en usage dans le traitement du prolapsus du rectum est la meilleure preuve qu'aucun d'eux ne satisfait pleinement à toutes les indications et ne donne des résultats constamment bons.	The number of methods and operative procedures in use for the treatment of rectal prolapse is the best proof that none of them completely satisfies all of the particulars or provides consistently good results.

His words still ring true today.

References

1. Allingham W. Procidentia Recti. In: Fistula, Hæmorrhoids, Painful Ulcer, Stricture, Prolapsus, and Other Diseases of the Rectum, Their Diagnosis and Treatment, Ch. 12. 2nd ed. Philadelphia: Lindsay & Blakiston. 1873, pp. 209–17.
2. Wu JS. Rectal prolapse: a historical perspective. Curr Probl Surg. 2009;46:598–600, 602–716.
3. Auffret. Un cas de procidence du gros intestin d'une longueur de 90 centimètres. —Opération par excision. — Double rangée de suture. — Mort. Progr Méd. 1882;10:650–2.
4. Mikulicz J. Zur operativen Behandlung des Prolapsus recti et coli invaginati. Arch Klin Chir. 1889;38:74–97.
5. Miles WE. Recto-sigmoidectomy as a method of treatment for procidentia recti. Proc R Soc Med. 1933;26:1445–8.
6. Gabriel WB. The treatment of complete prolapse of the rectum by rectosigmoidectomy (Auffret-Mikulicz-Miles procedure). Dis Colon Rectum. 1958;1:241–50.
7. Altemeier WA, Giuseffi J, Hoxworth P. Treatment of extensive prolapse of the rectum in aged or debilitated patients. Arch Surg. 1952;65:72–80.
8. Auguste T, Dubreuil A, Bost R, Bonaz B, Faucheron J-L. Technical and functional results after laparoscopic rectopexy to the promontory for complete rectal prolapse. Gastroenterol Clin Biol. 2006;30:659–63.
9. Lenormant C. La colopexie. Contribution a l'étude thérapeutique du prolapsus du rectum. Rev Chir Paris. 1907;35:191–216. 443–470.

Rectal Prolapse-Rectopexy

71

James S. Wu

Presentation

An 84-year-old female presented for repair of rectal prolapse (Fig. 71.1). She did not have a history of constipation.

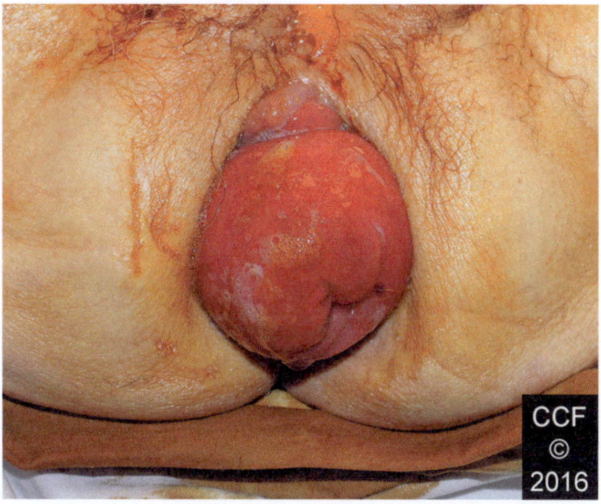

Fig. 71.1 True procidentia

J. S. Wu (✉)
Department of Colon and Rectal Surgery, Cleveland Clinic, Cleveland, OH, USA

J. S. Wu, M. D. Inkster (eds.), *Cleveland Clinic Colorectal Case Studies*,
https://doi.org/10.1007/978-3-031-39880-3_71

Management

The patient underwent laparotomy with sutured rectopexy. The lateral avascular peritoneal attachments of the rectum were divided. The rectum was mobilized posteriorly down to the tip of the coccyx. Pexing sutures were placed into the sacral promontory (Fig. 71.2). Proximal traction was placed on the rectosigmoid to reduce the prolapse. The sacral promontory sutures were sewn to the avascular lateral peritoneal attachments of the rectum (Fig. 71.3).

Figure 71.4 shows the position of bilateral pexing sutures. Gentle traction has been applied to the rectum during suture placement. The postoperative appearance of the anus is shown in Fig. 71.5.

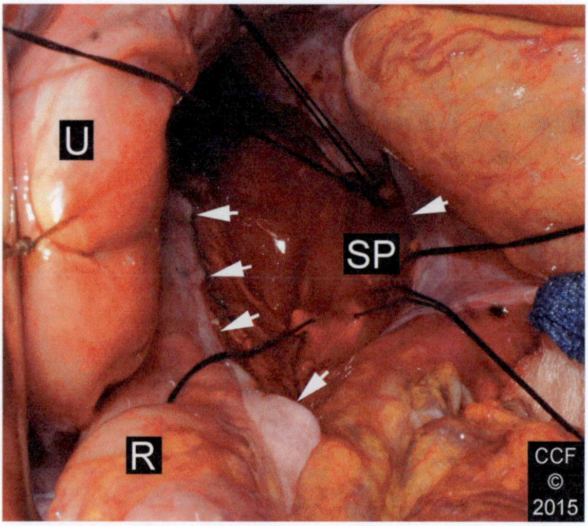

Fig. 71.2 The uterus (U) has been elevated and suspended out of the pelvis with suture. The rectum (R) has been mobilized from the sacrum. The divided peritoneum on the right side of the rectum is indicated with arrows. Silk sutures have been placed into the sacral promontory (SP)

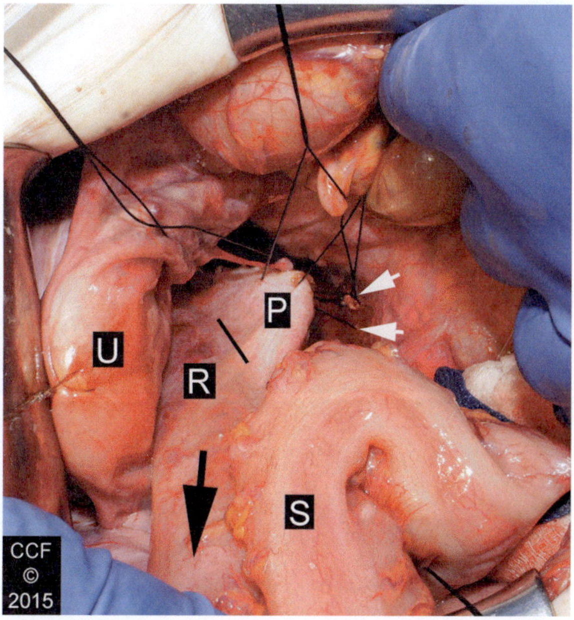

Fig. 71.3 Traction (black arrow) is placed on mobilized rectum (R) so that the procidentia is reduced. The sutures from the sacral promontory (white arrows) are sewn to the avascular lateral peritoneal attachments of the rectum (P). The border between the rectal wall and the lateral peritoneal attachments is marked by a black line. The sigmoid colon (S) is seen at the lower part of the photograph. The uterus is anterior (U)

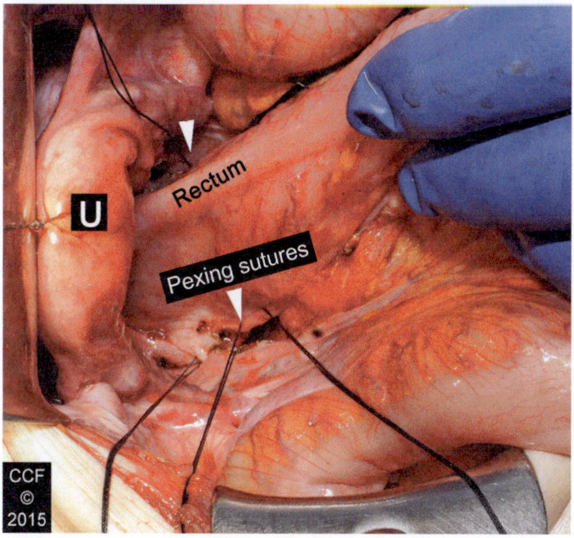

Fig. 71.4 The mobilized rectum is suspended with manual traction. The avascular lateral peritoneal attachments of the mobilized rectum are secured to the sacral promontory with bilateral pexing sutures (arrow heads). The uterus (U) is anterior

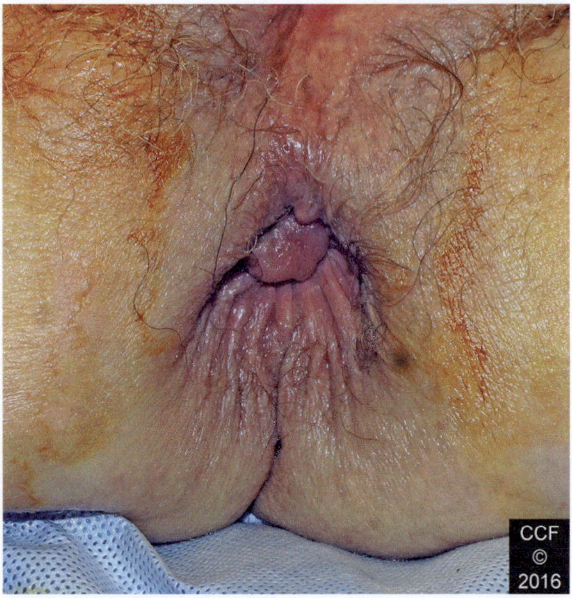

Fig. 71.5 The postoperative appearance of the anus

Comment

The operation performed here is a variation of abdominal rectopexy described in 1919 by Kümmell. In Kümmell's operation, the rectum is pulled up taut and then fixed to the anterior longitudinal ligament in the region of the sacral promontory as shown in Fig. 71.6.[1]

Zur Operation des hochgradigen Mastdarmvorfalls. Von Hermann Kümmell in Hamburg-Eppendorf. Befestigung des Rektums an das Lig. longitud. ant. nach Beseitigung des Prolapses in Seitenansicht	**Operation for high grade rectal prolapse. By Hermann Kümmell, Hamburg-Eppendorf.** Securing the rectum to the anterior longitudinal ligament after elimination of the prolapse (side view).

In the case presented, the sutures were placed through the lateral peritoneal attachments instead of the rectal wall.

The goal of abdominal rectopexy is to prevent prolapse by securing the rectum to the pelvis [2]. Fixation is done with suture or prosthetic material. Potential

[1]Georg Thieme Verlag KG was contacted regarding republication of Figure 6. The publisher replied that: "due to the age of the publication we cannot grant you any licenses for material from this book. However, we do not object to your using any content from Kümmell H. Zur Operation des hochgradigen Mastdarmvorfalls. Zentralbl Chir."

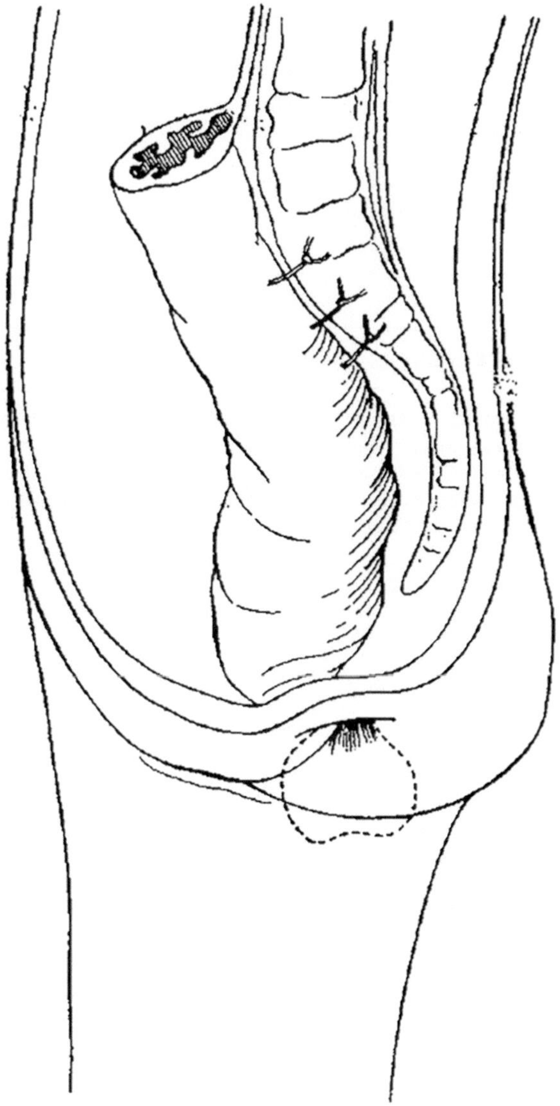

Fig. 71.6 Securing the mobilized rectum after reduction of the prolapsus to the sacral anterior longitudinal ligament as drawn by Kümmell, 1919 [1]

complications include injury to the intestine, blood vessels, vagina, ureter, and autonomic nerves associated with sexual function. Recurrence always is possible. Rectopexy is but one of many operations for the correction of rectal prolapse.

"Clear evidence demonstrating the superiority of one surgical technique over the others for the treatment of total rectal prolapse is yet to come forward despite the description of more than three hundred different procedures [3]."

Thomas Auguste, Alain Dubreuil,
Richard Bost, Bruno Bonaz,
Jean-Luc Faucheron,
Hôpital Albert Michallon,
Clinique du Mail,
Grenoble
2006

References

1. Kümmell H. Zur Operation des hochgradigen Mastdarmvorfalls. Zentralbl Chir. 1919;46:465–9.
2. Wu JS. Rectal prolapse. A historical perspective. Curr Prob Surg. 2009;46:602–716.
3. Auguste T, Dubreuil A, Bost R, Bonaz B, Faucheron J-L. Technical and functional results after laparoscopic rectopexy to the promontory for complete rectal prolapse. Gastroenterol Clin Biol. 2006;30:659–63.

72 Mitigating Death from Rectal Cancer

Jacques Lisfranc de Saint-Martin

James S. Wu

Jacques Lisfranc de St. Martin (1787–1847) [1]

In his obituary, Jacques Lisfranc is credited with the first successful ablation of rectal cancer [2].

Il est le premier à réussir une ablation du carcinome du rectum.	He is the first to successfully complete an ablation of carcinoma of the rectum.

Lisfranc's 1830 memoir describes rectal cancer *ablation* by transanal excision [3].

Mémoire. sur l'excision. de la partie inférieure du rectum, devenue carcinomateuse. Par J. Lisfranc Chirurgien en chef de l'hôpital de la Pitié 1830	Memoir on excision of the distal rectum for cancer by J. Lisfranc Surgeon in chief, Hospital of Pity 1830
Je l'ai tenté et j'ai réussi, comme on l'a vu, contre les cancers de la verge, de la langue et du vagin: l'art prescrivait l'ablation complète de ces organes,… Mais la chirurgie tendait au moins une main secourable à ces malades; car quoiqu'elle leur imposât un grand sacrifice, elle leur conservait la vie. Il n'en est pas ainsi dans les cancers confirmés qui affectent la partie inférieure du canal intestinal; l'art avait reconnu et proclamé son impuissance à ce sujet; les malades étaient voués à une mort inévitable: et quelle mort! quelle douleur!	I have tried and successfully used against cancer of the penis, the tongue and the vagina, the prescribed treatment of complete removal of these organs. Surgery at least offered a helping hand for these illnesses; even though it imposes a great sacrifice, it does preserve life. This has not been the case for confirmed cancers of the distal intestinal canal. The healing arts recognized and proclaimed its impotence with regard to this subject. The afflicted were regarded as doomed to inevitable death: and what a death! What pain!

J. S. Wu (✉)
Department of Colon and Rectal Surgery, Cleveland Clinic, Cleveland, OH, USA

J. S. Wu, M. D. Inkster (eds.), *Cleveland Clinic Colorectal Case Studies*,
https://doi.org/10.1007/978-3-031-39880-3_72

Lisfranc created an operation for the removal of some distal mobile tumors.

Avant tout examinons les circonstances dans lesquelles nous croyons l'opération praticable. On s'assurera, autant que possible, de l'épaisseur du cancer autour du rectum: quand le tissu cellulaire qui environne la partie inférieure du canal intestinal est sain, l'intestin est mobile et se laisse abaisser; notre opinion est qu'alors on doit opérer.	Before everything, we examine the circumstances which lead us to think that operation is practical. As much as possible, one determines the cancer thickness around the rectum: when the tissue in the region of the distal intestinal canal is healthy, the intestine is mobile and can be pulled down, it is our opinion that one should operate.

The conduct of surgery was as follows.

Le malade est placé comme si on voulait pratiquer l'opération de la taille latéralisée. …il est fort aisé, avec les ciseaux courbes sur le plat ou avec le bistouri, d'en réséquer une très-grande étendue, et lors même que le cancer occuperait toute l'épaisseur des parois de l'intestin, pourvu qu'il ne s'élevât pas à plus d'un pouce au-dessus de l'anus, on pourrait encore renverser le rectum sur lui-même, de manière à mettre toute la maladie à découvert. On incise alors parallèlement à l'axe du tronc la portion renversée de l'intestin, et on l'excise avec de forts ciseaux courbes sur le plat.	The patient was positioned for surgery in the lateral position. It is very easy with curved scissors or with the scalpel, to resect a very large tumor even when the cancer occupies the entire thickness of the walls of the intestine provided that it is not more than an inch above the anus. The rectum could still be everted so that all the disease is discovered. We incise parallel to the trunk of the inverted portion of the intestine and excise it with heavy curved scissors.

The epitaph on Lisfranc's tomb raises in all surgeons awareness not only of benefits, but also of potential adverse consequences of their work [2]:

SI LA CHIRUGIE EST BRILLANTE QUAND ELLE OPÈRE, ELLE L'EST ENCORE BIEN D'ADVANTAGE LORSQUE SANS FAIRE COULER LE SANG ET SANS MUTILATION, ELLE OBTIENT LA GUÉRISON DU MALADE	IF SURGERY IS BRIGHT WHEN SHE IS OPERATING, SHE IS AGAIN MUCH MORE WHEN BLOOD IS NOT SPILLED AND WITHOUT MUTILATION, SHE OBTAINS THE HEALING OF THE SICK

References

1. Fischer L-P. Jacques Lisfranc De Saint-Martin (1787-1847). Hist Sci Méd. 2005;39:17–34.
2. Jacques Lisfranc de Saint-Martin – napoleon-monuments.eu.
3. Lisfranc J. Mémoire sur l'excision de la partie inférieure du rectum, devenue carcinomateuse. Imprimerie de Ch. Dezauche, Faubourg Montmartre, N°. 11, 1830:3–7.

Rectal Cancer-Abdominoperineal Resection, Lithotomy

73

James S. Wu and Katharine L. Jackson

Presentation

A 77-year-old male underwent colonoscopy because of rectal bleeding (Fig. 73.1). A low rectal mass was found. Biopsy showed moderately differentiated adenocarcinoma. The serum carcinoembryonic antigen was slightly elevated. Computed

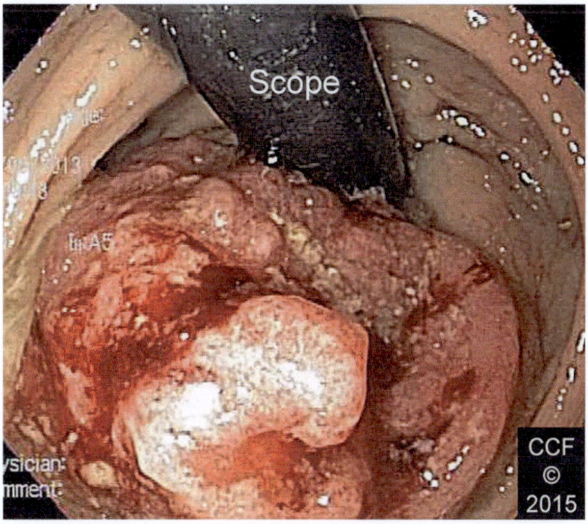

Fig. 73.1 Endoscopic examination of the rectum showed a distal rectal mass. The mass was posterior on digital examination. The endoscope (scope) is labelled

J. S. Wu (✉)
Department of Colon and Rectal Surgery, Cleveland Clinic, Cleveland, OH, USA

K. L. Jackson
Department of Colorectal Surgery, Department of Surgery, Duke University, Durham, NC, USA

J. S. Wu, M. D. Inkster (eds.), *Cleveland Clinic Colorectal Case Studies*,
https://doi.org/10.1007/978-3-031-39880-3_73

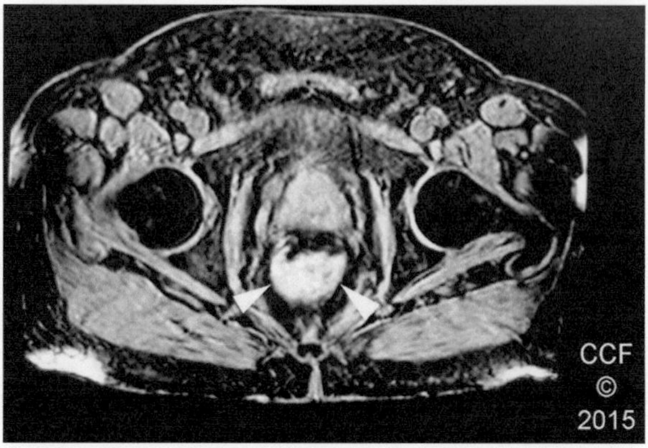

Fig. 73.2 Axial CT view of the pelvis shows a posterior rectal mass (arrowheads)

tomography showed a posterior rectal mass (Fig. 73.2) but no evidence of metastatic disease. Transrectal ultrasonic staging (TRUS) showed that the tumor was T3N0.

Management

Following preoperative chemotherapy and radiation, abdominoperineal resection was done (Fig. 73.3).

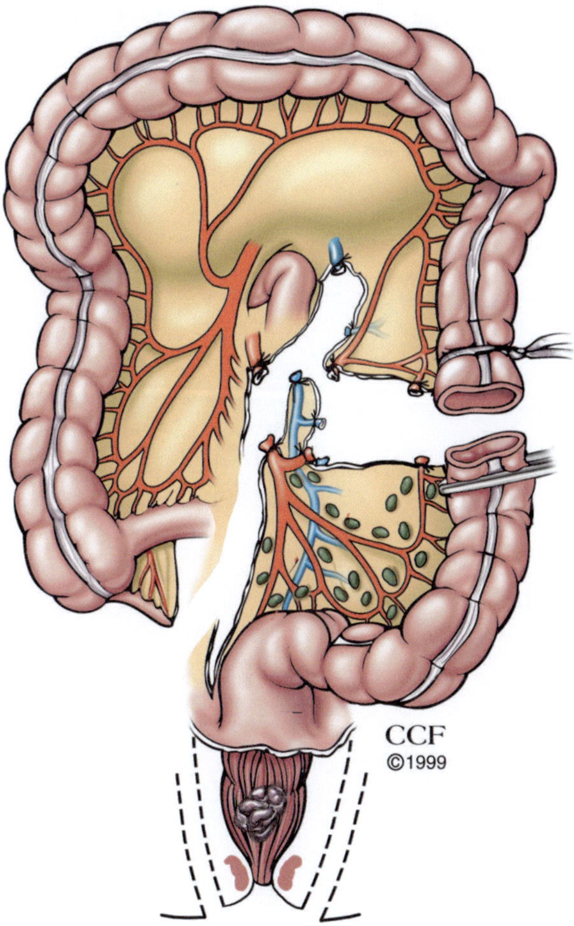

Fig. 73.3 Abdominoperineal resection. The anus, rectum, and sigmoid colon with associated lymphatics are removed. The operation results in a permanent colostomy

Abdominal Portion

The permanent colostomy location was marked at predetermined site with indelible ink (Fig. 73.4).

The abdomen was entered through a midline incision. Exploration did not reveal metastatic disease. As shown in Fig. 73.5, the inferior mesenteric artery (IMA) and vein (IMV) were identified, isolated and divided.

Following division of the colon at the left colon-sigmoid colon junction, the rectosigmoid colon was mobilized to the pelvic floor. As shown in Fig. 73.6, posteriorly, the mesorectum with its fascia was dissected from the presacral fascia along a bloodless plane. Next, the lateral ligaments were divided. Finally, the anterior rectum was mobilized. Since this was a posterior rectal tumor, the anterior rectal dissection was done posterior to Denonvillier's fascia.

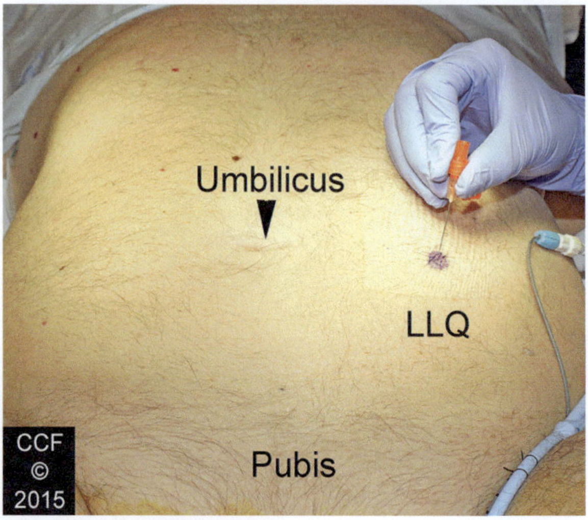

Fig. 73.4 The patient had been marked for a permanent colostomy before surgery. The site was marked with three needle punctures before skin preparation

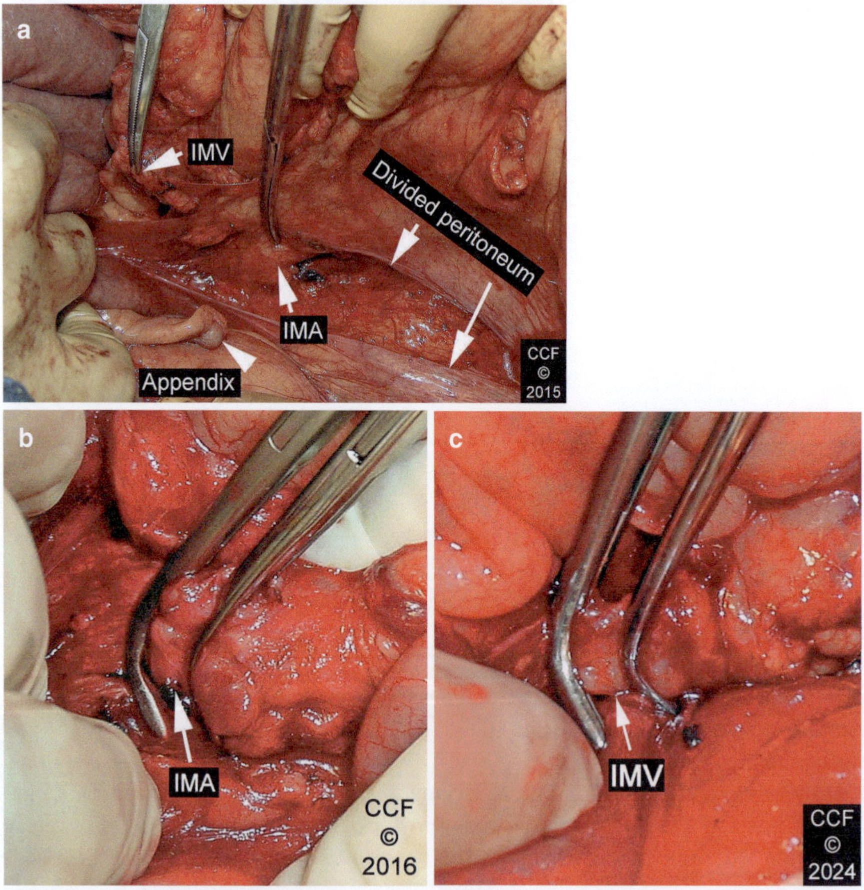

Fig. 73.5 (**a**) The peritoneum overlying the retroperitoneum was divided allowing identification of the IMA and IMV; (**b**) the IMA was isolated and divided between clamps close to its origin at the aorta; (**c**) the IMV was divided close to the lower border of the pancreas

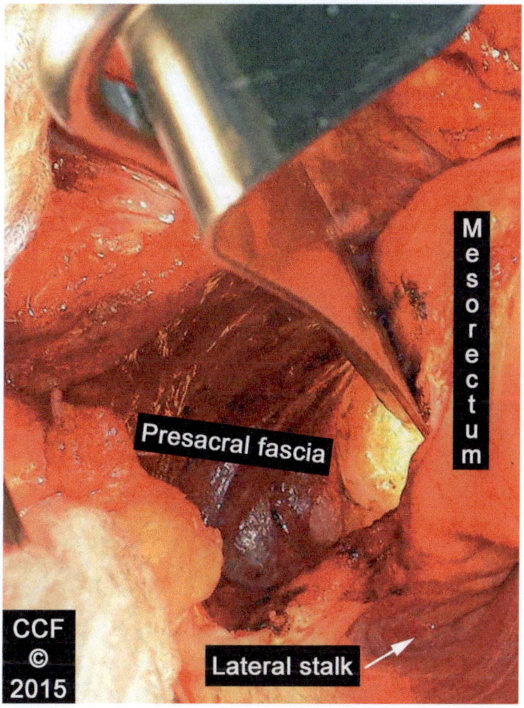

Fig. 73.6 Posterior rectal mobilization was done by sharp dissection to the pelvic floor. The arrow identifies the right lateral ligament. The mesorectum and the presacral fascia are labelled

Perineal Portion

Following rectal washout, the anus was sewn closed with a circumferential purse-string suture as shown in Fig. 73.7. The surgical site was prepared sterilely. A circumferential incision was made around the external sphincter (Fig. 73.8).

The pelvis was entered first by dividing the anococcygeal ligament. The lateral levator attachments then were divided. The anterior attachments adjacent to the genital structures were divided last after exteriorization of the rectosigmoid (Fig. 73.9).

Finally, the perineal wound was closed (Fig. 73.10). The pelvis was filled with an omental pedicle graft.

The resected specimen was opened at the end of the case (Fig. 73.11). No residual tumor was seen on final pathology.

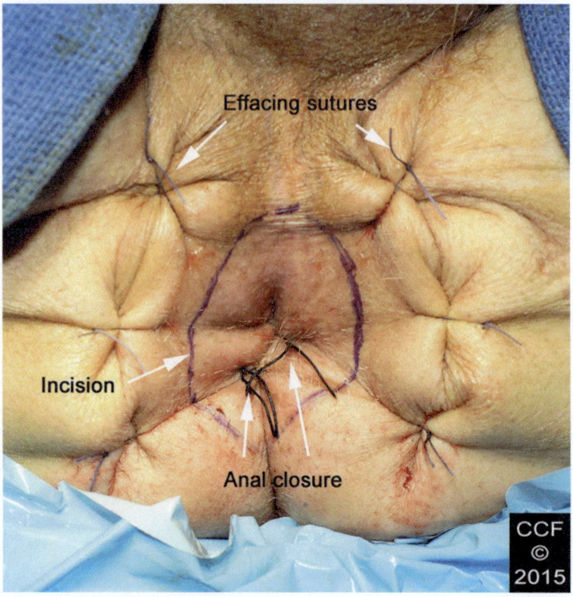

Fig. 73.7 In the lithotomy position, the anus was closed with two purse-string sutures. The surgical field was cleansed. The anal area was effaced with retracting sutures (arrows). The path of a circumferential incision has been marked

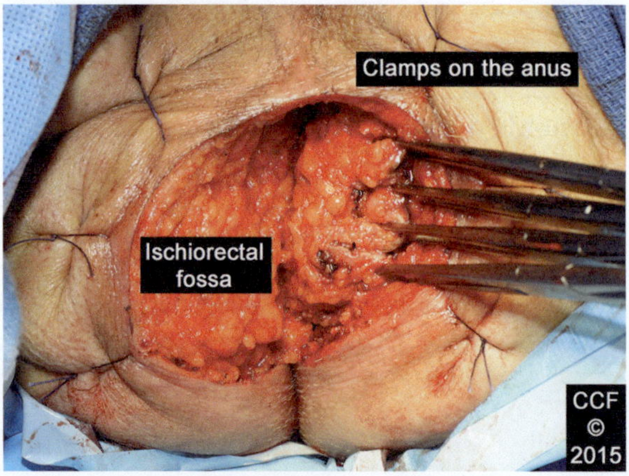

Fig. 73.8 An elliptical incision was made around the external anal sphincter. The dissection was carried to the pelvic floor

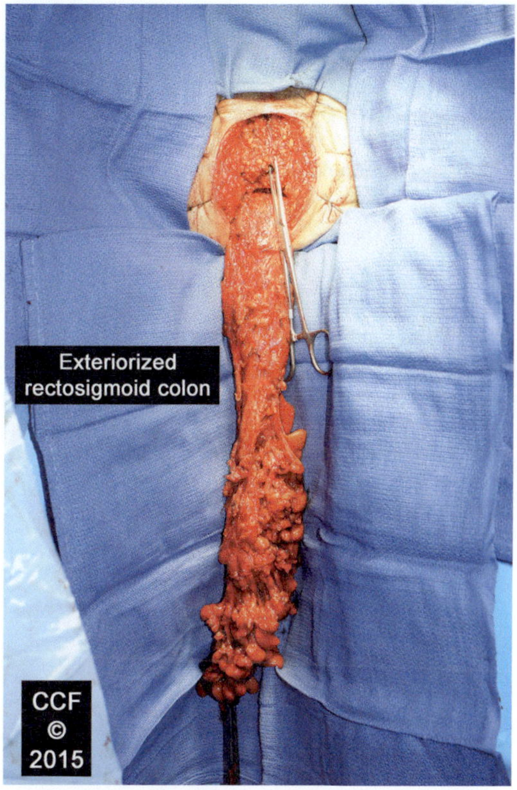

Fig. 73.9 Exteriorized rectosigmoid colon following division of the anococcygeal ligament and the lateral levator ani muscles

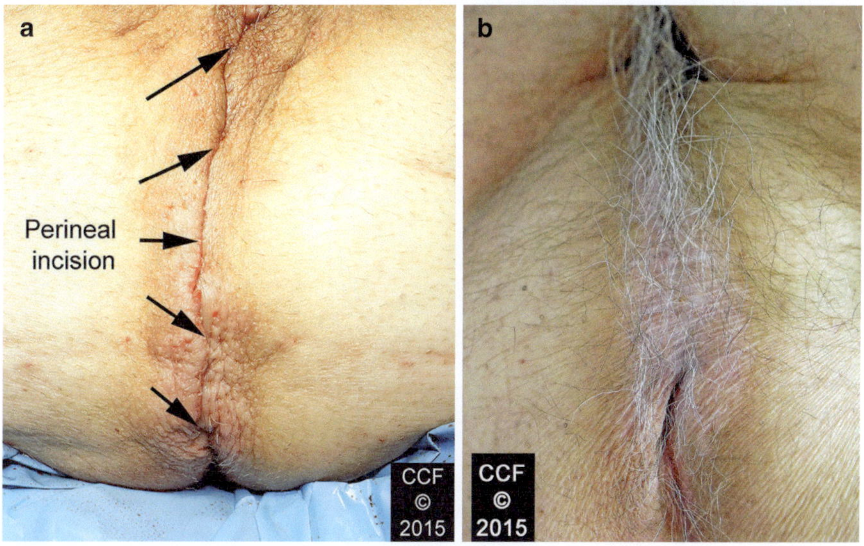

Fig. 73.10 (**a**) The perineal wound was closed in layers; (**b**) The perineal wound 1 year after surgery

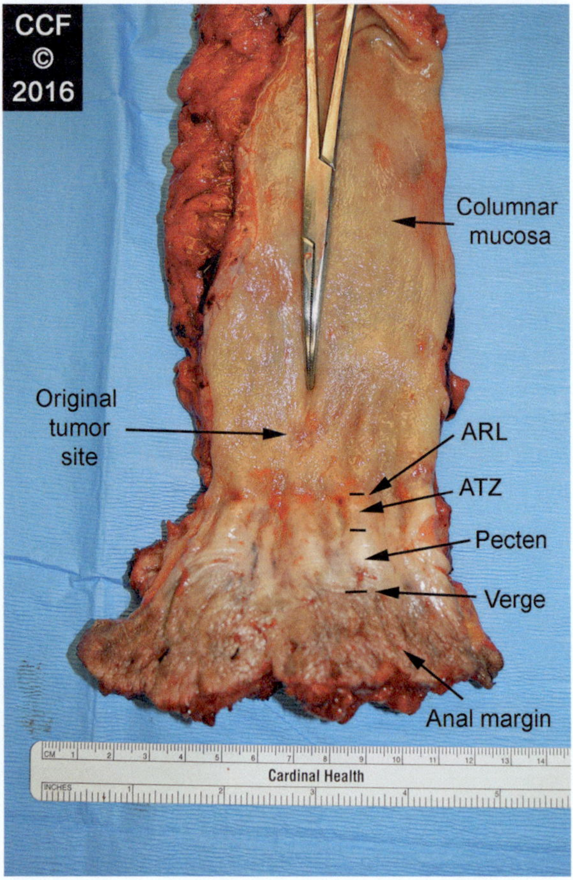

Fig. 73.11 No residual tumor was found at the original tumor site. The columnar mucosa, anorectal line (ARL), anal transitional zone (ATZ), pecten, anal verge, and anal margin are labeled

Rectal Cancer Abdominoperineal Resection, Prone

74

Thomas E. Garofalo and James S. Wu

Presentation

An elderly male with a low rectal cancer underwent abdominoperineal resection of the rectum. The abdominal portion of the operation was done in the lithotomy position. The patient was then repositioned prone. The operative steps of the perineal excision in the prone position are described in Figs. 74.1, 74.2, 74.3, 74.4, 74.5, 74.6, 74.7, and 74.8.

T. E. Garofalo · J. S. Wu (✉)
Department of Colon and Rectal Surgery, Cleveland Clinic, Cleveland, OH, USA

J. S. Wu, M. D. Inkster (eds.), *Cleveland Clinic Colorectal Case Studies*,
https://doi.org/10.1007/978-3-031-39880-3_74

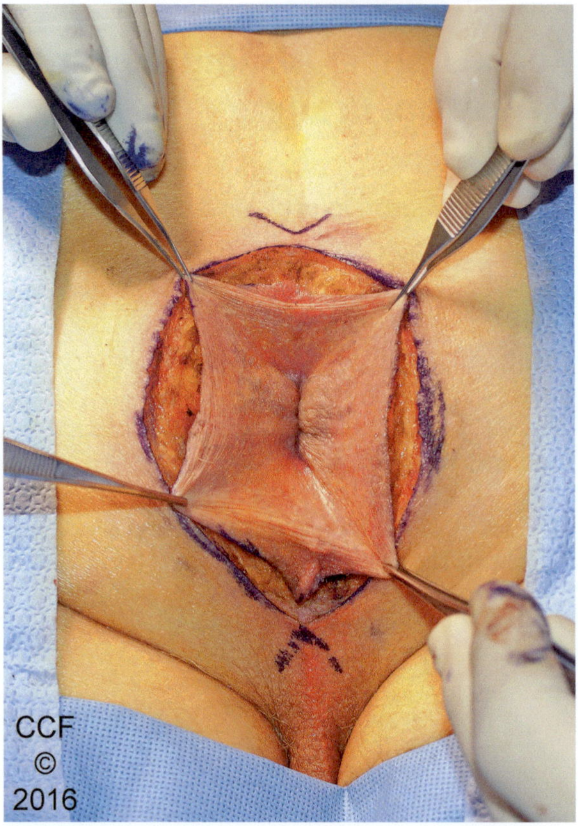

Fig. 74.1 In the prone position, after suture closure of the anus and sterile preparation, a circumferential incision was made in the perianal skin

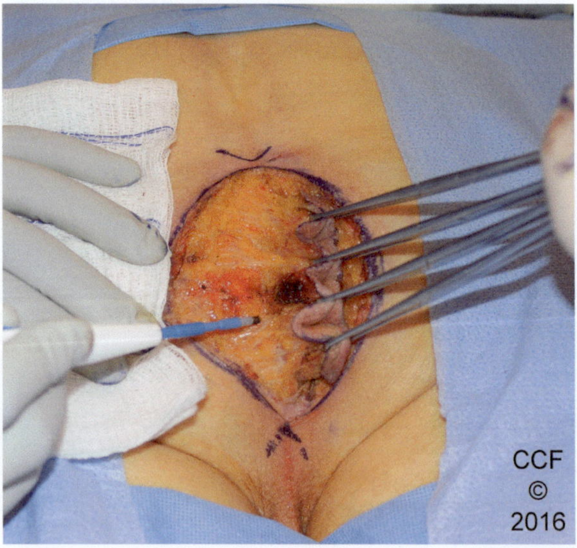

Fig. 74.2 The anus was dissected free from surrounding soft tissue

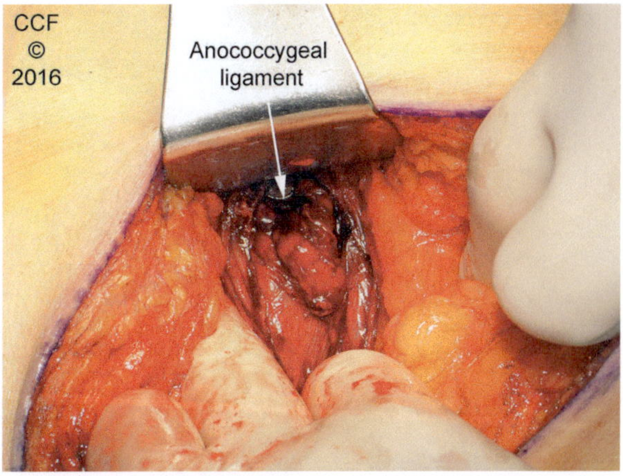

Fig. 74.3 The anococcygeal ligament is identified and divided, providing entry into the pelvis

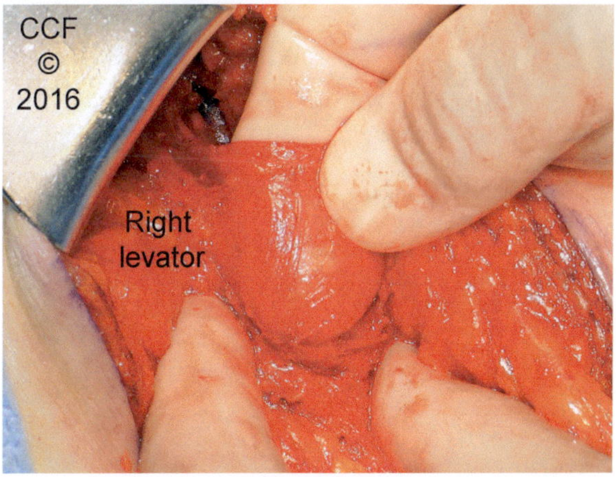

Fig. 74.4 The right levator muscle is identified and divided. The underlying forefinger and thumb provide traction

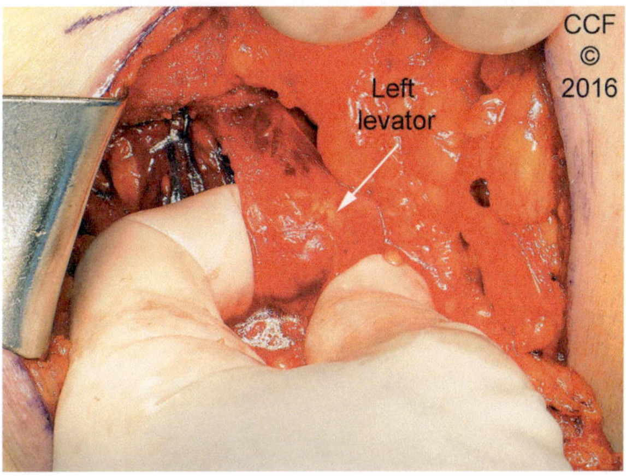

Fig. 74.5 The left levator muscle is isolated and divided

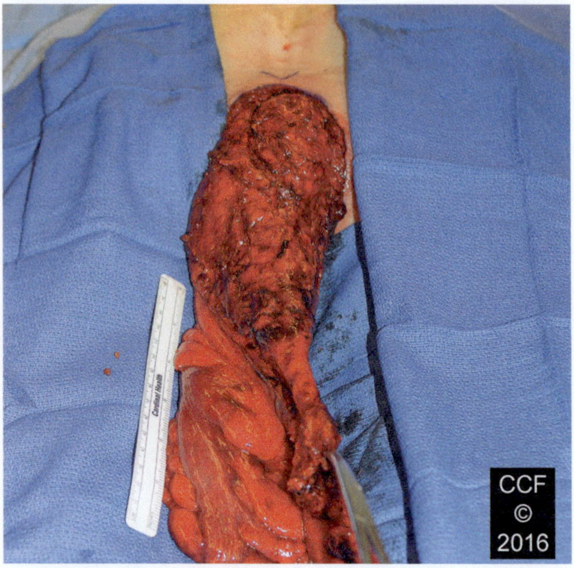

Fig. 74.6 The rectum and sigmoid colon are exteriorized

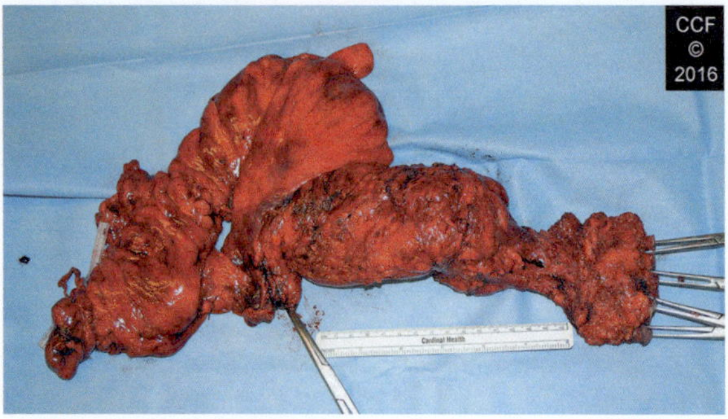

Fig. 74.7 Following the division of the anterior attachments, the specimen is removed. Clamps are seen on the inferior mesenteric artery (center left) and on the anus (right)

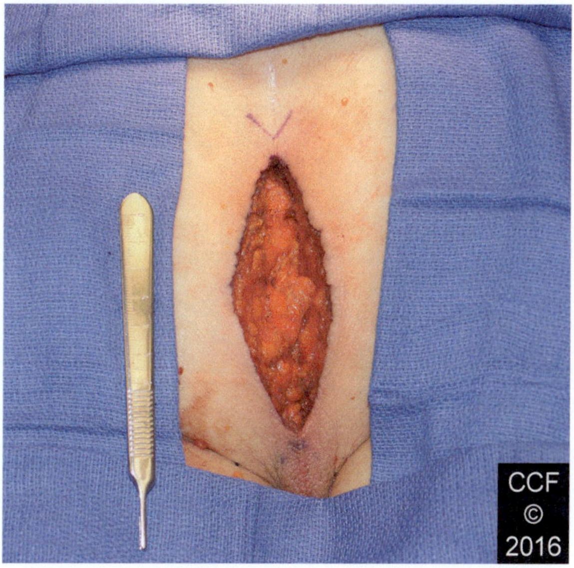

Fig. 74.8 The perianal wound is prepared for closure

Comment

Performance of the perineal portion of abdominoperineal excision in the prone position has dual advantages. First, exposure is excellent. Second, the surgeon can take full advantage of an assistant who stands on the opposite side of the operating table.

Abdominoperineal Resection for Rectal Cancer-Comment

75

James S. Wu

Presentation

Abdominoperineal resection for rectal cancer was developed at the beginning of the twentieth century. The operation removes the tumor-bearing segment, the anus, and lymphatic routes of spread upwards along the superior rectal vessels, laterally along the middle rectal vessels and inferiorly. The operation results in a permanent colostomy.

Surgery is divided into two parts. The abdominal portion involves the mobilization of the rectosigmoid colon and its mesenteries down to the pelvic floor. The perineal portion mobilizes the anus from the pelvic floor and perianal soft tissue. In 1904, Mayo described the principles of abdominoperineal resection of the rectum for carcinoma as follows:

Cancer of the Large Bowel
Read at the Oregon State Medical Society,
Portland August 30-31, 1904
By C. H. Mayo, M.D.
Rochester, Minn.
Surgeon to St. Mary's Hospital of Rochester, Minn.

> "The block removal of the rectum and glands where possible from below and in high location of the cancer, the combined abdominal and perineal methods of removing rectum, glands, and all malignant tissue en masse, is the surgery for the cancer of this region. This method is merely the application of principles of the surgery of cancer, regardless of location, as exemplified by Halstead's operation for the removal of cancer of the breast [1]."

J. S. Wu (✉)
Department of Colon and Rectal Surgery, Cleveland Clinic, Cleveland, OH, USA

J. S. Wu, M. D. Inkster (eds.), *Cleveland Clinic Colorectal Case Studies*,
https://doi.org/10.1007/978-3-031-39880-3_75

In introducing the 1908 operation eponymously associated with his name, Miles modestly gives credit to surgeons who preceded him.[1]

A Method of Performing Abdominoperineal Excision for Carcinoma of the Rectum and of the Terminal Portion of the Pelvic Colon
By W. Ernest Miles, F.R.C.S. Eng., L.R.C.P. Lond.,
Surgeon to the Cancer Hospital, Brompton, S.W., and to the Gordon Hospital for diseases of the rectum. Vauxhall Bridge-Road, S.W.

"Removal of the rectum by a combined abdominal and perineal operation was first performed by Czerny in 1884. Since that time several other surgeons, notably Maunsell, Chaput, Gaudier, Challot, Weir, Boechal, Giordino, Quénu, Reverdin, Tuttle, Gant, Mathews, Sir Charles Ball, Wallis, and Aldrich-Blake have employed the method with certain modifications of procedure and with varying success in regard to mortality. So far as I have been able to gather from the literature of the subject, however, the technique of these operators seems to have failed in one important respect —namely, the complete eradication of *the zone of upward spread* of cancer from the rectum, whereby the chance of recurrence of the disease, above the field of operation, can be diminished if not entirely obviated.

Until the close of the year 1906 I had relied solely upon the perineal methods of excision of the rectum, but I found that, even after the most complete and extensive removal possible, recurrence of the disease was a rule to which there were few exceptions. Moreover, I found that although perfection of technique had reduced the proportion of recurrences in the immediate vicinity of the field of operation, recurrence nevertheless appeared in situations that were beyond the scope of a removal from the perineum. Post-mortem examination showed that these situations were (a) the pelvic peritoneum, (b) the pelvic mesocolon, and (c) the lymph nodes situated over the bifurcation of the left common iliac artery.

From these observations it is obvious that the abovementioned structures constitute *the zone of the upward spread* of cancer from the rectum, the removal of which is just as imperative as in the thorough clearance of the axilla in cases of cancer of the breast if freedom from recurrence is to be hoped for.

The study of the spread of cancer from the rectum has led me to formulate certain essentials in the technique of the operation which must be strictly adhered to if satisfactory results are to be obtained—namely: (1) that an abdominal anus is a necessity; (2) that the whole of the pelvic colon, with the exception of the part from which the colostomy is made, must be removed because its blood-supply is contained in the zone of upward spread; (3) that the whole of the pelvic mesocolon below the point where it crosses the common iliac artery, together with a strip of peritoneum at least an inch wide on either side of it, must be cleared away; (4) that the group of lymph nodes situated over the bifurcation of the common iliac artery are in all instances to be removed; and lastly (5), that the perineal portion of the operation should be carried out as widely as possible so that the lateral and downward zones of spread may be effectively extirpated."

[1] Miles [2]. Permission to reproduce this excerpt was generously provided by Elsevier Science & Technology journals, CCC|Marketplace™, License Number 5404871109347, License date Oct 09, 2022.

Biographical Note

William Ernest Miles

At his memorial service, Sir Gordon Gordon-Taylor gave the following eulogy [3]:

> 'I had the privilege of working alongside him for several months during the autumn of 1917 at the advanced abdominal centre just outside the wall of Ypres, where was collected together much of the "abdominal talent" of the British Expeditionary Force. It was an international group in very truth for there were surgeons from the U.S.A., Canada, Australia, and New Zealand, as well as English, Scots, and Irish, and Miles was largely responsible for the wonderful friendship, the good fellowship and camaraderie that prevailed amidst that group, working "at the back of the front," on 16-hour "shifts" for months on end, in unpleasant, noisy, and sleepless surroundings, and he made of us a "brotherhood-in-arms."
>
> He had a genius for friendship, and the deft fingers from which skill and pity flowed added adoring patients to the circle of his friends.

His philosophy of life might be briefly, yet imperfectly, expressed in the following lines:

From quiet home and first beginning
Out to the undiscovered end
There's nothing worth the wear of winning
But laughter and the love of friends.

But for Miles, there was something else worth winning—the conquest of disease and the relief of pain and suffering.'

References

1. Mayo CH. Cancer of the large bowel. Med Sentinel. 1904;12:466–73.
2. Miles WE. A method of performing abdomino-perineal excision for carcinoma of the rectum and of the terminal portion of the pelvic colon. Lancet. 1908;2:1812–3.
3. Ernest Miles W. Obituary. Br Med J. 1947;ii:633–4.

76 Pelvic Omental Pedicle Flap

James S. Wu and Gwendolyn A. Fuller

Presentation

An 83-year-old male with low rectal cancer was treated by abdominoperineal resection. An omental pedicle flap graft was used to fill the pelvis (Fig. 76.1a–c).

After proctectomy, the mobilized omentum easily reaches into the pelvis, usually traveling along the left gutter.

Computed tomography (CT) of the pelvis shows the path of the omental pedicle flap graft along the left gutter and into the pelvis (Fig. 76.2).

Figure 76.3 is an illustration that shows the omentum positioned in the pelvis. Figure 76.4 is an operative photo showing the omentum filling the pelvis behind the bladder.

J. S. Wu (✉)
Department of Colon and Rectal Surgery, Cleveland Clinic, Cleveland, OH, USA

G. A. Fuller
Medical Illustration Team, Enterprise Creative Services, Cleveland Clinic, Cleveland, OH, USA

J. S. Wu, M. D. Inkster (eds.), *Cleveland Clinic Colorectal Case Studies*,
https://doi.org/10.1007/978-3-031-39880-3_76

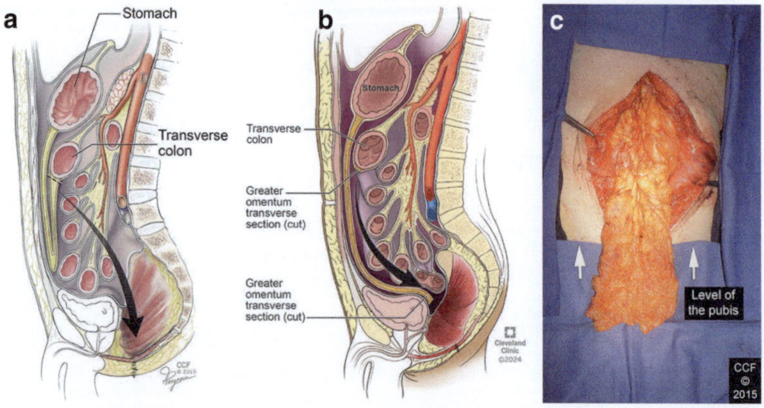

Fig. 76.1 Omental pedicle flap. (**a**) The avascular attachments of the omentum to the transverse colon are divided (dotted line); (**b**) The omentum previously attached to the transverse colon is moved into the pelvis (lateral view); (**c**) The mobilized omentum extends from the greater curvature of the stomach beyond the symphysis pubis

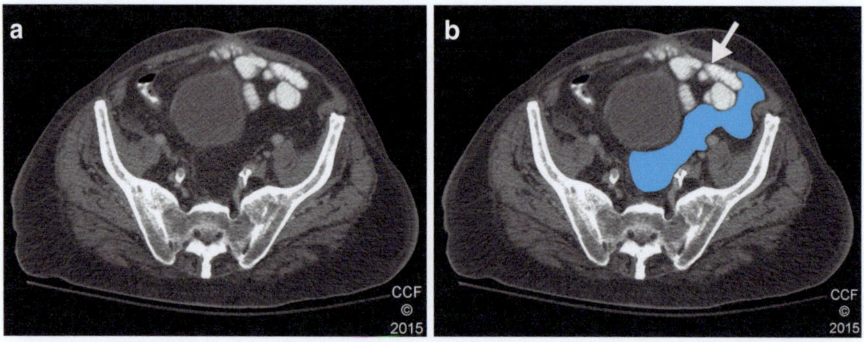

Fig. 76.2 (**a**). Computed tomogram of the pelvis demonstrating omental pedicle flap graft; (**b**). The fatty omental pedicle flap (blue high-light) fills the pelvis posterior to the bladder entering the pelvis from the left side. Small intestine (arrow) is excluded from the pelvis

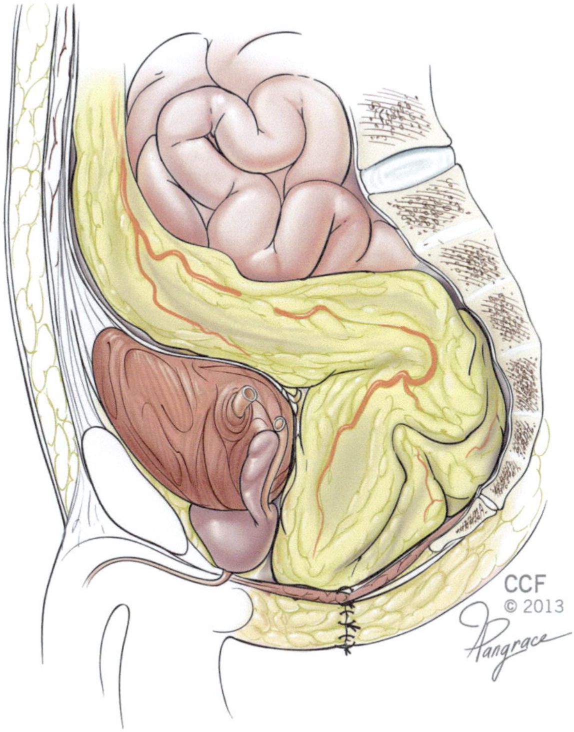

Fig. 76.3 Illustration showing an omental pedicle graft in the pelvis behind the bladder, excluding the small bowel from the pelvis

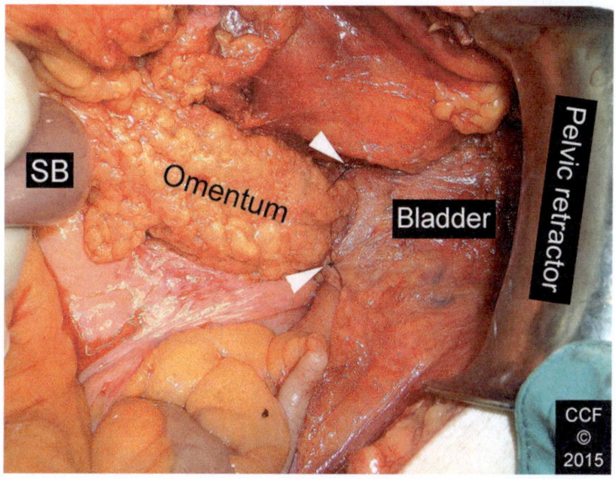

Fig. 76.4 Operative photo showing the omental pedicle flap secured in the pelvis behind the bladder with suture (arrowheads). The pelvic retractor and small bowel (SB) are identified

Comment

The greater or gastrocolic omentum is an adipose tissue layer, covered by peritoneum, that extends from the greater curvature of the stomach to the transverse colon [1]. The greater omentum receives its blood supply from the gastroepiploic arteries along the greater curvature of the stomach. The Arc of Barkow forms an

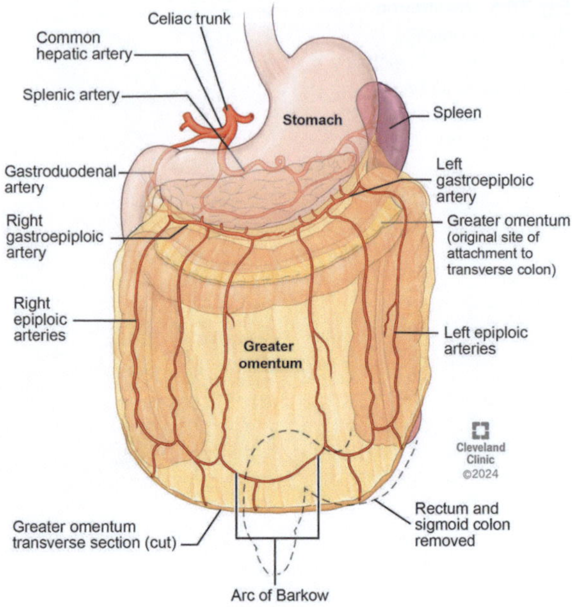

Fig. 76.5 Arterial supply of the omentum

anastomosis between the right and left gastroepiploic arteries (Fig. 76.5) [2]. Main arterial vessels descend from the left and right sides of the omentum.

The avascular omental connection to the transverse colon is divided to create the flap.

A pelvic omental pedicle flap has two purposes: (1) fill the pelvic dead space and (2) exclude small intestine from the pelvis. If postoperative radiation is needed, the small intestine will be kept out of the treatment field. In the event of perineal wound dehiscence, the small intestine will not be exposed, thus preventing the complication of perineal enterocutaneous fistula [3–6].

References

1. Di Nicola V. Omentum a powerful biological source in regenerative surgery. Regen Ther. 2019;11:182–91.
2. Bruzoni M, Steinberg GK, Dutta S. Laparoscopic harvesting of omental pedicle flap for cerebral revascularization in children with moyamoya disease. J Pediatr Surg. 2016;51:592–7.
3. Poston GJ, Smith SRG, Baker WNW. Retrocolic pelvic omentoplasty in abdominoperineal excision of the rectum. Ann R Coll Surg Engl. 1991;73:229–32.
4. Rice ML, Hay AM, Hurlow RH. Omentoplasty in abdominoperineal resection of the rectum. Aust N Z J Surg. 1992;62:147–9.
5. De Broux E, Parc Y, Rondelli F, Dehni N, Tiret E, Parc R. Sutured perineal omentoplasty after abdominoperineal resection for adenocarcinoma of the lower rectum. Dis Colon Rectum. 2005;48:476–82.
6. Killeen S, Devaney A, Mannion M, Martin ST, Winter DC. Omental pedicle flaps following proctectomy: a systematic review. Colorectal Dis. 2013;15:e634–45.

Rectal Cancer Resection with Preservation of Bowel Continuity: Historical Overview

77

James S. Wu

Presentation

In 1908, concerning excision for carcinoma of the rectum, Miles defined "essentials in the technique of the operation which must be strictly adhered to if satisfactory results are to be obtained." Among these was number five.

> …and lastly (5), that the perineal portion of the operation should be carried out as widely as possible so that the lateral and downward zones of spread may be effectively extirpated.

Miles' operation includes an "abdominal anus." [1] Subsequently, sphincter-sparing operations were introduced. The words of pioneers that provided evidence opposing or supporting this approach constitute the remainder of this section.

Handley: Cancer Surgery as a Branch of Lymphatic Surgery (1910) [2]

Hunterian Lectures
on
The Surgery of the Lymphatic System
By
W. Sampson Handley, M.S. F.R.C.S.
Hunterian Professor, Royal College of Surgeons of England

Cancer Surgery as a Branch of Lymphatic Surgery.

J. S. Wu (✉)
Department of Colon and Rectal Surgery, Cleveland Clinic, Cleveland, OH, USA

J. S. Wu, M. D. Inkster (eds.), *Cleveland Clinic Colorectal Case Studies*,
https://doi.org/10.1007/978-3-031-39880-3_77

'The whole field of the surgery of carcinoma belongs, in the strictest and most literal sense, to the ablational department of lymphatic surgery. When for instance, an operation is performed for breast cancer, its object is not the extirpation of an organ but, as I have expressed it elsewhere, "the removal intact of the permeated area of the lymphatic system which surrounds the primary growth." This permeated area often extends far beyond the limits of the breast.

With this anatomical preface, I may proceed to the case of rectal carcinoma in which I was able to demonstrate a mode of spread of the disease hitherto undetected.

Mrs. G, aged 32, was sent to me by Dr. Mervin Wilson, of Derby, and Dr. G. Kerr Grimmer, in September 1909, with a typical carcinoma of the rectum, a finger's length above the anus.

Early in October, 1909, by a combined abdominal and perineal operation, I removed the lowest 10 inches of the bowel, including the sphincters and the peri-anal skin.

A longitudinal strip along the whole length of the excised bowel, measuring 10 in., was submitted to microscopic examination by the hematoxylin-mucicarmine method. Conclusive evidence was obtained that the growth had spread by permeation along the mucous lymphatic plexus of the bowel …at least as far as the point of section of bowel 6 in. above the growth. How much further it had spread upwards, I am, of course, unable to say. A similar spread downward was traced as far as the region of the sphincters.

In view of the extent of mucous permeation revealed, excision of a considerable length of the bowel above the growth, and of the bowel below down to and including the sphincters, is evidently a right practice.'

Cripps: Discussion of the Surgical Treatment of Rectal Cancer (1912) [3]

Discussion on
The Surgical Treatment of Rectal
Cancer
Opening Paper
By Harrison Cripps, F.R.C.S
Consultant Surgeon to St. Bartholomew's Hospital

Pathology

"I do not propose to encroach upon the time allowed by discussing at length the pathology of rectal cancer, except in so far as it bears directly on surgical treatment. From this point of view it is so important that it is impossible to neglect it. Out of many hundreds of cases under my observation, with the rarest exceptions, the growth has always been of one type—namely, adenoid cancer.

Rectal cancer is essentially local in its early stage, and the method of its extension has an important bearing on the question of operation. When once started, it spreads at first by continuity, more so horizontally than in depth. This appears due to there being less resistance between the layers of muscle than there is in the muscles themselves. In this way, several square inches of the surface of the bowel are affected, while the whole thickness of the growth may for some time be less than half an inch. However, it eventually perforates into and through the muscular coats and invades the tissues outside. Owing presumably to the interruption of the blood supply by the pressure of the increasing growth, the mucous membrane over it soon falls into a necrotic state and ulcerates, the greatest depth of the ulceration being in the older part of the growth. After ulceration is established, the disease advances along the bowel by a hard everted edge which generally ends abruptly in sound mucous membrane. Lymphatic and glandular infection, in my experience, is quite a late stage of the disease, and thus affords the most hopeful prospect in operative treatment.

I must dwell a little longer upon this method of spreading. I do this on account of the recent researches of so eminent a pathologist as Mr. Sampson Handley. It will be remembered that Mr. Handley published 2 years ago in the British Medical Journal a paper with drawings taken from sections stained with muci-carmine, the object being to show how rectal cancer spreads along the submucous lymphatics for several inches or even feet beyond the original site without producing any tumor or hardness by which it could be detected. He further pointed out that it was in this spreading along the lymphatics parallel to the bowel that the explanation for recurrence was to be found, and from this he drew the inference that, for successful surgery, not only should the disease be removed, but long lengths of bowel, amounting to inches or feet, should be cut away. I believe this to be erroneous as bearing on the surgical treatment of rectal cancer. I have carefully studied his drawings and cannot accept the view that because cells in the lymphatics, feet away from the primary growth, stain a certain color with muci-carmine, this is, as he states, a conclusive proof of cancerous invasion. I have spent too many years in the histological study of rectal cancer to place the same reliance that Mr. Handley does on the significance of such stained cells, or that they invariably indicate cancerous infection. Before this dogma can be established, countless test experiments and methods of staining, both in normal and diseased tissues, must be undertaken and corroborated by clinical experience. Clinical experience is entirely opposed to the deduction that such an early dissemination of rectal cancer along the submucous lymphatics is common or even usual. That recurrence unfortunately takes place in a large number of cases is true; but let us consider how this growth would manifest itself if Mr. Handley's view was correct. He endeavors to show that the lymphatics are infected for many inches beyond the apparent margin of disease. If this were so, it would be merely a question of time before the whole of the infected area became thickened and hardened with the usual manifestations of adenoid cancerous growth. Then by the time that this had developed, the disease would be still spreading ahead, and if the patient lived long enough, many feet, or even the whole intestinal tract would become involved. It would also show the uselessness of removing the growth locally with only an area of an inch or less of apparently sound margin; in fact, it would make any reasonable local removal quite hopeless; but both the conditions just mentioned are inconsistent with clinical facts in the majority of cases.

It will be found that recurrence seldom takes place except at the extreme edge of the cut margin, and even this is exceptional, for in most cases recurrence is not in the remaining part of the bowel, but in the connective tissue and structures lying immediately external to the part removed. I have over and over again seen the recurrence in the neighborhood of the ischio-rectal fossa and skin near the anus, while the bowel itself at the cut margin and along the whole of its course upwards remained free from any visible infection up to the time of patient's death. I have always regarded an inch or so as a fair margin, and, when I have been able to secure this, can scarcely recall a case of recurrence in the cut margin itself. Again, if these widespread disseminations were usual, how would the many successful cases of removal be accounted for? In my own practice, I know of dozens of cases which remained perfectly well up to three to twenty-five years after removal where less than an inch of margin had been allowed. Lastly, amongst the most successful cases are those operations in which 2 or 3 in. of diseased bowel, with perhaps only a half-inch margin allowed, have been cleanly cut out, and an end-to-end anastomosis performed. Every surgeon may not be familiar with these cases in the rectum, but few can be without experience of the successful result that often follows an intra-abdominal section of a limited annular growth of the large intestine with an immediate end-to-end anastomosis. If the doctrine of the universal spread of cancer along long areas of the submucous tissue were generally accepted, I believe infinite harm would be done to operative surgery, for in every such case a grave increase of the danger of the operation would be entailed such as would be quite unnecessary and unjustifiable, and those brilliant cases of anastomosis made impossible, for you cannot join together in the rectum the ends if inches of the gut have been removed, and I believe that an operation, now invaluable in properly selected cases, would soon fall into discredit if such wholesale removals became the fashion in deference to an unproved pathological theory.

Recurrence

When this takes place it generally does so in the tissue lying external to the excised portion or in the glands and lymphatics lying in the sacral neighborhood. Occasionally, the recurrence takes place in the cut edges of the bowel itself."

Cole: The Intramural Spread of Rectal Carcinoma 1913 [4]

The Intramural Spread of Rectal Carcinoma
By Percival P. Cole. M.D., CH.B., F.R.C.S.Eng.,
Assistant Surgeon to the Dreadnought Hospital, Greenwich;
Surgical Registrar to the Cancer Hospital; Surgeon
to the West Ham and Eastern General Hospital
(From the Cancer Hospital Pathological Laboratory)

"Operative measures for the eradication of cancer must be planned according to the pathological findings. That widely divergent views are held as to the particular operative treatment applicable to cancer of the rectum and pelvic colon is sufficiently evidenced by recent papers on the subject by Harrison Cripps, Paul, Miles, and Sampson Handley. It may reasonably be assumed that corresponding differences of opinion exist as to the pathological conditions which obtain; and, indeed, such assumption is amply confirmed by the perusal of these papers, as well as by the remarks made by speakers during the discussion on rectal cancer at the Royal Society of Medicine in 1910.

A convenient classification—adopted by Miles—of the pathologic factors which must be considered in planning any radical operation for cancer of the rectum is as follows: (1) The spread of disease in the bowel wall—intramural; and (2) that which occurs in the in surrounding or distinct tissues—extramural.

This communication is concerned with the first factor, and an attempt has been made to determine its extent and significance."

Material

This comprises 20 cases, in 18 of which the bowel investigated was removed by operation.

Technique

The bowel was slit up immediately after operation, stretched by nailing to a piece of board, and placed in a fixative solution…. After fixation a strip the whole length of the bowel was taken and cut into inches. Each inch of tissue was embedded in paraffin, sectioned, and stained….

Nature of Growth

The growth in every case was an adeno-carcinoma. In 18 cases the appearance presented was that of a typical carcinomatous ulcer,…

Spread and Ulceration

Microscopical examination throws some light on this process of ulceration.

It is assumed that carcinoma commences as a downgrowth of glandular epithelium which pierces the muscularis mucosa and invades the submucous coat.

It will be gathered that the carcinoma spreads more widely in the submucous coat than is indicated by the surface ulceration. The muscular coat is invaded to an equal, and frequently to a greater, extent."

Cheatle: The Spread of Cancer in the Lower Part of the Intestine (1914) [5]

The Spread of Cancer in the Lower
Part of the Large Intestine
By G. Lenthal Cheatle, C.V.O., C.B., F.R.C.S.,
Surgeon and Joint Lecturer on Surgery
King's College Hospital

"In the British Medical Journal, 1910, vol i, pp. 853 and 922, Mr. Sampson Handley published a case of very extensive spread of cancer in the lymphatic vessels of the submucous tissue in the lower intestine. Like many others, I was at once struck with the importance of this observation, and at the same time realized from my own clinical experience that this extensive spread in the lymphatics of the submucous tissue of the large intestine could not be applicable to all cases. Therefore I determined to examine all my subsequent cases with a view to the determination of this point.

The cases which I publish are all cancers of the lower part of the large intestine, and they show how strictly limited is the growth of the primary focus of disease. Very little spread can be seen in the submucous tissue of any of them. Indeed, there is no spread to be observed in any other part of the bowel wall.

In one of my cases…there is a most alarming diffuse spread in all directions, namely, in the submucous tissue, the intramuscular tissue, the intermuscular tissue, and subperitoneal tissue, as well as in the lymphatic glands of the mesocolon. Even the appendices epiploicae are loaded with it; in fact, every available lymphatic space seems to be occupied. This appears to be an exceptional case.

Before publishing these cases I made a point of informing Mr. Sampson Handley of their nature, and he informed me that he has had the same experience in cases he has examined since the one which caused such disturbance in the minds of surgeons who read his paper.

In the majority of my cases I have not seen the submucous spread greater than that seen in the extramural lymphatic distribution.

I have no doubt that the publication of Mr. Sampson Handley's case has influenced surgeons to remove a greater length of bowel than is absolutely necessary in most cases. On the other hand, I quite agree that extensive removal is the main indication, for two reasons.

First, the operator can never be sure from clinical observation whether he be dealing with a case of extensive or limited distribution, although the presence of enlarged and discrete lymphatic glands may help him to decide the matter in favour of the presence of extensive spread of cancer.

Secondly, an extensive removal of the intestine enables the operator to deal more effectively with the lymphatic area in direct communication with the diseased parts."

Gabriel, Dukes, and Bussey: Lymphatic Spread of Cancer of the Rectum (1935) [6]

Lymphatic Spread of Cancer of the Rectum
By W. B. Gabriel
Surgeon, St. Mark's Hospital, London
Cuthbert Dukes
Pathologist, St. Mark's Hospital, London
and H.J.R. Bussey
Research Assistant, St. Mark's Hospital, London

Gabriel, Dukes, and Bussey performed 100 gland dissections on rectums removed for malignant disease: 70 perineo-abdominal and 30 perineal excisions. They found:

> "As a rule the regional lymph glands are the first to be affected by metastases in cancer of the rectum. Lymphatic spread then proceeds from below upwards along the chain of glands accompanying the superior hemorrhoidal artery. Irregular or interrupted spread is very uncommon. Lateral or downward lymphatic spread is only found in the late stage of the disease when the hemorrhoidal lymphatics are blocked by metastases."

Gilchrist and David: Lymphatic Spread of Carcinoma of the Rectum (1938) [7]

Lymphatic Spread of Carcinoma of the Rectum
Richard K. Gilchrist, M.D., and
Vernon C. David, M.D.
Chicago, Ill

Gilchrist and David undertook a study to determine the lymph node metastases and the extent of removal needed to eradicate all involved nodes. With regard to distal lymphatic spread the authors found:

> "Where the upward lymph channels are blocked by metastases, there may be a retrograde metastasis downward as shown in Figure. 5. The patient, age 65, had had symptoms for at least 6 months. The tumor involved about 65 percent of the circumference of her bowel. Twenty-seven nodes were found by gross dissection, 22 of them having metastases. The lowest of the five nodes below the tumor was 4 cm. below the lowest edge of the tumor."

The authors opined that the Miles operation seemed ideal regarding wide removal of the lymphatic node bearing area (Fig. 77.1).

"*Fig. 5.*—Hosp. No. 33779: Showing an instance of retrograde metastases. The lowest of the involved nodes being 4 cm below the inferior edge of the tumor [8]."

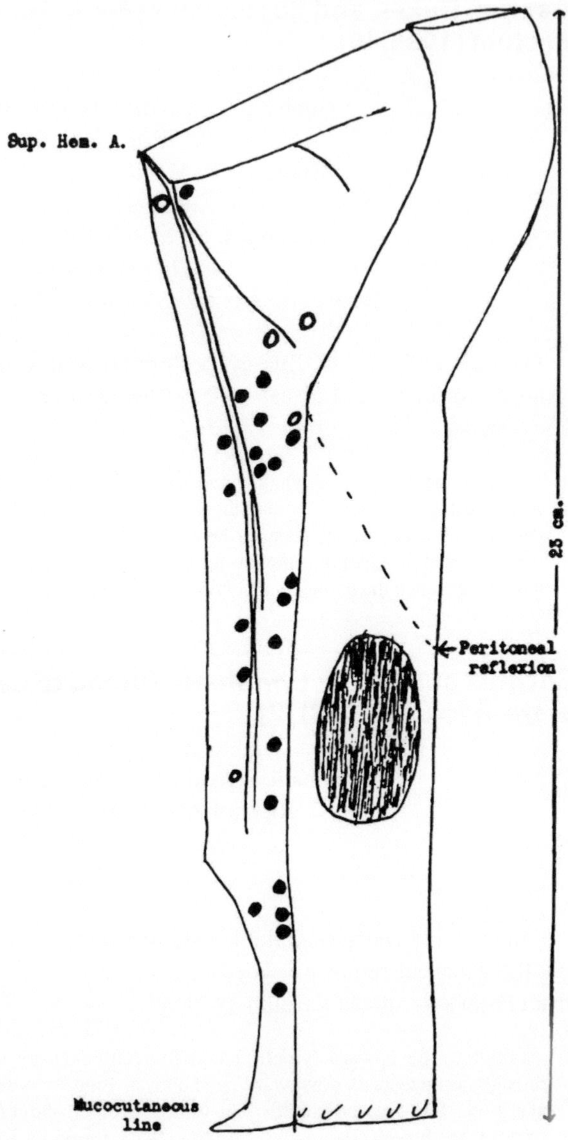

Fig. 77.1 Gilchrist and David's Fig. 5, see preceding quote

Dukes: The Surgical Pathology of Rectal Cancer (1944) [9]

The Surgical Pathology of Rectal Cancer:
President's Address
By Cuthbert E. Dukes, O.B.E., M.D., M.Sc., D.P.H.

"There is not much to be said about the extent to which a rectal cancer may spread within the bowel above or below its naked-eye boundaries except that such intramural spread is rare. A rectal cancer seems generally to enlarge equally in all directions superficially from a central focus in the mucous membrane, but as a rule the lateral surface spread in the transverse axis proceeds faster than the upward and downward spread in the long axis, thus accounting for the oval shape. The limits of the growth within the submucosa are often a little wider than in the mucous membrane but apart from this it is rare to find any extension within the rectum itself, either above or below the margin of the surface growth."

Connell and Rottino: Retrograde Spread of Carcinoma in the Rectum and Rectosigmoid (1949) [10]

The authors examined nine cancers of the rectum and rectosigmoid for retrograde spread (tumor spread from the primary lesion in the direction of the anal canal). Retrograde spread was not found in five specimens. In one specimen, retrograde extension was seen for 6.4 cm below the main lesion. In two specimens, extensive retrograde involvement of lymph channels and lymph nodes was found.

Dunphy, Broderick: A Critique of Anterior Resection in the Treatment of Cancer of the Rectum and Pelvic Colon (1951) [11]

A Critique of Anterior Resection in the Treatment
of Cancer of the Rectum and Pelvic Colon
J. Englebert Dunphy, M.D., and Earl G. Broderick, M.D.,
Boston, Mass.
(From the Surgical Service, Peter Bent Brigham Hospital, and
the Department of Surgery, Harvard Medical School)

"The term anterior resection has been applied to abdominal resection of the rectum for such a long time that it should be retained but because it is sometimes misconstrued as implying a segmental resection of the pelvic colon it requires definition. Properly executed it includes mobilization of the pelvic colon and rectum to the coccyx behind and the prostate or vagina anteriorly, a high ligation of the inferior mesenteric artery, and an excision of the same extent of mesentery and nodes as is accomplished in the abdominal part of a Miles resection. The variable branches of the middle hemorrhoidal artery may or may not be divided, depending largely upon their relation to the position of the lesion being resected.

The Indications for Anterior Resection

There is an aggregate of evidence which warrants caution in accepting anterior resection as an adequate cancer operation. It is a technically difficult operation and from the standpoint of removing the cancer may not be as well performed in the hands of the occasional operator as an abdominoperineal resection. Pathologic studies are not entirely reassuring in regard to the validity of limiting the resection of normal bowel distal to the growth. The high incidence of local recurrence is particularly disturbing and in the occasional case the evidence indicates that an abdominoperineal resection might have prevented such recurrence.

In the face of this evidence we feel that the use of anterior resection should be restricted to the following specific indications:

1. *To extend the scope of resection in cancer of the sigmoid.*
2. *To avoid colostomy in the presence of distant metastases from cancer of the upper rectum or rectosigmoid colon provided the local disease can be extirpated.*
3. *To avoid colostomy in the elective surgery of cancer of the lower pelvic colon and upper rectum, provided a 10 cm. operative margin of normal bowel can be resected distal to the tumor, the pelvic fascia is not invaded by neoplasm, and there are no obvious lymph node metastases."*

Quer, Dahlin, Mayo: Retrograde Intramural Spread of Carcinoma of the Rectum and Rectosigmoid (1953)

Retrograde Intramural Spread of Carcinoma
of the Rectum and Rectosigmoid
A Microscopic Study
Erich A. Quer, M.D., David C. Dahlin, M.D.,
and
Charles W. Mayo, M.D., F.A.C.S.
Rochester, Minnesota

In 1953, Quer et al. [12] described 91 cases of adenocarcinoma of the rectum. Retrograde intramural spread was found in only 5/91 cases. The authors concluded:

"On the basis of our results, it can be recommended that from the standpoint of retrograde intramural spread a margin of 2.5 to 3 centimeters of grossly uninvolved intestinal wall below the lowest grossly palpable or visible edge of the carcinoma is sufficient to make the operation adequate. Eighty-eight of our 91 patients could have been treated successfully by removal of that much distal intestinal wall."

Grinnell: Distal Intramural Spread of Carcinoma of the Rectum and Rectosigmoid (1954) [13]

Distal Intramural Spread of Carcinoma of the
Rectum and Rectosigmoid
Robert S. Grinnell, M.D., F.A.C.S.,
From the Department of Surgery,
Presbyterian Hospital, and The Laboratory of Surgical Pathology,
College of Physicians and Surgeons,
Columbia University,
New York, New York

"Of the 126 carcinomas studied, 93 whose lower margin above was from 5 to 18 centimeters inclusive above the dentate line were used as the main basis of this report as it is this area of the bowel which is most concerned in the present controversy. In 76 of the 93 tumors the operation in which they were removed was considered curative by the surgeon and in 17 it was considered palliative. Definite retrograde mural spread was found in 18 specimens. It occurred in 9, or over one-half, of the 17 specimens removed by palliative resection and in 9, or 12 per cent, of the 76 curative resections.

The extent of downward spread varied from 1 to 7 centimeters. The maximum spread of 7 centimeters occurred in a specimen from a palliative resection. The greatest extension in a curative resection was 4.0 cm. In 67 of the 76 curative resections there was no retrograde spread.

Comment

On the basis of our results on retrograde extension of tumors lying between 5 to 18 centimeters from the dentate line and found to be curative at operation, a margin of 5 cm below the tumor would have been adequate in all."

Pollett and Nicholls: The Relationship Between the Extent of Distal Clearance and Survival and Local Recurrence Rates After Curative Anterior Resection for Carcinoma of the Rectum (1983) [14]

The Relationship Between the Extent of Distal Clearance and Survival and Local Recurrence Rates after Curative Anterior Resection for Carcinoma of the Rectum.
William G. Pollett. F.R.C.S.(C), R. J. Nicholls, M.Chir, F.R.C.S.
from St. Mark's Hospital,
London, England

In 1983, Pollet and Nicholls examined the influence of the distal margin of resection on survival. This study involved 334 patients who had undergone radical restorative operations for single rectal adenocarcinoma. The authors' results and conclusions were as follows:

"The length of rectum below the tumor measured on fixed pinned-out pathologic specimens was 2 cm or less in 55 patients (group 1), 2 to 5 cm in 177 (group 2), and 5 cm or more in 102 (group 3). The Dukes' classification, histologic grade, and extent of local spread of the tumors were similar in the three groups. Overall crude 5-year survival rates for groups 1, 2, and 3 were 69.1%, 68.4%, and 69.6%, respectively. Corresponding cancer-specific death rates were 25.5%, 23.2%, and 21.6%. These rates were also similar in matching pathologic subgroups of the three main groups. Of 23 observed or suspected local recurrences, there were four recurrences in group 1 (7.3%), 11 in group 2 (6.2%), and eight in group 3 (7.8%). These results suggest that a margin less than 2 cm below a rectal carcinoma does not affect survival or local recurrence adversely."

Williams, Dixon, and Johnston: Reappraisal of the 5 cm Rule of Distal Excision for Carcinoma of the Rectum: A Study of Distal Intramural Spread and of Patients' Survival (1983)

Reappraisal of the 5 centimetre rule of distal excision for carcinoma of the rectum: a study of distal intramural spread and of patients' survival
N. S. Williams, M. F. Dixon, and D. Johnston
University Departments of Surgery and Pathology,
The General Infirmary,
Leeds

In 1983, Williams et al. [15] reported:

"Fifty consecutive specimens, obtained in the course of potentially curative abdominoperineal resection for rectal carcinoma situated 5–10 cm from the anal verge, were examined for the presence of microscopic distal intramural spread. Thirty-eight patients (76 per cent) were found to have no intramural spread. Seven patients (14 per cent) had spread for 1 cm or less and only 5 patients (10 per cent) had spread for more than 1 cm. Each of these 5 patients had a poorly differentiated Dukes C carcinoma and each was dead or dying from distant metastases within 3 years of the operation. The results of anterior resection for carcinoma of the rectum were reviewed a minimum of 5 years after operation, to find out whether patients with a wide distal margin of resection had fared better than patients with a small margin. Seventy-nine patients had undergone a potentially curative resection, 48 with a distal margin of less than 5 cm (mean 2·8 cm; group 1) and 31 with a distal margin greater than 5 cm (mean 6·5 cm; group 2). The two groups were well matched for age, sex, degree of differentiation of the tumors and distance of the lesion from the anal verge, but 54 per cent of patients in group 1 had Dukes' grade C tumor whereas only 23 per cent of the patients in group 2 had Dukes' C tumors. Despite the higher proportion of unfavorable tumors in group 1, the outcome, in terms both of survival and of recurrence, was as good in patients with the small distal margin as in the patients with the wide distal margin of clearance. The rigid, routine application of the '5 centimetre rule' of distal excision may cause patients with low rectal cancer to lose their anal sphincter unnecessarily."

Heald and Ryall: Recurrence and Survival After Total Mesorectal Excision for Rectal Cancer (1986) [16]

Recurrence and Survival after Total Mesorectal Excision for Rectal Cancer

R. J. Heald, R. D. H. Ryall

Colorectal Research Unit,

Basingstoke District Hospital,

Basingstoke, Hampshire

"A 7 1/2-year consecutive series is presented from a district hospital with a policy of referring all rectal carcinomas to one surgical firm.

Of 115 patients in whom curative resection was attempted, 69 had anastomoses below 5 cm and 39 had mural resection margins of less than 2·5 cm. Surgical priority, however, was given to complete excision of the visceral rectal mesentery or mesorectum. At an average of 4.2 years postoperatively, three pelvic recurrences have developed but there have been no staple-line recurrences in patients who had 'curative' surgery. The corrected cumulative probability of survival at 5 years is 87% and the tumor-free survival by Dukes stage is A 94%, B 87%, and C 58%. Patients with low tumours did no less well than those with high tumours, when treated by anterior resection. On this evidence, it is often safe to limit mural clearance and thus preserve the anal sphincters, provided that the mesorectum is excised intact with the cancer."

Shirouzou, Isomoto, Kakegawa: Distal Spread of Rectal Cancer and Optimal Distal Margin of Resection for Sphincter-Preserving Surgery (1995) [17]

In 1995, Shirouzo and coworkers examined distal spread of rectal cancer and optimal distal margin of resection for sphincter-preserving surgery.

Distal Spread of Rectal Cancer and Optimal Distal Margin of Resection for Sphincter-Preserving Surgery

Kazuo Shirouzu, M.D., Hirohara Isomoto, M.D., and Teruo Kakegawa, M.D.

"Background. Ascertaining the optimal distal margin of resection in sphincter-preserving surgery has become an important problem. This study was designed to examine distal spread of rectal carcinoma and to determine the optimal distal margin or resection for sphincter preserving surgery.

Methods. Six hundred ten consecutive specimens of resected rectal carcinomas were analyzed retrospectively and pathologically.

Distal spread was not found in patients with Stage I disease (0/150), according to the International Union Against Cancer stage. Only 1.2% (2/162) of patients with Stage II disease and 5.1% (10/195) with Stage III disease had slight spread but this was confined to within a 1 cm length. Most patients with distal spread had a lower survival rate and died of distant metastasis rather than local recurrence, even after curative surgery.

Conclusions. Distal spread seems to be an important risk factor for distant metastasis. Distal margin of resection of 1 cm may be appropriate clearance for most rectal cancers."

Sir Charles Gordon-Watson: Origin and Spread of Cancer of the Rectum (1938) [18]

Origin and Spread of Cancer of the Rectum
In Relation to Surgical Treatment
By Sir Charles Gordon-Watson, K.B.E., C.M.G., F.R.C.S. Eng., F.A.C.S.
Consulting Surgeon, St. Bartholomew's Hospital,
St. Mark's Hospital for Diseases of the Rectum,
and the Metropolitan Hospital, London

Relation to Surgical Treatment

"For many years there has been considerable controversy about the ideal methods for radical treatment of malignant disease of the rectum.

Radical operations as distinct from conservative methods have attained a high measure of efficiency but will always be tainted with the stigma of an artificial anus. The revival in recent years of conservative methods, which allow complete eradication, may help to remove this stigma.

Conclusion

Sir James Paget in his Bradshaw lecture observed that "better treatment will follow better diagnosis and better diagnosis will certainly follow a more exact pathology."

References

1. Miles WE. A method of performing abdomino-perineal excision for carcinoma of the rectum and of the terminal portion of the pelvic colon. Lancet. 1908;2:1812–3.
2. Handley WS. The surgery of the lymphatic system. Br Med J. 1910;1:922–8.
3. Cripps H. Discussion on the surgical treatment of rectal cancer. Br Med J. 1912;2:843–55.
4. Cole PP. The intramural spread of rectal carcinoma. Br Med J. 1913;1:431–3.
5. Cheatle GL. The spread of cancer in the lower part of the large intestine. Br Med J. 1914;1:303.
6. Gabriel WB, Dukes C, Bussey HJR. Lymphatic spread in cancer of the rectum. Br J Surg. 1935;23:395–413; This excerpt is reused with permission from the British Journal of Surgery, CCC|Marketplace™, Order License ID 1146489-1, Order Date: 09 Sep 2021.
7. Gilchrist RK, David VC. Lymphatic spread of carcinoma of the rectum. Ann Surg. 1938;108:621–42; This excerpt was reused with the generous permission of Wolters Kluwer Health, Inc., CCC|RightsLink®, License Number 5153121195460, License date Sep 20, 2021.
8. Gilchrist RK, David VC. Lymphatic spread of carcinoma of the rectum. Ann Surg 1938;108:621–642.
9. Dukes CE. The surgical pathology of rectal cancer. Proc R Soc Med. 1944;37:131–44; The excerpt is reused with permission from SAGE Publications, CCC|RightsLink®, Order Number 501680576, Order date Sep 20, 2021.
10. Connell JF Jr, Rottino A. Retrograde spread of carcinoma in the rectum and rectosigmoid. Arch Surg. 1949;59:807–13.
11. Dunphy JE, Broderick EG. A critique of anterior resection in the treatment of cancer of the rectum and pelvic colon. Surgery. 1951;30:106–15; This excerpt is reused with the permission of Mr. Thomas Rexson Yesudoss, Copyrights Coordinator, ELSEVIER | HCV – Health Content Management, October 10, 2022.
12. Quer EA, Dahlin DC, Mayo CW. Retrograde intramural spread of carcinoma of the rectum and rectosigmoid. A microscopic study. Surg Gynecol Obstet. 1953;96:24–30; Reprinted with permission from the Mr. Spencer Dimmick, the Journal of the American College of Surgeons, formerly Surgery Gynecology & Obstetrics, Sep 21, 2021.
13. Grinnell RS. Distal intramural spread of carcinoma of the rectum and rectosigmoid. Surg Gynecol Obstet. 1954;99:421–30; Reprinted with permission from the Mr. Spencer Dimmick, the Journal of the American College of Surgeons, formerly Surgery Gynecology & Obstetrics, Sep 21, 2021.
14. Pollett WG, Nicholls RJ. The relationship between the extent of distal clearance and survival and local recurrence rates after curative anterior resection for carcinoma of the rectum. Ann Surg. 1983;198:159–63; This excerpt is reused with the generous permission of Wolters Kluwer Health, Inc., CCC|RightsLink®, License Number 5153450260590, License date Sept 21, 2021.
15. Williams NS, Dixon MF, Johnston D. Reappraisal of the 5 centimetre rule of distal excision for carcinoma of the rectum: a study of distal intramural spread and patients' survival. Br J Surg. 1983;70:150–4; This excerpt was reused with the generous permission of John Wiley and Sons, CCC|Rightslink®, License Number 5153460453490, License date Sep 21, 2021.
16. Heald RJ, Ryall RDH. Recurrence and survival after total mesorectal excision for rectal cancer. Lancet. 1986;1:1479–82; This excerpt is reused with the generous permission of Elsevier, CCC|RightLink®, License number 5153470131044, License date Sep 21, 2021.
17. Shirouzu K, Isomoto H, Kakegawa T. Distal spread of rectal cancer and optimal distal margin of resection for sphincter-preserving surgery. Cancer. 1995;76:388–92; This excerpt was reused with the with the generous permission of John Wiley and Sons, CCC|Rightslink®, License Number 5153471117219, License date Sep 21, 2021.
18. Gordon-Watson C. Origin and spread of cancer of the rectum in relation to surgical treatment. Lancet. 1938;1(5970):239–45; This excerpt is reused with the generous permission of Elsevier, CCC|RightLink®, License number 5153480821776, License date Sep 21, 2021.

Griffiths' Point

78

James S. Wu

Presentation

In 1956, Griffiths[1] described the surgical anatomy of the blood supply of the distal colon by dissection and radiopaque injection of 100 embalmed-dissecting room cadavers and necropsy subjects.

Surgical Anatomy of the Blood Supply of the Distal Colon
J. D. Griffiths, F.R.C.S.
Chief Assistant, St. Bartholomew's Hospital, London

> "The recent and progressive adoption of the procedure of high ligation of the inferior mesenteric artery in colonic resection for carcinoma of the rectum and distal colon has occasioned this present re-examination of the precise vascular pattern underlying such techniques. In particular, information has been sought regarding the all-important subject of the nature and extent of anastomosis between the superior and inferior mesenteric arteries.
>
> A truly critical point exists, however, at the splenic flexure, where the marginal artery is often small."

He also noted that the marginal artery:

> "…lies often 1 to 1½ inches from the medial border of the colon, and in obese patients is very difficult to identify. The greatest care must be taken not to damage it during operative mobilisation of the colon."

[1] Griffiths [1]. These excerpts were reused with permission from the ROYAL SOCIETY OF MEDICINE PRESS LTD. Except (up to 400 words), CCC Marketplace™, Order License ID 1179086-1, Order Date 18-Jan-2022.

J. S. Wu (✉)
Department of Colon and Rectal Surgery, Cleveland Clinic, Cleveland, OH, USA

J. S. Wu, M. D. Inkster (eds.), *Cleveland Clinic Colorectal Case Studies*,
https://doi.org/10.1007/978-3-031-39880-3_78

In 1961, Griffiths investigated the marginal artery in necropsy bodies by injecting through the aorta a barium suspension containing gelatin. His experiments

> "demonstrate the free anastomosis between the superior and inferior mesenteric arteries afforded by the marginal artery, thus enabling any colic branch to be ligated without danger of ischaemia occurring in the colon of a fit patient" [2].

He also noted that:

> "Many post-operative fistulae occurring after anastomosis in the colon are in part due to the inadvertent devascularization of the ends of the bowel following misplaced ligature of the marginal artery. It has been emphasized by Naunton Morgan (personal communication) that the marginal artery should be ligated 1 in. (2.5 cm) beyond the site of section of the colon, thus obviating the danger of the marginal artery being distorted after mobilization of the colon."

In 1976, Meyers observed that:

> "Clinical experience has shown repeatedly that the inferior mesenteric artery may be ligated or removed with impunity, and yet at times its occlusion will give rise to infarction of the descending colon."

Meyers studied 46 patients with selective arteriograms that identified the vascularization of the splenic flexure [3]. Analysis of the arteriographic studies showed that the anastomosis at Griffiths' point was present in 48%, poor or tenuous in nine percent, and absent in 43%. Meyer's concluded:

> "This critical point is of significance in occlusive vascular impairment of the left colon, both in spontaneous instances and following surgical ligation of the inferior mesenteric artery, and in "nonocclusive" ischemic colitis.
>
> Individuals with absence of dependable anastomoses at Griffiths' point at the splenic flexure many be particularly vulnerable to low perfusion states and develop the syndrome of ischemic colitis".

The best guarantee of adequate perfusion of the left colon after inferior mesenteric artery ligation and splenic flexure mobilization is the observation of brisk pulsatile bleeding from the marginal artery at the end of the colon.

References

1. Griffiths JD. Surgical anatomy of the blood supply of the distal colon. Ann R Coll Surg Engl. 1956;19:241–56.
2. Griffiths JD. Extramural and intramural blood-supply of colon. Br Med J. 1961;1:323–6.
3. Meyers MA. Griffith's point: critical anastomosis at the splenic flexure. Significance in ischemia of the colon. Am J Roentgenol. 1976;126:77–94. Reprinted from the abstract: Copyright© 1976; the copyright owner is specified as in the American Journal of Radiology.

Rectal Cancer-Total Mesorectal Excision 79

Hermann Kessler and James S. Wu

Total Mesorectal Excision (TME)

In 1982, Heald et al. [1] postulated that the mesorectum in rectal cancer surgery was the key to pelvic recurrence. The authors described five cases where minute foci of adenocarcinoma were demonstrated in the mesorectum several centimeters distal to the apparent lower edge of a rectal cancer. The authors noted that in "orthodox" anterior resection, much of this lymphatic tissue remains in the pelvis and suggested that these foci might lead to suture-line or pelvic recurrence. They reported total mesorectal excision (TME) as a part of over 100 consecutive anterior resections (Fig. 79.1). Fifty of these, which were classified as "curative" or "conceivably curative" operations, were followed for over 2 years with no pelvic or staple-line recurrence.

In Fig. 79.2, three examples of TME are shown. Specimen 1 on the left demonstrates the appearance of the mesorectum after adequate resection. Specimen 2 shows sites where the mesorectal fascia has been violated (arrows). Specimen 3 shows sites exemplified by the arrow where pieces of the rectal mesentery have been carved away from the specimen.

The incorrect technique for mesorectal dissection is shown in Fig. 79.3.

H. Kessler · J. S. Wu (✉)
Department of Colon and Rectal Surgery, Cleveland Clinic, Cleveland, OH, USA

J. S. Wu, M. D. Inkster (eds.), *Cleveland Clinic Colorectal Case Studies*,
https://doi.org/10.1007/978-3-031-39880-3_79

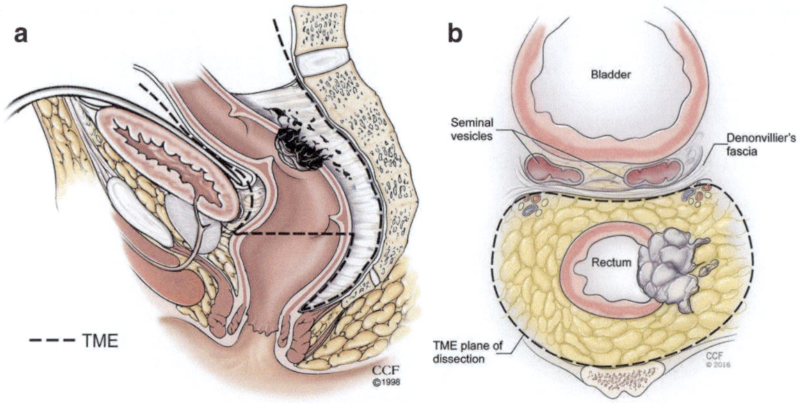

Fig. 79.1 (**a**) The suggested plane of excision (after Heald, 1982), sagittal view; (**b**) axial view

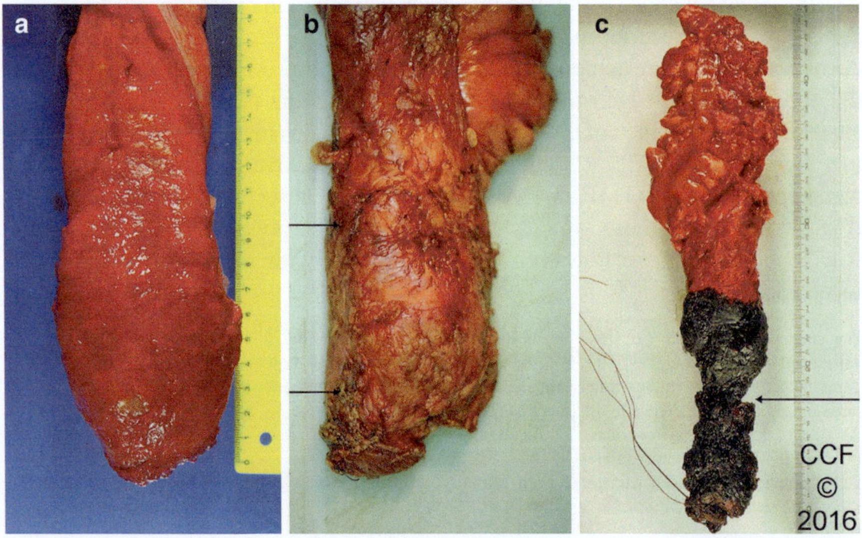

Fig. 79.2 (**a**) The mesorectum with its fascia has been removed intact; (**b**) the mesorectal fascia has been violated (arrows); (**c**) the mesorectum has been incompletely removed. The specimen has been prepared with India ink to identify the surgical margins

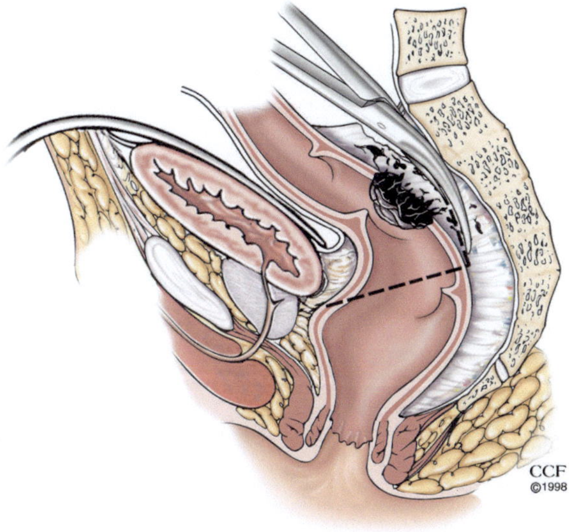

Fig. 79.3 Total mesorectal excision: incorrect: the tumor-associated mesorectal envelope is violated, in this case, by the surgeon's scissors. This distal margin is too close to the tumor

Reference

1. Heald RJ, Husband EM, Ryall RDH. The mesorectum in rectal cancer surgery—the clue to pelvic recurrence? Br J Surg. 1982;69:613–6.

Reference

Rectal Cancer-Reconstitution of Bowel Continuity After Low Anterior Resection

80

James S. Wu, Hani B. Baradi, and Erika B. Woodrum

Presentation

A case of restitution of bowel continuity after low anterior resection for rectal cancer is presented. Selected operative details are shown [1].

Excision[1]

Following high ligation of the inferior mesenteric artery (IMA) and inferior mesenteric vein (IMV), the sigmoid colon and rectum were excised with a clear distal margin (Fig. 80.1).

Following excision of the rectum and sigmoid colon, the left colon, the splenic flexure, and the distal transverse colon are mobilized from the left upper quadrant so that a tension-free low colorectal or coloanal anastomosis with an adequate blood supply can be made. Factors that contribute to a successful anastomosis are shown in Table 80.1.

The marginal artery of Drummond is seen in the mesentery close to the colon (Fig. 80.2).

The left colic artery triangular arcade can be preserved by dividing the left colic artery near its origin (Fig. 80.3). The importance of this concept was stressed by

[1] As previously described for abdominoperineal resection of the rectum.

J. S. Wu (✉)
Department of Colon and Rectal Surgery, Cleveland Clinic, Cleveland, OH, USA

H. B. Baradi
Mercy Colon and Rectal Surgery, Oklahoma City, OK, USA

E. B. Woodrum
Medical Illustration Team, Enterprise Creative Services, Cleveland Clinic, Cleveland, OH, USA

J. S. Wu, M. D. Inkster (eds.), *Cleveland Clinic Colorectal Case Studies*,
https://doi.org/10.1007/978-3-031-39880-3_80

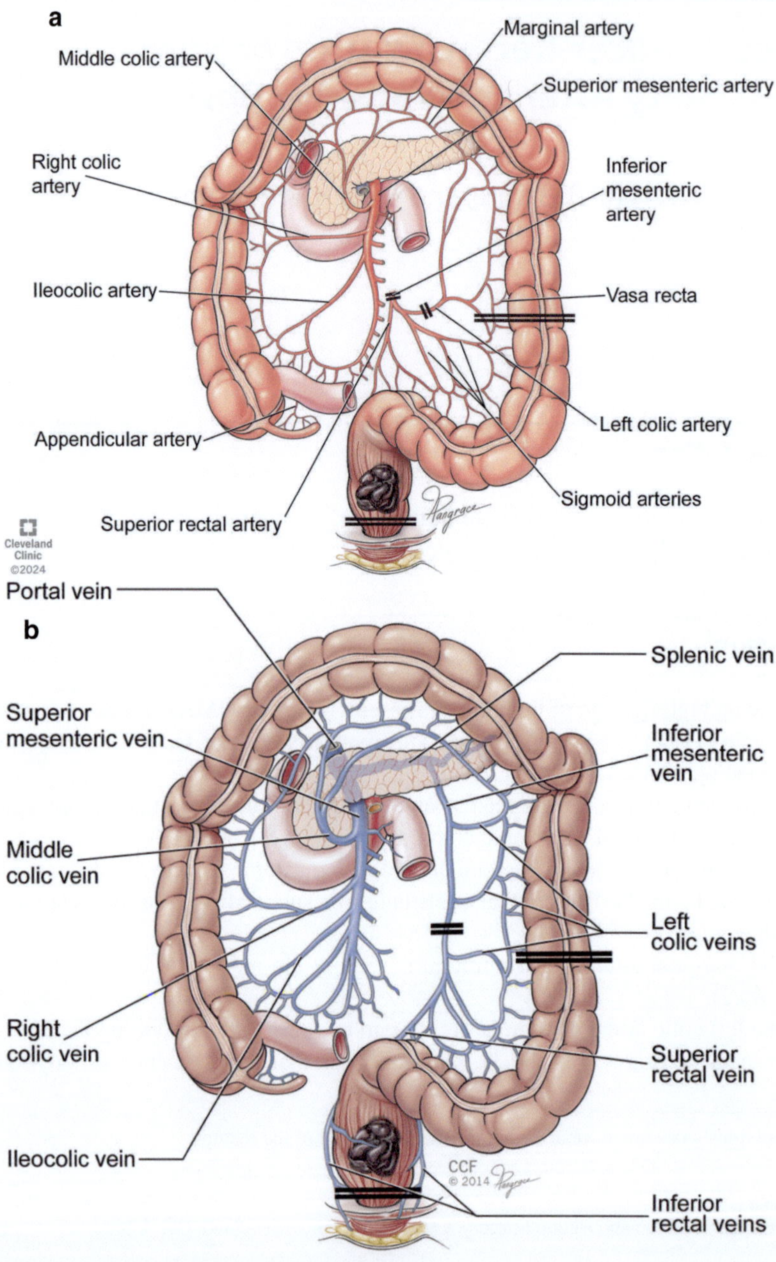

Fig. 80.1 (**a**) The inferior mesenteric artery is divided close to its origin on the aorta. The left colic artery is divided close to its origin on the IMA. The proximal and distal lines of resection are marked; (**b**) the IMV is divided in the vicinity of the IMA. As in (**a**), the proximal and distal lines are marked; (**c**) the postresection appearance of the colon and its arterial supply. The left colon is perfused by the marginal artery. (**d**) The resected specimen. The distal line of resection is 2 cm removed from the tumor

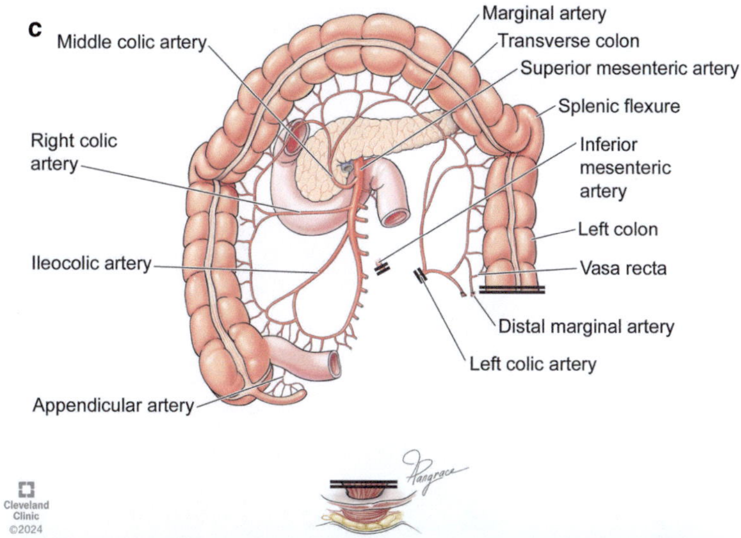

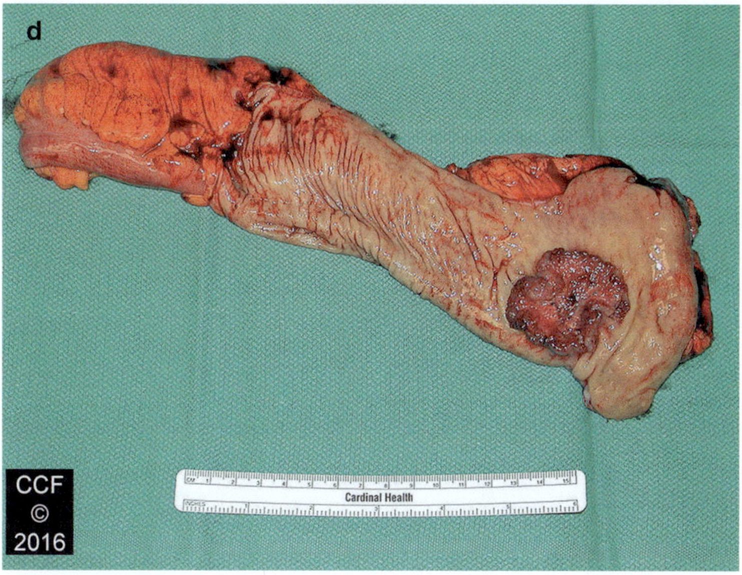

Fig. 80.1 continued

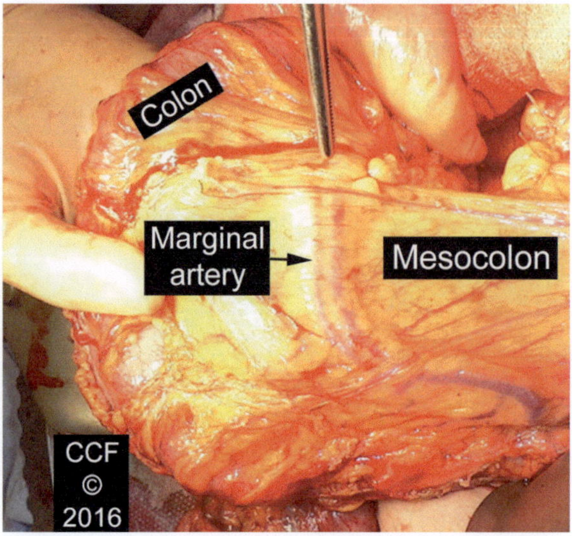

Fig. 80.2 The marginal artery of Drummond provides collateral circulation from the superior mesenteric artery to the left colon. The end of the marginal artery is identified by forceps

Table 80.1 Factors that contribute to a successful low colorectal or coloanal anastomosis

Mobilization of the splenic flexure
Preservation of the marginal artery of Drummond
Preservation of the left colic artery triangular arcade
Division of the inferior mesenteric vein near the lower border of the pancreas

Griffiths in his 1956 landmark paper, *Surgical Anatomy of the Blood Supply of the Distal Colon* [2], in which he stated:

> "The terminal form of the left colic artery should always be preserved after ligation of the inferior mesenteric at its origin, since it forms a secondary marginal artery, otherwise the distal colon is dependent solely on the very fine marginal artery of the splenic flexure."

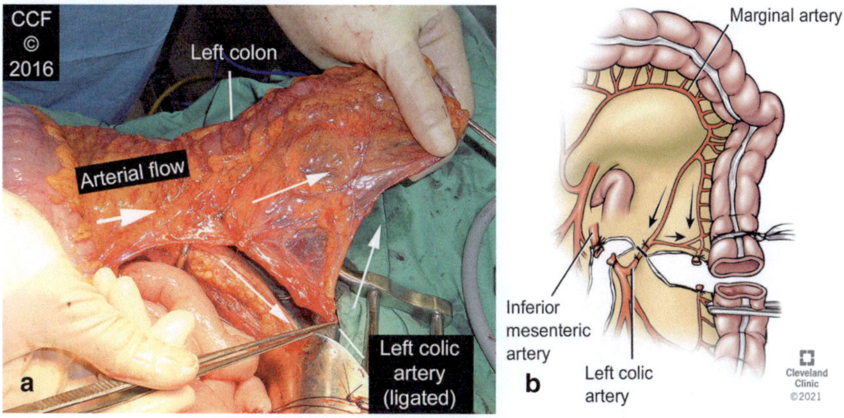

Fig. 80.3 Preservation of the left colic artery triangular arcade. (**a**) The left colic artery is divided proximal to its bifurcation. Inflow from the marginal artery passes retrograde through the proximal bifurcation branch and antegrade through the distal bifurcation branch to increase perfusion of the left colon terminus; (**b**) illustration showing the concept of retrograde blood flow down the preserved left colic bifurcation (after Jagelman)

Despite mobilization, the colon might not reach the pelvis. One possible cause is the remaining IMV that tethers the left colon to the left upper quadrant. Division of the IMV near the lower border of the pancreas allows the distal transverse colon, splenic flexure, and the left colon to move into the pelvis without tension (Fig. 80.4) [3].

Ultimately, the best sign of adequate perfusion of the left colon is pulsatile arterial bleeding from the cut end of the marginal artery at the end of the left colon (Fig. 80.5).

An example of adequate left colon, splenic flexure, and distal transverse colon mobilization is shown in Fig. 80.6. Attached omentum identifies the transverse colon. The location of the symphysis pubis is marked by the pelvic retractor. A colonic reservoir (coloplasty) has been added to the colonic terminus.

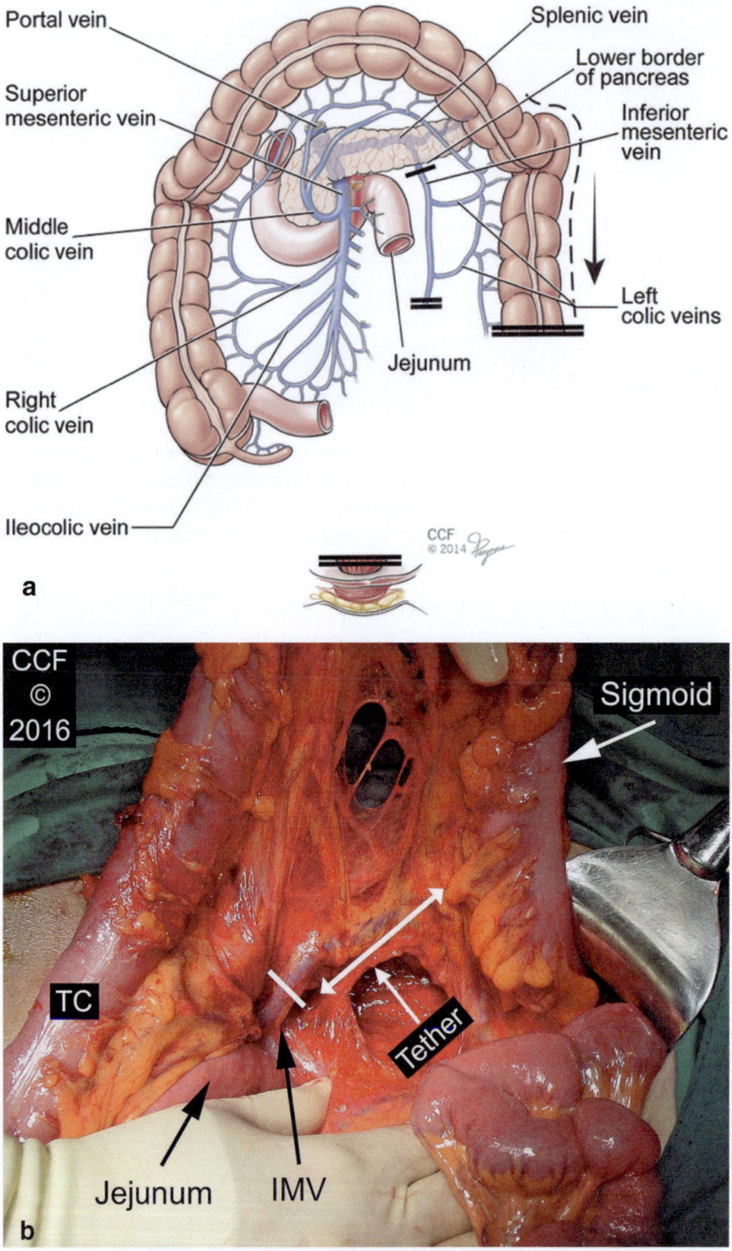

Fig. 80.4 (**a**) The lateral peritoneal and splenic flexure attachments are divided to free the colon from the left upper quadrant. Despite this, colonic mobility is hindered by tethering caused by the inferior mesenteric vein. Division of the inferior mesenteric vein close to the lower border or the pancreas allows the left colon, splenic flexure, and the distal transverse colon to move into the pelvis with a good blood supply and without tension (arrow); (**b**) operative photo showing the IMV at the lower border of the pancreas. The tethering effect on the sigmoid colon is evident. The neighboring jejunum and transverse colon (TC) are labelled. The IMV is divided (white line) close to the lower border of the pancreas to allow the left colon to reach the low pelvis

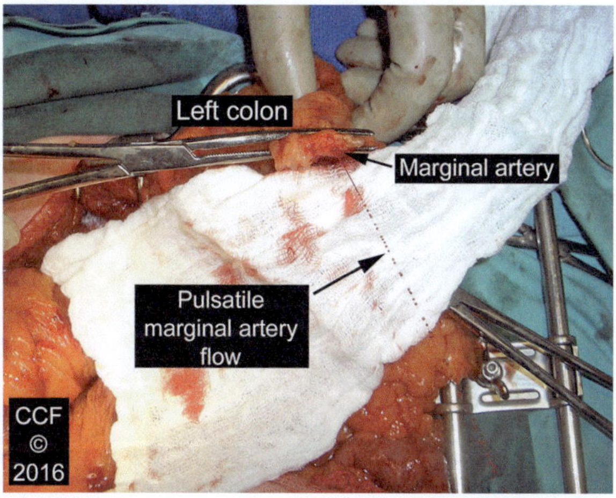

Fig. 80.5 Pulsatile arterial bleeding is seen from the cut end of marginal artery at the end of left colon

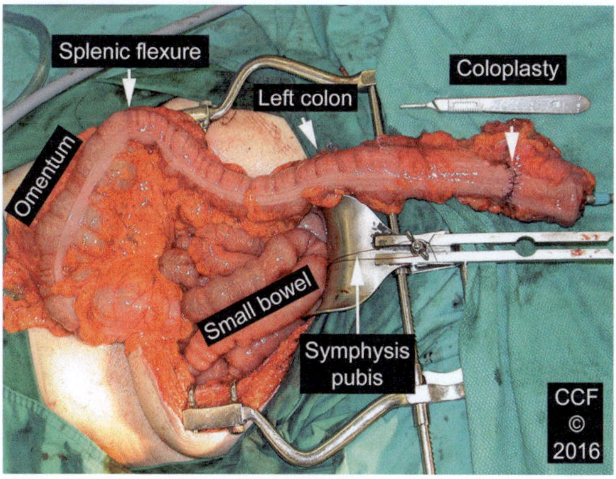

Fig. 80.6 Successful reconstitution of bowel continuity after low anterior resection depends on the creation of a left colon conduit with adequate length and excellent blood supply. In this figure, the transverse colon, splenic flexure, and left colon have been mobilized so that the end of the colon reaches well beyond the symphysis pubis identified by the attachment to Balfour's pelvic retractor

Reconstitution of Intestinal Continuity

Bowel continuity was restored by stapled colorectal anastomosis with a "coloplasty" reservoir first described by Z'Graggen in 1999 and coworkers in pigs and later applied to humans by Fazio et al. in 2000 (Fig. 80.7) [4, 5].

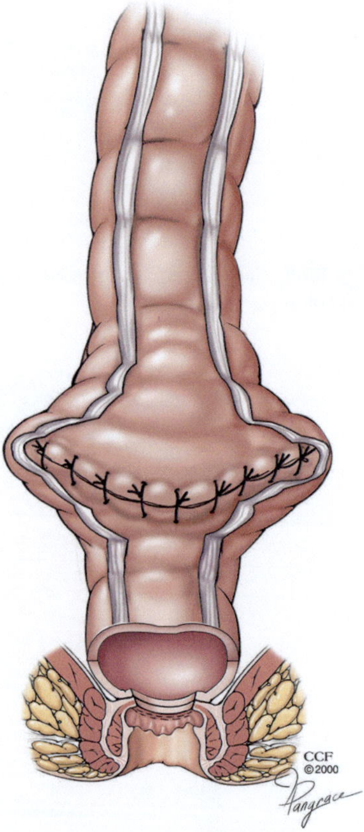

Fig. 80.7 Enhancement of low colorectal anastomosis by "coloplasty"

Technique

1. Adequate blood supply to the end of the colon is ensured by observing brisk bleeding from the cut end of the colon.
2. An 8–10 cm longitudinal colotomy is made between the taenia in the colon destined to become the coloplasty. The colotomy begins 4–6 cm from the cut end of the colon (Fig. 80.8).

The longitudinal colostomy is closed transversely (Fig. 80.9).
The complete coloplasty with attached stapling anvil is shown in Fig. 80.10.

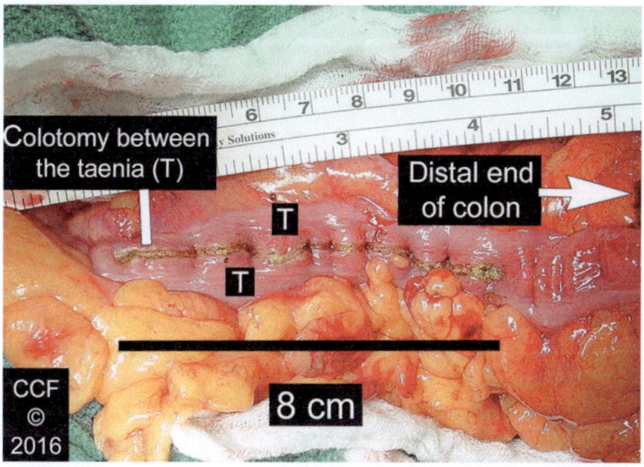

Fig. 80.8 Four to six cm from the distal end of the colon, an 8 cm colotomy is made between the taenia (T). In this image, the serosa has been marked with electrocautery

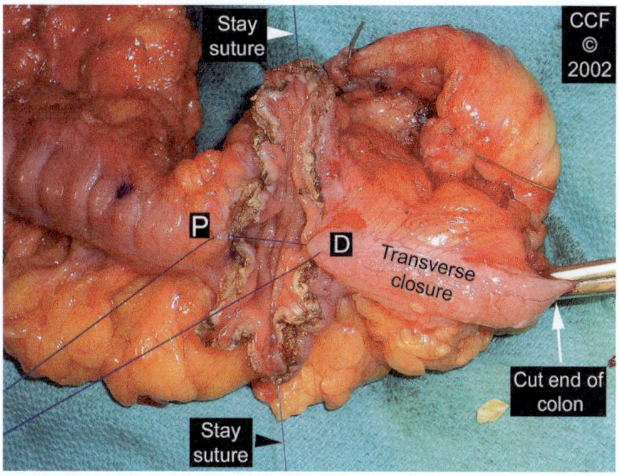

Fig. 80.9 The longitudinal colotomy is closed transversely. The proximal (P) and distal (D) ends of the colotomy are united. Lateral stay sutures are shown

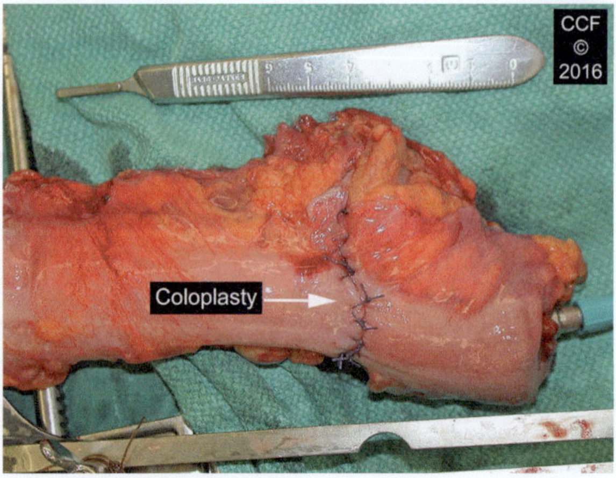

Fig. 80.10 The end of the left colon was converted from a straight tube into a reservoir by coloplasty. An 8–10 cm longitudinal incision was made 4–6 cm from the end of the colon. The incision was closed transversely

References

1. Jagelman DG. Colectomy for malignant disease of the colon: the 'no touch' isolation technique. In: Fielding LP, Goldberg SM, editors. Rob and Smith's Operative Surgery. Surgery of the Colon, Rectum, and Anus. 5th ed. Oxford: Butterworth-Heinemann, LTD; 1993. p. 359–68.
2. Griffiths JD. Surgical anatomy of the blood supply of the distal colon. Ann R Coll Surg Engl. 1956;19:241–56.
3. Augestad KM, Cranshaw B, Delaney CP. Cancer of the rectum. Operative management. In: Fazio VW, Church JM, Delaney CP, Kiran RP, editors. Current Therapy in Colon and Rectal Surgery. 3rd ed. Philadelphia: Elsevier; 2017. p. 147.
4. Z'graggen K, Mauer CA, Mettler D, Stoupis C, Wildi S, Büchler MW. A novel colon pouch and its comparison with straight coloanal and colon J-pouch-anal anastomosis: Preliminary results in pigs. Surgery. 1999;125:105–12.
5. Fazio VW, Mantyh CR, Hull TL. Colonic "Coloplasty": novel technique to enhance low colorectal or coloanal anastomosis. Dis Colon Rectum. 2000;43:1448–50.

Rectal Cancer-Posterior Pelvic Exenteration with Vertical Rectus Abdominis Myocutaneous Flap Reconstruction

81

Chad M. Michener, Thomas E. Garofalo, and James S. Wu

Presentation

A 35-year-old female presented with locally advanced low rectal cancer involving the anus and, secondarily, the posterior vaginal wall. After neoadjuvant therapy, she underwent posterior pelvic exenteration with *en bloc* removal of the rectum, anus, uterus, cervix, and posterior vaginal wall[1]. The resulting perineal wound is shown in Fig. 81.1.

Figure 81.2 shows the mobilized rectus abdominis myocutaneous (VRAM) flap that will be used to reconstruct the vagina after posterior vaginectomy.

Figure 81.3 shows the vagina and the perineal wound with the VRAM flap sewn into place.

[1] The patient's ovaries were left at her request.

C. M. Michener
Ob/Gyn and Women's Health Institute, Cleveland Clinic, Cleveland, OH, USA

T. E. Garofalo · J. S. Wu (✉)
Department of Colon and Rectal Surgery, Cleveland Clinic, Cleveland, OH, USA

J. S. Wu, M. D. Inkster (eds.), *Cleveland Clinic Colorectal Case Studies*,
https://doi.org/10.1007/978-3-031-39880-3_81

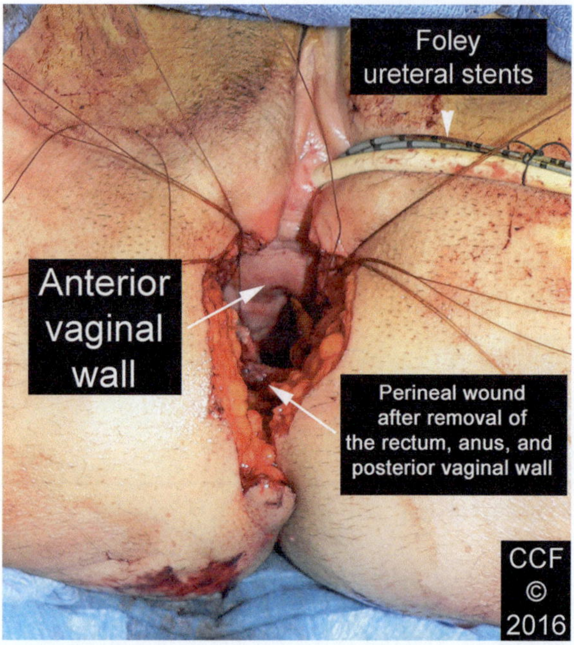

Fig. 81.1 Perineal wound following removal of the rectum, anus, and posterior wall of the vagina. The anterior wall of the vagina is seen (arrow)

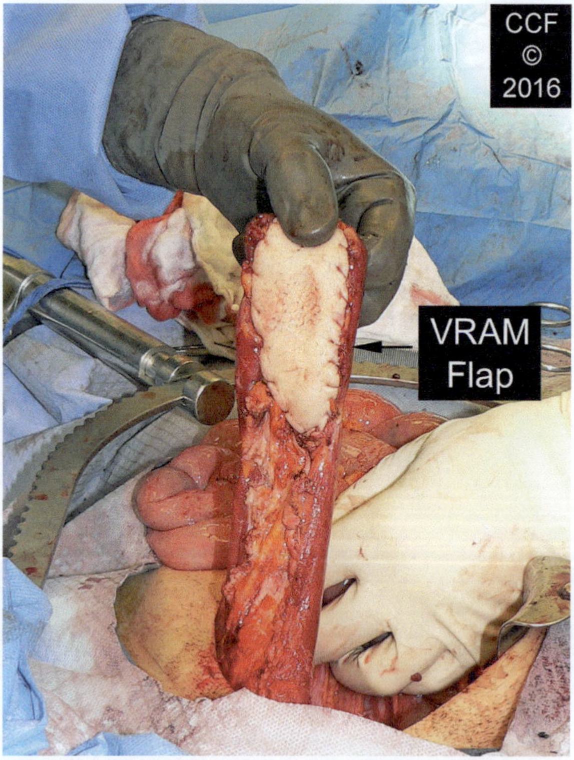

Fig. 81.2 Vertical rectus abdominis myocutaneous (VRAM) flap: An elliptical island of skin 8 cm × 5 cm was created superior and to the right of the umbilicus. The VRAM flap was based on the rectus muscle and inferior epigastric artery

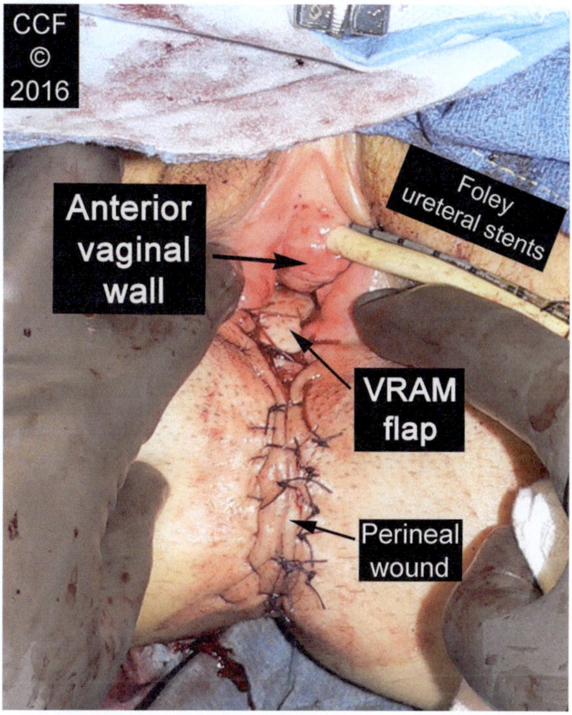

Fig. 81.3 The perineal skin incision was closed with interrupted sutures. The 7 cm × 4 cm defect caused by excision of the posterior vaginal wall was reconstructed with a VRAM flap. The anterior vaginal wall and bladder catheter (Foley) with ureteral stents also are identified

Comment

En bloc excision is an appropriate therapy for rectal cancer with posterior vaginal wall involvement. The operation leaves a gaping defect where the posterior wall of the vagina has been removed. In 1979, Robbins reported rectus abdominis myocutaneous flap for breast reconstruction [1]. VRAM flap reconstruction in the setting of vaginectomy and prior pelvic irradiation, demonstrated in this case, effectively closed the vaginal defect with a flap that replaces the posterior vaginal wall [2]. In this multidisciplinary case, rectal resection was done by colorectal surgery. The VRAM reconstruction of the posterior wall defect was done by gynecologic surgical oncology (CMM). Postoperatively, the perineal surgical site is cleansed by sitz baths. Prolonged pressure on the perineal area, e.g., long periods of upright sitting, was avoided.

References

1. Robbins TH. Rectus abdominis myocutaneous flap for breast reconstruction. Aust NZ J Surg. 1979;49:527–30.
2. Bell SW, Dehni N, Chaouat M, Lifante JC, Parc R, Tiret E. Primary rectus abdominis myocutaneous flap for repair of perineal and vaginal defects after extended abdominoperineal resection. Br J Surg. 2005;92:482–6.

Stage IV Rectal Cancer

82

Carolyn L. Power, Hermann Kessler, and James S. Wu

Presentation

A 42-year-old male presented with a one-year history of bloody stool. Digital rectal exam revealed a left anterolateral mass at the top of the levator muscles. Flexible sigmoidoscopy revealed a friable near-obstructing adenocarcinoma of the rectum. Metastatic workup included pelvic Magnetic Resonance Imaging (MRI) (Fig. 82.1) and Computed Tomography (CT)/Positron Emission Tomography (PET) scan (Fig. 82.2).

C. L. Power · H. Kessler · J. S. Wu (✉)
Department of Colon and Rectal Surgery, Cleveland Clinic, Cleveland, OH, USA

J. S. Wu, M. D. Inkster (eds.), *Cleveland Clinic Colorectal Case Studies*,
https://doi.org/10.1007/978-3-031-39880-3_82

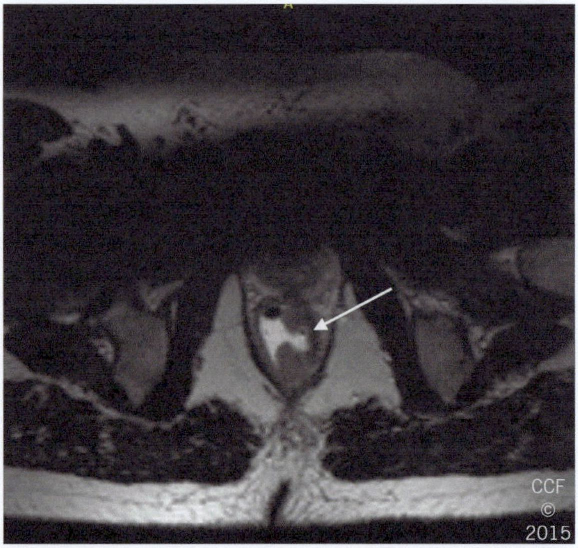

Fig. 82.1 T2-weighted axial MRI shows a near-obstructing lesion in the rectum (arrow)

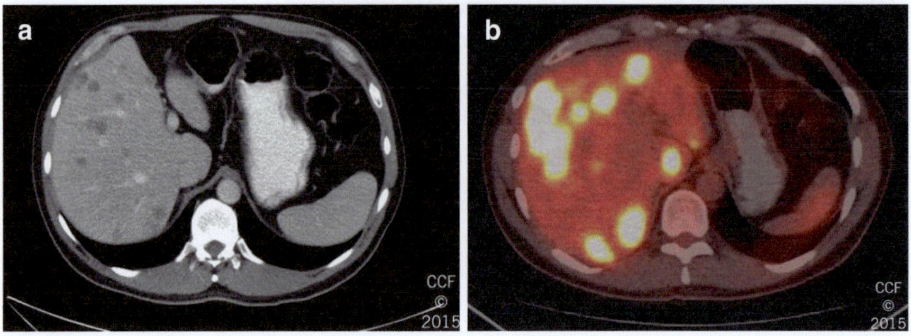

Fig. 82.2 (**a**, **b**) CT and PET scan, respectively, shows multiple metastases throughout the liver (M1a: metastases in one distant organ)

Management

At the Multidisciplinary Tumor Board, the following management possibilities were discussed:

1. Resection of the primary tumor, surgical resection for the liver metastases,
2. Upfront chemotherapy and radiation therapy (CRT) for the primary tumor: local radiation therapy (50 Gy/5fx) and FOLFOX (FOL = Leucovorin Calcium, F = Fluorouracil, OX = Oxaliplatin) plus bevacizumab.

The decision of the Tumor Board was the second option.

Repeat CT/PET scanning 6 months after treatment showed total resolution not only of liver metastases but also of the rectal tumor (Fig. 82.3).

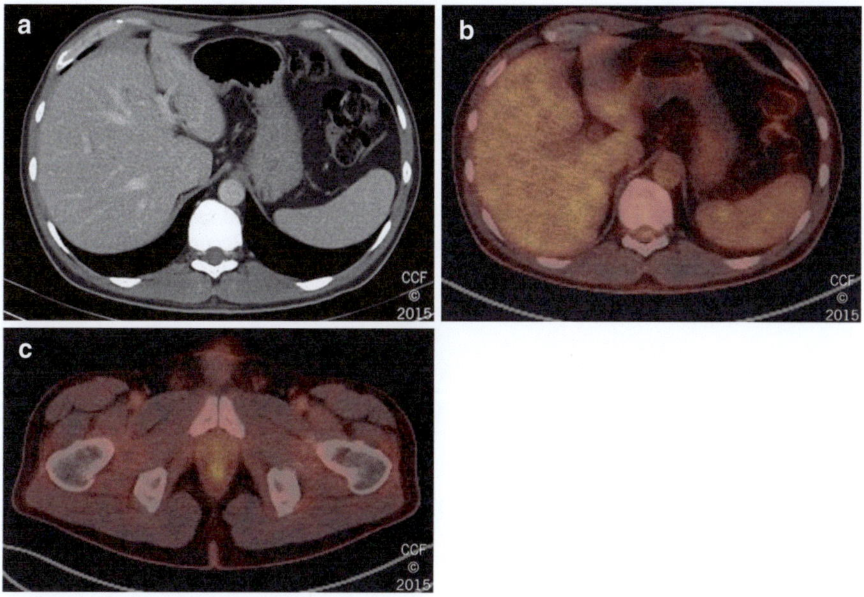

Fig. 82.3 (**a**, **b**) CT and PET scan, respectively, shows resolution of liver metastases. (**c**) PET image showing resolution of index lesion

Flexible sigmoidoscopy with retroflexion revealed the absence of tumor. As findings appeared to show complete remission, a program of maintenance chemotherapy and observation was initiated. Primary surgical resection was not recommended.

Comment [1–3]

For rectal cancer, the risk of local recurrence is high even following local therapy that initially seems successful. In general, the mainstay of curative treatment is oncologic surgical resection with Total Mesorectal Excision and lymph node dissection. However, the treatment of rectal cancer is evolving continuously.

Stage IV cancer, which has the worst prognostic outlook, is assessed in terms of local symptoms and patient comorbidities. Local therapy with radiation and surgery may be considered, particularly for patients with significant local symptoms such as bleeding, obstruction, and pain. Chemotherapy is the one treatment modality that has been shown to improve overall survival. In this particular case, neoadjuvant chemoradiotherapy was administered with the option for surgery if indicated. After completion of neoadjuvant CRT, tumor restaging revealed no residual tumor. A program of observation and maintenance chemotherapy was started. Surgical resection was not done.

References

1. Ronnekleiv-Kelly SM, Kennedy GD. Management of stage IV rectal cancer: Palliative options. World J Gastroenterol. 2011;17:835–47.
2. O'Neil BH, Tepper JE. Current options for the management of rectal cancer. Curr Treat Options in Oncol. 2007;8:331–8.
3. Habr-Gama A, Perez RO, Wynn G, Marks J, Kessler H, Gama-Rodrigues J. Complete clinical response after neoadjuvant chemoradiation therapy for distal rectal cancer: characterization of clinical and endoscopic findings for standardization. Dis Colon Rectum. 2010;53:1692–8.

Malignant Urorectal Fistula

83

Sanford S. Luria, David Hernandez Gonzalo, Eric W. Willis, and James S. Wu

Presentation

An 83-year-old man complained of watery stool and fecaluria (Fig. 83.1). Colonoscopy revealed an anterior rectal mass (Fig. 83.2). Biopsies were obtained (Fig. 83.3).

S. S. Luria
Glickman Urological & Kidney Institute, Cleveland Clinic, Cleveland, OH, USA

D. Hernandez Gonzalo
Department of Pathology, Immunology and Laboratory Medicine, University of Florida, Gainesville, FL, USA

E. W. Willis
Department of Pathology, CORPath, Columbus, OH, USA

J. S. Wu (✉)
Department of Colon and Rectal Surgery, Cleveland Clinic, Cleveland, OH, USA

J. S. Wu, M. D. Inkster (eds.), *Cleveland Clinic Colorectal Case Studies*,
https://doi.org/10.1007/978-3-031-39880-3_83

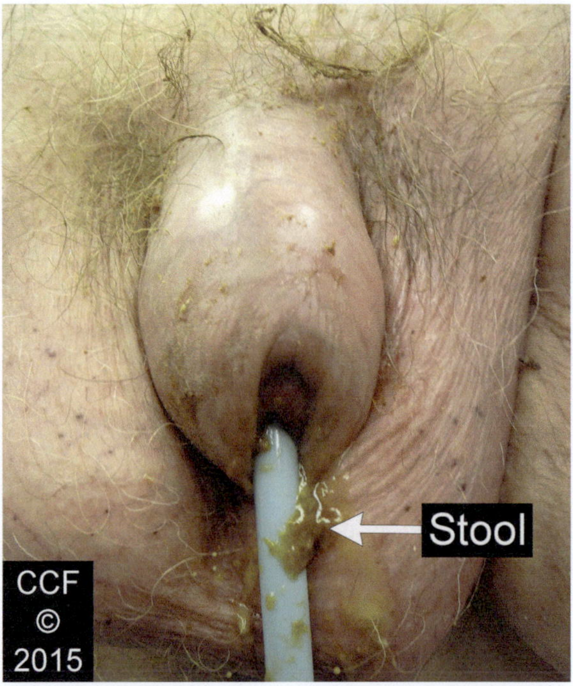

Fig. 83.1 Fecaluria

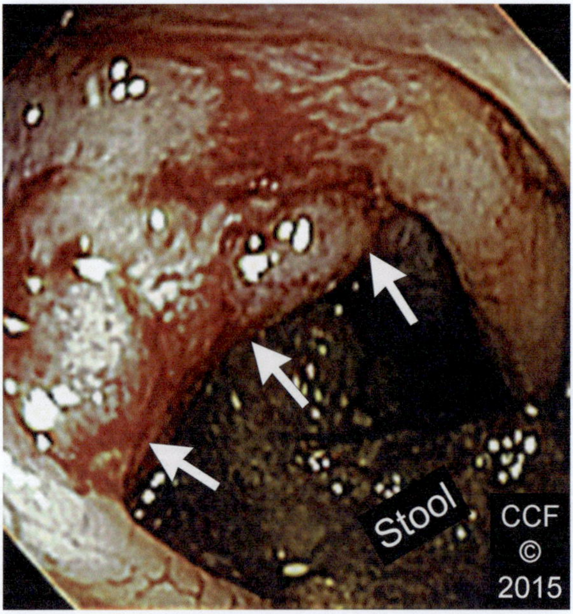

Fig. 83.2 Anterior rectal mass (arrows)

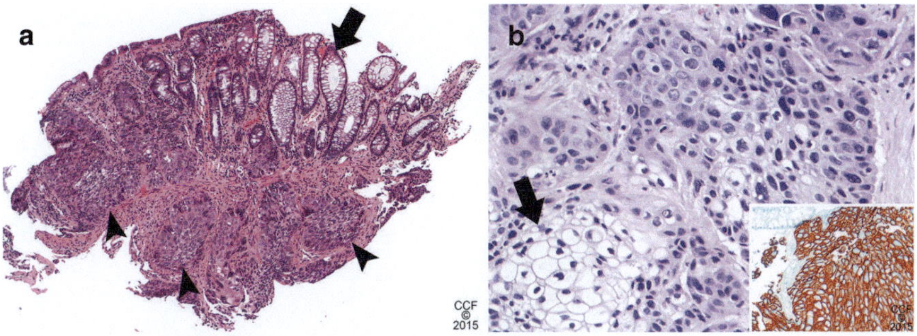

Fig. 83.3 (**a**) Rectal biopsy showing tumor nests (arrowheads) underlying unremarkable colonic mucosa (arrow). The nests are present mainly within the submucosa. Tumor cells contain enlarged and hyperchromatic nuclei and eosinophilic cytoplasm (hematoxylin–eosin original magnification ×50); (**b**) Nests of malignant squamous epithelium, characterized by polygonal cells with dyskeratosis and intercellular bridges. The squamous component has also clear cell features (arrow). Tumor cells are positive for CK5/6 and p63 and are negative for CK7 and CDX-2 (hematoxylin–eosin, original magnification ×200; CK5/6 stain, original magnification × 100 [inset])

Comment

A biopsy of the anterior rectal mass revealed a high-grade urothelial carcinoma with squamous differentiation as supported by positive CK5/6 and p63 stains and negative CK7 and CDX2. Brachytherapy used to treat prostate cancer has been associated with the development of secondary bladder malignancies (Fig. 83.4) [1, 2]. The patient has developed a rectovesical fistula. Transverse colostomy was done to divert feces away from the rectum and thereby stop urinary contamination with feces (Fig. 83.5). Bilateral nephrostomy tubes were placed in order to relieve urinary obstruction caused by the tumor. The procedures were palliative.

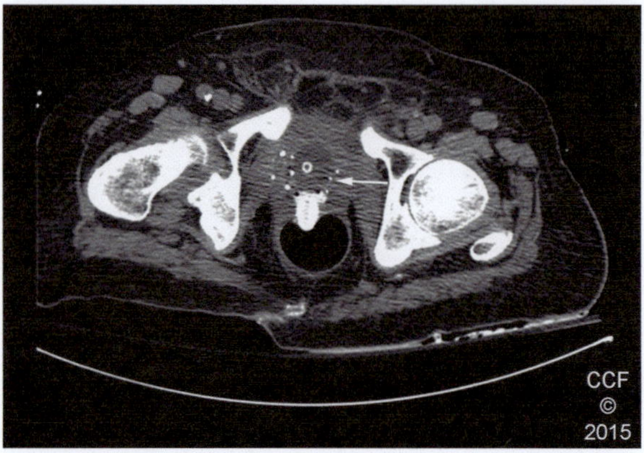

Fig. 83.4 CT scan shows prostate brachytherapy seeds (arrow)

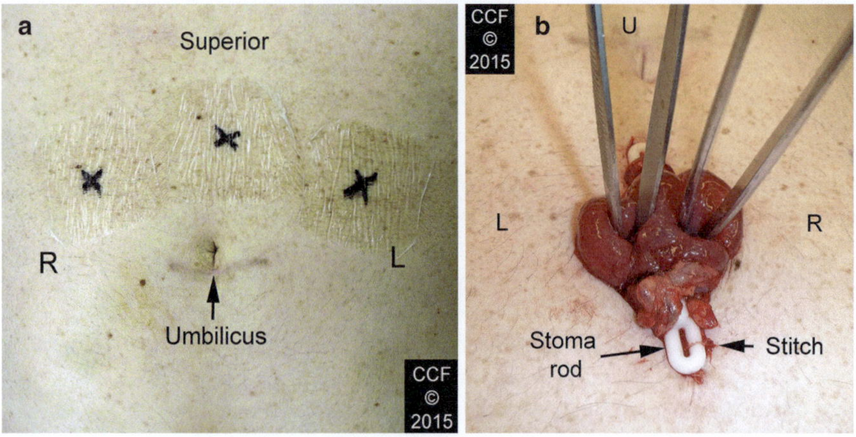

Fig. 83.5 (**a**) The upper abdomen has been marked for upper quadrant and midline ostomies. A small incision was made in the midline. The mobile apex of the transverse colon was exteriorized, suspended over a stoma rod (3" Ostomy rod with eyelets, Marlen Manufacturing & Development Co., 5150 Richmond road, Bedford, Ohio. 44146), and matured primarily; (**b**) forceps identify the two limbs of the colostomy. The umbilicus is labeled (U). Right (R), Left (L)

References

1. Sountoulides P, Koletsas N, Kikidakis D, Paschalidis K, Sofikitis N. Secondary malignancies following radiotherapy for prostate cancer. Ther Adv Urol. 2010;2:119–25.
2. Liauw SL, Sylvester JE, Morris CG, Blasko JC, Grimm PD. Second malignancies after prostate brachytherapy: Incidence of bladder and colorectal cancers in patients with 15 years of potential follow-up. Int J Radiat Oncol Biol Phys. 2006;66:669–73.

Prostate Cancer-Rectal Stricture

84

James S. Wu, Jing-Jing Yang, and Eric W. Willis

Presentation

An 85 year-old man presented with obstipation. Digital rectal examination revealed a firm mass. No blood was detected on the examining finger. Flexible sigmoidoscopy, pelvic MRI, and biopsy were done (Figs. 84.1, 84.2, and 84.3).

J. S. Wu (✉)
Department of Colon and Rectal Surgery, Cleveland Clinic, Cleveland, OH, USA

J.-J. Yang
Departments of Pathology, Medical Diagnostic Laboratories, LLC, Hamilton, NJ, USA

E. W. Willis
Department of Pathology, CORPath, Columbus, OH, USA

J. S. Wu, M. D. Inkster (eds.), *Cleveland Clinic Colorectal Case Studies*,
https://doi.org/10.1007/978-3-031-39880-3_84

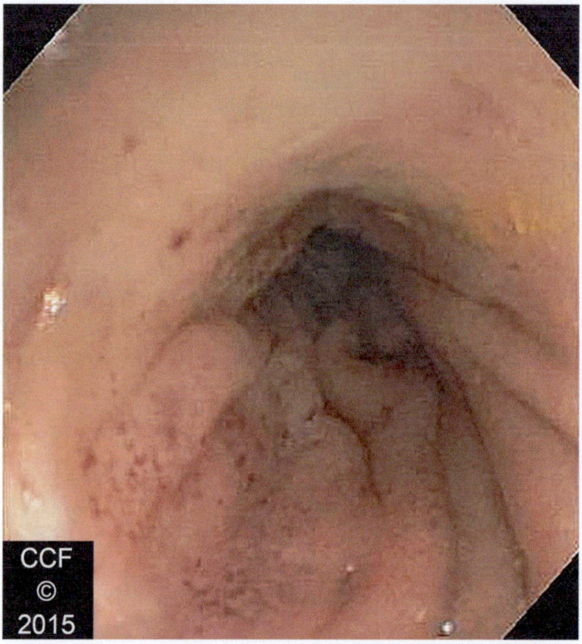

Fig. 84.1 Flexible sigmoidoscopy revealed a smooth rectal stricture. The mucosa appeared normal

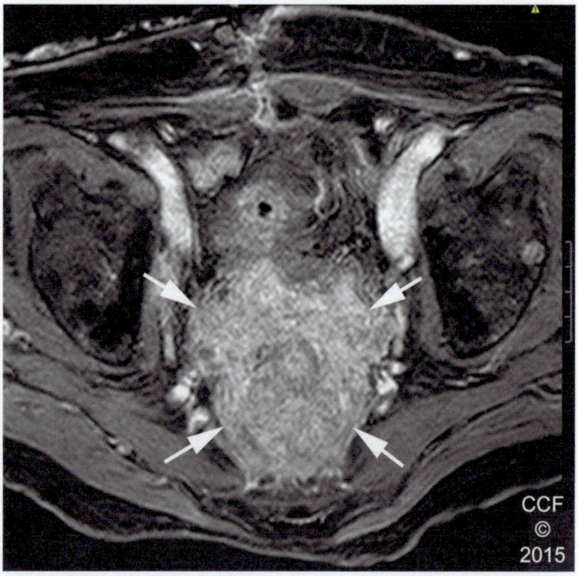

Fig. 84.2 Pelvic magnetic resonance imaging shows a mass (arrows) stricturing the rectum

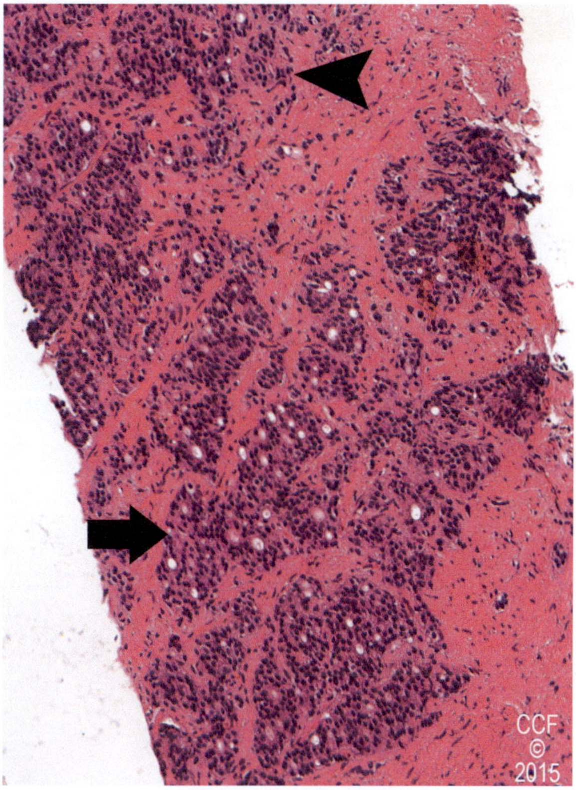

Fig. 84.3 Biopsy showing predominantly poorly-formed glands with cribriforming, corresponding to Gleason pattern 4 (arrow). Focal solid sheets of tumor were present, corresponding with Gleason pattern 5 (arrowhead). (H&E, original magnification, 400 ×)

Diagnosis

Transrectal biopsy (Fig. 84.3) revealed Gleason's grade 4 + 5 = 9 prostate cancer. Osseous metastases were seen on bone scan (Fig. 84.4).

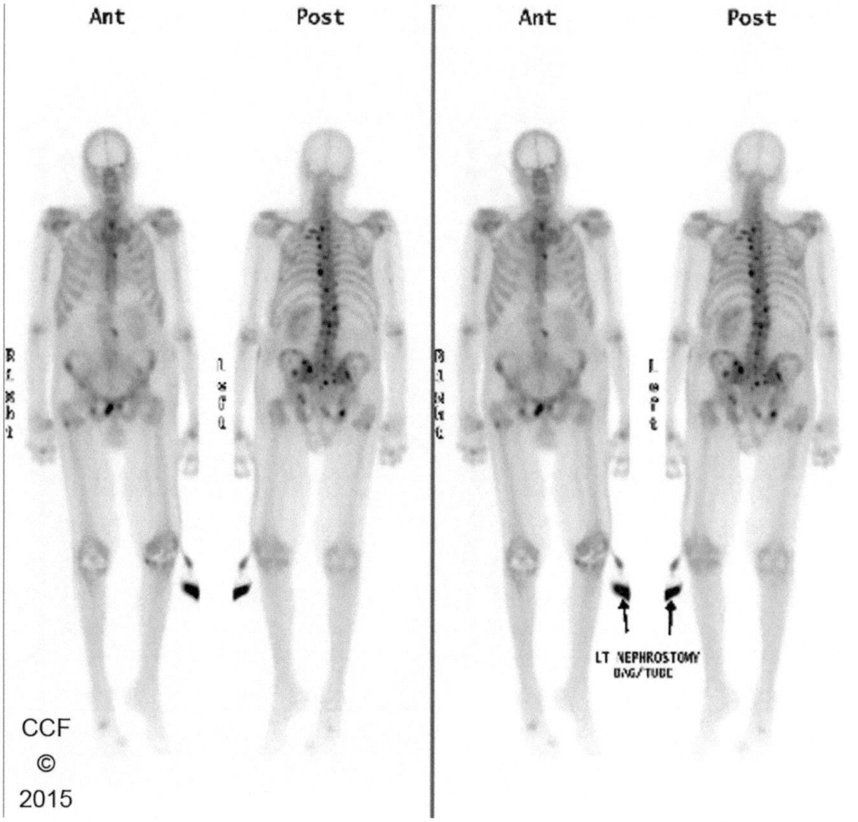

Fig. 84.4 Bone scan reveals multiple sites of radionuclide uptake consistent with multiple osseous metastases

Discussion

Adenocarcinoma of the rectum is an intraluminal lesion that bleeds easily on contact. Palpation of a rectal mass that does not show blood suggests an extraluminal origin[1]. In males, the prostate is suspect. In this case, magnetic resonance imaging showed that the rectal lumen was severely constricted circumferentially by neighboring prostate cancer.

[1]Personal communication: Rupert B. Turnbull, Jr, MD to Victor W. Fazio, MD to one of the authors (JSW).

85 Prostate to Rectal Fistula-Pelvic Exenteration

Craig D. Zippe and James S. Wu

Presentation

An otherwise healthy 63-year old male was treated for prostate cancer with both external beam radiotherapy and brachytherapy. Following treatment, the patient developed fecaluria, rectal bleeding requiring blood transfusion, and pelvic pain requiring continuous narcotic medication. A cystogram was obtained (Fig. 85.1a, b).

C. D. Zippe
Glickman Urological & Kidney Institute, Cleveland Clinic, Cleveland, OH, USA

J. S. Wu (✉)
Department of Colon and Rectal Surgery, Cleveland Clinic, Cleveland, OH, USA

J. S. Wu, M. D. Inkster (eds.), *Cleveland Clinic Colorectal Case Studies*,
https://doi.org/10.1007/978-3-031-39880-3_85

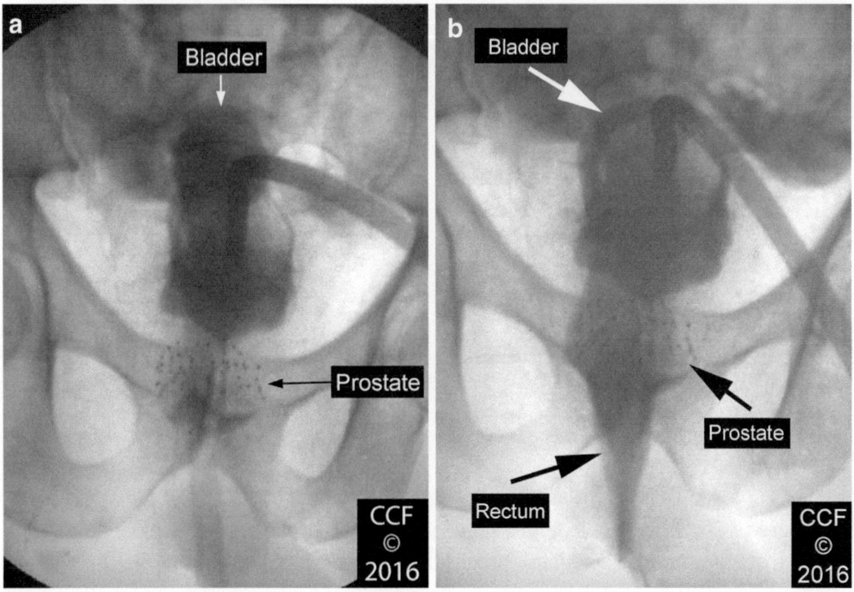

Fig. 85.1 Fluoroscopic spot views over the pelvis demonstrate contrast opacification of a small volume urinary bladder *via* a balloon-tipped catheter. Multiple small densities are seen in the region of the symphysis pubis/prostate (radiation implant seeds). In (**a**), contrast is seen in the bladder. (**b**) shows subsequent opacification of the rectum

Management

The patient has a fistula between the prostate and the rectum. An interdisciplinary urologic and colorectal surgery team performed pelvic exenteration with urinary ileal conduit and end colostomy (Fig. 85.2).

Marks for both urostomy and colostomy were placed preoperatively (Fig. 85.3).

The bladder, prostate, and rectum joined at the fistula site are mobilized *en bloc* (Fig. 85.4). The resected specimen is shown in Fig. 85.5.

Urinary diversion was through an ileal conduit (Fig. 85.6). The fecal stream was diverted through an end colostomy.

Pathology showed adenocarcinoma of the prostate with coloprostatic fistula. Margins were negative for carcinoma.

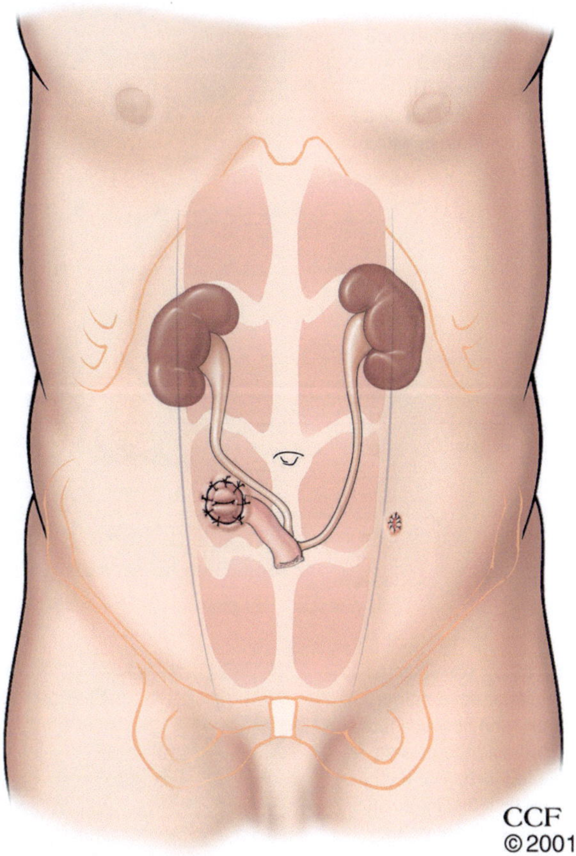

Fig. 85.2 Ileal conduit (Bricker, 1950) after removal of the bladder, prostate, and rectum. A colostomy is seen in the left lower quadrant. In this illustration, the colostomy has been drawn lateral to the rectus muscle. In practice, the colostomy is brought through the rectus muscle

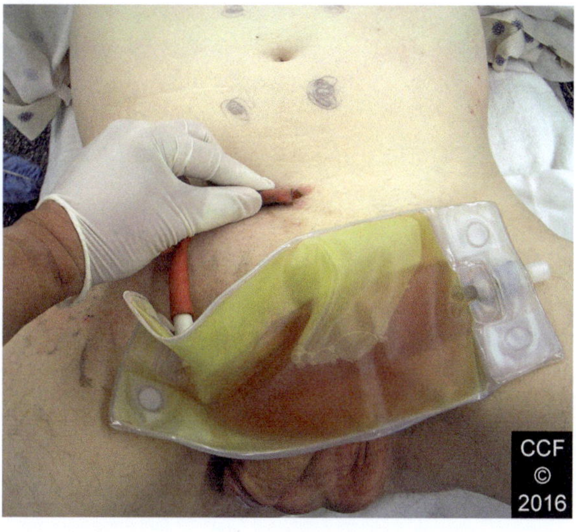

Fig. 85.3 Sites for urostomy and colostomy have been selected. The bladder is drained via a suprapubic catheter

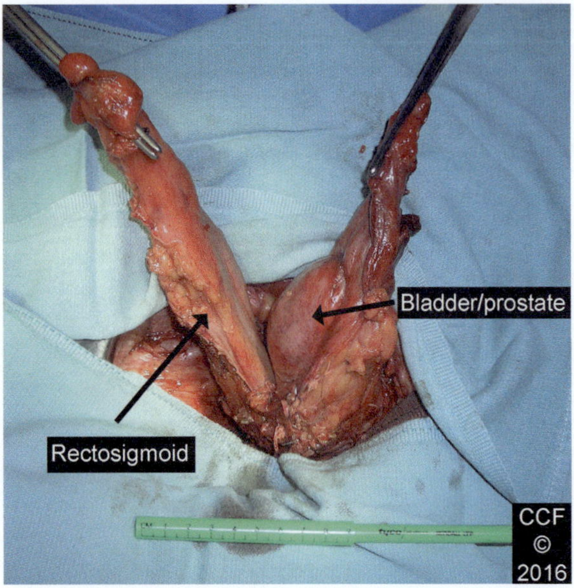

Fig. 85.4 The rectum and sigmoid colon (left) and the bladder (right) have been mobilized. The rectum was divided distal to the fistula flush with the pelvic floor

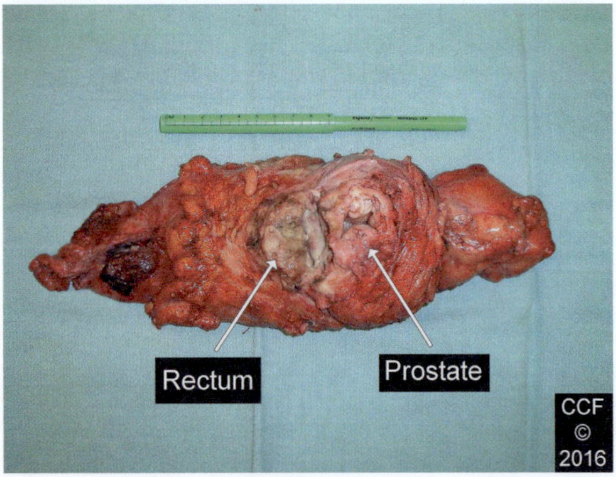

Fig. 85.5 The resected specimen: the fistulous connection between the rectum and the prostate has been divided. The rectum is on the left. The bladder and prostate are on the right

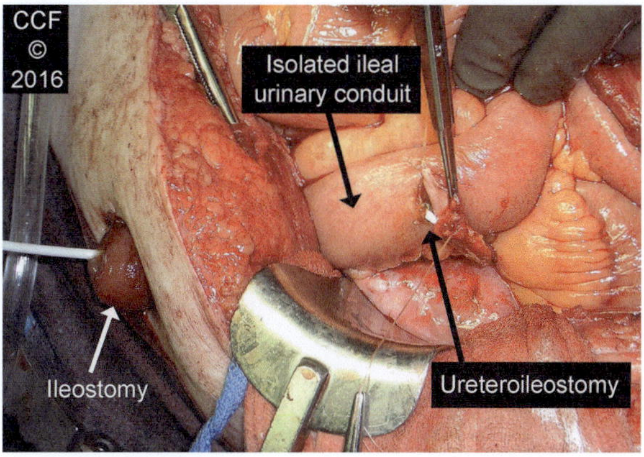

Fig. 85.6 The urine is diverted through an ileal conduit. An isolated segment of ileum has been brought to the skin as an ileostomy. The ureters are anastomosed to the ileal conduit over urinary stents

Comment

The importance of total exenteration is that a urologic cancer that has eroded into the rectum or a rectal cancer that has extended into the urologic structures potentially can be resected *en bloc* for cure [1]. Even if a curative outcome is not achieved, complete exenteration provides local cancer control and palliative relief of urinary obstruction, fecal obstruction, and intractable pelvic pain.

Following cystectomy, ureteral disposal previously had been by implantation of the ureters into the skin or the colon [2, 3]. In 1950, Bricker introduced a different approach in which the ureters are implanted into an isolated segment of terminal ileum that is exteriorized through the anterior abdominal wall as an ileostomy[1] [4–6].

> "Our interest in pelvic evisceration and disposal of the ureters was interrupted by the war and it was not until 1946 that the problem was again attacked. This time the stimulus was afforded by a case of carcinoma of the rectum in a male with involvement of the trigone of the bladder. The case, with operation on July 5, 1947 and a subsequent one, with operation on April 15, 1948, were reported before the Ewing Society at Memorial Hospital on January 15, 1949…. The procedure of reconstruction as applied to this type of extensive carcinoma of rectum requires a slightly different approach than that which we had previously employed, since for this lesion it is necessary to do a high resection of the sigmoid colon and its mesentery, making it difficult or impossible to use an isolated segment of the sigmoid colon as a receptacle for the ureters. Our solution…has been to transplant the ureters into the terminal ileum or into the cecum itself. In each instance, the terminal ileum and cecum were isolated from the remainder of the intestinal tract,…"
>
> Eugene M. Bricker, M.D.
> Department of Surgery
> Washington University School of Medicine
> and Barnes Hospital
> St. Louis

[1] Bricker [4]. The excerpt was reproduced with the generous permission of Elsevier Science & Technology Journals, CCC|Marketplace™, order license ID 1143991-1; order date 28 Aug 2021.

References

1. Bricker EM, Butcher HR, McAfee A. Results of pelvic exenteration. Arch Surg. 1956;73:661–70.
2. Verhoogen J, deGraeuwe A. La cystectomie totale. Folia Urol. 1908/9;iii:629–73.
3. Walters W. Implantation of the ureters into the colon. Surgery. 1937;2:12–7.
4. Bricker EM. Bladder substitution after pelvic evisceration. Surg Clin North Am. 1950;30:1511–21.
5. Bricker EM. Functional results of small intestinal segments as bladder substitutes following pelvic evisceration. A progress report. Surgery. 1952;32:372–83.
6. Bricker EM. Bladder substitution with isolated small intestine segments. A progress report. Am Surg. 1952;18:654–64.

Fecal Disimpaction

86

James S. Wu

Presentation

A 61-year-old female was admitted to the hospital because of abdominal pain and tenesmus. She was taking narcotic pain medication following recent shoulder surgery. Digital examination revealed anal sphincter hypertonicity and posterior anal canal tenderness. A solid mass was palpated with the finger tip. Colonoscopy within the last year was normal. Computed tomography revealed a large rectal mass consistent with feces (Fig. 86.1a, b).

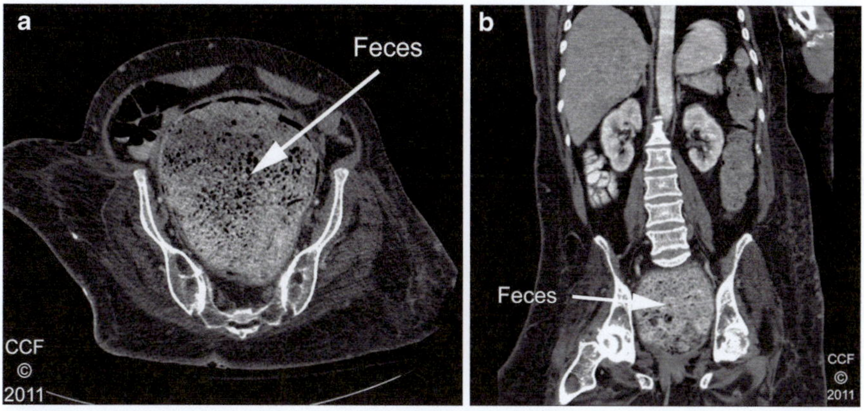

Fig. 86.1 CT scan images of the pelvis show a large rectal mass consistent with feces (arrows): (**a**) axial view; (**b**) coronal view

J. S. Wu (✉)
Department of Colon and Rectal Surgery, Cleveland Clinic, Cleveland, OH, USA

J. S. Wu, M. D. Inkster (eds.), *Cleveland Clinic Colorectal Case Studies*,
https://doi.org/10.1007/978-3-031-39880-3_86

Comment [1, 2]

Impacted feces cannot be eliminated from the rectum. The condition commonly is seen in elderly and hospitalized patients. Causes include medications that decrease gut motility, immobility, and decreased cognition. Associated complaints include constipation, abdominal pain, anal pain, anorectal bleeding, tenesmus, and incomplete evacuation. Diarrhea may be seen due to liquid feces flowing around the impacted feces. Inspection may reveal liquid feces at the anal outlet. Digital examination commonly reveals a hypertonic sphincter and anal canal tenderness due to stercorally induced anal fissure. A hard fecal mass is commonly encountered at the tip of the examining finger. A more thorough examination and fecal disimpaction are done in the operating room under anesthesia.

Technique

With a well-lubricated gloved hand, using the index and middle fingers, the solid feces in the distal rectum are broken up and removed. Removal of the distal solid fecal load was followed by elimination of a large volume of liquid stool (Fig. 86.2). The fingers are highly suitable instruments for fecal disimpaction because they have excellent tactile sense and lack of sharp edges (Fig. 86.3). Figure 86.4 shows another case in which the rectum was filled with a large mass of desiccated stool that had a clay-like consistency. The stool could not be eliminated because of sphincter hypertonicity due to a fissure.

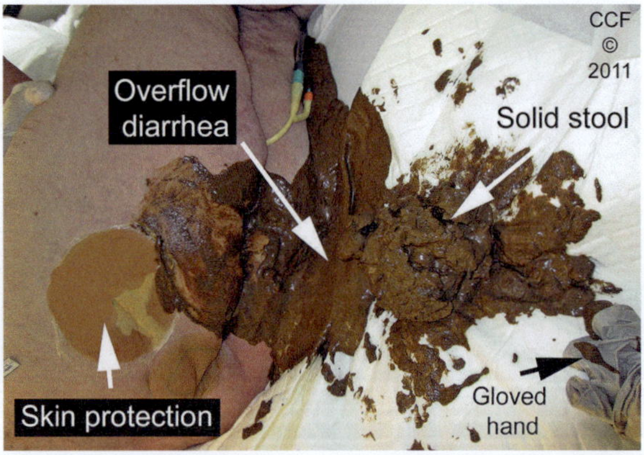

Fig. 86.2 In this case, removal of a distal plug of solid inspissated stool is followed by a surge of liquid stool

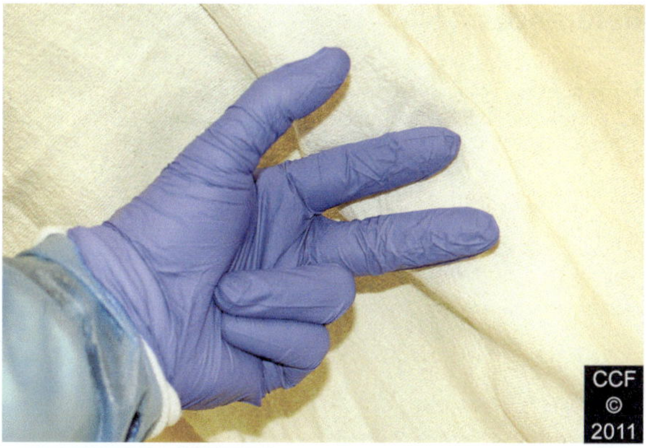

Fig. 86.3 Fecal disimpaction was done with well-lubricated, gloved, index, and middle fingers

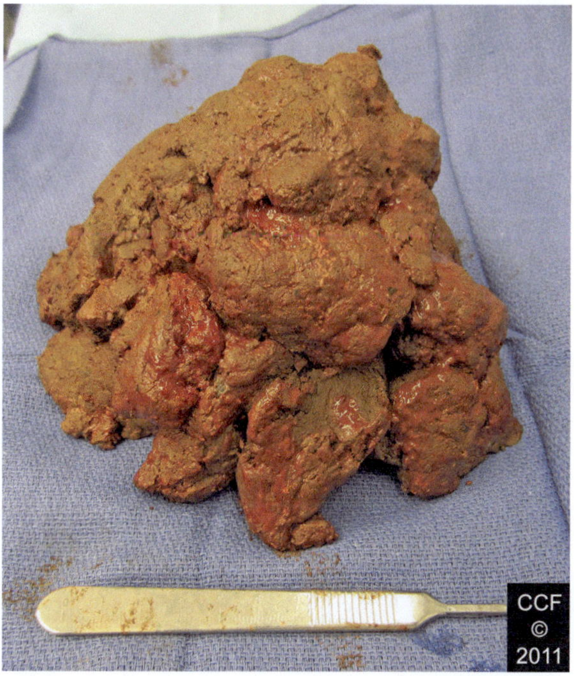

Fig. 86.4 In this case, the disimpacted feces formed a large solid mass with a clay-like consistency that was impossible to eliminate, especially in the presence of an anal fissure

Postdisimpaction Follow-Up

Stool proximal to distal solid feces usually is softer and will pass with enemas or a cathartic agent. Postdisimpaction treatment includes elimination of the remaining fecal load and treatment of the accompanying anal fissure, if present. Disimpaction may best be performed under anesthesia. Diagnostic studies are done to exclude a mechanical or neoplastic problem. Steps are taken to ensure future bowel regularity.

References

1. Wrenn K. Fecal impaction. New Engl J Med. 1989;321:658–62.
2. Araghizadeh F. Fecal impaction. Clin Colon Rectal Surg. 2005;18:116–9.

Rectal Submucosal Lesion

87

Samuel Ruskin and James S. Wu

Presentation

A rectal polyp was seen on colonoscopy (Fig. 87.1). Biopsy showed lymphoid aggregates. The site was marked with India ink. Examination of the submucosa was achieved by magnetic imaging (MRI) (Fig. 87.2).

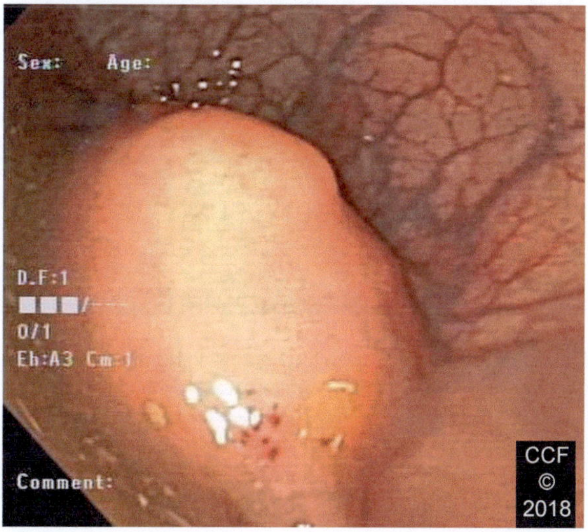

Fig. 87.1 Rectal mass seen on colonoscopy

S. Ruskin
Radiology & Diagnostic Imaging Institute, Cleveland Clinic, Cleveland, OH, USA

J. S. Wu (✉)
Department of Colon and Rectal Surgery, Cleveland Clinic, Cleveland, OH, USA

J. S. Wu, M. D. Inkster (eds.), *Cleveland Clinic Colorectal Case Studies*,
https://doi.org/10.1007/978-3-031-39880-3_87

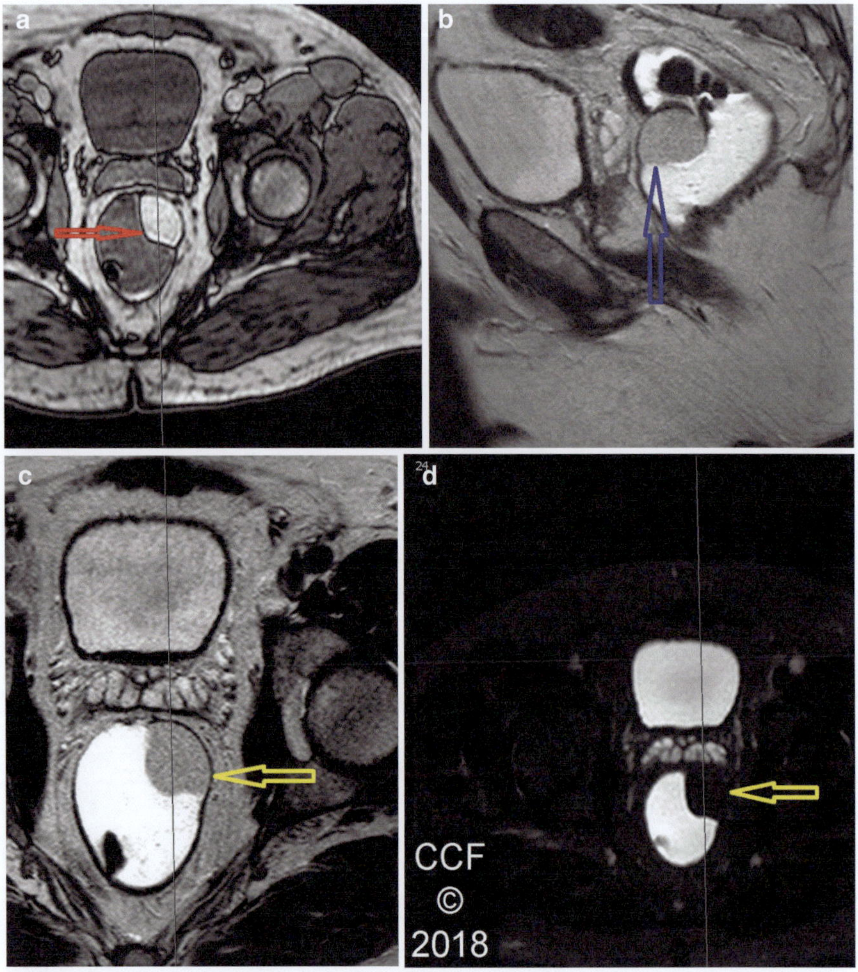

Fig. 87.2 (**a**) Axial T1-weighted out-of-phase image through the rectum demonstrates a well-circumscribed, mildly T1 hyperintense mass with associated "India-ink" artifact (red arrow) consistent with macroscopic fat; (**b/c**) sagittal (**b**) and axial (**c**) T2-weighted images through the rectum demonstrate a T2 intermediate intensity submucosal anterior midrectal mass (blue arrow in (**b**) and yellow arrow in (**c**)) that does not invade the muscularis propria; (**d**): axial T2-weighted fat saturated image through the rectum demonstrates that the mass loses signal diffusely with fat saturation (yellow arrow)

Comment

The evaluation of rectal submucosal lesions may involve a combination of complementary tests including optical colonoscopy, histopathology, and radiologic studies. In this case, colonoscopy revealed a large rectal lesion. The mucosa appeared normal. Its size raised concerns of a submucosal lesion. Lesions may be intramural or extramural. Both benign and malignant lesions are possible (Table 87.1) [1, 2].

Table 87.1 Classification of rectal submucosal lesions that present as a mass

Intramural lesions	Extramural lesions
Leiomyoma	Endometriosis
Lipoma	Tailgut cyst
Neuroendocrine tumor	Rectal duplication
Gastrointestinal stromal tumor	Retrorectal developmental cysts
Schwannoma	Epidermoid cyst
Lymphoma	Dermoid cyst
Melanoma	Extramural tumor
Metastasis	

This case was presented at a tumor board. Magnetic resonance imaging revealed a well-circumscribed lesion that does not invade the muscularis consistent with a benign lipoma. No other therapy was offered.

References

1. Pickhardt PJ, Kim DH, Menias CO, Gopal DV, Arluk GM, Heise CP. Evaluation of submucosal lesions of the large intestine. Part 2. Nonneoplastic causes. Radiographics. 2007;27:1693–703.
2. Kim H, Kim JH, Lim JS, Choi JY, Chung YE, Park M-S, et al. MRI findings of rectal submucosal tumors. Korean J Radiol. 2011;12:487–98.

88 Gastrointestinal Stromal Tumor

Carolyn L. Power, Michael A. Valente, Abraham Ahmed, Eric W. Willis, Michelle D. Inkster, and James S. Wu

Presentation

A 70-year-old male complained of rectal pain. Digital examination revealed a posterior mass. Colonoscopy showed a bulging of the posterior rectal mucosa (Fig. 88.1). Magnetic Resonance Imaging (MRI) showed a retrorectal mass (Fig. 88.2).

Anterior resection of the rectum with coloanal anastomosis and protecting loop ileostomy was done. Histopathology is shown in Fig. 88.3.

C. L. Power · M. A. Valente · J. S. Wu (✉)
Department of Colon and Rectal Surgery, Cleveland Clinic, Cleveland, OH, USA

A. Ahmed
Diagnostic Imaging and Interventional Radiology, H. Lee Moffitt Cancer Center & Research Institute, Tampa, FL, USA

E. W. Willis
Department of Pathology, CORPath, Columbus, OH, USA

M. D. Inkster
Department of Gastroenterology, Cleveland Clinic, Cleveland, OH, USA

J. S. Wu, M. D. Inkster (eds.), *Cleveland Clinic Colorectal Case Studies*,
https://doi.org/10.1007/978-3-031-39880-3_88

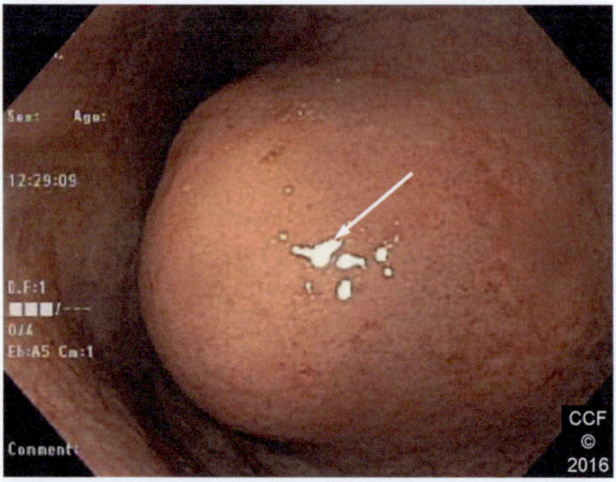

Figs. 88.1 Colonoscopic retroflexion shows an extraluminal mass effect (arrow)

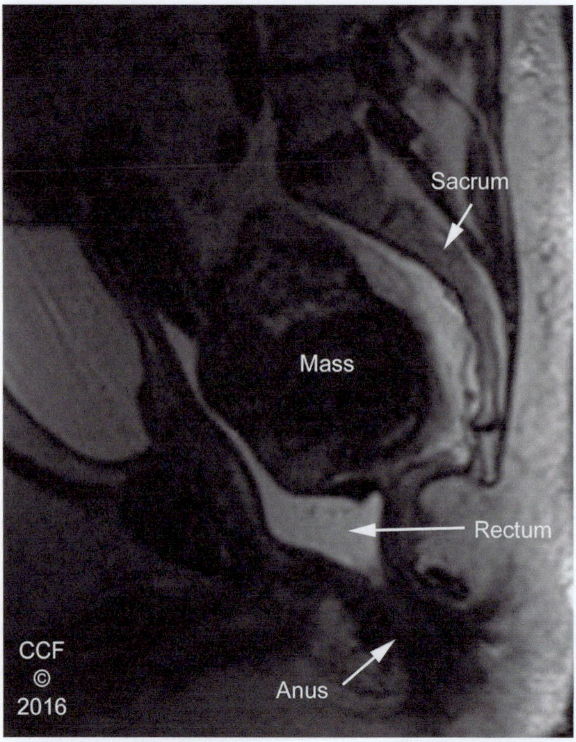

Fig. 88.2 MRI (sagittal view) shows a mass displacing the rectum anteriorly. The rectal lumen is narrowed markedly

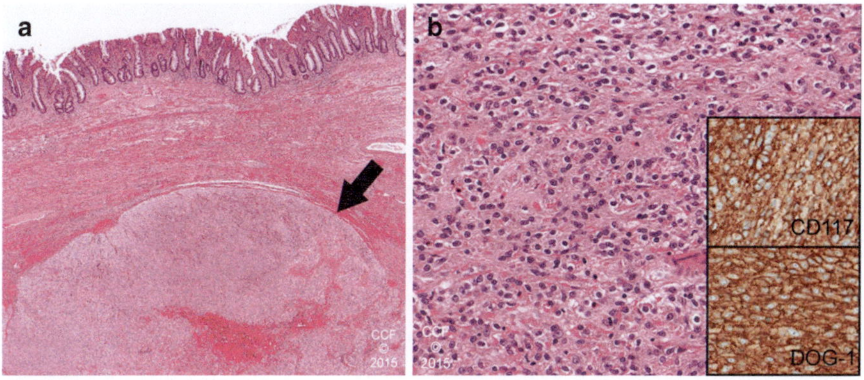

Fig. 88.3 (**a**) Submucosal mass with a pushing border (arrow) displaying epithelioid and spindled morphology (Original magnification, H&E, 20×); (**b**) High-power view showing eosinophilic tumor cells with perinuclear vacuoles in a fibrillary matrix (Original magnification, H&E, 200×). The neoplastic cells are strongly and diffusely positive for CD117 (c-KIT) and DOG-1

Comment

In 1983, Mazur and Clark described 28 gastric wall tumors classified by light microscopy as leiomyomas or leiomyosarcomas that were re-evaluated for histogenesis [1]. They called the tumors gastric stromal tumors, and it appeared that some may be of neural origin. In 1998, Hirota and colleagues reported that gastrointestinal stromal tumors (GISTs) are the most common mesenchymal neoplasm arising in the digestive tract and proposed that GISTs may arise from the interstitial cells of Cajal (ICC) [2]. Also in 1998, Kindblom et al. [3] reported that gastrointestinal stromal tumors show phenotypic characteristics of the ICCs. A review by Takaki discussed the role of ICCs as the gut pacemaker cells [4].

GISTs overexpress the tyrosine kinase receptor, KIT. DOG-1 is a protein, the antibodies to which are highly specific for GISTs and when used in conjunction with immunohistological staining for KIT/CD117, virtually confirms the diagnosis of GIST [5] Amato recommends surgery as the first-line treatment for resectable nonmetastatic colorectal GISTs [6]. In 2006, Min and Leabu [7] described the role of the interstitial cells of Cajal as follows:

> "Interstitial cells of Cajal (ICC) is a peculiar cell network composed of cells having processes described by the eminent Spanish neuroanatomist of the 19th century, S. Ramon y Cajal. Now is it is widely accepted that ICC are pace maker cells of the gut and probable progenitor cells of gastrointestinal stromal tumors (GIST)."

Biographical Note

Santiago Ramón y Cajal (1852–1934)

The study of GIST cells is incomplete without studying the life of Santiago Ramón y Cajal, after whom the interstitial cells of Cajal are named. Santiago Ramón y Cajal received his medical degree from the University of Saragossa in 1873. After serving as an army medic during an expedition to Cuba, he earned a doctorate from Madrid in 1877. He held professorships at the Universities of Valencia, Barcelona, and Madrid. He shared the 1906 Nobel Prize in Physiology or Medicine with Camillo Golgi "in recognition of their work on the structure of the nervous system." [8] Upon his death in 1934, his obituary in the British Medical Journal read [9]:

> "Cajal was entirely self-taught. His father, who was a professor of anatomy at Zaragoza, first turned his attention to the structure of the human body, and his intense love of beauty and skill in drawing stimulated his interest in histology. He owed to Golgi's publications and to photographic methods the use of silver impregnation in histological work. But apart from Golgi, he had no teachers."

References

1. Mazur MT, Clark HB. Gastric stromal tumors: Reappraisal of histogenesis. Am J Surg Pathol. 1983;7:507–19.
2. Hirota S, Isozaki K, Moriyama Y, Hashimoto K, Nishida T, Ishiguro S, et al. Gain-of-function mutations of *c-kit* in human gastrointestinal stromal tumors. Science. 1998;279:577–80.
3. Kindblom L-G, Remotti HE, Aldenborg F, Meis-Kindblom JM. Gastrointestinal pacemaker cell tumor (GIPACT). Gastrointestinal stromal tumors show phenotypic characteristics of the interstitial cells of Cajal. Am J Pathol. 1998;152:1259–69.
4. Takaki M. Gut pacemaker cells: the interstitial cells of Cajal (ICC). J Smooth Muscle Res. 2003;39:137–61.
5. DOG-1. Segen's medical dictionary. © 2012 Farlex, Inc.;. http://medical-dictionary.thefreedictionary.com/DOG-1. Accessed 21 Oct 2018.
6. Amato A. Colorectal gastrointestinal stromal tumor. Tech Coloproctol. 2010;14(Suppl 1):S91–5.
7. Min KW, Leabu M. Interstitial cells of Cajal (ICC) and gastrointestinal stromal tumor (GIST): facts, speculations, and myths. J Cell Mol Med. 2006;10:995–1013.
8. Santiago Ramón y Cajal – Biographical. NobelPrize.org. Nobel media AB 2019. 2019. <https://www.nobelprize.org/prizes/medicine/1906/cajal/biographical/.
9. Cajal R y. Obituary. Br Med J. 1934;ii:794–5.

Rectal Carcinoid

89

James S. Wu, David Hernandez Gonzalo, and Eric W. Willis

Presentation

A smooth raised rectal lesion was seen on routine colonoscopy and anoscopy (Fig. 89.1). A biopsy showed carcinoid.

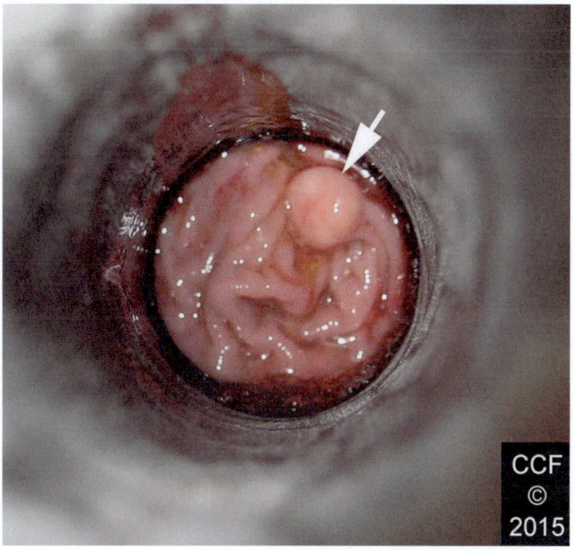

Fig. 89.1 A raised rectal lesion visualized with an anoscope (arrow). The estimated diameter was less than 1 cm

J. S. Wu (✉)
Department of Colon and Rectal Surgery, Cleveland Clinic, Cleveland, OH, USA

D. Hernandez Gonzalo
Department of Pathology, Immunology and Laboratory Medicine, University of Florida, Gainesville, FL, USA

E. W. Willis
Department of Pathology, CORPath, Columbus, OH, USA

J. S. Wu, M. D. Inkster (eds.), *Cleveland Clinic Colorectal Case Studies*,
https://doi.org/10.1007/978-3-031-39880-3_89

Management

The lesion was removed completely with a negative margin by transanal excision (Fig. 89.2a, b).

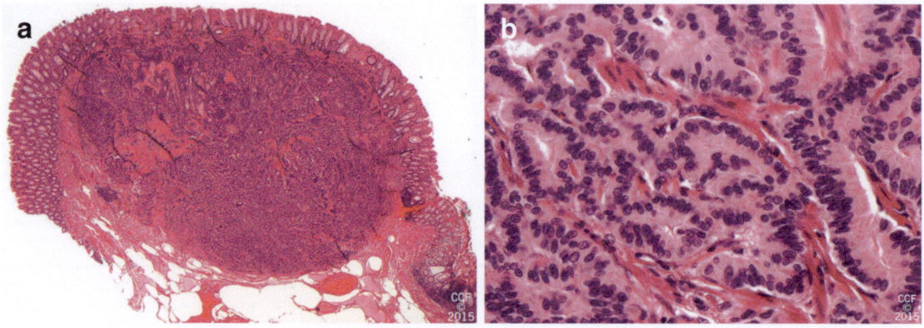

Fig. 89.2 (**a**) At low power, a well-circumscribed 6.5 mm submucosal rectal tumor undermining unremarkable rectal epithelium. The tumor is characterized by uniform cells arranged in solid nests, trabeculae and ribbons (hematoxylin-eosin, original magnification × 50). (**b**) At higher magnification, uniform bland tumor cells with eosinophilic cytoplasm and nuclei displaying characteristic "salt-and-pepper" chromatin pattern. Nucleoli are not prominent. Low mitotic index (hematoxylin-eosin, original magnification × 200)

Comment

The first histologic description of carcinoid tumors is credited to Lubarsch who in 1888 drew the microscopic appearance of two ileal cancers [1]. In 1907, Oberndorfer described carcinoid or "cancer-like" tumors of the small intestine. Histologically, the tumors looked like cancer; however, their clinical behavior suggested a more benign character. Therefore, Oberndorfer called the tumors, "Karzinoide" [2].

Karzinoide Tumoren des Dünndarms *Von* *Siegfried Oberndorfer.*	*Carcinoid tumors of the small intestine* *By* *Siegfried Oberndorfer.*
Im Laufe der letzen Jahre fand ich verschiedene Male kleine Tumoren in Dünndarm…	During the passage of the last few years, several times, I found small tumors in the small intestine...
Um nochmals die Hauptcharaktere dieser Geschwülstchen zusammenfassen:	Summarizing, once again the main characteristics of these small tumors:
1. Sie sind meistens klein, treten sehr häufig multipel auf.	1. Most are small and frequently are multiple.
2. Ihre Zellen liegen meist in undifferenzierten Verbänden, höchstens mit Andeutung von Drüsenbildungen.	2. Their cells mostly are undifferentiated groups, most with hint of glandular formation.
3. Sie sind umschrieben und haben keine Tendenz, infiltrativ in die Umgebung vorzudringen.	3. They are circumscribed and have little tendency to infiltrate the environment.
4. Sie metastasieren nicht.	4. They don't metastasize.
5. Sie wachsen anscheinend äusserst langsam, erreichen keine wesentliche Grösse und sind demzufolge anscheinend harmloser Natur.	5. They apparently grow very slowly, do not achieve a large size, and seem to have a harmless nature
Sind nun die Geschwülstchen überhaupt Krebse? Histologisch zweifellos, obwohl auch hier schon auffallen muss, dass ihr Stroma vielfach zahlreiche, von der Muscularis mucosae abstammende, glatte Muskelfasern enthält, die zum Teil sogar allein die Umrahmung der Zellennester bilden. Klinisch können sie mit grosser Einschränkung als Krebse angesehen werden, denn sie haben zweifellos kein besonderes Wachstumsvermögen, sie haben noch niemals zu schwereren Erscheinungen geführt, sie haben noch nie Metastasen gesetz, sie sind scharf umschrieben.	Now, are these small tumors cancers at all? Histologically without doubt, but it must be noted that the stroma is mostly derived from the muscularis mucosa, contains smooth muscle fibers, which in some cases form nests of cells. Clinically, one can look upon these tumors as cancer with some reservation because they don't have particular growth assets, they have never led to more severe phenomena, they have never metastasized, they are sharply circumscribed.
Vielleicht könnte man sie als Karzinoide bezeichnen.	Perhaps one could call them cancer-like.

The similarity between the carcinoid histology seen in Figs. 89.2 a, b and Oberndorfer's illustrations of two cases shown in Fig. 89.3a, b, is striking.

In 1914, Gosset and Masson described two types of appendiceal tumors [3].

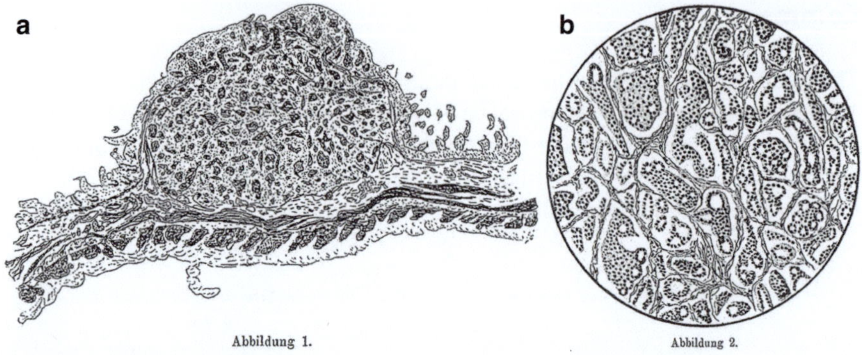

Fig. 89.3 (**a**) and (**b**) Abbildung 1, 2. Oberndorfer's histologic description reads as follows

Mikroskopisch boten sie alle dasselbe Bild: dicht stehende, grössere und kleinere Nester kleiner, dichtgedrängter, mit rundlichem Kern versehener Zellen, die ihren Haupsitz in der Submukosa haben, die Muscularis mucosae aber verschiedentlich durchbrechen und auch hier Nester bilden, untereinander anastomosieren.	Microscopically, they all presented the same picture: densely packed, larger and smaller nests of small, densely packed cells with a round nucleus, which have their main seat in the submucosa, but break through the muscularis mucosae occassionally and also form nests here, anastomosing with one another.

TUMEURS ENDOCRINE DE L'APPENDICE Par MM A. Gosset, Professeur agrégé à la Faculté, Chirurgien de la Salpêtrière et P. Masson, Assistant à L'Institut Pasteur	ENDOCRINE TUMORS OF THE APPENDIX By A. Gosset, Associate Professor at the Faculty, Surgeon at the Salpêtrière and P. Masson, Assistant to the Pasteur Institute
Conclusion.-Dans le groupe de ce qu'on appelle les cancers appendiculaires, il faut donc établir deux catégories L'une comprend les épithéliomas du type intestinal, cylindrique banal. L'autre... comprend des adénomes, des < < carcinoïdes >>, des épithéliomas vrais que la réaction de l'argent rattache à la glande endocrine de l'intestin. Ces tumeurs ne sont certainement pas l'apanage exclusif de l'appendice. Logiquement, on doit les rencontrer partout où l'épithélium endodermique contient des cellules argentaffines. Et de fait, les carcinoïdes intestinaux de Lübarsch, Oberndorfer, etc., semblent devoir être reliés au groupe endocrin de l'intestin.	Conclusion. In the group of appendiceal cancers, one must establish two categories. The first comprises epitheliomas of the intestinal type, common cylindrical The other are the adenomas, the << carcinoids >>, the epitheliomas which show a reaction with silver in the endocrine glands of the intestine. The tumors certainly are not the exclusive prerogative of the appendix Logically, one must consider all of the endodermal epithelia that react with silver. And in fact, the intestinal carcinoids of Lūbarsch, Obenerdorfer, etc. seem to make an intestinal endocrine group.

Table 89.1 Characteristics of carcinoid tumours derived from different embryonic divisions of the gut (Willliams and Sandler, 1963) [6]

	Foregut	Midgut	Hindgut
Histologic structure	Tendency to be trabecular	Characteristic	Tendency to be trabecular
Argentaffin and diazo reactions	Usually negative	Positive	Often negative
Association with the carcinoid syndrome	Frequent	Frequent	None
Tumor 5-H.T. content	Low	High	Not detected
Urinary 5-hydroxyindole-acetic acid	High	High	Normal
5-H.T.P. Secretion	Frequent	Rare	Not detected
Metastases to bone and skin	Common	Unusual	Common

5-HTP (5-hydroxytryptophan), *5-HT* (5-hydroxytryptamine)

In 1952, Erspamer et al. [4] identified 5-Hydroxytryptamine (enteramine or serotonin) as a specific storage product of enterochromaffin cells.

In 1954, Thorson and colleagues described a syndrome associated with carcinoid disease characterized by metastases to the liver, valvular disease of the right side of the heart, peripheral vasomotor symptoms and bronchoconstriction (carcinoid syndrome) [5]. The authors proposed that "5-hydoxytryptamine (enteramine or serotonin) is the one which in its effects seems most likely to correspond with the signs and symptoms of the syndrome."

In 1963, Williams and Sandler described a classification of carcinoid tumors based on gut embryonic origin, histologic structure, chemical reactivity, production of bioactive amine derivatives, and metastatic potential as shown in Table 89.1 [6].

In 1987, Moertel stated for carcinoids of the rectum size relates to metastasis: <1 cm never; >2 cm, always [7]. In 2007, Fahy et al. [8], stated that predicting rectal carcinoid behavior exclusively on tumor size was imprecise. They found that poor prognostic features include: large size, deep invasion, lymphovascular invasion, and elevated mitotic rate. In 2019, the World Health Organization noted a transition in classification from carcinoid tumors occurring in the GI tract to neuroendocrine tumors (NET) [9]. The prognosis of rectal neuroendocrine tumors is dependent on several factors including: tumor size, muscularis invasion, lymph node and distant metastases, and tumor grade [10].

References

1. Lubarsch O. Ueber den primären Krebs des ileum nebst Bemerkungen űber das gleichzeitige Verkommen von Krebs and Tuberculose. Archiv Pathol Anat Phys klin Med. 1888;111:280–317.
2. Oberndorfer S. Karzinoide Tumoren des Dünndarms. Frankf Z Pathol. 1907;1:426–32.
3. Gosset A, Masson P. Tumeurs endocrines de l'appendice. Press Med. 1914;22:237–40.
4. Erspamer V, Asero B. Identification of enteramine, the specific hormone of the enterochromaffin cell system, as 5-hydroxytryptamine. Nature. 1952;169:800–1.
5. Thorson Å, Biörck G, Björkman G, Waldenström J. Malignant carcinoid of the small intestine with metastases to the liver, valvular disease of the right side of the heart (pulmonary stenosis

and tricuspid regurgitation without septal defects), peripheral vasomotor symptoms, bronchoconstriction, and an unusual type of cyanosis. Am Heart J. 1954;47:795–817.

6. Williams ED, Sandler M. The classification of carcinoid tumours. Lancet. 1963;281(7275):238–9; This table is reused with the generous permission of Elsevier Ltd, CCC | RightsLink®, License Number 5170811432932, License date Oct 16, 2021.
7. Moertel CG. An odyssey in the land of small tumors. J Clin Oncol. 1987;5:1503–22.
8. Fahy BN, Tang LH, Klimstra D, Wong WD, Guillem JG, Paty PB, et al. Carcinoid of the rectum risk stratification (CaRRs): A strategy for preoperative outcome assessment. Ann Surg Oncol. 2007;14:1735–43.
9. Klimstra DS, Klöppel G, LaRosa S, Rindi G. Classification of neuroendocrine neoplasms of the digestive system. In: World Health Organization Classification of Tumours, 5E, WHO Classification of Tumours Editorial Board. Digestive system tumours, vol. 1. Lyon: IARC Press; 2019. p. 16–9.
10. Rodriques A, Castro-Poças F, Pedroto I. Neuroendocrine rectal tumors: main features and management. GE Port J Gatroenterol. 2015;22:213–20.

Solitary Rectal Ulcer

90

James S. Wu and Homer O. Wiland

Presentation

A 30-year-old male presented with bright red bleeding per rectum and mucous discharge.

Digital rectal examination revealed an anterior rectal mass. Pelvic magnetic resonance imaging (MRI) and flexible endoscopy with biopsy were done (Figs. 90.1, 90.2, and 90.3).

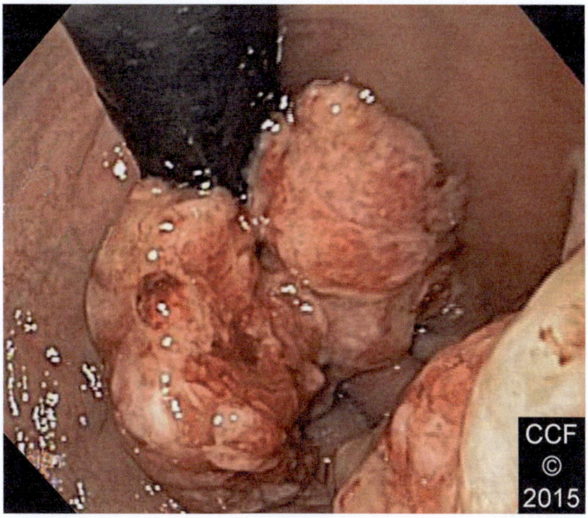

Fig. 90.1 Flexible endoscopy with retroflexed view shows a multilobulated friable mass in the anterior distal rectum

J. S. Wu (✉)
Department of Colon and Rectal Surgery, Cleveland Clinic, Cleveland, OH, USA

H. O. Wiland
Department of Pathology, OhioHealth Mansfield Hospital, Mansfield, OH, USA

J. S. Wu, M. D. Inkster (eds.), *Cleveland Clinic Colorectal Case Studies*,
https://doi.org/10.1007/978-3-031-39880-3_90

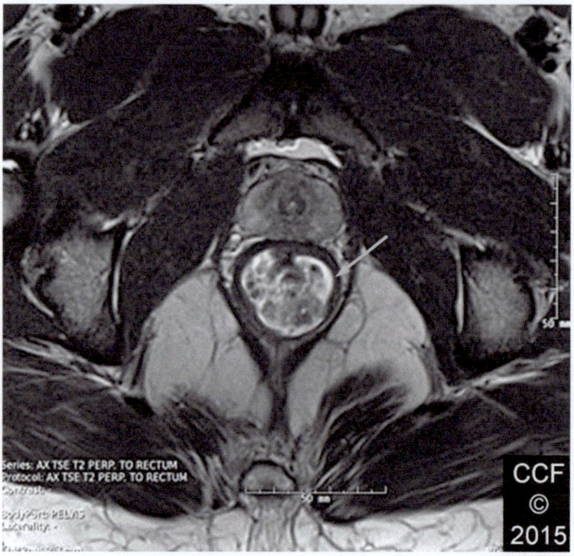

Fig. 90.2 Pelvic MRI shows an anterior rectal mass (arrow) that does not penetrate the rectal muscular wall. The mass is situated in the rectum adjacent to the prostate

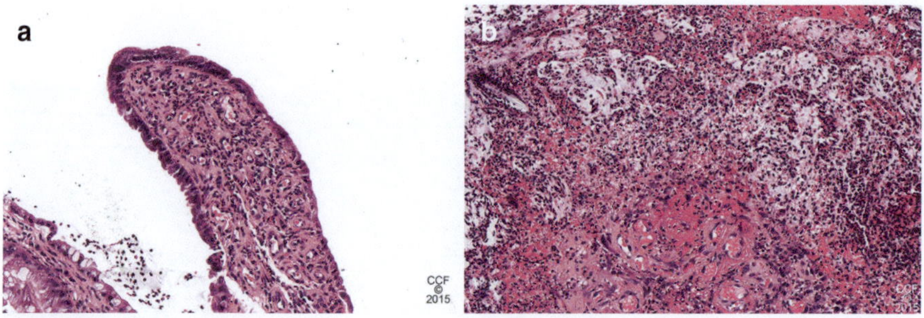

Fig. 90.3 (**a**, **b**) Description: Several of the rectal biopsy fragments consist only of ulcer and associated granulation tissue (H-E, original magnification ×100). All other fragments show portions of villiform colonic mucosa with cores of granulation tissue characterized by small, proliferating capillaries and admixed inflammatory cells. The epithelial lining shows mucin loss with well polarized, uniform, basally located nuclei, in keeping with regenerative epithelial changes (H-E, original magnification ×100). There is no evidence of dysplasia

Comment

In 1830, Cruveilhier described chronic ulceration with cicatrization of the rectum that could be mistaken for malignancy [1].

Ulcère chronique du rectum avec rétrécissement de cet intestin, pris pour un cancer de cet organe. —Mort avec les symptômes de l'étranglement. *Jean Cruveilhier* *Réflexions.* –Cette malade est donc morte avec les symptômes de l'étranglement: il est probable que si l'inflammation chronique, source de l'ulcération de l'intestin rectum avait été traitée convenablement dans le principe, le rétrécissement fibreux, conséquence presque nécessaire d'une ulcération circulaire de l'intestin qui tend à se cicatriser, aurait été prévenu. Dans l'oberservation suivante, il était bien facile de prendre l'inflammation chronique du rectum pour un cancer de cet organe, vu le désordre considérable qui existait tout autour de l'intestin.	*Chronic ulcer of the rectum with narrowing of that intestine taken as a cancer of that organ. -Death with symptoms of strangulation.* *Jean Cruveilhier* *Reflections.* -This patient died with symptoms of strangulation: it is likely that if the chronic inflammation, the source of ulceration of the rectum, had been treated properly, in principle, the fibrotic stricture, almost a necessary consequence of circular ulceration of the intestine which is predisposed to cicatrization, may have been prevented. In the following observation, it was easy to take chronic rectal inflammation for cancer of this organ, given the considerable disorder that existed around the intestine.

Rutter states that the term "solitary rectal ulcer" (SRU) was introduced by Lloyd-Davies in 1937 [2]. In 1969, Madigan and Morson described 68 patients with SRU [3]. They found that the disease is found most commonly in young adults and that it is equally common among men and women. The majority complained of bleeding and the passage of mucous on defecation. Ulceration was found with the greatest frequency on the anterior aspect of the rectal wall. Most were located at 7 to 10 cm. Ulcers frequently were situated astride a valve of Houston. More than one ulcer was seen in 30%. In five of 51 biopsies, the authors found misplaced mucosa including epithelial elements and lamina propria in the submucosa. This misplaced tissue gave appearances that may be confused with adenocarcinoma.

Tjandra et al. [4] described 80 patients with SRU. The macroscopic appearance of the lesions varied widely and included polypoid lesions, ulcerated lesions, edema, and hyperemia. The authors found that surgery was required in only one-third. Surgical procedures were performed in patients who had persistent severe symptoms causing a major alteration in lifestyle and in whom conservative measures had failed.

Vaizey et al. [5] discussed treatment options that include fiber, biofeedback behavioral retraining, and surgery. Operations include suturing, local excision, anterior resection, rectopexy, and fecal diversion. Overall, they emphasized that there is no specific cure for solitary rectal ulcer syndrome.

Biographical Note

Jean Cruveilhier (1791–1874)

Cruveilhier was a French physician and anatomist. He studied medicine at the University of Montpellier and rose to the position of Professor of Anatomy (1825) and first chair of Pathology (1836) at the University of Paris. He wrote extensively on normal and morbid anatomy [6]. His celebrated work, Anatomie Pathologiqe du Corps Human (Pathological Anatomy of the Human Body), was published in two volumes (1829–1842) [7].

In a memorial to his mentor, *Dupuytren*, Cruveilhier cautioned against ignorance and indifference [8].

L'ignorance en courant fait sa ronde homicide; L'indifférence observe, et le hasard décide.	Ignorance makes his homicidal rounds; Indifference observes, and hazard decides.

References

1. Cruveilhier J. Ulcère chronique du rectum avec rétrécissement de cet intestin, pris pour un cancer de cet organe. — Mort avec les symptômes de l'étranglement. Maladies du Rectum. Anatomie Pathologique du Corps Humain. Tome 2, 1ère partie. Paris: JB Ballière; 1842. p. 4. Accessed from Google Books November 06, 2023.
2. Rutter KRP. Solitary rectal ulcer syndrome. Proc R Soc Med. 1975;68:22–6.
3. Madigan MR, Morson BC. Solitary ulcer of the rectum. Gut. 1969;10:781–881.
4. Tjandra JJ, Fazio VW, Church JM, Lavery IC, Oakley JR, Milson JW. Clinical conundrum of solitary rectal ulcer. Dis Colon Rectum. 1992;35:227–34.
5. Vaizey CJ, van den Bogaerde JB, Emmanuel AV, Talbot IC, Nicholls RJ, Kamm MA. Solitary rectal ulcer syndrome. Br J Surg. 1998;85:1617–23.
6. Jean Cruveilhier. Britannica.com. Accessed November 21, 2023.
7. Cruveilhier J. Anatomie pathologique du corps humain. Paris: JB Bailliére; 1829/1842.
8. Cruveilhier. Vie de Dupuytren. Paris: Bechet Jeune & Labé; 1844. p. 19.

Entamoeba histolytica

91

Michelle D. Inkster, James M. Hekman, Eric W. Willis, and James S. Wu

Presentation

A 40-year-old sexually active HIV-positive homosexual male receiving highly active antiretroviral therapy complained of diarrhea. A battery of tests was sent. A test for *Entamoeba histolytica* was positive.

An image of *Entamoeba histolytica* trophozoites is shown in Fig. 91.1.

M. D. Inkster
Department of Gastroenterology, Cleveland Clinic, Cleveland, OH, USA

J. M. Hekman
Department of Internal Medicine, Cleveland Clinic, Cleveland, OH, USA

E. W. Willis
Department of Pathology, CORPath, Columbus, OH, USA

J. S. Wu (✉)
Department of Colon and Rectal Surgery, Cleveland Clinic, Cleveland, OH, USA

J. S. Wu, M. D. Inkster (eds.), *Cleveland Clinic Colorectal Case Studies*,
https://doi.org/10.1007/978-3-031-39880-3_91

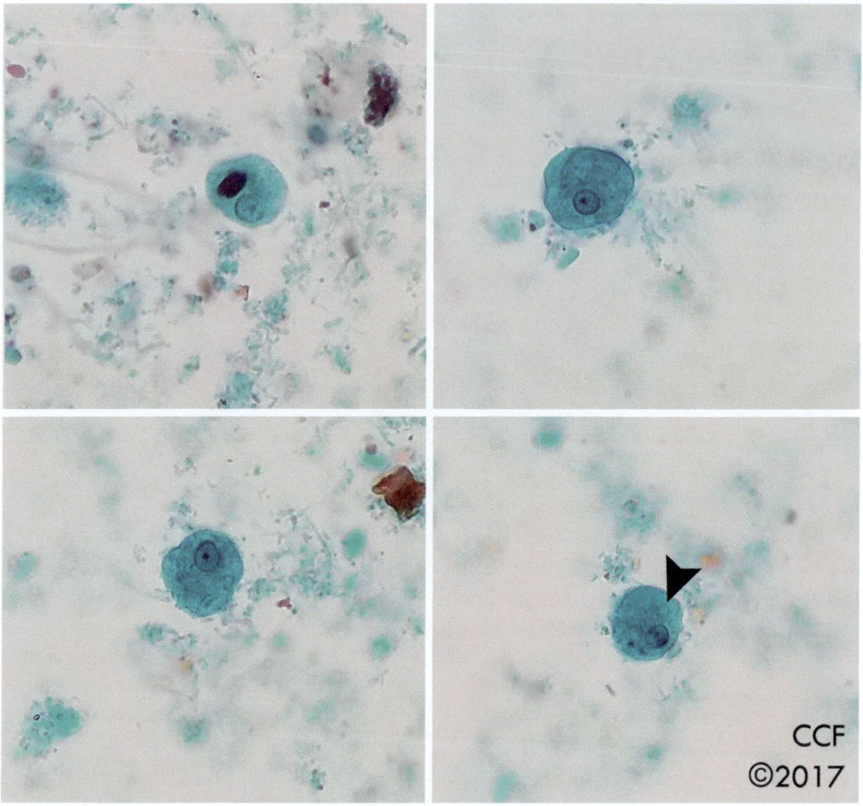

Fig. 91.1 The trichrome-stained stool sample shows multiple trophozoites with single nuclei containing a small, central karyosome. The cytoplasm contains clear spaces, representing partially digested red blood cells (arrowhead), which is consistent with *Entamoeba histolytica*

Comment [1]

Entamoeba histolytica seropositivity is more commonly seen in patients who are men who have sex with men (MSM) than in heterosexual individuals with a seroprevalence of 1–21% among MSM compared with 0–7% of heterosexuals and is diagnosed more frequently in people with HIV than those without HIV presenting with gastrointestinal symptoms. Moreover, seropositivity rates for HIV patients are higher in those with CD4 values <200 cells/uL [2].

Watanabe et al. [3] note that invasive amebiasis caused by *Entamoeba histolytica* is the second most common cause of parasitic infections worldwide. In developing countries, amebiasis usually is contracted by ingestion of contaminated water or food. Among men who have sex with men, amebiasis may be contracted by the oral anal sexual contact. Most infected patients are asymptomatic. However, amebic colitis may lead to diarrhea, perforation, or hemorrhage. In addition, abscesses may form in the liver, lungs, and brain [4].

When a patient, who is at high risk for sexually transmitted diseases, presents with diarrhea, gas, and bloating, a high index of suspicion for parasitic infection should be considered. *Entamoeba*, *Giardia,* and *Cryptosporidium* may be present in up to 20% of persons with these symptoms, especially in a population that has a high rate of HIV infection. Routine yearly testing for these organisms is recommended by some authorities.

References

1. Kazal HL, Sohn N, Carrasco JI, Robilotti JG Jr, Delaney WE. The gay bowel syndrome: Clinico-pathologic correlation in 260 cases. Ann Clin Lab Sci. 1976;6:184–92.
2. Hung CC, Chang SY, Ji DD. Entamoeba histolytica infection in men who have sex with men. Lancet Infect Dis. 2012;12(9):729–36. https://doi.org/10.1016/S1473-3099(12)70147-0. PMID: 22917103
3. Watanabe K, Gatanaga H, Escueta-de Cadiz A, Tanuma J, Nozaki T, Oka S. Amebiasis in HIV-1 infected Japanese men: clinical features and response to therapy. PLoS Negl Trop Dis. 2011;5:e1318. https://doi.org/10.1371/journal.pntd.0001318.
4. Reed SL. Amebiasis: an update. Clin Infect Dis. 1992;14:385–93.

Herpes Simplex Virus Proctitis

92

James S. Wu, Homer O. Wiland, and Eric W. Willis

Presentation

A 22-year-old male developed severe rectal pain two weeks following anoreceptive intercourse. Examination and endoscopy were done under sedation. The rectal mucosa appeared inflamed (Fig. 92.1). A biopsy was taken (Fig. 92.2).

J. S. Wu (✉)
Department of Colon and Rectal Surgery, Cleveland Clinic, Cleveland, OH, USA

H. O. Wiland
Department of Pathology, OhioHealth Mansfield Hospital, Mansfield, OH, USA

E. W. Willis
Department of Pathology, CORPath, Columbus, OH, USA

J. S. Wu, M. D. Inkster (eds.), *Cleveland Clinic Colorectal Case Studies*,
https://doi.org/10.1007/978-3-031-39880-3_92

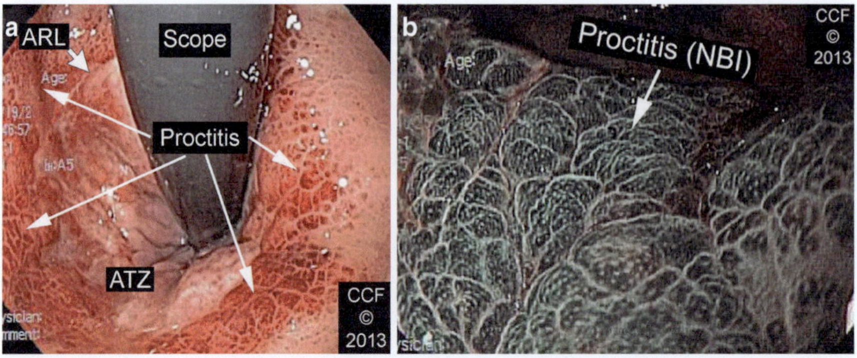

Fig. 92.1 (**a**) Flexible proctoscopy, retroflexed view, with white light shows distal rectal inflammation (proctitis). There is a sharp demarcation between the anal transitional zone (ATZ) and the columnar mucosa at the anorectal line (ARL); (**b**) the inflamed area appears green-black under illumination with narrow band imaging (NBI)

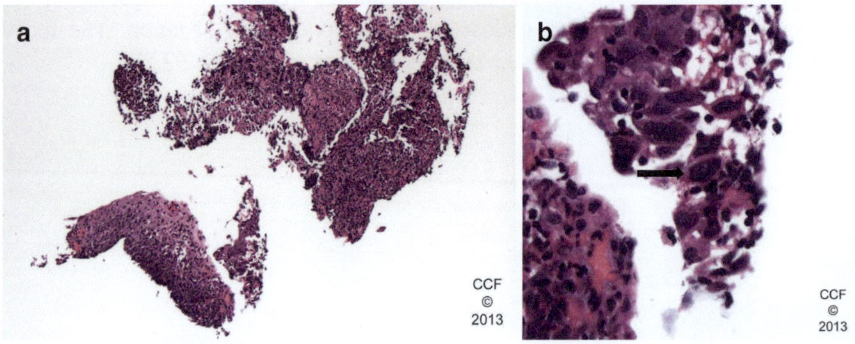

Fig. 92.2 (**a**) Biopsy of the anal transitional zone shows fragments of acutely inflamed squamous mucosa and detached fragments of fibrinopurulent debris, consistent with ulcer; (**b**) higher-power view of the squamous mucosa showed evidence of viral intranuclear inclusions. The affected epithelial cells are enlarged and show evidence of nuclear chromatin margination, nuclear molding, and multinucleation (arrow) (H-E, original magnification x 400)

Management

Tests for sexually transmitted pathogens showed Herpes simplex 1 and 2. The viral nuclear inclusion seen on biopsy was consistent with Herpes simplex infection. As shown in Fig. 92.1, the inflammation involving the distal rectum is consistent with viral introduction through intimate contact. Treatment with oral acyclovir was initiated.

Comment [1–5]

Herpes viruses have a double-stranded DNA genome. Herpes simplex virus 1 (HSV-1) transmission is primarily oral. Herpes simplex virus 2 (HSV-2) transmission is primarily genital. Replication occurs in the host cell nucleus. HSV can set up a latent infection in the ganglia of the spinal cord. Infection is by person-to-person contact. Herpes proctitis follows anoreceptive intercourse. Symptoms include fever, anorectal pain, difficulty urinating, tenesmus, and sacral dermatome paresthesia. Sigmoidoscopy shows mucosal inflammation in the distal rectum. Biopsy shows intranuclear inclusion bodies. Current therapy includes acyclovir, a synthetic antiviral that functions as an DNA polymerase inhibitor.

References

1. Diseases & Conditions, Proctitis. http://my.clevelandclinic.org/disorders/proctitis/hic_proctitis.aspx, Accessed 29 Nov 2013.
2. Goodell SE, Quinn TC, Mkrtichian E, Schuffler MD, Holmes KK, Corey L. Herpes simplex virus proctitis in homosexual men. Clinical, sigmoidoscopic, and histopathologic features. N Engl J Med. 1983;308:868–71.
3. Lamb CA, Lamb EIM, Mansfield JC, Sankar KN. Sexually transmitted infections manifesting as proctitis. Frontline Gastroenterol. 2013;4:32–40. https://doi.org/10.1136/flgastro-2012-100274.
4. Whitley RJ, Kimberlin DW, Roizman B. Herpes simplex viruses. Clin Infect Dis. 1998;26:541–55.
5. Acyclovir. Prescribers digital reference. pdr.net. Accessed 11 Jul 2021.

Histoplasma capsulatum Colitis

93

Michelle D. Inkster, Gary W. Procop, Keith K. Lai,
Erick M. Remer, Adarsh Bhimraj, Ryan M. Miller,
Marisa Tungsiripat, and James S. Wu

Presentation A

A 54-year-old HIV-positive male complained of fatigue, weakness, right lower quadrant pain, and diarrhea. He had lost 70 pounds of weight over the last year. His white blood cell count was 21.56 k/μL (3.0–11.00 k/μL). Additional diagnoses included cachexia, severe protein calorie malnutrition, and skin lesions, biopsy of which showed Kaposi's sarcoma. At presentation, he was not taking highly active retroviral therapy (HAART); his $CD4^{+}$ cell count was 15 cells/μL. Diagnostic colonoscopy with biopsy was done (Fig. 93.1).

Colon biopsies showed numerous noncaseating granulomas and yeast, highly suggestive of disseminated histoplasmosis (Fig. 93.2).

M. D. Inkster
Department of Gastroenterology, Cleveland Clinic, Cleveland, OH, USA

G. W. Procop · K. K. Lai
Pathology & Laboratory Medicine Institute, Cleveland Clinic, Cleveland, OH, USA

E. M. Remer
Radiology & Diagnostic Imaging Institute, Cleveland Clinic, Cleveland, OH, USA

J. S. Wu (✉)
Department of Colon and Rectal Surgery, Cleveland Clinic, Cleveland, OH, USA

A. Bhimraj · R. M. Miller · M. Tungsiripat
Department of Infectious Diseases, Cleveland Clinic, Cleveland, OH, USA

J. S. Wu, M. D. Inkster (eds.), *Cleveland Clinic Colorectal Case Studies*,
https://doi.org/10.1007/978-3-031-39880-3_93

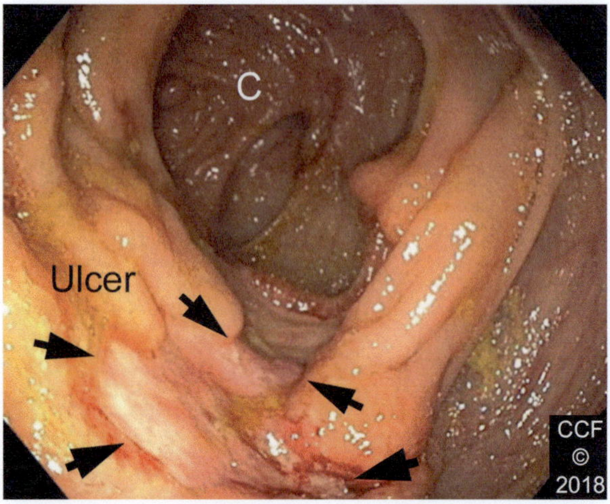

Fig. 93.1 Colonoscopy showed a proximal right colon ulcer (arrows). The cecum (C) is labeled

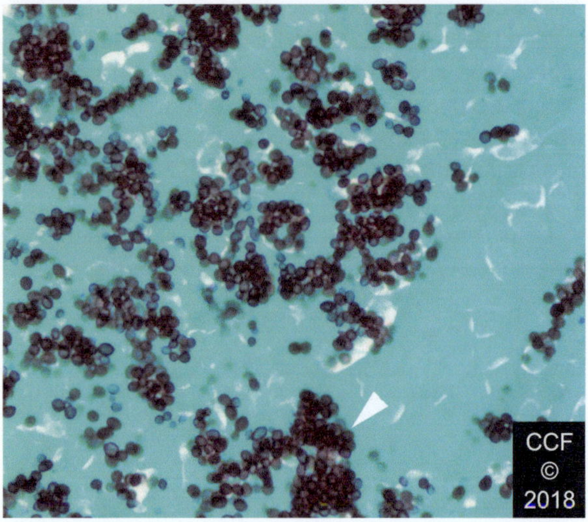

Fig. 93.2 Numerous small yeasts that were uniform in size and often appearing in clusters (white arrowhead) were seen on Grocott–Gomori's methenamine silver (GMS) stain consistent with *Histoplasma capsulatum*

Management

The *Histoplasma* urinary antigen test for this patient was positive. The patient was treated with highly active antiretroviral therapy (HAART) and antifungal medication: liposomal amphotericin B induction for 4 weeks followed by Itraconazole for one year. The patient's abdominal pain and diarrhea resolved. The *Histoplasma* urinary antigen level normalized. Follow-up colonoscopy showed resolution of the cecal ulceration.

Presentation B

A 38-year-old HIV-positive male was referred for weight loss, fever, and diarrhea. Computed tomography showed wall thickening of the cecum, ascending colon, and hepatic flexure (Fig. 93.3a, b).

Colonoscopy showed ulceration of the right colon and transverse colon (Fig. 93.4a, b).

Histologic sections showed cryptitis, granulation tissue, and noncaseating granulomas (Fig. 93.5a, b).

Because the patient was at high risk for human papilloma virus injection, rectal retroflexion was done with narrow-band imaging. Multiple raised anal transitional zone lesions were seen. Biopsies showed low-grade squamous intraepithelial lesions (LSIL).

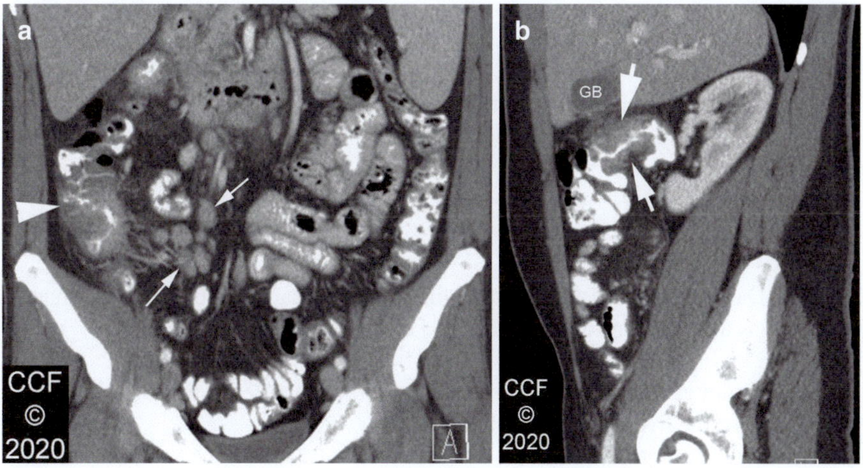

Fig. 93.3 Computed tomography: (**a**) Wall thickening of the cecum and right colon (arrow head) and a cluster of enlarged lymph nodes (arrows), coronal view; (**b**) Thickening of the hepatic flexure (arrows), sagittal view. The adjacent gallbladder (GB) also is labeled

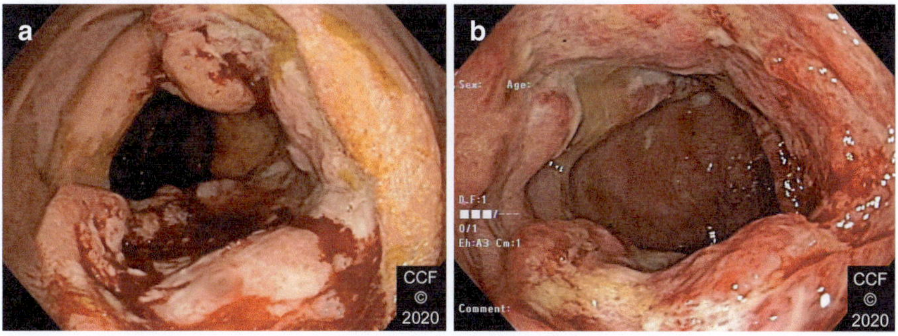

Fig. 93.4 Colonic ulceration seen at colonoscopy; (**a**) Right colon; (**b**) Transverse colon

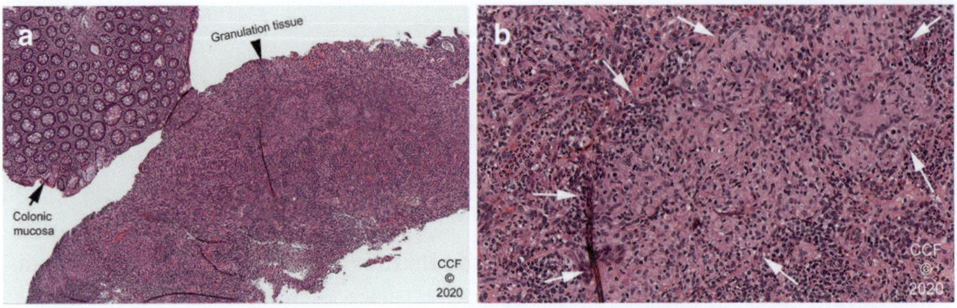

Fig. 93.5 (**a**) Low-resolution histologic sections from the ascending colon biopsy specimen demonstrated colonic mucosa with neutrophilic cryptitis (arrow) and prominent granulation tissue consistent with ulcer (arrowhead); (**b**) In high-resolution histologic sections, multiple noncaseating granulomas (arrows) were seen

Management

The patient was treated with the antifungal drug, Itraconazole. He was referred for endoscopic ablation of anal dysplasia.

Comment

In 1906, Darling reported the autopsy findings of a patient who died of what he thought was a unique protozoan infection [1].

> A protozoön general infection producing pseudotubercles in the lungs and focal necroses in the liver, spleen and lymphnodes.
> Samuel L. Darling, M.D.
> Pathologist, Ancon Hospital
> Ancon, Canal Zone, Isthmus of Panama

> On Dec. 7, 1905, while examining smears from the lungs, spleen and bone marrow, in a case that appeared to be miliary tuberculosis of the lungs, I found enormous numbers of small bodies generally oval or round.
>
> Intestines: There were a few small superficial circular ulcers from 2 to 4 mm. in diameter in the cecum and ileum.
>
> There is seen to be a general infection by a parasite having a predilection for endothelial and epithelial cells.
>
> For the parasite, the name *Histoplasma capsulata* is proposed.

The etymology of this name appears to be derived from histo (Greek, histos, tissue), plasma (fluid), and capsule (enclosing structure). In 1908, Darling described three cases of histoplasmosis [2].

"Histoplasmosis is a term applied to a fatal infection by a protozoon, *Histoplasma capsulatum*, which has been encountered three times during the past two and one-half years in Ancon Hospital, Canal Zone, Panama.

The most striking clinical features are splenomegaly, emaciation, irregular remittent temperature and leukopenia.

The microorganism was found in endothelial cells lining blood and lymph vessels and in areas of necrosis and pseudo-granulomata, in the intestinal tract, spleen, liver, lungs, lymph nodes and rib marrow.

The bodies are round and oval. There is among the larger forms a tendency toward an oval outline. An average-sized spherical body is 3 microns in diameter. The bodies are always surrounded by a clear, refractile, achromatic zone or capsule, giving the impression at once of an encysted protozoon. The body does not stain hemogenously but very irregularly, hardly any two parasites looking exactly alike. The body consists of a deeply staining substances, or chromatin, a faintly staining substance staining light blue with polychrome stains; and achromatic spaces.

Twenty-four hours after the death of the host, the chromatin and faintly staining basophilic substance of the micro-organism stains beautifully."

In 1934, Dodd and Tompkins described a case of Darling's disease in an infant who subsequently died.[1]

A case of histoplasmosis of Darling in an infant
Katharine Dodd and Edna H. Tompkins
From the Departments of Pediatrics and Anatomy, Vanderbilt University School of Medicine, Nashville, Tennessee

"A six-month-old, white, male infant, a native of Tennessee, was brought to the Vanderbilt Hospital on November 11, 1932. He had been gaining and developing normally until three weeks before admission, when he developed what was called a "cold." One week after the onset of the illness, he began to cough paroxysmally and to vomit with coughing. Two days before admission, his mother noticed a "lump" in the left upper abdomen. The baby became drowsy and feverish and refused to nurse.

The day after admission, after receiving a transfusion of blood, the child was taken home against advice. He was readmitted on November 20, 1932.

The laboratory findings on this admission were:… white blood cells, 17,700…. The pH of the blood was 7.04;…

The supravital studies of the blood,… did reveal a parasitic invasion of the large mononuclear cells,… The parasitic inclusions were oval or round and strikingly uniform in size. Including the capsule, they measured about 5 by 3 microns.

Treatment of the overwhelming parasitic invasion of the body was problematical and seemed almost hopeless. Symptomatic treatment was, however, given. The child received sodium bicarbonate and a transfusion of blood intravenously, but showed only temporary improvement. He died suddenly on November 23, 1932, three days after his second admission."

[1] Dodd and Tompkins [3]. Permission to reproduce this excerpt was generously provided by Ms. Cathi Siegel, Managing Editor, American Journal of Tropical Medicine and Hygiene, August 24, 2021.

At autopsy, De Monbreun obtained material from which *Histoplasma capsulatum* successfully was cultivated.[2]

The cultivation and cultural characteristics of Darling's Histoplasma capsulatum
W. A. De Monbreun
From the Department of Pathology, Vanderbilt University Medical School, Nashville, Tennessee

"The autopsy of the case whose clinical disease was Darling's histoplasmosis was done within two hours following the death of the patient. As soon as the spleen was removed its surface was seared and pieces of tissue were obtained from it as aseptically as possible. In smears of this tissue there occurred large numbers of endothelial cells within which could be seen enormous numbers of the yeast-like organisms previously described.

…culture media were immediately inoculated with minute fragments of the splenic tissue:…

Examination of the cultures…, after eighteen days incubation at room temperature, revealed pure cultures of a fungus….

By means of intravenous injections of cultures of the yeast-like form of the fungus, a fatal disease, possessing all the important clinical and pathologic features exhibited by all the reported cases of Darling's histoplasmosis, has been induced in two monkeys (*M. rhesus*). Following an intravenous injection of 5 cc. of a broth suspension of a three day culture from a blood agar slant, each animal rapidly became emaciated and anemic, and showed marked enlargement of their superficial lymph nodes. Both animals developed a bloody diarrhea. Three days before death, which, in each instance occurred on the fourteenth day following the injection, the parasites were demonstrated within the mononuclear cells in smears of the peripheral blood. The lesions characteristic of the human disease were observed at autopsy of these animals.

The fungus cultivated from the sixth case, and described in this paper, fulfils all of Koch's postulates."

Colitis due to fungal infection with *Histoplasma capsulatum* is illustrated in Presentations A and B (above).

In their 2007 review of colonic histoplasmosis, Psarros and Kauffman state that:[3]

"All gastrointestinal (GI) forms of histoplasmosis are likely manifestations of disseminated disease.

H. capsulatum has the ability to remain within the host for years after the initial infection. This presence allows reactivation to occur when cellular immunity is diminished, sometimes long after the individual has left the endemic region.

[2] DeMonbreun [4]. Permission to reproduce this excerpt was generously provided by Ms. Cathi Siegel, managing editor, American journal of tropical medicine and hygiene, October 19, 2021.

[3] Psarros and Kauffman [5]. This excerpt is reused with the generous permission of Ms. Christina Lesica, senior managing editor, gastroenterol hepatology, New York, June 14, 2022.

The pathologic findings of GI tract histoplasmosis include mucosal ulceration, diffuse lymphohistiocytic infiltration of the bowel wall, submucosal nodules, polypoid lesions, and obstructing masses.

The terminal ileum and the colon are the most frequently involved organs, and bowel perforation and hemorrhage are noted as the most common serious complications.

Unremitting diarrhea with malabsorption has been noted, as has bloody diarrhea mimicking inflammatory bowel disease."

Georgios Psarros, MD and
Carol A. Kauffman, MD
Division of Infectious Diseases
Department of Internal Medicine
Veterans Affairs, Ann Arbor Healthcare System
Univeristy of Michigan Medical School
Ann Arbor, Mich.

The differential diagnosis for patients with colonic strictures is listed in Table 93.1. Colonic stricturing raises the possibility of neoplasm. Colonoscopy with biopsy helps to make the diagnosis.

Diagnostic tests that make the diagnosis of histoplasmosis are listed in Table 93.2.

Table 93.1 Differential diagnosis for colonic stricture

Malignancy
Tuberculosis
Crohn's disease
Ischemia
Anastomotic
Histoplasmosis

Table 93.2 Diagnostic tests for histoplasmosis

Component	Reference range	Results
Histoplasma Ag, blood	None detected (ng/mL)	2.56
Histo yeast—CF	<1:8 dilutions	1:64
Histo mycelial Ab—CF	<1:8 dilutions	1:128
Histoplasma Ag, urine	None detected (ng/mL)	1.29
Histoplasma Ab, ID	Negative	Positive

References

1. Darling ST. A protozoön general infection producing pseudotubercles in the lungs and focal necrosis in the liver, spleen and lymphnodes. J Am Med Assoc. 1906;46:1283–5.
2. Darling ST. Histoplasmosis: a fatal infectious disease resembling kala-azar found among natives of tropical America. Arch Intern Med. 1908;ii:107–23.
3. Dodd K, Tompkins EH. A case of histoplasmosis of Darling in an infant. Am J Trop Med. 1934;14:127–37.
4. DeMonbreun WA. The cultivation and cultural characteristics of Darling's Histoplasma capsulatum. Am J Trop Med. 1934;S1–14:93–125.
5. Psarros G, Kauffman CA. Colonic histoplasmosis: a difficult diagnostic problem. Gastroenterol Hepatol. 2007;3:461–3.

Koch's Postulates

94

James S. Wu

Presentation

The causal relationship between an infectious agent and disease was defined by Jakob Henle and his pupil, Robert Koch [1]. Their ideas were presented in an 1884 lecture by Koch on the etiology of tuberculosis.

Die Aetiologie der Tuberkulose	*The Etiology of Tuberculosis*
von Dr. R. Koch, 1884 [2]	*By Dr. R. Koch, 1884* [3]
Oft wird dieser Einwand allerdings eine gewisse Berechtigung haben und es gehört deswegen zur vollständigen Beweisführung, dass man sich nicht allein damit benügt, das Zusammentreffen der Krankheit und der Parasiten zu constatiren, sondern dass ausserdem direct diese Parasiten als die eigentlche Ursache der Krankheit nachgewiesen werden. Dies kann nur in der Weise geschehen, dass die Parasiten von dem erkrankten Organismus vollständig abgetrennt und von allen Produkten der Krankheit, welchen etwa ein krankmachender Einfluss zugeschrieben werden könnte, befreit werden, und dass durch Einführung der isolirten Parasiten in den gesunden Organismus die Krankheit mit Allen ihren eigenthümlichen Eigenschaften von Neuem hervorgerufen wird.	The facts obtained in this manner can in every possible way serve as proof to which only extreme skepticism can still raise the objection that the organisms found are not the cause but only concurrent phenomena of the disease. To be sure, this objection often has a real justification and therefore it is not sufficient to establish only the concomitant occurrence of disease and parasite but the parasite must be shown to be the real cause. This can be done only by fully isolating the parasite from the body and all products of disease which might be considered as having a deleterious effect and producing the disease again with all its characteristics by the introduction of the isolated organisms into a normal host.

The Nobel Prize in Physiology or Medicine 1905 was awarded to Robert Koch "for his investigations and discoveries in relation to tuberculosis" [4].

J. S. Wu (✉)
Department of Colon and Rectal Surgery, Cleveland Clinic, Cleveland, OH, USA

J. S. Wu, M. D. Inkster (eds.), *Cleveland Clinic Colorectal Case Studies*,
https://doi.org/10.1007/978-3-031-39880-3_94

References

1. Evans AS. Causation and disease: The Henle-Koch postulates revisited. Yale J Biol Med. 1976;49:175–95.
2. Koch R. Die Aetiologie der Tuberkulose. Mitt Kaiser Gesund, vol. 2; 1884. p. 1–88.
3. Rivers TM. Viruses and Koch's postulates. J Bacteriol. 1937;33:1–12.
4. Robert Koch. The Nobel Prize in physiology or medicine 1905. NobelPrize.org. Nobel Media AB 2020. 2020. <https://www.nobelprize.org/prizes/medicine/1905/summary/>.

Colonoscopic Electrosurgical Snare Polypectomy

95

James S. Wu and Michelle D. Inkster

Presentation

A 50-year-old patient underwent screening colonoscopy. A sessile polyp, seen near the hepatic flexure, was removed by electrosurgical snare polypectomy (Fig. 95.1).

Pathology showed tubular adenoma.

J. S. Wu (✉)
Department of Colon and Rectal Surgery, Cleveland Clinic, Cleveland, OH, USA

M. D. Inkster
Department of Gastroenterology, Cleveland Clinic, Cleveland, OH, USA

J. S. Wu, M. D. Inkster (eds.), *Cleveland Clinic Colorectal Case Studies*,
https://doi.org/10.1007/978-3-031-39880-3_95

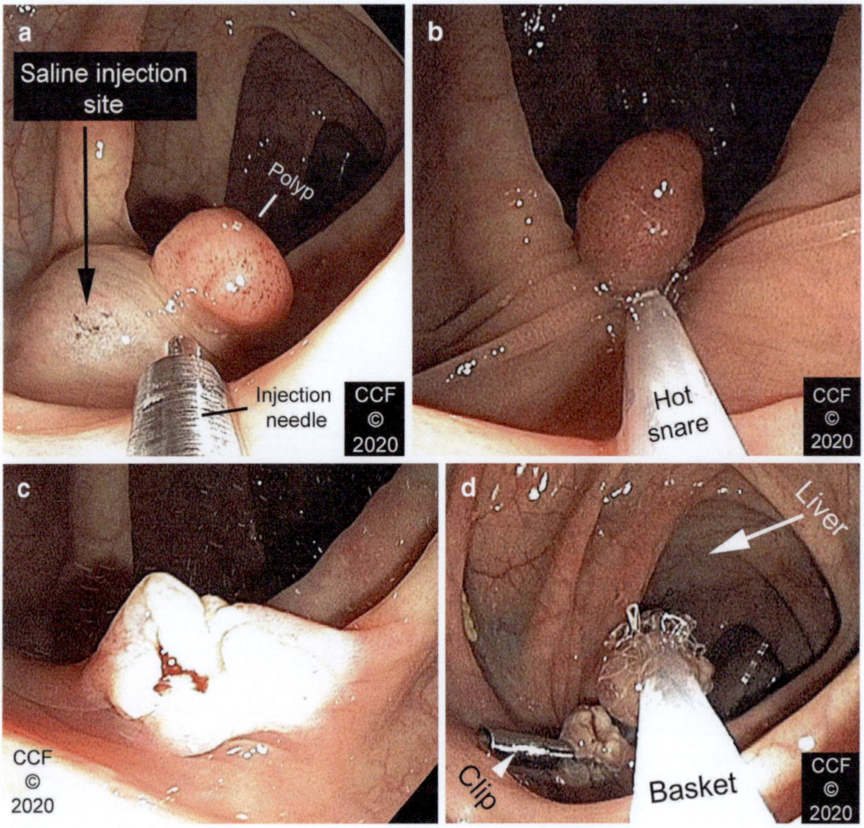

Fig. 95.1 (**a**) The polyp is raised with saline. The saline injection needle and the saline injection site are labelled; (**b**) The polyp is removed by electrosurgical snare polypectomy; (**c**) the postpolypectomy base; (**d**) The postpolypectomy base was closed with a clip. The polyp was retrieved with a basket. The liver is seen through the wall of the hepatic flexure

Comment

In 1948, Cattell published a review on the then current standards for the treatment of polyps of the large intestine.[1]

> "The discovery and treatment of intestinal polyps while still in a benign or premalignant state is of the utmost importance. The destruction of polyps in the lower segments by fulguration or their removal from the proximal segments by laparotomy permits local removal without the necessity for removal of large segments of the intestine which becomes necessary when malignant degeneration has occurred."
>
> Richard B. Cattell, M.D.
>
> The Department of Surgery, The Lahey Clinic, Boston, Massachusetts

[1] Cattell [1]. This excerpt is reused with the generous permission of Elsevier, CCC|RightsLink®, License number 5207241245657, License date Dec 13, 2021.

Table 95.1 Management of colon and rectal polyps (Cattell, 1948)

Location	Detection	Management
Rectum and rectosigmoid	Sigmoidoscopy	Transanal fulguration, Transanal excision, Endotherm snare Resection
Colon	Air contrast enema Manual palpation	Colotomy and excision, colonic resection

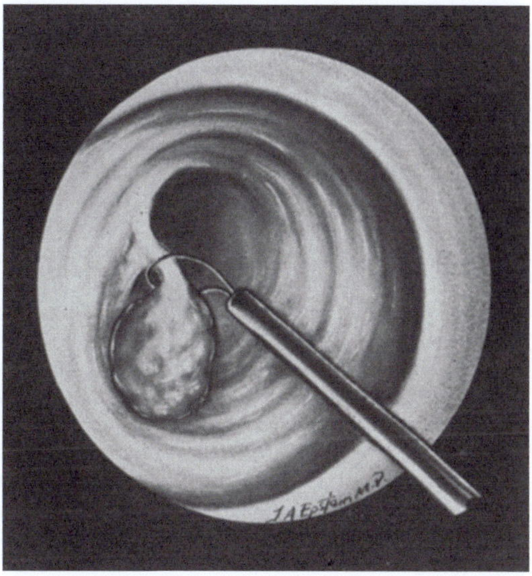

Fig. 95.2 Position of wire of electric snare around the stalk of pedunculated polyp (Turell, 1948). This figure is reused with the generous permission of Elsevier, CCC|RightsLink®, license number 5207680885915, license date Dec 14, 2021

Polyp detection was primarily by barium contrast study and rigid proctosigmoidoscopy. Methods for the management of colon and rectal polyps (not due to congenital polyposis) discussed by Cattell are listed in Table 95.1.

In the same December 1948 issue of the American Journal of Surgery, Turell described a sigmoidal electrosurgical snare that was designed to remove rectosigmoid polyps (Fig. 95.2).[2]

> "The pedunculated polyp may or may not be grasped at its tip with a suitable forceps before a wire snare is applied to the pedicle about 0.5 cm from the base. After the electric activation of the wire loop of the snare, the stalk of the polyp is strangulated by pulling the wire loop slowly into the hollow of the shaft of the snare, thus electrically amputating the tumor cleanly and efficiently."
>
> Robert Turell, M.D.
>
> New York

[2]Turell [2]. This excerpt is reused with the generous permission of Elsevier, CCC|RightsLink®, License number 5207690165024, License date Dec 14, 2021.

In his review of snare polypectomy, Sivak[3] states that it was Dr. Hiromi Shinya who performed the first colonoscopic electrosurgical snare polypectomy in September 1959.

Polypectomy: Looking Back

> "The only thing new in the world is the history you don't know"
> Harry S. Truman
>
> 'Colonoscopic polypectomy as practiced today is essentially the invention of a young resident in surgery, Dr. Hiromi Shinya, who enlisted the assistance of a junior engineer, Mr. Hiroshi Ichikawa.
>
> Shinya: "In the beginning, I sometimes had the opportunity to do colonoscopy during surgery when the abdomen was open, mainly to search for additional polyps during operations to remove polyps. The allowed me to observe the effects of pushing and pulling on the colon and the mesentary. The secret of success was right- and left-hand coordination. The key was to 'widen' the sigmoid-descending colon junction. I discovered the alpha loop maneuver by accident, but this seemed to open the junction, and so I began to do the maneuver on purpose. I found that rotation and pulling back, hooking a fold, was helpful, and then, as a third thing, I realized the importance of 'telescoping' the colon."
>
> The first report of colonoscopic polypectomy (11 cases) was by Dr. Shinya, then still a fellow in surgery, to the New York Surgical Society in 1970. He presented his experience with colonoscopic polypectomy to the American Society for Gastrointestinal Endoscopy (ASGE) in May 1971 at its plenary session in Miami Beach, Florida. Dr. Shinya and Mr. Ichikawa never applied for a patent on the polypectomy snare.
>
> Why is colonoscopic polypectomy the "most important" achievement of the great era of GI endoscopy? It is the prototypic endoscopic therapeutic procedure, the basic blueprint for many significant endoscopic devices that followed. That which was once labeled "very dangerous" now surpasses all other endoscopic therapeutic procedures in terms of numbers performed, and it surely impacts the lives of millions of people throughout the world. As we now know, removal of colon polyps prevents colorectal cancer, and colonoscopic polypectomy is the "most important" achievement, because it is preventative medicine at its best.'
>
> Michael V. Sivak Jr., MD
> Cleveland, Ohio

References

1. Cattell RB. Surgical treatment of polyps of the large intestine. Am J Surg. 1948;76:733–47.
2. Turell R. Colonic adenomas. Am J Surg. 1948;76:783–9.
3. Sivak MV Jr. Polypectomy: looking back. Gastrointestinal Endos. 2004;60:977–82.

[3] Sivak [3] . Permission to reuse these excerpts was granted by Elsevier, CCC|RightLink®, License number 5155160483636, License date Sep 24, 2021.

Endoscopic Submucosal Dissection

96

Emre Gorgun, Kelsey E. McHugh, Sami S. Judeeba, Tasadooq Hussain, and James S. Wu

Presentation

An 80-year-old man underwent colonoscopy. A 40-mm sessile polyp was seen on retroflexion (Fig. 96.1). The patient was referred for endoscopic submucosal dissection (ESD).

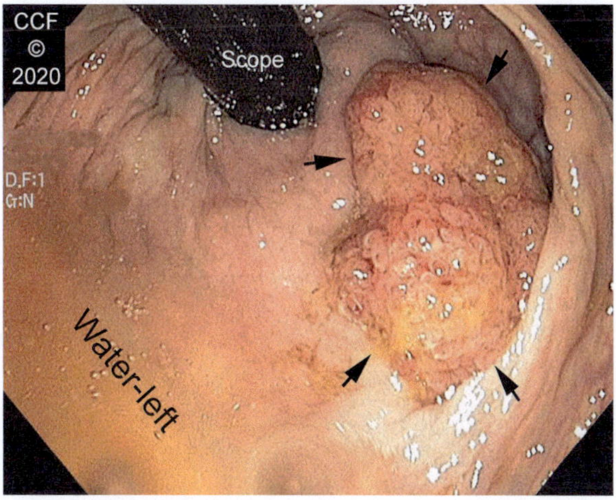

Fig. 96.1 With the patient in the left lateral decubitus position, the polyp is seen at location in the distal rectum opposite the water. The polyp was not biopsied or tattooed

E. Gorgun · S. S. Judeeba · J. S. Wu (✉)
Department of Colon and Rectal Surgery, Cleveland Clinic, Cleveland, OH, USA

K. E. McHugh
Department of Laboratory Medicine and Pathology, Mayo Clinic, Phoenix, AZ, USA

T. Hussain
Department of General and Colorectal Surgery, Wrightington Wigan & Leigh Teaching Hospitals NHS Foundation Trust, Manchester, UK

J. S. Wu, M. D. Inkster (eds.), *Cleveland Clinic Colorectal Case Studies*,
https://doi.org/10.1007/978-3-031-39880-3_96

Endoscopic Submucosal Dissection

The lesion was raised by submucosal injection of saline in order to lift the polyp from the muscularis propria (Fig. 96.2a). A circumferential incision around the lesion into the submucosa was performed with a dual knife. The lesion was then dissected from the underlying deep layers (Fig. 96.2b) with an electrocautery knife and retrieved. The area resected was 50 mm in total. To repair the defect, the tissue edges were approximated with four hemostatic clips (Fig. 96.2c). There was no bleeding during the procedure. The resected specimen was submitted intact (Fig. 96.2d).

Surveillance examination at six months and at three years showed no residual tumor.

Surgical pathology showed tubulovillous adenoma with extensive high-grade dysplasia, completely excised. There was no evidence of invasive adenocarcinoma (Fig. 96.3a–d).

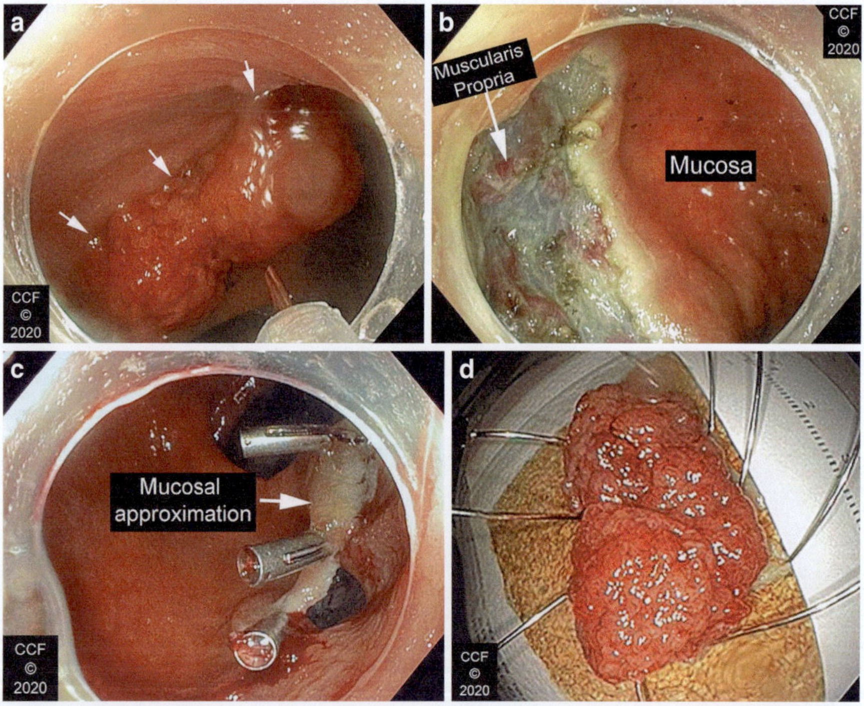

Fig. 96.2 (**a**) The lesion is raised by submucosal injection of saline at the polyp base (arrows); (**b**) The mucosal lesion is lifted off of the muscularis (arrow); (**c**) Following lesion removal, the mucosal defect is approximated with clips; (**d**) The resected polyp is submitted for histologic examination in one piece

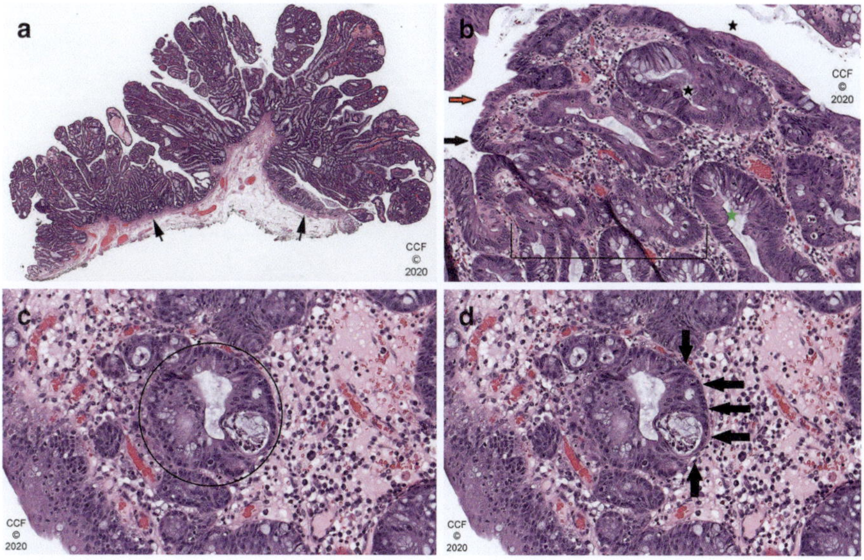

Fig. 96.3 Endoscopic submucosal dissection of a tubulovillous adenoma with high-grade dysplasia. (**a**) Low-power view. The dissection margin is clear of the muscularis mucosae (arrows); (**b**) This focus of high-grade dysplasia is characterized by severe cytologic and architectural atypia. Cytologic atypia includes nuclear rounding, nuclear enlargement, coarse (black arrow) to open (red arrow) nuclear chromatin, variably prominent nucleoli, nuclear pseudostratification (green star), and loss of nuclear polarity (black star) from the base to the surface of the mucosa. The glands lined by this severe cytologic atypia demonstrate architectural complexity characterized by evolving intraluminal cribriforming (bracket) as well as focal intraluminal necroinflammatory debris; (**c**) The circle delineates the location of the basement membrane surrounding the colonic crypts; (**d**) The arrows point to the intact basement membrane

Comment [1]

In 2004, Yahagi et al. [2] described endoscopic submucosal dissection for *en bloc* resection of colorectal mucosal tumors.

> "Endoscopic submucosal dissection (ESD) has been developed for the en bloc resection of mucosal tumors of gastrointestinal tract and widely applied, especially to gastric lesions. However, the large intestine involves the following issues that are not seen in the upper gastrointestinal tract:
>
> 1. Very thin walls present a high risk of perforation;
> 2. Enterobacterium-induced, serious peritonitis, may develop in the event of perforation; and
> 3. Lumen is narrow and angulated, causing poor operability of an endoscope and generating higher difficulty in endoscopic procedure."
>
> Naohisa Yahagi, Mitsuhiro Fujishiro,
> Atsushi Imagawa, Naomi Kakushima,
> Mikitaka Iguchi, Masao Omata
> The University of Tokyo,
> Wakayama Medical University, Japan

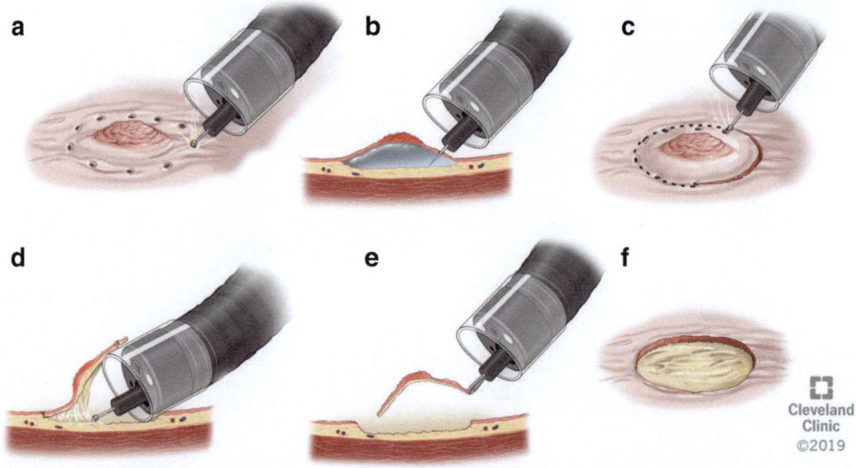

Fig. 96.4 (**a**) A 2–3-mm circumferential border around the polyp is scored using an electrosurgical knife; (**b**) Lifting agents, dilute epinephrine, and dyes are injected into the submucosal space; (**c**) Dissection around the border is started and continued along the first half of the lesion to enter deep into the submucosal space; (**d**) The submucosal space is visualized clearly; (**e**) *en bloc* removal is done; (**f**) Following specimen removal, hemostasis is achieved, and the wound is closed with clips

In addition, the authors state that

> "The strict indications for ESD are lesions that cannot be resected en bloc by conventional procedures, but requires a precise histopathologic evaluation;…"

In 2013, Nakajima et al. [3] reported the results of a multicenter study in Japan surveying the then current status of endoscopic treatment for relatively large colorectal neoplasms (CRNs) and concluded that endoscopic submucosal dissection (ESD) is a feasible treatment for patients with mucosal CRN > 20 mm.

The steps involved in endoscopic submucosal dissection are summarized in Fig. 96.4 [4].

References

1. Sapci I, Gorgun E. Advanced colonic polypectomy. Surg Clin N Am. 2020;100:1079–89.
2. Yahagi N, Fujishiro M, Imagawa A, Kakushima N, Iguchi M, Omata M. Endoscopic submucosal dissection for the reliable en bloc resection of colorectal mucosal tumors. Dig Endosc. 2004;16(Suppl):S89–92.
3. Nakajima T, Saito Y, Tanaka S, Iishi H, Kudo S-e, Ikematsu H, et al. Current status of endoscopic resection strategy for large, early colorectal neoplasia in Japan. Surg Endosc. 2013;27:3262–70.
4. Yoshida N, Naito Y, Murakami T, Hirose R, Ogiso K, Inada Y, et al. Tips for safety in endoscopic submucosal dissection for colorectal tumors. Ann Transl Med. 2017;5:185.

Malignant Colon Polyp-3.0 mm Margin 97

James S. Wu and Homer O. Wiland

Presentation

A 50-year-old female underwent screening colonoscopy. A 1.5 cm pedunculated polyp was found. The polyp site was tattooed adjacent to the base, and the polyp was removed by snare polypectomy (Fig. 97.1). Resection and retrieval were complete. The pathologic diagnosis was invasive well-differentiated adenocarcinoma

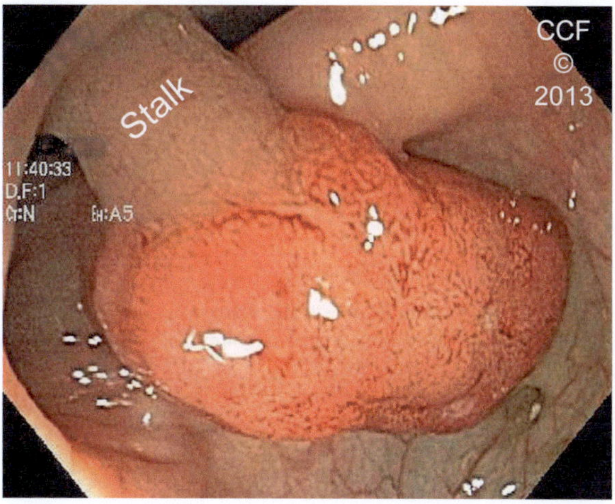

Fig. 97.1 5 cm pedunculated sigmoid colon polyp removed by snare

J. S. Wu (✉)
Department of Colon and Rectal Surgery, Cleveland Clinic, Cleveland, OH, USA

H. O. Wiland
Department of Pathology, OhioHealth Mansfield Hospital, Mansfield, OH, USA

J. S. Wu, M. D. Inkster (eds.), *Cleveland Clinic Colorectal Case Studies*,
https://doi.org/10.1007/978-3-031-39880-3_97

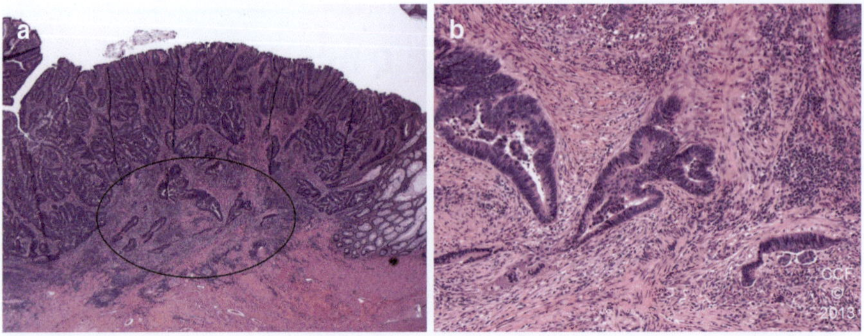

Fig. 97.2 (**a**) Low-power view of the polyp is remarkable for adenomatous change of the surface epithelium, characterized by a dark, hyperchromatic appearance (contrast with normal appearing colonic epithelium at the far right of the image). Several glands with an infiltrative appearance (circled) are identified within the stroma of the polyp's stalk, suspicious for invasive adenocarcinoma (H&E, original magnification ×20); (**b**) higher-power views of the suspicious areas seen on low-power highlight angulated glands (Fig. 97.2) as well as infiltrative single cells set within an altered, desmoplastic stroma, diagnostic of invasive adenocarcinoma (H&E, original magnifications ×400)

(Fig. 97.2). The lesion invaded into the submucosa. The tumor was 3.0 mm from the cauterized margin. The deep (stalk margin) was uninvolved by invasive carcinoma. Lymphovascular invasion was not identified. The carcinoma was microsatellite stable.

This malignant polyp had favorable histology (well-differentiation, >2 mm free margin) [1]. The patient was entered into a surveillance program. No recurrence has been seen after more than 10 years.

Reference

1. Volk EE, Goldblum JR, Petras RE, Carey WD, Fazio VW. Management and outcome of patients with invasive carcinoma arising in colorectal polyps. Gastroenterology. 1995;109:1801–7. See Comment in Chapter 98

Malignant Colon Polyp-0.725 mm Margin

98

Jean H. Ashburn, Gregory Zuccaro, Jr., Homer O. Wiland, Eric W. Willis, and James S. Wu

Presentation

A 63-year-old female presented for screening colonoscopy. A 1.5 cm pedunculated sigmoid colon polyp was identified and removed by snare polypectomy (Fig. 98.1a, b). The polypectomy site was marked with India ink. Specimen integrity was intact. The polyp size was 1.3 cm × 1.2 cm × 1 cm. Pathology showed invasive well-differentiated to moderately differentiated colonic adenocarcinoma arising in association with a tubular adenoma with high-grade dysplasia. The greatest dimension of the invasive carcinoma was 0.8 cm. Microscopic tumor extension was into the submucosa. The deep margin (stalk margin) was uninvolved by invasive carcinoma. Lymphovascular invasion was not identified. The carcinoma was microsatellite stable (MSS). The distance of invasive carcinoma from the deep margin was 0.725 mm as shown in Fig. 98.2a, b.

J. H. Ashburn
Department of Colon and Rectal Surgery, Atrium Health Wake Forest Baptist, Winston-Salem, NC, USA

J. S. Wu (✉)
Department of Colon and Rectal Surgery, Cleveland Clinic, Cleveland, OH, USA

G. Zuccaro, Jr.
Department of Gastroenterology, Cleveland Clinic, Cleveland, OH, USA

H. O. Wiland
Department of Pathology, OhioHealth Mansfield Hospital, Mansfield, OH, USA

E. W. Willis
Department of Pathology, CORPath, Columbus, OH, USA

J. S. Wu, M. D. Inkster (eds.), *Cleveland Clinic Colorectal Case Studies*,
https://doi.org/10.1007/978-3-031-39880-3_98

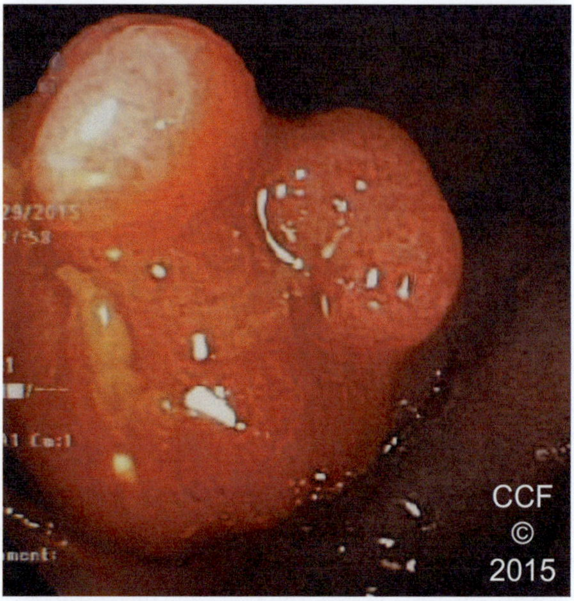

Fig. 98.1 Sigmoid colon polyp before snare polypectomy

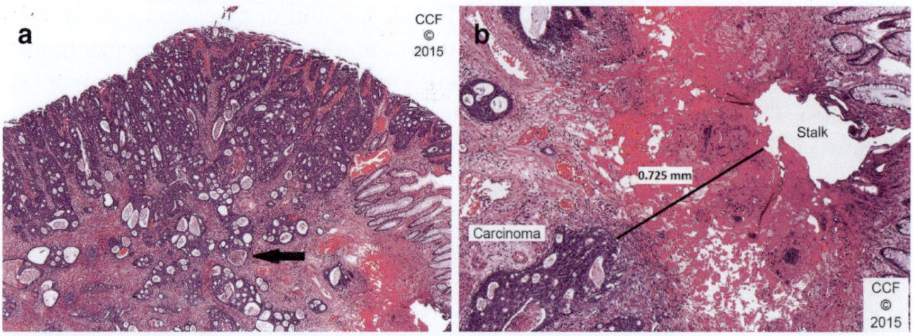

Fig. 98.2 (**a**) Sections of the polyp demonstrate, in part, a tubular adenoma with extensive high-grade dysplasia characterized by significant nuclear atypia and glandular crowding along surface epithelium. Within the stalk of the polyp, there appears to be an invasive moderately differentiated adenocarcinoma characterized by an irregular, haphazard glandular proliferation (arrow). (**b**) At the edge of the polyp stalk, the cauterized margin of excision is seen, and invasive adenocarcinoma is located 0.725 mm from the cauterized margin (line)

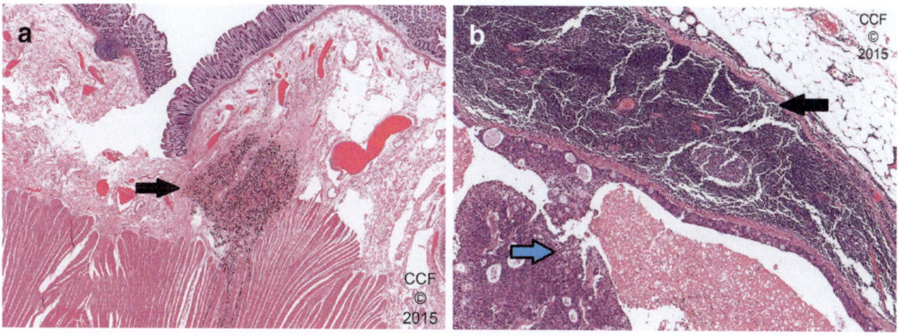

Fig. 98.3 (**a**) Histologic sections from the sigmoid resection demonstrate changes consistent with previous polypectomy site, as indicated by tattoo pigment (arrow). There is no evidence of residual dysplasia or carcinoma. (**b**) however, a total of 4 out of 25 regional lymph nodes (black arrow) show metastatic adenocarcinoma (blue arrow)

Management

The patient underwent laparoscopic sigmoid resection with colorectal anastomosis. Both surgery and convalescence were uneventful.

Pathology showed that the previous polypectomy and tattoo site were negative for residual carcinoma. However, metastatic adenocarcinoma was found in four of twenty-five (4/25) lymph nodes. A panel of immune-stains was performed on the lymph nodes containing metastatic adenocarcinoma. The lesion was positive for CDX2 and CK20 but negative for CK7 and PAX8. These stains help identify the primary as colonic rather than GYN (which would be PAX8 positive). The morphologic and immunophenotypic profile was consistent with a colorectal primary (Fig. 98.3a, b).

Comment

Netzer et al. state that, "Malignant colorectal polyps are defined as endoscopically removed polyps with cancerous tissue which has invaded the submucosa" [1, 2].

For patients found to have adenocarcinoma in a colorectal polyp removed endoscopically, the question is whether endoscopic polypectomy alone is adequate treatment or if resection of the Cancer-bearing segment of colon and its lymph node basin is needed. The risk of surgery is weighed against the risk of leaving behind metastases.

In 1995, Volk et al. designated malignant polyps as having favorable or unfavorable histology.[1]

[1]Volk et al. [3]. This excerpt was reproduced with the generous permission of Elsevier Inc., CCC|RightsLink® License number 5130990379142, License date Aug 16, 2021.

Management and Outcome of Patients with Invasive Carcinoma Arising in Colorectal Polyps
Emily E. Volk, John R. Goldblum, Robert E. Petras, William D. Carey, and Victor W. Fazio

"Malignant polyps were designated as having favorable histology (grade I or II carcinoma with at least a 2-mm free margin) or unfavorable histology (grade III invasive adenocarcinoma, invasive adenocarcinoma with an unassessable margin, or a margin of <2 mm). Malignant polyps with favorable histology were considered treated adequately by endoscopic polypectomy, whereas further therapy was recommended for malignant polyps with unfavorable histology.

Results: Of the 47 patients identified, 17 (36%) had favorable histology. Sixteen patients (94%) were treated with polypectomy alone. None had an adverse outcome (median follow-up, 70 months). Thirty patients (64%) had unfavorable histology,.... Ten of 30 patients with unfavorable histology had adverse outcomes that differed significantly from the favorable histology group *(P* = 0.03).

Conclusions: Endoscopic polypectomy alone is adequate therapy for malignant polyps with favorable histology."

These guidelines were followed in the preceding two presentations of malignant polyp. Other histopathologic guidelines exist [4, 5].

References

1. Netzer P, Forster C, Biral R, Ruchti C, Neuweiler J, Stauffer E, et al. Risk factor assessment of endoscopically removed malignant polyps. Gut. 1998;43:669–74.
2. Bujanda L, Cosme A, Gil I, Arenas-Mirave JI. Malignant colorectal polyps. World J Gastroenterol. 2010;16:3103–11.
3. Volk EE, Goldblum JR, Petras RE, Carey WD, Fazio VW. Management and outcome of patients with invasive carcinoma arising in colorectal polyps. Gastroenterology. 1995;109:1801–7.
4. Cooper HS, Deppisch LM, Gourley WK, Kahn EI, Lev R, Manley PN, et al. Endoscopically removed malignant colorectal polyps: Clinicopathologic correlations. Gastroenterology. 1995;108:1657–65.
5. Taylor JM, Hosie KB. The malignant polyp: Polypectomy or surgical resection. Chapter 6. In: Bustamante M, editor. Colonoscopy and colorectal cancer screening-future directions. London: IntechOpen. https://doi.org/10.5772/46055.

Malignant Colon Polyp-Haggitt Level 1

99

James S. Wu and Mohamed I. El Hag

Presentation

A 45-year-old female underwent screening colonoscopy. A 15 mm pedunculated sigmoid polyp (Fig. 99.1a) was identified and removed by snare polypectomy (Fig. 99.1b).

The colon adjacent to the polypectomy site was tattooed.

Pathology showed well-differentiated adenocarcinoma arising in a tubular adenoma. Lymphovascular and perineural invasion were not seen. The resection margin was 7 mm distant from the tumor margin. The cancer was confined to the polyp head (Haggitt level 1) (Fig. 99.2).

Management

This case was represented at tumor board. Tumor board recommendations included (a) genetic counseling and (b) surveillance colonoscopy. Factors affecting the management of this malignant polyp included favorable histology and Haggitt level 1 location.

J. S. Wu (✉)
Department of Colon and Rectal Surgery, Cleveland Clinic, Cleveland, OH, USA

M. I. El Hag
Pathology and Laboratory and Medicine Institute, Cleveland Clinic, Cleveland, OH, USA

J. S. Wu, M. D. Inkster (eds.), *Cleveland Clinic Colorectal Case Studies*,
https://doi.org/10.1007/978-3-031-39880-3_99

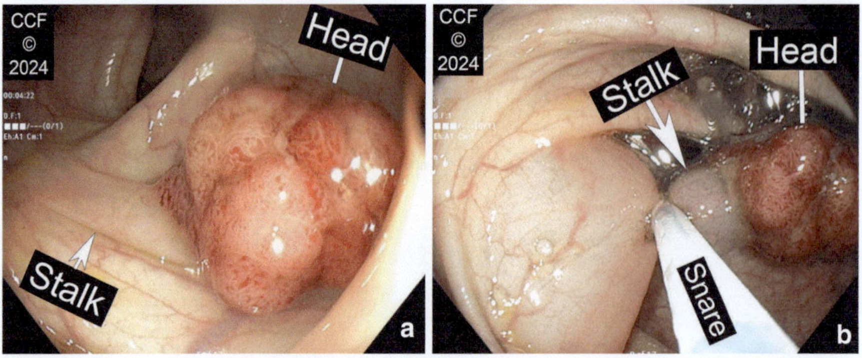

Fig. 99.1. (**a**) Pedunculated sigmoid colon polyp. The polyp head and stalk are labeled. (**b**) The polyp was removed by polypectomy using a hot snare. Again, the polyp head and stalk are labeled. Carbon black used to tattoo the wall opposite the polypectomy site is seen

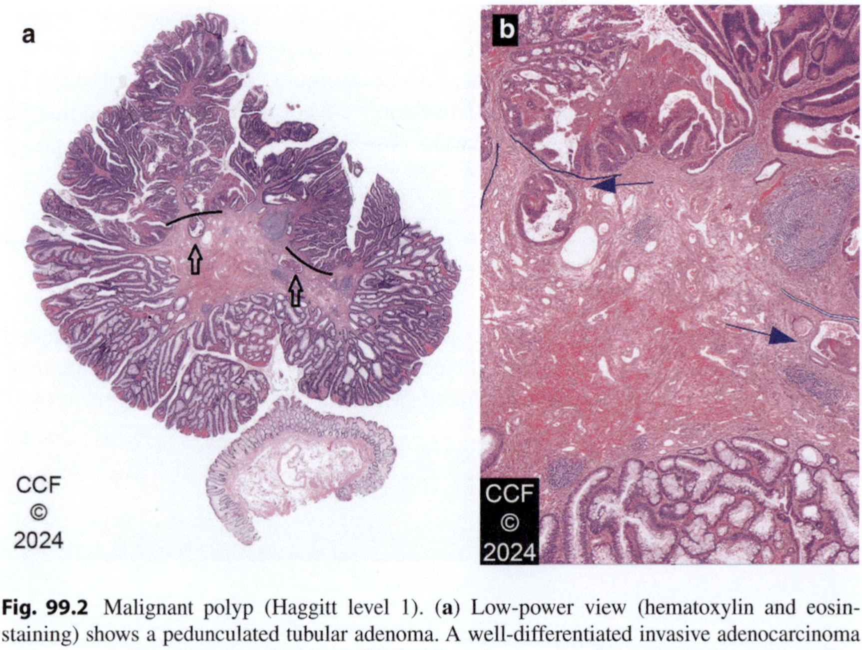

Fig. 99.2 Malignant polyp (Haggitt level 1). (**a**) Low-power view (hematoxylin and eosin-staining) shows a pedunculated tubular adenoma. A well-differentiated invasive adenocarcinoma arising within the tubular adenoma is confined to the polyp head (indicated by arrows). Black lines delineate the muscularis mucosae. (**b**) High-power view: arrows highlight the invasive glands, while the blue lines mark the muscularis mucosae

Comment

In addition to histology, carcinoma location within the polyp has a bearing on prognosis. In 1985, Haggitt et al. [1] studied prognostic factors in colorectal carcinomas arising in pedunculated and sessile adenomas removed by endoscopic polypectomy.

> "The best treatment for the patient whose polypectomy specimen discloses adenocarcinoma remains a controversial issue, primarily because there are insufficient data to predict when endoscopic polypectomy alone will provide as good a prognosis for cure as segmental colectomy with removal of regional lymph nodes. Theoretically, the decision for colectomy should be based on the risk of dying of unexcised malignant disease after polypectomy alone compared with the risks of death from the operation and from malignant disease after segmental colonic resection.
>
> We studied 129 colorectal carcinomas that arose in adenomas and in which invasion was no deeper than the submucosa of the underlying colonic wall. The following factors were evaluated: location; gross appearance (sessile versus pedunculated); histologic type of adenoma (tubular, villous, mixed); grade of carcinoma; level of invasion (0—carcinoma confined to the mucosa, 1—head, 2—neck, 3—stalk, 4—submucosa of underlying colonic wall); vascular invasion; and adequacy of excisional margins."

Haggitt levels of invasion for pedunculated and sessile malignant polyps are illustrated in Fig. 99.3.

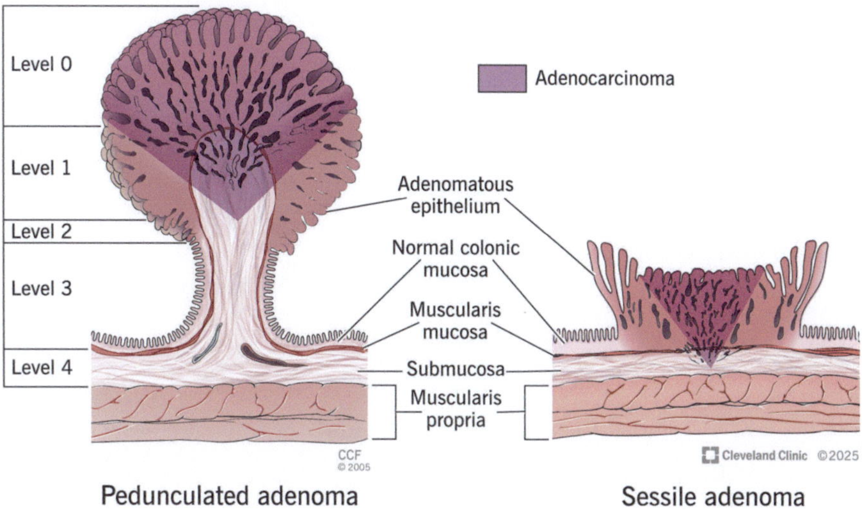

Fig. 99.3 Levels of invasion in a pedunculated adenoma (left) and a sessile adenoma (right) [after Haggitt]. Haggitt levels of invasion are as follows: level of invasion (0—carcinoma confined to the mucosa, 1—head, 2—neck, 3—stalk, 4—submucosa of underlying colonic wall). The purple areas represent zones of carcinoma. The maroon areas represent zones of adenomatous epithelium. Haggitt et al. state that "invasion below the muscularis mucosae in a sessile lesion represents level 4 invasion, i.e., invasion into the submucosa of the bowel wall. In contrast, invasive carcinoma in a pedunculated adenoma (*left*) must traverse a considerable distance before it reaches the submucosa of the underlying bowel wall." [1]

The authors found:

"…level 4 invasion is an independent variable that connotes a worse prognosis regardless of the size, gross aspect, or histologic type of the adenoma.

The risk of metastasis or local recurrence is very low when invasive carcinoma has not reached the submucosa of the bowel wall underlying the stalk of the polyp (level 4 invasion)." [1]

Reference

1. Haggitt RC, Glotzbach RE, Soffer EE, Wruble LD. Prognostic factors in colorectal carcinomas arising in adenomas: implications for lesions removed by endoscopic polypectomy. Gastroenterology. 1985;89:328–36. These excerpts were reused with the generous permission of Elsevier, CCC|RightsLink, License Number 5902650038311, License date Nov 05, 2024.

Proctosigmoiditis

100

James S. Wu and Eric W. Willis

Presentation

A 39-year-old female was referred for surgical management of proctosigmoiditis. She has had recurrent perirectal abscesses treated by surgical drainage and seton placement over 4 years. Colonoscopy revealed acute and chronic inflammation in the rectum and sigmoid colon plus a sigmoid stricture. Medical therapy was not beneficial. The patient agreed to the removal of the diseased rectum and sigmoid but requested that the anus be left behind so that reconstitution of bowel continuity might be done at a future date. Proctosigmoidectomy with low Hartmann pouch and end colostomy were done (Fig. 100.1).

Two years after surgery, the patient returned to see if her colon might be reattached to her anus. A small intestinal contrast study was normal. Colonoscopy showed an inflamed stricture at the colostomy. The patient agreed to have the remaining large intestine and the anorectum removed with the creation of a permanent ileostomy. The anus and distal rectum were excised by intersphincteric dissection. Pathology showed active inflammation with noncaseating granulomas and giant cells (Fig. 100.2). The operative specimen is seen in Fig. 100.3.

J. S. Wu (✉)
Department of Colon and Rectal Surgery, Cleveland Clinic, Cleveland, OH, USA

E. W. Willis
Department of Pathology, CORPath, Columbus, OH, USA1

J. S. Wu, M. D. Inkster (eds.), *Cleveland Clinic Colorectal Case Studies*,
https://doi.org/10.1007/978-3-031-39880-3_100

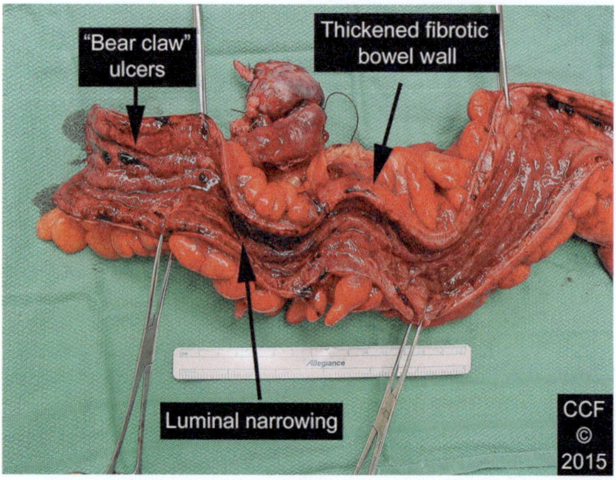

Fig. 100.1 Gross examination of the resected rectum shows hemorrhagic mucosa with prominent longitudinal deep "bear claw" ulceration, bowel wall thickening (up to 0.5 cm), and luminal narrowing

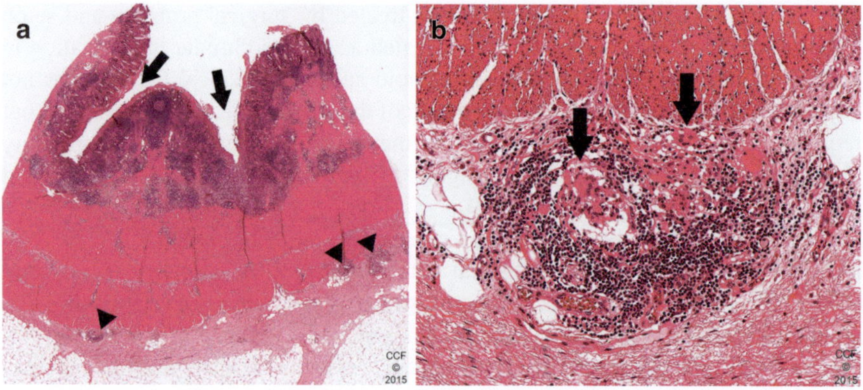

Fig. 100.2 Chronic active inflammation with granulomas: (**a**) Shows thickened bowel wall with alternating deep ulcerations (arrows) and intact mucosa; transmural inflammation (arrowheads) with granulomatous inflammation (Original magnification, H&E, 10×); (**b**) Is a higher power view showing granulomatous inflammation with multinucleated giant cells (arrows) (H&E, Original magnification, 200×)

Comment

In 1932, Crohn et al. reported terminal ileitis [1]. Inflammatory bowel disease of the large intestine has been divided into two categories, ulcerative colitis and Crohn's colitis. As pointed out by Wells, the characteristics of each are descriptive since the etiology is unknown [2].

Ulcerative colitis and Crohn's disease

> "If the aetiology of Crohn's disease and ulcerative colitis were known, a rational classification would be simple. Since we have no certain knowledge about causes, we can only hope to group the cases on a basis of descriptive pathology."

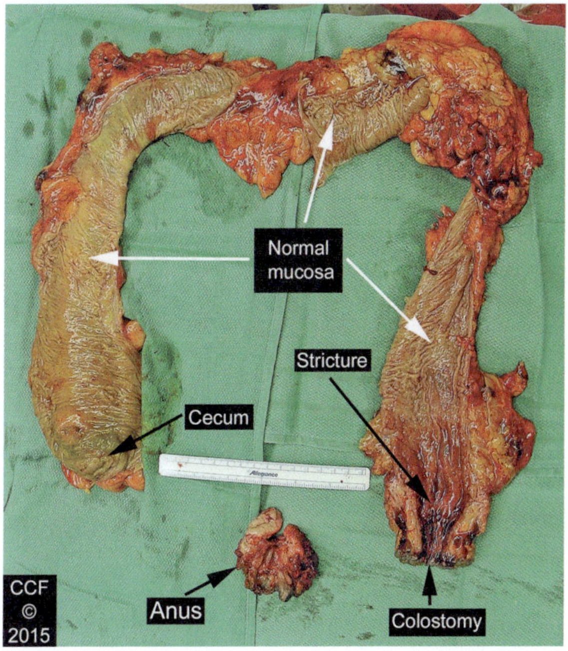

Fig. 100.3 Resected colon and anus. The strictured colon at the colostomy, normal colon proximal to the colostomy, and resected anus are highlighted with arrows

Charles Wells, F.R.C.S
Department of Surgery
University of Liverpool, 1952

In 1959, Brooke described *Granulomatous Diseases of the Intestine*.[1]

Nomenclature

"First let me take a problem—how can Crohn's disease be distinguished from ulcerative colitis? Moreover, is there any point in such a distinction? To answer the second question first: these two conditions may have entirely different origins despite contemporary opinion to the contrary, for one of the striking features of Crohn's disease is the severe hypertrophic type of reaction which is manifest in the thickened wall, seen microscopically to be due to œdema and what has been termed (but not determined as far as I know) as collagen. The very appearance makes hypersensitivity spring to mind. Per contra the intestinal wall in ulcerative colitis, though slightly thickened when the disease is not acutely active, becomes thinner and thinner as ulceration, starting in the mucosa, proceeds outwards; there is no macroscopic suggestion of a hypersensitivity reaction, though between muscularis mucosæ and smooth muscle what passes for collagen may sometimes be seen microscopically; the amount of this is less than in Crohn's disease.

Can, therefore, Crohn's disease be distinguished from ulcerative colitis? It is perhaps unfortunate that Crohn's disease was originally described in the small intestine and the title terminal ileitis applied to it; this was later changed to regional enteritis when the disease was detected higher in the intestine. In the land of its discovery, doubtless owing to the

[1] Brooke [3]. Permission to reuse this excerpt was generously granted by Elsevier Ltd., CCC|RightsLink®, License Number 5127741093679; License date 14 Aug 2021.

modesty of Dr. Burrill B. Crohn himself, it has never been termed "Crohn's disease"; this is a pity for the title regional ileitis has tended to separate the disease from the large intestine at least in the minds of those who work on the other side of the Atlantic."

Bryan N. Brooke,
M.D., Birm., M. Chir. Cantab, F.R.C.S.
Reader in Surgery,
University of Birmingham

In 1960, Lockhart-Mummery and Morson discussed Crohn's disease (regional enteritis) of the large intestine and its distinction from ulcerative colitis [4].

"Microscopically, the main difference between Crohn's disease and ulcerative colitis is that in the former there is granulomatous reaction extending through all layers of the bowel wall, whereas in colitis the inflammation is superficial and confined to the mucosa in the first place, with some later extension into the submucous tissue, but never any penetration of the muscularis externa except as the result of perforation in the acute fulminating form of the disease. Moreover, the intramural fissures of Crohn's disease are not seen in ulcerative colitis."

H.E. Lockhart-Mummery and B. C. Morson
From the Research Department
St. Mark's Hospital, London

Surgery for inflammatory bowel disease is indicated when medical therapy is not successful and is directed at treating complications [5, 6]. At presentation, this patient had intractable anal fistulae and stricturing proctosigmoiditis. Initially, the patient did not want a permanent stoma. Therefore, anterior resection of the rectum and sigmoid colon with colostomy and low Hartmann pouch preserving the anal sphincter was done. Two years later, the patient returned with recurrent stricturing disease at the colostomy. She initially requested reconstruction by colon to anal anastomosis but was persuaded to remove the entire large intestine and the anus because of the risk of recurrent structuring and fistulous disease. Additional surgery has not been required. In this case, an alternative operation in this would be colostomy resection with neo-end colostomy; the price paid, however, would be possible re-recurrence.

References

1. Crohn BB, Ginzburg L, Oppenheimer GD. Regional ileitis. A pathologic and clinical entity. J Am Med Assoc. 1932;99:1323–9.
2. Wells C. Ulcerative colitis and Crohn's disease. Ann R Coll Surg Engl. 1952;2:105–20.
3. Brooke BN. Granulomatous diseases of the intestine. Lancet. 1959;ii:745–9.
4. Lockhart-Mummery HE, Morson BC. Crohn's disease (regional enteritis) of the large intestine and its distinction from ulcerative colitis. Gut. 1960;1:87–105.
5. Williams JG, Hughes LE. Abdominoperineal resection for severe perianal Crohn's disease. Dis Colon Rectum. 1990;33:402–7.
6. Fazio VW, Wu JS. Surgical therapy for Crohn's disease of the colon and rectum. Surg Clin N Am. 1997;77:197–210.

Epiploic Appendagitis

101

Michelle D. Inkster and James S. Wu

Presentation

A 44-year-old male was referred for acute left lower abdominal pain. Computed tomography (CT) of the abdomen was done (Fig. 101.1a, b).

The radiologic diagnosis was epiploic appendagitis.

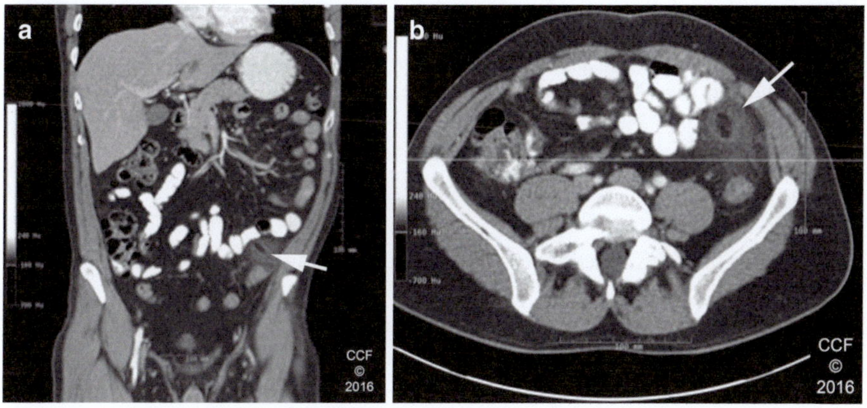

Fig. 101.1 Abdominal CT images of the abdomen. An oval-shaped "hyperattenuating ring sign" (arrows) ((**a**) axial view; (**b**) coronal view) is seen in both images [3]

M. D. Inkster
Department of Gastroenterology, Cleveland Clinic, Cleveland, OH, USA

J. S. Wu (✉)
Department of Colon and Rectal Surgery, Cleveland Clinic, Cleveland, OH, USA

J. S. Wu, M. D. Inkster (eds.), *Cleveland Clinic Colorectal Case Studies*,
https://doi.org/10.1007/978-3-031-39880-3_101

Comment

Epiploic appendagitis is a rare cause of acute abdominal pain. In 1917, Harrigan described *Torsion and Inflammation of the Appendices Epiploicæ* [1].

> "The appendices epiploicæ were first described by André Vesalius.
>
> The appendices epiploicæ are generally arranged in two rows along the wall of the large intestine. They are in intimate relations to the longitudinal bands of the colon. On the transverse colon, they spring almost entirely from the anterior surface, being attached between the two longitudinal bands—termed tænia mesocolica and tænia libera. They are absent from the rectum.
>
> An analysis of the literature discloses the fact that the essential and dominant lesion in the pathology of the appendices epiplociæ is torsion or twisting of the pedicle. If this is associated with infection, the conditions assume a practical and surgical importance, owing to the relief obtainable through operative intervention. If infection is absent, the pathology becomes of academic interest, for under these circumstances simple necrosis of the pedicle results in detachment of the distal end, which then becomes a foreign body of the peritoneal cavity.
>
> Virchow was the first pathologist to demonstrate the actual etiology and formation of the foreign bodies of the peritoneal cavity. He showed that as a result of obesity or an infection an increased amount of fat is deposited in the appendices epiploicæ. This fat undergoes saponification and calcification, which causes an increase in weight, and which in turn leads to gradual and progressive obliteration or obstruction of the blood-vessels of the pedicle. When the vascular obstruction or obliteration is complete, necrosis occurs and the freed and liberated epiploica then falls into the peritoneal cavity.
>
> Intra-abdominal torsion and inflammation may produce abdominal and peritoneal symptoms which are acute in onset and which simulate closely those of acute appendicitis."
>
> Anthony H. Harrigan, M.D.
> New York, N.Y.
> Assistant Visiting Surgeon,
> Fordham Hospital

In 1922, Frank described a case of torsion and gangrene of appendix epiploica necessitating operation [2].

In addition to appendicitis, epiploic appendagitis can also resemble diagnoses listed in Table 101.1 [3].

Seen in this case is the "hyperattenuating ring sign" consistent with acute epiploic appendagitis [4]. Recognizing appendagitis may avoid unnecessary surgery [5].

Table 101.1 Diagnoses that resemble appendagitis

Acute appendicitis
Acute diverticulitis
Sclerosing mesenteritis
Omental infarction
Metastases to the mesocolon

References

1. Harrigan AH. Torsion and inflammation of the appendices epiploicæ. Ann Surg. 1917;66:467–78.
2. Frank L. Torsion and gangrene of appendix epiploica necessitating operation. Am Med. 1922;28:42–6.
3. Singh AK, Gervais DA, Hahn PF, Sagar P, Mueller PR, Novelline RA. Acute epiploic appendagitis and its mimics. Radiographics. 2005;25:1521–34.
4. Han Q, Nair RT, DiSantis DJ. The hyperattenuating ring sign of acute epiploic appendagitis. Abdom Radiol. 2016;41:1431–2.
5. Hasbahceci M, Erol C, Seker M. Epiploic appendagitis: Is there need for surgery to confirm diagnosis in spite of clinical and radiological findings? World J Surg. 2012;36:441–6.

Sigmoid Volvulus: Endoscopic Decompression

102

Michelle D. Inkster, Emily Hromi, and James S. Wu

Presentation

A 76-year-old female was admitted from a nursing home with a 5-day history of progressively worsening abdominal pain, distension, and constipation. A flat film of the abdomen showed multiple loops of dilated intestine (Fig. 102.1). Computed tomography showed the characteristic "coffee bean" sign characteristic of sigmoid volvulus (Fig. 102.2). Emergent decompression of the volvulus was done (Figs. 102.3, 102.4, 102.5, and 102.6). Anatomic factors predisposing to sigmoid volvulus include sigmoid redundancy and an elongated mesenteric pedicle that is narrow at is parietal attachment (Fig. 102.7).

M. D. Inkster
Department of Gastroenterology, Cleveland Clinic, Cleveland, OH, USA

E. Hromi
Studio Hromi, LLC, Grand Rapids, MI, USA

J. S. Wu (✉)
Department of Colon and Rectal Surgery, Cleveland Clinic, Cleveland, OH, USA

J. S. Wu, M. D. Inkster (eds.), *Cleveland Clinic Colorectal Case Studies*,
https://doi.org/10.1007/978-3-031-39880-3_102

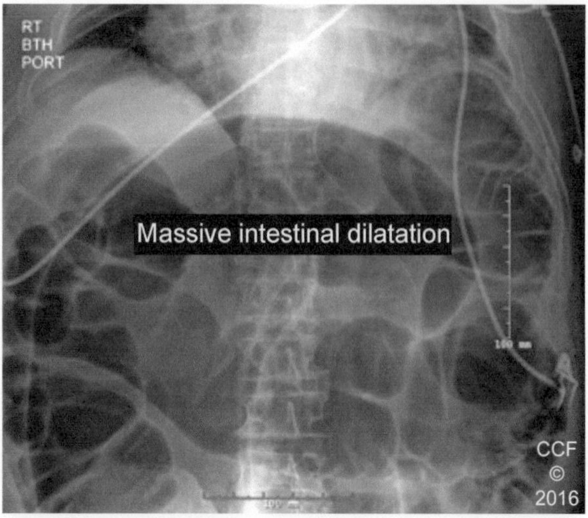

Fig. 102.1 Multiple overlying gas-filled loops of intestine are seen on this abdominal flat plate

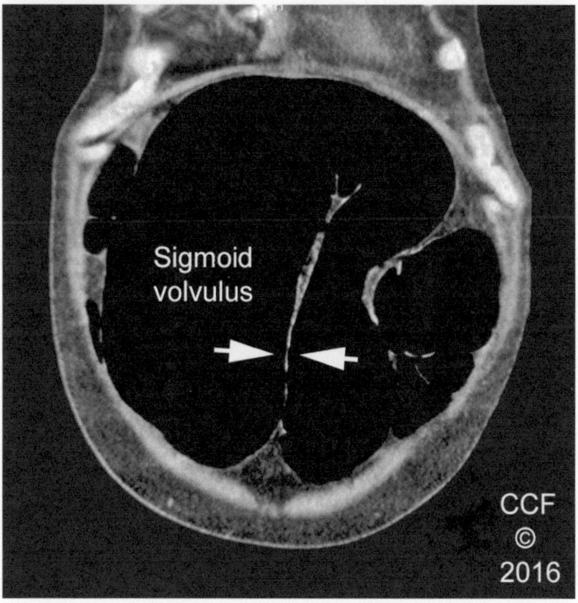

Fig. 102.2 Computed tomography showed shows massively dilated sigmoid colon that has the appearance of a "coffee bean" with a central cleft (arrows) [1]

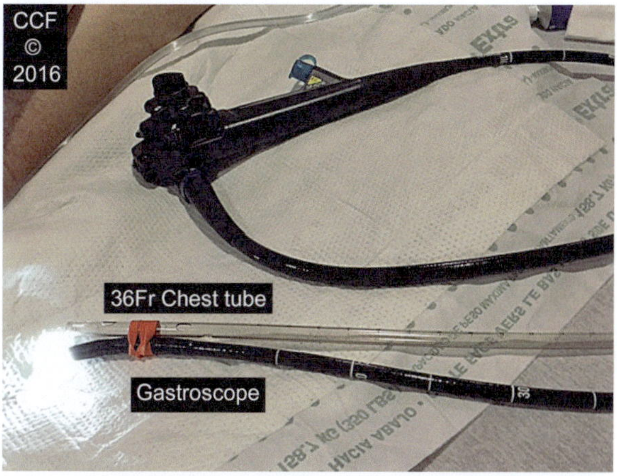

Fig. 102.3 A gastroscope with a 36 Fr chest tube attached to its tip with a rubber band

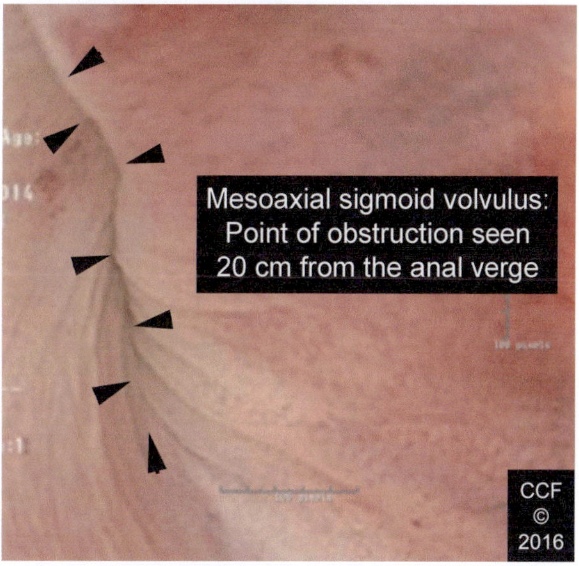

Fig. 102.4 Endoscopic view of the point of obstruction caused by the volvulus is seen 20 cm from the anal verge

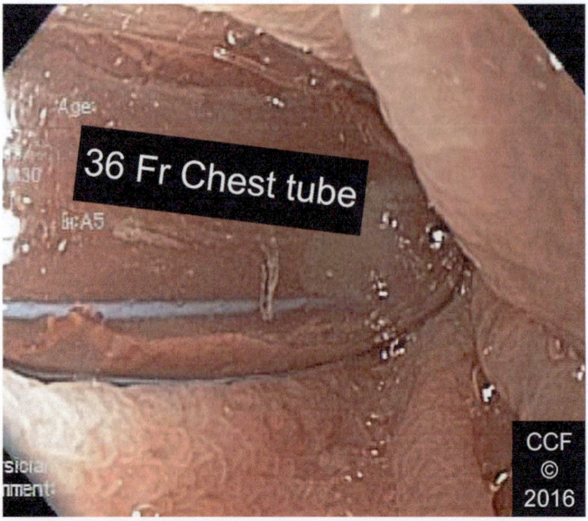

Fig. 102.5 Endoscopic view of the 36 Fr chest tube after passage through the point of obstruction into the sigmoid colon

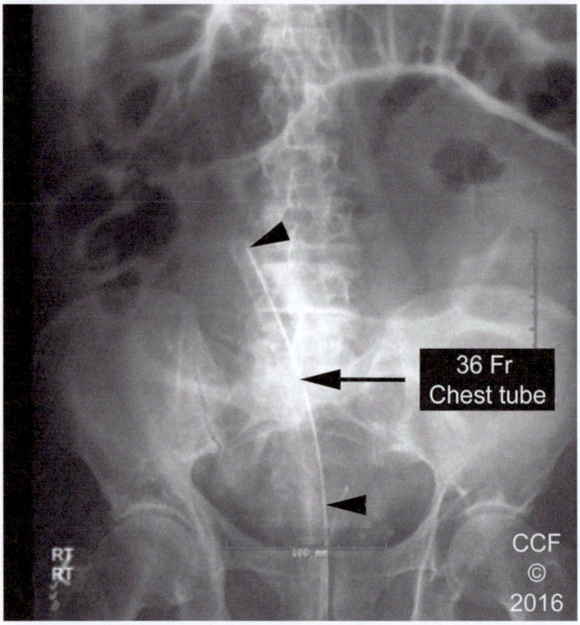

Fig. 102.6 The gastroscope passes proximal to the point of obstruction caused by the sigmoid volvulus. The chest tube (arrow and arrowheads), radiologically identified by its radiopaque marker stripe, is deployed with its tip in the mid-sigmoid colon. Decompression of the closed loop obstruction is immediate. The chest tube is secured to both buttocks with a generous amount of wide tape

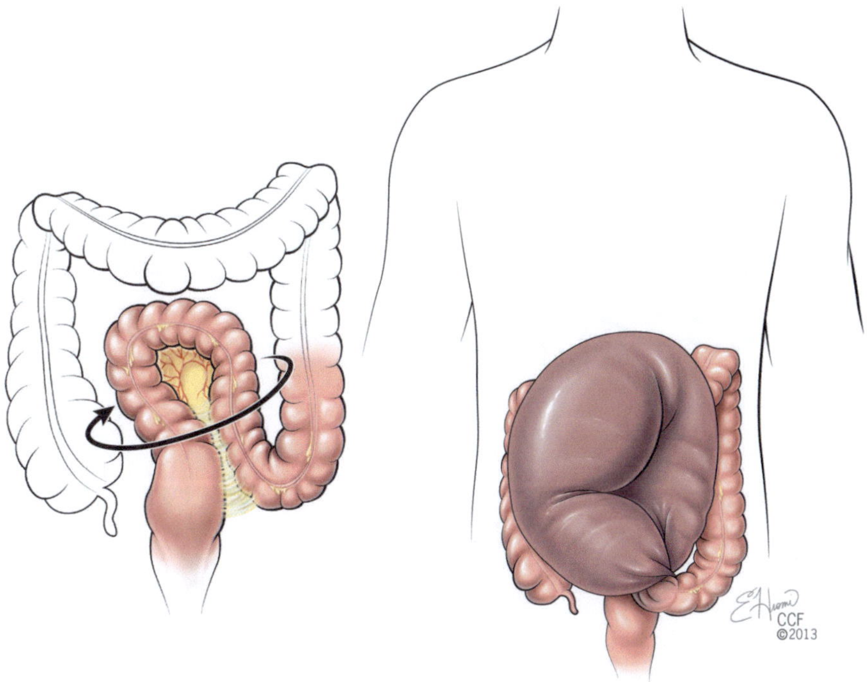

Fig. 102.7 As this illustration demonstrates, a redundant sigmoid colon with an elongated mesentery that is narrow at its parietal attachment undergoes mesoaxial rotation leading to volvulus. Volvulus results in closed-loop obstruction. The obstruction is relieved by the endoscopic placement of a wide-bore intraluminal stent, a 36 Fr chest tube, in this case

Comment [2–4]

In 1884, Treves published, *Intestinal Obstruction: Its varieties, with their pathology, diagnosis, and treatment* [5]. Chapter VII concerned itself with the subject of volvulus.

> "Under the general term "volvulus" may be included two distinct methods of producing obstruction. In one the bowel is so twisted about its mesenteric axis, or even in rare cases upon its own axis, that it becomes occluded. In the other form two suitable coils of intestine are so intertwined or knotted together as to cause also an obstruction in their lumina.
>
> 1. Volvulus of the sigmoid flexure.—This part of the bowel may be occluded by either of the two methods just named.
>
> (1) **The bowel is twisted about its mesenteric axis: Pathology.—**This is the most usual form of volvulus, and may, indeed, be said to be the only form that is at all common. If all the cases of volvulus of the intestine be considered collectively, it will be found that about two-thirds of the number are instances of twist of the sigmoid flexure about its mesenteric axis.

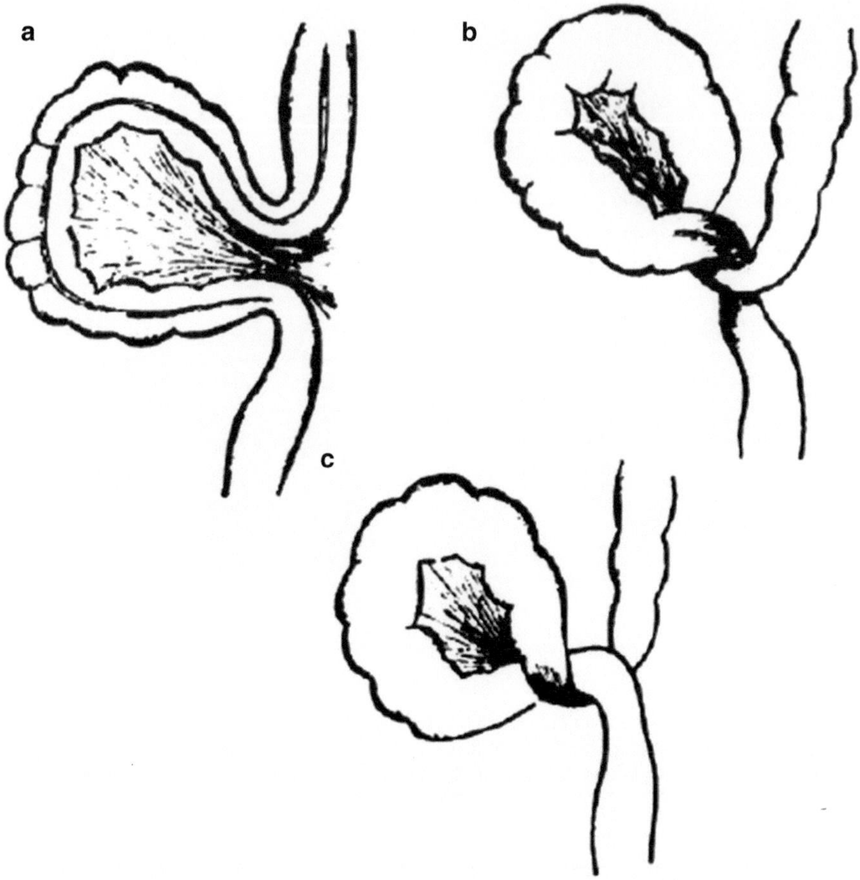

Fig. 102.8 (originally Fig. 27) Volvulus of the Sigmoid Flexure. From Treves [5]

The normal flexure forms a loop that is more like a capital C than a Greek ∑.

The arrangement of the gut that is necessary for the production of a volvulus is the following: The loop must be of considerable length, the meso-colon must be long and very narrow at its parietal attachment, so that the two ends of the loop may be brought as close together as possible. This condition is shown:

Fig. 102.8a, where it will be seen that the loose and free coil has practically a fixed pedicle around which it could with great ease be twisted.

According to Potain there are two kinds of twist. In one the superior part of the loop is carried from above downwards, and from behind forwards, in front of the lower half of the loop, so that the end of the descending colon is brought into contact with, and *in front* of, the commencement of the rectum ("type rectum en arrière"), Fig. 102.8b. In the second form the superior part of the coil is carried from above downwards, and from before backwards, behind the lower segment of the loop, so that the end of the descending colon is brought into contact with, and *behind*, the commencement of the rectum ("type rectum en avant"), Fig. 102.8c".

Frederick Treves, F.R.C.S.

Hunterian Professor of Anatomy at the Royal College of Surgeons of England

Unrelieved, sigmoid volvulus can result in the following complications:

1. Complete large bowel closed-loop obstruction
2. Vascular compromise to the sigmoid colon

This case illustrates emergency volvulus decompression and stenting. A 36 Fr chest tube was selected for this purpose for the following reasons: (a) wide bore, (b) stiffness, and (c) radiologic markings. Once the gastroscope travels proximal to the point of volvulus into the mid-sigmoid colon, the chest tube is secured to both buttocks with wide tape. The gastroscope is removed, leaving the chest tube in the sigmoid colon. The chest tube decompresses the colon, stents the lumen open, and prevents complete obstruction from recurring. This method transforms a potential surgical emergency into an elective operation.

Chest tube decompression of sigmoid volvulus can also be accomplished using a rigid proctoscope. The point of obstruction in sigmoid volvulus is usually encountered at about 20 cm from the anus, a distance within reach of the adult rigid proctoscope. After the proctoscope, with air insufflation, passes through the obstruction, the decompressing chest tube is passed through the lumen of the proctoscope. The proctoscope is then removed and the chest tube to secured to the buttocks. The flexible endoscopic method is advantageous because it provides a direct assessment of the sigmoid colon mucosa and its viability. Also, unlike the rigid sigmoidoscope, the flexible endoscope allows the operator's face to be distant from the point of gaseous fecal discharge when the obstruction is relieved.

References

1. Chung S-D, Chen K-H, Chen H-A, Tu C-C, Wu J-M. Acute abdomen with coffee bean sign. Emerg Med J. 2011;28:826.
2. Martin MJ, Steele SR. Twists and turns: A practical approach to volvulus and instussusception. Scand J Surg. 2010;99:93–102.
3. Ghazi A, Shinya H, Wolf WI. Treatment of volvulus of the colon by colonoscopy. Ann Surg. 1976;183:263–5.
4. Di Felice G. Sigmoid volvulus treated by colonoscopy. Gastrointest Endosc. 1986;32:244–5.
5. Treves F. Chapter VII. Volvulus. In: Intestinal Obstruction: Its Varieties with their Pathology, Diagnosis, and Treament. Philadelphia: Henry C. Lea's Son & CO.; 1884. p. 134–8.

103 Sudeck's Critical Point

James S. Wu and Erika B. Woodrum

Comment

In 1907, Sudeck reported two cases of fatal gangrene that followed trans-sacral rectal cancer resection. He identified inadequate perfusion of the colonic stump as the cause [1].

J. S. Wu (✉)
Department of Colon and Rectal Surgery, Cleveland Clinic, Cleveland, OH, USA

E. B. Woodrum
Medical Illustration Team, Enterprise Creative Services, Cleveland Clinic, Cleveland, OH, USA
e-mail: woodrue@ccf.org

J. S. Wu, M. D. Inkster (eds.), *Cleveland Clinic Colorectal Case Studies*,
https://doi.org/10.1007/978-3-031-39880-3_103

Ueber die Gefässversorgung des Mastdarmes in Hinsicht auf die operative Gangrän Von Dr. P. Sudeck, Oberarzt Krankenhaus St. Georg in Hamburg	On the vascular supply of the rectum with regard to operative gangrene By P. Sudeck, senior surgeon St. George's Hospital, Hamburg
Zwei eigene Fälle von operativer Gangrän des karzinomatösen Mastdarms, die beide male zum Tode führte, sowie die Diskussion des vorjährigen Chirurgenkongresses veranlassten mich, mich über die Ernährungsverhältnisse des Mastdarms genauer zu orientieren.	Two separate cases of gangrene following surgery to remove rectal cancer, which both led to death, as well as the discussion at the previous year's Congress of Surgeons, led me to focus more precisely on the nutritional (vascular) supply of the rectum.
Die anatomischen Lehrbücher zeigen uns die Ernährungsverhältnisse des Mastdarms so,...Die Art. meseraica inferior teilt sich in die A. colica sin. und die A. haemorrhoidalis superior. Die A. colica sin. versorgt das Colon descendens und anastomosiert mit der A. meseraica superior. Sie sendet ausserdem einen Ast zur Flexura sigmoidea.	The anatomic text books teach us the following about the vascular supply of the rectum....The inferior mesenteric artery divides into the left colic artery and the superior hemorrhoidal artery. The left colic artery supplies the descending colon and anastomoses with the superior mesenteric artery. In addition, it sends a branch to the sigmoid flexure.
Die A. haemorrhoidalis superior verläuft in situ in ziemlich gerader Fortsetzung des Stammes der A. meseraica inf. im Mesorectum an der hinteren Seite des Mastdarms, wo sie sich in 2 grösserer Aeste teilt. In ihrem Verlaufe gibt sie einen oder mehrere Aeste zu Flexura sigmoidea ab.	The superior hemorrhoidal artery is a straight continuation of the inferior mesenteric artery that divides into two large branches in the mesorectum on the posterior side of the rectum. Along its route it gives off one or several branches to the sigmoid flexure.
Alle diese Arterien sind durch Anastomosen miteinander verbunden, teilweise durch mehrere Gefässbogen übereinander, meistens nur durch einen Gefässbogen.	All of these arteries are bound together through anastomoses, sometimes through several vascular arches, most through only one vascular arch.
Diese Einrichtung der Vollanastomosen besteht nur an den beweglichen Darmteilen, nicht an dem unbeweglichen Rektum. Die letze grosse anastomose befindet sich...am Punkte X und an jedem der übrigen Präparate kann man mit aller Deutlichkeit die Einmündung der untersten Vollanastomose feststellen.	This arrangement of full anastomoses exists only on the mobile parts of the intestine, not on the immovable rectum. This last large anastomosis is located... at point X and on each of the other preparations, one can clearly see the opening of the lowest full anastomosis.

Sudeck states that "Punkte X" is a critical point (Kritische Punkt X) which is located at the junction between the superior hemorrhoidal (rectal) artery (SRA) and the last sigmoid artery (Fig. 103.1).

At Sudeck's critical point one arterial branch goes to the rectum as the SRA; a second arterial branch travels to the sigmoid colon as the last sigmoidal branch. In 2007, van Tonder et al. [2] determined the incidence of the presence of a macroscopic anastomosis between the SRA and the last sigmoidal branch by macroscopic dissection of 64 cadavers. A macroscopic anastomosis between the SRA and the last sigmoid artery was absent in 3 (4.7%) of the cadavers. The authors also found that although an anastomosis is present in the majority of cases, the vessel is very small in diameter and may not be sufficient to meet the demands of the caudal rectal stump.

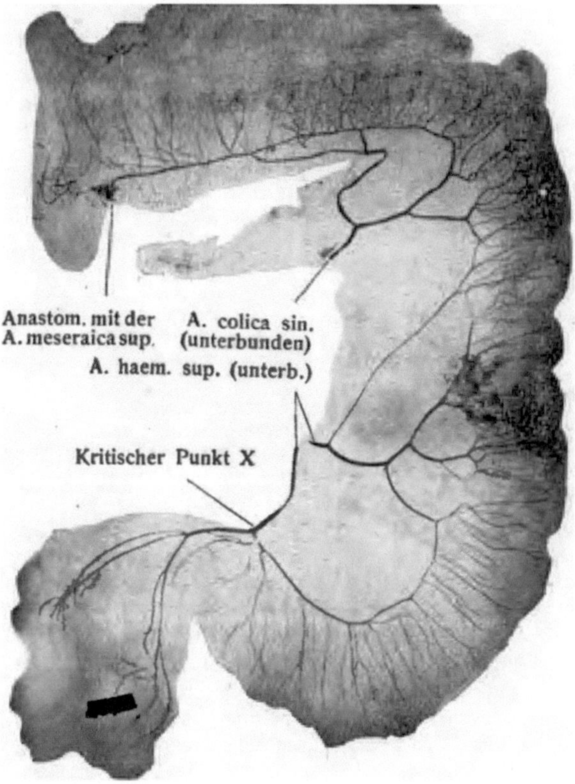

Fig. 103.1 Injection study by Sudeck identifying the critical point (Kritische Punkt X) at the rectosigmoid junction. Anastom. mit der A. meseraica sup. (Anastomosis with the superior mesenteric artery); A. colica sin. (unterbunden) Left colic artery (tied); A. haem. sup. (unterb.) Superior hemorrhoidal artery (tied)

In 1997, Yamazaki et al.[1] described a case of ischemic stricture, 6 cm in length, in the rectosigmoid colon distal to the anastomosis following radical sigmoidectomy with division of the SRA immediately distal to Sudeck's point (Fig. 103.2). The authors stressed the importance of Sudeck's point to surgery involving the sigmoid colon resection writing:

> "Despite Sudeck's cautionary report regarding the risk of colon necrosis following a pull-through procedure, published in 1907, most colorectal surgeons do not pay close attention to Sudeck's critical point when operating in the rectosigmoid region. We report herein the case of a patient who developed an ischemic stricture, 6 cm in length, in the rectosigmoid colon distal to the anastomosis following a radical sigmoidectomy with division of the superior rectal artery immediately distal to Sudeck's point. This is the first documentation of a patient developing an ischemic stricture attributable to sigmoidectomy. Division of the artery distal to Sudeck's point most probably impaired the blood supply to the rectosigmoid colon, which subsequently resulted in occlusive ischemic colitis. Thus, there is a risk that division of the superior rectal artery distal to Sudeck's point may lead to colonic ischemia in the remaining rectosigmoid region following sigmoidectomy.

[1] Yamazaki et al. [3]. These excerpts were reused with the generous permission of Springer Nature, CCC|RightsLink®, License number 5162740162001, License date Oct 05, 2021.

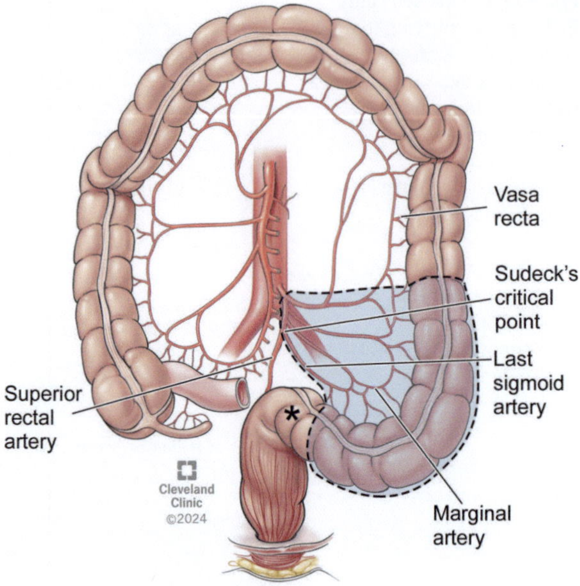

Fig. 103.2 Ischemia of the rectosigmoid colon (asterisk) caused by division of the superior rectal artery distal to Sudeck's point (after Yamazaki)

> In conclusion, the development of colonic ischemia in our patient reemphasizes the importance of Sudeck's point. This report suggests that an anastomosis in the rectosigmoid colon with the superior rectal artery divided below Sudeck's point carries the risk of impaired blood supply to the distal colon."

In order to avoid ischemia at a retained rectosigmoid stump after radical sigmoid colon resection, typically, the entire sigmoid is removed and the distal line of resection is at the rectum distal to the confluence of the taenia coli (Fig. 103.3).

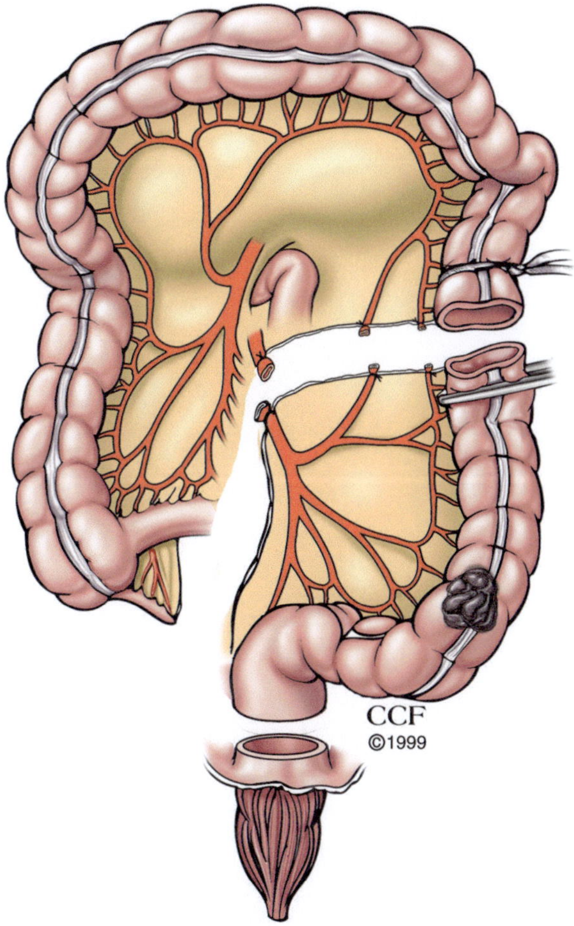

Fig. 103.3 Sigmoidectomy with high ligation of the inferior mesenteric artery. The distal line of resection at the rectum (distal to the confluence of the taenia coli) includes the rectosigmoid area that may have an impaired arterial blood supply

References

1. Sudeck P. Ueber die Gefässversorgung des Massdarmes in Hinsicht auf die operative Gangrän. Muench Med Wschr. 1907;54:1314–7.
2. van Tonder JJ, Boon JM, Becker JHR, van Schoor A-N. Anatomical considerations on Sudeck's critical point and its relevance to colorectal surgery. Clin Anat. 2007;20:424–7.
3. Yamazaki T, Shirai Y, Sakai Y, Hatakeyama K. Ischemic stricture of the rectosigmoid colon caused by division of the surperior rectal artery below Sudeck's point during sigmoidectomy: report of a case. Surg Today. Jpn J Surg 1997;27:254–6.

104 Sigmoid Volvulus-Resection

James S. Wu, Paul C. Janicki, and Michelle D. Inkster

Presentation

A 55-year-old female had abdominal pain for a year. She felt as though there was a balloon in her abdomen. There was no history of vomiting. She was passing flatus. Recent colonoscopy was normal. She had not had prior surgery. Examination revealed tympany without peritoneal signs. A plain abdominal film (Fig. 104.1) and a computed tomographic (CT) scan (Fig. 104.2) of the abdomen showed sigmoid volvulus.

J. S. Wu (✉)
Department of Colon and Rectal Surgery, Cleveland Clinic, Cleveland, OH, USA

P. C. Janicki
Radiology & Diagnostic Imaging Institute, Cleveland Clinic, Cleveland, OH, USA

M. D. Inkster
Department of Gastroenterology, Cleveland Clinic, Cleveland, OH, USA

J. S. Wu, M. D. Inkster (eds.), *Cleveland Clinic Colorectal Case Studies*,
https://doi.org/10.1007/978-3-031-39880-3_104

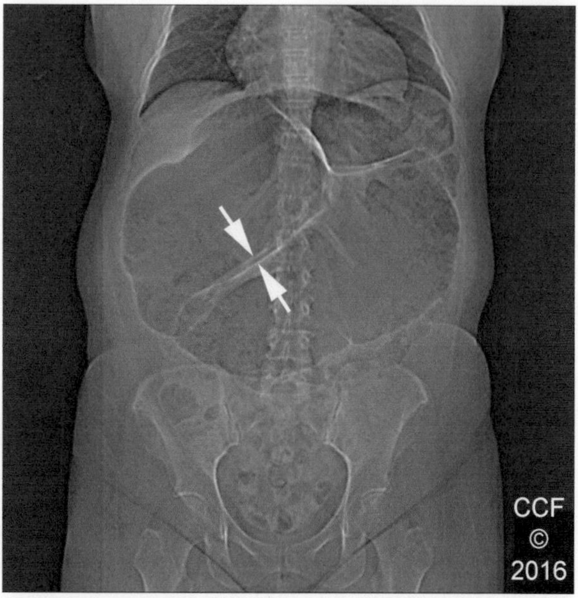

Fig. 104.1 Plain radiograph. Anterior–posterior view of the abdomen. The image shows the markedly distended sigmoid colon with a "U" shape, also known as the "coffee bean" sign [1]. The central cleft of the coffee bean (arrows) represents the proximal and distal segments of the sigmoid colon aligned side-by-side

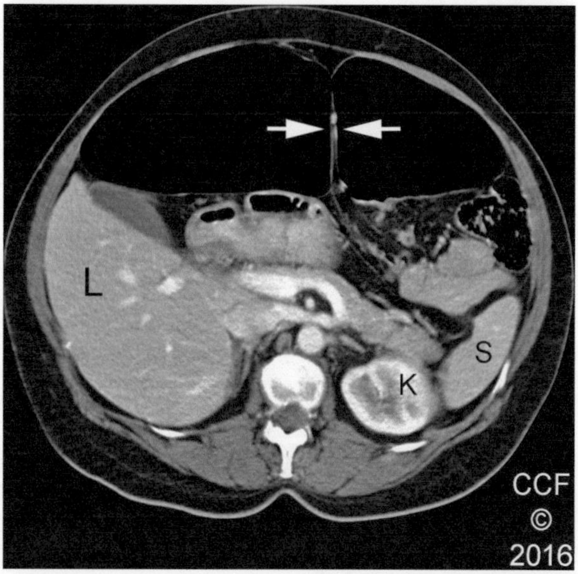

Fig. 104.2 CT scan of the abdomen, axial view. The apposed walls of the proximal and distal segments of the sigmoid colon with intervening mesentery are marked with arrows. The liver (L), left kidney, and spleen (S) are labeled

Management

At surgery, sigmoid volvulus was found (Figs. 104.3 and 104.4). Sigmoid colectomy (Fig. 104.5) was done.

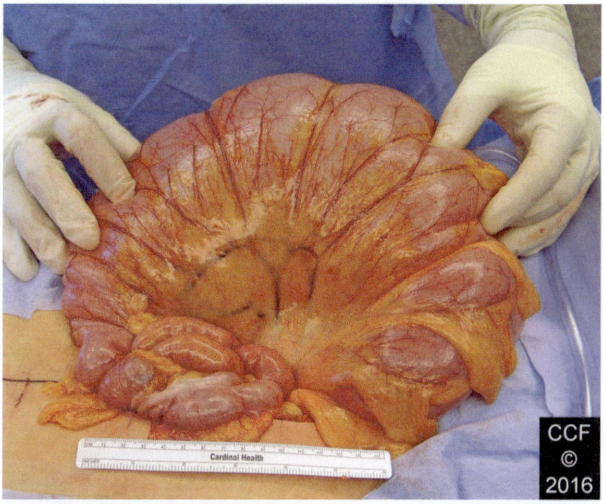

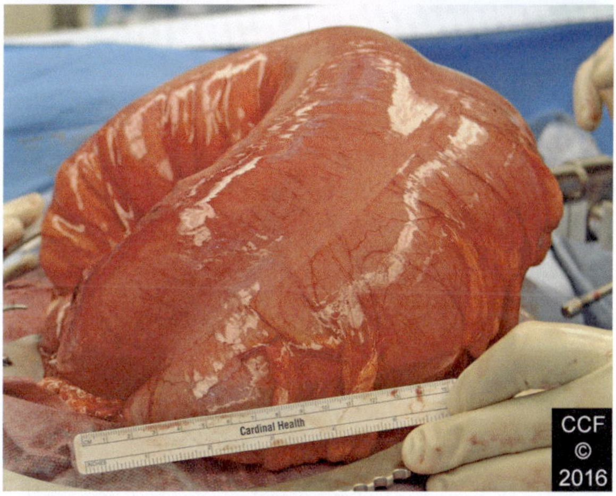

Figs. 104.3 and 104.4 Two views of the massively dilated exteriorized sigmoid colon. (Fig. 104.3) shows the colon and its mesentery; (Fig. 104.4) shows the colon viewed from a 90-degree perspective

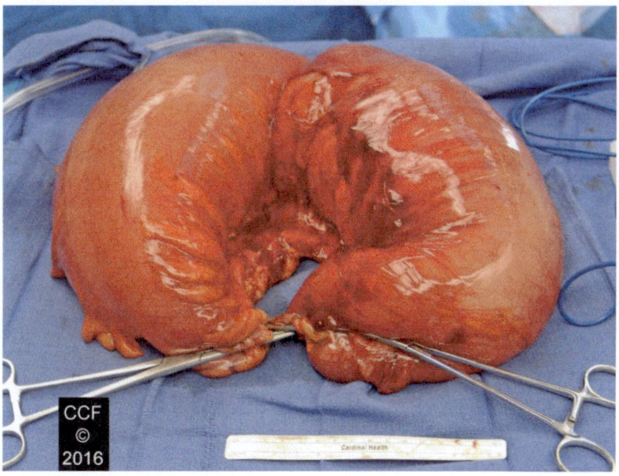

Fig. 104.5 Resected sigmoid colon

Comment [2–9]

Sigmoid volvulus occurs when the sigmoid colon twists on its mesenteric pedicle. Hellinger and Steinhagen [10] and Catalano [11] state the mesoaxial rotation may be "clockwise" or "anti-clockwise." Jones notes that the twist is usually "anticlockwise" [12]. Adverse sequelae include obstruction, ischemia, and perforation. Radiographic signs include marked dilatation of the sigmoid colon, the "bent inner tube," or "coffee bean" sign and the "whirl sign." In Fig. 104.1, the central cleft of the coffee bean is marked with arrows. Figure 104.2 shows the two apposed limbs of the volvulus in cross section. Without surgery, recurrence is common. Surgical options include stenting, pexy, and sigmoid resection with or without restoration of bowel continuity.

References

1. Chung S-D, Chen K-H, Chen H-A, Tu C-C, Wu J-M. Acute abdomen with coffee bean sign. Emerg Med J. 2011;28:826.
2. Halabi WJ, Jafari MD, Kang CY, Nguyen VQ, Carmichael JC, Mills S, Pigazzi A, Stamos MJ. Colonic volvulus in the United States. Trends, outcomes, and predictors of mortality. Ann Surg. 2014;259:293–301.
3. Swenson BR, Kwaan MR, Burkart NE, Wang Y, Madoff RD, Rothenberger DA, Melton GB. Colonic volvulus: Presentation and management in Metropolitan Minnesota, United States. Dis Colon Rectum. 2012;55:444–9.
4. Akinkuotu A, Samuel JC, Msiska N, Mvula C, Charles AG. The role of anatomy of the sigmoid colon in developing sigmoid volvulus: a case-controlled study. Clin Anat. 2011;24:634–7.
5. Martin MJ, Steele SR. Twists and turns: A practical approach to volvulus and intussusception. Scand J Surg. 2010;99:93–102.
6. Peterson CM, Anderson JS, Hara AK, Carenza JW, Menias CO. Volvulus of the gastrointestinal tract: Appearances at multimodality imaging. Radiographics. 2009;29:1281–93.
7. Blake MP, Mendelson RM. The whirl sign: A non-specific finding of mesenteric rotation. Australas Radiol. 1996;40:136–9.
8. Jones IT, Fazio VF. Colonic volvulus. Dig Dis. 1989;7:203–9.
9. Ghazi A, Shinya H, Wolf WI. Treatment of volvulus of the colon by colonoscopy. Ann Surg. 1976;183:263–5.
10. Hellinger MD, Steinhagen RM. Colonic volvulus. In: Wolff BG, Fleshman JW, Beck DE, Pemberton JH, Wexner SD, editors. The ASCRS Textbook of Colorectal Surgery. New York: Springer; 2007. p. 286–98.
11. Catalano O. Computed tomographic appearance of sigmoid volvulus. Abdom Imaging. 1996;21:314–7.
12. Jones DJ. Large bowel volvulus. Br Med J. 1992;305:358–60.

Diverticulosis/Diverticulitis-Introduction 105

James S. Wu and Michelle D. Inkster

Introduction

Diverticula are herniations through the muscular wall of the colon described by Cruveilhier in volume one of his seven-volume treatise on pathological anatomy published in 1849 [1].

TRAITÉ D'ANATOMIE PATHOLOGIQUE GÉNÉRALE, *Hernies tuniquaires du canal digestif.* Par J. Cruveilhier, Professor d'anatomie pathologique à la Faculté de médicine de Paris Mais c'est surtous dans le gros intestin, et particulièrement dans le rectum et l'S iliaque du colon, qu'on observe ce déplacement. On trouve la raison de cette espèce de prédilection dans l'inégalité de résistance des parois du gros intestin, les fibres longitudinale étant réunies en trois bandes parallèles, d'où résulte une force de résistance considérable à leur niveau, et une faiblesse relative dans les points intermédiares:...	*TREATISE ON GENERAL PATHOLOGICAL ANATOMY,* *Hernias of the tunics of the digestive canal* By J. Cruveilhier, Professor of Pathologic Anatomy of the Faculty of Medicine of Paris However, they (hernias) are principally made in the large intestine, especially in the rectum and sigmoid colon. One finds that the reason for this predilection is unequal strength of the walls of the large intestine, the longitudinal fibers being joined by three parallel strips, results in a considerable resistance force at their level, and a relative weakness in the points in between:...

J. S. Wu (✉)
Department of Colon and Rectal Surgery, Cleveland Clinic, Cleveland, OH, USA

M. D. Inkster
Department of Gastroenterology, Cleveland Clinic, Cleveland, OH, USA

J. S. Wu, M. D. Inkster (eds.), *Cleveland Clinic Colorectal Case Studies*,
https://doi.org/10.1007/978-3-031-39880-3_105

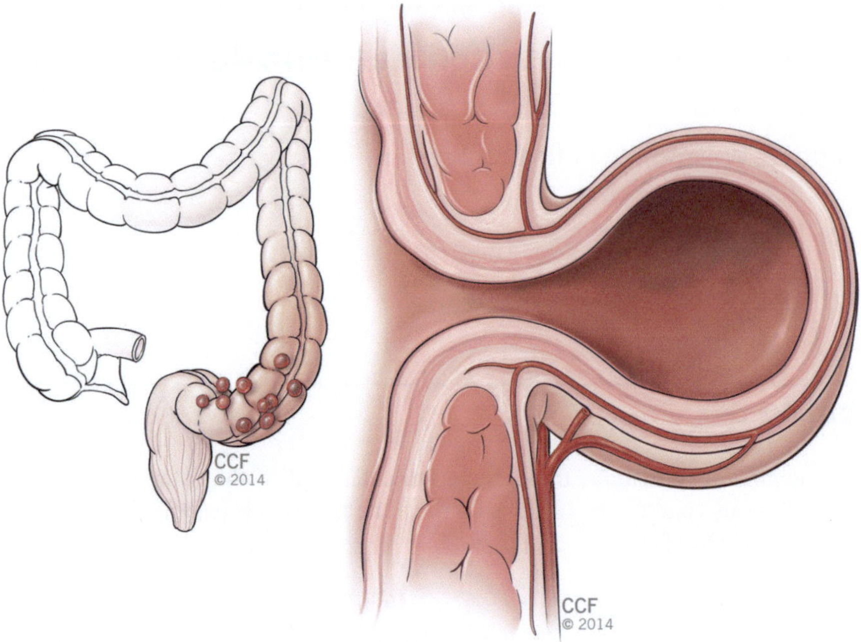

Fig. 105.1 Sigmoid colon diverticulosis. Diverticula (a) are outward herniations of colonic mucosa occurring at openings in the muscularis

They occur where nutrient vessels penetrate the intestinal wall in between the taenia coli to perfuse the intestinal mucosa (Figs. 105.1, 105.2, 105.3, and 105.4).

The appearance of diverticulosis on CT scanning, barium enema, and at surgery is shown in Figs. 105.5, 105.6, 105.7, and 105.8.

According to Hughes, Cutherbertson, and Carden:

> "Most frequently acute diverticulitis arises from inflammation or perforation of a single diverticulum." [2]
>
> E.S.R. Hughes, A.M. Cuthbertson, and
> A. B. G. Carden
> Melbourne

When the thin herniated colonic mucosa outside of the colon wall ruptures, enteric bacteria contaminate the normal sterile peritoneum causing inflammation. Diverticulitis with localized inflammation is defined as uncomplicated. Diverticulitis

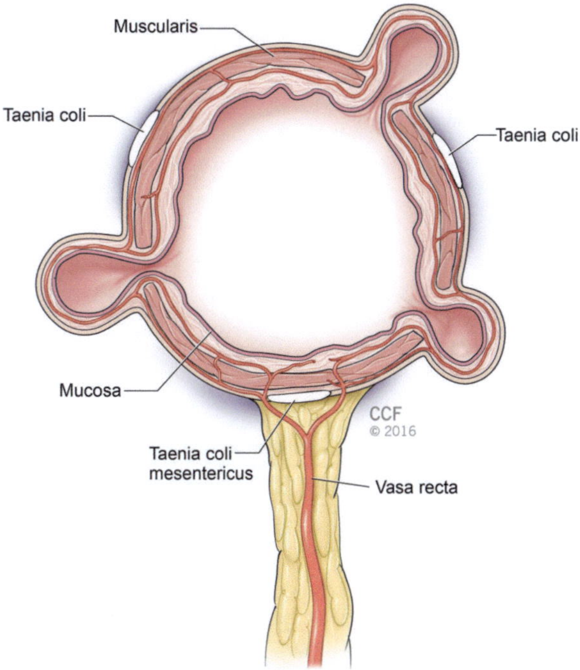

Fig. 105.2 Colon cross-section shows three taeniae. Diverticula occur where blood vessels penetrate to perfuse the mucosa. In the transverse colon, the taenia are identified by neighboring structures (e.g., *taenia mesentericus, taenia omentalis, taenia libera*)

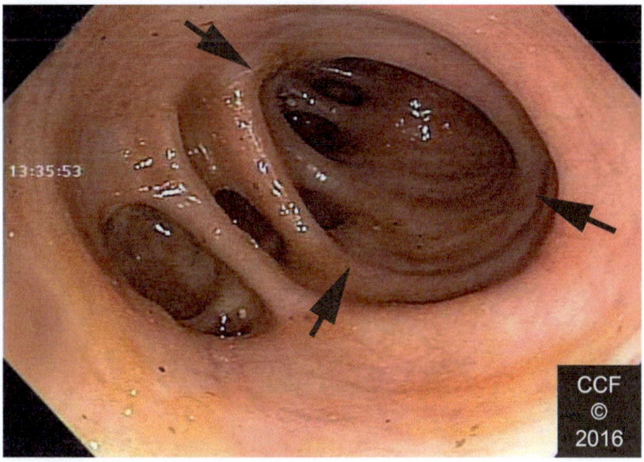

Fig. 105.3 Multiple sigmoid colon diverticula in a line. The location of the three taeniae is indicated by arrows. The diverticula are located in between the taenia

with abscess, fistula, obstruction, or free perforation are examples of complicated diverticulitis. Indications for operation are listed in Table 105.1.

Surgical options are shown in Table 105.2.

Factors that influence surgical management include patient fitness for surgery, risks of complications, plus surgeon and patient preferences.

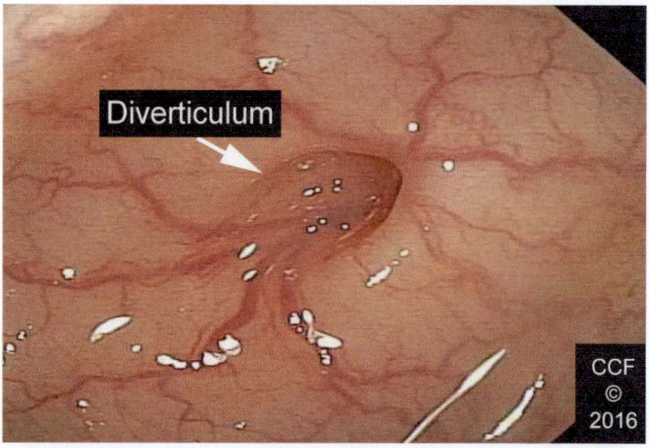

Fig. 105.4 Nutrient vessels to the colonic mucosa pass the through a diverticulum (arrow) as seen on colonoscopy

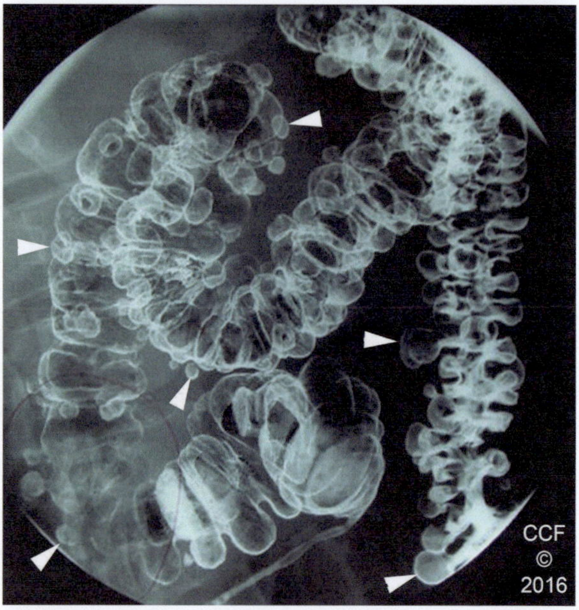

Fig. 105.5 Postevacuation barium enema shows pan-diverticulosis. Representative diverticula are marked by arrowheads

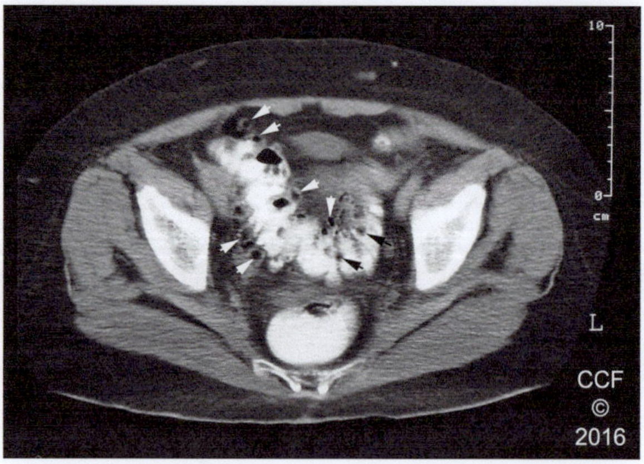

Fig. 105.6 Multiple sigmoid colon diverticula (arrows) seen on computed tomography

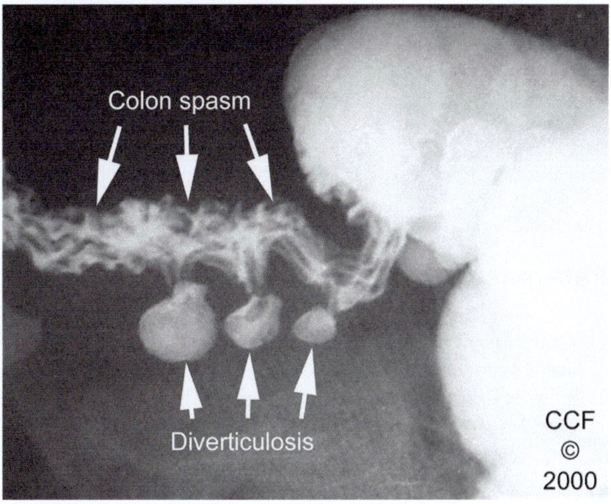

Fig. 105.7 Contrast enema shows three diverticula in the area of colonic spasm

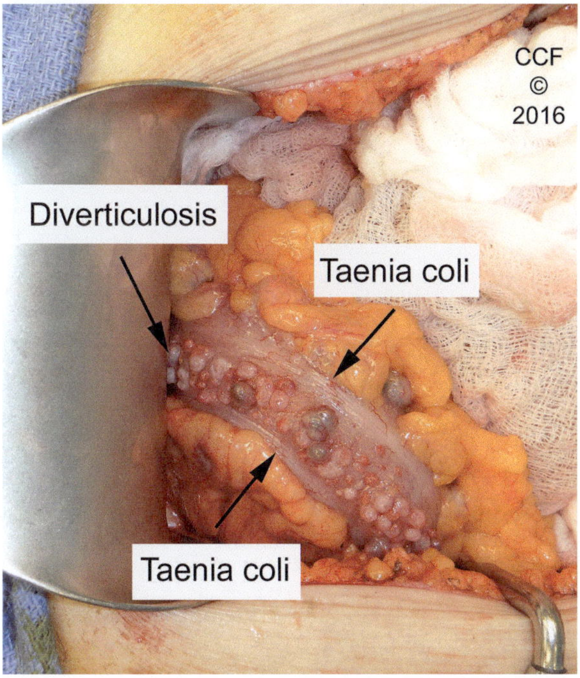

Fig. 105.8 In this operative view, multiple sigmoid colon diverticula are seen located between two longitudinal bands of taenia coli

Table 105.1 Indications for surgery in diverticulitis

Lack of improvement with medical therapy
Recurrent attacks of diverticulitis
Inability to exclude colon cancer
Fistula
Generalized peritonitis
Abscess
Large bowel obstruction

Table 105.2 Operations performed for diverticulitis

Operations
Resection with primary anastomosis
Resection with primary anastomosis and proximal diversion
Resection and proximal diversion
Proximal diversion
Drainage

References

1. Cruveilhier J. Hernies tuniquaires du canal digestif. Traité D'anatomie Pathologique Générale. Tome Premier, Paris: J. B. Baillière; 1849; p. 593.
2. Hughes ESR, Cuthbertson AM, Carden ABG. The surgical management of acute diverticulitis. Med J Aust. 1963;1(21):780–2.

Diverticulitis Complicated by Abscess: Drainage, Resection, and Primary Anastomosis

106

Jesus Flores and James S. Wu

Presentation

A 74-year-old female presented with chills and suprapubic lower abdominal pain. A computed tomographic (CT) scan was obtained (Fig. 106.1).

The patient's medical history is remarkable for prior hysterectomy. Colonoscopy 3 years earlier showed pan-diverticulosis.

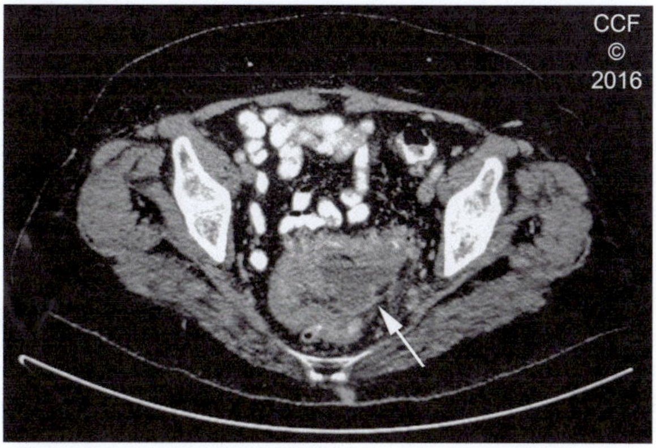

Fig. 106.1 Computed tomography shows a focal abscess (arrow) adjacent to the sigmoid colon in the lower pelvis measuring 5.4 cm × 3.8 cm × 3.6 cm consistent with sigmoid diverticulitis complicated by an abscess

J. Flores · J. S. Wu (✉)
Department of Colon and Rectal Surgery, Cleveland Clinic, Cleveland, OH, USA

J. S. Wu, M. D. Inkster (eds.), *Cleveland Clinic Colorectal Case Studies*,
https://doi.org/10.1007/978-3-031-39880-3_106

Management

The patient was admitted to the hospital. Intravenous antibiotics were administered. Percutaneous abscess drainage by a left trans-gluteal approach with a "pigtail" catheter returned 19 mL of purulent fluid. The patient's abdominal pain resolved. She was discharged home with the pelvic drain in place. Interval CT scan showed sigmoid wall thickening consistent with diverticulitis (Fig. 106.2). Subsequent colonoscopy was successful only up to the rectosigmoid colon.

Follow-up fistula/sinus track study showed a fistula between the pelvic abscess and the sigmoid colon. An opacified cavity in the left posterior pelvis was consistent with residual abscess (Fig. 106.3). A scout film showed pan-diverticulosis (Fig. 106.4).

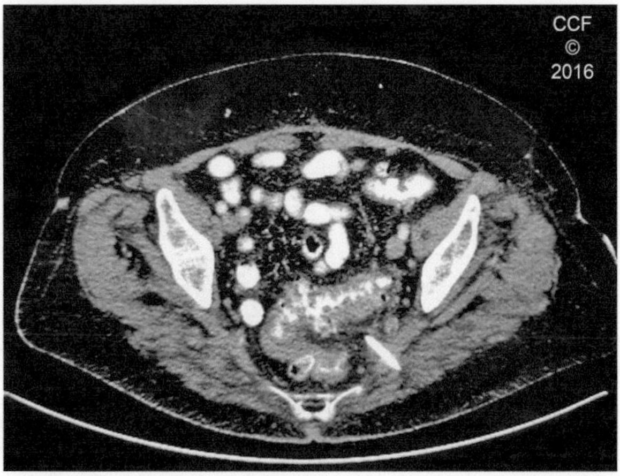

Fig. 106.2 The thickened wall of the sigmoid colon is seen adjacent to part of the percutaneous drain

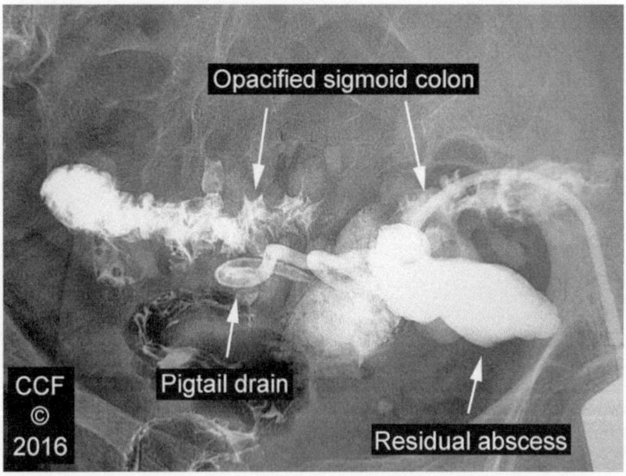

Fig. 106.3 Contrast injection of the pelvic drain shows a fistulous connection to the sigmoid colon and to a residual abscess cavity

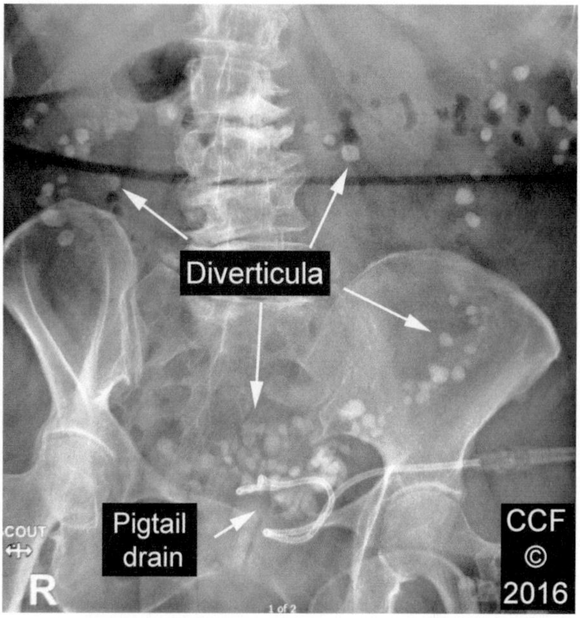

Fig. 106.4 Scout film shows contrast filled diverticula throughout the colon. The "pigtail" drain is shown in the pelvis

Surgery

Sigmoid colectomy with primary anastomosis was done. Bowel continuity was restored using an end-of-colon to side-of-rectum anastomosis (Figs.106.5, 106.6, 106.7, 106.8, and 106.9). Intraoperative colonoscopy cleared the colon of neoplasm.

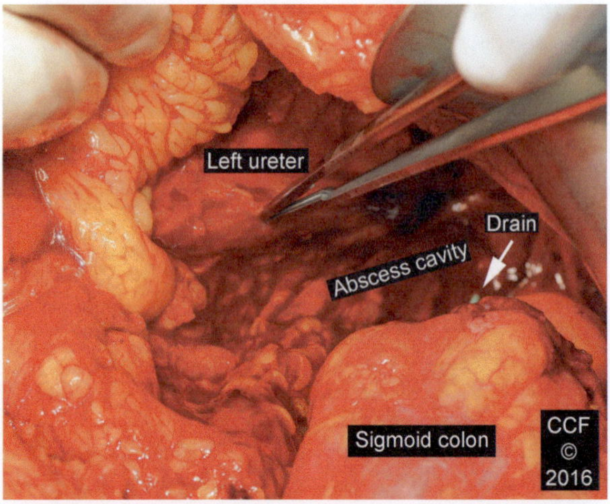

Fig. 106.5 The sigmoid colon has been mobilized. The left ureter was identified. The pelvis has been entered on the left exposing the abscess cavity and the percutaneous drain

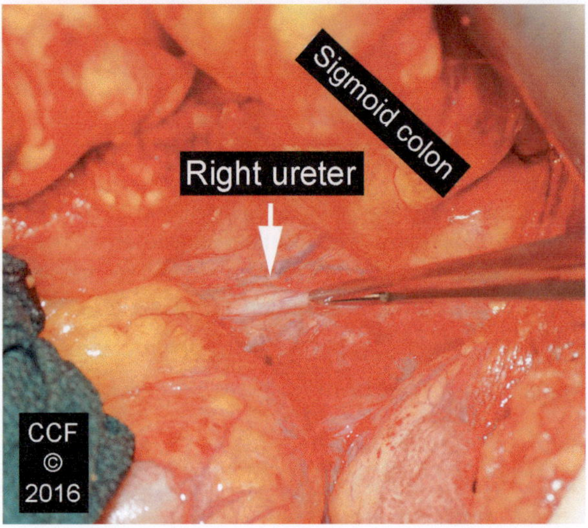

Fig. 106.6 The right ureter is identified

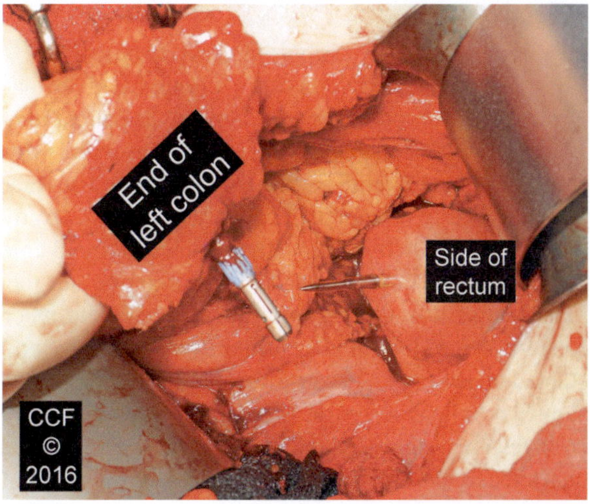

Fig. 106.7 Following sigmoid colon resection, bowel continuity was restored by end-of-left colon to side-of-rectum stapled anastomosis

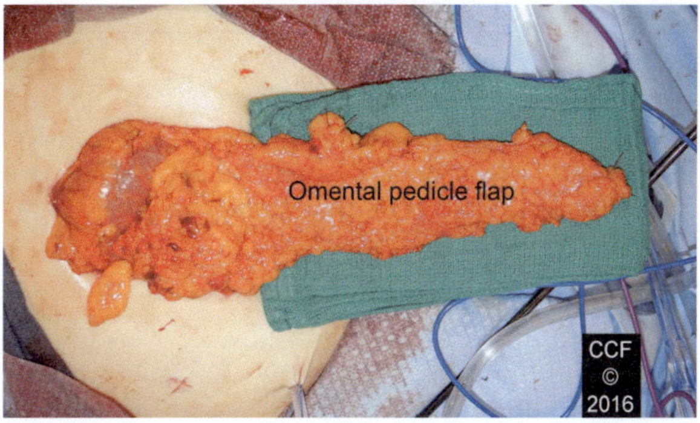

Fig. 106.8 An omental pedicle flap arising from the transverse colon was secured between the colorectal anastomosis and the vagina

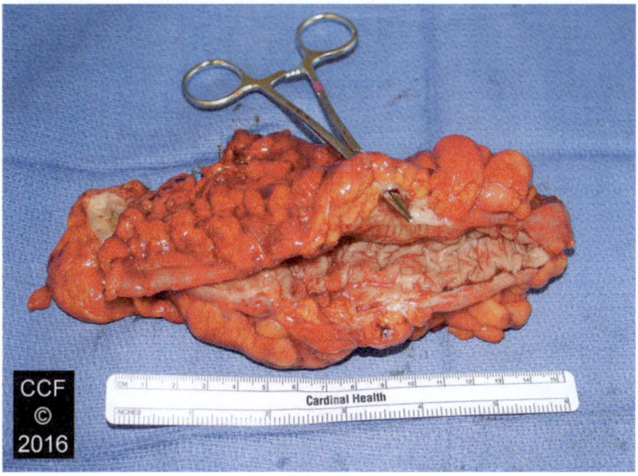

Fig. 106.9 The resected sigmoid colon. The hemostat identifies the origin of the colonic perforation. The resected specimen showed colonic wall and mesenteric thickening plus luminal narrowing

Comment [1]

This patient had diverticulitis complicated by a left-sided pelvic abscess. Percutaneous abscess drainage allowed the patient to recover from her acute illness. Elective single-stage sigmoid resection with primary anastomosis followed. Intraoperative ureteral catheters were placed to facilitate ureteral identification while operating in the inflamed, contaminated operative field. Although the patient had pan-diverticulosis, only the inflamed sigmoid colon was removed. Diverticula were present in the soft, pliable left colon used for the anastomosis. The distal line of resection was the rectum, the anatomic site where the taenia coli disappear. Restoration of intestinal continuity was done by end-of-colon to side-of-rectum stapled anastomosis because the stapling device could not be maneuvered to the stapled proximal end of the rectum. An omental pedicle flap was placed between the colorectal anastomosis and the vaginal cuff to prevent erosion of the colorectal anastomosis into the vagina with resultant colovaginal fistula. Intraoperative colonoscopy cleared the colon of proximal neoplasms.

Reference

1. Hall J, Hardiman K, Lee S, Lightner A, Stocchi L, Paquette IM, et al. The American Society of Colon and Rectal Surgeons Clinical Practice Guidelines for the treatment of left-sided colonic diverticulitis. Dis Colon Rectum. 2020;63:728–47.

Diverticulitis Complicated by Abscess: Drainage, Resection, Primary Anastomosis, and Loop Ileostomy

107

Carolyn L. Power, David Liska, Erick M. Remer, and James S. Wu

Presentation

An 88-year-old female presented with a 2-week history of right lower quadrant pain. On examination, she was afebrile, with normal vital signs. There was mild right lower quadrant tenderness. The white cell count was 17,000 cells per microliter. A computed tomographic scan of the abdomen and pelvis was obtained that showed a right-sided pelvic abscess adjacent to a pelvic phlegmon (Fig. 107.1).

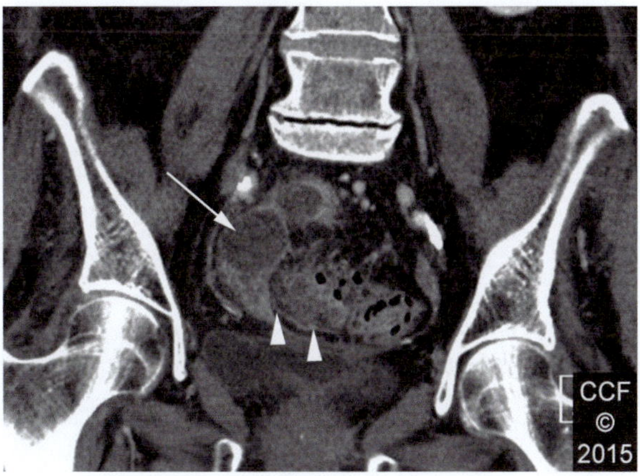

Fig. 107.1 Coronal computed tomographic view of the pelvis show a right-sided pelvic abscess (arrow) and an adjacent inflammatory mass (arrowheads). The findings were consistent with perforated diverticulitis

C. L. Power · D. Liska · J. S. Wu (✉)
Department of Colon and Rectal Surgery, Cleveland Clinic, Cleveland, OH, USA

E. M. Remer
Radiology & Diagnostic Imaging Institute, Cleveland Clinic, Cleveland, OH, USA

J. S. Wu, M. D. Inkster (eds.), *Cleveland Clinic Colorectal Case Studies*,
https://doi.org/10.1007/978-3-031-39880-3_107

Management

The patient was admitted to the hospital. Intravenous antibiotics were administered. The abscess was drained percutaneously with CT guidance (Fig. 107.2).

Cultures grew enteric organisms. Following abscess drainage, symptoms subsided, and the patient was discharged home on oral antibiotics. A drain injection study (1 week later) showed a fistulous connection to the sigmoid colon (Fig. 107.3).

Laparoscopic sigmoid resection with primary colorectal anastomosis and temporary diverting loop ileostomy was done.

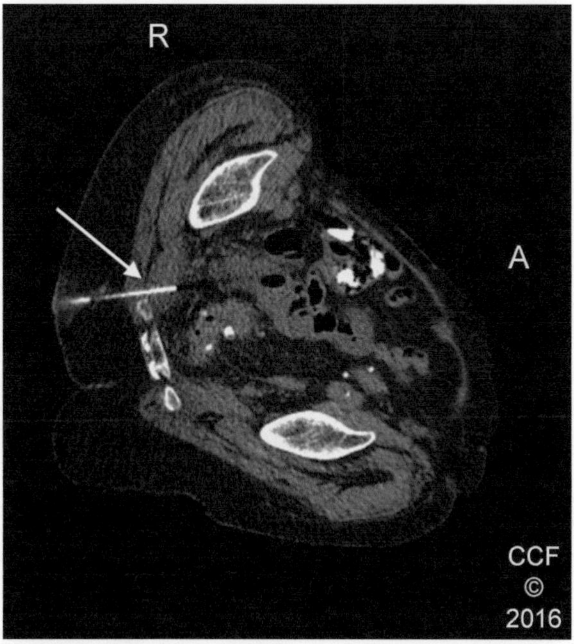

Fig. 107.2 The pelvic abscess is drained through the right buttock. The trocar needle is shown (arrow). A pigtail was placed. Right = R, anterior = A

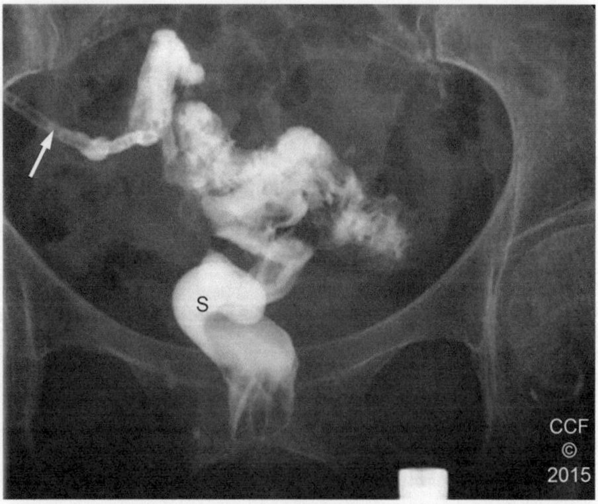

Fig. 107.3 Water-soluble contrast injected into the drain (arrow) opacifies the sigmoid colon (S)

Comment [1, 2]

This elderly patient had diverticulitis complicated by a right-sided pelvic abscess. Percutaneous abscess drainage allowed the patient to recover and avoid emergency surgery. The presence of a fistula detected by drain contrast injection led to the decision to operate. Laparoscopic resection decreased many of the problems associated with a large laparotomy incision (e.g., wound infection, pain, stress, hernia). Diversion of the fecal stream by loop ileostomy protected the anastomosis from immediate exposure to feces. The addition of a stoma, however, added potential problems related to stoma care, fluid and electrolyte losses,and future stoma closure.

References

1. Cauley CE, Patel R, Boudeianou L. Use of primary anastomosis with diverting ileostomy in patients with acute diverticultitis requiring urgent operative intervention. Dis Colon Rectum. 2018;61:586–92.
2. Lee JM, Chang JBP, El Hechi M, Kongkaewpaisan N, Bonde A, Mendoza AE, et al. Hartmann's procedure vs primary anastomosis with diverting loop ileostomy for acute diverticulitis: Nationwide analysis of 2,729 emergency surgery patients. J Am Coll Surg. 2019;229:48–55.

Diverticulitis Complicated by Colovesical Fistula-Hartmann's Procedure 108

James S. Wu

Presentation

A 55-year-old male complained of pneumaturia and brown colored urine. Computed tomography of the abdomen and pelvis was ordered (Fig. 108.1a, b). At colonoscopy, a sharp angulation in the sigmoid colon was encountered that could not be passed (Fig. 108.2). Contrast enema showed a focal narrowing of the sigmoid colon (Fig. 108.3).

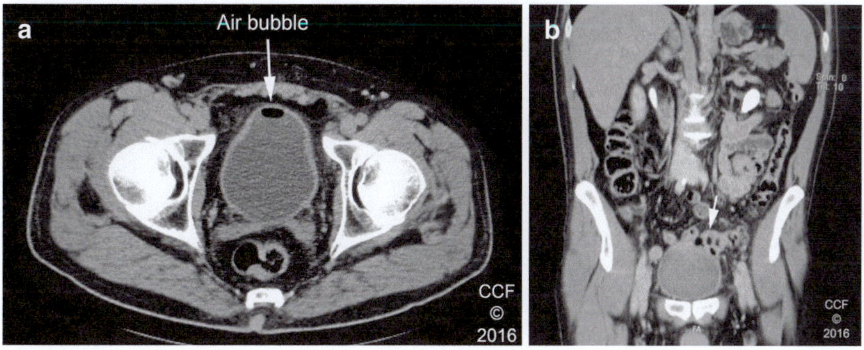

Fig. 108.1 (**a**) Computed tomography shows air in the bladder (arrow); (**b**) the sigmoid colon abuts the bladder (arrow); numerous sigmoid diverticula appear to be present

J. S. Wu (✉)
Department of Colon and Rectal Surgery, Cleveland Clinic, Cleveland, OH, USA

J. S. Wu, M. D. Inkster (eds.), *Cleveland Clinic Colorectal Case Studies*,
https://doi.org/10.1007/978-3-031-39880-3_108

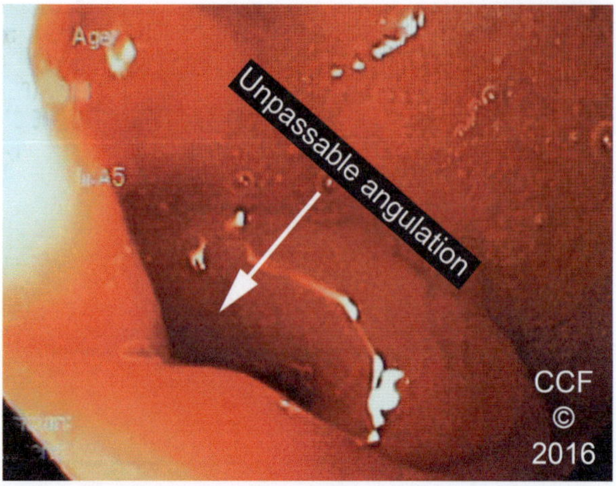

Fig. 108.2 Endoscopic examination of the colorectum reveals an unpassable angulation in the sigmoid colon (arrow)

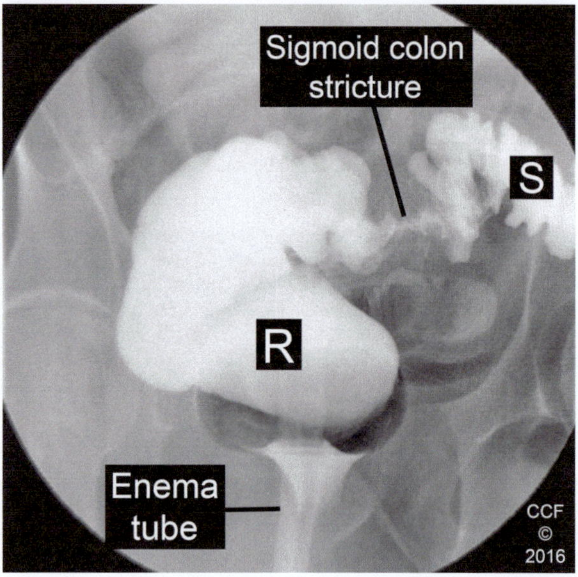

Fig. 108.3 Contrast enema showed a sigmoid colon stricture. *S* sigmoid colon, *R* rectum. The enema tube also is labelled

Management

A pelvic phlegmon was found at surgery. The sigmoid colon was attached to the dome of the bladder (Fig. 108.4). The attachments between the sigmoid colon and bladder were divided. The sigmoid colon was resected and inspected (Fig. 108.5).

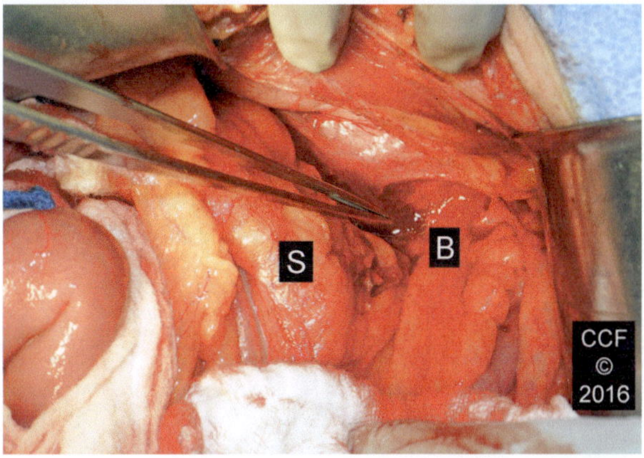

Fig. 108.4 Pelvic phlegmon. The sigmoid colon (S) was firm and adherent to the dome of the bladder (B). The site of colon to bladder attachment is indicated by forceps

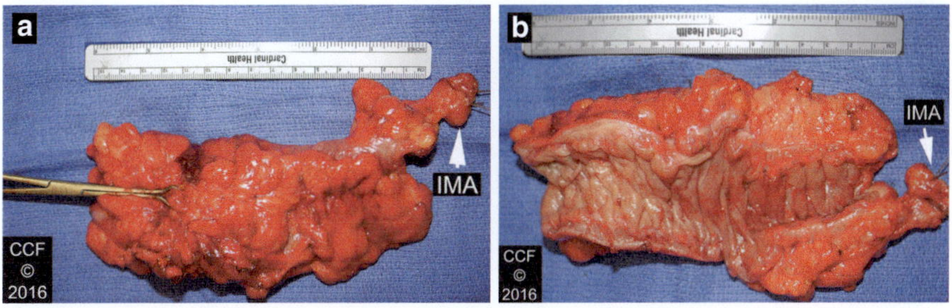

Fig. 108.5 (**a**) The resected sigmoid colon. The attachment of the colon to the bladder is marked by the clamp. High ligation of the inferior mesenteric artery (IMA) was done since the lumen of the sigmoid could not be inspected endoscopically before surgery. (**b**) Inspection of the sigmoid colon lumen excluded neoplasm

Comment

In the male, the mobile sigmoid colon inflamed from diverticulitis comes to rest on the bladder. The patient in this presentation underwent resection with a colostomy (Hartmann's procedure). This operation eliminated the colovesical fistula and avoided the risk of an anastomotic leak. However, for this operation, there is a significant risk that intestinal continuity will not be restored. Following division of the fistula, the bladder hole was closed with suture. Foley catheter bladder drainage was continued after surgery. Restoration of bowel continuity required two additional operations: Hartmann reversal with loop ileostomy followed by loop ileostomy closure.

Biographical Note

Henri Albert Hartmann (1860–1952)

In 1921, Hartmann described an operation for cancers of the sigmoid colon and the rectum that eponymously bears his name [1, 2]. His report was only two paragraphs. The tumor-bearing segment of colon is resected with the adjacent lymph nodes. The rectal stump is left in place in the pelvis and the fecal stream is exteriorized through a colostomy.

Nouveau procédé d'ablation des cancers de la partie terminale du colon pelvien, *Par M. Henri Hartmann, de Paris*	*New ablation procedure for cancers of the terminal end of the pelvic colon* *By Mr. Henri Hartmann, of Paris*
Il est de règle, pour l'extirpation des cancers de la partie terminale du côlon pelvien, de faire une opération actuellement encore très grave, l'amputation abdomino-périnéale du rectum. Chez deux malades, colostomisés pour des accidents d'occlusion, je me suis, dans un deuxième temps, borné à extirper le segment de côlon intermédiaire à l'anus artificiel et au rectum avec le territoire ganglionnaire correspondant. Puis j'ai fermé le bout supérieur du rectum et l'ai péritonisé, ne touchant pas au plancher périnéal.	An operation that is currently still very serious, abdominoperineal resection of the rectum, is standard practice for removing cancers of the distal pelvic colon. In two patients who underwent colostomy for occlusions, I was forced to perform a second operation to remove the segment of the colon between the artificial anus and the rectum, together with the corresponding lymph node area. I then closed the upper part of the rectum and peritonealized it without affecting the perineal floor.
Les suites de l'opération ont dans les deux cas été aussi simples que celles d'une opération d'appendicite à froid. La conservation d'un petit cul-de-sac rectal sus-sphinctérien n'a pas présenté le moindre inconvénient, mes opérations datent de 9 et de 10 mois; les malades vont très bien.	The consequences of the surgery in both cases have been as simple as those of an operation of appendicitis without anesthesia/preparation. The keeping of a small rectal cul-de-sac above the sphincter did not present the least inconvenience, my surgeries were done 9 months and 10 months ago, and the patients are doing very well.

In general, operations that remove the sigmoid colon leave a rectal stump and divert the fecal stream by colostomy are referred to as Hartmann's operation whether or not they are done for malignancy.

Hartmann's obituary in the British Medical Journal was written by Mr. V. Zachary Cope [3].

HENRI HARTMANN, M.D., F.R.C.S (Hon.)

> 'Probably no French surgeon has been, in his day, better known or more widely respected than Henri Hartmann, who as long ago as 1913 was thought worthy to be elected an honorary Fellow of the Royal College of Surgeons. Anatomists still describe the "pouch" which bears his name, and surgeons still, in selected cases, practise the operation he devised for some cases of carcinoma of the rectum.
>
> Hartmann succeeded in 1909 to the chair of surgery at The Hôtel Dieu, where he performed about a thousand operations yearly for 20 years or more. He kept personal notes of all his cases, and had a wealth of experience that he drew upon in his many published

works. He was a general surgeon in the best sense of the word. He wrote on tumours of the breast and on the treatment of war wounds, but his main work was within the abdomen.

Hartmann's clinic in Paris drew men from all parts of the world, and English surgeons regarded him as a man of outstanding surgical worth. The present generation furnishes few, if any, examples of such all-round surgical proficiency.'

References

1. Hartmann H. Nouveau procédé d'ablation des cancers de la partie terminale du colon pelvien. Congrès Francais de Chirurgie, Paris: Procès-Verbaux, Mémoires et Discussions; 1921;30:411.
2. Hotouras A. Henri Hartmann and his operation. Grand Rounds. 2008;8:L1–3. https://doi.org/10.1102/1470-5206.2008.9001.
3. Hartmann H, Cope Z. Obituary. Br Med J. 1952;i:167.

Diverticulitis Complicated by Colovaginal Fistula

109

James S. Wu and Mark E. Baker

Presentation

A 71-year-old female reported the passage of stool and flatus from her vagina. She has a history of diverticular disease. She had undergone hysterectomy. Contrast enema was obtained (Fig. 109.1).

J. S. Wu (✉)
Department of Colon and Rectal Surgery, Cleveland Clinic, Cleveland, OH, USA

M. E. Baker
Department of Radiology, Cleveland Clinic Lerner College of Medicine,
Case Western Reserve University, Cleveland, OH, USA

J. S. Wu, M. D. Inkster (eds.), *Cleveland Clinic Colorectal Case Studies*,
https://doi.org/10.1007/978-3-031-39880-3_109

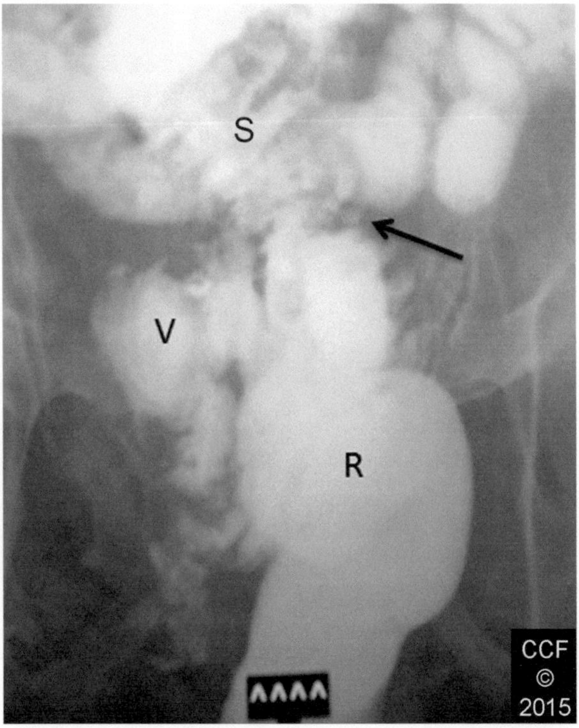

Fig. 109.1 Water-soluble contrast enema. After filling of the rectum (R) and sigmoid colon, contrast is seen within the vagina (V). The arrow highlights a sigmoid colon diverticulum

Management

Contrast enema showed a sigmoid colovaginal fistula. Sigmoid colectomy with colorectal anastomosis was done. The fistulous connection originating from the sigmoid colon is shown in Fig. 109.2. An omental pedicle graft Fig. 109.3 was positioned between the vaginal cuff and the colorectal anastomosis to prevent recurrent fistula formation.

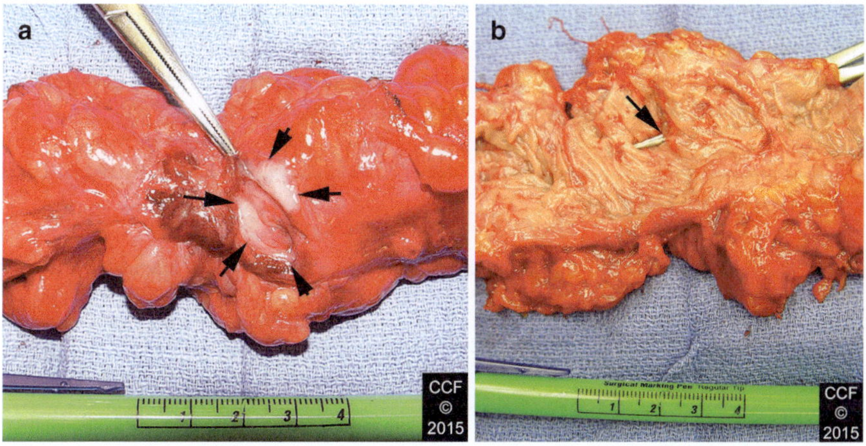

Fig. 109.2 Fistulous connection originating from the sigmoid colon: (**a**) The serosal side of the fistula indicated by a clamp. The serosal adhesions to the vagina are marked by arrows (**b**) the mucosal side of the fistula marked by the clamp tip (arrow)

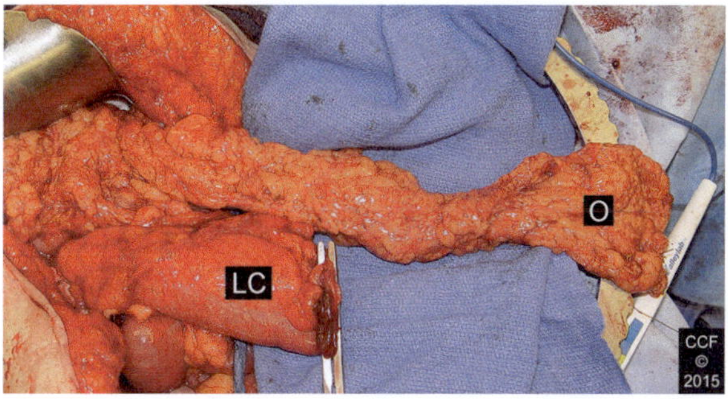

Fig. 109.3 Following sigmoid colon resection and mobilization of the splenic flexure, the left colon (LC) was anastomosed to the rectum. An omental pedicle graft (O) was secured between the colorectal anastomosis and the vaginal cuff

Comment

Causes of colovaginal fistula arising from the colon include: diverticulitis, pelvic or colonic malignancies, inflammatory bowel disease, and irradiated colon, especially after the uterus has been surgically removed [1–4]. Fistulae between the colon and vagina can also occur in pelvic operations where synthetic mesh is used. The diagnosis is suspected based on the history, physical examination, and radiographic studies that include vaginography, contrast enema, colonoscopy, and vaginal examination. Preoperative studies are done in order to define the fistula anatomy since the operative approach for anovaginal fistulas is different than that used for colovaginal fistulas. Ureteral catheters were used in order to facilitate intraoperative identification of the ureters. At surgery, sigmoid diverticulitis complicated by fistula to the vaginal cuff was found. Operative management included takedown of the fistula, resection of the sigmoid colon, mobilization of the splenic flexure, and colorectal anastomosis. An omental pedicle flap was placed in between the colorectal anastomosis and the vaginal cuff to prevent recurrent fistula. Proximal diversion may be used in selected cases. The prognosis for malignant fistulas is poor as complete surgical removal of tumor may not be possible.

References

1. Wu JS, Baker ME. Recognizing and managing acute diverticulitis for the internist. Cleve Clin J Med. 2005;72:620–7.
2. Yu NC, Raman SS, Patel M, Barbaric Z. Fistulas of the genitourinary tract: A radiographic review. Radiographics. 2004;24:1331–52.
3. Vasilevsky C-A, Belliveau P, Trudel JL, Stein BL, Gordon PH. Fistulas complicating diverticulitis. Int J Color Dis. 1998;13:57–60.
4. Bahadursingh AM, Longo WE, Rayburn WE. Colovaginal fistulas. Etiology and management. J Reprod Med. 2003;48:489–95.

Diverticular Disease Complicated by Stricture

110

James S. Wu

Presentation

A 52-year-old patient presented for screening colonoscopy. A stricture was encountered at the rectosigmoid colon that could not be traversed with the colonoscope. A barium enema was obtained (Fig. 110.1).

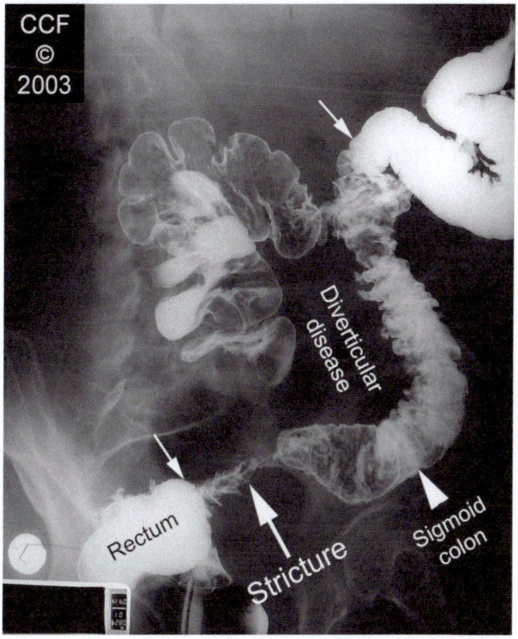

Fig. 110.1 Barium enema shows a stricture (large arrow) at the rectosigmoid colon. Sigmoid colon (arrowhead) diverticular disease is seen. The entire large intestine between the small arrows is abnormal

J. S. Wu (✉)
Department of Colon and Rectal Surgery, Cleveland Clinic, Cleveland, OH, USA

J. S. Wu, M. D. Inkster (eds.), *Cleveland Clinic Colorectal Case Studies*,
https://doi.org/10.1007/978-3-031-39880-3_110

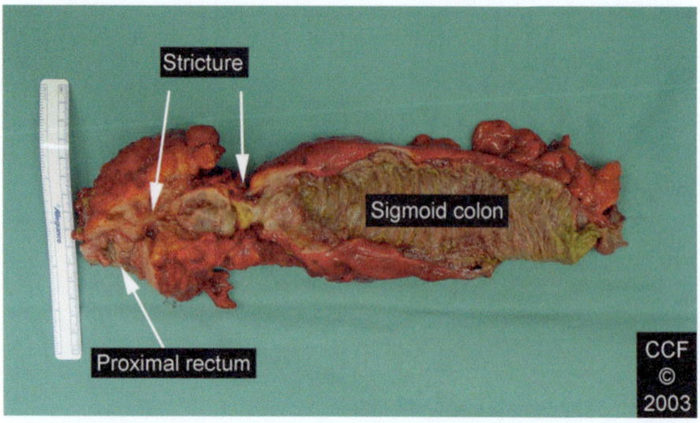

Fig. 110.2 Resected sigmoid colon, rectosigmoid stricture, and proximal rectum. Malignancy was not found

Management

Rectosigmoidectomy with high ligation of the inferior mesenteric artery, takedown of the splenic flexure, and colorectal anastomosis was done (Fig. 110.2).

Comment

This case involves a stricture adjacent to diverticular disease. Because the mucosa lining of the stricture could not be seen endoscopically, it was treated as if it might be cancer. Elective rectosigmoidectomy with lymph node clearance was done [1].

Reference

1. Venara A, Toqué L, Barbieux J, Cesbron E, Ridereau-Zins C, Lermite E, Hamy A. Sigmoid stricture associated with diverticular disease should be an indication for elective surgery with lymph node clearance. J Visc Surg. 2015;152:211–5.

Hartmann Reversal

111

James S. Wu

Presentation

A 68-year-old female developed peritonitis after attempted colonoscopy. Emergency sigmoid colectomy with end colostomy was done to treat rectosigmoid perforation with pelvic abscess. The patient was referred for reconstitution of bowel continuity.

Colostomy reversal surgery was done one year later. The patient was overweight (BMI 40). Preoperative colonoscopy through the end colostomy to the cecum and from the anus to the rectal stump did not reveal any mucosal lesions. The distance from the anus to the top of the rectal stump was 18 cm.

Operative Details

1. Urinary stents
2. Exploratory laparotomy
3. Extensive lysis of adhesions
4. Repair of small bowel injuries
5. Separation of left ureter from pelvic scar tissue
6. Rectal identification and mobilization
7. Attempted double-stapled colorectal anastomosis: unsuccessful due to split in the rectum
8. Further rectal mobilization
9. Division of the superior rectal artery 2 cm proximal to the rectal stump
10. Excision of the proximal rectum
11. Takedown colostomy
12. Colorectal anastomosis by single-stapled technique

J. S. Wu (✉)
Department of Colon and Rectal Surgery, Cleveland Clinic, Cleveland, OH, USA

J. S. Wu, M. D. Inkster (eds.), *Cleveland Clinic Colorectal Case Studies*,
https://doi.org/10.1007/978-3-031-39880-3_111

13. Control of pelvic sidewall hemorrhage
14. Pelvic drain
15. Loop ileostomy
    Operative time: 8 h
    Hospitalization: 10 days

Complications

1. Intraoperative blood loss requiring blood transfusion
2. Readmission for wound infection
   (a) Wound washout in the operating room
   (b) Placement of negative pressure dressing
3. Second readmission for pelvic abscess detected by computed tomographic (CT) scan
   (a) Percutaneous CT-guided abscess drainage
   (b) Intravenous antibiotics
   (c) Water-soluble contrast enema: no contrast extravasation
4. Third readmission for high ileostomy output, dehydration, and electrolyte imbalance
5. Ileostomy appliance leakage
6. Long-term rehabilitation: 6 weeks

Follow-Up 2 Months After Surgery

1. Wound healing complete: negative pressure dressing discontinued
2. Home intravenous antibiotics: completed
3. Pelvic drain removed
4. Eating solid food

Follow-Up 1 Year After Colostomy Takedown

1. Flexible sigmoidoscopy: patent anastomosis (Fig. 111.1)
2. Water-soluble contrast enema: patent colorectal anastomosis, no leak (Fig. 111.2)
3. Loop ileostomy closure done without incident

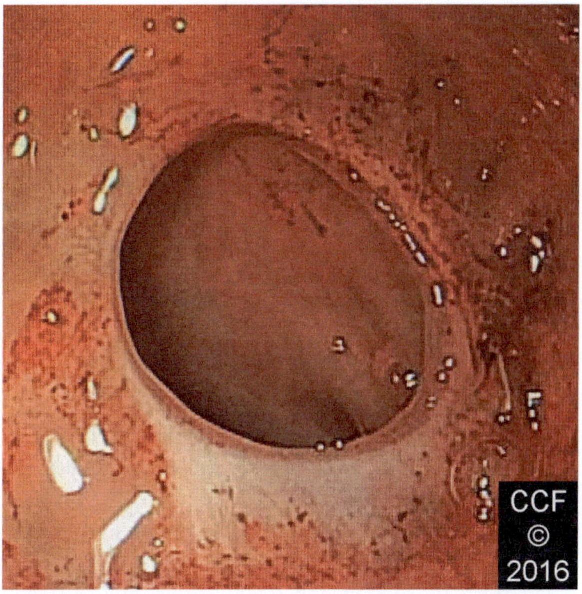

Fig. 111.1 Flexible endoscopic inspection showed a patent colorectal anastomosis

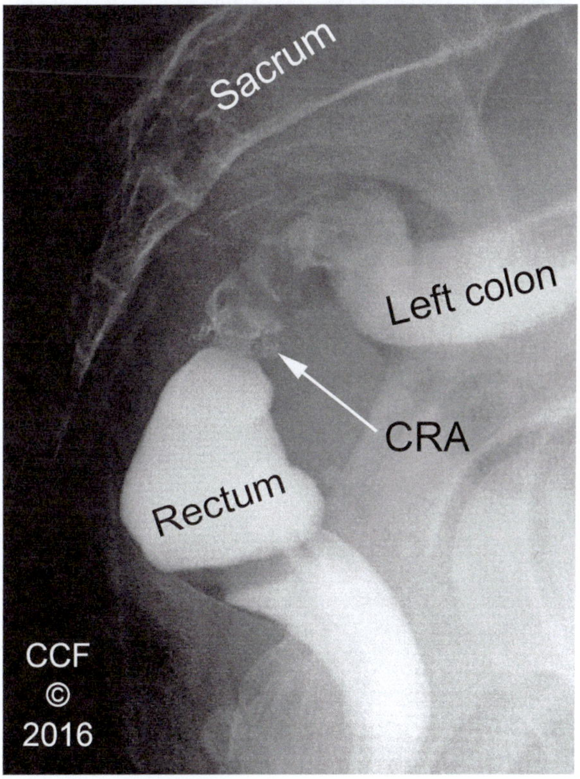

Fig. 111.2 Water-soluble contrast enema showed no contrast extravasation or obstruction across the colorectal anastomosis (CRA)

Comment

Among patients who undergo sigmoid colectomy with end colostomy and out of circuit rectum (Hartmann's operation), a large percentage will not have additional surgery to restore intestinal continuity. In 2009, Riansuwan and colleagues found that greater than 30% of patients undergoing Hartmann's procedure for diverticulitis will not have their stoma reversed within one year [1]. Predictors of nonreversal included: advanced age, elevated American Society of Anesthesiologists (ASA) score, pulmonary comorbidity, perforation, and need for anticoagulants. In the same year, Vermeulen et al. [2] discussed complications of Hartmann reversal. The authors found that Hartmann procedure reversal is a difficult operation with high postoperative morbidity and even mortality; in some cases it should not be performed at all.

As this case illustrates, colostomy reversal after Hartmann's operation can be difficult. Operative challenges are caused by adhesions, altered anatomy, and potential injury to neighboring structures (Table 111.1). The following operative images illustrate some of these obstacles. As shown in Fig. 111.3, dense adhesions often are a common feature of re-operative surgery. After the small intestine has been elevated from the pelvis, the rectal stump may be encased in inflammatory tissue (Fig. 111.4). Care is taken to avoid injury to the ureters, the left iliac vein, and the hypogastric nerves (Figs. 111.5 and 111.6). Rectal stump mobilization begins posteriorly next to the sacral promontory (Fig. 111.7). In this case, colorectal anastomosis was done by single-stapled end-to-end colorectal anastomosis (Figs. 111.8 and 111.9).

Familiarity with prior operations, the placement of ureteral catheters, and the allotment of ample operative time can be beneficial. In some cases, restoration of intestinal continuity may not be achievable. A plan to end surgery prematurely in a way that will leave the patient with the best postoperative situation is part of preoperative planning.

Table 111.1 Pelvic structures at risk for injury during Hartmann reversal

Small intestine
Rectum
Ureters
Iliac vein
Presacral fascia
Vagina
Pelvic sidewall
Nerves of sexual function
Urologic structures

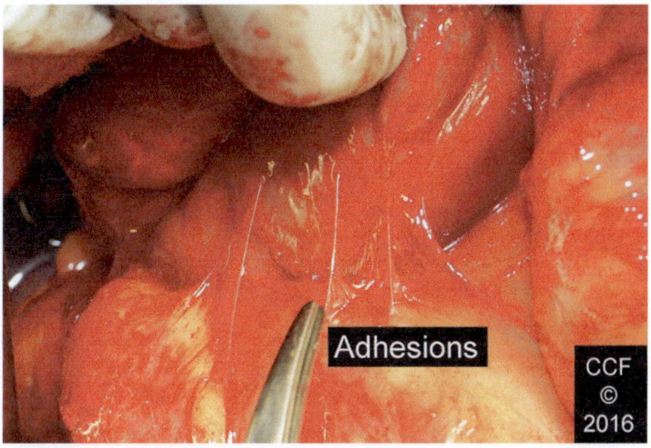

Fig. 111.3 Laparotomy revealed dense adhesions that had to be divided in order to expose the pelvis

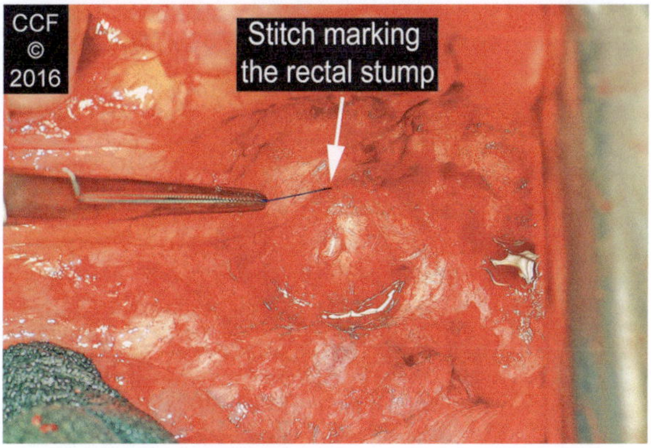

Fig. 111.4 After liberating the small bowel from the pelvis, the top of the rectal stump, embedded in pelvic scar tissue, is identified by a single stitch

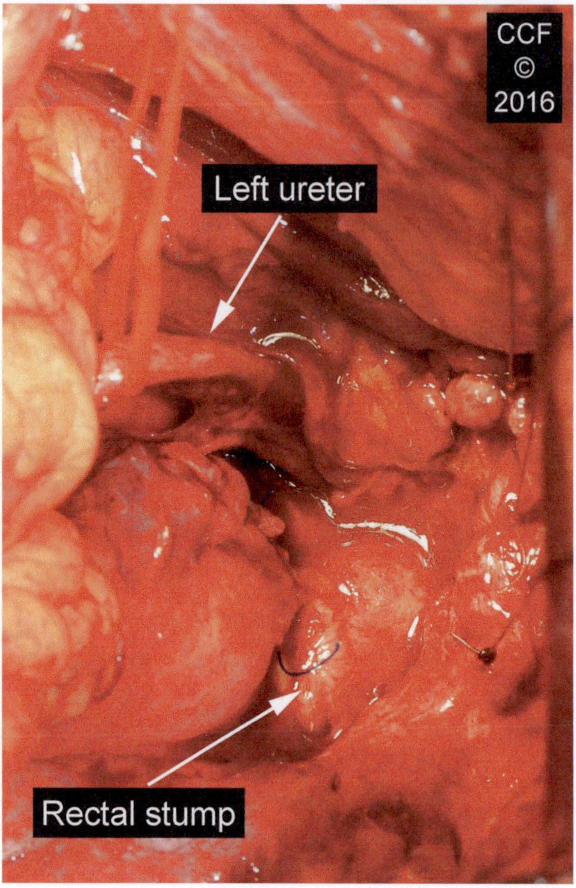

Fig. 111.5 The left ureter has been isolated and controlled with a vessel loop. The stitch identifies the top of the rectal stump

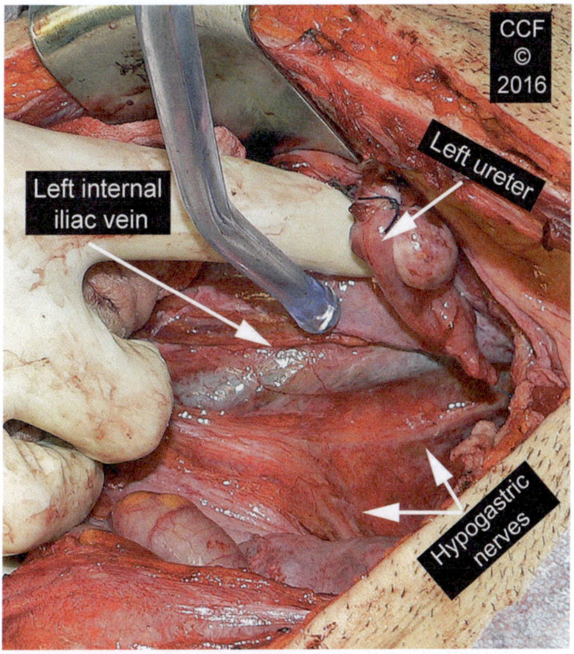

Fig. 111.6 The left iliac vein and the hypogastric nerves are demonstrated. Injury to the left iliac vein can lead to bleeding that is difficult to control. Injury to the hypogastric nerves can lead to sexual dysfunction. The left ureter is identified

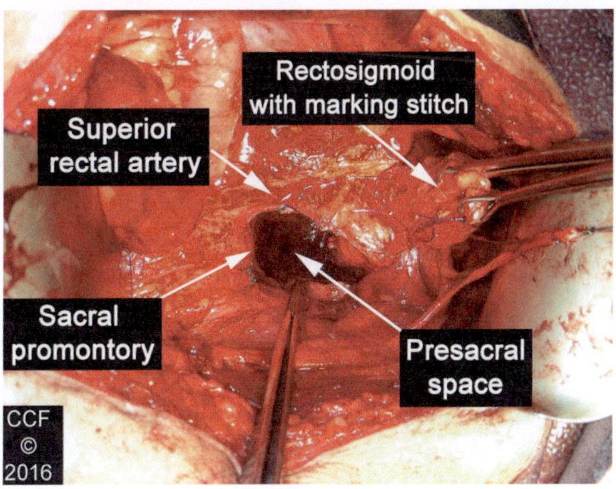

Fig. 111.7 Mobilization of the rectal stump begins posteriorly by entering the presacral space (forceps). The top of the rectal stump has been grasped with Babcock's clamps. Dissection proceeds laterally and finally anteriorly. The proximal rectum is mobilized and excised so that soft pliable rectum is used for the colorectal anastomosis

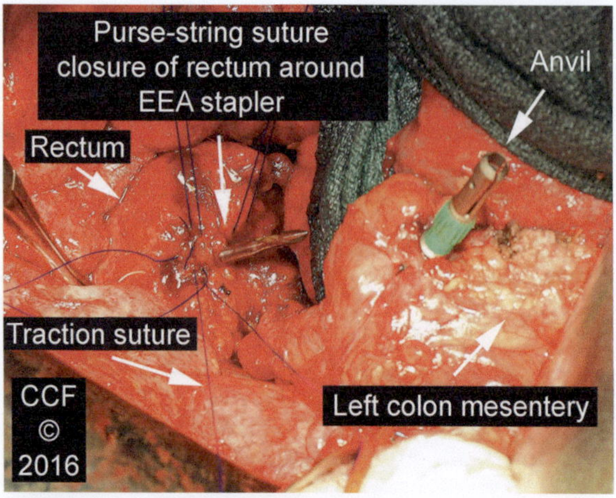

Fig. 111.8 The proximal end of the rectal stump, mobilized from surrounding structures, has been secured around the post of a circular stapling gun with a purse-string suture. The distal descending colon has been secured around the post of the anvil in preparation for single-stapled colorectal anastomosis

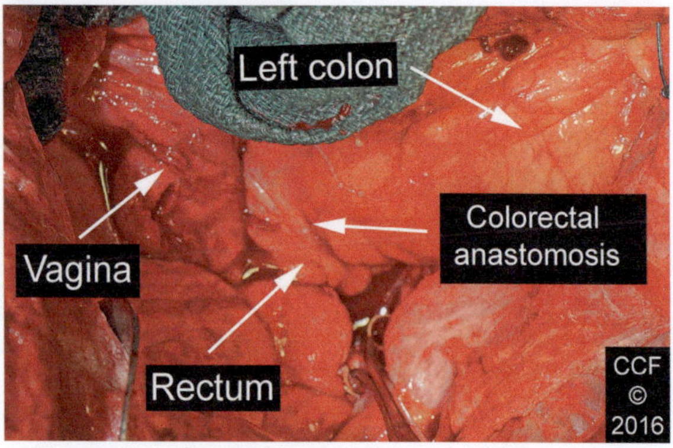

Fig. 111.9 Single-stapled colorectal anastomosis. The rectum used for the anastomosis is clear of the vagina. The anastomosis was watertight. The stapled "donuts" were intact. The left colon is identified

Technical Note

To separate loops of intestine that were intimately adhesed together, Dr. Fazio would inject saline in between the loops in order to create a fluid-filled space where he would cut and, in many cases, mitigate against intestinal injury. This idea is illustrated in Fig. 111.10.

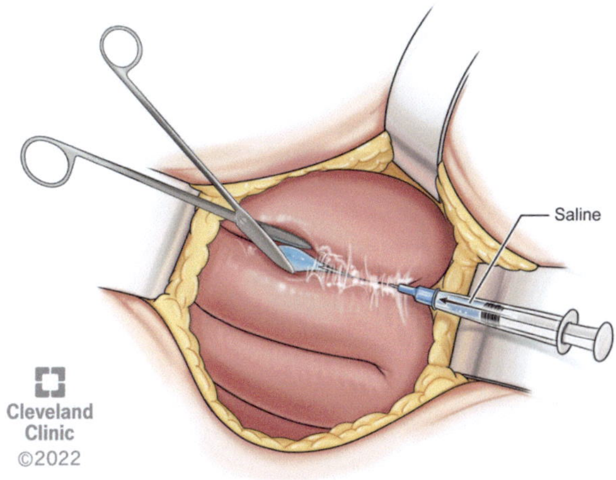

Fig. 111.10 Saline injection to separate closely adhesed loops of intestine. Saline is injected in between the intestinal loops. Using scissors, the adhesion overlying the fluid filled space between the intestinal loops is entered thus separating the loops

References

1. Riansuwan W, Hull TL, Millan MM, Hammel JP. Nonreversal of Hartmann's procedure for diverticulitis: Derivation of a scoring system to predict nonreversal. Dis Colon Rectum. 2009;52:1400–8.
2. Vermeulen J, Coene PPLO, Van Hout NM, van der Harst E, Gosselink MP, Mannaerts GHH, et al. Restoration of bowel continuity after surgery for acute perforated diverticulitis: should Hartmann's procedure be considered a one-stage procedure? Colorectal Dis. 2009;11:619–24.

Lymphocytic Colitis

112

Michelle D. Inkster, Homer O. Wiland, Eric W. Willis, and James S. Wu

Presentation

A 50-year-old female presented with profuse watery diarrhea.

Management

The patient underwent colonoscopy. The colonic mucosa appeared normal.

Random biopsies were taken of the terminal ileum and throughout the colon. Pathology showed lymphocytic colitis (Fig. 112.1).

M. D. Inkster
Department of Gastroenterology, Cleveland Clinic, Cleveland, OH, USA

H. O. Wiland
Department of Pathology, OhioHealth Mansfield Hospital, Mansfield, OH, USA

E. W. Willis
Department of Pathology, CORPath, Columbus, OH, USA

J. S. Wu (✉)
Department of Colon and Rectal Surgery, Cleveland Clinic, Cleveland, OH, USA

J. S. Wu, M. D. Inkster (eds.), *Cleveland Clinic Colorectal Case Studies*,
https://doi.org/10.1007/978-3-031-39880-3_112

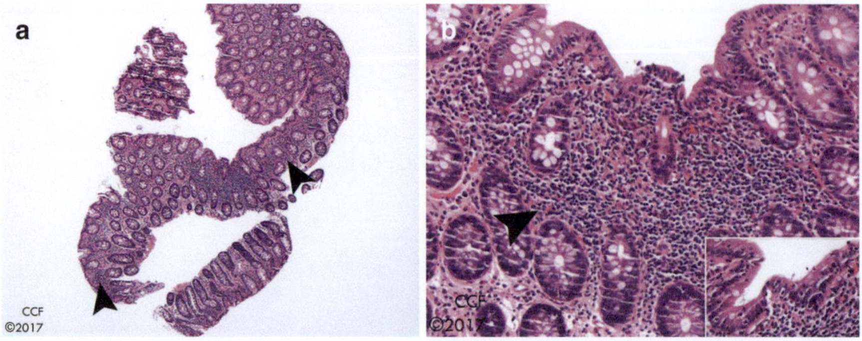

Fig. 112.1 (**a**) Low power view of colonic biopsies demonstrates overall preservation of crypt architecture with an increased inflammatory infiltrate in the lamina propria in a "top-heavy" distribution (arrowheads) (hematoxylin-eosin, original magnification ×40); (**b**) the lymphoplasmacellular infiltrate is associated with brisk lymphocytic-mediated epithelial injury noted in the crypt and surface epithelium (arrowhead). The subepithelial collagen table thickness is not significantly increased (hematoxylin-eosin, original magnification ×200, hematoxylin-eosin, original magnification ×400 [inset])

Comment

In 1989, Lazenby and colleagues defined lymphocytic colitis as follows:[1]

> "Lymphocytic colitis, previously termed "microscopic colitis", is a clinicopathologic syndrome of watery diarrhea, grossly normal colonoscopy, and mucosal inflammatory changes. The most distinctive feature of lymphocytic colitis was increased intraepithelial lymphocytes, particularly in the surface epithelium… Other prominent features of lymphocytic colitis included surface epithelial damage…, increased lamina propria chronic inflammation…, and minimal crypt distortion or active cryptitis."
>
> Audrey J. Lazenby, M.D., John H. Yardley, MD, Francis M. Giardiello, MD, Jose Jessurun, MD, and Theodore M. Bayless, MD
>
> Departments of Pathology and Medicine, The Johns Hopkins University School of Medicine, and The Johns Hopkins Hospital, Baltimore and the Unidad de Patologica, Hospital General de Mexico SS, UNAM, Mexico

Because the epithelium endoscopically appears normal, mucosal biopsy for histological examination is needed to make the diagnosis [2]. Treatments include discontinuation of medications which may cause diarrhea, such as serotonin uptake inhibitors (SSRI), proton pump inhibitors, statins and nonsteroidal medications (ibuprofen, naprosyn) [3]. Lymphocytic colitis can also be seen with celiac disease (can be distinguished by small bowel biopsy and serologic evaluation). Of note, about 30% of patients with Crohn's disease also test positive for celiac disease.

[1]Lazenby et al. [1]. Permission to reproduce this excerpt was generously granted by Elsevier Science & Technology Journals, CCC|Marketplace™; Order License ID 1140938-1; order date 16-Aug-2021.

Current treatment is usually the oral steroid, budesonide. Budesonide is resistant to gastric acid degradation and is mostly absorbed in the small intestine and proximal colon. This minimizes the side effects commonly seen in other steroids such as prednisone [4]. Edsbäcker et al. [5] showed that delivery from controlled release capsules of budesonide to the ileocolonic region was significantly greater than the standard capsules with the major fraction being released in the ileum and throughout the colon.

References

1. Lazenby AJ, Yardley JH, Giardiello FM, Jessurun J, Bayless TM. Lymphocytic ("Microscopic") colitis: a comparative histopathologic study with particular reference to collagenous colitis. Hum Pathol. 1989;20:18–28.
2. Münch A, Aust D, Bohr J, Bonderup O, Fernández Bañares F, Hjortswang H, et al. Microscopic colitis: Current status, present and futures challenges. Statements of the European Microscopic Colitis Group. J Crohn's Colitis. 2012;6:932–45.
3. Chande N, MacDonald JK, McDonald JWD. Interventions for treating microscopic colitis: A Cochrane Inflammatory Bowel Disease and Functional Bowel Disorders Review Group systematic review of randomized trials. Am J Gastroenterol. 2009;104:235–41.
4. O'Donnell S, O'Morain CA. Therapeutic benefits of budesonide in gastroenterology. Ther Adv Chronic Dis. 2010;1:177–86.
5. Edsbäcker S, Bengtsson B, Larsson P, Lundin P, Nilsson Å, Ulmius J, Wollmer P. A pharmacoscintigraphic evaluation of oral budesonide given as controlled-release (Entocort) capsules. Aliment Pharmacol Ther 2003;17:525–36.

Collagenous Colitis

113

James S. Wu, Rish K. Pai, Homer O. Wiland, and Michelle D. Inkster

A 74-year-old male presented with unexplained diarrhea. Colonoscopy showed a well-vascularized mucosa with diffuse surface irregularity as shown in Fig. 113.1. Random biopsies were taken (Fig. 113.2).

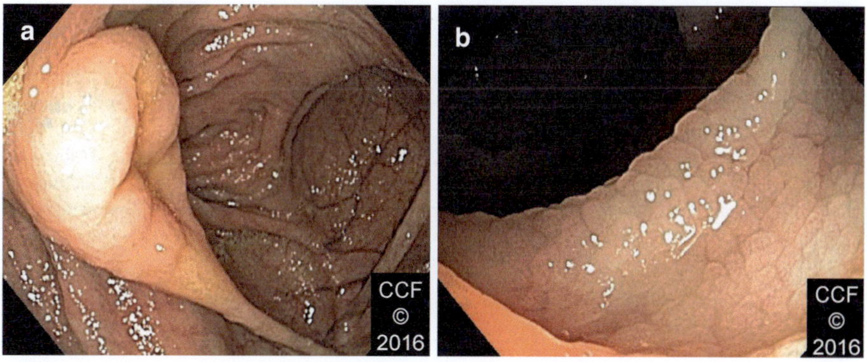

Fig. 113.1 Colonoscopy. Views of the cecum and ileocecal valve (**a**) and the transverse colon (**b**) show a diffuse surface nodular irregularity

J. S. Wu (✉)
Department of Colon and Rectal Surgery, Cleveland Clinic, Cleveland, OH, USA

R. K. Pai
Department of Laboratory Medicine and Pathology, Mayo Clinic, Phoenix, AZ, USA

H. O. Wiland
Department of Pathology, OhioHealth Mansfield Hospital, Mansfield, OH, USA

M. D. Inkster
Department of Gastroenterology, Cleveland Clinic, Cleveland, OH, USA

J. S. Wu, M. D. Inkster (eds.), *Cleveland Clinic Colorectal Case Studies*,
https://doi.org/10.1007/978-3-031-39880-3_113

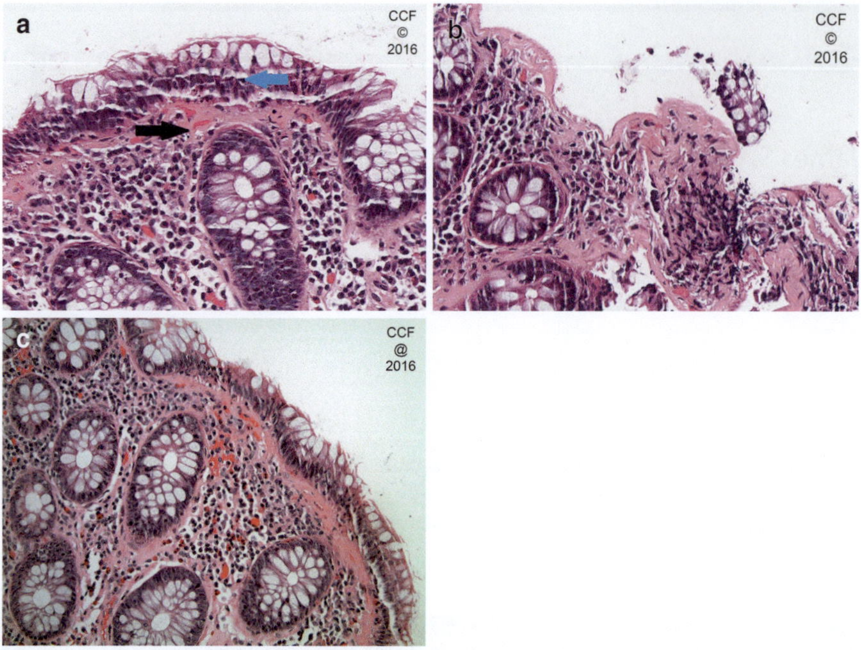

Fig. 113.2 (**a**) The colon biopsies show an intact crypt architecture, but there is a conspicuous thickening of the subepithelial collagen plate (black arrow), which harbors scattered inflammatory cells as well as entrapped capillaries. There are increased numbers of lymphocytes and plasma cells within the superficial aspect of the mucosa, and several intraepithelial lymphocytes are seen (blue arrow, H–E, original magnification ×200). (**b**) In other areas, there is epithelial denudation in areas of prominent collagen (H–E, original magnification ×200). (**c**) Congo red stains were negative for amyloid

Management

Treatment with Peptobismol™ was instituted with benefit.

Comment

In 1976, Lindström[1] and Freeman et al.[2] independently described collagenous colitis.

[1] Lindström [1]. Permission to reproduce this excerpt was generously granted, by John Wiley & Sons, Ltd, CCC|Marketplace®, Order License ID 1141246-1, Order Date 17-Aug-20221.

[2] Freeman et al. [2]. This text was adapted with the generous permission of Ms. Jessica Hertzog-grenier, director, communications, marketing and translation, Royal College of Physicians and Surgeons of Canada, October 19, 2021.

'Collagenous colitis' with watery diarrhea diarhhoea—A new entity?

C. G. Lindström

University Department of Pathology, Malmö General Hospital and Cytlab, Malmö, Sweden

"In 1970 Weinstein *et al.* described a special type of sprue—collagenous sprue—which was histologically characterized by a marked collagenous layer under the surface epithelium in the jejunal mucosa leading to a blocking of the intestinal resorption with the clinical picture of malabsorption. Earlier SCHEIN (1947) and HOURIHANE (1963) had published cases with the same histological picture.

We have had the opportunity to examine histologically a case with similar collagenous deposit but localized here in the colorectal mucosa with watery diarrhoea as a result. The combination of these manifestations seems not to have been described earlier. The term 'collagenous colitis' or 'collagenous proctocolitis' is proposed for this entity."

Watery diarrhea syndrome associated with a lesion of the colonic basement membrane (BM) — Lamina propria (LP) interface.

H. J. Freeman, W. M. Weinstein, T. K. Shnitka, R. H. Wensel, V. E. Sartor

Departments of Medicine and Pathology, University of Alberta, Edmonton

"In 2 patients with longstanding watery diarrhea, sigmoidoscopy examinations were normal but biopsies demonstrated a previously unreported mucosal abnormality. The most prominent feature was a marked thickening at the BM-LP interface.

The BM-LP abnormality was further characterized by electron microscopy, histochemistry and immunofluorescence. These studies revealed an accretion of LP collagen, microfibrils, ground substance, amorphous protein and small amounts of immunoglobulins to the BM,...

On salicylazosulfapyridine therapy, clinical and histological resolution occurred in one patient and partial resolution has occurred in the second patient. The rectal and colonic biopsy findings in our 2 patients clearly represent a unique histological marker in a form of inflammatory bowel disease."

Collagenous colitis is a form of microscopic colitis. Chronic profuse watery diarrhea, abdominal pain, and weight loss are common presentations. Elderly females are most commonly affected. Peritonitis due to colonic perforation has been reported. Causes include nonsteroidal anti-inflammatory medications, selective serotonin reuptake inhibitors, duloxetine, and proton pump inhibitors. Therapy includes: bulking agents, 5-aminosalicylic acid agents, bismuth, steroids, anticytotics, and discontinuation of suspected inciting agents [3]. Collagenous colitis traditionally has been associated with "normal" appearing mucosa at colonoscopy with characteristic histologic features of collagen deposition in the subepithelial layer. Reports of distinct endoscopic findings have emerged which describe pseudomembranes, mucosal vascular pattern alteration, erythema, nodularity, and fractures [4]. The mucosa in this case was nodular. Epithelial denudation in areas of prominent collagen is a common finding in collagenous colitis. Congo red staining was done to exclude amyloid as thickened collagen can mimic amyloid [5]. Submucosal collagen deposition also can be caused by medication such as the antihypertensive medication olmesartan medoxodil [6].

References

1. Lindström CG. 'Collagenous colitis' with watery diarrhoea—A new entity? Path Europ. 1976;11:87–9.
2. Freeman HJ, Weinstein WM, Shnitka TK, Wensel RH, Sartor VE. Watery diarrhea syndrome associated with a lesion of the colonic basement membrane (BM)—lamina propria (LP) interface. Ann R Coll Phys Surg Can. 1976;9:45.
3. Temmerman F, Baert F. Collagenous and lymphocytic colitis: Systematic review and update of the literature. Dig Dis. 2009;27((suppl) 1):137–45.
4. Koulaouzidis A, Saeed AA. Distinct colonoscopy findings of microscopic colitis: Not so microscopic after all? World J Gastroenterol. 2011;17:4157–65.
5. Mahajan D, Goldblum JR, Xiao S-Y, Shen B, Liu X. Lymphocytic colitis and collagenous colitis: A review of clinicopathologic features and immunologic abnormalities. Adv Anat Pathol. 2012;19:28–38.
6. Rubio-Tapia A, Herman ML, Ludvigsson JF, Kelly DG, Mangan TF, Wu T-T, Murray JA. Severe spruelike enteropathy associated with olmesartan. Mayo Clin Proc. 2012;87:732–8.

Breast Cancer Metastatic to Colon

114

Michelle D. Inkster, Homer O. Wiland, Eric W. Willis, and James S. Wu

Presentation

A 70-year-old female underwent colonoscopy because of chronic diarrhea. Random biopsies were taken. Pathology is shown in Fig. 114.1.

The patient underwent an esophagogastroduodenoscopy because of nausea. Random biopsies were taken. In addition to chronic Helicobacter pylori infection, the following was seen (Fig. 114.2).

M. D. Inkster
Department of Gastroenterology, Cleveland Clinic, Cleveland, OH, USA

H. O. Wiland
Department of Pathology, OhioHealth Mansfield Hospital, Mansfield, OH, USA

E. W. Willis
Department of Pathology, CORPath, Columbus, OH, USA

J. S. Wu (✉)
Department of Colon and Rectal Surgery, Cleveland Clinic, Cleveland, OH, USA

J. S. Wu, M. D. Inkster (eds.), *Cleveland Clinic Colorectal Case Studies*,
https://doi.org/10.1007/978-3-031-39880-3_114

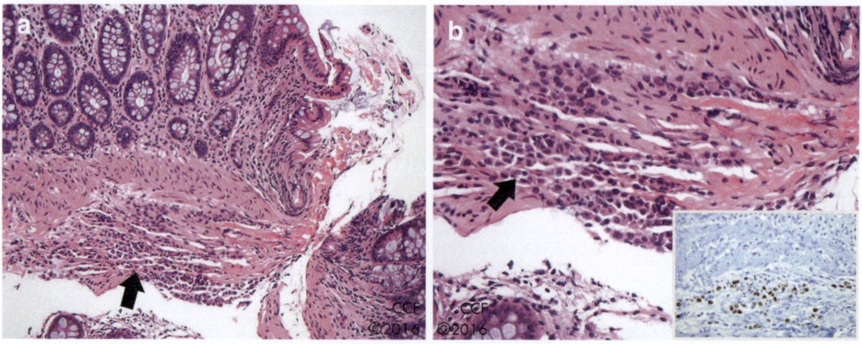

Fig. 114.1 (**a**) Random colon biopsy demonstrating a 1 mm focus of epithelioid cells with increased nuclear to cytoplasmic ratios within the superficial submucosa, (arrow) (hematoxylin–eosin, original magnification x200); (**b**) malignant epithelioid cells at higher magnification (arrow). An immunohistochemical stain for estrogen receptor (ER) is positive (expressed in greater than 90% of nuclei) (hematoxylin–eosin, original magnification ×400; ER stain, original magnification ×200 [inset])

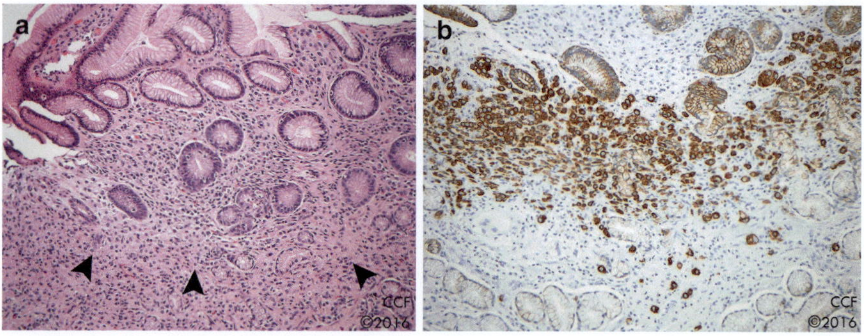

Fig. 114.2 (**a**) Epithelioid cells expanding the lamina propria (arrowheads) of this gastric biopsy distorting its normal glandular architecture (hematoxylin–eosin, original magnification ×200); (**b**) an immunohistochemical stain for cytokeratin AE1/E3 highlights the cells of interest, confirming their epithelial origin (AE1/E3 stain, original magnification ×200)

Comment

The most common sites of metastatic breast cancer are lung, bone, lymph nodes, and liver [1]. Metastasis to the large intestine is rare. This case demonstrates breast cancer metastatic to the colon detected incidentally on random biopsies taken because of diarrhea. She had had a mammogram 10 years earlier that was reported as normal. Subsequent mammography showed two lesions in the right breast as well as enlarged lymph nodes in the right axillary tail; biopsy showed lobular carcinoma. Lobular carcinoma tends to spread to bones, gynecological organs, peritoneum, retroperitoneum, and the gastrointestinal tract [2]. Computed tomography for this patient showed ascites with probable carcinomatosis, bilateral hydronephrosis, and diffuse skeletal blastic metastases.

Breast cancer metastases to the gastrointestinal tract are under-recognized. Lesions in the colon can be confused with a primary colonic neoplasm. A high level of suspicion that a colonic lesion may be metastatic from the breast is required especially when a patient has a history of breast cancer. Patients with lobular breast carcinoma have a poor prognosis and rarely survive longer than two years after the diagnosis of gastrointestinal involvement [3]. This case emphasizes the benefit of ongoing screening when appropriate.

References

1. Klein MS, Sherlock P. Gastric and colonic metastases from breast cancer. Dig Dis. 1972;17:881–6.
2. Black M, Hakam A, Harris C, Jiang K. Metastatic breast carcinoma uncovered in an otherwise unremarkable "random colon biopsy". Hum Pathol Case Rep. 2016;4:23–31.
3. Molina-Barea R, Rios-Peregrina RM, Slim M, Calandre EP, Hernández-García MD, Jimenez-Rios JA. Lobular breast cancer metastasis to the colon, the appendix and the gallbladder. Breast Care. 2014;9:428–30.

Colonic Amyloidosis

115

Michelle D. Inkster, Eric W. Willis, and James S. Wu

Presentation

A 62-year-old female presented with a 2-week history of diarrhea, nausea, vomiting, bloody stools, and a 10-pound weight loss.

Flexible sigmoidoscopy with random biopsies was done. Pathology showed amyloid Fig. 115.1.

M. D. Inkster
Department of Gastroenterology, Cleveland Clinic, Cleveland, OH, USA

E. W. Willis
Department of Pathology, CORPath, Columbus, OH, USA

J. S. Wu (✉)
Department of Colon and Rectal Surgery, Cleveland Clinic, Cleveland, OH, USA

J. S. Wu, M. D. Inkster (eds.), *Cleveland Clinic Colorectal Case Studies*,
https://doi.org/10.1007/978-3-031-39880-3_115

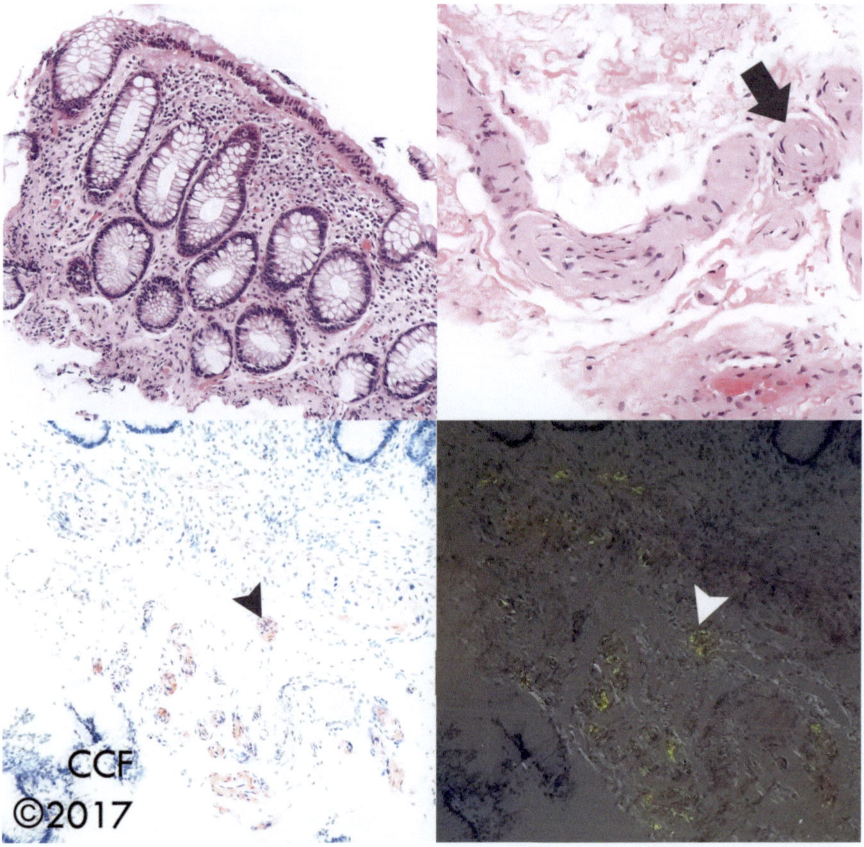

Fig. 115.1 Upper left: sections from the colon biopsy demonstrate an unremarkable mucosa; upper right: the submucosal vessels show subtle hyalinization (arrow); lower left: a congo red stain shows the presence of orange-red amyloid in the submucosal vessels (black arrowhead); lower right: apple-green birefringence under polarized light (white arrowhead) is seen. Ancillary immunohistochemical stains (not shown) were positive for kappa and negative for lambda, AA1, and transthyretin. The background lamina propria plasma cells were polytypic

Comment

In 1854, Virchow described amyloid bodies [1]:

Ueber eine im Gehirn und Rückenmark des Menschen aufgefundene Substanz mit der chemischen Reaction der Cellulose Von Rud. Virchow Glucklicher war ich, als ich vor kurzer Zeit meine Aufmersamkeit auf die sogenannten *Corpora amylacea* des Gehirns richtete, über deren genaure Natur ich gegenüber den sonstigten Amyloidkörpern des Menschen früher kein genaues Urtheil gewonnen hatte.	Concerning a substance found in the human brain and spinal cord with the chemical reaction of cellulose By Rudolf Virchow I was happier when, a short time ago, I focused my attention on the so-called *corpora amylacea* of the brain, the exact nature of which I had previously failed to obtain from the other amyloid bodies of humans.

In 2012, Desport et al. [2] described amyloid light-chain (AL) amyloidosis as follows:

> "AL amyloidosis results from extra-cellular deposition of fibril-forming monoclonal immunoglobin (Ig) light chains (LC) (most commonly of lambda isotype) usually secreted by a small plasma cell clone. The key event in the development of AL amyloidosis is the change in secondary or tertiary structure of an abnormal monoclonal LC,....
>
> The diagnosis of amyloid is based on the finding, by light microscopic examination, of amorphous extracellular Congo red positive deposits, which display characteristic dichroism and apple green birefringence under polarised light."

Chronic diarrhea and weight loss can be the presenting sign of gastrointestinal amyloidosis and is considered in the differential diagnosis [3, 4]. In this patient, renal biopsy also showed amyloidosis (Fig. 115.2).

Bone marrow biopsy showed plasma cell neoplasm with associated amyloidosis (Fig. 115.3).

The final diagnosis, in this case, was light chain amyloidosis. The amyloid was characterized as IgG kappa immunoglobulin.

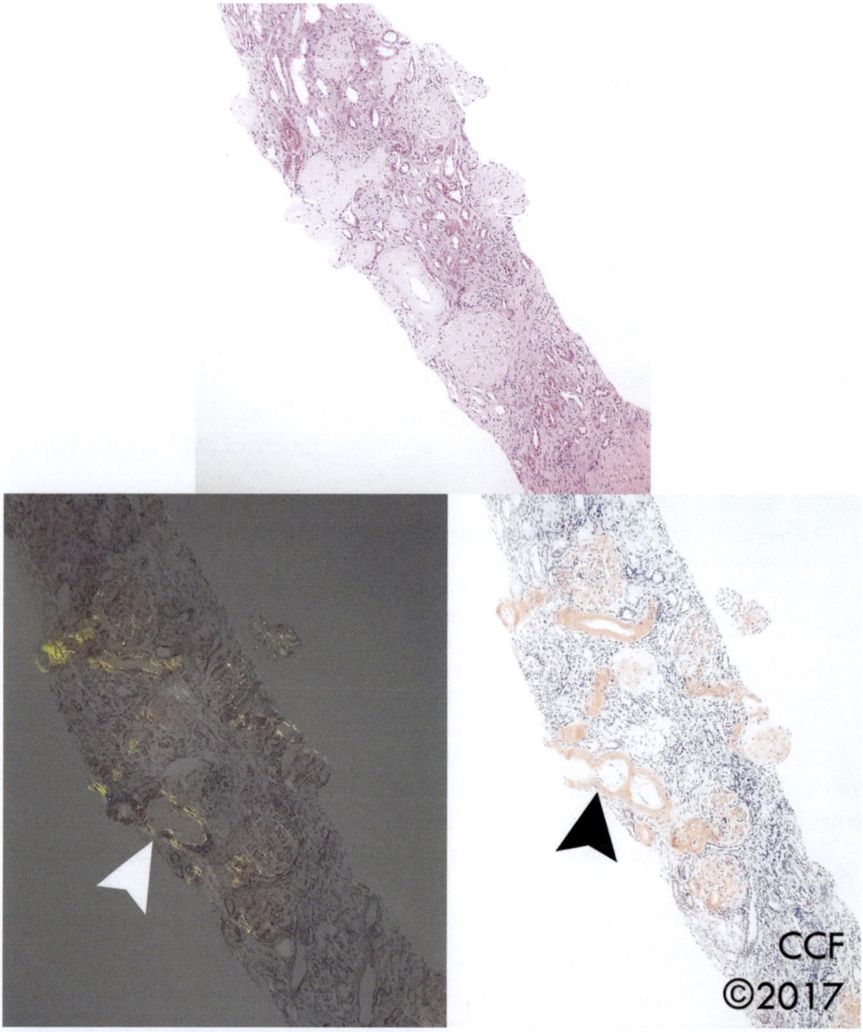

Fig. 115.2 Sections from the kidney biopsy show an amorphous, hyaline material within the glomerular capillaries and renal vasculature (top). The amyloid stains red-orange with congo red (black arrowhead) [lower right] and shows similar apple-green birefringence under polarized light (white arrowhead) [lower left]

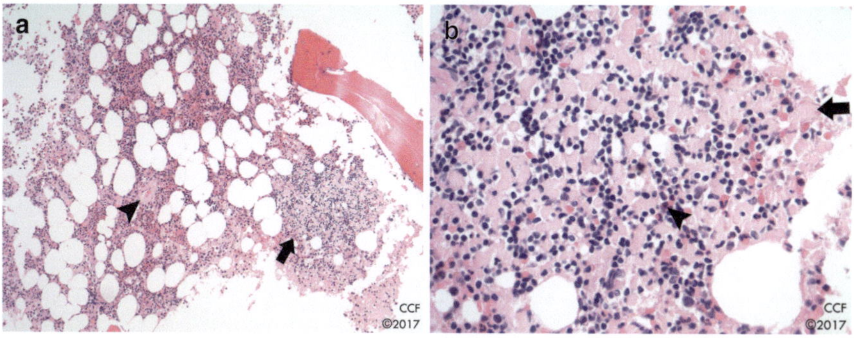

Fig. 115.3 (**a**) Low power view shows a normocellular bone marrow with trilineage hematopoiesis. A nodular aggregate of lymphocytes, plasma cells, and amorphous eosinophilic material is seen (arrow). Thickened arterioles are also identified (arrowhead); (**b**) higher power view of the nodular aggregate of lymphocytes, plasma cells (arrowhead), and amorphous eosinophilic material (arrow), consistent with amyloid

References

1. Virchow R. Ueber eine im Gehirn und Rückenmark des Menschen aufgefundene Substanz mit der chemischen Reaction der Cellulose. Arch Pathol Anat Physiol Klin Med. 1854;6:135–7.
2. Desport E, Bridoux F, Sirac C, Delbes S, Bender S, Fernandez B, et al. AL amyloidosis. Orphanet J Rare Dis. 2012;7:54.
3. Wang C, Li Y, Jin Y, Zhou W, Zhu Y, Yao F, Qian J. Chronic diarrhea as the presenting feature of primary systemic AL amyloidosis: serendipity or delayed diagnosis? BMC Gastroenterol. 2013;13:71.
4. Biswas S, Iqbal J, Makin A. Gastric amyloidosis presenting with severe weight loss. BMJ Case Rep. 2010; https://doi.org/10.1136/bcr.01.2010.2650.

Blue Rubber Bleb Nevus Syndrome 116

Michelle D. Inkster and James S. Wu

Presentation

A 61-year-old female was referred for evaluation of iron deficiency anemia. Colonoscopy (Fig. 116.1) and a small bowel capsule study (Fig. 116.2) were done. Small cutaneous nevi were noted on examination of the skin.

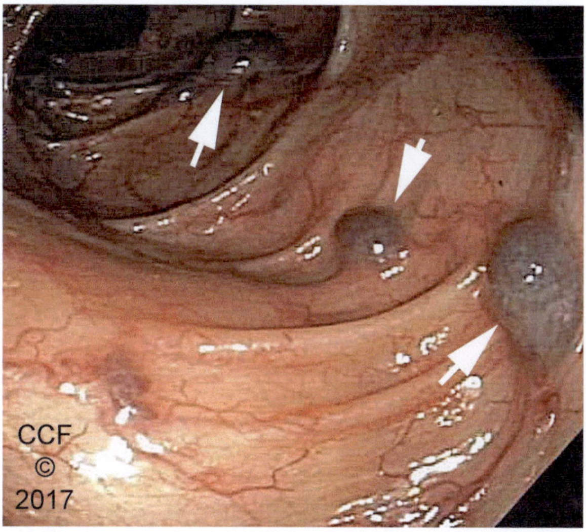

Fig. 116.1 Colonoscopy shows multiple nevi (arrows)

M. D. Inkster
Department of Gastroenterology, Cleveland Clinic, Cleveland, OH, USA

J. S. Wu (✉)
Department of Colon and Rectal Surgery, Cleveland Clinic, Cleveland, OH, USA

J. S. Wu, M. D. Inkster (eds.), *Cleveland Clinic Colorectal Case Studies*,
https://doi.org/10.1007/978-3-031-39880-3_116

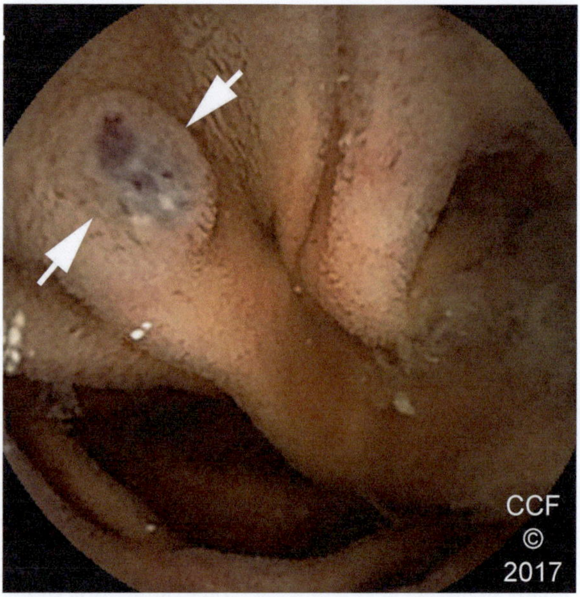

Fig. 116.2 Small intestinal mucosal nevus (arrows) seen on a small bowel capsule study

Comment

The cause of this patient's anemia was attributed to "Blue rubber bleb nevus syndrome (BRBNS)." In 1860, Gascoyen described a case of a 44-year-old man who died from suffocation because of a parotid gland nevus [1].

> "The tumour was congenital and always very large…. For many years the man had suffered comparatively little from it; latterly, however, it had been increasing rapidly, so as to occupy the whole of the parotidean region,….
>
> Numerous other nævi were scattered over various parts of the body and limbs, forming tumours of greater or less size.
>
> The various symptoms increased with the growth of the tumour, till death resulted from suffocation.
>
> *Post-mortem examination.*—Several nævi were seen studding the surface of the intestines, and a small one existed on the liver.
>
> The portion of the tumour which was exhibited consisted of tortuous and dilated blood-vessels,…
>
> The vessels appeared to be capillary veins of the gland enormously distended, which opened into large pouches and thus formed a true erectile tissue;…
>
> In the case of the small intestine having a nævus visible beneath its peritoneal coat, the growth had originated in the submucous cellular tissue, and projected considerably into the cavity of the bowel, but the mucous membrane covering it was still entire."

In 1930, McClure and Ellis described a patient with vascular tumors on the skin and tongue who underwent exploratory operation because of gastrointestinal bleeding. Hemangiomas on the liver, stomach, and small intestine were found [2]. Intussusception of a jejunal lesion was seen. Sections showed a "tumor mass composed of large dilated blood vessels filled with red blood cells and lined by a single layer of epithelium." In 1958, Bean described "blue rubber-bleb nevi of the skin and gastrointestinal tract."

> "There is a characteristic variety of bluish nevus of the skin found in association with angiomas of the gastrointestinal tract which cause serious bleeding. The larger angiomas have some of the feel and look of rubber nipples, are compressible and refill fairly promptly from their rumpled compressed state. I have called then rubber-bleb nevi…" [3].

In 1960, Berlyne and Berlyne established an inherited transmission of cutaneous cavernous hemangiomas through five generations [4].

Although blue rubber bleb nevi most commonly are seen in the skin and gastrointestinal tract, any part of the body may be affected [5]. Diarrhea secondary to gastrointestinal bleeding occurs since blood is a purgative. Treatment for BRBNS includes support, management of anemia, laser ablation, sclerotherapy, and surgical intervention [6].

References

1. Gascoyen GG. Case of nævus involving the parotid gland and causing death from suffocation. Nævi of the viscera. Trans Path Soc London. 1860;11:267–70.
2. McClure RD, Ellis SW. Hemangiomata of the intestine. Am J Surg. 1930;10:241–4.
3. Bean WB. Blue rubber bleb nevi of the skin and gastrointestinal tract. In: Vascular Spiders and Related Lesions of the Skin. Springfield: Thomas CC; 1958. pp. 178–85.
4. Berlyne GM, Berlyne N. Anæmia due to "Blue-Rubber-Bleb" nævus disease. Lancet. 1960;276:1275–7.
5. Kassarjian A, Fishman SJ, Fox VL, Burrows PE. Imaging characteristics of blue rubber bleb nevus syndrome. AJR. 2003;181:1041–8.
6. Browning J, Siddiqui F. Blue rubber bleb nevus syndrome (Bean syndrome). Clin Advisor Dermatol. 2019. www.dermatologyadvisor.com Accessed 20 Sep 2022.

117 Colonic Ulceration Due to the Phosphate Binder, Sevelamer

Michelle D. Inkster, Michael W. Cruise, and James S. Wu

Presentation

A 42-year-old female underwent colonoscopy because of diarrhea. She had end-stage renal disease for which she was taking sevelamer (a phosphate binder). Erythematous areas were seen (Fig. 117.1). Random biopsies were nondiagnostic. One year later, repeat colonoscopy was done because of continuing diarrhea. Colonoscopy showed deep ulceration and exudates (Fig. 117.2). Histopathology of biopsies is shown in Fig. 117.3.

M. D. Inkster
Department of Gastroenterology, Cleveland Clinic, Cleveland, OH, USA

M. W. Cruise
Pathology & Laboratory Medicine Institute, Cleveland Clinic, Cleveland, OH, USA

J. S. Wu (✉)
Department of Colon and Rectal Surgery, Cleveland Clinic, Cleveland, OH, USA

J. S. Wu, M. D. Inkster (eds.), *Cleveland Clinic Colorectal Case Studies*,
https://doi.org/10.1007/978-3-031-39880-3_117

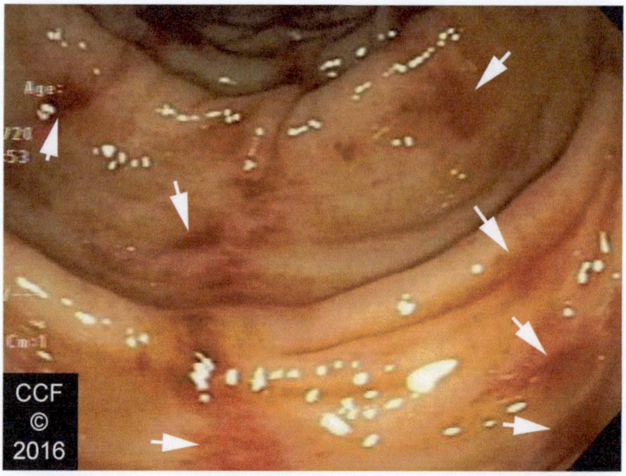

Fig. 117.1 Erythematous areas on initial colonoscopy (arrows)

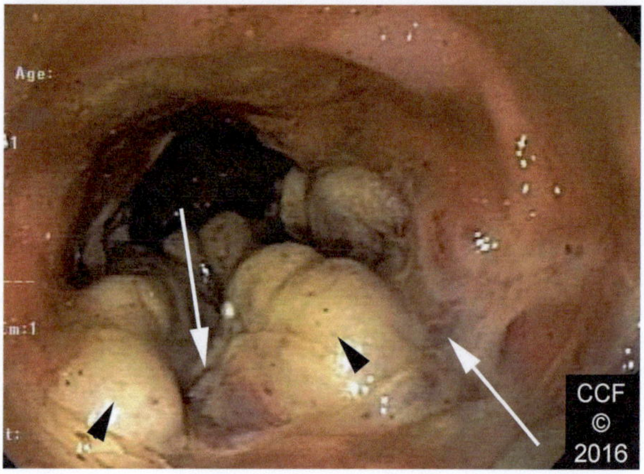

Fig. 117.2 Rectal ulceration (arrows) and exudates (arrowheads) seen on colonoscopy a year later

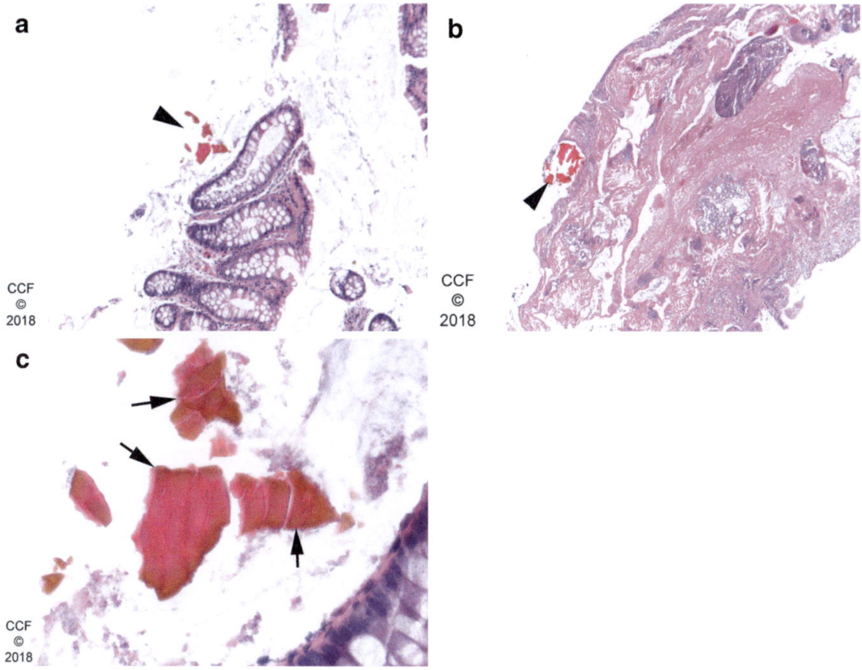

Fig. 117.3 (**a**–**c**) Colon biopsies show sevelamer crystals in the mucosa (arrows and arrowheads)

Comment

Sevelamer is a nonabsorbed anion exchange resin phosphate binder used for the control of serum phosphate in patients with chronic kidney disease [1]. Gastrointestinal side effects include constipation, fecal impaction, and stercoral ulceration [2]. A characteristic histopathologic finding is sevelamer induced mucosal injury and crystal deposition in the mucosa [3–8]. In this case, the ulceration resolved following cessation of the Sevelamer.

References

1. Rastogi A. Sevelamer revisited: pleiotropic effects on endothelial and cardiovascular risk factors in chronic kidney disease and end-stage renal disease. Ther Adv Cardiovasc Dis. 2013;7:322–42.
2. Madan P, Bhayana S, Chandra P, Hughes JI. Lower gastrointestinal bleeding: Association with Sevelamer use. World J Gastroenterol. 2008;14:2615–6.
3. Swanson BJ, Limketkai BN, Liu T-C, Montgomery E, Nazari K, Park JY, et al. Sevelamer crystals in the gastrointestinal tract (GIT): a new entity associated with mucosal injury. Am J Surg Pathol. 2013;37:1686–93.

4. Chintamaneni P, Das R, Kuan S-F, Kermanshahi TR, Hashash JG. Hematochezia associated with sevelamer-inducted mucosal injury. ACG Case Rep J. 2014;1:145–7.
5. Amer S, Nguyen C, DePetris G. Gastric pneumatosis due to sevelamer-mediated necrosis. Am J Gastroenterol. 2015;110:799.
6. Tieu C, Moreira RK, Song LMWK, Majumder S, Papadakis KA, Hogan MC. A case report of sevelamer-associated recto-sigmoid ulcers. BMC Gastroenterol. 2016;16:20.
7. Kim J, Olson K, Butani L. Sevelamer crystals in the mucosa of the gastrointestinal tract in a teenager with end-stage renal disease. Pediatr Nephrol. 2016;31:339–41.
8. Desai M, Reiprich A, Khov N, Yang Z, Mathew A, Levenick J. Crystal-associated colitis with ulceration leading to hematochezia and abdominal pain. Case Rep Gastroenterol. 2016;10:332–7.

Colonic Spirochetosis

118

Michelle D. Inkster, David Hernandez Gonzalo, Eric W. Willis, and James S. Wu

Presentation

A 50-year-old female underwent colonoscopy because of chronic diarrhea. The colon appeared macroscopically normal. Random biopsies were taken from the mucosa (Fig. 118.1a, b). Pathology showed the presence of spirochetes. Infectious disease consultation was requested regarding management.

M. D. Inkster
Department of Gastroenterology, Cleveland Clinic, Cleveland, OH, USA

D. Hernandez Gonzalo
Department of Pathology, Immunology and Laboratory Medicine, University of Florida, Gainesville, FL, USA

E. W. Willis
Department of Pathology, CORPath, Columbus, OH, USA

J. S. Wu (✉)
Department of Colon and Rectal Surgery, Cleveland Clinic, Cleveland, OH, USA

J. S. Wu, M. D. Inkster (eds.), *Cleveland Clinic Colorectal Case Studies*,
https://doi.org/10.1007/978-3-031-39880-3_118

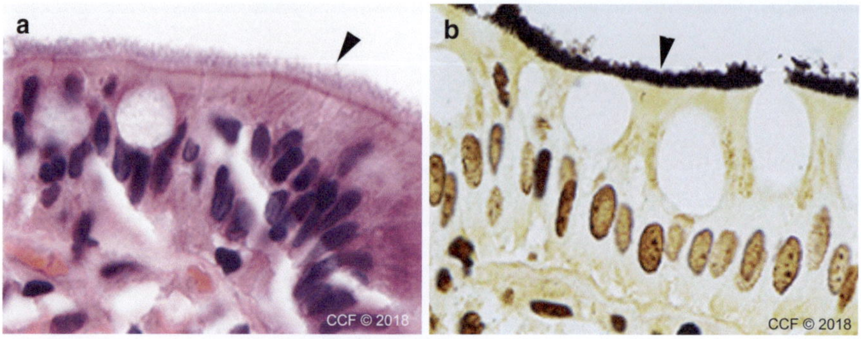

Fig. 118.1 (**a**) Random colon biopsy. The surface epithelium appears unremarkable except for the presence of a fuzzy basophilic fringe (arrowhead) in the luminal surface of the colonic mucosa (hematoxylin–eosin, oil immersion microscopy, original magnification ×1000). (**b**) Numerous tangled organisms staining dark brown to black (arrowhead) with modified Steiner stain (silver stain) carpet the mucosal surface (Steiner stain, oil immersion microscopy, original magnification ×1000)

Comment [1–5]

In humans, intestinal spirochetosis (IS) is seen in immunosuppressed patients, including HIV-positive patients, where the causative organisms *Brachyspira pilosicoli* and *Brachyspira aalborgi* predominate. Common symptoms include abdominal pain, watery diarrhea, and bleeding. However, in many cases, IS is found incidentally on colonoscopy in asymptomatic patients. Inflammation is not seen endoscopically in most patients. Biopsies are needed in order to make the diagnosis. The spirochetes can be confirmed with Warthin-Starry stain or with immunohistochemical stain for *Treponema pallidum*, which crossreacts with *Brachyspira* species. Histologically, biopsy shows a fuzzy purplish appearance on the colonic lumen where spirochetal organisms attach to the apical cell membrane of the colorectal epithelium. Treatment with metronidazole can eliminate the spirochetes; however, treatment may not improve symptoms. Because of this observation, no treatment may be necessary, particularly in asymptomatic patients.

References

1. Harland WA, Lee FD. Intestinal spirochaetosis. Br Med J. 1967;3:718–9.
2. van Mook WNKA, Koek GH, van der Ven AJAM, Ceelen TL, Bos RP. Human intestinal spirochaetosis: any clinical significance? Eur J Gastroenterol Hepatol. 2004;16:83–7.
3. Lin RK, Miyai K, Carethers JM. Symptomatic colonic spirochaetosis in an immunocompetent patient. J Clin Pathol. 2006;59:1100–1.
4. Tsinganou E, Gebbers J-O. Human intestinal spirochetosis-a review. Ger Med Sci. 2010;8:ISSN 1612–3174.
5. Anthony NE, Blackwell J, Ahrens W, Lovell R, Scobey MW. Intestinal spirochetosis: An enigmatic disease. Digestive Dis Sci. 2013;58:202–8.

Kaposi's Sarcoma

119

Michelle D. Inkster, Eric W. Willis, and James S. Wu

Presentation

The patient is a 23-year-old male with oropharyngeal lesions, severe facial swelling, cervical lymphadenopathy, and skin lesions (Fig. 119.1) that were consistent with Kaposi's sarcoma (KS). He was referred for upper endoscopy, colonoscopy, and small bowel capsule to determine if he had visceral involvement.

Multiple lesions were found in the stomach and small bowel by upper endoscopy and capsule endoscopy (Fig. 119.2). Colonoscopy showed multiple lesions (Fig. 119.3). Histopathology showed Kaposi's sarcoma (Fig. 119.4).

M. D. Inkster
Department of Gastroenterology, Cleveland Clinic, Cleveland, OH, USA

E. W. Willis
Department of Pathology, CORPath, Columbus, OH, USA

J. S. Wu (✉)
Department of Colon and Rectal Surgery, Cleveland Clinic, Cleveland, OH, USA

J. S. Wu, M. D. Inkster (eds.), *Cleveland Clinic Colorectal Case Studies*,
https://doi.org/10.1007/978-3-031-39880-3_119

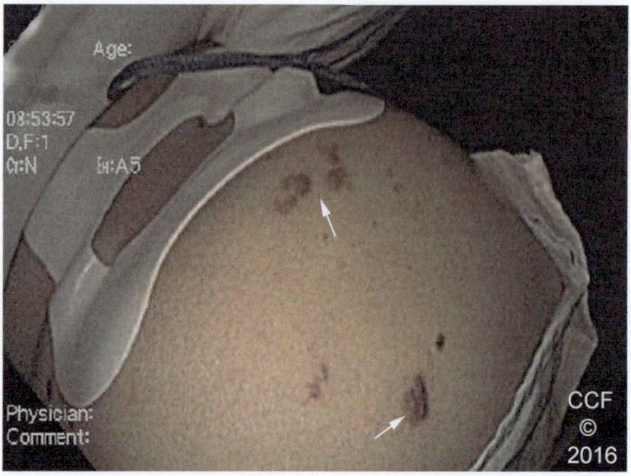

Fig. 119.1 Cutaneous Kaposi's sarcoma (arrows)

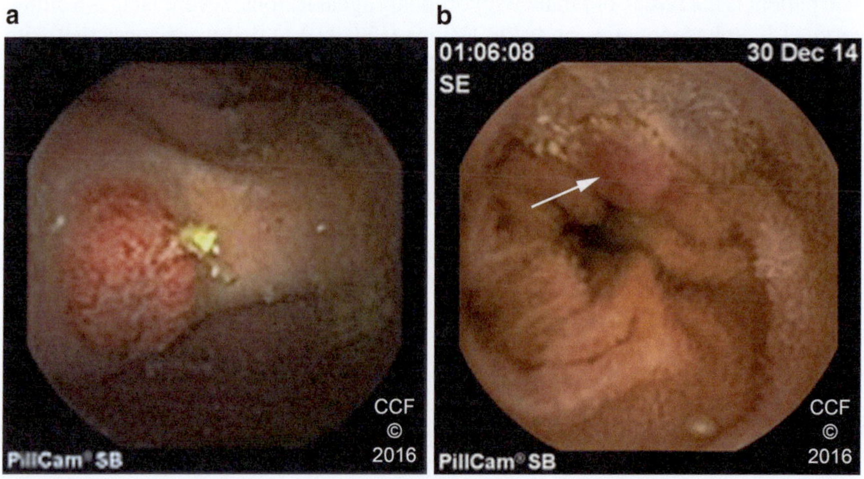

Fig. 119.2 Kaposi's sarcoma seen on capsule examination: (**a**) Gastric lesion and (**b**) small intestinal lesion (arrow)

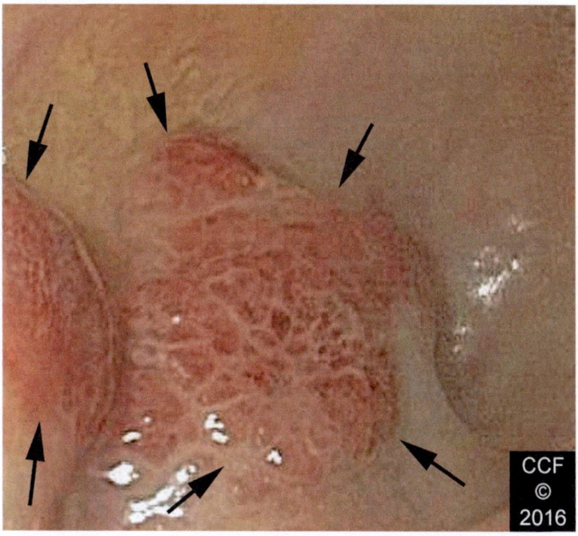

Fig. 119.3 Colonic Kaposi's sarcoma (arrows)

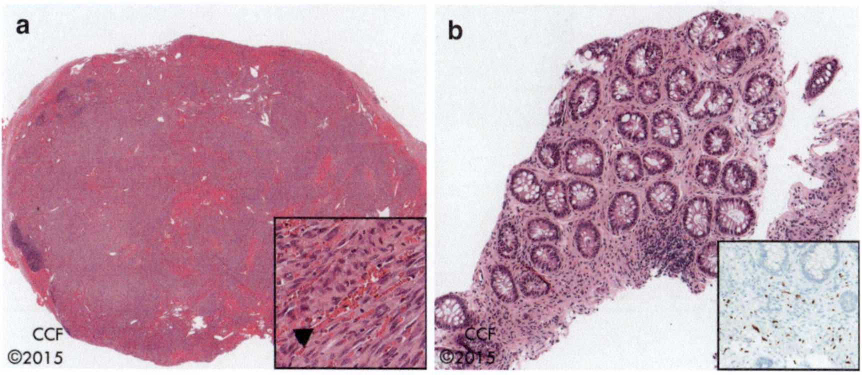

Fig. 119.4 (**a**) Tumor nodule composed of bland fascicles of spindle cells with slit-like vascular spaces (arrowhead) (Original magnification, H&E, 10×, 200×). (**b**) Separate biopsy showing a pink, spindle cell lesion in-between benign glands. Immunohistochemistry for human herpesvirus 8 (HHV-8) is positive in the spindled cells (inset) (Original magnification, H&E, HHV-8, 100×)

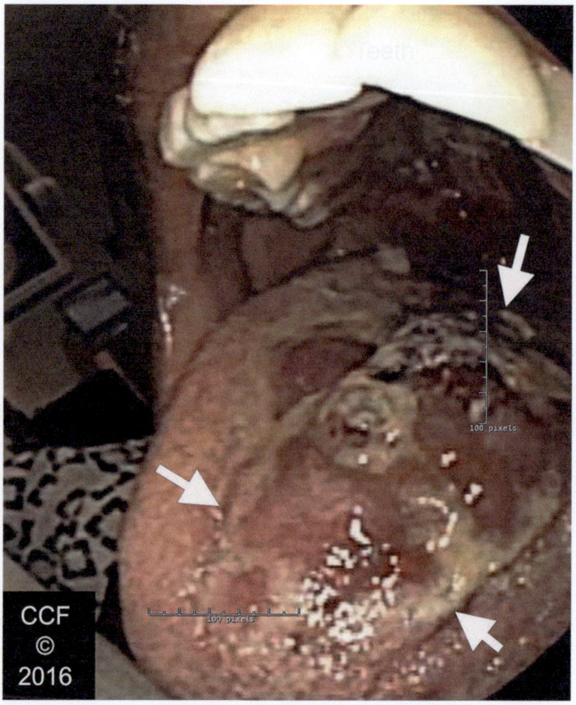

Fig. 119.5 KS of the tongue. The tumor (arrow) is labelled for reference

Comment

In 1872, Moritz Kaposi reported five idiopathic cases of multiple pigmented skin sarcomas [1]. The syndrome that he described was seen in older men. Involving the skin, the airway, the gut, and the liver, it was fatal within a few years.

Idiopathisches multiples Pigmentsarkom der haut
von
Dr. Kaposi,
Docent an der Universität in *Wien*

Wir können die Charaktere der Krankheit, … in Folgendem zusammen fassen:

Es entwickeln sich in der haut ohne bekannte, allgemeine oder locale Veranlassung, schrottkorn-, erbsen- bis haselnuss-grosse, braunroth bis blauroth gefärbte Knoten. Ihre Oberfläche ist glatt, ihre Consistenz derb-elastisch, manchmal schwellend, wie ein Blutschwamm. Sie stehen isolirt und ragen dann, wenn grösser geworden, kugelig hervor; oder sie gruppiren sich und bleiben mehr flach. In letzterem Falle involviren sich die centralen Knoten des plaque und veranlassen da eine narbige, dunkel pigmentirte Depression. Sie entstehen regelmässig zuerst in der Fusssohle und auf den Fussrücken, bald darauf auch auf den Händen, und sind an diesen Theilen auch überhaupt in der grössten Zahl enwickelt und mit diffuser Verdickung der Haut und Entstellung der Hände und Füsse gepaart.

Im weiteren Verlaufe erscheinen isolirte und gruppirte Knoten, aber immerhin in geringerer Zahl und in unregelmässiger Anordnung auch an den Armen und Beinen, im Gesichte and am Stamme.

Die Lymphdrüsen sind nicht erheblich geschwellt.

Endlich kommt es auch zur Bildung der gleichen Knoten auf der Schleimhaut des Kehlkopfes, der Trachea, des Magens und Darmes; besonders reichlich des Dickdarms, bis herab an den After, und zu Knoten in der Leber.

Die Krankenheit führt zum Tode, and zwar innerhalb einer kurzen Frist von 2–3 Jahren.

Die beobachteten Fälle betrafen nur Männer vom 40. Jahre aufwärts…

Idiopathic multiple pigmented sarcomas of the skin
By
Dr. Kaposi,
Lecturer, University of Vienna

We can summarize the character of the disease,… in the following way:

It develops in the skin without any known, general, or local cause, corn grain-, pea-, to hazelnut-sized, brown-red to blue-red colored knots. Their surface is smooth; their consistency is elastic, sometimes swollen, like a blood-filled sponge. They are isolated and then protrude when they become larger, spherical; or they cluster and remain flatter. In the last case, the central knot of the plaque develops a scarred, dark pigmented depression. They regularly arise first on the soles of the foot and on the back of the foot, soon thereafter, on the hands, and in these places develop in the greatest number and with diffuse thickening of the skin and disfigurement of the hands and feet.

In the further course of the disease, isolated and group knots appear, but in lesser number and in an irregular arrangement also on the arms and legs, on the face and on the trunk.

The lymph glands are not greatly swollen.

Finally, the same knots appear on the mucous membranes of the larynx, trachea, stomach and the intestines; particularly the large intestine to the anus, and to knots in the liver.

This disease leads to death within a short period of time, 2–3 years.

The cases observed occur only in men older than 40 years of age…

In 1959, Cox et al. [2]. described KS involvement of lymph nodes, gastrointestinal tract, lungs, heart, liver, spleen, and bone marrow. Figure 119.5 shows an example of KS of the tongue.

In 1986, Shiels reported that KS is associated with immunosuppression from drugs or AIDS [3]. KS associated with immunosuppressive drugs was identified in patients undergoing renal transplant. AIDS-related KS was found in association with AIDS chiefly in homosexual men. Rezende and colleagues report that KS is the most common neoplasm among HIV-infected individuals. Among those with gastrointestinal KS, concomitant skin lesions are common [4]. Kaposi's sarcoma is associated with human herpesvirus 8 (HHV-8) [5, 6]. It is proposed that Kaposi's sarcoma-associated herpes virus is highly oncogenic in HIV-1-infected and iatrogenically immunosuppressed individuals. In this case, immunohistochemistry for HHV 8 was positive. Treatment with chemotherapy resulted in lesion regression. No KS lesions were found on follow-up upper endoscopy and colonoscopy.

References

1. Kaposi. Idiopathisches multiples Pigmentsarkom der Haut. Arch f. Dermat Syph. 1872;4:265–73.
2. Cox FH, Helwig EB. Kaposi's sarcoma. Cancer. 1959;12:289–98.
3. Shiels RA. A history of Kaposi's sarcoma. J Roy Soc Med. 1986;79:532–4.
4. Rezende REF, Kahwage RL, da Costa TV, Machado AA, Brunaldi MO, Kemp R, Módena JLP. Upper gastrointestinal Kaposi's sarcoma in HIV-infected patients: ten years of endoscopy observation at a single Brazilian center. Int J Infect Dis. 2015;39:110–5.
5. Schulz TF. Kaposi's sarcoma-associated herpesvirus (human herpes virus 8): epidemiology and pathogenesis. J Antimicrob Chemother. 2000;45(Topic T3):15–27.
6. Wang HW, Trotter MWB, Lagos D, Bourboulia D, Henderson S, Mäkinen T, et al. Kaposi sarcoma herpesvirus-induced cellular reprogramming contributes to the lymphatic endothelial gene expression in Kaposi sarcoma. Nature Genet. 2004;36:687–93.

120 Colonic Hepato-Diaphragmatic Interposition

James S. Wu, Arthur A. Parsee, and Michelle D. Inkster

Presentation

A patient had a radiograph of the abdomen taken in which the colon was seen interposed between the diaphragm and the liver (Fig. 120.1).

J. S. Wu (✉)
Department of Colon and Rectal Surgery, Cleveland Clinic, Cleveland, OH, USA

A. A. Parsee
Department of Diagnostic Radiology, H. Lee Moffitt Cancer Center and Research Institute, Tampa, FL, USA

M. D. Inkster
Department of Gastroenterology, Cleveland Clinic, Cleveland, OH, USA

J. S. Wu, M. D. Inkster (eds.), *Cleveland Clinic Colorectal Case Studies*,
https://doi.org/10.1007/978-3-031-39880-3_120

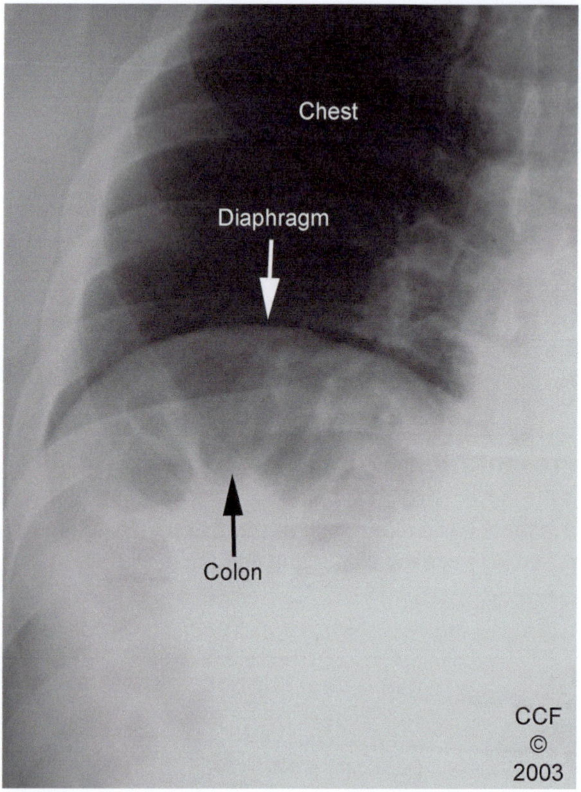

Fig. 120.1 Plain film of the abdomen shows a loop of colon interposed between the right hemidiaphragm and the liver (Chilaiditi's sign)

Biographical Note

Demetrius Chilaiditi

In 1910, Demetrius Chilaiditi described three cases in which the colon was interposed between the liver and the diaphragm (hepato-diaphragmatic interposition).[1]

Zur Frage der Hepatoptose und Ptose in allgemeinen im Anschluss an drei Fälle von temporärer, partieller Leberverlagerung.	On the question of hepatoptosis and ptosis in general connected to three cases of temporal, partial liver displacement.
Von	by
Dr. Demetrius Chilaiditi	Dr. Demetrius Chilaiditi
Aus der III. medizinischen Universitätsklink und dem Röntgeninstitut des allgemeinen Krankenhauses in Wien	From the 3rd University Medical Clinic and the Röntgen Institute of the General Hospital of Vienna
Im Anschluss an drei Fälle von partieller temporärer Leberverlagerung, mit interposition von Darm zwischen Leber und Zwerchfellkuppe,…	In connection to three cases of partial temporal liver displacement, with interposition of the intestine between liver and the dome of the diaphragm, …

[1]Chilaiditi [1]. The publisher of Fortschritte auf dem Gebiete der Röntgenstrahlen und der Nuklearmedizin, Georg Thieme Verlag, Stuttgart, did not object to republication of this excerpt and figure (August 24, 2021).

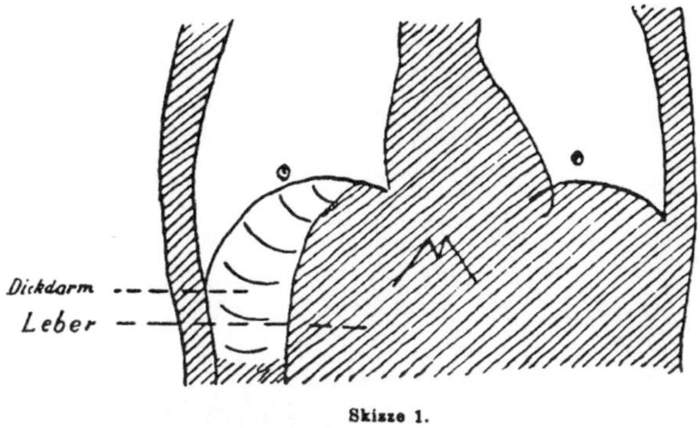

Fig. 120.2 The anatomic relationship between the diaphragm, colon (Dickdarm) and the liver (Leber) as illustrated by Chilaiditi in 1910

Chilaiditi's sign is defined as objective evidence (often radiologic) of colonic interposition between the right hemidiaphragm and the liver, as shown in Fig. 120.1. Chilaiditi's illustration showing the anatomic relationships between the diaphragm, liver, and colon is shown in Fig. 120.2. Predisposing factors include laxity of the hepatic suspensory ligaments and a redundant colon with a long mesentery [2]. Chilaiditi's syndrome refers to subjective symptoms attributed to hepato-diaphragmatic colon interposition. Symptoms of hepato-diaphragmatic interposition (e.g., pain, nausea, vomiting, alteration of bowel habits) are subjective features of Chilaiditi's syndrome. Chilaiditi's sign may be an incidental finding that causes no symptoms and may not require operative intervention. Hepato-diaphragmatic interposition can lead to intestinal obstruction, perforation, and ischemia; in these situations, surgery may be required. Chilaiditi's sign also has led to the erroneous diagnoses of pneumoperitoneum, subphrenic abscess, and diaphragmatic hernia [3–6]. Yin et al. [7] report a case of Chilaiditi's syndrome precipitated by colonoscopy.

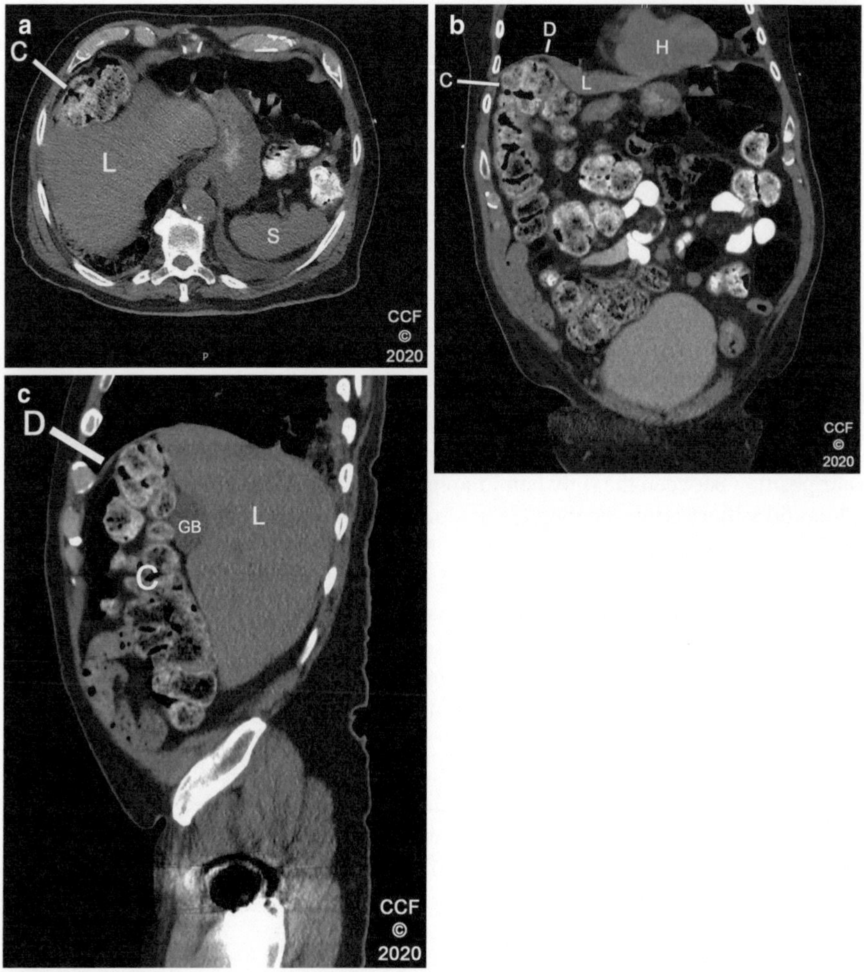

Fig. 120.3 Computed tomogram showing colon hepato-diaphragmatic interposition. (**a**) Axial view shows the colon (C) located anterior to the liver (L). The spleen (S) also is seen; (**b**) coronal view shows the colon (C) positioned inferior to the diaphragm (D) and lateral to the liver (L). The heart (H) also is seen; (**c**) sagittal view shows the colon (C) inferior to the diaphragm (D) and anterior to the liver (L) and gall bladder (GB)

The relationships between the colon, the liver, and the diaphragm seen in axial, coronal, and sagittal views are demonstrated by computed tomography (Fig. 120.3a–c).

References

1. Chilaiditi D. Zur Frage der Hepatoptose und Ptose in allgemeinen im Anschluss an drei Fälle von temporärer, partieller Leberverlagerung. Fortschr Röntgenstr. 1910;16:173–208.
2. Orangio GR, Fazio VW, Winkelman E, McGonagle BA. The Chilaiditi syndrome and associated volvulus of the transverse colon: an indication for surgical therapy. Dis Colon Rectum. 1986;29:653–6.
3. Sohal RJ, Adams SH, Phogat V, Durer C, Harish A. Chilaiditi's sign: A Case Report. Cureus. 2019;11:e6230. https://doi.org/10.7759/cureus.6230.
4. Taha A. Chilaiditi's syndrome: correct diagnosis can save the patient from unnecessary and life threatening surgery. J Adv Surg Res. 2017;2:45–7.
5. Rohman L, Jones A. Chilaiditi's sign. Emerg Med J. 2012;29:86.
6. Kamiyoshihara M, Ibe T, Takeyoshi I. Chilaiditi's sign mimicking a traumatic diaphragmatic hernia. Ann Thorac Surg. 2009;87:959–61.
7. Yin AX, Park GH, Garnett GM, Balfour JF. Chilaiditi syndrome precipitated by colonoscopy: A case report and review of the literature. Hawai'I J Med Pub Health. 2012;71:158–62.

121 Colonic Endometriosis

Catherine L. Forse and James S. Wu

Presentation

A 49-year-old female underwent diagnostic evaluation for gastrointestinal bleeding. Colonoscopy was incomplete. Computed tomography (CT) showed a cecal mass (Fig. 121.1).

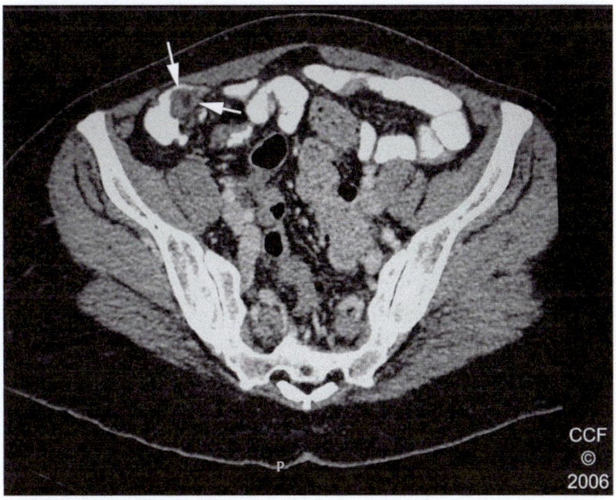

Fig. 121.1 Abdominal CT scan. Arrows point to a cecal mass

C. L. Forse
Department of Pathology and Laboratory Medicine, Faculty of Medicine, University of Ottawa, Ottawa, ON, Canada

J. S. Wu (✉)
Department of Colon and Rectal Surgery, Cleveland Clinic, Cleveland, OH, USA

J. S. Wu, M. D. Inkster (eds.), *Cleveland Clinic Colorectal Case Studies*,
https://doi.org/10.1007/978-3-031-39880-3_121

Management

Abdominal exploration showed a mass intimately attached to the cecum. Right hemicolectomy was done. The opened operative specimen showed that the mass had eroded into the intestinal lumen (Fig. 121.2).

Pathology showed endometriosis, whose features are shown in Figs. 121.3, 121.4, 121.5, and 121.6.

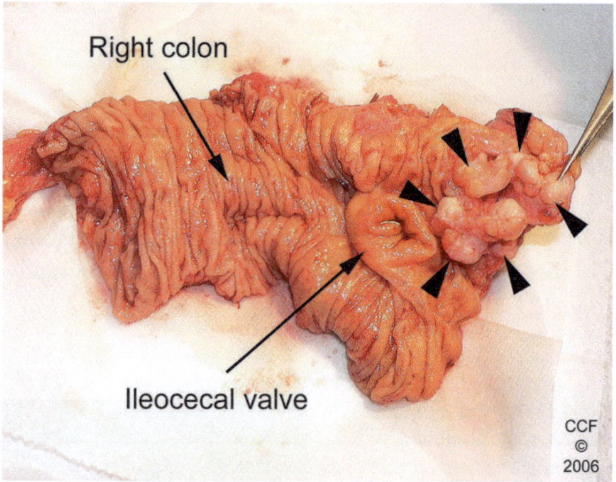

Fig. 121.2 Right colectomy specimen shows a mass (arrowheads and forceps) that has eroded through the intestinal wall into the lumen. The ileocecal valve is labelled

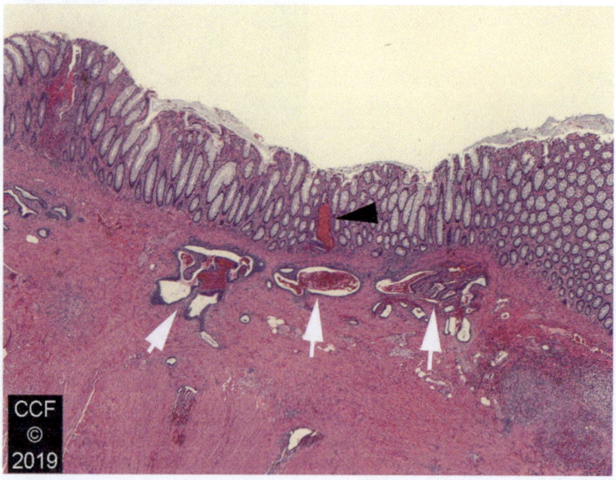

Fig. 121.3 Endometriosis involving the colon. Note the presence of tubular glands surrounded by hemorrhage involving the submucosa (white arrows) and mucosa (black arrowhead) of the colon. 20× mag, H&E

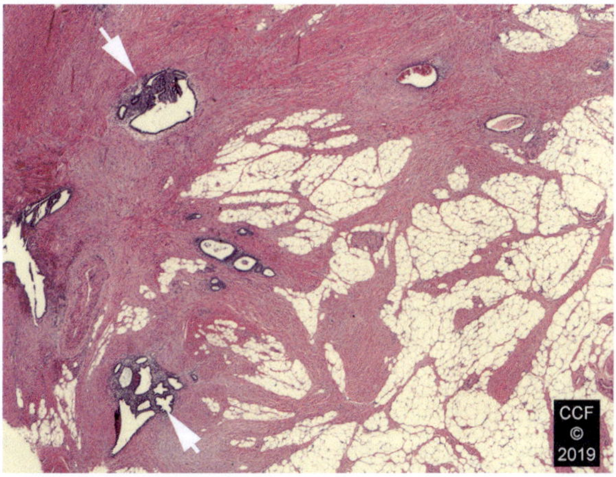

Fig. 121.4 Endometriosis involving the pericolonic soft tissues. Haphazardly arranged tubular glands (arrows) surrounded by fibrosis and adipose tissue. 20× mag, H&E

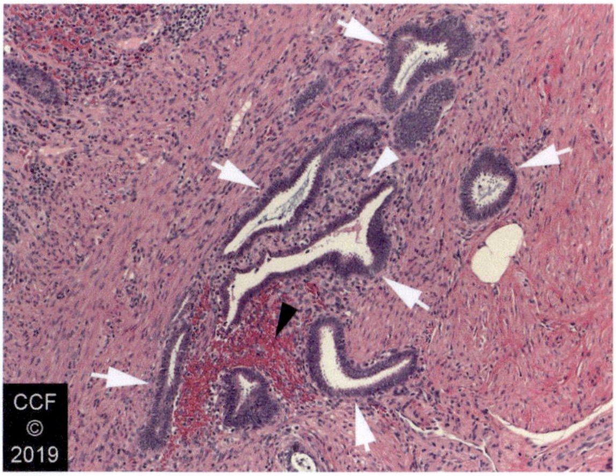

Fig. 121.5 High magnification view of endometriosis involving the submucosa of the colon. Note the presence of glands lined by simple columnar epithelium (white arrows) and surrounded by endometrial-type stroma (white arrowhead). Note the stromal hemorrhage associated with the glands (black arrowhead). 100× mag, H&E

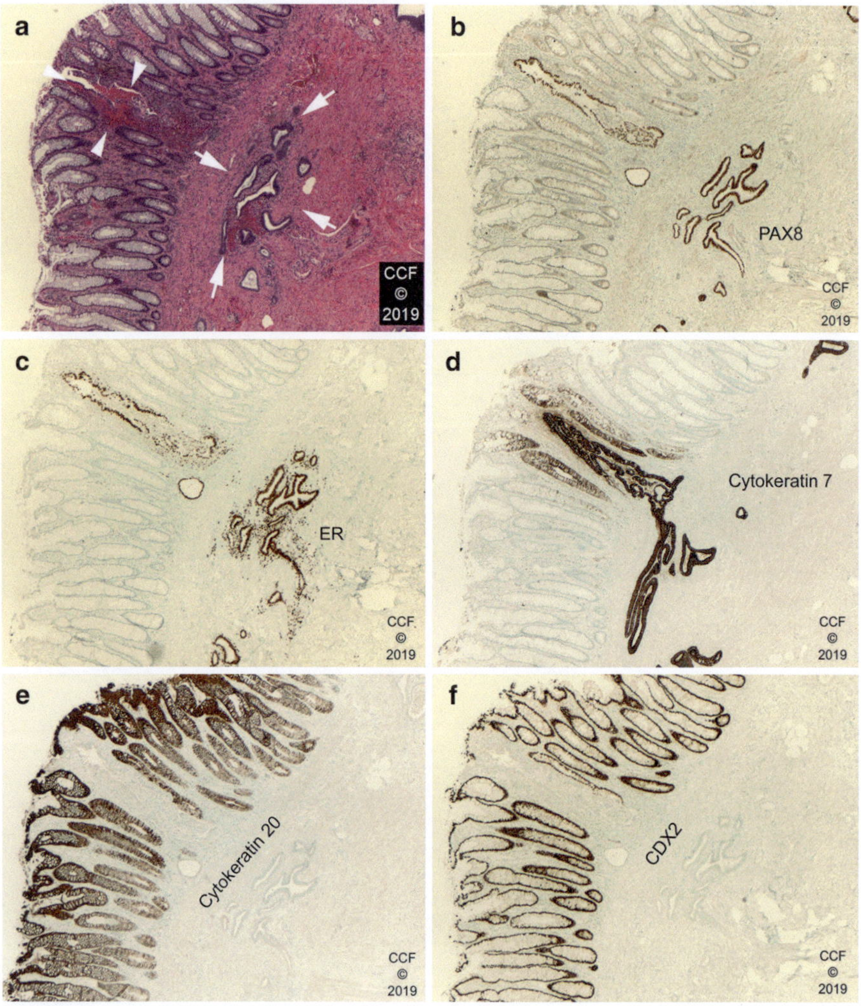

Fig. 121.6 (**a**) Endometriosis involving the submucosa (arrows) and mucosa (arrowhead) of the colon. 40× mag, H&E. (**b**) Immunohistochemistry demonstrates that the endometrial glands are strongly positive for PAX8. (**c**) Immunohistochemistry demonstrates that the endometrial glands and associated stromal cells are strongly positive for estrogen receptor (ER). (**d**) Immunohistochemistry demonstrates that the endometrial glands are strongly positive for cytokeratin 7. (**e**) The overlying colonic mucosa is negative for PAX8, ER and cytokeratin 7 but is strongly positive for cytokeratin 20. (**f**) The overlying colonic mucosa is strongly positive for CDX2

Comment

Merriam-Webster's dictionary defines endometriosis as: "the presence and growth of functioning endometrial tissue in places other than the uterus [1]." In this case, endometrial tissue attached to and then grew through the wall of the cecum leading to large intestinal bleeding and surgical resection. One of the issues with endometriosis is that it can be mistaken for colonic adenocarcinoma. Just like colon cancer, endometriosis presents with a haphazard arrangement of glands with hemorrhage and altered stroma. PAX-8 is a transcription factor which is expressed predominantly in thyroid and gynecological tissues and is not expressed by the gastrointestinal tract. Being strongly PAX-8 positive lets the pathologists know that these glands are not originating in the gastrointestinal tract [2]. Cytokeratin 7 (CK7) and cytokeratin 20 (CK20) are general keratins expressed by epithelial organs in certain patterns of expression [3]. The colon is CK20 positive and CK7 negative, while gynecological tissues are CK7 positive and CK20 negative. In this case, this is more evidence that the glands are not from the GI tract. Expression of the homeobox intestinal differentiation factor CDX2 suggests that a carcinoma may be of gastrointestinal origin [4].

In order not to miss the diagnosis of gastrointestinal endometriosis, a high index of suspicion is needed especially in the setting of cyclic pain with defecation, cyclic constipation, dyschezia, and rectal bleeding [5].

References

1. "Endometriosis." Merriam-Webster.com; Dictionary, Merriam Webster, https://www.merriam-webster/com/dictionary/endometriosis. Accessed 2 Sep 2022.
2. Arakawa T, Fukuda S, Hirata T, Neriishi K, Wang Y, Takeuchi A, et al. PAX8: A highly sensitive marker for the glands in extragenital endometriosis. Reprod Sci. 2019:193371911982809. https://doi.org/10.1177/1933719119828095.
3. Rekhtman N, Bishop J. Chapter 1. Immunostains: Introduction. In: Quick Reference Handbook for Surgical Pathologists. Berlin: Springer; 2011. pp. 1–21.
4. Kaimaktchiev V, Terracciano L, Tornillo L, Spichtin H, Stoios D, Bundi M, et al. The homeobox intestinal differentiation factor CDX2 is selectively expressed in gastrointestinal adenocarcinomas. Mod Pathol. 2004;17:1392–9.
5. Abrão MS, Petraglia F, Falcone T, Keckstein J, Osuga Y, Chapron C. Deep endometriosis infiltrating the rectosigmoid: critical factors to consider before management. Hum Reprod Update. 2015;21:329–39.

Massive Lower Gastrointestinal Hemorrhage

122

James S. Wu and Michelle D. Inkster

Presentation

A 73-year-old male presented to the emergency department following multiple episodes of massive painless rectal bleeding over a 6-h period. He felt light-headed.

Past History

Polycythemia vera for which he takes Coumadin.

Emergency Room Examination

Vital signs: T 36.6 °C, Pulse 131 bpm, Respirations 24/min, BP 100/66 mmHg.

The patient was awake and alert. The abdomen was soft and nontender. Rectal examination revealed maroon colored blood.

Laboratory

Sodium 139 (136–146 mmol/L)
Potassium 3.8 (3.5–5.0 mmol/L)

J. S. Wu (✉)
Department of Colon and Rectal Surgery, Cleveland Clinic, Cleveland, OH, USA

M. D. Inkster
Department of Gastroenterology, Cleveland Clinic, Cleveland, OH, USA

J. S. Wu, M. D. Inkster (eds.), *Cleveland Clinic Colorectal Case Studies*,
https://doi.org/10.1007/978-3-031-39880-3_122

Chloride 106 (98–110 mmol/L)
CO2 18 (23–32 mmol/L)
WBC 21.67 (3.760–11.00 k/μL) Neut% 86.7 (39.5–74.0%)
Abs Neut (ANC) 18.81 (1.45–7.50 k/μL)
Lymph % 5.6 (15.9–47.3%)
Anisocytosis present
Hb 10.8 (13.0–17.0 g/dL)
Platelet count 342 (150–400 k/μL)
PT 28.7 (8.4–13.0 s)
PT INR 2.6 (0.8–1.2)
PTT 31.8 (23.0–43.2 s)
Troponin T < 0.01 (0.00–0.10 ng/mL)
Mg 1.6 (1.7–2.6 mg/dL)
Albumin 3.3 (3.5–5.0 g/dL)

Emergency Room Interventions

- Central venous access established,
- Foley urinary bladder catheter placed,
- Transfusion
  - Six units of packed red blood cells
  - Two units of fresh frozen plasma,
- Vitamin K,
- Amicar,
- Protonix.
  The patient was admitted to intensive care.

Intensive Care

On arrival:
Vital signs: Temperature 36.6 °C, pulse 115 bpm, respirations 20/min
Blood pressure 129/56 mmHg
Hb 11.3 g/dL
PT 19.6 s
PT INR 1.8

Interventions

Gastroenterology

1. Esophagogastroduodenoscopy: normal.

2. Colonoscopy on the unprepared colon revealed blood and diverticula throughout the colon. Nonbloody bile was noted at the ileocecal valve. No active bleeding was noted.

Interventional Radiology

Mesenteric angiogram

1. Inferior mesenteric artery: extensive diverticulosis mostly in the sigmoid and descending colon, without evidence of active extravasation. No evidence of arteriovenous (AV) fistula or aneurysms,
2. Middle colic artery: diverticulosis in the splenic flexure and the distal transverse colon without evidence of extravasation,
3. Superior mesenteric artery: normal branching pattern; no evidence of active extravasation or AV fistula.

Management

Following initial resuscitation, the possibility of surgery to eliminate the bleeding source in the event of recurrent bleeding was discussed. The patient was marked for a stoma and given ostomy education by a Wound Ostomy Care nurse.

Twenty-four hours following admission to the intensive care unit, the patient passed 1.5 L of red bloody bowel movement. His blood pressure abruptly fell to 80/40 mmHg and his heart rate rose to 114 bpm. The hemoglobin was 7.4 g/dL. Transfusion with an additional four units of packed red blood cells was administered.

Without further testing, the patient was taken to surgery. The entire colon from the cecum to the rectum was removed. The resected colon is shown in Fig. 122.1. Examination of the rectum and terminal ileum did not show active bleeding. Following surgery, bleeding stopped.

Comment

The 2016 American College of Gastroenterology (ACG) Clinical Guideline regarding the management of patients with acute lower gastrointestinal bleeding defines lower gastrointestinal bleeding as the onset of hematochezia (maroon or red blood passed per rectum) originating from either the colon or the rectum [1]. Common sources include diverticular disease, vascular ectasia, colitis, postpolypectomy hemorrhage, neoplasia, and anorectal lesions. Sources proximal to the colon may also cause hematochezia.

Initial evaluation includes history and physical examination, complete blood count, electrolytes, type and cross match, and coagulation profile. The goals of resuscitation are the restoration of euvolemia, stabilization of vital signs, and

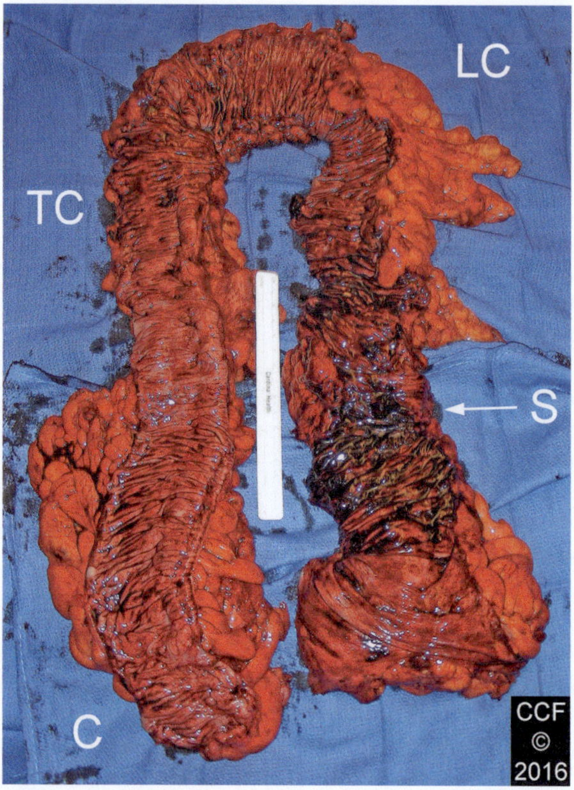

Fig. 122.1 Total abdominal colectomy specimen removed for massive lower GI bleeding. The large adherent clot in the sigmoid colon (S, arrow) suggests that this was the origin of bleeding. C (cecum), TC (transverse colon), LC (left colon)

correction of coagulopathy. Determination of the bleeding source is accomplished by one or more tests that may include: endoscopy, arteriography, and nuclear medicine.

Persistent or recurrent lower gastrointestinal bleeding may require surgery. Accurate localization of the bleeding source is preferred. However, when preoperative localization is not successful, and exsanguination is life threatening, "blind" total colectomy is considered [2].

The decision to proceed with total colectomy in this case was prompted by the following factors: recurrent massive hemorrhage with hemodynamic instability, transfusion of 10 units of blood, failure of preoperative localization tests, pancolonic diverticular disease (the most common cause), and non-bloody bile drainage from the ileocecal valve (suggesting a colonic origin). Before surgery, stoma marking and education was done. At surgery, the colon was removed. Bleeding was not seen from the terminal ileum. Following surgery, the bleeding stopped; the patient recovered and was discharged. The resected colon was full of blood with clot adherent to the mid-sigmoid colon suggesting that this was the site of bleeding.

References

1. Strate LL, Gralnek IM. ACG clinical guideline: Management of patients with acute lower gastrointestinal bleeding. Am J Gastroenterol. 2016;111:459–74.
2. Baker R, Senagore A. Abdominal colectomy offers safe management for massive lower GI bleed. Am Surg. 1994;60:578–81. discussion p. 582.

References

Gallstone Ileus

123

Douglas W. Yoder and James S. Wu

Presentation

A 52-year-old female presented with a 3-day history of progressive abdominal bloating, nausea, and vomiting. Physical examination was notable for abdominal distension without abdominal tenderness. An abdominal plain film was obtained (Fig. 123.1).

D. W. Yoder
Department of Surgery, Blanchard Valley Health System, Findlay, OH, USA

J. S. Wu (✉)
Department of Colon and Rectal Surgery, Cleveland Clinic, Cleveland, OH, USA

J. S. Wu, M. D. Inkster (eds.), *Cleveland Clinic Colorectal Case Studies*,
https://doi.org/10.1007/978-3-031-39880-3_123

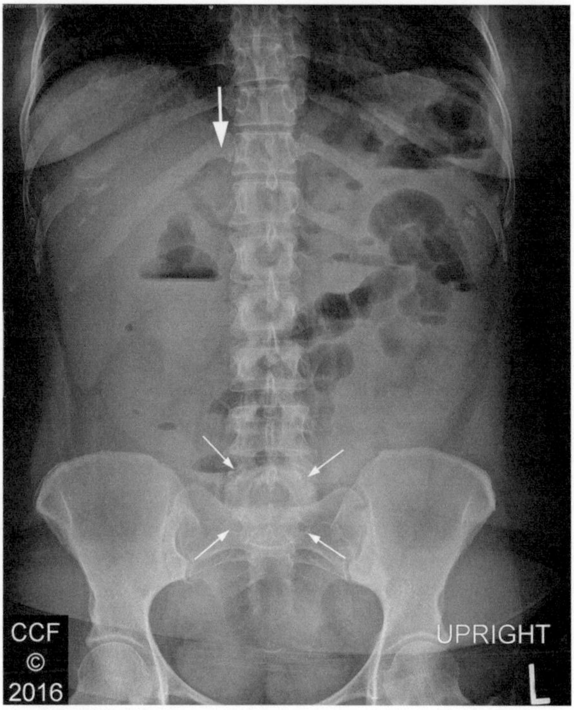

Fig. 123.1 Plain abdominal film shows air in the biliary tree (large arrow) and a calcified mass in the pelvis (small arrows)

Management

The patient was taken to surgery. A large obstructing calculus was palpated in the sigmoid colon. An inflammatory mass was present between the gallbladder and the proximal transverse colon. A hard mass was palpated in the sigmoid colon. (Fig. 123.2). A sigmoid colotomy was performed, and a calculus was extracted (Fig. 123.3). Cholecystectomy with *en-bloc* removal of the adjacent transverse colon (containing the gallbladder to colon fistula) was resected. Figure 123.4 shows the extracted gallstone reunited with the excised gallbladder. Colon continuity was restored by primary repair of the colotomy. The patient recovered and was discharged on the fifth postoperative day.

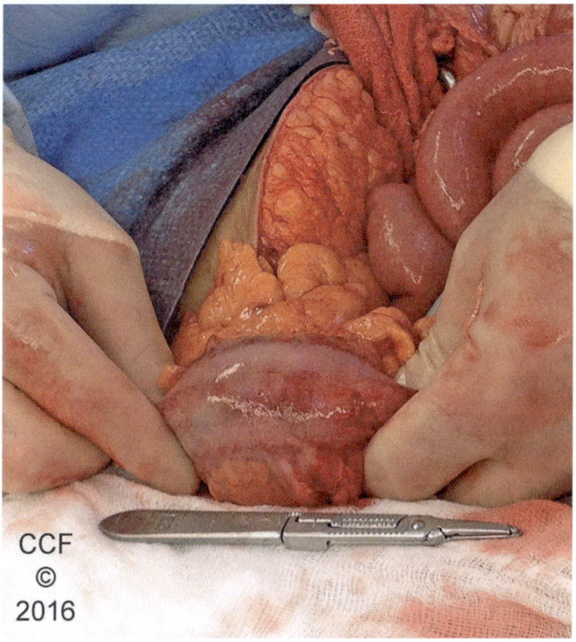

Fig. 123.2 Obstructing gallstone within the sigmoid colon

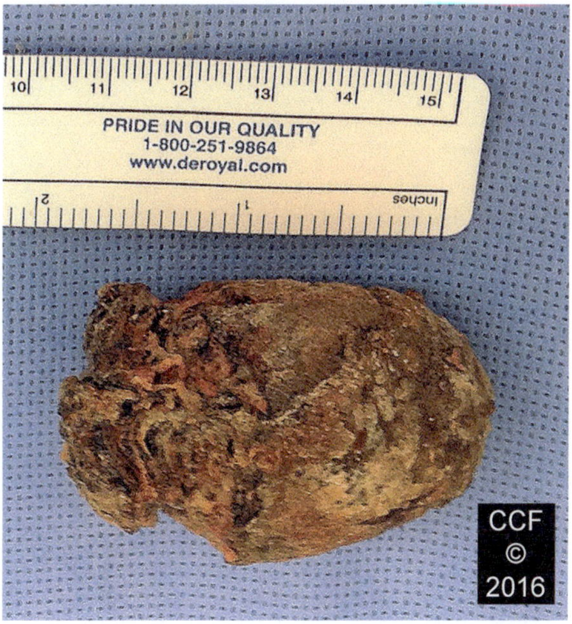

Fig. 123.3 The gallstone after extraction from the sigmoid colon

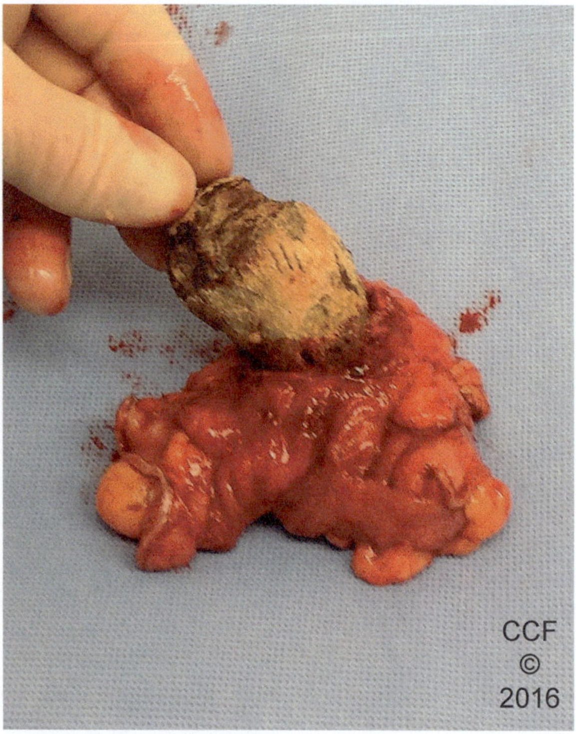

Fig. 123.4 The gallstone reunited with the excised gallbladder at the site of the fistula to the colon

Comment

Gallstone ileus is a condition in which intestinal obstruction is caused by a gallstone that has traveled from the gallbladder to the gut through a fistula [1–3]. Although the most common site of fistulization is the duodenum, fistulas to the colon have also been reported. In this case, a fistula developed between the gallbladder and adjacent transverse colon. Obstruction occurred at the rectosigmoid colon, a point of relative narrowing. Treatment by colotomy to remove the gallstone, plus *en-bloc* resection of the gallbladder and affected neighboring transverse colon eliminated the fistula and the obstruction in a single operation.

References

1. Rigler LG, Borman CN, Noble JF. Gallstone obstruction. Pathogenesis and Roentgen manifestations. J Am Med Assoc. 1941;117:1753–9.
2. Reisner RM, Cohen JR. Gallstone ileus: A review of 1001 reported cases. Am Surg. 1994;60:441–6.
3. Ravikumar R, Williams JG. The operative management of gallstone ileus. Ann R Coll Surg Engl. 2010;92:279–81.

Amyand's Hernia

124

William J. O'Brien, Michelle D. Inkster, and James S. Wu

Presentation

An 82-year-old male presented with right-sided abdominal and scrotal pain. Computed tomography showed a narrow-necked right inguinal hernia containing the appendix (Fig. 124.1).

W. J. O'Brien
Department of Surgery, Cleveland Clinic, Cleveland, OH, USA

M. D. Inkster
Department of Gastroenterology, Cleveland Clinic, Cleveland, OH, USA

J. S. Wu (✉)
Department of Colon and Rectal Surgery, Cleveland Clinic, Cleveland, OH, USA

J. S. Wu, M. D. Inkster (eds.), *Cleveland Clinic Colorectal Case Studies*,
https://doi.org/10.1007/978-3-031-39880-3_124

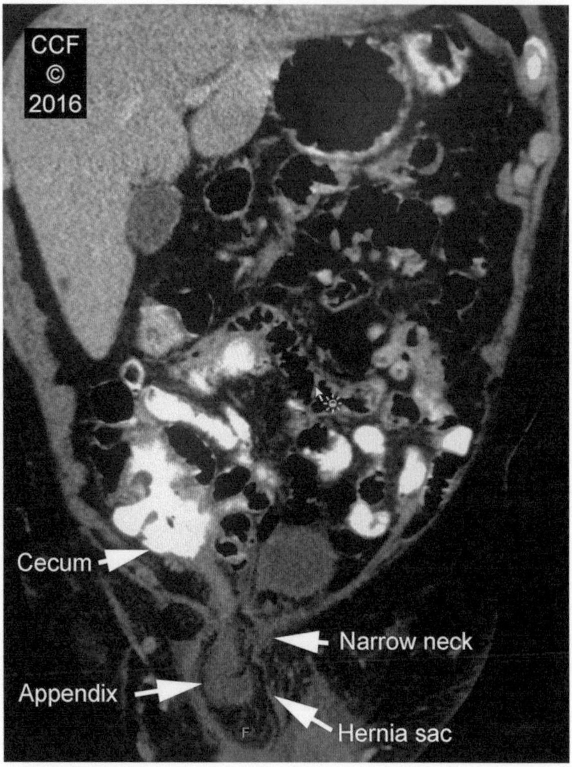

Fig. 124.1 Computed tomography shows a right inguinal hernia. The appendix and the site of its origin, the cecum, are marked with arrows. The base of the appendix remains in the abdomen. The distal half of the appendix is located within the hernia sac beyond a narrow neck

Management

Laparoscopy revealed the appendix trapped in the inguinal canal (Fig. 124.2). The appendix was liberated and removed. The tip of the appendix that had been incarcerated was gangrenous (Fig. 124.3).

A drain was placed in the scrotum. The excised appendix showing gangrene at its tip is shown in Fig. 124.4.

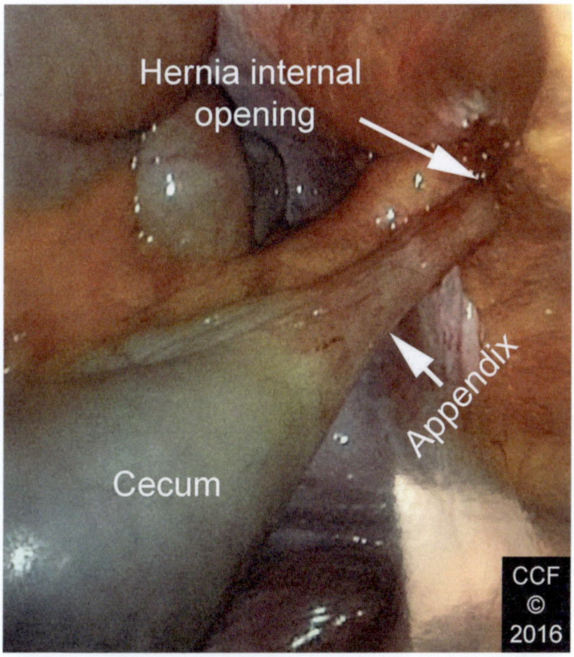

Fig. 124.2 Laparoscopic image showing the base of the appendix. The tip of the appendix has been trapped by the narrow entrance into the inguinal canal

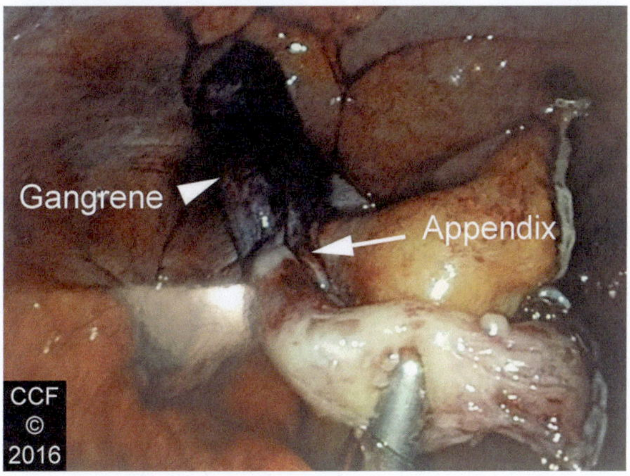

Fig. 124.3 The gangrenous tip of the appendix is seen after liberation from the inguinal canal

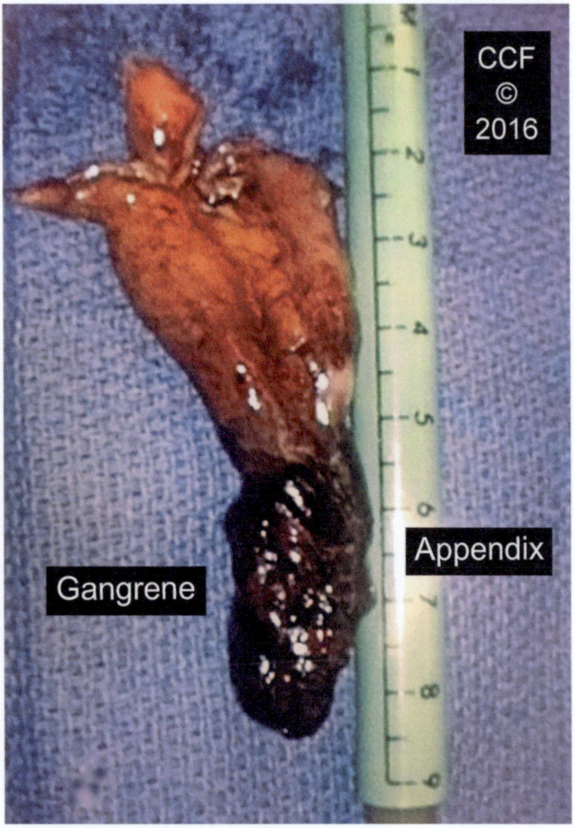

Fig. 124.4 The excised appendix. Gangrene is seen at the tip of the appendix which had been entrapped in the inguinal canal

Comment

The first appendectomy, a case associated with *Hernia Scrotalis*, is attributed to Claudius Amyand [1].

Philosophical Transactions [2]:[1]

Of an inguinal rupture, with a pin in the appendix cœci, incrusted with stone; and some observations on wounds in the guts

By

Claudius Amyand, Esq; Serjeant Surgeon to his Majesty and F. R. S.

[1] The font used by Dr. Amyand's publisher was changed to a modern font. For example, the phrase, "faving it was obferved to keep a ftrong and conftant Preffure over the Abdominal Aperture," was changed to "saving it was observed to keep a strong and constant pressure over the abdominal aperture."

"October 8, 1735. *Hanvil Anderson*, a boy, 11 years of age, was admitted to St. *George's Hospital* near *Hyde-Park* Corner, for the cure of a *Hernia Scrotalis*, which he had from his infancy, and a fistula between the scrotum and thigh terminating into it, which for a month last past had discharged a great quantity of an unkindly sort of matter. The rupture was small, and not troublesome, and part of it could be replaced, but as it appeared that the sinuous ulcer sprung from that part that could not; so 'twas evident that the cure of the fistula depended upon the cure of the hernia, which latter could be obtained by no other operation than that for the *Bubonocele*, which was agreed to, and performed the 6th day of *December* following.

This operation proved the most complicated and perplexing I ever met with, many unsuspected oddities and events concurring to make it as intricate as it proved laborious and difficult.

This tumor, principally composed of the omentum, was about the bigness of a small pippin: in it was found the appendix cœci perforated by a pin incrusted with stone towards the head, the point of which having perforated that gut, gave way to a discharge of fæces through the fistulous opening therein, as the portion of the pin obturating the aperture in it shifted its situation. The abscess formed in the hernial bag occasionally, and the suppuration for two months last past from this place outwardly, had knit and confounded, and, as it were, inbodied together the gut and omentum with the hernial bag, and these with the spermatick vessels and the testicule, so that it was as difficult to distinguish them from each other, as it was to separate them without wounding them; this pin, whose point was fixed in the omentum, continually shifting its situation, and occasioning a discharge of fæces. The pin frequently lying in the way of the knife, and starting out of the wounded gut, as a shot out of a gun, the inundation of fæces upon this occasion from a gut we could not well distinguish, were so many difficulties in the way: but the greatest yet was, what to do with the gut, which all this while was unknown, and of which we could not come to the knowledge, till the operation was over; for this appendix cœci, which was the only gut found in the rupture, was so contracted, carnous, duplicated, and changed in its figure and substance, that it was impossible to determine what kind of gut it was, or to find out that it was only this appendix elongated, and in disguise.

We apprehended none of these difficulties, when we undertook this operation, in which we proceeded as usual: The omentum lying uppermost in the hernial bag was dissected from the parts it was knit to, and particularly the gut it was imbodied with, and afterwards cut off close to the abdominal muscles without any previous ligature, the vessels in it being small, and the substance of it more like a sweet-bread than the caul.

Much time was spent in this dissection; we were streightened for room, and greatly disturbed by the discharge of the fæces coming out from the gut, upon every motion the pin lodged in it and the omentum suffered, upon the separation of these from each other. The gut forming a double tube, like a double-jointed syphon, continuing in the curve as it passed over the testicule and spermaticks, was separated one part from the other and from the adjacent parts, as far as the aperture in the abdominal muscles, where the unperforated end of it was separated therefrom, and thence stretched out and unfolded, which brought in view the aperture made in it by the pin hitherto concealed, through which that part of it, which was incrusted with chalk, had just made its way out upon an occasional pressure, as a cork out of a bottle. It was the opinion of the physicians and surgeons present, to amputate this gut: to which end a circular ligature was made about the sound part of it, two inches above the aperture, and this being cut off an inch below the ligature, was replaced in the abdomen, in such a manner that an artificial anus might be made there, if the patient's case should require it. Afterwards so much of the hernial bag as had been detached from the skin, the spermaticks, etc. was cut off, which, as they appeared in the sound state, were preserved *in Situ*. The fistulous opening adjoining to the thigh, and answering to the aperture in the gut, was opened; some angles of skin in the way removed; the aperture in the muscles, which had been inlarged by incision, was stopped up with a tent; and the rest of the

Table 124.1 Pathological types of Amyand's hernia and their respective management (Losanoff and Basson)

Type	Salient features	Surgical management
I	Normal appendix	Reduction or appendectomy (depending on age), mesh hernioplasty
II	Acute appendicitis localized in the sac	Appendectomy through hernia, endogenous repair
II	Acute appendicitis, peritonitis	Appendectomy though laparotomy, endogenous repair
IV	Acute appendicitis, other abdominal pathology	Appendectomy, diagnostic workup, and other procedures as appropriate

dressings and the situation of the patient ordered so, as to remove from the wound all such pressure from within as might disturb the cure.

'Tis easy to conceive that this operation was as painful to the patient as laborious to me: it was a continued dissection; attended with danger on parts not well distinguished: it lasted near half an hour, and the patient bore it with great courage. During it the patient vomited largely, and had several stools but was soon composed by half an ounce of diacodium, and emollient embrocations and fomentations, frequently applied warm on the belly: he was blooded, and an emollient carminative oily clyster was ordered to be applied in the evening; but as he was easy, and the belly not tense, that was omitted. He was confined to a very sparing diet, and his body kept open by clysters, injected every 2d day, when stools were wanted, to prevent straining. When dressed upon the 4th day after the operation, everything appeared well, and we had good reason to hope for a cure, especially as the discharge by the anus was natural. The tent put into the abdominal aperture was not removed till the 8th. Upon the 10th the ligature round the appendix cœci, where it had been amputated, dropt off, and no fæces followed it; and as it was then plain they had taken the natural course, from that time the wound was treated like an ordinary one, saving it was observed to keep a strong and constant pressure over the abdominal aperture, as well to fence against the intrusion of the viscera into the wound, as by a strong incarnation and cicatrix, effectually to secure the patient against a rupture. During the time of the cure, he was confined to his bed, always kept to sparing diet, and ordered never to go to stool but in a bed-pan; by these means the wound was completely healed up in less than a month, and the patient soon discharged with a truss, which he was ordered to wear some time, to confirm the cure.

That the appendix cœci should be the only gut found in this rupture, is a case singular in practice."

Milanchi and Allins [3] define Amyand's hernia as an "inguinal hernia containing vermiform appendix." In 2008, Losanoff and Basson described four types of Amyand's hernia and recommendations for management[2] (Table 124.1) [4, 5].

Creese's biography of Amyand includes the following details of his life [1]. Claudius was born in Paris and naturalized in London on April 11, 1700. He was "Sergeant-Surgeon to King George II, …Fellow of the Royal Society,… a founder

[2]Losanoff and Basson [4]. This table was reproduced with the generous permission of Springer Verlag France, Order License ID 1143992-1. Order date 28 Aug 2021.

and first Principal Surgeon to St. George's Hospital, Master of the Barber Surgeons—one of the leading London surgeons of his day—and the first surgeon to do an appendectomy."

References

1. Creese PG. The first appendectomy. Surg Gynecol Obstet. 1953;97:643–52.
2. Amyand C. Of an inguinal rupture, with a pin in the appendix coeci, incrusted with stone: and some observations on wounds in the guts. Phil Trans R Soc. 1736 VIII;39:329–42.
3. Milanchi S, Allins AD. Amyand's hernia: history, imaging, and management. Hernia. 2008;12:321–2.
4. Losanoff JE, Basson MD. Amyand hernia: a classification to improve management. Hernia. 2008;12:325–6.
5. Green J, Gutwein LG. Amyand's hernia: a rare inguinal hernia. J Surg Case Rep. 2013;9:2 (pages) https://doi.org/10.1093/jscr/rtj043.

125 Colonic Pseudo-Obstruction (Ogilvie's Syndrome)

Michelle D. Inkster and James S. Wu

Presentation

A 72-year-old male underwent chest surgery. He received narcotics for pain. One week after surgery, he developed abdominal pain and distension. A plain abdominal film was obtained (Fig. 125.1). Recent colonoscopy was normal.

A nasogastric tube was placed. Methylnaltrexone, a narcotic reversal agent, was given. Enemas were administered. There was no clinical or radiological improvement.

M. D. Inkster
Department of Gastroenterology, Cleveland Clinic, Cleveland, OH, USA

J. S. Wu (✉)
Department of Colon and Rectal Surgery, Cleveland Clinic, Cleveland, OH, USA

J. S. Wu, M. D. Inkster (eds.), *Cleveland Clinic Colorectal Case Studies*,
https://doi.org/10.1007/978-3-031-39880-3_125

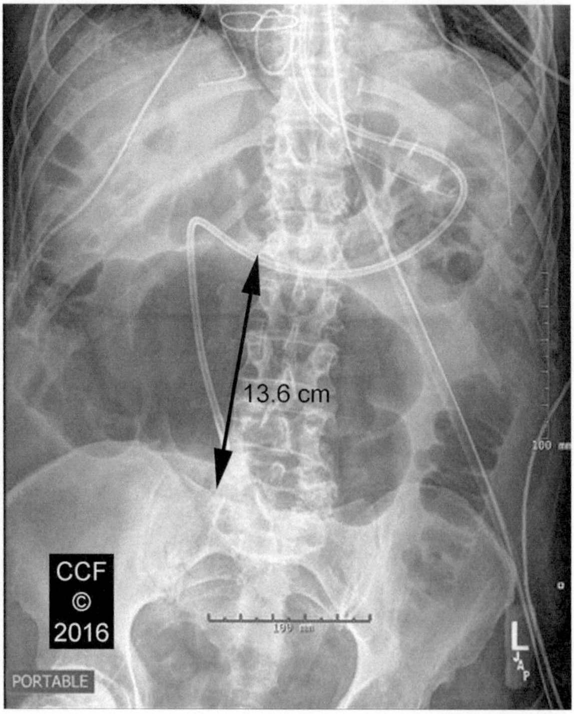

Fig. 125.1 Plain abdomen abdominal film shows cecal dilatation (13.6 cm). A feeding tube is in position. Unlike the right colon, the posterior wall of the cecum is not retroperitoneal. This anatomic feature allowed the cecum to move across the midline to the left side of the abdomen

Management

In intensive care, with cardiac monitoring, anesthesia standby, and atropine at the bedside, 2 mg of neostigmine was given intravenously. Within 5 min, 900 mL of liquid stool was expelled accompanied by large flatus. A repeat abdominal film was obtained (Fig. 125.2).

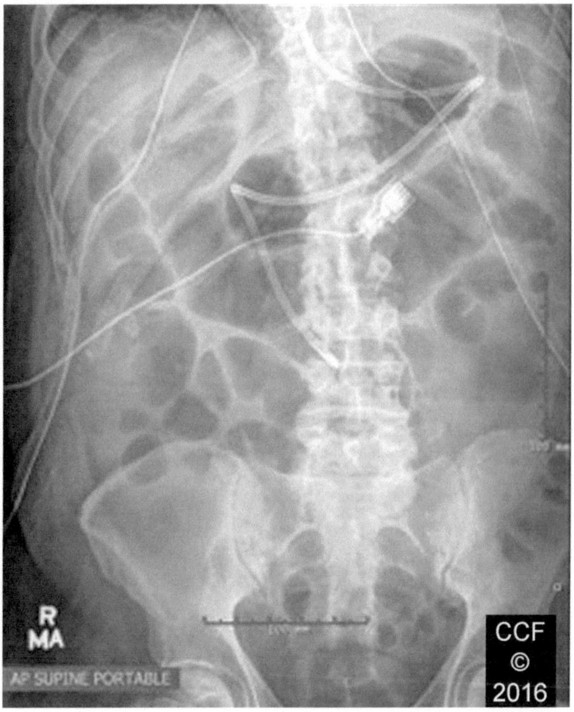

Fig. 125.2 Plain film after neostigmine shows marked decompression of the cecum

Comment

In 1948, Ogilvie reported a new clinical syndrome [1].

Large-intestine colic due to sympathetic deprivation
A new clinical syndrome
By
Sir Heneage Ogilvie, K.B.E., M.Ch., F. R. C. S.
Surgeon to Guy's Hospital

> "The subtitle of this note is intentionally provocative. Two cases are described, presenting essentially similar features. In each case the symptoms so strongly suggested obstruction of the distal colon by a carcinoma that laparotomy was eventually undertaken in spite of normal findings in a barium enema. In each case the operation disclosed a normal colon and extensive and entirely unsuspected malignant disease involving the region of the crura of the diaphragm and the coeliac axis and semilunar ganglia."

Ogilvie proposed:

> "The subdiaphragmatic growth had interrupted the sympathetic supply to the large intestine, so that the parasympathetic innervation, which in the distal colon comes from the second and third sacral nerves, was allowed to act unopposed."

In 1958, Dudley and co-workers described 13 patients in whom many of the symptoms and signs of intestinal obstruction were found but in whom mechanical intestinal obstruction was not present [2]. They introduced the term "pseudo-obstruction" to form the basis of an etiological classification. Therapies to treat this condition include drugs, endoscopic decompression, and surgery [3–5]. In 1927, Ritvo and Weiss reported the use of physostigmine to increase peristalsis in the gastrointestinal tract for the purpose of aiding in radiologic diagnosis [6]. Atropine was used as an antidote for toxic symptoms. This case illustrates the use of intravenous neostigmine to relieve acute colonic pseudo-obstruction [7–9]. Neostigmine competes with acetylcholine for attachment to acetylcholinesterase and increases levels of acetylcholine thus facilitating smooth muscle contraction. Colonoscopy has been and is used for decompression but is potentially dangerous because it is done in the unprepped colon, air insufflation must be kept to a minimum, and a long time is needed to complete the procedure. Given these potential problems, a pharmacolocical approach in selected patients often is more effective and has a faster result. Prior to neostigmine treatment, conservative treatment with nasogastric decompression and correction and fluid/electyrolyte imbalance are done. Mechanical obstruction and contraindications to therapy are excluded. The administration of neostigmine is done in an intensive care unit with cardiac monitoring. Side effects include nausea, vomiting, hypotension, and bradycardia. Atropine is made available to reverse bradycardia and hypotension if needed.

Biographical Note

Sir William Heneage Ogilvie, K.B.E., M.Ch., F.R.C.S.

William Heneage Ogilvie was born in Chile in 1887. He was educated at Oxford and received his medical training at Guy's Hospital [10]. In World War II, Ogilvie served with the British Army and advocated mandatory exteriorization of colon injuries.[1]

> "*The exteriorization of colon injuries.* A step which I have repeatedly advocated since the outbreak of war, the exteriorization of colon injuries, is, perhaps the greatest single factor in the improved results we are able to record. The principle that all damaged parts of the large intestine must be excluded till the process of repair is complete applies to all injuries even suspected ones, and to all parts of the large bowel, particularly the extraperitoneal portion of the rectum."
>
> W.H. Ogilvie, Major-General, R.A.M.C.
> Abdominal wounds in the Western Desert, 1944

His description of the syndrome that bears his name was reported 4 years later.

[1] Ogilvie [11]. Reprinted with permission from Mr. Spencer Dimmick, The Journal of the American College of Surgeons, formerly Surgery Gynecology & Obstetrics, August 30, 2021.

References

1. Ogilvie H. Large-intestine colic due to sympathetic deprivation. A new clinical syndrome. Br Med J. 1948;2:671–3.
2. Dudley HAF, Sinclair ISR, McLaren IF, McNair TJ, Newsam JE. Intestinal pseudo-obstruction. J R Coll Surg Edinb. 1958;49:206–17.
3. Maldonado JE, Gregg JA, Green PA, Brown AL. Chronic idiopathic intestinal pseudo-obstruction. Am J Med. 1970;49:203–12.
4. Murr MM, Sarr MG, Camilleri M. The surgeon's role in the treatment of chronic intestinal pseudoobstruction. Am J Gastroenterol. 1995;90:2147–51.
5. Kukora JS, Dent TL. Colonoscopic decompression of massive nonobstructive cecal dilation. Arch Surg. 1977;112:512–7.
6. Ritvo M, Weiss S. Physostigmine as an aid in gastrointestinal Roentgen-ray diagnosis. Am J Roentgenol Rad Ther. 1927;18:301–14.
7. Stephenson BM, Morgan AR, Salaman JR, Wheeler MH. Ogilvie's syndrome: a new approach to an old problem. Dis Colon Rectum. 1995;38:424–7.
8. Trevisani GT, Hyman NH, Church JM. Neostigmine: safe and effective treatment for acute colonic pseudo-obstruction. Dis Colon Rectum. 2000;43:599–603.
9. De Giorgio R, Barbara G, Stanghellini V, Toninis M, Vasina V, Cola B. Review article: the pharmacological treatment of acute colonic pseudo-obstruction. Aliment Pharmacol Ther. 2001;15:1717–27.
10. Ogilvie H. Large-intestine colic due to sympathetic deprivation. a new clinical syndrome. Classical Articles in Colon and Rectal Surgery. Dis Colon Rectum. 1987;30:984–7.
11. Ogilvie WH. Abdominal wounds in the Western Desert. Surg Gynecol Obstet. 1944;78:225–38.

MIX
Papier aus verantwortungsvollen Quellen
Paper from responsible sources
FSC® C105338

If you have any concerns about our products,
you can contact us on
ProductSafety@springernature.com

In case Publisher is established outside the EU,
the EU authorized representative is:
Springer Nature Customer Service Center GmbH
Europaplatz 3, 69115 Heidelberg, Germany

Printed by Libri Plureos GmbH
in Hamburg, Germany

Cleveland Clinic Colorectal Case Studies

James S. Wu • Michelle D. Inkster
Editors

Cleveland Clinic Colorectal Case Studies

Volume II

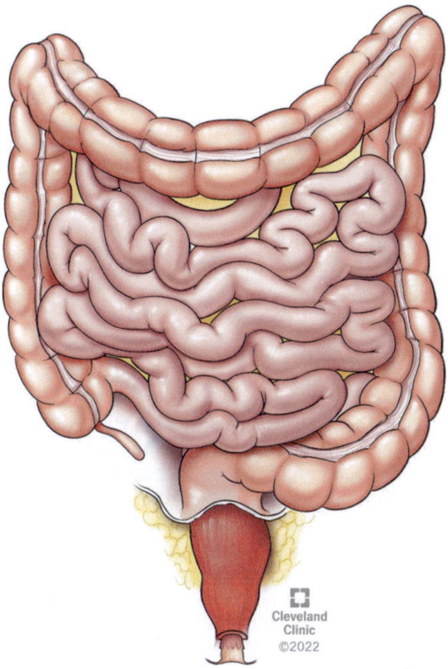

Springer

Editors
James S. Wu
Department of Colon and Rectal Surgery
Cleveland Clinic
Cleveland, OH, USA

Michelle D. Inkster
Department of Gastroenterology
Cleveland Clinic
Cleveland, OH, USA

ISBN 978-3-031-39882-7 ISBN 978-3-031-39880-3 (eBook)
https://doi.org/10.1007/978-3-031-39880-3

This Springer imprint is published by the registered company Springer Nature Switzerland AG
The registered company address is: Gewerbestrasse 11, 6330 Cham, Switzerland

Paper in this product is recyclable.

To our daughter, Margaret, the light of our lives.

Foreword

Dr. Wu and Dr. Inkster have written and recruited respected clinical and academic physicians to contribute to this work on colon and rectal surgery. Anatomy, pathology, radiology, endoscopy, and medical illustrations support a collection of case studies selected from decades of clinical experience. The presentations are arranged distal to proximal starting at the perianal and anal areas then move in sequence to the rectum, the colon, and finally the small intestine. The cases are a mixture of the common and the unusual reflecting their origin from a tertiary medical center. The intention of the book is the introduction of fundamental principles to those who are beginning their journey. Each clinical presentation is followed by a discussion centered on history, especially on contributions of early practitioners who not only did but also recorded what they did for the benefit of generations that would follow long after they were gone. Included are not only their words but also their visual impressions preserved from woodcuts, engravings, and pen/ink drawings. Chronologically, the discussions end short of the present. The "latest and the greatest" is not the point. How we got here and who led us here is. Notable is the inclusion of cases that most would recognize as failures or complications. By including these, we are reminded, sometimes painfully, that the results of our decisions and our actions do not always end the way we would like.

The book is dedicated to my friend and colleague, Vic Fazio. He preceded me from Australia to work with Dr. Rupert Turnbull in the early 1970s. Both of us never left. We, like others, came here because of the Cleveland Clinic's reputation for excellence in intestinal surgery. Dr. Tom Jones in the 1940s achieved the lowest mortality rate for abdominoperineal resection for his time. Dr. Turnbull came on as Dr. Jones' Fellow. In that role, although he assisted in hundreds of operations, he only performed one himself. Following Dr. Jones' untimely passing in 1949, Dr. Turnbull performed almost 100 operations in one year, achieving the same low mortality as his mentor. Dr. Turnbull was a world authority on ulcerative colitis, Crohn's disease, colorectal cancer, ostomy surgery, and nursing ostomy education. Under his guidance, the specialty of colorectal surgery blossomed slowly at first then inexorably. Among his first recruits were Drs. Frank Weakley, Victor Fazio, and David Jagelman. In 1951, with Dr. George "Barney" Crile, he championed subtotal colectomy and ileostomy for toxic ulcerative colitis resulting in reduced mortality. In 1953, he described an operation to prevent ileostomy dysfunction. In the same year, he introduced Karaya as a barrier to protect the skin of ostomates. In the 1950s and

60s, he advocated the "no-touch" isolation technique for the operative treatment of colon cancer. In 1958, a former patient, Ms. Norma Gill, became the Clinic's first full-time "enterostomal" therapist. The School of Enterostomal Therapy subsequently was created and produced its first graduates in 1961. The Department of Colorectal Surgery was formed in 1968 with Dr. Turnbull serving as its chairman from 1968 to 1975. Those of us who trained with him learned operative techniques that we used our entire careers. We in turn shared this information with many Fellows and trainees whom we have had the honor of teaching. I have been told that there is a "Cleveland" way of doing certain things that if seen in the operating room even from a distance identifies the operator as having passed through here. Many of these techniques are represented in this work. I expect that, like everything, some things will last because they continue to be useful while others will fall by the wayside as they are replaced by something better. For the moment, I think what is presented here still has merit. Hopefully, that will continue to be the case for a while longer.

The book ends with recollections written by the nurses, secretaries, and staff who kept Vic's practice afloat. Their memories emote feelings of dedication, respect, pride, and love.

Congratulations to Dr. Wu and Dr. Inkster and the contributing authors.

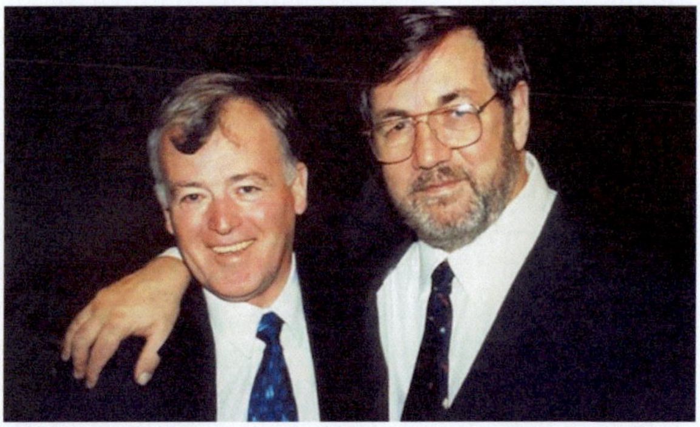

Drs. Ian Lavery and Victor Fazio at the 21st Annual Turnbull Symposium on the occasion of Dr. Fazio's 25th anniversary as Chairman of the Department of Colon and Rectal Surgery.[1]

[1]Access to this photo was provided by Ms. Joyce Balliet.

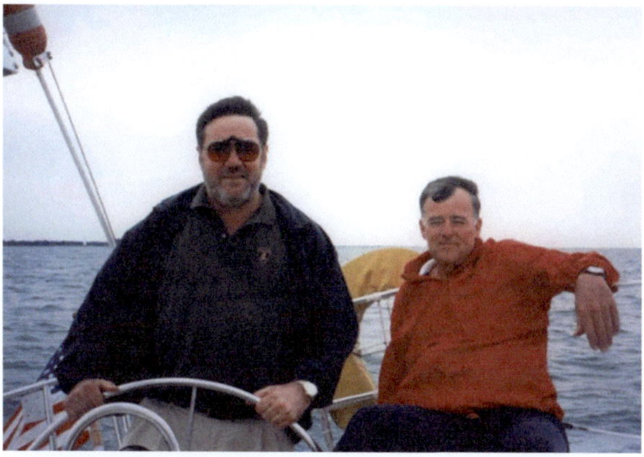

Aussies on the water.[1]

Cleveland, OH, USA
March, 2023

Ian C. Lavery

Preface

This work is dedicated to Dr. Victor W. Fazio, formerly the Chairman of the Department of Colon and Rectal Surgery, who served as a mentor to a generation of physicians and surgeons from around the world. The book introduces colorectal surgery and gastroenterology concepts using a case study format. All cases were contributed by practitioners associated with the Cleveland Clinic. Operative photographs, radiographs, endoscopic images, histology, illustrations, and historical perspective are emphasized. Also included are sections on anatomy, embryology, intestinal anastomoses, and surgical instruments. The intended audience is students and residents. Each case contains a teaching point. The artwork, created under the direction of the Cleveland Clinic medical illustration team, provides cohesion to the whole.

This project began in 2005, when one of us (MDI) suggested that we should collect cases that we encounter during our daily practices at the Cleveland Clinic for publication at some future date for the purpose of education regarding disease, diagnostic evaluation, management, and complications of therapy. A few of these are presented for the benefit of students and trainees, current and future.

The presentations are followed by comments that emphasize historical origins as much as possible. In 1985, a medical school classmate (of JSW) presented a case of breast cancer to Dr. Samuel A. Wells, Jr, Chairman of the Department of Surgery at Washington University in St. Louis. The student referred to Dr. William Halsted. Dr. Wells stopped the presentation and asked, "Who was Halsted?" The message to us in the audience was clear: you have to know where you come from. Our decision to avoid editorialization when possible follows the approach of Mr. Harlow Giles Unger, preeminent author of American historical biographies, who states: "As a former reporter, I never editorialize (when writing historical biographies). I let the characters speak for themselves."

Reference

1. Unger Harlow G., The Taft School, *Taft Bulletin;* Fall 2019. https://www.taftschool.org>bulletin>fall-2019. p. 42–47; published Nov 25, 2019. We thank Mr. Unger for his permission to quote him and Ms. Linda Hedman Beyus, Editor of the Taft School Bulletin, The Taft School Alumni Office, for her kind introduction to Mr. Unger.

Warrensville Hts, OH, USA — James S. Wu
Cleveland, OH, USA — Michelle D. Inkster

Origins

During World War I, three surgeons, Drs. Frank Bunts, George Crile Sr., and William Lower all served at the U.S. Army's Base Hospital No. 4 (the Lakeside Unit) at Rouen, France. They were joined by Dr. John Phillips, an internist, who during the war had served as a Captain in the medical corps. At war's end, following the military model, these four citizen-soldiers conceived a unified practice that would encompass all medical and surgical specialties. The Cleveland Clinic was incorporated on February 5, 1921.

What is now termed General Surgery was the parent of all the surgical departments. George Crile, Sr. was famous for thyroid surgery, particularly for goiters, and that was what kept the Clinic flourishing for its first 20 years. As chiefs of surgery, Dr. Crile and later Dr. Thomas Jones established standards that allowed the Clinic as a whole to achieve surgical mortality that was among the lowest in the country. Although gastroenterology was practiced at the Clinic from the beginning as part of internal medicine, a formal department was not officially founded until 1936. The first chairman was Dr. Everett Collins, who originally came here in 1931 as a radiologist and who was very interested in gastrointestinal disease. Having observed his interest, the founders asked him to start a specialized gastroenterology program. Within that department, he emphasized inflammatory bowel diseases. Rigid endoscopy, practiced by Dr. R. J. F. Renshaw in the 1930s was followed by flexible fiberoptic endoscopy by Dr. Benjamin Sullivan in the 1960s. Intestinal surgery was practiced as part of general surgery from the clinic's inception. However, it was Dr. Jones who showed that surgery for colon and rectal cancer could be achieved with consistently low mortality.

Over the next half-century, Drs. Edgar Achkar, Charles Brown, George Crile, Jr., Richard Farmer, Thomas Jones, George Rankin, Eugene Winkelman, Rupert Turnbull, and Frank Weakley set the cornerstones of an institutional focus on inflammatory bowel disease and colorectal cancer. Following the untimely death of Dr. Jones in 1949, Dr. Turnbull continued his legacy, becoming the first Chairman of a separate Colon and Rectal Surgery Department in 1968. Dr. Turnbull's contributions focused on intestinal stomas, colon cancer, and inflammatory bowel disease. In 1961, with Ms. Norma Gill, a former patient, Dr. Turnbull created a school dedicated to the discipline of enterostomal therapy. This program has benefited ostomy patients worldwide. Dr. Victor Fazio succeeded Dr. Turnbull as Chairman of the Department of Colon and Rectal Surgery in 1975. Dr. Fazio's team partnered with, recruited, and trained like-minded surgeons, physicians, and specialists from around the world to meet the needs of the ever-expanding discipline of colon and rectal surgery. The clinic motto, "To act as a unit," continues to guide and to inspire us today [1, 2].

Comment

The Cleveland Clinic was founded based on the military experience of its founders in France during WWI. It was there that Dr. George Crile coined the Clinic's motto, "To act as a unit." That is, out of battlefield necessity, to act as a unit for the benefit of many. A few of Dr. Crile's recollections from that conflict are presented [3].

Paris, September 16th [4]

"Military surgery has its shadows and its highlights. The highlights are romantic, for in a brief season, whole areas of the body are conquered; great principles are worked out; foundation stones laid.

Patients come in volleys. The surgeon is barraged with fractures, shelled with broken heads: bombed with bellies; gassed with wounds.

Mobile Hospital No. 5, October 4th [5]

This morning our troops went over. The war goes on. Off with peace! Roads are all but impassable; automobiles are mired everywhere; wreckage is on every side. Guns are booming; mile of convoys, ammunition and food are going up; trains of wounded are coming down. The Argonne forest is sprouting wooden crosses.

Mobile Hospital No. 5, October 17th

Everything is overflowing with patients. Our divisions are being shot up; the wards are full of machine gun wounds.

I have been operating on 12-hour shifts here. One hundred and twenty cases are waiting for operation this morning. In one night I had sixty deaths.

Rain, rain; mud, blood; blood, death! All day, all night we hear the incessant tramp of troops—troops going in, wounded coming back, Even in our dreams we hear it. If it ceases for a few hours it is so insistent in our conditioned brain that the incessant rhythmic tramp continues.

Autumn in the beautiful Argonne! Rolling hills, green meadows, shepherd dogs, sheep, lazy cows, brown oak leaves, yellow linwood, red gum, grey and velvety beeches, the rocks and the ground brilliantly blotched with blood—all color blending with the dying and the dead!

C.C.S. 17, September 30th [6, 7]

Ed Lower and I are convinced from our experience with war wounds that there exists no basic distinction between the war patient and the civilian patient; between the man exhausted of days and weeks of intensive fighting waiting, dirty, wet, hungry, and thirsty, and the starved patient exhausted by the ravages of disease.

No. 9, August 27th [8, 9]

Frank Bunts came today to be the C.O. in the place of Ed who has returned to the United States. Frank will make a good C.O. I am more delighted that I can express to have him here, for I have missed Ed sorely. What a remarkable record Bunts,

Crile and Lower have had all of these years. We have been rivals in everything, yet could differ in opinion about anything and through all the vicissitudes of personal, financial, and professional relations we have been able to think and act as a unit" [10].

References

1. Clough JD, Studer PG, Szilagyi S, editors. To act as a unit. The story of the Cleveland Clinic. 5th ed. Cleveland, OH: Cleveland Clinic Foundation; 2011.
2. We are indebted to Mr. Frederick K. Lautenzenheiser and Mr. John E. Bowen, Cleveland Clinic Archivists, for providing us with access to and direction towards the individuals mentioned above.
3. Crile GW. George Crile. An autobiography, edited with sidelihts, by Grace Crile. Philadelphia, PA: J.B. Lippincott Company; 1947.
4. Crile GW. George Crile. An autobiography, edited with sidelights, by Grace Crile. Philadelphia, PA: J.B. Lippincott Company; 1947. p. 312.
5. Crile GW. George Crile. An autobiography, edited with sidelights, by Grace Crile. Philadelphia, PA: J.B. Lippincott Company; 1947. p. 350–351.
6. Crile GW. George Crile. An Autobiography, edited with sidelights, by Grace Crile. Philadelphia, PA: J.B. Lippincott Company; 1947. p. 337; C. C. S 17 refers to Casualty Clearing Center No. 17.
7. Crile GW. George Crile. An Autobiography, edited with sidelights, by Grace Crile. Philadelphia, PA: J.B. Lippincott Company; 1947. p. 315.
8. Crile GW. George Crile. An Autobiography, edited with sidelights, by Grace Crile. Philadelphia, PA: J.B. Lippincott Company; 1947. p. 344.
9. Crile GW. George Crile. An Autobiography, edited with sidelights, by Grace Crile. Philadelphia, PA: J.B. Lippincott Company; 1947. p. 326; No 9 refers to General Hospital No. 9.
10. These excerpts were taken from a copy of Dr. Crile's two volume autobiography that was given to Dr. Inkster by one of her patients.

James S. Wu
Michelle D. Inkster

Vesalius-The intestines

Brevis intestinorum historia enumeratio.

Intestina invicem variant, omnia tamen inter ventriculum, et qua excrementa egerimus.

Andreas Vesalius

De Humani Corporis Fabrica [1]

Brief account of the intestines

The intestines follow one after another but all [are located] between the stomach and where we discharge the excrements.

Andreas Vesalius

On the Fabric of the Human Body

Revised Version of 1555 [2, 3]

References

1. Vesalius A. De Humani Corporis Fabrica, A Facsimile of the revised version of 1555, Vol II of II. Leopold Publishing; 2014. p. 135.
2. This translation was by Transperfect. www.transperfect.com.
3. Richardson WF, Carman JB. ON THE FABRIC OF THE HUMAN BODY. A translation of De Humani Corporis Fabrica Libri Septem. Book V. The Organs of Nutrition and Generation. Novato, CA: Norman Publishing; 2007. p. 87.

Chinese Proverb

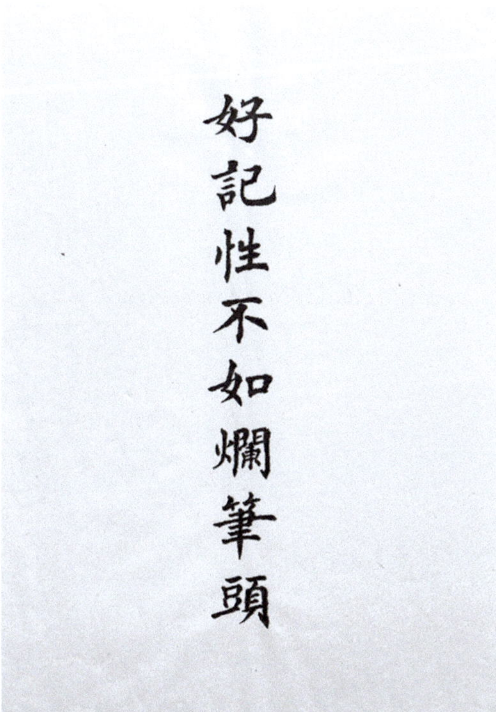

好記性不如爛筆頭
Hǎo jì xìng bù rú làn bǐtóu
“The palest ink is more powerful than the sharpest memory.”
Chinese proverb
Calligraphy by: Jian Ma, mamin@frontier.com

In Remembrance

Victor Warren Fazio, A.O., M.B.M.S., F.R.A.C.S., F.R.C.S., Eng (Hon), F.R.C.S., Edin (Hon), F.A.C.S., F.R.A.C.S. (Hon), M.D. Lodz (Hon), F.R.C.S.I. (Hon)

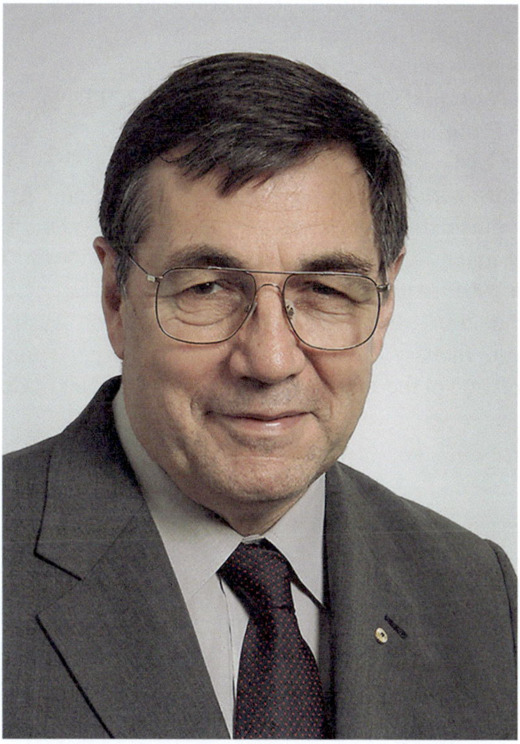

Victor Warren Fazio, A.O., M.B.M.S.
Master surgeon, preeminent educator and pioneer in the field of Colon and Rectal Surgery
Victor Warren Fazio
1940 Born in Sydney, New South Wales

- Secondary School-St. Joseph's College, Hunter's Hill

  1965 M.B.B.S., University of Sydney

- Postgraduate training at St. Vincent's Hospital, Sydney

  under the direction of Dr. Noel C. Newton

- Additional training with Sir E. S. R. Hughes

  1970 Fellow Royal Australasian College of Surgeons (F.R.A.C.S.) by examination
  1971 Service in Bien Hoa (Vietnam) under Dr. Fred Collins
  1972 Lahey Clinic, Hepatobiliary service of Dr. Ken Warren;
  Colorectal Surgery service of Dr. Malcolm Veidenheimer
  1973 Cleveland Clinic, Colorectal service of Dr. Rupert Turnbull, Jr.
  1974 Cleveland Clinic, Staff Surgeon
  1975 Cleveland Clinic, Chairman, Colon & Rectal Surgery
  1995 Master of Surgery (honoris causa)
  The University of Sydney
  2004 Order of Australia, Officer (A.O.) in the General Division
  2013 Emeritus Professor of Surgery

Awards, Short List

Honorary Fellowship European Surgical Association, April 2007 -Fifth N.E.C.R.S. Distinguished Recognition Award, 2006 -Cleveland Clinic Teacher of the Year Award Winner, 2005-6 -Distinguished Alumnus Award Cleveland Clinic Foundation, June 2005 -America's Top Doctors 2004 (Castle Connolly Ltd. Peer Nomination), June 2004, June 2002 -Officer, Order of Australia (Services to colorectal surgery), January 2004 -Al and Norma Lerner Humanitarian Award, October 2002 -Creation of the Victor W. Fazio Endowed Chair in Colorectal Surgery.

Acknowledgments

First and foremost, we thank the Cleveland Clinic for its unreserved support of this work. We express our heartfelt gratitude to the Cleveland Clinic Library staff for providing access to the world literature for more than 20 years. We thank the Cleveland Clinic Department of Medical Art and Photography for extraordinary artwork. Mr. Joe Pangrace and his staff, Mr. Tony Christovich, Ms. Gwen Fuller, Ms. Emily Hromi, Mr. Ken Kula, Ms. Amanda Mendelsohn, Ms. Maribel Ruiz, and Ms. Erika Woodrum, created illustrations that communicate that which words alone are inadequate to express. We thank Ms. Kathy Miller for preparing and then teaching us to prepare for ourselves digital images suitable for publication. We thank Mr. Fred Lautzenheiser and Mr. John Bowen of the Cleveland Clinic Archives for teaching us Cleveland Clinic History. We thank Professors Richard Drake and Jennifer McBride for co-writing the chapters on anatomy. We gratefully acknowledge Dr. John Goldblum, Chairman of the Cleveland Clinic Department of Anatomic and Surgical Pathology, and members of his staff, present and former, including: Ms. Kathleen Ranney, Drs. Daniela Allende, Ana Bennett, Michael Cruise, Mohamed El Hag, Clifton Fulmer, Ilyssa Gordon, Scott Kilpatrick, James Lapinski, Kelsey McHugh, Mark Melaragno, Rish Pai, Melissa Piliang, Scott Robertson, Erica Savage, Sebouh Setrakian, Charles Sturgis, Jacob Sweeney, Ralph Tuthill, and Jing-Jing Yang. In particular, we thank Drs. David Hernandez Gonzalo, Keith Lai, Homer Wiland, Eric Willis, and Catherine Forse, who, when Fellows in the department, volunteered to provide the majority of the histopathologic images used in this book. They performed this work during their own time before and after regular hours. We acknowledge their generosity and collegiality. We thank Dr. Carolyn Power, Research Fellow in the Department of Colon and Rectal Surgery, for her dedicated and selfless contribution to this book over two years. We thank Drs. Abraham Ahmed, Joseph Azok, Mark Baker, Ajay Bhardwaj, Sean Carlson, Michael Christian, Mark Cohen, Bradley Cole, David Einstein, Ihab Haddadin, Paul Janicki,

Leonard Kahn, Paresh Mahajan, Patrick O'Keefe, Charles O'Malley, Jr., Arthur Parsee, Erick Remer, Samuel Ruskin, Todd Stultz, and Ryan Ward of the Radiology Institute for selection and description of diagnostic images. We thank Ms. Joyce Balliet, medical photographer, for photographing Dr. Fazio's operations and preserving the details of each operation in 35 mm and digital formats. We thank Mr. Apollo Draco for technical expertise in the preparation of videos. We thank Drs. Tracy Hull, Scott Steele, Conor Delaney, and Matthew Walsh of the Digestive Diseases and Surgery Institute for their continuous support. We thank the case contributors. Without their experience, generosity, and commitment to education, this book would not have been possible. We thank Dr. Ian Lavery for reviewing this work and writing its foreword. We thank Mr. Robert Yonchak, Esq., Mr. Michael Michetti, Esq., Ms. Rose Wenstrup, Esq, and Mr. Gregory Stein, Esq. for guiding this work to publication. We thank the Springer Nature Publishing Company and our project editors, Mr. Richard Hruska, Ms. Anila Vijayan, Ms. Shaik Jainul Safha, Ms. Jananee Ravichandran, Ms. Patricia Gutierrez, Mr. Dhanapal Palanisamy, and Mr. Kristopher Spring for putting this book into print. Finally, we thank Drs. Kenneth Bennett, Robert Fry, and Ira Kodner, surgeons at the Washington University School of Medicine, all prior Fellows of the Cleveland Clinic, for mentorship and friendship over many years.

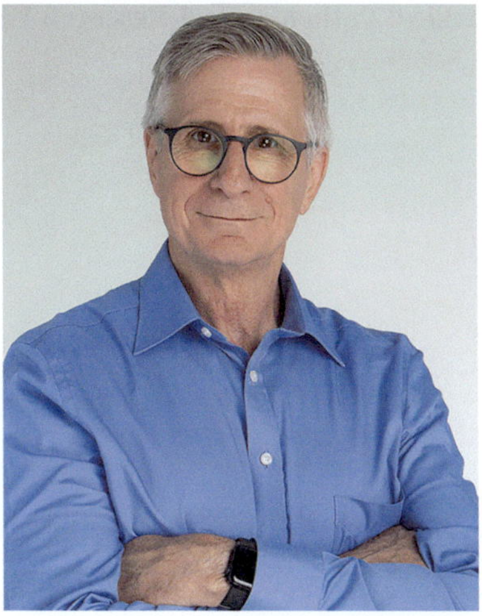

For the past 37 years, Mr. Joseph A. Pangrace has applied his knowledge and skill as a medical illustrator for the Cleveland Clinic. He began working at the Cleveland Clinic immediately following his graduation from the Medical Illustration Program at the Cleveland Institute of Art. Mr. Pangrace's work has been published in medical journals, textbooks, and atlases. In 2005, he was awarded the Medical Illustrator's Max Bröedel prize for continuous-tone illustration. He currently acts as the Medical Illustration Section Leader for the Center for Medical Art and Photography and Medical Art Director for the Cleveland Clinic Journal of Medicine.

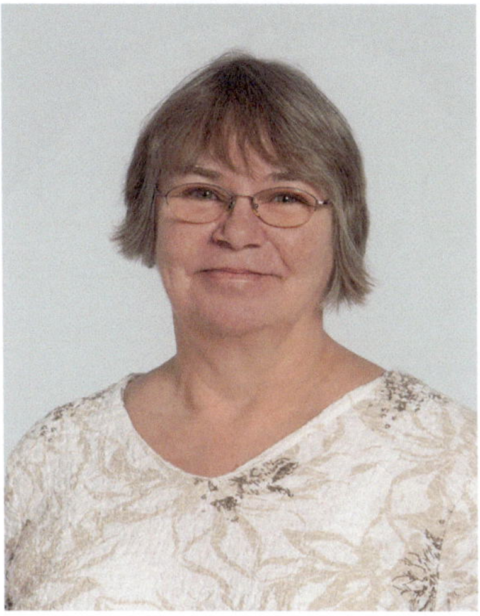

Ms. Kathleen Miller, Digital Technologist, Cleveland Clinic Department of Medical Art and Illustration, prepared the majority of photographs and illustrations used in this work for publication. This work was done with painstaking attention to detail, with many revisions, over many years. Her steadfast commitment to this book is warmly acknowledged.

Cleveland Clinic Surgical Pathology and Research Fellows

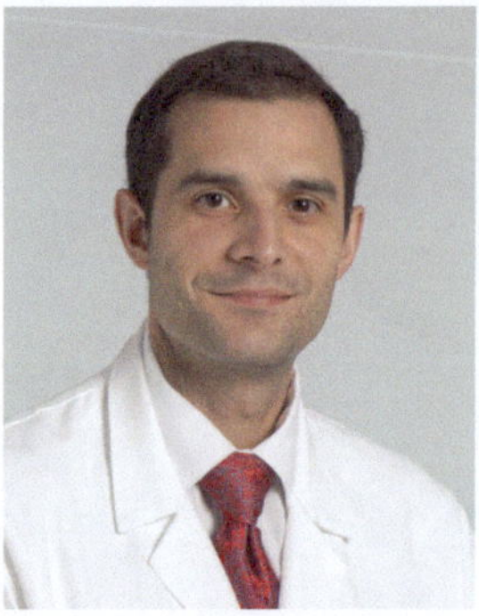

David Hernandez Gonzalo, MD

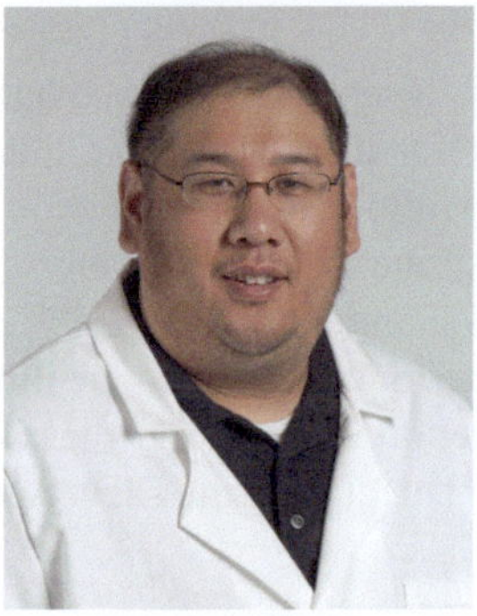

Keith K. Lai, MD

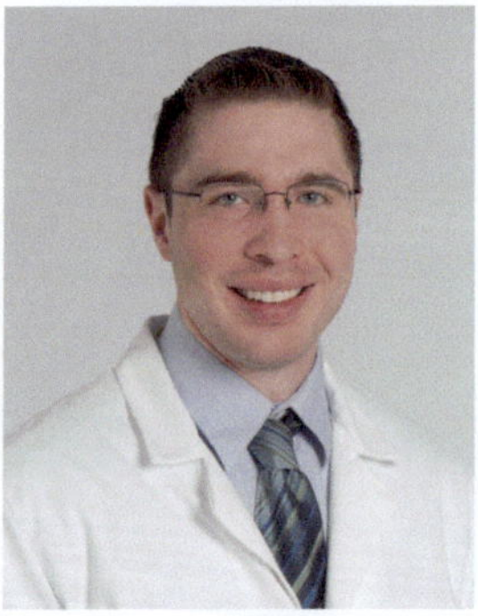

Homer O. Wiland, MD

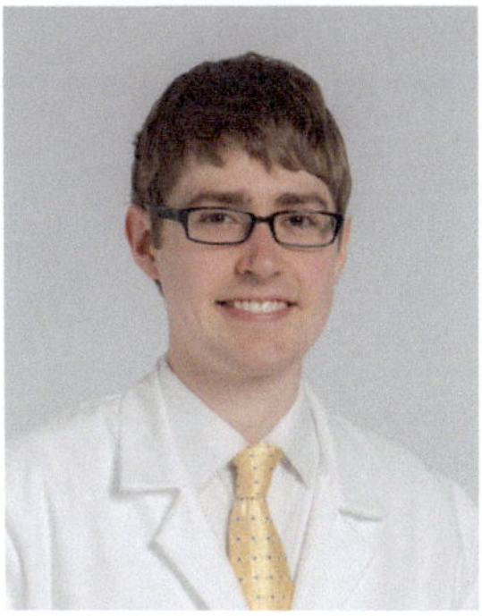

Eric W. Willis, MD

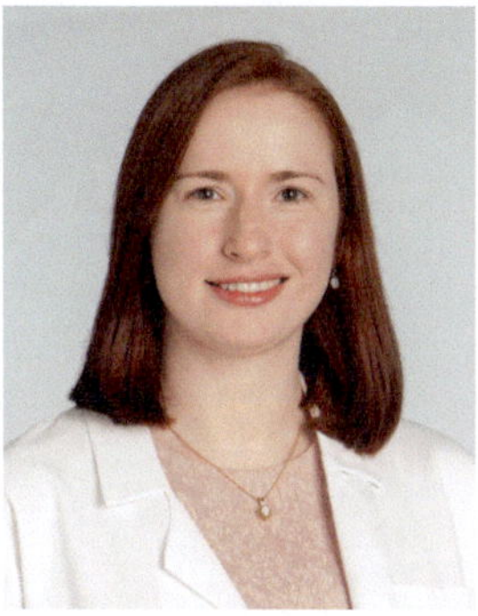

Catherine L. Forse, MD

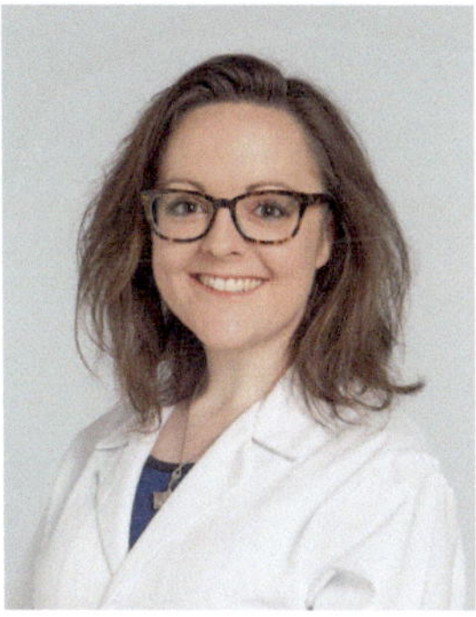

Carolyn L. Power, MD

Cleveland Clinic Library Staff (1994–2025)
"Without whom, this work would not have been possible."
Previous Staff
Gretchen Hallerberg
Jodith Janes
Kevin Kennedy
Javan Jackson
Devera Kastner
Marian Simonson
Marlene Englander
Cindy Avallone
Barb Anderson
Brian Hanna
Doug Bazdar
Antoinette Bolden
Mina Chercourt
Lorelei Woody
Kate Kretschmann
Evone Jeffries
Laura Migneco-Fretnzko
Jill Moorman
Kim Brady
Current Staff
Rosa Blackburn
Latoya Lee
Matt Weaver
Michelle Kraft
Snezana Lebinac
Loren Hackett
Theresa Kline
Neil Nero
LaDonna Pierce
DeAnna Camara
Mary Pat Harnegie
Mary Schleicher
Shelby Stuart
Olivia Davis
Shelley Ivary
Ethan Haas

James S. Wu
Michelle D. Inkster

Contents of Volume II

Contents of Volume I

Contributors

Armen Aboulian Department of Colon and Rectal Surgery, Kaiser Permanente Woodland Hills Medical Center, Woodland Hills, CA, USA

Amelia Agostinelli WOC Nursing Department, Cleveland Clinic, Cleveland, OH, USA

Eberechi S. Agwa Hematology & Medical Oncology, Cleveland Clinic, Cleveland, OH, USA

Abraham Ahmed Diagnostic Imaging and Interventional Radiology, H. Lee Moffitt Cancer Center & Research Institute, Tampa, FL, USA

Matthew T. Allemang Department of Surgery, Cleveland Clinic, Cleveland, OH, USA

Daniela Allende Pathology & Laboratory Medicine Institute, Cleveland Clinic, Cleveland, OH, USA

Jean H. Ashburn Department of Colon and Rectal Surgery, Atrium Health Wake Forest Baptist, Winston-Salem, NC, USA

H. Nail Aydin Department of Colon and Rectal Surgery, Cleveland Clinic, Cleveland, OH, USA

Joseph T. Azok Radiology & Diagnostic Imaging Institute, Cleveland Clinic, Cleveland, OH, USA

Mark E. Baker Department of Radiology, Cleveland Clinic Lerner College of Medicine, Case Western Reserve University, Cleveland, OH, USA

Joyce M. Balliet Department of Colon and Rectal Surgery, Cleveland Clinic, Cleveland, OH, USA

Hani B. Baradi Mercy Colon and Rectal Surgery, Oklahoma City, OK, USA

David C. Baringer Department of General Surgery, Cleveland Clinic, Cleveland, OH, USA

Ana E. Bennett Pathology & Laboratory Medicine Institute, Cleveland Clinic, Cleveland, OH, USA

Douglas D. Benson Rocky Mountain Colon and Rectal Surgeons, Lone Tree, CO, USA

Ajay Bhardwaj Radiology and Diagnostic Imaging Institute, Cleveland Clinic, Cleveland, OH, USA

Adarsh Bhimraj Department of Infectious Diseases, Cleveland Clinic, Cleveland, OH, USA

Vladimir Bolshinsky Department of Colorectal Surgery, Surgical Health Specialists, Melbourne, Australia

Stephen Brandstetter Department of Colon and Rectal Surgery, Cleveland Clinic Akron General Hospital, Akron, OH, USA

Aaron Brzezinski Department of Gastroenterology, Cleveland Clinic, Cleveland, OH, USA

Sean W. Carlson Department of Radiology, UPMC Children's Hospital of Pittsburgh, Pittsburgh, PA, USA

Christi M. Cavaliere Department of Surgery, Section of Plastic Surgery, Louis Stokes Cleveland VA Medical Center, Cleveland, OH, USA

Sricharan Chalikonda Department of Surgery Allegheny Health Network, Pittsburgh, PA, USA

Michael O. Christian Radiology & Diagnostic Imaging Institute, Cleveland Clinic, Cleveland, OH, USA

James M. Church Department of Colon and Rectal Surgery, Cleveland Clinic, Cleveland, OH, USA

Michael S. Cline Department of Gastroenterology, Cleveland Clinic, Cleveland, OH, USA

Mark A. H. Cohen Radiology & Diagnostic Imaging Institute, Cleveland Clinic, Cleveland, OH, USA

Bradley L. Cole Radiology & Diagnostic Imaging Institute, Cleveland Clinic, Cleveland, OH, USA

Michael W. Cruise Pathology & Laboratory Medicine Institute, Cleveland Clinic, Cleveland, OH, USA

John P. Cullen Department of Colon and Rectal Surgery, Cleveland Clinic, Cleveland, OH, USA

Christopher R. Daigle Department of Surgery, Cleveland Clinic Akron General Hospital, Akron, OH, USA

Amber N. Dalton Dermatology & Plastic Surgery Center, Cleveland Clinic, Cleveland, OH, USA

Robert L. DeBernardo, Jr. Ob/Gyn & Women's Health Institute, Cleveland Clinic, Cleveland, OH, USA

Sandra Dellaportas Department of Internal Medicine, Cleveland Clinic, Cleveland, OH, USA

David W. Dietz Department of Surgery, NYU Langone Medical Center, New York, NY, USA

Lewis A. Diulus III Crystal Plastic Surgeons, Akron, OH, USA

Apollo A. Draco Information Technology Institute, Cleveland Clinic, Cleveland, OH, USA

Richard L. Drake Department of Anatomy, Cleveland Clinic Lerner College of Medicine, Cleveland, OH, USA

John A. Dumot Department of Gastroenterology, University Hospitals of Cleveland, Cleveland, OH, USA

David M. Einstein Radiology & Diagnostic Imaging Institute, Cleveland Clinic, Cleveland, OH, USA

Mohamed I. El Hag Pathology and Laboratory Medicine Institute, Cleveland Clinic, Cleveland, OH, USA

Charis Eng Genomic Medicine Institute and Center for Personalized Genetic Healthcare, Cleveland Clinic, Cleveland, OH, USA

Victor W. Fazio Department of Colon and Rectal Surgery, Cleveland Clinic, Cleveland, OH, USA

Jesus Flores Department of Colon and Rectal Surgery, Cleveland Clinic, Cleveland, OH, USA

Catherine L. Forse Department of Pathology and Laboratory Medicine, Faculty of Medicine, University of Ottawa, Ottawa, ON, Canada

Robert D. Fry Department of Colon and Rectal Surgery, University of Pennsylvania, Philadelphia, PA, USA

Gwendolyn A. Fuller Medical Illustration Team, Enterprise Creative Services, Cleveland Clinic, Cleveland, OH, USA

Clifton G. Fulmer Pathology & Laboratory Medicine Institute, Cleveland Clinic, Cleveland, OH, USA

Thomas E. Garofalo Department of Colon and Rectal Surgery, Cleveland Clinic, Cleveland, OH, USA

Susan L. Gearhart Department of General and Colon & Rectal Surgery, Johns Hopkins Bayview Medical Center, Baltimore, MD, USA

John R. Goldblum Pathology & Laboratory Medicine Institute, Cleveland Clinic, Cleveland, OH, USA

David Hernandez Gonzalo Department of Pathology, Immunology and Laboratory Medicine, University of Florida, Gainesville, FL, USA

Ilyssa O. Gordon Pathology & Laboratory Medicine Institute, Cleveland Clinic, Cleveland, OH, USA

Emre Gorgun Department of Colon and Rectal Surgery, Cleveland Clinic, Cleveland, OH, USA

Ihab S. Haddadin Radiology & Diagnostic Imaging Institute, Cleveland Clinic, Cleveland, OH, USA

Amer A. Hanano Radiology and Diagnostic Imaging Institute, Cleveland Clinic Florida, Weston, FL, USA

James M. Hekman Department of Internal Medicine, Cleveland Clinic, Cleveland, OH, USA

Alexander G. Heriot Department Colorectal Surgery, Peter MacCallum Cancer Centre, Melbourne, Australia

Brian T. Hill Cleveland Clinic Taussig Cancer Institute, Cleveland Clinic, Cleveland, OH, USA

Barbara J. Hocevar Rupert B. Turnbull, Jr., School of WOC Nursing Education, Cleveland Clinic, Cleveland, OH, USA

David A. Horvath Plastic and Cosmetic Surgery, Abbington, PA, USA

Emily Hromi Cleveland Clinic Center for Medical Art and Photography, MI, USA

Emina H. Huang Department of Surgery, University of Texas Southwestern, Dallas, TX, USA

Tracy L. Hull Department of Colon and Rectal Surgery, Cleveland Clinic, Cleveland, OH, USA

Tasadooq Hussain Department of General and Colorectal Surgery, Wrightington Wigan & Leigh Teaching Hospitals NHS Foundation Trust, Manchester, UK

Michelle D. Inkster Department of Gastroenterology, Cleveland Clinic, Cleveland, OH, USA

Katharine L. Jackson Department of Colorectal Surgery, Department of Surgery, Duke University, Durham, NC, USA

Deepa Jagadeesh Cleveland Clinic Taussig Cancer Institute, Cleveland, OH, USA

David G. Jagelman Department of Colon and Rectal Surgery, Cleveland Clinic, Cleveland, OH, USA

Paul C. Janicki Radiology & Diagnostic Imaging Institute, Cleveland Clinic, Cleveland, OH, USA

Sami S. Judeeba Department of Colon and Rectal Surgery, Cleveland Clinic, Cleveland, OH, USA

Leonard A. Kahn Radiology & Diagnostic Imaging Institute, Cleveland Clinic, Cleveland, OH, USA

Hermann Kessler Department of Colon and Rectal Surgery, Cleveland Clinic, Cleveland, OH, USA

Scott E. Kilpatrick Pathology and Laboratory Institute, Cleveland Clinic, Cleveland, OH, USA

Ira J. Kodner Department of Colon and Rectal Surgery, Washington University School of Medicine, St. Louis, MO, USA

Matthew D. Kroh Department of General Surgery, Digestive Diseases Institute, Cleveland Clinic, Cleveland, OH, USA

Kenneth G. Kula Center for Medical Art and Photography, Cleveland Clinic, Cleveland, OH, USA

Keith K. Lai Pathology & Laboratory Medicine Institute, Cleveland Clinic, Cleveland, OH, USA

Irene C. Lalak Department of Dermatology, Cleveland Clinic, Cleveland, OH, USA

James E. Lapinski Pathology & Laboratory Medicine Institute, Cleveland Clinic, Cleveland, OH, USA

Ian C. Lavery Department of Colon and Rectal Surgery, Cleveland Clinic, Cleveland, OH, USA

Brandie Leach Genomic Medicine Institute and Center for Personalized Genetic Healthcare, Cleveland Clinic, Cleveland, OH, USA

Jason E. Leedy Cleveland Plastic Surgery Institute, Mayfield Heights, OH, USA

Jennifer J. Liang Department of Colon and Rectal Surgery, Cleveland Clinic, Cleveland, OH, USA

Susan A. Lintala Department of Gastroenterology, Cleveland Clinic, Cleveland, OH, USA

David Liska Department of Colon and Rectal Surgery, Cleveland Clinic, Cleveland, OH, USA

Careen Y. Lowder Cole Cye Institute, Cleveland Clinic, Cleveland, OH, USA

Sanford S. Luria Glickman Urological & Kidney Institute, Cleveland Clinic, Cleveland, OH, USA

Paresh Mahajan Radiology & Diagnostic Imaging Institute, Cleveland Clinic, Cleveland, OH, USA

Christian G. Massier Department of General Surgery, Cleveland Clinic, Cleveland, OH, USA

Jennifer M. McBride Department of Anatomy, Cleveland Clinic Lerner College of Medicine, Cleveland, OH, USA

Kelsey E. McHugh Department of Laboratory Medicine and Pathology, Mayo Clinic, Phoenix, AZ, USA

Mark J. Melaragno Pathology & Laboratory Medicine Institute, Cleveland Clinic, Cleveland, OH, USA

Amanda C. Mendelsohn Medical Illustration Team, Enterprise Creative Services, Cleveland Clinic, Cleveland, OH, USA

Carla R. Merrick Department of Colon and Rectal Surgery, Cleveland Clinic, Cleveland, OH, USA

Chad M. Michener Ob/Gyn and Women's Health Institute, Cleveland Clinic, Cleveland, OH, USA

Ryan M. Miller Department of Infectious Diseases, Cleveland Clinic, Cleveland, OH, USA

William J. O'Brien Department of Surgery, Cleveland Clinic, Cleveland, OH, USA

Patrick J. O'Keefe Radiology & Diagnostic Imaging Institute, Cleveland Clinic, Cleveland, OH, USA

Charles M. O'Malley, Jr. Radiology & Diagnostic Imaging Institute, Cleveland Clinic, Cleveland, OH, USA

Robert S. O'Shea Department of Gastroenterology and Hepatology, Cleveland Clinic, Cleveland, OH, USA

Rish K. Pai Department of Laboratory Medicine and Pathology, Mayo Clinic, Phoenix, AZ, USA

Joseph A. Pangrace CMI, Medical Illustration Team, Enterprise Creative Services, Cleveland Clinic, Cleveland, OH, USA

Arthur A. Parsee Department of Diagnostic Radiology, H. Lee Moffitt Cancer Center and Research Institute, Tampa, FL, USA

Theodore E. Partridge Department of Surgical Services, South Pointe Hospital, Warrensville Heights, OH, USA

Jessica R. Philpott Department of Gastroenterology, Cleveland Clinic, Cleveland, OH, USA

Melissa Piliang Dermatology & Plastic Surgery Center, Cleveland Clinic, Cleveland, OH, USA

Carolyn L. Power Department of Colon and Rectal Surgery, Cleveland Clinic, Cleveland, OH, USA

Gary W. Procop Pathology & Laboratory Medicine Institute, Cleveland Clinic, Cleveland, OH, USA

Andrei S. Purysko Department of Diagnostic Radiology, Cleveland Clinic, Cleveland, OH, USA

Erick M. Remer Radiology & Diagnostic Imaging Institute, Cleveland Clinic, Cleveland, OH, USA

Feza H. Remzi Inflammatory Bowel Disease Center, NYU Langone Health, New York, NY, USA

Florian Rieder Department of Gastroenterology, Hepatology and Nutrition, Digestive Disease Institute, Cleveland Clinic, Cleveland, OH, USA

Alain G. Rizk Radiology and Diagnostic Imaging Institute, Cleveland Clinic, Cleveland, OH, USA

Scott A. Robertson Pathology & Laboratory Medicine Institute, Cleveland Clinic, Cleveland, OH, USA

Samuel Ruskin Radiology & Diagnostic Imaging Institute, Cleveland Clinic, Cleveland, OH, USA

Chizu Sakai-Imoto WOC Nursing Department, Cleveland Clinic, Cleveland, OH, USA

Janice M. Santisi Digestive Diseases and Surgery Institute, Cleveland Clinic, Cleveland, OH, USA

Erica C. Savage Pathology & Laboratory Medicine Institute, Cleveland Clinic, Cleveland, OH, USA

Thomas K. Schroeder Department of Colon and Rectal Surgery, Cleveland Clinic, Cleveland, OH, USA

Dawn M. Schultz Department of Nursing, Cleveland Clinic, Cleveland, OH, USA

Sebouh Setrakian Pathology & Laboratory Medicine Institute, Cleveland Clinic, Cleveland, OH, USA

Nafis Shafizadeh Department of Pathology, Kaiser Permanente Woodland Hills Medical Center, Woodland Hills, CA, USA

Sherief Shawki Department of Colon and Rectal Surgery, Mayo Clinic Rochester, Rochester, MN, USA

Shu-Jane Shen Radiology and Diagnostic Imaging Institute, Cleveland Clinic, Cleveland, OH, USA

Lena J. Slater-Everhart Department of Surgical Services, South Pointe Hospital, Warrensville Heights, OH, USA

Luca Stocchi Department of Colon and Rectal Surgery, Mayo Clinic, Jacksonville, FL, USA

Todd W. Stultz Radiology & Diagnostic Imaging Institute, Cleveland Clinic, Cleveland, OH, USA

Charles D. Sturgis Hospital Pathology Associates/Allina, Minneapolis, MN, USA

Jacob R. Sweeney Pathology & Laboratory Medicine Institute, Cleveland Clinic, Cleveland, OH, USA

Ursula M. Szmulowicz Department of Colon and Rectal Surgery, Cleveland Clinic, Cleveland, OH, USA

Marisa Tungsiripat Department of Infectious Diseases, Cleveland Clinic, Cleveland, OH, USA

Ralph J. Tuthill Pathology & Laboratory Medicine Institute, Cleveland Clinic, Cleveland, OH, USA

Michael A. Valente Department of Colon and Rectal Surgery, Cleveland Clinic, Cleveland, OH, USA

Ryan D. Ward Radiology & Diagnostic Imaging Institute, Cleveland Clinic, Cleveland, OH, USA

Kenneth D. Webster Department of Obstetrics and Gynecology, Cleveland Clinic, Cleveland, OH, USA

Homer O. Wiland Department of Pathology, OhioHealth Mansfield Hospital, Mansfield, OH, USA

Eric W. Willis Department of Pathology, CORPath, Columbus, OH, USA

Erika B. Woodrum Medical Illustration Team, Enterprise Creative Services, Cleveland Clinic, Cleveland, OH, USA

James S. Wu Department of Colon and Rectal Surgery, Cleveland Clinic, Cleveland, OH, USA

Jing-Jing Yang Departments of Pathology, Medical Diagnostic Laboratories, LLC, Hamilton, NJ, USA

Douglas W. Yoder Department of Surgery, Blanchard Valley Health System, Findlay, OH, USA

Craig D. Zippe Glickman Urological & Kidney Institute, Cleveland Clinic, Cleveland, OH, USA

Gregory Zuccaro, Jr. Department of Gastroenterology, Cleveland Clinic, Cleveland, OH, USA

Massarat Zutshi Department of Colon and Rectal Surgery, Cleveland Clinic, Cleveland, OH, USA

The original version of the book has been revised. A correction to this book can be found at https://doi.org/10.1007/978-3-031-39880-3_236

Colonic Inertia

126

James S. Wu

Presentation

A 58-year-old female reported constipation of 20-year duration. She had one bowel movement every 2 weeks.

An evaluation was initiated.

1. *Marker transit study*

   A SITZMARKS® capsule (24 rings each) [1] was ingested on days 1, 2, and 3. Plain abdominal films taken on days 4 and 7 showed 58 markers on each film.
2. *Fluoroscopic defecography*: [2]

   Defecography was done after administration of oral, vaginal, and rectal contrast. Findings:
   (a) Evacuation was initiated rapidly.
   (b) There was 0% residual after rectal evacuation.
   (c) A small rectocele was seen.
3. *Anal manometry* [3] showed normal resting and squeeze pressures. The recto-anal inhibitory reflex was present. There was no evidence of paradoxical contraction.
4. *Colonoscopy* revealed no abnormality.
5. *Thyroid-stimulating hormone level*:

   3.6 mU/L (0.4-4.0 mU/L).
6. Consultations with internal medicine, endocrinology, and psychiatry revealed no contraindications for surgery.

J. S. Wu (✉)
Department of Colon and Rectal Surgery, Cleveland Clinic, Cleveland, OH, USA

J. S. Wu, M. D. Inkster (eds.), *Cleveland Clinic Colorectal Case Studies*,
https://doi.org/10.1007/978-3-031-39880-3_126

Interpretation of Tests

Marker transit: The SITZMARKS® colonic transit diagnostic test has single capsule and three capsule versions (1 capsule: each capsule with 24 markers). Prior to the test, laxatives, enemas, and suppositories are avoided for 5 days. In the single capsule version, one capsule is ingested on day 1. A flat plate abdominal X-ray is done on day 5. Patients who expel at least 80% (19 or more) markers have normal colonic transit. In the three-capsule version, capsules are taken on days 1, 2, and 3. An abdominal flat plate X-ray is taken on day 4. If more than 50 markers are present on day 4, transit time is abnormal. This patient's marker transit study was abnormal. A representative abnormal marker transit abdominal plain film is shown in Fig. 126.1.

Defecography: Defecography is a real-time test that evaluates both rectal structure and function. Barium paste is instilled in the rectum; its evacuation is evaluated by cine radiography (Fig. 126.2a, b). Simultaneous contrast in the small intestine and vagina allows for the assessment of the rectocele and enterocele.

Anorectal manometry assesses anorectal reflexes, rectal compliance, and defecatory function. Colonoscopy excludes mechanical causes of constipation such as neoplasm or stricture. Consultation is obtained to identify and treat medical/psychiatric causes of constipation (medication, autonomic failure, endocrine disorder, mental disorder), and to determine fitness for surgery.

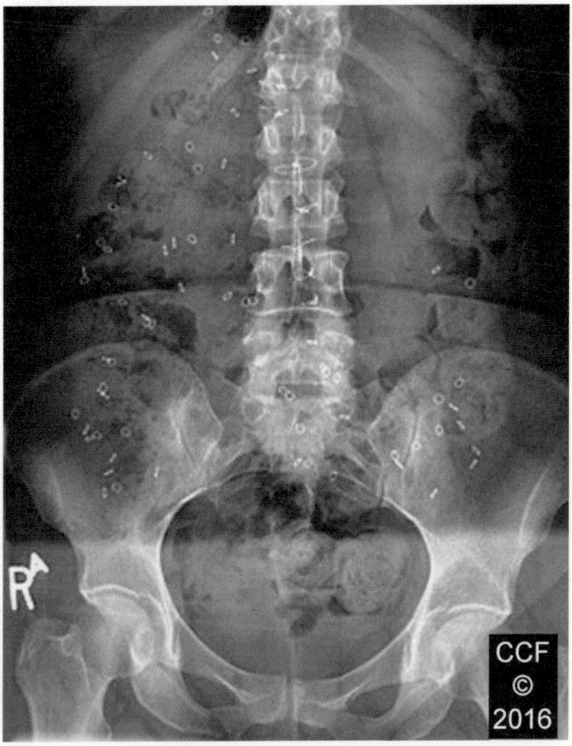

Fig. 126.1 This representative abdominal plain film shows SITZMARKS® rings distributed around the colon

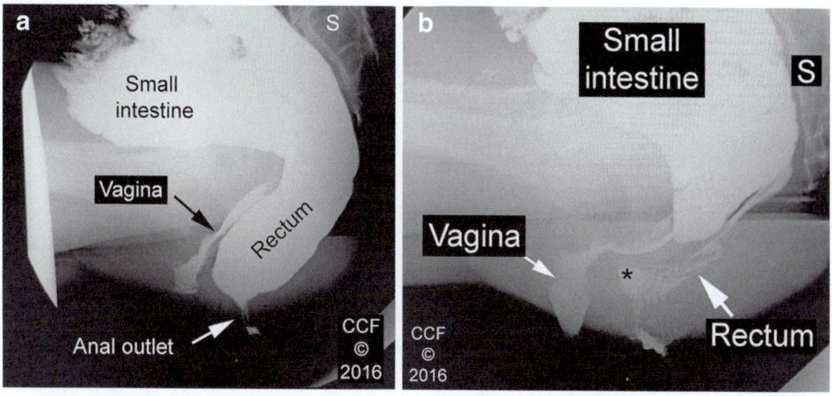

Fig. 126.2 (**a**) Contrast is seen in the rectum, vagina, and small intestine; S identifies the sacrum (**b**) postevacuation spot film showed complete rectal emptying. A small rectocele is seen (asterisk)

Operation

Total abdominal colectomy (Fig. 126.3a, b) with ileorectal anastomosis (IRA) (Fig. 126.4) was done.

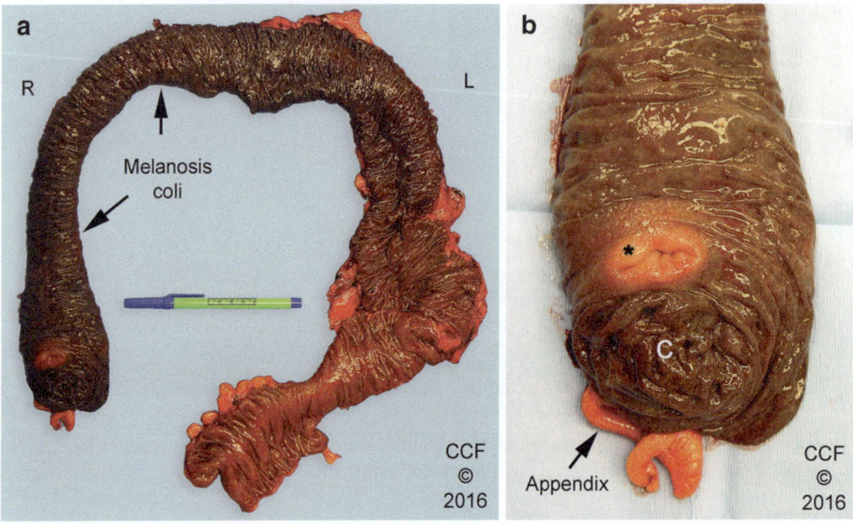

Fig. 126.3 (**a**) Abdominal colectomy specimen shows melanosis coli, a consequence of anthraquinone cathartic use; (**b**) the ileocecal valve (asterisk), appears normal. The cecum (letter C) and appendix are labeled

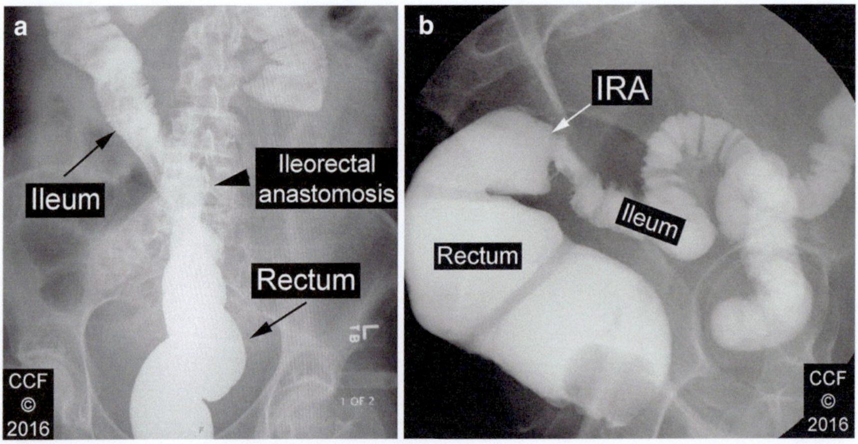

Fig. 126.4 (**a**) Ileorectal anastomosis IRA, anterior–posterior view; (**b**) IRA lateral view. The rectum and ileum are labelled in both radiographs

Comment

In 2013, the American Gastroenterological Association defined chronic constipation:[1]

> "Constipation is a syndrome that is defined by bowel symptoms (difficult or infrequent passage of stool, hardness of stool, or a feeling of incomplete evacuation) that may occur either in isolation or secondary to another underlying disorder…."
>
> Adil E. Bharucha, John H. Pembrerton,
> and G. Richard Locke III
> Division of Gastroenterology and Hepatology
> Division of Colon and Rectal Surgery
> Mayo Clinic
> Rochester, Minnesota.

Most patients can be treated medically. However, a small group of patients benefit from surgery.

In his landmark paper from 1913, Lane defined chronic intestinal stasis:

> "By chronic intestinal stasis I mean that the passage of the contents of the intestinal canal is delayed sufficiently long to result in the production, in the small intestine especially, of an excess of toxic material, and in the absorption into the circulation of a greater quantity of poisonous products than the organs which convert and excrete them are able to deal with." [5].
>
> Chronic Intestinal Stasis
> By Sir W. Arbuthnot Lane, Bart., M.S., F.R.C.S,
> Senior Surgeon, Guy's Hospital, London

In his remarks on chronic intestinal stasis, Bainbridge described his investigation of patients operated on by Sir Arbuthnot Lane. Removal of the colon was done in 52 cases [6]. McCoy and Beck define colonic inertia "as the inability of the colon to modify stool to an acceptable consistency and move the stool from the cecum to the rectosigmoid area at least once every three days" [7]. Selection of patients who will benefit from surgery is done based on history, physical examination, laboratory tests, anatomic assessment of the colon, transit study, assessment of anorectal function, and medical fitness for surgery. Total abdominal colectomy with ileorectal anastomosis has been used for patients with colonic inertia without rectal emptying problems [8–10].

[1]Bharucha [4]. This excerpt is reused with the generous permission of Elsevier, Inc. CCC |RightsLink® License Number 5156501358606, License Date Sep 26, 2021.

References

1. How to interpret a SITZMARKS® test https://www.sitzmarks.com. Accessed 1 Nov 2016.
2. Kim AY. How to interpret a functional or motility test-defecography. J Neurogastroenterol Motil. 2011;17:416–20.
3. Kim J-H. How to interpret conventional anorectal manometry. J Neurogastroenterol Motil. 2010;16:437–9.
4. Bharucha AE, Pemberton JH, Locke GR III. American Gastroenterological Association technical review on constipation. Gastroenterology. 2013;144:218–38.
5. Lane WA. Chronic intestinal stasis. Br Med J. 1913;2:1125–8.
6. Bainbridge S. Remarks on chronic intestinal stasis. Br Med J. 1913;2:1129–30.
7. McCoy JA, Beck DE. Surgical management of colonic inertia. Clin Colon Rectal Surg. 2012;25:20–3.
8. Beck DE, Jagelman DG, Fazio VW. The surgery of idiopathic constipation. Gastroenterol Clin N Am. 1987;16:143–56.
9. Pilarsky AJ, Singh JJ, Weiss EG, Noguerus JJ, Wexner SD. Long-term follow-up of patients undergoing colectomy for colonic inertia. Dis Colon Rectum. 2001;44:179–83.
10. Hassan I, Pemberton JH, Young-Fadok TM, You YN, Drelichman ER, Rath-Harvey D, Schleck CD, Larson DR. Ileorectal anastomosis for slow transit constipation: Long-term functional and quality of life results. J Gastrointest Surg. 2006;10:1330–7.

Hemorrhagic Colonic Lipoma

127

James S. Wu, Catherine L. Forse, and Arthur A. Parsee

Presentation

A 65-year-old patient underwent colonoscopy because of lower GI bleeding. An ulcerated lobulated mass occupying two thirds of the lumen at the hepatic flexure was seen. Computed tomography showed a polypoid lesion at the hepatic flexure (Fig. 127.1). Extended right hemicolectomy was done (Fig. 127.2). The opened specimen is shown in Fig. 127.3.

Histopathology showed submucosal lipoma (Fig. 127.4a, b).

J. S. Wu (✉)
Department of Colon and Rectal Surgery, Cleveland Clinic, Cleveland, OH, USA

C. L. Forse
Department of Pathology and Laboratory Medicine, Faculty of Medicine, University of Ottawa, Ottawa, ON, Canada

A. A. Parsee
Department of Diagnostic Radiology, H. Lee Moffitt Cancer Center and Research Institute, Tampa, FL, USA

J. S. Wu, M. D. Inkster (eds.), *Cleveland Clinic Colorectal Case Studies*,
https://doi.org/10.1007/978-3-031-39880-3_127

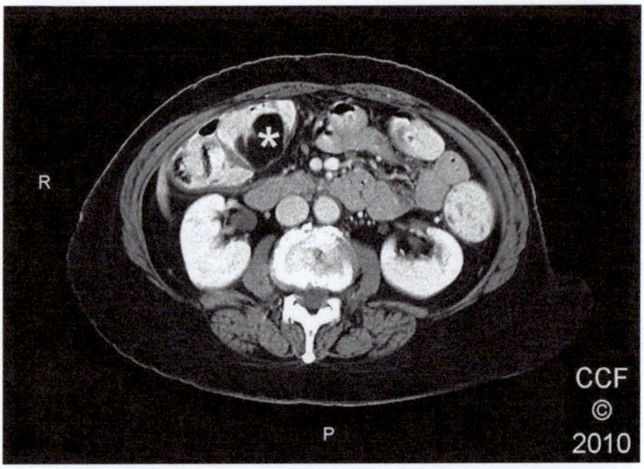

Fig. 127.1 Computed tomography, axial view shows a mass in the hepatic flexure (asterisk) with fat attenuation

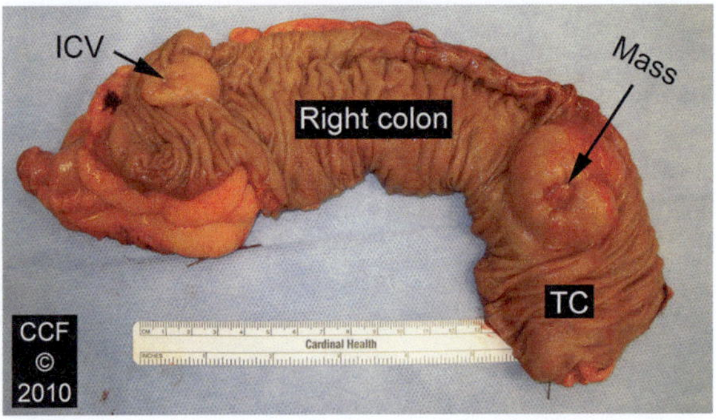

Fig. 127.2 Extended right hemicolectomy specimen showing a mass with a central ulceration, the source of bleeding. The ileocecal valve (ICV) is labeled as a point of reference

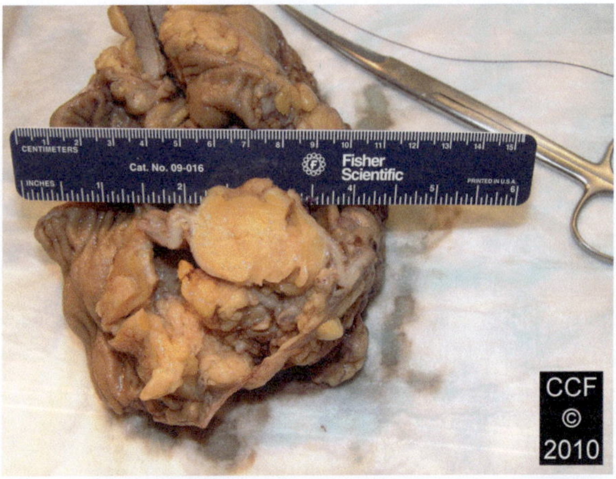

Fig. 127.3 The opened mass showed fat

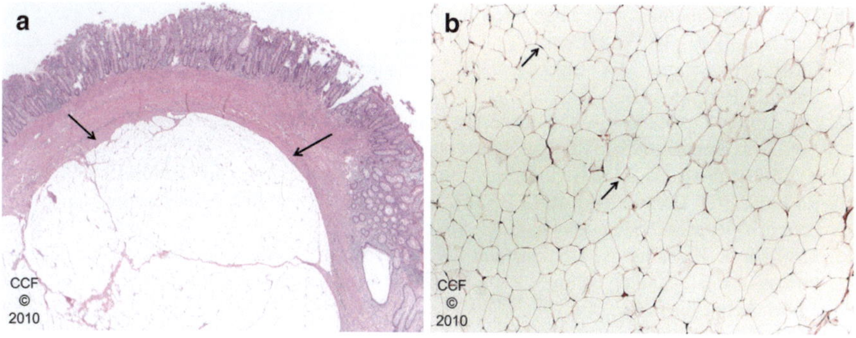

Fig. 127.4 (**a**) Submucosal lipoma in a colon resection. Note the well-circumscribed lobulated architecture of the adipose tissue (black arrows). H&E, 20× magnification; (**b**) submucosal lipoma. Note the equal size and shape of the adipocytes and their small eccentric nuclei (black arrows). H&E, 200× magnification

Comment

Lipomas are nonepithelial benign fatty tumors that are found throughout the gastrointestinal tract, most frequently in the colon [1, 2]. Most are submucosal and found incidentally. Most are asymptomatic and are left untreated. Colonic lipomas have minimal malignant potential [3]. Complications of colonic lipomas include hemorrhage, obstruction, and intussusception [4, 5]. Massive hemorrhage from colonic lipomas, although rare, can lead to life-threatening blood loss [6–11]. Massive hemorrhage from the hepatic flexure colon lipoma described in this case was treated by extended right hemicolectomy with ileocolic anastomosis. Recovery was uneventful.

References

1. Lipomas of the colon. El Salvador Atlas of Gastrointestinal Video Endoscopy. Gastrointestinalatlas.com. Accessed 15 Sep 2019.
2. Nallamothu G, Adler DG. Review. Large colonic Lipomas. Gastroenterol Hepatol. 2011;7:490–2.
3. Kouritas VK, Baloyiannis I, Koukoulis G, Mamaloudis I, Zacharoulis D, Efthimiou M. Spontaneous expulsion from rectum: a rare presentation of intestinal lipomas. World J Emerg Surg. 2011;6:19.
4. Boyce S, Khor YP. A colonic submucosal lipoma presenting with recurrent intestinal obstruction attacks. BMJ Case Rep. 2009;2009:bcr1120081199. https://doi.org/10.1136/bcr.11.2008.1199.
5. Eglinton T, Bagshaw P, Bayliss S. Colo-colonic intussusception secondary to a colonic lipoma diagnosed with preoperative CT scan. NZ Med J. 2005;118 No 1214. http://www.nzma.org.nz/journal/118-1214/1442/

6. D'Javid IF. Lipomas of the large intestine: Review of the literature and report of a case. J Int Coll Surg. 1960;33:639–68.
7. Castro EB, Stearns MW. Lipoma of the large intestine: A review of 45 cases. Dis Colon Rectum. 1972;15:441–4.
8. Hovelius L. Lipomatosis of the ileocecal valve: An uncommon cause of melena. Case Report. Acta Chir Scand. 1973;139:673–6.
9. Key JC, Roberts JW. Massive bleeding from colonic lipoma. Arch Surg. 1980;115:889–90.
10. Rodriquez DI, Drehner DM, Beck DE, McCauley CE. Colonic lipoma as a source of massive hemorrhage: report of a case. Dis Colon Rectum. 1990;33:977–9.
11. Vasiliadis K, Katsamakas M, Nikolaidou A, Christoforidis E, Tsalis K, Tsalikidis A. Submucosal lipoma of the ascending colon as a source of massive lower gastro-intestinal bleeding: a case report. Acta Chir Belg. 2008;108:356–9.

Colonic Giant Venous Malformation

128

Michelle D. Inkster, Eric W. Willis, and James S. Wu

Presentation

A large vascular lesion was found on screening colonoscopy in an asymptomatic 51-year-old female without risk factors for colorectal cancer (Fig. 128.1). Biopsies were not taken. Computed tomography showed a right-sided mass (Fig. 128.2). Right hemicolectomy was done. The pathologic diagnosis was giant venous malformation (Fig. 128.3a, b).

M. D. Inkster
Department of Gastroenterology, Cleveland Clinic, Cleveland, OH, USA

E. W. Willis
Department of Pathology, CORPath, Columbus, OH, USA

J. S. Wu (✉)
Department of Colon and Rectal Surgery, Cleveland Clinic, Cleveland, OH, USA

J. S. Wu, M. D. Inkster (eds.), *Cleveland Clinic Colorectal Case Studies*,
https://doi.org/10.1007/978-3-031-39880-3_128

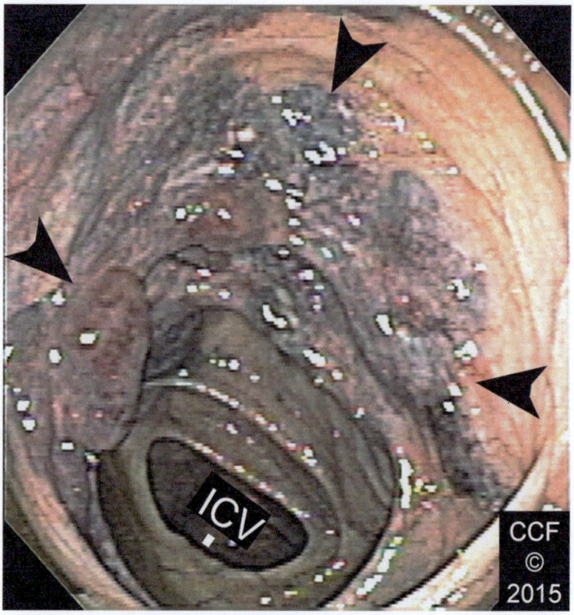

Fig. 128.1 A two-thirds circumference vascular lesion (arrow heads) was found on screening colonoscopy in the right colon. Its proximity to the ileocecal (ICV) valve is seen

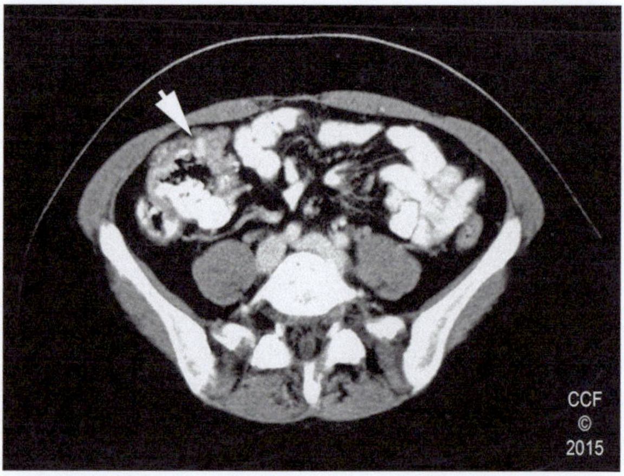

Fig. 128.2 Computed tomography shows a right colon mass (arrow)

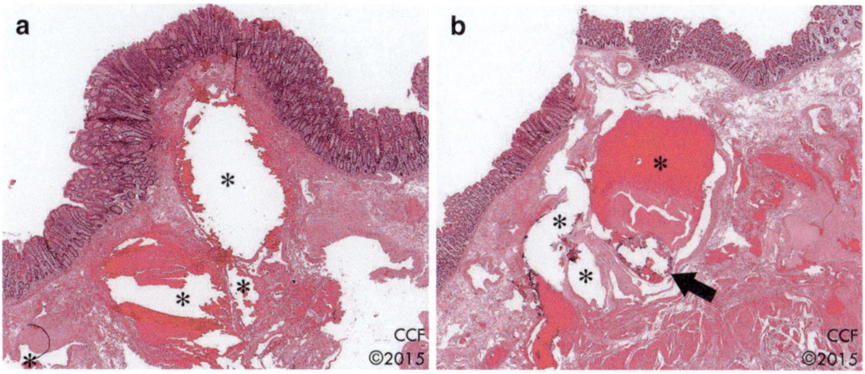

Fig. 128.3 (**a**) Clusters of large, cavernous vascular channels (asterisks) in the submucosa (original magnification, H&E, 20×); (**b**) occasional calcified, organizing thrombi (arrow) are present in the ectatic vessels (asterisks) original magnification H&E, 15×

Comment

In 1960, Margulis et al. [1] described two cases where operative mesenteric arteriography demonstrated the site of colonic bleeding. One case involved "multiple vascular malformations in the cecum." In 1974, a case was presented to Dr. Margulis at the Weekly Clinicopathological Exercises at the Massachusetts General Hospital [2]. Dr. Alexander R. Margulis's diagnosis was "arteriovenous malformation of ascending colon." Dr. James J. Galdabini in his discussion of the case used the term "angiodysplasia" (AD) in place of "vascular malformation" to avoid the connotation of a congenital origin. ADs may be asymptomatic but can be a cause of gastrointestinal bleeding. In a review of gastrointestinal angiodysplasia, Sami et al. [3] reported that most AD lesions are detected in the cecum and ascending colon. In this case, the vascular lesion was detected by colonoscopy and computed tomography [4].

References

1. Margulis AR, Heinbecker P, Bernard HR. Operative mesenteric arteriography in the search for the site of bleeding in unexplained gastrointestinal hemorrhage: a preliminary report. Surgery. 1960;48:534–9.
2. Case Records of the Massachusetts General Hospital. Case 36-1974. New Engl J Med. 1974;291:569–75.
3. Sami SS, Al-Araji SA, Ragunath K. Review article: gastrointestinal angiodysplasia — pathogenesis, diagnosis and management. Aliment Pharmacol Ther. 2014;39:15–34.
4. Yoo S. GI-associated hemangiomas and vascular malformations. Clin Colon Rectal Surg. 2011;24:193–200.

Gastrointestinal Bleeding and Aortic Stenosis (Heyde's Syndrome)

129

Michelle D. Inkster and James S. Wu

Presentation

A 69-year-old female with severe aortic stenosis was admitted to the hospital after having syncopal events and gastrointestinal bleeding. Upper endoscopy and colonoscopy were uninformative. Small bowel capsule enteroscopy showed an arteriovenous malformation (AVM) in the proximal jejunum. Subsequent push enteroscopy showed the lesions (Fig. 129.1). These were ablated endoscopically with argon plasma coagulation (APC).

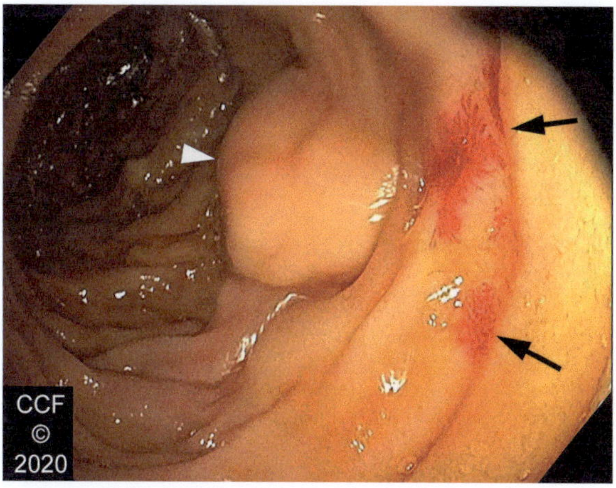

Fig. 129.1 Push enteroscopy showed jejunal vascular lesions (black arrows) that were ablated. The raised area is consistent with a lipoma (white arrowhead)

M. D. Inkster
Department of Gastroenterology, Cleveland Clinic, Cleveland, OH, USA

J. S. Wu (✉)
Department of Colon and Rectal Surgery, Cleveland Clinic, Cleveland, OH, USA

J. S. Wu, M. D. Inkster (eds.), *Cleveland Clinic Colorectal Case Studies*,
https://doi.org/10.1007/978-3-031-39880-3_129

Comment

In 1958, Heyde, a practitioner at the Vancouver Clinic in Washington State, in a one paragraph letter to the editor of the *New England Journal of Medicine* noted that patients with aortic stenosis developed gastrointestinal lesions that can bleed [1]. In 2012, Gupta et al. reported that acquired von Willebrand's disease is associated with gastrointestinal angiodysplasia [2]. In a subsequent 2012 article concerning Heyde's syndrome, Loscalzo related that Heyde's observation was the spark that lead to the identification of the mechanism of bleeding, namely, fragmentation of high-molecular-weight multimers of von Willebrand factor resulting in acquired von Willebrand's disease [3].

References

1. Heyde EC. Gastrointestinal bleeding in aortic stenosis. New Eng J Med. 1958;259:196.
2. Gupta PJ, Kannan M, Chatterjee T, Dixit A, Mahapatra M, Choudhry VP, et al. Acquired von Willebrand's disease associated with gastrointestinal angiodysplasia: a case report. Haemophilia 2006;12:452–5.
3. Loscalzo J. From clinical observation to mechanism — Heyde's syndrome. New Eng J Med. 2012;367:1954–6.

Hereditary Hemorrhagic Telangiectasia (Osler-Weber-Rendu Disease)

130

Michelle D. Inkster, Gregory Zuccaro, Jr., and James S. Wu

Presentation

A 34-year-old female with hereditary hemorrhagic telangiectasia (Osler-Weber-Rendu disease) presented on multiple occasions with gastrointestinal bleeding. Examination of the skin and mucous membranes revealed numerous telangiectasias. The condition was inherited from the maternal side of her family. Endoscopy revealed multiple telangiectasias (Fig. 130.1) that were ablated as they were found.

M. D. Inkster · G. Zuccaro, Jr.
Department of Gastroenterology, Cleveland Clinic, Cleveland, OH, USA

J. S. Wu (✉)
Department of Colon and Rectal Surgery, Cleveland Clinic, Cleveland, OH, USA

J. S. Wu, M. D. Inkster (eds.), *Cleveland Clinic Colorectal Case Studies*,
https://doi.org/10.1007/978-3-031-39880-3_130

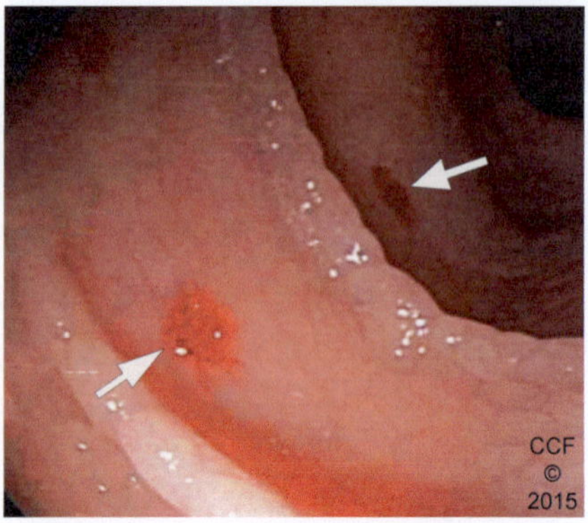

Fig. 130.1 Duodenal telangiectasias (arrows) seen on esophagogastroduodenoscopy

Comment

In 1865, Babington [1] described hereditary epistaxis.

Hereditary Epistaxis

To the Editor of The Lancet

"SIR,—The following history of an hereditary tendency to epistaxis, you may, perhaps, deem sufficiently remarkable to merit insertion in The Lancet:—.

Mrs. L—, a native of Lincolnshire, was, during all her early life and up to the period of her marriage, the subject of frequent and violent epistaxis. She had four children, two of whom (a male and a female) likewise had habitual and severe epistaxis. The male, Mr. L.—, died of this disease; the female, Mrs. C.—, had six female children, of whom three, suffered from epistaxis during all the earlier period of their lives. One of them, who is my informant, Mrs. K.—, has six children; two of them (females) have habitual and very severe epistaxis. The elder has a son now about nineteen years of age, who has had frequent and very severe epistaxis. The younger is not married, and has always been subject to violent epistaxis; her age is twenty-eight. One of Mrs. K—'s sisters, Mrs. C—, mentioned above as one of the three daughters who suffered from epistaxis, has two sons, both subject to violent epistaxis. One is married and has children; and one of them, a boy about six years old, has epistaxis. Mrs. K—'s other sister, Mrs. B, now dead, but not through her hereditary disease, had one daughter, who suffered from violent epistaxis, and is dead. Thus epistaxis, violent and habitual, has been observed in five consecutive generations, and for the last three generations in two branches. I have myself at different times attended Mrs. K—, her two daughters, and her grandson, and in all the haemorrhage was on more than occasion so violent as to necessitate the operation of plugging; and in the cases of the daughters and grandson to give rise to the apprehension of a fatal result."

I am, Sir, yours very truly,

B. G. Babington, M.D.

In 1896, Rendu [2] described repeated epistaxis and angiomas of the skin and mucous membranes.

Epistaxis répétées chez un sujet porteur de petitis angiomes cutanés et muqueux Par M. Rendu Agrégé, médecin de l'hôpital Necker Le symptôme prédominant actuellement est la disposition quotidienne que présente le malade à saigner du nez. Depuis trois semaines, les épistaxis se succèdent tous les jours, et souvent plusieurs fois par jour. Il existe sur la peau du nez, des joues, de la lèvre supérieure et du menton de petites taches pourprées, grandes comme une tête d'épingle, les plus grosses atteignant les dimensions d'une lentille, et qui sont de véritables angiomes cutanés, produit par une dilatation de vaisseaux superficiels de la peau.	Repeat epistaxis in a subject who had small cutaneous and mucous angiomas By Mr. Rendu Professor of Medicine, Necker Hospital The patient's main symptom actually was daily nose bleeding. For 3 weeks, the epistaxis occurred every day, sometimes several times a day. On the skin of the nose, cheeks, upper lip and chin, there are small purplish spots, as large as the head of a pin, the largest with dimensions of a lentil, which are true cutaneous angiomas, products of dilation of the superficial vessels of the skin.

In 1901, Ostler [3] described a family form of recurring epistaxis, associated with multiple telangiectasias of the skin and mucous membranes.

> "The association here described is rare, as, after a careful search through the literature, I can find but one reference to a similar case.
>
> An hereditary form of epistaxis has been well described by Babbington.
>
> In the three cases here described, two belonged to a family in which epistaxis had occurred in seven members. Both of my patients had had bleeding at the nose from childhood, and both presented numerous punctiform angiomata on the skin of the face and of the mucous membrane of the nose, lips, cheeks and tongue."
>
> William Osler, M.D.
> Professor of Medicine
> Johns Hopkins University

In 1907, Weber [4] described *Multiple hereditary developmental angiomata (telanfiectases) of the skin and mucous membranes associated with recurring hemorrhages*. Concerning the familial nature of the condition, he wrote:

> "The study of families affected with multiple angiomata of the skin and mucous membranes might help to throw light on the general subject of pathological inheritance in man."
>
> F. Parkes Weber, M.D. Cantab., F.R.C.P Lond.

Hereditary hemorrhagic telangiectasia (HHT) also known as Osler-Weber-Rendu disease (OWRD) is now recognized as an autosomal dominant condition that is associated with vascular abnormalities of mutiple organs (skin, mucous membranes, lung, liver, and brain) [5, 6].

References

1. Babington BG. Hereditary epistaxis. Lancet. 1865;86(2195):362–3.
2. Rendu H. Epistaxis répétées chez un sujet porteur de petitis angiomes cutanés et muqueux. Bull Mem Soc Méd (Paris). 1896:13:731–3.

3. Osler W. On a family form of recurring epistaxis, associated with multiple telangiectases of the skin and mucous membranes. Bull Johns Hopkins Hosp. 1901;12:333–7.
4. Weber FP. Multiple hereditary developmental angiomata (telangiectases) of the skin and mucous membranes associated with recurring hæmorrhages. Lancet. 1907;170(4377):160–2.
5. Abdalla SA, Letarte M. Hereditary Haemorrhagic telangiectasia: current views on genetics and mechanism of disease. J Med Genet. 2006;43:97–110.
6. Jackson SB, Villlano NP, Benhammou JN, Lewis M, Pisegna JR, Padua D. Gastrointestinal manifestations of hereditary hemorrhagic telangiectasia (HHT): A systematic review of the literature. Dig Dis Sci. 2017;62:2623–30.

Colonic Sessile Serrated Lesion

131

Michelle D. Inkster, David Hernandez Gonzalo,
Eric W. Willis, and James S. Wu

Presentation

A 61-year-old female underwent screening colonoscopy with polypectomy (Fig. 131.1). Pathology showed luminal serrations (Fig. 131.2).

M. D. Inkster
Department of Gastroenterology, Cleveland Clinic, Cleveland, OH, USA

D. Hernandez Gonzalo
Department of Pathology, Immunology and Laboratory Medicine, University of Florida, Gainesville, FL, USA

E. W. Willis
Department of Pathology, CORPath, Columbus, OH, USA

J. S. Wu (✉)
Department of Colon and Rectal Surgery, Cleveland Clinic, Cleveland, OH, USA

J. S. Wu, M. D. Inkster (eds.), *Cleveland Clinic Colorectal Case Studies*,
https://doi.org/10.1007/978-3-031-39880-3_131

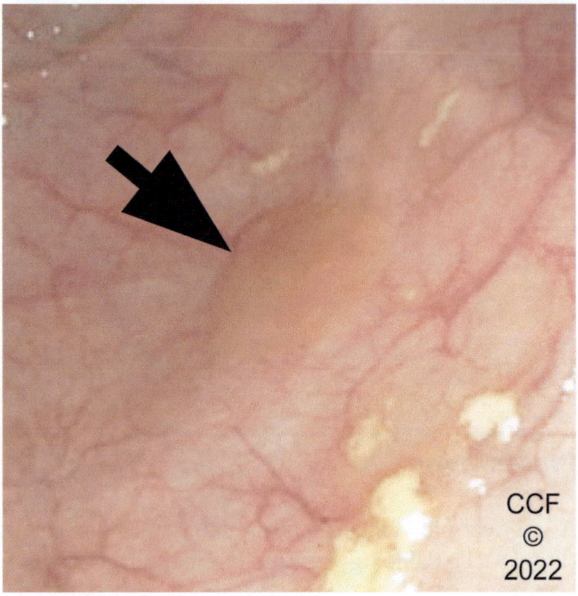

Fig. 131.1 A sessile colon lesion was removed at colonoscopy. The polyp was small (about 2 mm) and difficult to see. It shows vascular pattern loss

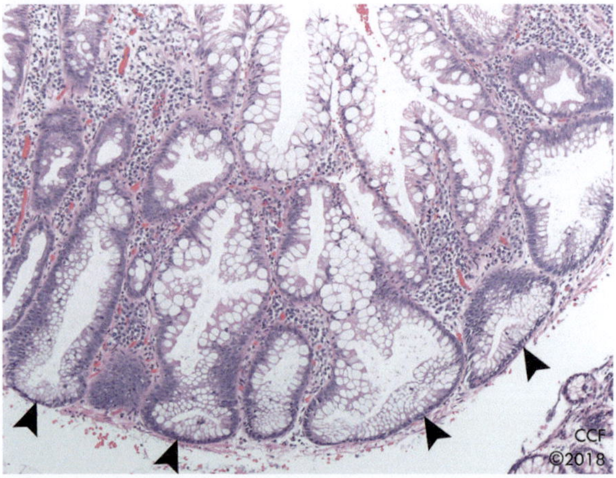

Fig. 131.2 Sections show colonic mucosa with proliferative crypts which are lined by cells with basally located nuclei and abundant cytoplasmic mucin. There are pronounced luminal serrations and lateral branching at the base of the crypts (arrowheads). The histologic changes are most consistent with a colonic sessile serrated lesion (SSL)

Comment

Additional histopathologic examples of colonic SSLs are shown in Figs. 131.3 and 131.4.

The term "metaplastic polyposis" was introduced by Williams et al. [1] in 1980 to describe the endoscopic or gross appearance of polyposis coli but in which the polyps appeared to be metaplastic.

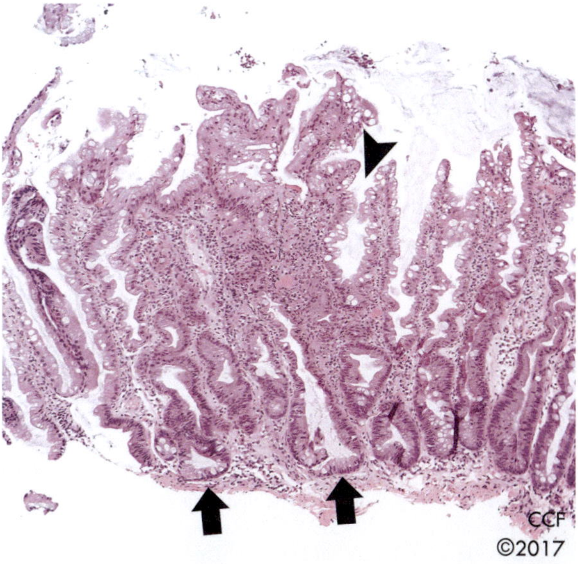

Fig. 131.3 The biopsy demonstrates serrated epithelium (arrowhead) with dilation and branching of the crypt bases (arrows)

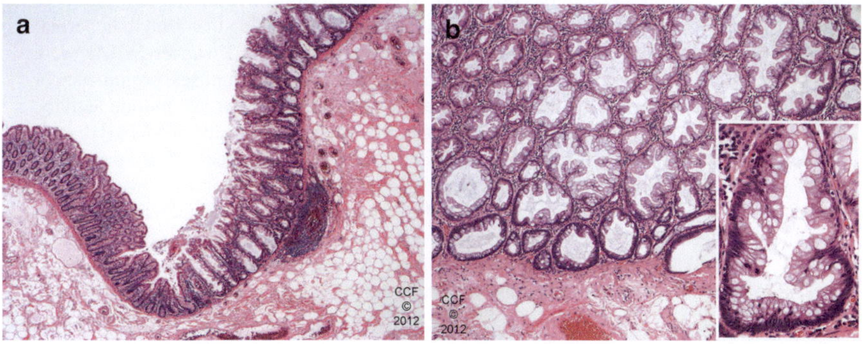

Fig. 131.4 (**a**) Low-power view of SSL (right) in contrast to normal colon (left). Note the serrated appearance of the lesion throughout the entire thickness of the epithelium (hematoxylin–eosin, original magnification ×50); (**b**) High-power view of SSL demonstrating basal dilation of the crypts, basal crypt serration, and crypts horizontal to the basement membrane. Inset showing "L or boot"-shaped gland at the base (hematoxylin–eosin, original magnification ×200, hematoxylin–eosin, original magnification ×400 [inset])

> "Five hundred and fifty-four colorectal metaplastic polyps have been studied histologically. A structural similarity between the larger metaplastic polyps and colorectal adenomas is illustrated and the importance of the distinction of metaplastic from dysplastic epithelium in the differentiation of these lesions is stressed. ...The possibility that 'metaplastic polyposis' is a pathologic entity is discussed."

In 1984, Urbanski et al. [2] reported a case of adenocarcinoma arising within a mixed hyperplastic adenomatous polyp. Recognition of a subset of hyperplastic polyps as a distinct form of colorectal neoplasia was reported by Longacre and Fenoglio-Preiser in 1990.[1]

Mixed Hyperplastic Adenomatous Polyps/Serrated Adenomas
A Distinct Form of Colorectal Neoplasia
Teri A. Longacre, M.D., and Cecelia M. Fenoglio-Preiser, M.D.
From the VA Medical Center, Albuquerque,
and the Department of Pathology,
University of New Mexico School of Medicine,
Albuquerque, New Mexico

"We present the clinicopathologic characteristics of 110 colorectal mixed hyperplastic adenomatous polyps (MHAP) that exhibited the architectural but not the cytologic features of a hyperplastic polyp. They are compared with 60 traditional adenomas, 40 hyperplastic polyps, and five colonic polyps that contained admixed but well-defined hyperplastic and adenomatous glands (HP/AD). The patients with MHAP ranged in age from 15 to 88 years (mean, 63 years). Five patients had two or more (up to seven) lesions. MHAP measured 0.2-7.5 cm in diameter. They were distributed throughout the colorectum, but a slight preponderance of large lesions (more than 1.0 cm) occurred in the cecum and appendix. All MHAP were characterized by a serrated glandular pattern simulating that seen in hyperplasia (27% of MHAP were initially diagnosed as hyperplastic polyps). However, MHAP were distinguished by the presence of goblet cell immaturity, upper zone mitoses, prominence of nucleoli, and the absence of a thickened collagen table. Although surface mitotic activity, nuclear pseudostratification, and nuclear cytoplasmic ratio were greater in MHAP than in hyperplastic polyps, they were slightly less than in traditional adenomas. Thirty-seven percent of MHAP contained foci of significant dysplasia; 11% contained areas of intramucosal carcinoma. We conclude that these lesions reflect a morphologically unique variant of adenoma and suggest that they be termed "serrated adenoma" in order to emphasize their neoplastic nature. We further offer the hypothesis that MHAP may arise from the neoplastic transformation of a more differentiated cell in the crypt than the traditional adenoma."

Features of SSLs include those listed on Table 131.1 [4–6]. They are precursors to colorectal cancer. They occur commonly in the right side of the colon. They progress to cancer by a pathway that is distinct from the adenoma sequence. Associated

Table 131.1 Features of colonic sessile serrated lesions

Precursors of colorectal cancers
More common in the right colon but can occur distally
Pathway to cancer that is distinct from the adenoma to carcinoma sequence
Genetic changes associated with development of dysplasia and progression to cancer: *BRAF* mutation
Serrated histologic appearance
May be more difficult to detect endoscopically than adenomas. Narrow band imaging (NBI) facilitates their detection during endoscopy

[1]Longacre and Fenoglio-Preiser [3]. This abstract is reused with the generous permission of Wolters Kluwer Health, Inc., CCC|RightsLink®, License Number 5171721103196, License date Oct 18, 2021.

genetic changes occur in the *BRAF* gene. They have a distinct histologic appearance. They may be more difficult to detect endoscopically.

References

1. Williams GT, Arthur JF, Bussey HJR, Morson BC. Metaplastic polyps and polyposis of the colorectum. Histopathology 1980;4:155–70. Permission to reuse this excerpt was generously granted by John Willey and Sons, CCC|RightsLink, License Number 5901910090206, License date Nov 04, 2024.
2. Urbanski SJ, Kossakowska AE, Marcon N, Bruce WR. Mixed hyperplastic adenomatous polyps—an underdiagnosed entity. Report of a case of adenocarcinoma arising within a mixed hyperplastic adenomatous polyp. Am J Surg Pathol. 1984;8:551–6.
3. Longacre TA, Fenoglio-Preiser CM. Mixed hyperplastic adenomatous polyps/serrated adenomas. A distinct form of colorectal neoplasia. Am J Surg Pathol. 1990;14:524–37.
4. Rex DK, Ahnen DJ, Baron JA, Batts KP, Burke CA, Burt RW, et al. Serrated lesions of the colorectum: Review and recommendations from an expert panel. Am J Gastroenterol. 2012;107:1315–29.
5. Ashburn JH, Plesec TP, Kalady MF. Serrated polyps and serrated polyposis syndrome. Clin Colon Rectal Surg 2016;29:336–44.
6. Mesteri I, Bayer G, Meyer J, Capper D, Schoppmann SF, von Deimling A, et al. Improved molecular classification of serrated lesions of the colon by immunohistochemical detection of BRAF V600E. Mod Pathol 2014;27:135–44.

Mesenteric Mesothelioma

132

Michelle D. Inkster, Sricharan Chalikonda, Eric W. Willis, and James S. Wu

Presentation

An abdominal lymph node biopsy showed well-differentiated papillary mesothelioma. Histopathology is shown in Fig. 132.1.

M. D. Inkster
Department of Gastroenterology, Cleveland Clinic, Cleveland, OH, USA

S. Chalikonda
Department of Surgery Allegheny Health Network, Pittsburgh, PA, USA

E. W. Willis
Department of Pathology, CORPath, Columbus, OH, USA

J. S. Wu (✉)
Department of Colon and Rectal Surgery, Cleveland Clinic, Cleveland, OH, USA

J. S. Wu, M. D. Inkster (eds.), *Cleveland Clinic Colorectal Case Studies*,
https://doi.org/10.1007/978-3-031-39880-3_132

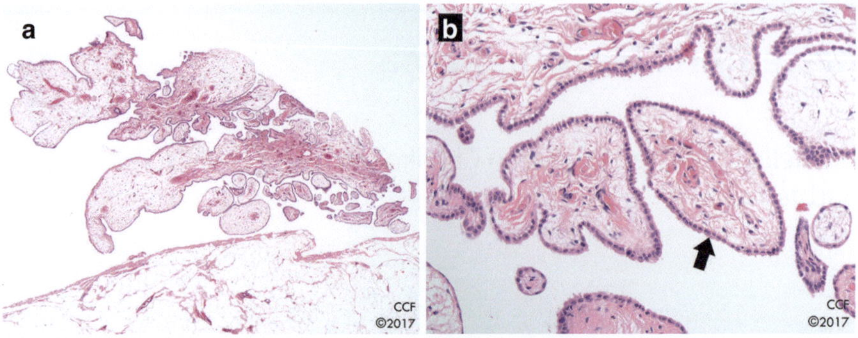

Fig. 132.1 (**a**) The low-power image shows finger-like papillary projections arising from the peritoneal surface; (**b**) The high-power image shows that the papillary proliferation is lined by a single layer of cuboidal mesothelial cells (arrow) with bland nuclei and eosinophilic cytoplasm. Features of malignant mesothelioma such as stromal invasion are absent

Management

Diagnostic laparoscopy was done for staging of this finding. No intra-abdominal evidence of malignancy was seen. The patient has been followed with computed tomographic scans since then without recurrence for 3 years.

Comment

Churg et al. [1] report on the entity formerly known as well-differentiated papillary mesothelioma (now referred to as well-differentiated papillary mesothelial tumor WDPMT), which shows differing mutations and behavior than malignant mesothelioma. It is characterized by papillary architecture with fibrovascular cores lined by cytologically bland cuboidal mesothelial cells. Mesothelioma in-situ can show morphologic overlap with WDPMT, and BAP1 staining can be helpful to differentiate the two.

Reference

1. Churg A, Galateau-Salle F. Well differentiated papillary mesothelial tumor: a new name and new problems. Mod Pathol. 2022;35:1327–33. https://doi.org/10.1038/s41379-022-01082-y.

Early Observations on Heredity

133

Michelle D. Inkster and James S. Wu

Presentation

In 1653, Dr. William Harvey, Physician to the Kings Majesty, published *The Anatomical Exercises Concerning the Motion of the Heart and Blood* [1]. In the preface to this work, Zachariah Wood, Physician of Rotterdam, wrote that fundamental to Harvey's method was that:

> "…*Harvey* did not trust other mens writings, but his own faithfull eyes, the truest reporters of Anatomy, because Anatomy is better gaind by ocular inspection than by long reading, and profound meditation.[1, 2]

Nehemiah Grew (1641–1712)

In 1672, Nehemiah Grew described the anatomy of seeds highlighting their central importance to vegetation [2].[3]

[1] The font used by Dr. Harvey's publisher was changed to a modern font. For example, the letter f in the word trueft was changed to s making the word truest.

[2] The font used by Dr. Wood's publisher was changed to a modern font. For example, the letter f in the word truft was changed to s making the word trust.

[3] The font used by Dr. Grew's publisher was changed to a modern font. For example, the letter f in the word fo was changed to s making the word so.

M. D. Inkster
Department of Gastroenterology, Cleveland Clinic, Cleveland, OH, USA

J. S. Wu (✉)
Department of Colon and Rectal Surgery, Cleveland Clinic, Cleveland, OH, USA

J. S. Wu, M. D. Inkster (eds.), *Cleveland Clinic Colorectal Case Studies*,
https://doi.org/10.1007/978-3-031-39880-3_133

The Anatomy of Vegetables
Nehemiah Grew, M.D.
Chap. VII
Of the Seed

"As the original, so the Ultimate end & Perfection of *Vegetation* is the *Seed*."

In 1682, Grew published, *The Anatomy of Plants with an Idea of a Philosophical History of Plants,* in which he likened the relationship between a seed matured within an apricot fruit to that between a fetus and the uterus [3].

"CHAP. VI.

Of the GENERATION of the SEED.

…so I shall take an *Aprecock*, as very apt and convenient, to observe and represent the *Method* which *Nature* taketh in its *Generation.*

2. In order to this, the first thing that is to be done, is to make a fit *Uterus*. Both to keep the *Membranes* of the *Foetus* warm, and succulent, till it be formed: and to preserve and secure the Foetus itself afterwards, till it comes to be born into the *Ground*."

Dr. Grew communicated this idea through a series of cross-sectional illustrations (TAB. LXXXI, Fig. 133.1).

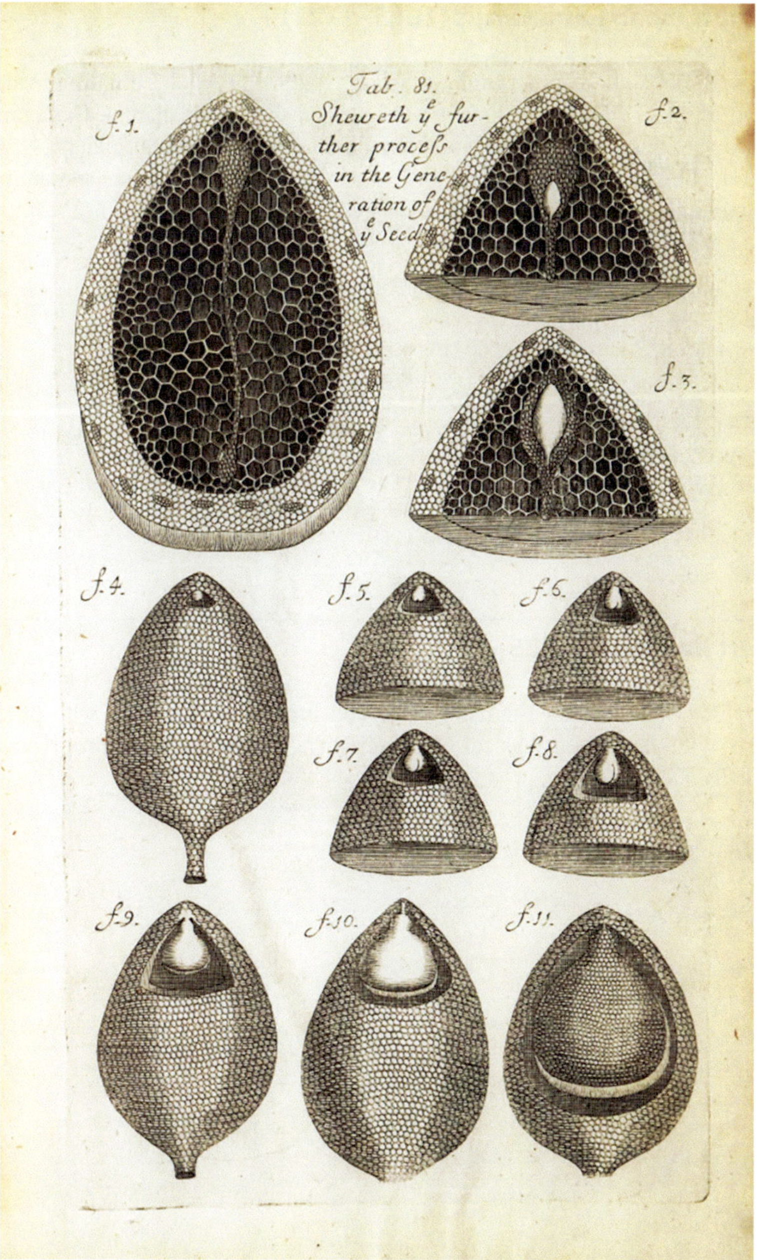

Fig. 133.1 (Grew's TAB. LXXXI. F.1) *The outer and midle coats or Membranes; with the Chanel, oval at both ends, now formed in the latter.* f. 2, *Part of the same, with the upper Oval grown larger, and the inmost Cover now also formed therein.* f. 3. *the same with the inmost cover grown larger.* f. 4. *the Inmost Cover more magnified, and the hollow in the smaller end, laid open, to shew the Seed itself, newly begun in a round Node.* f. 5. *the same; in which the Node begins to be divided into two Lobes.* f. 6,7, 8, *the gradual forming of the Lobes.* f. 9, *next the forming of the Radicle.* f. 10. 11, *Its gradual contraction at the point, into a short and slender Navle string. Which in the further growth of the Seed, breaks and disappears*

Rudolph Jacob Camerarius (1665–1721)

In 1694, Rudolf Jakob Camerarius published a letter to D. Mich Bernardum Valentini entitled *De Sexu Plantarum Epistola* (a letter on the sex of plants). Camerarius is credited with description of male and female reproductive parts of plants [4]. At the end of the epistle, Camerarius concludes that reproduction in plants and animals is the same. This idea is summarized in an Ode, one stanza of which is accompanied with a translation by Möbius.[4]

De Sexv Plantarvm Epistola Rudolphi Jacobi Camerarii, Professoris Tubingensis [5] Ode O mira plantis atque animalibus Quod vivit, & prolem propagat, Omne modo generator uno.	Ueber das Geschlecht der Planzen (De sexu plantarum epistola.) 1694. von R.J. Camerarius Uebersetzt und herausgegeben von M. Möbius (1899) [6] Ode Für Thier' und Pflanzen gleiche Geschlectlichkeit! Was lebt, was Nachkommen hervorbringt, Alles ensteht auf dieselbe Weise.

Robert Bakewell (1725–1795)

Robert Bakewell was an English farmer and breeder of livestock who produced animals with favorable physical characteristics. Youatt, in his *Library of useful knowledge* [7], published:

[4]An English translation might read:
"Oh, wonderful plants and animals
That which lives and propagates
All only generate in one way."

SHEEP:
Their Breeds, Management, and Diseases.

> "The cultivation of the sheep and the manufacture of the fleece have, from the earliest period of history, formed the most important branches of the agriculture and the commerce of Great Britain. Many years did not pass after the subjugation of our island by the Romans, ere the most valuable and expensive woollen robes, and worn on days of ceremony alone, were furnished by the British factories.
>
> No fewer than 32,000,000 of these useful animals graze on our pastures. Exclusive of the value of the carcase, that of the fleece alone cannot be less than seven millions of pounds sterling, employing nearly 350,000 individuals, and ultimately yielding manufactures to the amount of at least twenty-one millions of pounds annually.
>
> As a lowland sheep, and destined to live on good pasture, the New Leicester is without a rival—in fact he has improved, if he has not given the principal value to, all the other long-wooled sheep.
>
> This account combines the main excellencies of both Bakewell's own breed.... It is precisely the form for a sheep provided with plenty of good food and without any great distance to travel or exertion to make in gathering it." Fig. 133.2.

In an obituary, William Housman stated that Bakewell's operating principle was "Like will produce like [8]."

Imre Festetics (1764–1847)

Imre Festetics was a Moravian sheep breeder and geneticist. His contribution to genetics was summarized by Szabó and Poczai [9]. Festetics formulated four rules to distinguish heredity from nature that were published in *Oekonomische Neuigkeiten und Verhandlungen* (Economic News and Announcements) in 1819 [10, 11].

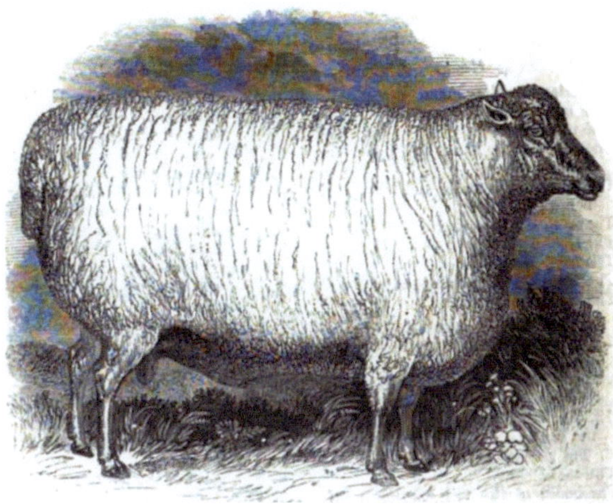

Fig. 133.2 The New Leicester sheep. Copied from Youatt. Sheep: their Breeds, Management, and Diseases, 1837, page 110. Accessed from Google Books, September 3, 2022

Weitere Erklärungen des Herrn Grafen Emmerich Festetics über Inzucht	Further clarification by count Emmerich von Festetics on inbreeding.
Diese 5 Paragraphen enthalten meiner Meinung nach, die genetischen Gesetze der Natur.	These 5 paragraphs contain my thoughts on the genetic laws of nature.
(a) Die Thiere von Gesundheit und robuster Constitution pflanzen, und vererben ihre charakteristichen Eigenschaften fort.	(a) Healthy and robust animals are able to propagate and pass on their specific characteristics;
(b) Eigenschaften der Voraltern, welche von den Eigenschaften ihrer Nachkommen unterschieden sind, kommen in folgenden Generationen wieder zum Vorschein.	(b) Traits of grandparents that are different from those of the immediate progeny may reappear in later generations;
(c) Von Thieren, welche durch viele Generationen die namlichen sich angeeignete Eigenschaften besessen haben, fallen mit unter Abkömmlinge, die abweichende Charactere haben. Diess sind Varietäten, Spiel der Natur, zur Fortpflanzung, wenn die Vererbung der Eigenschaften der Zweck ist, untauglich.	(c) Animals possessing desirable traits that have been inherited over many generations can sometimes have offspring with divergent traits. Such progeny are variants or freaks of nature and are unsuitable for further propagation if the aim is the heredity of specific traits.
(d) Bedingniss bleibt bei der Inzucht die scrupulöseste Auswahl der Stammthiere.	(d) A precondition for successful application of inbreeding is scrupulous selection of stock animals.

Szabó and Poczai credit Festetics with the introduction of the word *Genetics* (genetische Gesetze) the transmission of "charakteristichen Eigenschaften" (characteristic traits), and the possibility of "abweichende Charactere" (different characteristics).

Gregor Mendel (1822–1884)

In 1866, Mendel published his paper, *Versuche über Planzen-Hybriden (Experiments in Plant Hybridization)*, using various peas belonging to the species *Pisum sativum.*

Versuche über Pflanzen-Hybriden [12]
von
Gregor Mendel
(Vorgelegt in den Sitzungen vom 8. Februar und 8. März 1865.) Verhandlungen des naturforschenden Vereines in Brünn
Einleitende Bemerkungen

Künstliche Befruchtungen, welche an Zierpflanzen desshalb vorgenommen wurden, um neue Farben-Varianten zu erzielen, waren die Veranlassung zu den Versuchen, die her besprochen werden sollen. Die auffallende Regelmässigkeit, mit welcher dieselben Hybridformen immer wiederkehrten, so oft die Befruchtung zwischen gleichen Arten geschah, gab die Anregung zu weiteren Experimenten, deren Aufgabe es war, die Entwicklung der Hybriden in ihren Nachkommen zu verfolgen.

Schluss-Bemerkungen

Bei Pisum wurde es durch Versuche erwiesen, dass die Hybriden verschiedenartige Keim—und pollen-Zellen bilden, und dass hierin der Grund für die Veränderlichkeit ihrer Nachkommen liegt. Auch bei anderen Hybriden, deren Nachkommen sich ähnlich verhalten, dürfen wir eine gleiche Ursache voraussetzen; für jene hingegen, welche constant bleiben, scheint die Annahme zulässig, dass ihre Befruchtungszellen gleichartig sind und mit der Hybriden-Grundzelle ühereinstimmen

Experiments in plant hybridization [13]
By
Gregor Mendel
Read at the February 8th, and March 8th, 1865,
Meetings of the Brünn Natural History Society
Introductory remarks

Experience of artificial fertilization, such as is effected with ornamental plants in order to obtain new variations in color, has led to the experiments which will here be discussed. The striking regularity with which the same hybrid forms always reappeared whenever fertilization took place between the same species induced further experiments to be undertaken, the object of which was to follow up the developments of the hybrids in their progeny

Concluding Remarks

With *Pisum* it was shown by experiment that the hybrids form egg and pollen cells of *different kinds*, and that herein lies the reason of the variability of their offspring. In other hybrids, likewise, whose offspring behave similarly we may assume a like cause; for those, on the other hand, which remain constant the assumption appears justifiable that their reproductive cells are all alike and agree with the foundation–cell of the hybrid.

Pliny Earle II (1809–1892)

In 1845, Earle published an article on the inability to distinguish colors in which he diagnosed red/green color blindness, in part, based on his own family. Earle's maternal grandfather and two of his brothers had this condition. There were 17 descendants who, with one exception, were all male. In order to show the relationship between the disease, individual patients, and relatives over many generations, he used a pedigree chart (Fig. 133.3) [14] (e.g., see [15]). The squares and circles in his pedigree chart were black for those who cannot distinguish colors.

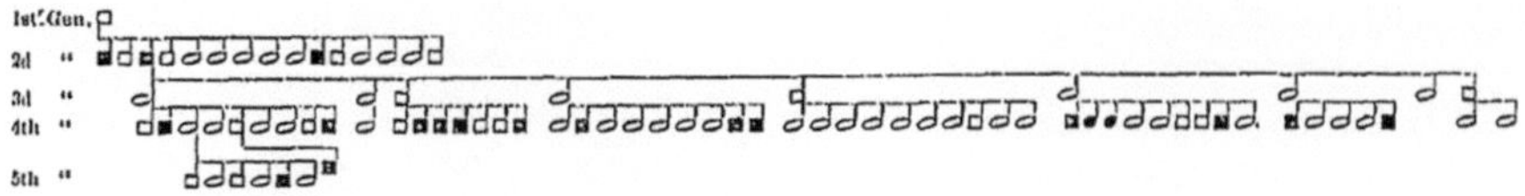

Fig. 133.3 Genealogical Chart of Pliny Earle's family covering five generations. Males are represented by squares and females by circles. For those who cannot distinguish colors, the squares or circles are wholly black

On the Inability to distinguish Colours.
By
Pliny Earle, M. D.,
Physician to Bloomingdale Asylum for the Insane
Peculiarities heretofore observed

"(a) The inability to distinguish colours is hereditary, and
(b) When thus entailed, it sometimes everleaps one generation or more.
(c) Males are more frequently affected than females.
(a) In several of the cases reported in foreign publications, the truth of this proposition is demonstrated; but in none of their families did the peculiarity prevail so extensively as in that of which the author of this article is a member. My maternal grandfather and two of his brothers were characterized by it, and among the descendants of the first mentioned, there are *seventeen* persons in whom it is found. I have not been able to extend my inquires among the collateral branches of the family, but have heard of one individual, a female, in one of them who was similarly affected.

For the purpose of clearly illustrating the prevalence of this physiological peculiarity in the family, I have prepared the subjoined genealogical chart. Males are represented by squares and females by circles. For those who cannot distinguish colours the squares or circles are wholly black.

The chart includes five generations. Nothing is known of the first generation, in regard to the power of perception in colours. In the second, of a family consisting of seven brothers and eight sisters, three of the brothers, one of whom, as before mentioned, was the grandfather of the writer, had the defect in question."

Charles Darwin (1809–1882)

In his *Introduction* to *On the Origin of Species*, published in 1859, Darwin wrote: [16]
On
The Origin of Species
By Means of Natural Selection,
Or the
Preservation of Favoured Races in the Struggle
For life.
By Charles Darwin, M.A.,
Fellow of the Royal, Geological, Linnæan, Etc., Societies

Introduction

> "In considering the Origin of Species, is quite conceivable that a naturalist, reflecting on the mutual affinities of organic beings, on their embryological relations, their geographical distribution, geological succession, and other such facts, might come to the conclusion that each species had not been independently created, but had descended, like varieties, from other species. Nevertheless, such a conclusion, even if well founded, would be unsatisfactory, until it could be shown how the innumerable species inhabiting this world have been modified, so as to acquire that perfection of structure and coadaptation which most justly excites our admiration."

Eduard Strasburger (1844–1912)

In 1878, Eduard Strasburger used the words gamete and zygote in his discussion of the copulation process of Acetabularia (a green algae) [17, 18].

Ueber Befruchtung und Zelltheilung von Dr. Eduard Strasburger Professor an der Universität Jena Die Copulationvergänge bei Acetabularia Diese Pflanze hatte ich Gelegenheit im verflossenen Herbst und Winter in la Spezia und in Nizza to beobachten. Die Resultate meiner Untersuchungen sollen demnächst in der botan. Zeitung publicirt werden, hier sei nur der Copulation zwischen den schwärmenden Gameten dieser Pflanze erwähnt. Die Gameten werden in Grösserer Anzahl aus dem Inhalte der Dauersporen erzeugt und copuliren nur dann, wenn sie verschiedenen Dauersporen enstammen. Die copulation erfolgt normaler Weise in der art, dass zwei Gameten mit ihren farblosen Enden auf einander stossen, dann aber sich rasch gegen einander umlegen und nun mit ihren Längsseiten in Berührung kommen. Bei jetz erfolgender Copulation verschmelzen die gleichwerthigen Theile beider Schwärmer mit einander. Die Cilieninsertionen liegen dann neben einander und längerer Zeit hindurch sieht man die Zygote noch mit ihren vier Cilien schwärmen. Endlich kommt sie zur Ruhe, die farblose Stelle wird eingezogen, die Cilien schwinden, eine Cellulosemembran wird auf der Oberfläche der Zygote kenntlich.	On Fertilization and Cell Division By Dr. Eduard Strasburger Professor, University of Jena The Copulation Process of Acetabularia I had the opportunity of observing this plant last autumn and winter in La Spezia and in Nice. The results of my investigations soon will be published in the Botanical Journal; here, only the copulation between the swarming gametes of these plants will be mentioned. The gametes are produced in larger numbers from the contents of the permanent spores and only copulate when when they arise from different permanent spores. When copulation normally occurs the two gametes meet at their colorless ends, but then quickly they fold and come into contact with each other along their long sides. When copulation occurs, the similar parts of the two swarmers fuse with each other. The cilia insertions then lie next to each other and for a long time the zygote can still be seen swarming with its four cilia. Finally, it comes to rest, the colorless area is retracted, the cilia disappear, a cellulose membrane becomes recognizable on the zygote.

Walther Flemming (1843–1905)

In 1882, Walther Flemming described cell division by mitosis staining dividing salamander cells; [19–21].

Zellsubstanz, Kern Und Zelltheilung von Walther Flemming Professor der Anatomie in Kiel	Cell Substance, Nucleus and Cell division By Walther Flemming Professor Anatomy, University of Kiel

An illustration from Flemming's work depicting cell division is shown in Fig. 133.4 (Fleming's Tafel VII).

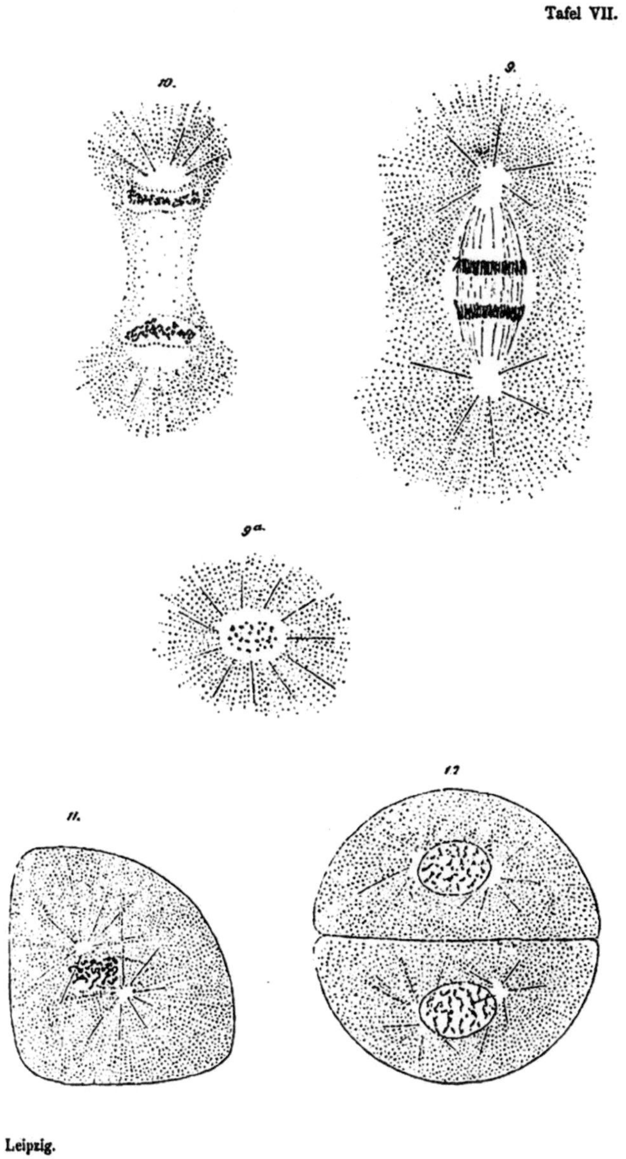

Fig. 133.4 (Fleming's Tafel VII)
(9) Trennung der chromatischen Figur ist erfolgt.
(9a) eine solche Tochtergruppe vom Pol aus gesehen.
(10) Der Knäuelform der Tochterkerne correspondirend.
(11) Zelle dritter Generation, schräg vom Pole gesehen, wieder in Theilung, Knäuelform.
(12) Die zwei ersten Tochterzellen, im Wieder Anfang der Theilung...

Flemings Board VII
(9) Separation of the chromatic figure is successful.
(9a) such a daughter group seen from the pole.
(10) Corresponding ball-shaped daughter nucleus
(11) Third generation cell, seen obliquely from the pole, again dividing.
(12) The first two daughter cells, beginning division again...

Hugo M. de Vries (1848–1935)

In 1889, Hugo de Vries, a Dutch botanist, published *Intracellulare Pangenesis* in which he states that individual hereditary traits are represented by *Theilchen* (particles).

Intracellulare Pangenesis [22] von Hugo de Vries Prof. der Botanik an der Universität von Amsterdam Für mich besteht **Darwin**'s provisorische Hypothese der Pangenesis aus den beiden folgenden Sätzen: 1. In jeder Keimzelle (Eizelle, Pollenkorn, Knospe u.s.w.) sind die einselnen erblichen Eigenschaften des ganzen Organismus durch bestimmte stoffliche Theilchen vertreten. Diese vermehren sich durch Theilung und gehen bei der Zelltheilung von der Mutterzelle auf ihre Töchter über. 2. Ausserdem werfen die sämmtlichen Zellen des Körpers zu verschiednen Zeiten ihrer Etwicklung solche Theilchen ab; diese fliessen den Keimzellen zu und übertragen auf diese die ihnen etwa fehlenden Eigenschaften des Organismus (Transporthypothese).	Intracellular Pangenesis [23] by Hugo de Vries Professor of Botany in the University of Amsterdam Translated from the German by C. Stuart Gager, Professor of Botany in the University of Missouri To my mind Darwin's provisional hypothesis of pangenesis consists of the following two propositions: 1. In every germ cell (egg-cell, pollen grain, bud, etc.) the individual hereditary qualities of the whole organism are represented by definite material particles. These multiply by division and are transmitted during cell-division from the mother-cell to the daughter-cells. 2. In addition, all the cells of the body, at different stages of their development, throw off such particles; these flow into the germ-cells, and transmit to them the qualities of the organism, which they are possibly lacking. (Transportation-hypothesis).

In a series of lectures delivered at the University of California in 1904, de Vries discussed the origin of species and varieties by mutation [24].

Species and Varieties
Their origin by mutation
Lectures delivered at the University of California
By
Hugo de Vries
Professor of Botany in the
University of Amsterdam
Mutations
Lecture XVI
The Origin of the Peloric Toad-flax

"I have tried to show previously that species, in the ordinary sense of the word, consist of distinct groups of units. In systematic works these groups are all designated by the name of varieties, but it is usually granted that the units of the system are not always of the same value. Hence we have distinguished between elementary species and varieties proper. The first are combined into species whose common original type is now lost or unknown, and from their characters is derived an hypothetical image of what the common ancestor is supposed to have been. The varieties proper are derived in most cases from still existing types, and therefore are subjoined to them. A closer investigation has shown that this derivation is ordinarily produced by the loss of some definite attribute, or by the re-acquisition of an apparently lost character. The elementary species, on the other hand, must have arisen by the production of new qualities, each new acquisition constituting the origin of a new elementary form."

William Bateson (1861–1926), Edith R. Saunders (1865–1945), Reginald C. Punnett (1875–1967)

William Bateson, Edith Saunders, and Reginald Punnett were coworkers. Independently and together, they advanced the field of Mendelian genetics.

In 1906, Bateson delivered an address before the Neurological Society of London [25].

An Address on
Mendelian Heredity and its Application to Man.
by W. Bateson, M.A., F.R.S.

'Mr. President and Gentleman, —Though I venture to call my paper "Mendelian Heredity and its Application to Man,“ I ought to say that that application is rather for the future than for the present. We do know cases in man where the rules of inheritance traced in other animals and plants must certainly apply, but those cases are very few. On the other hand, I feel sure that if members of your profession were to take the matter up and study the phenomena of inheritance with due regard to those points which we now know to be critical, the list will be very soon increased.

The advance in knowledge which I am about to describe is the outcome of the work of Mendel. I have not time to tell you who Mendel was, or how it came about that his paper, published in 1865 was completely ignored until 1900, when De Vries and others simultaneously rediscovered it.'

Bateson then described the transmission of discriminating points (e.g., color) following the cross match of peas.

"Such segregating characters, or *allelomorphs*, as they are called, are, so far as we know, always constituted in pairs. In respect of each pair, therefore, there are only three kinds of individuals—the pure or *homozygous*, of each kind, and the impure, or *heterozygous*, containing both.

It is often found that one member of the allelomorphic pair is so conspicuous in the heterozygotes that these impure individuals may pass for pure. The character which thus prevails is then called the dominant (D), the other being the recessive (R)."

Fig. 133.5 Punnett's Fig. 133.5. Diagram to illustrate the nature of the F_2 generation from the cross of rose comb x pea comb. Reproduced from Punnett. Mendelism, 3E., The MacMillan Company, New York, 1911, p.37

RP RP Walnut	RP Rp Walnut	RP rP Walnut	RP rp Walnut
Rp RP Walnut	Rp Rp Rose	Rp rP Walnut	Rp rp Rose
rP RP Walnut	rP Rp Walnut	rP rP Pea	rP rp Pea
rp RP Walnut	rp Rp Rose	rp rP Pea	rp rp Single

Both Bateson and Punnett published books on Mendel's ideas (Bateson, *Mendel's Principles of Heredity*; Punnett, *Mendelism*) [26, 27]. Punnett devised the square, eponymously named after him, as a means of explaining the number and variety of genetic combinations. For example, in his chapter entitled *The Presence and Absence of Theory*, in the third edition of his text, *Mendelism*, Punnett describes his method [28].

Mendelism
By
R. C. Punnett
Fellow of Gonville and Caius College
Professor of Biology in the University of Cambridge

"In this case we are concerned with the transmission of the two factors, rose (*R*) and pea (*P*), the presence of each of which is alternative to its absence. The rose-combed bird contains the factor for rose but not that for pea, and the pea-combed bird contains the factor for pea but not that for rose. When both factors are present in a bird, as in a hybrid made by crossing rose with pea, the result is a walnut. For convenience of argument we may denote the presence of a given factor by a capital letter and its absence by the corresponding small letter. The use of the small letter is merely a symbolic way of intimating that a particular factor is absent in a gamete or zygote. Represented thus the zygote constitution of a pure rose-combed bird is *RRpp*; for it has been formed by the union of two gametes both of which contained *R* but not *P*. Similarly we may denote the pure pea-combed bird as *rrPP*. On crossing the rose with the pea union occurs between a gamete *Rp* and a gamete *rP*, resulting in the formation of a heterozygote of the constitution *RrPp*. The use of small letters here informs us that such a zygote contains only a single dose of each of the factors *R* and *P*, although, of course, it is possible for a zygote, if made in a suitable way, to have a double dose of any factor. Now when such a bird comes to form gametes a separation takes place between the part of the zygotic cell containing *R* and the part which does not contain it (*r*). Half of its gametes, therefore, will contain *R* and the other half will be without it (*r*). Similarly half of its gametes will contain *P* and the other half will be without it (*p*). It is obvious that the chances of *R* being distributed to a gamete with or without *P* are equal. Hence the gametes containing *R* will be of two sorts, *PR* and *Rp,* and these will be produced in equal numbers. Similarly the gametes without *R* will also be of two sorts, *rP* and *rp*, and these again, will be produced in equal numbers. Each of the hybrid walnut-combed birds, therefore, gives rise to a series consisting of equal numbers of gametes of the four difference types *RP*, *Rp*, *rP*, and *rp*; and the breeding together of such F_1 birds means the bringing together of two such series of gametes. When this happens an ovum of any one of the four types has an equal chance of being fertilized by a spermatozoon of any one of the four types. A convenient and simple method of demonstrating what happens under such circumstances is the method sometimes termed the "chessboard" method. For two series each consisting of four different types of gamete we require a square divided up into 16 parts. The four terms of the gametic series are first written horizontally across the four sets of four squares, so that the series is repeated four times. It is then written vertically four times, care being taken to keep to the same order. In this simple mechanical way all the possible combinations are represented and in their proper proportions. Fig. 133.5 shows the result of applying this method to our series *RP*, *Rp*, *rP*, *rp*, and the 16 squares represent the different types of zygotes formed and the proportions in which they occur."

In 1905, Bateson, Saunders, and Punnett published an observation while performing crosses of sweet pea plants [29].

Sweet Pea (Lathyrus odoratus).
(Experiments carried out by W. Bateson,
E. R. Saunders, and R. C. Punnett (in 1904).)

"Light axil commonly behaves as a simple recessive to dark axil. The figures frequently show that the result 3 dark : 1 light appears in the *coloured* plants alone, whites never having dark axil, thence it is might be suggested that there is a correlation or "coupling" between light axil and white."

This exception to the principle of independent assortment suggested that certain alleles were linked [30].

Abbie Lathrop (1868–1918), Leo Loeb (1869–1959)

Animals are used as models to study human diseases. Abbie Lathrop owned and operated a mouse farm in Granby, Massachusetts. When one breed developed mammary tumors, she sent samples to Leo Loeb [31].

The incidence of cancer in various strains of mice
By A. E. C. Lathrop and Leo Loeb.
[From the Department of Pathology, Barnard Free Skin and Cancer
Hospital, St. Louis]

"The principal results of our investigations which, after a few preliminary observations were begun more than three years ago, and which we hope to be able to continue, may be summarized as follows:

1. Mice raised in the same breeding establishment, under the same conditions of climate and feeding show a very different incidence of cancer of the mammary gland among female mice depending on the strain or family to which the mice belong.
2. The tumor rate in the different strains remains approximately constant in the succeeding generations.
9. From our investigations we may conclude that hereditary factors play a great part in the incidence of cancer among mice and that hereditary transmission is to a great extent responsible for the so-called endemic occurrence of cancer among animals."

References

1. Harvey W. The anatomical exercises of Dr. William Harvey, professor of physick and physician to the Kings Majesty, concerning the motion of the heart and blood. London: Francis Leach for Richard Lowndes; 1653. Translation of: De motu cordis/William Harvey; Dissertatio de corde/Jacobus de Back; and De circulatione sanguinis/William Harvey. The preface of Zacharie Wood, Physician at Rotterdam, upon the anatomical excercise of Doctor WILLIAM HARVEY. The United States Library of Congress Rare Book Collection, http://hdl.loc.gov/loc.rbc/General.19309.1; Accessed 2 Jul 2022
2. Grew N. The anatomy of vegetables begun with a general account of vegetation founded thereon. Printed for Spencer Hickman, Printer to the R. Society, at the Rose in S. Pauls Church-Yard, 1672. The font used by Dr. Grew's publisher was changed to a modern font. The letter f in the word fo was changed to s making the word so.
3. Grew N. The anatomy of plants. With an idea of a philosophical history of plants. W. Rawlins, 1682. Accessed from Google Books, December 26, 2023; pp. 209, Tab. 81, The Explication of the Tables. TAB. LXXXI.
4. Camerarius RJ. Britannica, the editors of encyclopaedia. In: Encyclopedia Britannica; 2022. https://www.britannica.com/biography/Rudolph-Jacob-Camerarius. Accessed 11 Jul 2022.
5. Camerarri, RJ. De Sexu Plantarum Epistola. Tvbingæ, Typis Viduæ Rommeii, A. MDCXCIV; from Archive.org. Accessed 10 Jul 2022.
6. Camerarius RJ. Ueber das Geschlecht der Pflanzen. (De sexu plantarum epistola.) 1694. Uebersetzt und herausgegebn von M. Möbius. Leipzig: Verlag von Wilhelm Engelmann; 1899. p. 51–4. babel.hathitrust.org. Accessed 10 Jul 2022.
7. Youatt W. Sheep: their breeds, management, and diseases. London: Baldwin and Cradock. Paternoster Row, MDCCCXXXVII. Accessed 3 Sep 2022.
8. Housman W. Robert Bakewell. J. Roy Agricultural Soc Eng, third series. 1894;5:1–31.
9. Szabó AT, Poczai P. The emergence of genetics from Festetics' sheep through Mendel's peas to Bateson's chickens. J Genet. 2019;98:63.
10. Festetics E. Weitere Erklärungen des Herrn Grafen Emmerich von Festetics über Inzucht. Oekon Neuigk Verhandl. 1819;22:169–70.
11. Poczai P, Santiago-Blay JA, Sekerák J, Bariska I, Szabó AT. Mimush sheep and the spectre of inbreeding: historical background for Festetic's organic and genetic laws four decades before Mendel's experiments in peas. J Hist Biol. 2022;55(3):495–536. https://doi.org/10.1007/s10739-022-09678-5. Published online: 07 Jun 2022.
12. Mendel G. Versuche über Plflanzen-Hybriden. Verhandlungen des naturforschenden Vereines, in Brünn. IV. Band 1865. Sitzung am 8. März. Seite 25. Brünn: Im Verlage des Vereines; 1866. Archive.org. Accessed 15 Apr 2023; b. Mendel G. Versuche über Plflanzen-hybriden. Mendel. Versuche. http://www.mendelweb.org. Accessed 15 Apr 2023.
13. Mendel G. Experiments in plant hybridization (1865). © 1996, Electronic Scholarly Publishing Project. https://www.esp.org. Reproduced for educational purposes. Accessed 11 Apr 2018.
14. Earle P. On the inability to distinguish colours. Am J Med Sci. 1845;9:346–54.

15. Gardner EJ, Richards RC. Multiple cutaneous and subcutaneous lesions occurring simultaneously with hereditary polyposis and osteomatosis. Am J Hum Genet. 1953;5:139–47. This type of pictorial display of family relationships or genealogical chart, is still used today. Aldred Scott Warthin's Family "G", (Warthin AS. Heredity with reference to carcinoma as shown by the study of the cases examined in the pathological laboratory of the University of Michigan, 1895-1913. Arch Intern Med 1913; 12: 546–555) and Kindred 109.
16. Darwin C. On the Origin of Species by Means of Natural Selection. Introduction. London: John Murray, Albemarle Street, 1859. p. B3.
17. Strasburger E. Die Copulationsvorgänge bei Acetabularia. In: Ueber Befruchtung und Zelltheilung. Jena: Verlag von Hermann Dabis; 1878. p. 9. Archive.org, Digitalizing sponsor: Google, Accessed 3 Jul 2022.
18. Herranz G. Origin of the terms embryo, gamete and zygote. Zygote. 2012;20:313–20.
19. Flemming W. Zellsubstanz, Kern und Zelltheilung. Leipzig: Verlag von F. C. W. Vogel; 1882. Internet Archive, Archive.org, Digitalizing sponsor: Google, Accessed 3 Jul 2022.
20. Paweletz N. Walther Flemming: pioneer of mitosis research. Nat Rev Mol Cell Biol. 2001;2:72–5.
21. Dröscher A. Flemming, Walther. Wiley Online Library; 2015. https://doi.org/10.1002/9780470015902.a0002790.
22. DeVries H. Intracellulare Pangenesis. Jena: Verlag von Gustav Fischer; 1889. p. 3. Internet Archive, archive.org, Accessed 3 Jul 2022.
23. De Vries H. Intracellular Pangenesis. Translated from the German by C. Stuart Gager, Chicago. The Open Court Publishing Co.; 1910, p. 5. The Electronic Scholarly Publishing Project, Accessed 3 Jul 2022.
24. De Vries H. Mutations. Lecture XVI. In: species and varieties. their origin by mutation. lectures delivered at the University of California. Edited by Daniel T. MacDougal. 3E, Chicago, The Open Court Publishing Company, 1912. Accessed from Archive.org, April 15, 2023.
25. Bateson W. An address on Mendelian heredity and its application to man. Br Med J 1906;2:61–67.
26. Bateson W. Mendel's Principles of Heredity. Cambridge: at the University Press, New York: G. P. Putnam's Sons, 1909.
27. Punnett RC. Mendelism, Cambridge, MacMillan and Bowes. London: MacMillan and Co., LTD; 1905.
28. Punnett RC. Mendelism. The MacMillan Company, New York, 1911, Ch. IV, pp. 29–38.
29. Bateson W, Saunders ER, Punnett RC, Sweet Pea (*Lathyrus odoratus*). In: Report II. Experimental Studies in the Physiology of Heredity. Reports to the Evolution Committee of the Royal Society. London: Harrison & Sons, St. Martin's Lane, 1905, p. 97.
30. Lobo I, Shaw K. Discovery and types of genetic linkage. Nat Edu. 2008;1:139.
31. Lathrop AEC, Loeb L. The incidence of cancer in various strains of mice. Proc Soc Exp Biol Med (New York) 1913;11;34–38.

Cronkhite–Canada Syndrome

134

Jessica R. Philpott, Carolyn L. Power, Eric W. Willis,
Robert S. O'Shea, Michelle D. Inkster, and James S. Wu

Presentation

A 77-year-old male presented with weight loss and bloody diarrhea. He noted progressive severe edema, changes in his skin, and dysgeusia. He had been treated at an outside facility for inflammatory colitis with mesalamine, zinc, and diuretics. Esophagogastroduodenoscopy and colonoscopy were done (Figs. 134.1 and 134.2). Pathology of biopsies showed hamartomas with inflammation.

He was seen in follow-up clinic. In addition to the generalized colonic polyposis seen on colonoscopy, physical examination showed skin hyperpigmentation, alopecia, and onychatrophia (Fig. 134.3a–d). The lower extremities were edematous.

Based on the constellation of signs, symptoms, and colon pathology, Cronkite-Canada syndrome (CCS) was diagnosed. Treatment with steroids was started with marked improvement in his symptoms.

J. R. Philpott · M. D. Inkster
Department of Gastroenterology, Cleveland Clinic, Cleveland, OH, USA

C. L. Power · J. S. Wu (✉)
Department of Colon and Rectal Surgery, Cleveland Clinic, Cleveland, OH, USA

E. W. Willis
Department of Pathology, CORPath, Columbus, OH, USA

R. S. O'Shea
Department of Gastroenterology and Hepatology, Cleveland Clinic, Cleveland, OH, USA
e-mail: oshear@ccf.org

J. S. Wu, M. D. Inkster (eds.), *Cleveland Clinic Colorectal Case Studies*,
https://doi.org/10.1007/978-3-031-39880-3_134

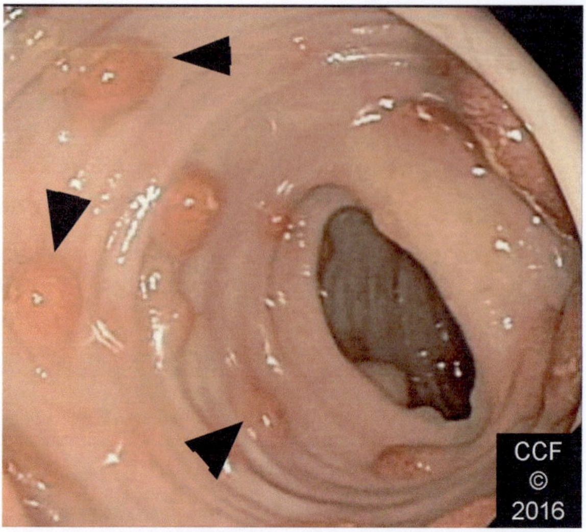

Fig. 134.1 Diffuse colonic polyposis

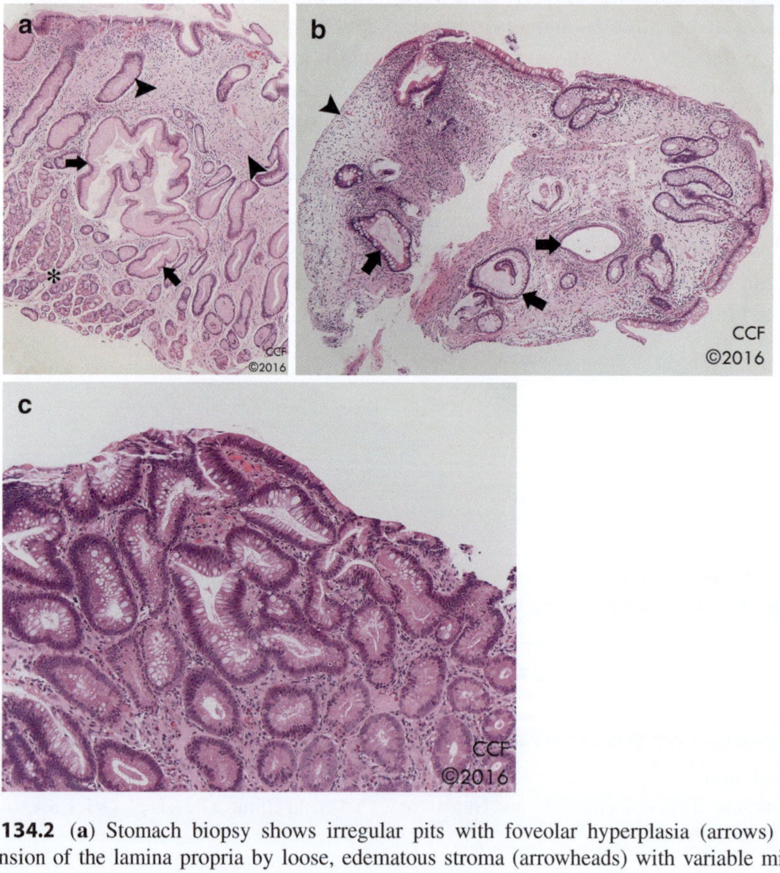

Fig. 134.2 (**a**) Stomach biopsy shows irregular pits with foveolar hyperplasia (arrows) and expansion of the lamina propria by loose, edematous stroma (arrowheads) with variable mixed inflammatory cells. Oxyntic glands (asterisk) indicate that the biopsy was likely taken from the body or fundus. (**b**, **c**) Colonic mucosa with irregular, cystically dilated crypts with inspissated mucin (arrows). The lamina propria is edematous and inflamed (arrowhead). The polypoid and background mucosa show similar histologic findings

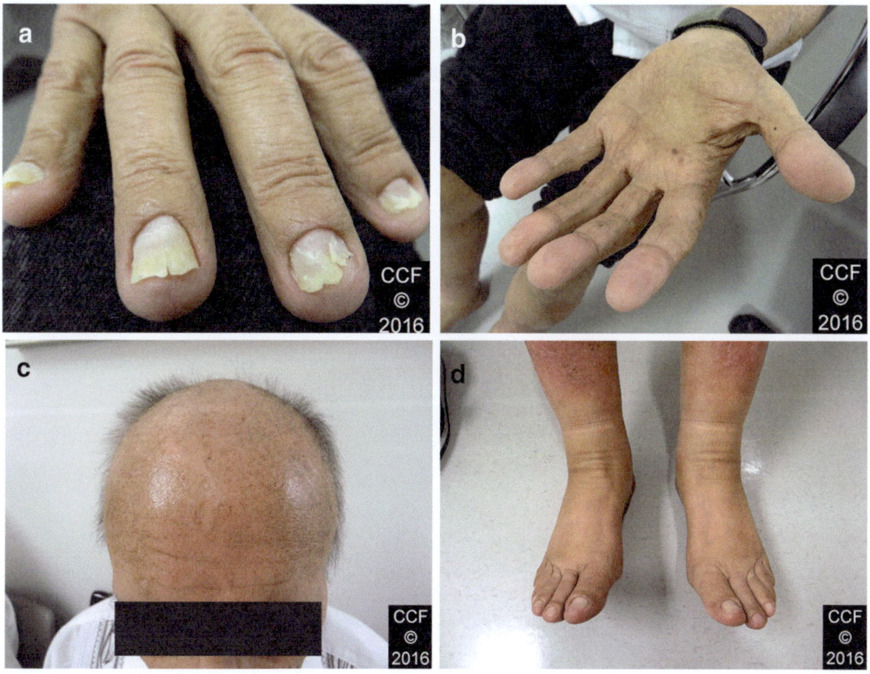

Fig. 134.3 (**a**) Onychatrophia. (**b**) Hyperpigmentation of the palmar surface of the hands. (**c**) Hair loss and hyperpigmentation of the scalp. (**d**) Lower extremity edema and hyperpigmentation

Comment

The syndrome that bears their names was described by Cronkhite and Canada in 1955 [1]. The authors presented two cases with distinct clinical features. The constellation of generalized gastrointestinal polyposis, skin hyperpigmentation, alopecia, and onychatrophia were prominent features thought to be part of a generalized nutritional deficiency state.

About 400 cases have been reported worldwide [2, 3]. The etiology is unknown, and there is no consistently effective treatment. The condition is not familial. The average age at onset is 60 years, and there is a slightly increased male:female ratio of 3:2. The differential diagnosis includes Peutz–Jeghers syndrome, juvenile polyposis, familial polyposis of the colon, Gardner's syndrome, and Turcot's syndrome. Pathological types seen in CSS include inflammatory, hyperplastic, hamartomatous, and adenomatous polyps [4].

References

1. Cronkhite LW Jr, Canada WJ. Generalized gastrointestinal polyposis. An unusual syndrome of polyposis, pigmentation, alopecia and onychotrophia. N Engl J Med. 1955;252:1011–5.

2. Wen X-H, Wang L, Wang Y-X, Qian J-M. Cronkhite-Canada syndrome: Report of six cases and review of literature. World J Gastroenterol. 2014;20:7518–22.
3. Zhao R, Huang M, Benafea O, Zhao J, Cheng L, Zou K, Zhu L. Cronkhite-Canada syndrome: a rare case report and literature review. BMC Gastroenterol. 2016;16:23.
4. Wu Z-Y, Sang L-X, Chang B. Cronkite-Canada syndrome: from clinical features to treatment. Gastroenterol Rep. 2020;8:333–42.

Peutz–Jeghers Syndrome

135

Aaron Brzezinski, Erica C. Savage, Janice M. Santisi,
Erick M. Remer, Michelle D. Inkster, and James S. Wu

Presentation

A patient was seen in gastroenterology clinic because of small intestinal polyposis. Distinctive melanin spots on the patient's lips were noted (Fig. 135.1).

A. Brzezinski · M. D. Inkster
Department of Gastroenterology, Cleveland Clinic, Cleveland, OH, USA

J. M. Santisi
Digestive Diseases and Surgery Institute, Cleveland Clinic, Cleveland, OH, USA

E. C. Savage
Pathology & Laboratory Medicine Institute, Cleveland Clinic, Cleveland, OH, USA

E. M. Remer
Radiology & Diagnostic Imaging Institute, Cleveland Clinic, Cleveland, OH, USA

J. S. Wu (✉)
Department of Colon and Rectal Surgery, Cleveland Clinic, Cleveland, OH, USA

J. S. Wu, M. D. Inkster (eds.), *Cleveland Clinic Colorectal Case Studies*,
https://doi.org/10.1007/978-3-031-39880-3_135

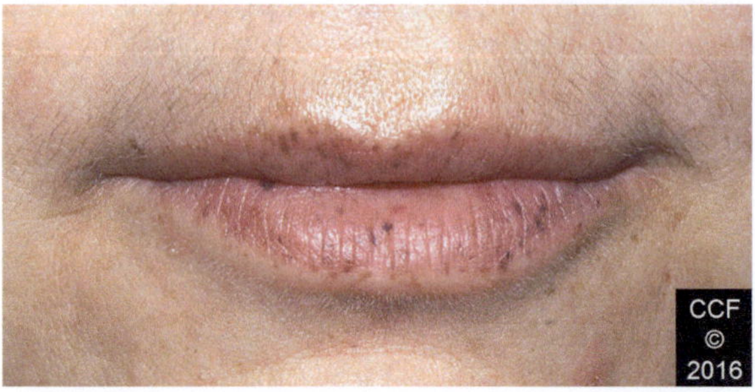

Fig. 135.1 Pigmented spots are seen on this patient's lips

Comment

> "Dr. J. T. Conner showed two cases of Pigmentation of the Lips and Mouth in twins, both girls, aged twelve years, of dark complexion and anæmic. The pigment spots, which were only noticed two years ago, were of ink-black colour, mostly of very small size, and scattered over the lips (especially the lower), gums, and hard palate, but not on the tongue [1]."
> Æsculapian Society of London, 1895

In 1896, Hutchinson [2] presented portraits of the twins.
PLATE CXLI.
Pigmented Spots on the Lips, &c., in Twin Sisters.
(Dr. Conner's Cases.)

> "The faces here represented are those of twin sisters, who were so much like each other that it was with difficulty that they were distinguished. Both were very dark brunettes. They were nine years of age when, in 1894, the portrait was taken. They were in good health, and had not suffered from any illness. The interesting feature in the case was this, that both the sisters had at exactly the same age developed a number of black pigmented spots on the lips and inside the mouth. It was at about the age of three that these spots had first been noticed, and the evidence was definite that none had been present at birth. The spots had increased in number and size at exactly parallel rates in the two, and the conditions presented were just the same in each. The arrangement and size of the spots are well shown in the Plate, so far as the skin, the lips, and prolabia are concerned. Inside the mouth, on the lining of the lips and cheeks, were many spots, some of them considerably larger than those on the skin. There were none on the gums or tongue. The figure representing the mucous membrane of the lips may be taken to illustrate both cases, for they were exactly alike.
> I am indebted to my friend Dr. Conner for the opportunity of seeing these girls, and for permission to have the portrait taken."

The portrait of Dr. Conner's patients is shown in Fig. 135.2.

In 1921, Peutz described a syndrome of familial polyposis of the mucous membranes of the nasopharynx and intestinal tract associated with peculiar pigmentation of the skin and mucous membranes [3].[1]

[1] Peutz [4]. This excerpt is reused with the generous permission of Dr. Douglas L. Riegert-Johnson, 10 Oct 2022.

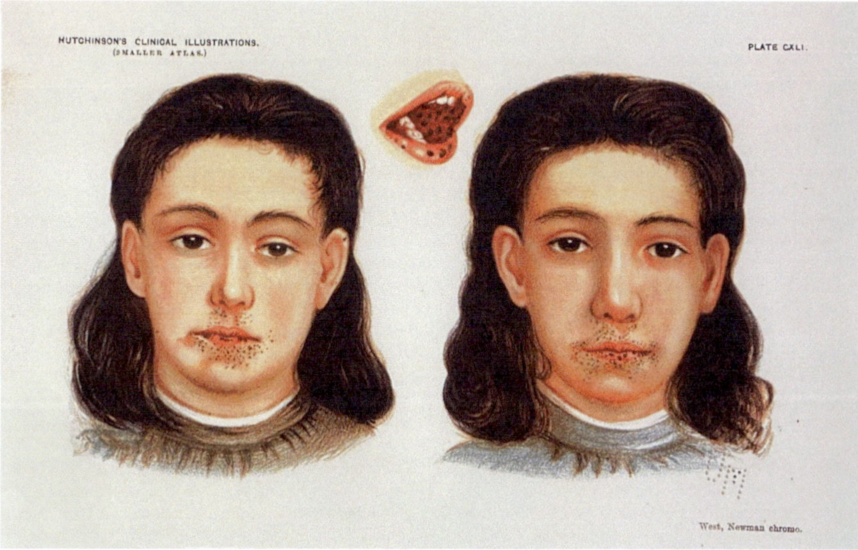

Fig. 135.2 PLATE. Portrait of twin sisters described by Conner and presented by Hutchinson. The pigmented spots around the lips, Hutchinson referred to as a "peculiar form of freckles"

Over een zeer merkwaardige, gecombineerde familiaire polyposis van de slijmvliezen van den tractus intestinalis met die van de neuskeelholte en gepaard met eigenaardige pigmentaties van huid- en slijmvliezen. Door J. L. A. Peutz 1e geneesheer van het ziekenhuis. Uit het R. K. Ziekenhuis, Westeinde, den Haag. Het vinden bij één familie van, zoowel neus- en keelpolypen als tegelijkertijd ook polypen van den tractus intestinalis deed mij besluiten tot de volgende mededeeling. Ik ontleen het recht hiertoe vooral aan het feit, dat wel neus-keelpolypen evenals darm-polypen afzonderlijk zijn beschreven, maar—voor zoover mij althans bekend is —niet gecombineerd bij één en denzelfden patient en bovendien bij meerdere leden uit één familie. De zeer opvallende pigmentaties die dezelfde leden uit het gezin tevens vertoonden, verhoogen m. i. de belangwekkendheid van deze familie nog zeer aanmerkelijk. Ter illustratie moge nu het volgende dienen. Op 6 Dec. 1920 werd op de inwendige afdeeling opgenomen W. v. d. S., oud 15 jaren. Sinds den zomer klaagde de jongen over slechte eetlust, een hevig gevoel van onpasselijkheid, in de buik af en toe steken. Eén keer was de buikpijn zoo sterk geweest, dat hij er door ging braken. Aan de ontlasting was nooit iets bijzonders bemerkt. Al eenige jaren lang had deze patient er slecht uitgezien, in de laatste maanden was hij ook zichtbaar vermagerd. Tevoren was hij altijd gezond geweest, wel was de eetlust nooit groot. De ouders zijn gezond; de moeder is den laatsten tijd onder mijn behandeling voor vethart; er zijn zeven kinderen, waaronder een tweeling; de oudste is 25, de jongste 4 jaar. Patient is eenige jaren geleden hier poliklinisch behandeld voor herhaaldelijk *recidiveerende en zeer uitgebreide neuspolypen.* Toen ik den jongen voor het eerst zag, meende ik een bekende in hem te zien, zoo sprekend geleek hij op een in den gepasseerden zomer door mij onderzochten jongen J. van ongeveer elf jaren, die mij door collega KUYNDERS werd toegezonden wegens *allermerkwaardigste pigmentaties van het gelaat en van de slijmvliezen van de mondholte en* met de opmerking, dat *anamnestisch* ook andere familieleden dergelijke vlekjes vertoonden. Het bewijs werd inderdaad thans geleverd, beide jongens bleken broers te zijn. Evenals het elfjarig broertje had ook W. ontelbaar vele pigmentvlekjes in het gelaat, kleiner en donkerder dan de bekende zomersproeten, welke aan het gelaat een zonderling grauw-zwart aanzien gaven. Reeds zonder meer was het te zien, dat deze pigmentvlekken ook de slijmvliezen der lippen bedekten; bij het openen van den mond zag men het verrassende feit, dat *ook in de mondholte de slijmvliezen* dergelijke vlekken vertoonden. Deze waren wat minder in aantal en iewat grooter en bruiner dan die van het gelaat. Bij mijn verder onderzoek der familie bleek deze pigmentatie te bestaan bij vijf der kinderen; twee kinderen en ook beide ouders waren zonder vlekken. De moeder deed mij nog opmerken, dat alleen die kinderen, die op den vader geleken, die pigmentaties bezaten en verder, dat bij die kinderen de pigmentatie steeds opgetreden was in het vijfde levensjaar in het gelaat, te voren echter reeds in de mondholte; de jongste heeft ze bijv. nu reeds op de lippen.	Very remarkable case of familial polyposis of mucous membrane of intestinal tract and nasopharynx accompanied by peculiar pigmentations of the skin and mucous membrane. By J. L. A. Peutz [4] First physician to the hospital From the R. K. Hospital, Westeinde, the Haag (Translated by Wytske M. Westra, M. D.) Encountering—within one family—both nasopharyngeal as well as gastrointestinal polyps, motivated me to write this paper. I feel entitled to do so since nasopharyngeal and gastrointestinal polyps, although described separately, never (at least to my knowledge) were described combined in one and the same patient and moreover in more than one member of the same family. The peculiar pigmentations found in these patients only further contributed to my conviction that this is an important observation. To illustrate the above I would now like to present you with the following case. On December 6th of 1920, W. v. d. S. was admitted to the internal medicine wards. This 15-year-old boy had been complaining of lack of appetite, serious nausea, and occasional abdominal pain since the summer. Once, the abdominal pain took such serious proportions that it caused him to vomit. He never noticed anything abnormal in his feces. However, he had been a rather unhealthy-looking child for a number of years, and lost visible weight in the previous months. Otherwise he had always been relatively healthy, although never with a big appetite. His parents are both in good health; the mother is a patient of mine as a result of a 'fatty' heart; there are seven children, two twins, the eldest is 25 and the youngest child is currently 4 years of age. The boy had been treated as an outpatient for recurrent extensive nasal polyps a number of years ago. When I saw the boy for the first time, I thought I had met him before, as he looked so much like another patient of mine, an 11-year-old boy that was sent to me in the summer of 1919 by my colleague Dr. Kuynders because of 'extremely peculiar pigmentations of the face and the oral mucosa'. According to the patient there were other members in his family suffering from the same type of pigmentations. This was confirmed when it became clear the two boys were brothers. W. just like his 11-year-old brother, had numerous skin discolorations in his face-smaller and darker then the well-known summer freckles—which gave his face a peculiar gray-black appearance. Immediately also it was evident that these pigmentations were also present on the lips; however, it was not until examination of the oral cavity that the surprising fact appeared that these strange discolorations were also present in the oral mucosa, although they were somewhat less numerous and slightly larger and darker than those on the boy's face. After an in-depth family history it appeared that five of the seven children suffered from these pigmentations; the two remaining children and both of the parents did not. The mother also made the observation that the pigmentations only seemed to occur in the children that resembled their father, and furthermore that these pigmentations consistently started to appear in the face around the age of five. Prior to this however, evident discolorations of the oral mucosa become noticeable; in the youngest child for example abnormalities are already clearly present on the "lips".

Peutz adds that W's sister underwent surgery because of bowel obstruction due to intestinal intussusception caused by a "nut"-sized polyp. Two of the father's sisters died of "ileus" at ages 11 and 20. The patient, W, underwent surgery for small bowel obstruction; findings included multiple small and large intestinal polyps. Small intestinal polyps located by palpation were removed.

The microscopic appearance of one resected specimen showed malignant degeneration.

Conclusie: Klierpolypen met maligne degeneratie, n.l. een beginnende vorming van een adenocarcinoom.	Conclusion: Adenomatous polyps with malignant degeneration, i.e., early adenocarcinoma [4]

Peutz concluded that the disease was congenital, was associated with malignant degeneration of intestinal polyps.

In 1949, Jeghers, McKusick and Katz [5] defined the two key features of the syndrome:

1. distinctive melanin spots of the buccal mucosa and lips,
2. polyposis of the small intestine.

An increased risk of both gastrointestinal and nongastrointestinal cancers for Peutz–Jeghers syndrome has been documented [6, 7].

In 1997, Hemminki et al. [8] reported a susceptibility locus for Peutz–Jeghers syndrome to 19p. Jenne et al. [9] found that Peutz–Jeghers syndrome is caused by mutations in a serine threonine kinase. Laparotomy has been recommended for Peutz–Jeghers' syndrome for irretrievable symptomatic polyps and polyp-related complications [10]. Currently, in addition to upper endoscopy and colonoscopy, small bowel capsule (PillCam®) and magnetic resonance (MR) enterography have been shown to be excellent procedures for the diagnosis and surveillance of small bowel polyps (Figs. 135.3a–b and 135.4a–b).

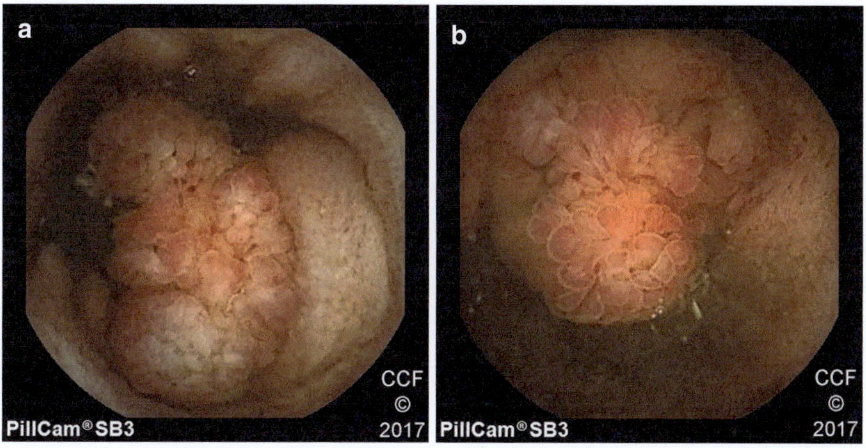

Fig. 135.3 Two PillCam® views (**a** and **b**) of the same small intestinal polyp

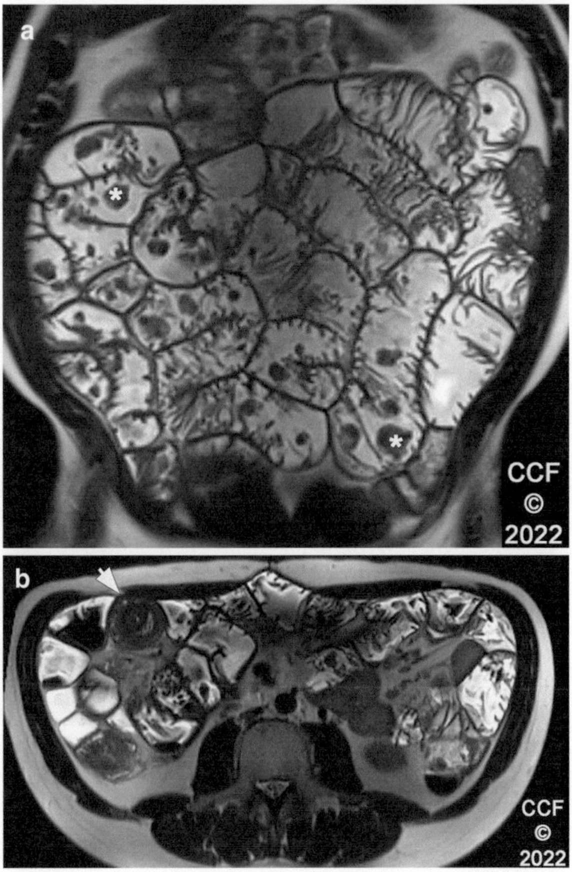

Fig. 135.4 MR enterography, T2-weighted images of a patient with Peutz–Jeghers syndrome. (**a**) a spectacular coronal view shows multiple intraluminal small intestinal polyps (two have been labeled with asterisks); (**b**) an axial view shows a point of small bowel intussusception caused by a polyp (arrow)

Histopathology of a Peutz-Jeghers polyp is shown in Fig. 135.5

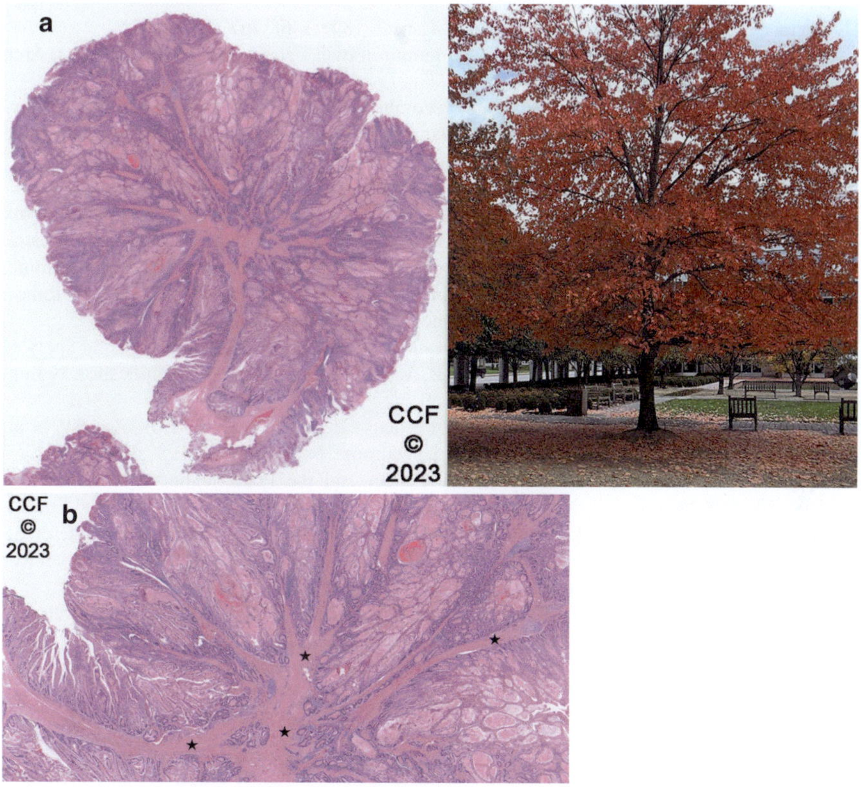

Fig. 135.5 Histopathology of a small intestinal Peutz–Jeghers polyp. (**a**) Peutz–Jeghers polyp, low power. At low magnification, Peutz–Jeghers polyps frequently are compared to a tree in which the arborizing smooth muscle resembles the trunk of a tree and its branches (upper left panel). The upper right panel shows a maple tree in the quadrangle of the Lerner Research Institute at the Cleveland Clinic during the fall. Each shows multiple limbs projecting from a central trunk. (**b**) Peutz–Jeghers polyp, 2X. The polyp is composed of benign small intestinal mucosa separated by an arborizing overgrowth of benign smooth muscle (stars) arising from the muscularis mucosae

References

1. Connor JT. Aesculapian Society of London. Lancet. 1895;146(3767):1168–9.
2. Hutchinson J. Pigmentation of the lips and mouth in twin sisters. (Dr. Conner's Cases). Arch Surg. 1896;7:290.
3. Peutz JLA. Over een zeer merkwaardige, gecombineerde familiaire polyposis van de slijmvliezen van den tractus intestinalis met die van de neuskeelholte en gepaard met eigenaardige pigmentaties van huid-en slijmvliezen. Nederl Maandschr Geneesk. 1921;10:134–46.
4. Peutz JLA. Appendix: Peutz's original report on Peutz-Jeghers syndrome. Peutz J. Very remarkable case of familial polyposis of mucous membrane of the intestinal tract and nasopharynx associated by peculiar pigmentations of skin and mucous membrane. Translated by Westra, Wytske M, MD. Riegert-Johnson D, Gleeson FC, Westra W. et al. Peutz-Jeghers syndrome. In: Riegert-Johnson DL, Boardman LA, Hefferon T, Roberts M, editors. Cancer syndromes. Bethesda, MD: National Center for Biotechnology Information (US); 2009. p. 187–95.
5. Jeghers H, McKusick VA, Katz KH. Generalized intestinal polyposis and melanin spots of the oral mucosa, lips and digits (concluded)* A syndrome of diagnostic significance. N Engl J Med. 1949;241:1031–6.
6. Giardiello FM, Welsh SB, Hamilton SR, Offerhaus GJA, Gittelsohn AM, Booker SV, et al. Increased risk of cancer in the Peutz- Jehgers syndrome. N Engl J Med. 1987;316:1511–4.
7. Spigelman AD, Murday V, Phillips RKS. Cancer and the Peutz-Jeghers syndrome. Gut. 1989;30:1588–90.
8. Hemminki A, Tomlinson I, Markie D, Järvinen H, Sistonen P, Björkqvist A-M, et al. Localization of a susceptibility locus for Peutz-Jeghers syndrome to 19p using a comparative genomic hybridization and targeted linkage analysis. Nat Genet. 1997;15:87–90.
9. Jenne DE, Reimann H, Nezu J-I, Friedel W, Loff S, Jeschke R, et al. Peutz-Jeghers syndrome is caused by mutations in a novel serine threonine kinase. Nat Genet. 1998;18:38–43.
10. Oncel M, Remzi FH, Church JM, Connor JT, Fazio VF. Benefits of 'clean sweep' in Peutz-Jeghers patients. Color Dis. 2004;6:332–5.

Familial Adenomatous Polyposis Coli 136

Carolyn L. Power, Homer O. Wiland, Eric W. Willis,
and James S. Wu

Presentation

A patient was referred for surgery because colonoscopy had revealed adenomatous polyps that were too numerous to count. Histopathology of representative biopsies is shown in Fig. 136.1 (a and b).

C. L. Power · J. S. Wu (✉)
Department of Colon and Rectal Surgery, Cleveland Clinic, Cleveland, OH, USA

H. O. Wiland
Department of Pathology, OhioHealth Mansfield Hospital, Mansfield, OH, USA

E. W. Willis
Department of Pathology, CORPath, Columbus, OH, USA

J. S. Wu, M. D. Inkster (eds.), *Cleveland Clinic Colorectal Case Studies*,
https://doi.org/10.1007/978-3-031-39880-3_136

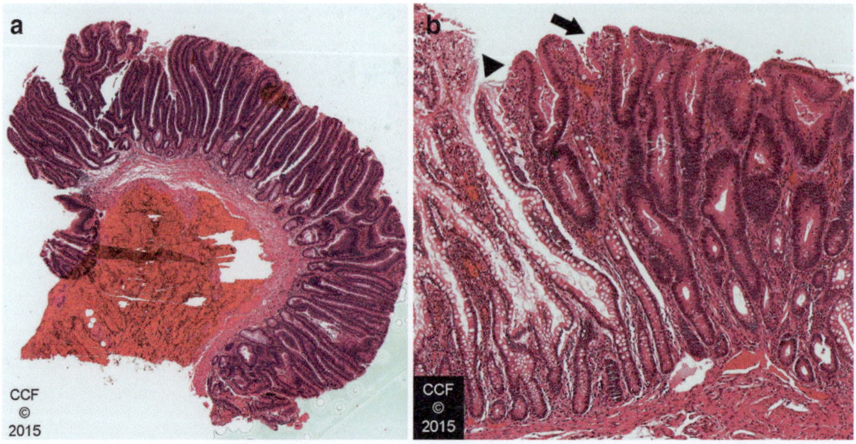

Fig. 136.1 (**a**) Tubular adenoma (H&E, original magnification, 20x) (**b**) Adenomatous epithelium with dark, overlapping pencil-shaped nuclei to the right (arrow) compared with normal epithelium to the left (arrowhead) (H&E, original magnification, 50×)

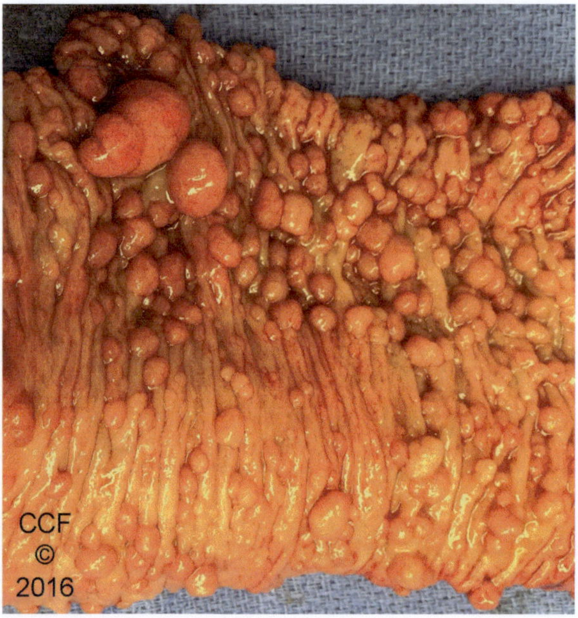

Fig. 136.2 The resected colon of a patient with familial adenomatous polyposis; the mucosal surface is covered with multiple polyps (This image was generously donated by Matthew F. Kalady, MD) (The authors acknowledge with gratitude members of the Sanford R. Weiss, MD Center for Hereditary Colorectal Neoplasia for offering several images of operative specimens from patients with FAP)

Management

The patient underwent proctocolectomy. An example of multiple polyps in a patient with familial polyposis coli is shown in Fig. 136.2.

Comment

In 1882, Cripps described two cases of disseminated rectal polyposis in a brother and a sister, aged 19 and 17 [1].

Two Cases of Disseminated Polypus of the Rectum
By W. Harrison Cripps.

"CASE 1. —The patient, a boy, aged 19, gave the following history. So far as was known he was a healthy child until 9 years of age. It was then noticed that, after being exposed to cold one day, he had considerable hæmorrhage from the rectum. Six months after this a bleeding protrusion was occasionally observed after defecation. He was admitted into a hospital, and the protrusion removed when he was 11 years of age. The symptoms of bleeding were temporarily relieved, but returned again in a couple of years. He was again subjected to an operation, which only afforded temporary relief. Since that period he has on three occasions, at St. Bartholomew's and other hospitals, had growths removed from the rectum under chloroform, but without any real benefit. When admitted into St. Bartholomew's under the care of Mr. Smith he was extremely anæmic, having suffered severely from hæmorrhage during the last few months. His pulse was rapid and feeble, and he seemed scarcely in a condition to bear even an examination. After a few days' rest in bed he recovered considerably from his collapsed condition, no more hæmorrhage having occurred. He was examined under chloroform and the following condition found. On dilating the sphincter several mulberry-looking masses of growth were observed, varying in size from a small pea to a good-sized nut. Some of these had little or no pedicle, while others had well-marked stalks half an inch in length. The growths were very soft, nor was there any induration about the mucous membrane from which they sprang. By the aid of a duck-bill speculum from twenty to thirty distinct and separate polypoid growths could be seen pretty equally distributed about the last three inches of the rectum. Besides the growths which could be observed, others could be felt higher up by the finger, which failed to define any limit to the diseased condition of the bowel. A few of the more prominent outgrowths were removed by ligature and immediately transferred to chromic-acid solution, forming the specimens from which the accompanying drawings were taken.

CASE 2. —The second case corresponded so nearly in its symptoms with that just related that further details are scarcely necessary, the patient in this case being a girl, aged 17. She had noticed the symptoms for seven years, and had twice been operated upon. In her case the visible growths were rather larger, but not quite so numerous as in the boy; others could, however, be felt with the finger besides those visible by the speculum. But the most extraordinary and interesting part of the case consisted in the fact that she was sister of the patient whose case we have just described.

Polypus of the rectum is by no means a rare disease, and, moreover, cases have been described in which two or three growths have been found in the same individual, but as a rule, polypus is single.

Instances of such wide dissemination of the disease must be extremely rare.

A section of the growth cut at right angles to the mucous membrane, and longitudinally divided with its pedicle, showed the following structure: a central stalk of fibrous tissue, continuous with that forming the submucous network, which when followed towards the free margin of the tumour, divides and subdivides dicotyledonously like the branches of a tree." (Fig. 136.3).

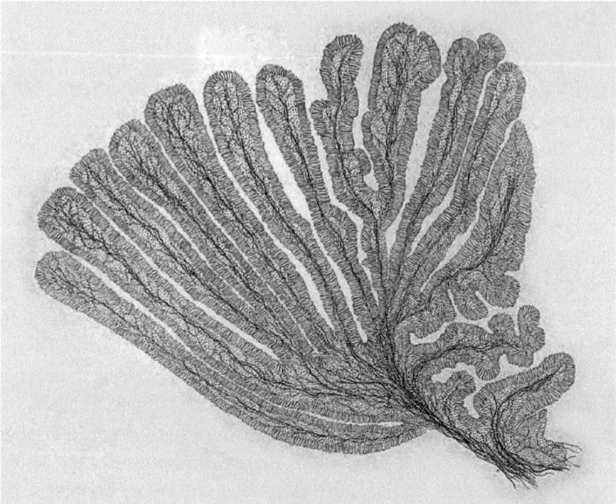

Fig. 136.3 Illustration of Mr. W. Harrison Cripps' case of Mucous Polypi of Rectum (1882)

Cripps' description: "Section of growth under low power. The epithelium forms a single layer, resting upon a reticulated tissue, the fibers of which converge toward the pedicle. The reticulated tissue is filled with small round cells."

This report suggested that disseminated polyposis of the rectum might be familial and appear at a young age. In 1890, Cripps reviewed cases involving polyps of the large intestine. In the postmortem examination of a 19-year-old male (likely the same as above), he noted and documented an association between adenoid polyposis and cancer [2].

Polypus of the Rectum
By Harrison Cripps, F.R.C.S.
Assistant Surgeon to St. Bartholomew's Hospital, etc.

"A. C., aged nineteen, was admitted under the care of my colleague Mr. T. Smith, in 1881. So far as was known, he was a healthy child until nine years of age. It was then noticed that, after being exposed to cold one day, he had considerable hæmorrhage from the rectum.

March 15, 1887. He was brought in in a moribund condition, his friend stating that since his last discharge from the hospital, he had suffered dull, aching pain in the abdomen; that two days since he was seized with violent cramping pain in the lower abdomen and sickness. He had taken no food for two days. He had had constant hiccough. One examination he was found to be moribund, with the signs of peritonitis, and he died the next day.

On post-mortem examination he was found to be suffering from adenoid cancer of the lower part of the sigmoid flexure, and there was at this point an almost impervious stricture of the bowel. The rectum below this contained a large number of polypoid growths similar to those that had been removed during the patient's lifetime; above the seat of the cancer there were but few to be found, and in the ascending and transverse colon not more than three or four, and these were small and rudimentary.

On microscopic examination the polypi proved to be well-marked examples of the adenoid variety."

In this 1890 paper, Cripps also reported a family of six, three of whom had polyposis hinting at the mode of transmission.

Also in 1890, Handford described a case of disseminated colon polyposis with cancer and liver metastasis [3].

Disseminated polypi of the large intestine becoming malignant; strictures (malignant adenoma) of the rectum and of the splenic flexure of the colon; secondary growths in the liver.

By H. Handford, M.D.

'E. F—, a cachetic-looking woman, aged 34, was transferred from the surgical side of the General Hospital, Nottingham, to my care in September, 1889, on account of some lung affection which was diagnosed during life and proved *post mortem* to be bronchiectasis of the left lung. A week previously my surgical colleague, Mr. A. R. Anderson, had removed the accompanying polypus (measuring in the spirit preparation 3.75 cm. by 3 cm., rounded in shape, and weighing 180 grains), which was attached by a long narrow pedicle just above a stricture of the rectum, extending from about two inches above the sphincter upwards for about two inches. The stricture would admit the index finger readily, but it was only by a great effort that the finger could be passed beyond it.

On surgical grounds it had been decided that the case was not suitable for excision of the rectum, and the passage of fæces was so free that colotomy was not at that time necessary. She went home, and was readmitted in February, 1890, five months later with the stricture very tight, great abdominal distension, especially of the cæcum and ascending colon, and a greatly enlarged nodular liver, reaching from the fourth space in the nipple line to the level of the umbilicus. She died ten days after readmission.

At the inspection, fourteen hours *post mortem*, a tight stricture of the rectum was found, commencing four cm. from the sphincter and extending upwards for six cm. The mucous membrane was ulcerated, and had in great part disappeared. The thickness of the walls of the stricture was nearly one inch. From the middle of the transverse colon to the stricture of the rectum the intestine was studded with polypi, about 170 in number in all—most numerous in the sigmoid flexure and in the rectum. Most were sessile, from 1 mm. to 1 cm. long, and from 1 mm. to 5 mm. broad. Others were pedunculated, from 5 mm. to 4 cm. long, and with a globular, raspberry-shaped mass at the end, from 1 cm. to 3 cm. in diameter. (These measurements were taken in the spirit preparation.) At the middle of the transverse colon there was a sessile polypus about the size of a small walnut. The base of it was infiltrating the intestinal wall, and had given rise to a puckered stricture which would admit one finger. The liver weighed 7 lbs. 12 oz., and contained several enormous masses of secondary growth and innumerable smaller ones.

On microscopic examination of the rectal stricture the growth was found to involve chiefly the muscular coat. The peritoneal coat was unaffected. The mucous membrane, together with a portion of the submucous coat, had disappeared by ulceration. The growth was what is often called a "cylindrical epithelioma;" but, from the very evident way in which the gradual changes in structure could be traced in this case, from the simple adenoid polypus to the malignant growth with secondary deposits, I think it is better termed a "malignant adenoma." The secondary deposits in the liver were of the same nature as the rectal growth,…'

Figure 136.4 (a and b) depicts Handford's drawings of a simple and malignant adenoma.

Fig. 136.4a.—Vertical section of a simple sessile polypus (simple adenoma) of the transverse colon. There is a central core of connective tissue containing blood vessels, &c., covered by a thickened mucous membrane, consisting of multiple tubular crypts (Lieberkühn's follicles). Just beneath the mucous membrane are four solitary glands.

Fig. 136.4 From drawings by Handford, 1890. Figures 136.4a, 136.4b

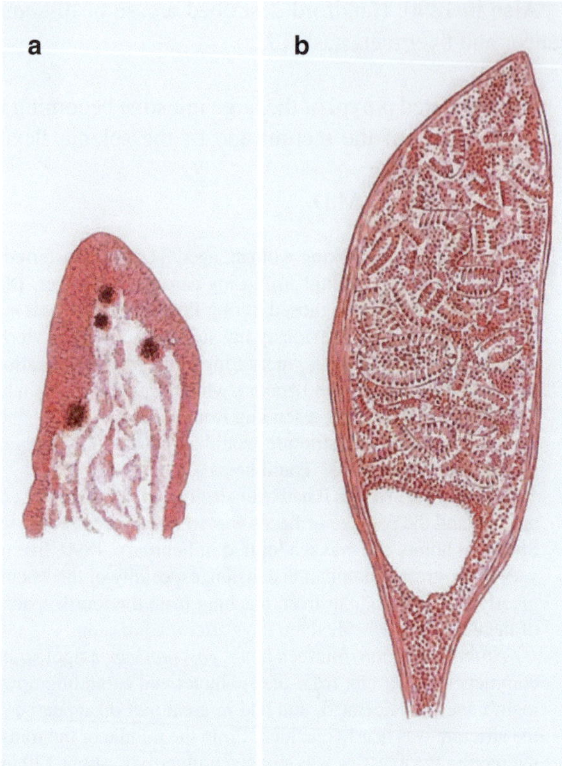

Fig. 136.4b—Portion of a section of a much larger sessile polypus of the splenic flexure of the colon in the same case. The growth is becoming malignant (malignant adenoma), has infiltrated the wall of the bowel, and caused a stricture. (Portions of this section were indistinguishable from sections of the secondary growths in the liver.)

Thus, in 1890, by using the term "malignant adenoma," Handford recognized the progression of adenoma to malignancy. He also recognized the association of colon cancer and hepatic metastasis.

In meticulous autopsy studies of polyposis patients published in 1907, Doering documented the association of colonic polyposis and cancer. In addition, he demonstrated that while the jejunum and ileum were not involved, numerous polyps could develop in the duodenum as well as the stomach [4].

Die Polyposis intestini und ihre Beziehung zur carcinomatösen Degeneration Von Privatdocent Dr. Hans Doering Assistentarzt der Klinik der chirurgischen Universitätsklink zu Göttingen.	Intestinal polyposis and its relation to carcinomatous degeneration By Private lecturer Dr. Hans Doering Assistant physician From the Surgical University Clinic in Göttingen.
Eigene Beobachtung 1. Hermann O., 16 Jahre alt. Zum ersten Mal aufgenommen am 27. 3. 1900.	Personal observations 1. Hermann O., 16 years old. First encounter on 3. 27. 1900.
Nach Mittheilung der überweisenden Arztes soll die Mutter und deren Bruder an Rectumkrebs gestorben sein. Ob neben den Tumoren noch Polypenbildung vorhanden war, ist unbekannt. Der Pat. selbst leidet schon seit langer Zeit an lästigem Stuhldrang. Dabei kommt es oft zum Vorfall weicher, leicht blutender Polypen, die nach der Defäcation meist von selbst ins Rectum zurückschlüpfen. Im Allgemeinen sind die Blutungen gering; alle 4—5 Wochen erfolgt jedoch ein stärkerer Blutabgang.	According to the referring doctor, the mother and brother both died of rectal cancer. Whether polyps were found in addition to the cancer is not known. The patient himself has been suffering for a long time with an annoying urge to defecate. This often results in the prolapse of soft, easily bleeding polyps, which usually slip back into the rectum on their own. The bleeding is mostly slight however, every 4—5 weeks, there is a greater loss of blood.
4.1.1907. Bei der Digitaluntersuchung des Rectums findet man etwa 2 cm oberhalb des Anus eine derbe, circuläre, nur wenig verschiebliche Resistenz, die ulcerirt ist und an deren oberes Ende man nicht gelangen kann.	1. 4. 1907: On digital examination of the rectum, one finds about 2 cm above the anus a firm circular, only slightly displaceable resistance which is ulcerated and the upper end of which cannot be reached.
12.1 Operation: Da eine Exstirpation des Carcinoms wegen seiner festen Verwachsungen unmöglich, Anlegung eines Anus praeternaturalis.	12.1. operation: Since extirpation of the cancer is not possible due to firm adhesion, application of an artificial anus.

Following the patient's death, an autopsy was performed.

Autopsie:	Autopsy:
Das ganze colon oberhalb der Geschwulst, also bis zur Ileocoecalklappe, is geröthet. An der geschwollenen Schleimhaut sitzen massenhaft hirsekorn- bis haselnussgrosse, mehr oder weniger deutlich gestielte, weiche Knoten von röthlicher Farbe. Die grösseren sind an ihrer Oberfläche leicht ulcerirt und mit graugelblichen Belage bedeckt. In Coecum finden sich ebenfalls zahlose, aber nur linsengrosse Knötchen. Ileum und Jejunum sind davon frei. Im Duodenum finden sich wieder zahlreiche, zum Theil ziemlich lang gestielte bis haselnussgrosse Auswüchse der Schleimhaut, die an ihrer Oberfläche ein zerklüftetes Aussehen haben. Sie besitzen Hanfkorn- bis Wallnussgrösse. Die Papille ist durchgängig und entleert dunkelgelbe Galle. Magenschleimhaut mit vielen Längsfalten versehen, ist an einigen Stellen deutlich grobhöckerig. Pathol. -anatom. Diagnose: Polyposis intestinalis vorzugsweise im Duodenum und Colon. Carcinom in der Ampulle des Rectums und an der Flexura hepatica coli. Mehere krebsige Geschwüre im Colon. Beginnende Polypenbildung im Magen, chronische Gastritis.	The entire colon above the tumor; i.e., up to the ileocecal valve is reddened. Masses of millet grain to hazel nut sized, more or less clearly stalked, soft nodules of a reddish color are attached to the swollen membrane. The larger sides are slightly ulcerated on their surface and covered with greyish-yellow coatings. In the cecum there are also numerous, but only lentil-sized nodules. Ileum and jejunum are free from it. In the duodenum there are again numerous outgrowths of the mucous membrane, some of which have quite long pedicles up to the size of a hazelnut and which have a fissured appearance on their surface. They are hemp seed to walnut size. The papilla is patent and drains yellow bile. The gastric mucosa with many longitudinal folds, is clearly rough in some places. Pathological anatomical diagnosis: Intestinal polyposis primarily in the duodenum and colon. Carcinoma in the ampulla of the rectum and at the flexura hepatica coli. Several cancerous ulcers in the colon. Incipient formation of polyps in the stomach, chronic gastritis.

In 1925, the familial nature of colonic adenomatous polyposis and the progression from adenoma to cancer were succinctly stated by Lockhart-Mummery.

Cancer and Heredity
By P. Lockhart-Mummery, F.R.C.S. Eng,
Senior Surgeon to St. Mark's Hospital
for Diseases of the Rectum.
Clinical and Family Records

Case 1.—A young woman, aged 31, came into my ward at St. Mark's Hospital with multiple polypi of the colon. Examination showed that she had a vast number of simple adenomatous polypi throughout the visible part of the rectum and colon, when examined with the sigmoidoscope. I removed her colon, as the only feasible means of relieving her, and she made a good recovery. The colon removed was found to be studded with adenomata as far as the ascending colon.

I was already aware that this condition of multiple adenomata was invariably antecedent to carcinoma, one or more of the adenomata sooner or later undergoing malignant change. I also knew that the condition of multiple adenomata is often hereditary in a marked degree, and with this view I asked my house surgeon, Mr. J. C. Anderson, to make careful inquiries into this patient's family history, and as a result the following extraordinary family history was obtained.

The patient is one of a family of four, and on her mother's side had nine uncles and aunts. Seven of these, including her mother, have died of cancer of the bowel at ages between 30 and 54, and her maternal grandfather also died of cancer of the bowel." (Chart 1, Figure 136.5).

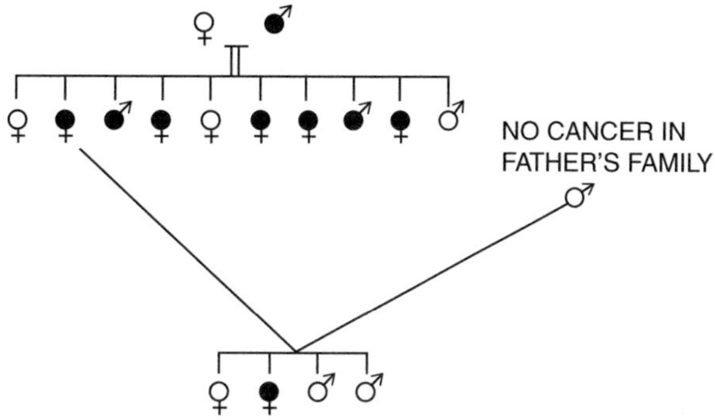

Fig. 136.5 Lockhart-Mummery's Chart 1.—Family History of Case 1. Cases indicated in black had either cancer or multiple adenomatous polyps of the bowel or both. This Figure is reused with the generous permission of Elsevier, CCC | RightsLink, License Number 5714390505982, License Date Jan 22, 2024

[This excerpt is reused with the generous permission of Elsevier, CCC | RightsLink, License Number 5714360882676, License date Jan 22, 2024]

Lockhart-Mummery's conclusion regarding colorectal cancer and heredity was as follows[5]:

Conclusion

1. Adenomatosis of the large bowel is a condition which tends to develop in succeeding generations in the same family.
2. Individuals with multiple adenomata of the large bowel almost invariably develop cancer in one or more of the adenomata after a few years.
3. The members of families with an hereditary tendency to multiple adenomata tend to die of cancer of the large bowel, and at an early age.
4. Simple adenomata of the large bowel are a common antecedent of cancer.

In 1928, Jüngling [6] described a kindred in which intestinal polyposis is inherited through generations. The dominant nature of intestinal polyposis and its tendency toward death from rectal carcinoma was noted (Fig. 136.6).

In 1950, Gardner and Stephens described familial cancer of the lower digestive tract.

Cancer of the Lower Digestive Tract in One Family Group
Eldon J. Gardner and Fayette E. Stephens
Laboratory of Human Genetics,
University of Utah,
Salt Lake City 1, Utah

> "Nine cases of carcinoma of the lower digestive tract have been detected among the descendants of one couple. A total of 45 members are included in the group. The primary site in eight of these cases was localized in the bowel or rectum. The evidence indicates an inherited tendency favoring carcinoma of the lower digestive tract coming through the mother's side of the family."

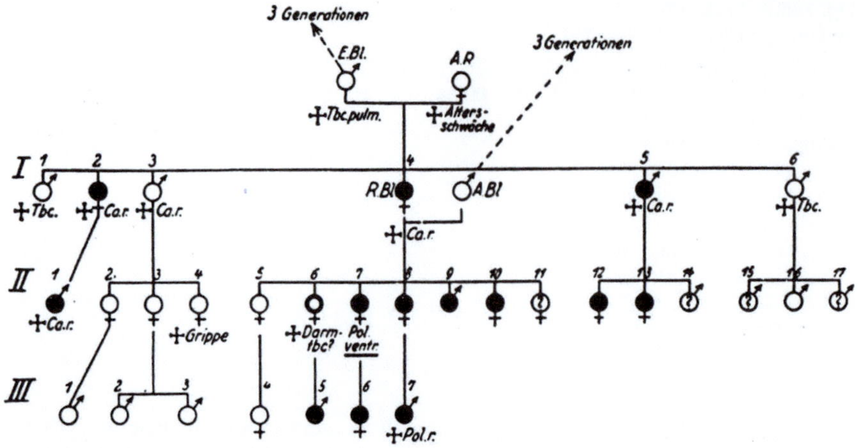

Fig. 136.6 Three generation kindred described by Jüngling in 1928 showing the incidence of intestinal polyposis (black discs); deceased (Cross); rectal carcinoma (Ca.r.); tuberculosis (Tbc); Flu (Grippe); intestine (Darm); Pol (polyp); Polyposis ventriculi (Pol. ventr)

Polyposis intestini
Hereditäre Verhältnisse und Beziehungen zum Carcinom
Von
Prof. Dr. Otto Jüngling
Aus der Chirurgischen Universitätsklinik zu Tübingen und der Chirurgischen Abteilung des Städtischen Katharinenhospitals zu Stuttgart

Eine von mir seit dem Jahre 1912 verfolgte Familienkrankengeschichte scheint auf einige der angeschittenen Fragen Licht zu werfen. Ich habe im vergangenen Jahre Herrn Hüchtemann veranlaßt, der Familiengeschichte weiter nachzugehen und alle erreichbaren, auch die seitdem geborenen Mitglieder der Familie nachzuuntersuchen. Herr Hüchtemann hat seine Beobachtungen in einer Dissertation niedergelegt. Ich beziehe mich im Folgenden im wesentlichen auf die Ergebnisse seiner Nachforschung.

In dem Stammbaum sind die Fälle von nachgewiesener Polyposis intestini mit schwarzen Scheiben, die Fälle, bei denen keine Polyposis vorlag, mit Kreisen bezeichnet. Nicht nachuntersuchte Fälle der jetzt noch lebenden Generationen haben ein Fragezeichen im Kreise.

Dieser Stammbaum läßt keine andere Deutung als die einer dominanten Vererbung zu. Durchweg is mehr als die Hälfte der kinder erkrankt,…

Die Prognose der polyposis intestini ist sehr traurig. Von unserem material sind sämtliche Fälle der I. Generation an Rectumcarcinom gestorben. Von den 8 Kranken der II. Generation is ein Mann an Rectumcarcinom gestorben,... Von der III. Generation ist ein Knabe im Alter von 15 Jahren an Verblutung im Laufe einiger Jahre zugrunde gegangen.

Intestinal polyposis
Hereditary conditions and relationships to carcinoma
By
Prof. Dr. Otto Jüngling
From the Surgical University Clinic in Tübingen and the Surgical Department of the State Katharinen Hospitals in Stuttgart

A family case history that I have followed since 1912 seems to throw light on some of the questions raised. In the past year I have persuaded Mr. Hüchtemann to further investigate the family history and to examine all the family members who can be contacted including those who have been born since then. Mr. Hüchtemann has laid down his observations in a dissertation. In the following, I essentially refer to the results of his investigations.

In the pedigree, cases of detected intestinal polyposis are denoted by black discs, cases without polyposis by circles. Unexamined cases of the now living generations have a questions mark in a circle.

This pedigree allows no other interpretation than that of dominant inheritance. More than half of the children always are affected,…

The prognosis of intestinal polyposis is very sad. From our material, all of the first-generation cases have died of rectal cancer. Of the eight affected in the second-generation, one man died of rectal cancer. From generation III, a 15-year-old boy died from bleeding that occurred over a year.

Fig. 136.7 Kindred 109 Chart 1 showing descendants of man and his first wife described by Gardner and Stephens in 1950 (Permission to reproduce this figure was generously received from Elsevier Science and technology journals license terms and conditions. License number 4250771077848, license date, Dec. 16, 2017)

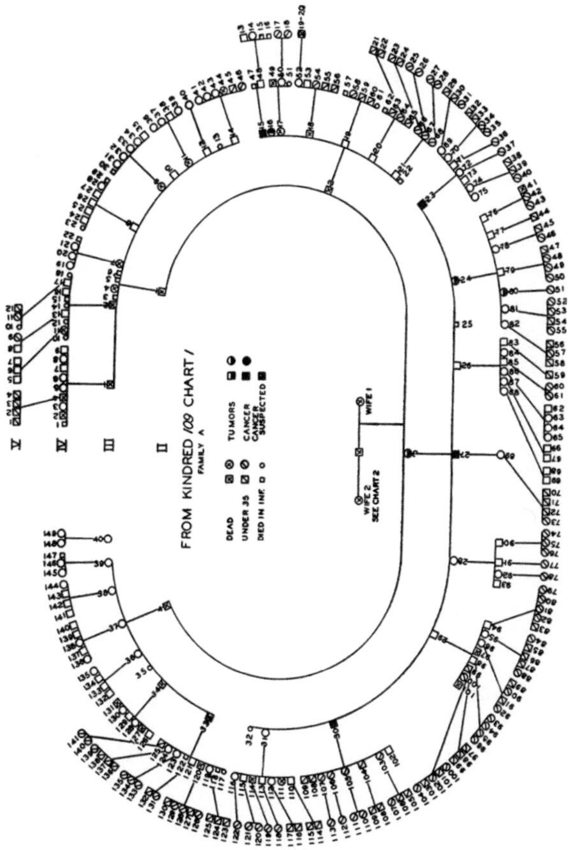

FIG. 1. Pedigree of Kindred 109, showing descendents of *I-2*'s first wife.

Part of the family (Kindred 109) is shown in Fig. 136.7.

In subsequent articles, Gardner and colleagues described hereditary polyposis and extraintestinal manifestations of abnormal growth including epidermoid cysts, fibromas, and osteomatosis, a syndrome now referred to as Gardner's syndrome [7, 8].

"Classical" FAP has been defined by the presence of >100 synchronous colorectal adenomas [9, 10]. However, the number of polyps in FAP actually varies from less than one hundred to thousands [11].

The first clue as to the location of the gene responsible for FAP was provided by Herrera et al. [12] who, in 1986, reported a case of a 42-year-old male with mental retardation, colon carcinoma, horseshoe kidney, absence of left lobe of the liver, agenesis of the gallbladder, and possible Gardner's syndrome. Chromosome analysis revealed an interstitial deletion of 5q. Shortly after that, in 1987, Bodmer et al. [13] demonstrated that the FAP gene is located on chromosome 5. In the same year, Leppert and coworkers [14] studied five kindreds segregating a gene for adenomatous polyposis coli. Linkage analysis determined that the defective gene was located on the long arm of chromosome

5. In 1991, Groden et al. [15] reported the identification and characterization of the familial adenomatous polyposis coli gene. A less severe form of familial polyposis, attenuated adenomatous polyposis coli (AAPC), is characterized by a low number of adenomatous polyps (usually less than 100), and with an elevated colon cancer risk. In 1993, Spirio et al. [16] described mutations near the 5′ end of APC gene that provided the molecular basis for AAPC. The identification of mutations of the APC gene led to presymptomatic diagnosis by screening for truncated APC gene products. The mechanism by which cancer develops in patients with FAP follows the model of Knudson who, in 1971, proposed that certain cancers are caused by two mutational events [17, 18].

> Mutation and Cancer: Statistical Study of Retinoblastoma
> Alfred G. Knudson, Jr.
> Graduate School of Biomedical Sciences and
> M.D. Anderson Hospital and Tumor Institute,
> The University of Texas at Houston
> Houston, Texas
>
> "Based on observations on 48 cases of retinoblastoma and published reports, the hypothesis is developed that retinoblastoma is a cancer caused by two mutational events. In the dominantly inherited form, one mutation is inherited via germinal cells and the second occurs in somatic cells. In the nonhereditary form, both mutations occur in somatic cells."

A heterozygous condition is created when a mutated and a normal allele are present. An alteration in the remaining normal allele produces two abnormal alleles and a loss of heterozygosity (LOH) [19]. The APC gene product is a protein that serves as a tumor suppressor [20].

Surgical Management

One of the primary aims of colorectal surgery in the treatment of patients with FAP is the prevention of colorectal cancer. Several colorectal surgical options for FAP are listed in Table 136.1 [21–23].

Thomson attributes the practice of performing colectomy with ileorectal anastomosis (IRA) to Lloyd-Davies in 1948 [21]. The continent ileostomy was reported by Kock in 1975 for reconstruction after proctocolectomy for ulcerative colitis [22]. Restorative proctocolectomy was reported by Parks and Nicholls in 1978 [23]. Each of these surgical approaches has advantages as well as disadvantages. Total proctocolectomy removes all large intestinal mucosa at risk for cancer, but the patient has a permanent ileostomy. IRA leaves rectal mucosa which might later develop cancer. Continent ileostomy has a nipple valve that frequently requires revision. Restorative

Table 136.1 Surgical options for FAP

Surgical options
Proctocolectomy with end ileostomy
Ileorectal anastomosis
Continent ileostomy
Restorative proctocolectomy

proctocolectomy continues to be used widely by surgeons familiar with pelvic surgery.

Looking forward to the day when means other than surgery may be found for the treatment of polyposis and the prevention of cancer, Dukes, in his Hunterian Lecture delivered at the Royal College of Surgeons of England on March 25th, 1952, provoked his audience to think of the possibilities of new methods of investigation and treatment reciting a poem, imagining a young surgeon addressing an elderly nonaffected member of a polyposis family [24]:[1]

"You are old, Father William," the young surgeon said,
  "And your colon from polyps is free.
Yet most of your siblings are known to be dead –
  A really *bad* family tree."

"In my youth," Father William replied with a grin,
  "I was told that a gene had mutated,
That all who carried this dominant gene
  To polyps and cancer were *fated.*

"I sought for advice from a surgical friend,
  Who sighed and said – 'Without doubt
Your only escape from an untimely end
  Is to have your intestine *right out.*'

It seemed rather bad luck – I was then but nineteen –
  So I went and consulted a quack,
Who took a firm grip on my dominant gene
  And promptly *mutated it back.*"

"This," said the surgeon, "is something quite new
  And before we ascribe any merit
We must see if the claims of this fellow are true,
  And observe what your *children* inherit!"
Cuthbert E. Dukes, O.B.E., M.D., F.R.C.S.
Pathologist, St. Mark's and St. Peter's Hospitals, London

References

1. Cripps WH. Two cases of disseminated polypus of the rectum. Trans Pathol Soc London. 1882;33:165–8.
2. Cripps H. Polypus of the rectum. Illustrated Med News. 1890;18:51–53, 80–82.
3. Handford H. Disseminated polypi of the large intestine becoming malignant; strictures (malignant adenoma) of the rectum and of the splenic flexure of the colon; secondary growths in the liver. Trans Pathol Soc London. 1890;41:133–7.

[1] Permission to reproduce this poem was obtained from the Royal College of Surgeons of England, Order License ID 1327044-1; Copyright Clearance Center. Invoice number: TRX20044394, Fri 2/24/2023.

4. Doering H. Die Polyposis intestini und ihre Beziehung zur carcinomatösen Degeneration. Archiv Klin Chir. 1907;83:194–227.
5. Lockhart-Mummery P. Cancer and heredity. Lancet. 1925;205(5296):427–9.
6. Jüngling O. Polyposis intestini. Hereditäre Verhältnisse und Beziehungen zum Carcinom. Bruns Beitr klin Chir. 1928;143:476–83.
7. Gardner EJ. A genetic and clinical study of intestinal polyposis, a predisposing factor for carcinoma of the colon and rectum. Am J Hum Genet. 1951;3:167–76.
8. Gardner EJ, Richards RC. Multiple cutaneous and subcutaneous lesions occurring simultaneously with hereditary polyposis and osteomatosis. Am J Hum Genet. 1953;5:139–47.
9. Ellis CN. Colonic adenomatous polyposis syndromes: Clinical management. Clin Colon Rectal Surg. 2008;21:256–62.
10. Bussey HJR. Familial Polyposis Coli. Family Studies, Histopathology, Differential Diagnosis, and Results of Treatment. Baltimore, MD: Johns Hopkins University Press, 1975. p. 89.
11. Cleveland Clinic. Familial adenomatous polyposis coli. myclevelandclinic.org/health/diseases/16993-familial-adenomatous-polyposis-fap. Accessed 6 Mar 2023.
12. Herrera L, Kakati S, Gibas L, Pietrzak E, Sandberg AA. Brief clinical report: Gardner syndrome in a man with an interstitial deletion of 5q. Am J Med Genet. 1986;25:473–6.
13. Bodmer WF, Bailey CJ, Bodmer J, Bussey HJR, Ellis A, Gorman P, et al. Localization of the gene for familial adenomatous polyposis on chromosome 5. Nature. 1987;328:614–6.
14. Leppert M, Dobbs M, Scambler P, O'Connell P, Nakamura Y, Stauffer D, et al. The gene for familial polyposis coli maps to the long arm of chromosome 5. Science. 1987;238:1411–3.
15. Groden J, Thliveris A, Samowitz W, Carlson M, Gelbert L, Albertsen H, et al. Identification and characterization of the familial adenomatous polyposis coli gene. Cell. 1991;66:589–600.
16. Spirio L, Olschwang S, Groden J, Robertson M, Samowitz W, Joslyn G, et al. Alleles of the *APC* gene: An attenuated form of familial polyposis. Cell. 1993;75:951–7.
17. Knudson AG Jr. Mutation and cancer: statistical study of retinoblastoma. Proc Natl Acad Sci. 1971;68:820–3.
18. Knudson AG Jr. Genetics of human cancer. Annu Rev Genet. 1986;20:231–51.
19. Fearnhead NS, Britton MP, Bodmer WF. The ABC of APC. Hum Mol Genet. 2001;10:721–33.
20. Lesko AC, Goss KH, Yang FF, Schwertner A, Hulur I, Onel K, Prosperi JR. The APC tumor suppressor is required for epithelial cell polarization and three-dimensional morphogenesis. Biochim Biophys Acta. 2015;1854:711–23.
21. Thomson JPS. Familial adenomatous polyposis: the large bowel. Ann R Coll Surg Engl. 1990;72:177–80.
22. Kock NG. Intra-abdominal "reservoir" in patients with permanent ileostomy. Preliminary observations on a procedure resulting in fecal "continence" in five ileostomy patients. Arch Surg. 1969;99:223–31.
23. Parks AG, Nicholls RJ. Proctocolectomy without ileostomy for ulcerative colitis. Br Med J. 1978;2:85–8.
24. Dukes CE. Familial intestinal polyposis. Hunterian Lecture delivered at the Royal College of Surgeons of England on 25th March, 1952. Ann R Coll Surg Engl. 1952;10:293–304.

Lynch Syndrome

137

James S. Wu, Brandie Leach, Charis Eng,
David Hernandez Gonzalo, and Eric W. Willis

Presentation

A right colon moderately differentiated adenocarcinoma was found in a 50-year-old male on screening colonoscopy. He has a first-degree relative who had colon cancer. PCR-based testing of the tumor for microsatellite instability showed that all five of the tested loci were unstable and that MSH2 showed no expression. Computed tomography (CT) showed the location of the carcinoma (Fig. 137.1).

Histopathology is shown in Fig. 137.2.

J. S. Wu (✉)
Department of Colon and Rectal Surgery, Cleveland Clinic, Cleveland, OH, USA

B. Leach · C. Eng
Genomic Medicine Institute and Center for Personalized Genetic Healthcare, Cleveland Clinic, Cleveland, OH, USA

D. Hernandez Gonzalo
Department of Pathology, Immunology and Laboratory Medicine, University of Florida, Gainesville, FL, USA

E. W. Willis
Department of Pathology, CORPath, Columbus, OH, USA

J. S. Wu, M. D. Inkster (eds.), *Cleveland Clinic Colorectal Case Studies*,
https://doi.org/10.1007/978-3-031-39880-3_137

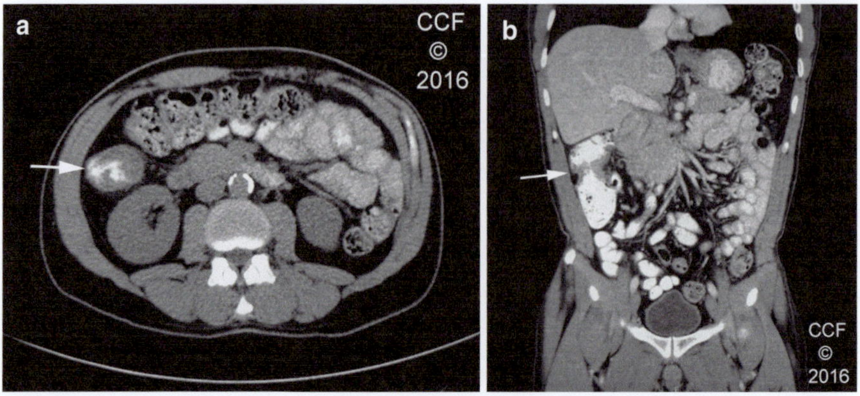

Fig. 137.1 (**a**, **b**) CT scans show a near obstructing ascending colon cancer (arrows)

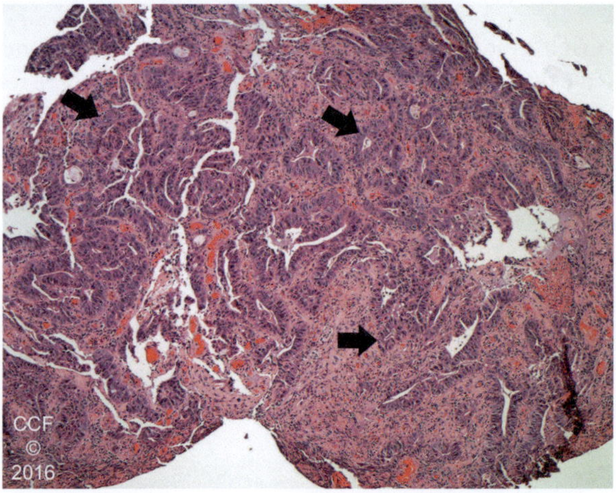

Fig. 137.2 Ascending colon biopsy showing angular and infiltrative neoplastic glands (arrows) penetrating into the submucosa surrounded by a desmoplastic stroma (hematoxylin–eosin, original magnification ×50)

Management

Subtotal colectomy with ileorectal anastomosis was done (Fig. 137.3).

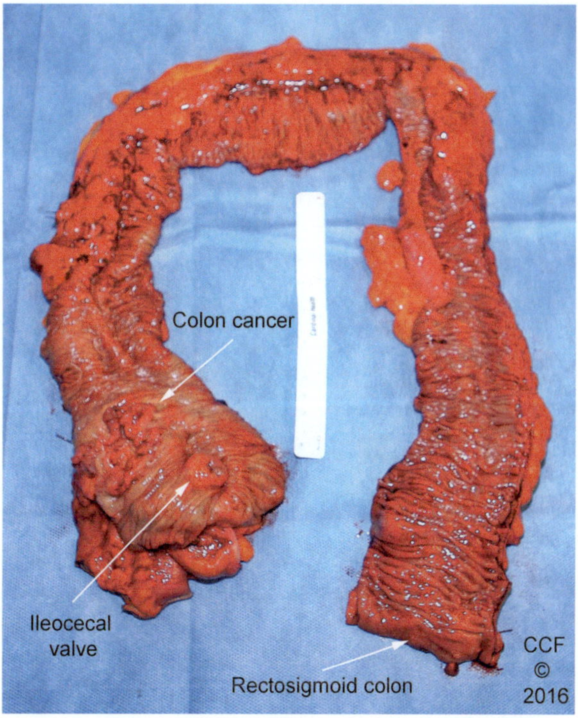

Fig. 137.3 The terminal ileum and colon from the cecum to the rectum have been removed. The specimen contained a right-sided colon cancer (arrow). The ileocecal valve and rectosigmoid colon have been marked as points of reference

Comment

In 1913, Warthin described "Family G," a kindred in which cancers of the stomach, uterus, and intestine appeared in three successive generations (Fig. 137.4) [1, 2].

In 1971, Lynch and Krush revisited Family G and found 95 individuals who had developed cancer predominantly of the colon, endometrium, and stomach [3]. Now called Lynch syndrome, this is a hereditary condition that accounts for about 1–5% of colorectal cancers [4]. Clinical features are shown in Table 137.1.

This patient's colorectal adenocarcinoma was found to have high levels of microsatellite instability [5]. There was no evidence of a *BRAF* mutation. Germline analysis of the *MLH1* and *MSH2* genes revealed the deleterious mutation c.1226_1227delAG in *MSH2*, which confirmed the diagnosis of Lynch syndrome [5–12].

Genetic testing of this patient's colon cancer before surgery changed management. Without the information provided by genetic testing, he would have undergone right hemicolectomy alone. Knowing the diagnosis of Lynch syndrome, his entire colon was removed to decrease the risk of metachronous colorectal cancer. His diagnosis also led to screening of his family for gene carriers. He continues to undergo yearly endoscopic examination of the remaining rectum.

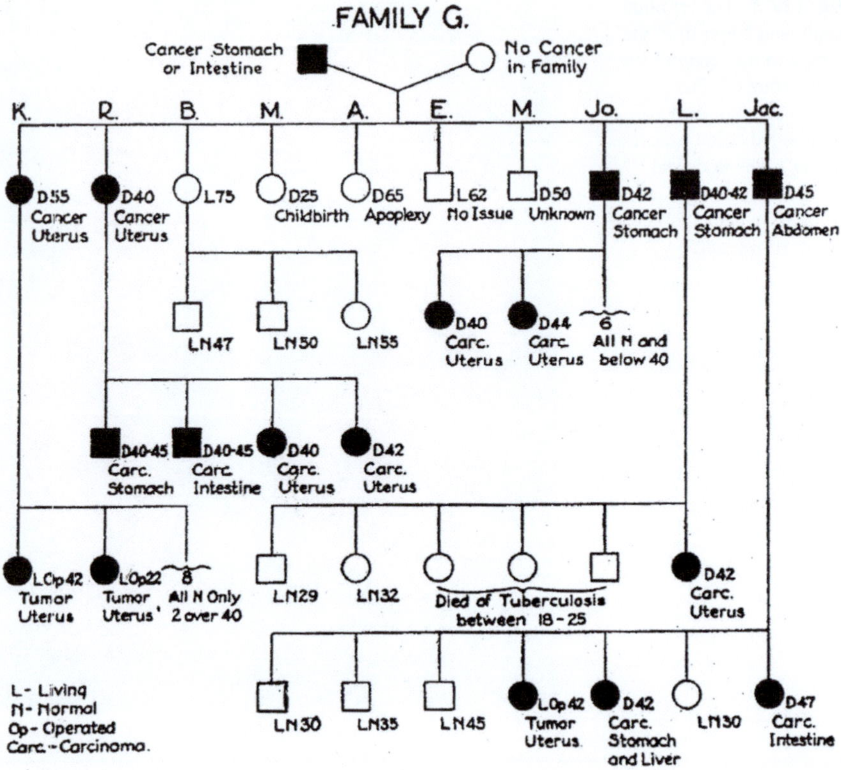

Fig. 137.4 Warthin's "Family G" documenting cancers of the stomach, uterus, and intestine in three successive generations

Table 137.1 Clinical features of Lynch syndrome

Clinical features
Autosomal dominant
Early onset of colon cancer (~44 years)
Excess cancers proximal to the splenic flexure (~70%)
Synchronous and metachronous cancers
Extracolonic malignancies (endometrial, ovary, stomach, small intestine, renal pelvis, ureter, pancreas, skin, brain)
Lifetime colorectal cancer risk of 15–80%
Mismatch repair genes
MLH1, chromosome 3
MSH2, chromosome 2
EPCAM, chromosome 2
MSH6, chromosome 2
PMS2, chromosome 7

In 2019, Ami MacKay published a memoir entitled, *Daughter of Family G: A Memoir of Cancer Genes, Love, and Fate* [13], in which she recounts her family's legacy of hereditary cancer, a story that begins with the 1895 fateful meeting between Dr. Warthin and Ms. Pauline Gross, a dressmaker, of a family in which cancer of the gastrointestinal and female organs was common.

References

1. Warthin AS. Heredity with reference to carcinoma as shown by the study of the cases examined in the pathological laboratory of the University of Michigan, 1895–1913. Arch Intern Med. 1913;12:546–55.
2. Warthin AS. The further study of a cancer family. J Cancer Res. 1925;9:279–86.
3. Lynch HT, Krush AJ. Cancer family "G" revisited: 1895–1970. Cancer. 1971;27:1505–11.
4. Lynch HT, Smyrk T. Hereditary nonpolyposis colorectal cancer (Lynch syndrome), an updated review. Cancer. 1996;78:1149–67.
5. Thibodeau SN, Bren G, Schaid D. Microsatellite instability in cancer of the proximal colon. Science. 1993;260:816–9.
6. Papadopoulos N, Nicolaides NC, Wei Y-F, Ruben SM, Carter KC, Rosen CA, et al. Mutation of a *mutL* homolog in hereditary colon cancer. Science. 1994;263:1625–9.
7. Bronner CE, Baker SM, Morrison PT, Warren G, Smith LG, Lescoe MK, et al. Mutation in the DNA mismatch repair gene homologue *hMLH1* is associated with hereditary non-polyposis colon cancer. Nature. 1994;368:258–61.
8. Leach FS, Nicolaides NC, Papadopoulos N, Liu B, Jen J, Parsons R, et al. Mutations of a *mutS* homolog in hereditary nonpolyposis colorectal cancer. Cell. 1993;75:1215–25.
9. Fishel R, Lescoe MK, Rao MRS, Copeland NG, Jenkins NA, Garber J, et al. The human mutator gene homolog *MSH2* and its association with hereditary nonpolyposis colon cancer. Cell. 1993;75:1027–38.
10. Nicolaides NC, Papadopoulos N, Liu B, Wei Y-F, Carter KC, Ruben SM, et al. Mutations of two *PMS* homologues in hereditary nonpolyposis colon cancer. Nature. 1994;371:75–80.
11. Ligtenberg MJL, Kuiper RP, Chan TL, Goossens M, Hebeda KM, Voorendt M, et al. Heritable somatic methylation and inactivation of *MSH2* in families with Lynch syndrome due to deletion of the 3′ exons of *TACSTD1*. Nat Genet. 2009;41:112–7.
12. Kovacs ME, Papp J, Szentirmay Z, Otto S, Olah E. Deletions removing the last exon of TACSTD1 constitute a distinct class of mutations predisposing to Lynch syndrome. Hum Mutat. 2009;30:197–203.
13. McKay A. Daughter of Family G: A memoir of cancer genes, love and fate. Canada: Knopf; 2019.

138 Colon Cancer-Principles of Oncologic Resection

James S. Wu

Presentation

> "In the large intestine the growth itself must be removed, a length of bowel on each side of the growth, the lymph vessels which drain the bowel, the glands in which those vessels end (all the primary glands, that is, and as many of the secondary as are accessible), and finally all the tissue in which those glands and vessels lie."
> Berkeley G. A. Moynihan, M.D., F.R.C.S., Leeds, 1908 [1]

In 1909, Jamieson and Dobson published an article entitled, *The Lymphatics of the Colon*. The concepts presented were so important that they were published twice, once in the Proceedings of the Royal Society of Medicine [2] and again in the Annals of Surgery [3]. In each, the authors defined the operative treatment of colon cancer in different anatomic locations based on the necessity of removing draining lymphatic glands.

> The lymphatics of the colon. With special reference to the operative treatment of cancer of the colon.
>
> 'To minimize as far as possible the likelihood of recurrence, it is necessary to remove with the primary growth those glands which are likely to have become affected.
>
> The ideal operation consists in removing a considerable length of gut on each side of the growth, the primary glands, together with the vessels running to them from the gut, and the tissues in which these vessels lie—i.e., the so-called "lymphatic area."'
>
> J. Kay Jamison, M.B., University of Leeds
>
> J. F. Dobson, M.S., F.R.C.S., Leeds General Infirmary

J. S. Wu (✉)
Department of Colon and Rectal Surgery, Cleveland Clinic, Cleveland, OH, USA

J. S. Wu, M. D. Inkster (eds.), *Cleveland Clinic Colorectal Case Studies*,
https://doi.org/10.1007/978-3-031-39880-3_138

References

1. Moynihan BGA. The surgical treatment of cancer of the sigmoid flexure and rectum. Surg Gynecol Obstet. 1908;6:463–6.
2. Jamieson JK, Dobson JF. The lymphatics of the colon. Proc R Soc Med 1909;2(Surg Sect):149–74.
3. Jamieson JK, Dobson JF. The lymphatics of the colon. With special reference to the operative treatment of cancer of the colon. Ann Surg. 1909;50:1077–90. These excerpts were reused with the generous permission of Wolters Kluwers Health, Inc., CCC | RightsLink®, License number 5156560086402, License date Sep 26, 2021

Sigmoid Colon Cancer

139

James S. Wu

Presentation

A patient was referred for colon adenocarcinoma found at the mid-sigmoid colon at colonoscopy.

Management

Sigmoid colectomy was done. A conceptual drawing showing the relation of the colon to external abdominal landmarks is shown in Fig. 139.1.

Principles of surgery include: [1, 2]

1. Vascular ligation of the inferior mesenteric artery and vein (Fig. 139.2).
2. Mobilization of the colon distal transverse colon, splenic flexure, left colon, sigmoid colon, and the proximal rectum. The inferior mesenteric vein is divided twice; first close to the inferior mesenteric artery and secondly close to the lower border of the pancreas. This second division allows the left colon to reach to the rectum for colorectal anastomosis.
3. The proximal line of resection is at the left colon–sigmoid colon junction.
4. The distal line of resection is at the proximal rectum.

The operative specimen is shown in Fig. 139.3.

J. S. Wu (✉)
Department of Colon and Rectal Surgery, Cleveland Clinic, Cleveland, OH, USA

J. S. Wu, M. D. Inkster (eds.), *Cleveland Clinic Colorectal Case Studies*,
https://doi.org/10.1007/978-3-031-39880-3_139

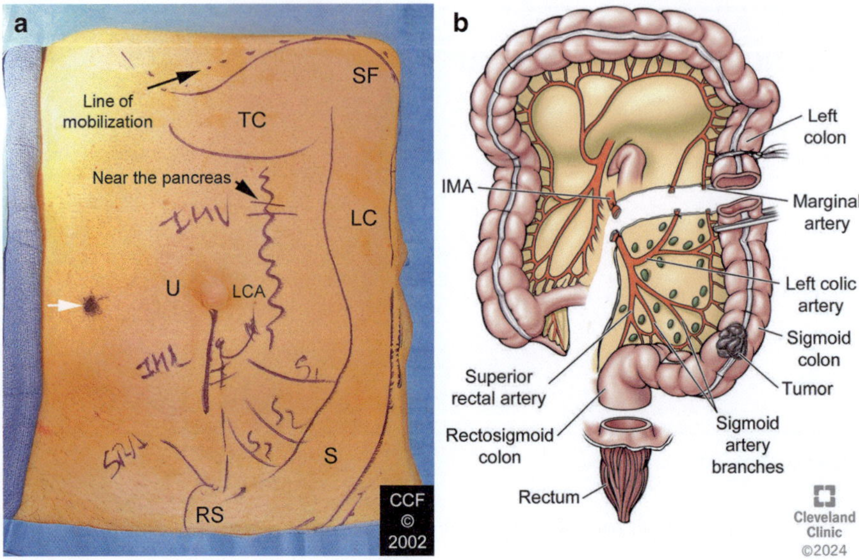

Fig. 139.1 (**a**) Conceptual drawing showing the relation of the colon to external abdominal landmarks. The transverse colon (TC), splenic flexure (SF), left colon (LC), sigmoid colon (S), and rectosigmoid (RS) junction are labeled. The inferior mesenteric artery (IMA), inferior mesenteric vein (IMV), and left colic artery (LCA) are divided. The IMV (squiggle) is divided near the IMA and close to the lower border of the pancreas. The umbilicus (U) and a stoma site (white arrow) also are shown. The abdomen was entered through a midline incision. The inferior mesenteric artery (IMA) plus branches of the sigmoid artery are labeled (S1, S2, and S3). The superior rectal artery (SRA) is marked adjacent to the proximal rectum; (**b**) Illustration showing sigmoid colon cancer resection. High ligation of the inferior mesenteric artery is done. In addition, the left colic artery and the marginal artery (adjacent to the left colon-sigmoid colon junction) are divided. Proximally, the colon is divided at the left-colon-sigmoid colon junction. Distally, the line of resection is at the proximal rectum. The tumor, the sigmoid colon, and the accompanying lymph node bearing mesentery are resected. Additional labelled landmarks include the superior rectal and sigmoid arteries. To prevent fecal spillage, the left colon has been gently encircled with an umbilical tape; the proximal sigmoid colon has been closed with a clamp

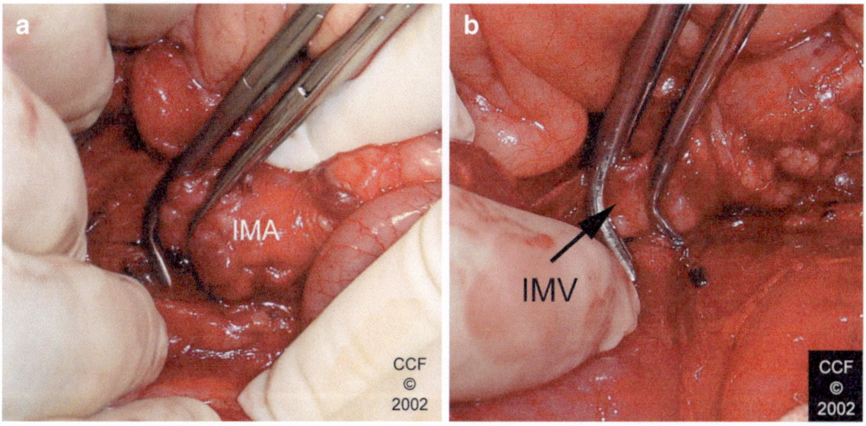

Fig. 139.2 (**a**) The inferior mesenteric artery (IMA) is isolated, divided, and ligated close to its aortic origin; (**b**) The inferior mesenteric vein is isolated, divided near the IMA. In both cases, vascular division is done between two tonsil clamps aligned in parallel. The tonsil clamp is suited for this purpose because it is curved and small. The parallel alignment allows the two clamps to fit into a confined space deep in the abdominal cavity. The tips curve away from the vessel origin on the side that will be ligated and toward the specimen on the side that will be removed

Fig. 139.3 Mid-sigmoid colon cancer. The entire sigmoid colon with its associated mesentery was resected. The lines of resection were the left colon proximally and the proximal rectum distally. The cancer was bisected during opening of the specimen

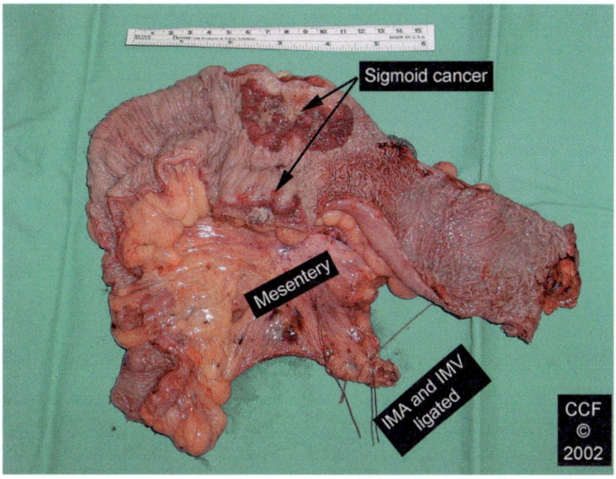

References

1. Jagelman DG. Colectomy for malignant disease of the colon: the 'no touch' isolation technique. In: Fielding LP, Goldberg SM, editors. Rob and Smith's Operative Surgery. Surgery of the Colon, Rectum and Anus. 5th ed. Oxford: Butterworth-Heinemann, Ltd; 1993. p. 359–68.
2. Jamieson JK, Dobson JF. The lymphatics of the colon. With special reference to the operative treatment of cancer of the colon. Ann Surg. 1909;50:1077–90.

Splenic Flexure Cancer

140

James S. Wu

Presentation

An 82-year-old man underwent colonoscopy because of a positive fecal occult blood test. Colonoscopy showed a mass at the splenic flexure (Fig. 140.1). Biopsy showed moderately differentiated adenocarcinoma. Evaluation for metastatic disease was negative.

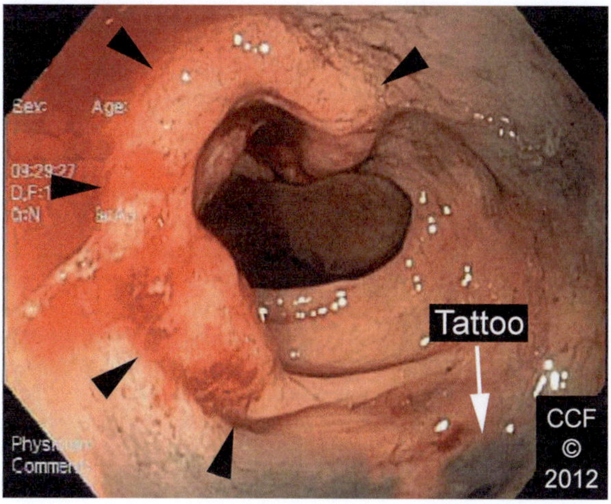

Fig. 140.1 Colonoscopy shows a cancer (arrowheads) encompassing 50% of the luminal circumference at the splenic flexure. The tumor site is marked with a tattoo (arrow)

J. S. Wu (✉)
Department of Colon and Rectal Surgery, Cleveland Clinic, Cleveland, OH, USA

J. S. Wu, M. D. Inkster (eds.), *Cleveland Clinic Colorectal Case Studies*,
https://doi.org/10.1007/978-3-031-39880-3_140

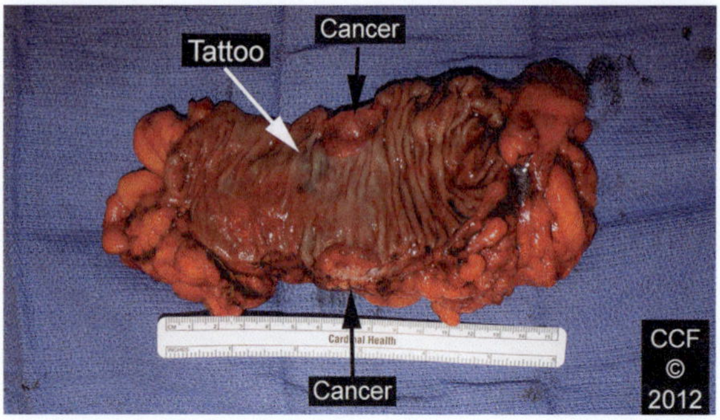

Fig. 140.2 Splenic flexure cancer. The distal transverse colon, splenic flexure, and left colon were excised. The cancer was bisected when the specimen was opened. The tattoo placed at colonoscopy is seen

Management

The left transverse colon, splenic flexure, and left colon along with the accompanying mesentery contained between the ligated left middle colic artery and the left colic artery were excised. The omentum attached to the left transverse colon also was excised. Pulsatile bleeding was seen both from the right transverse colon and the proximal sigmoid colon prior to anastomosis. Pathology showed moderately differentiated adenocarcinoma, T2N0 with 0/12 lymph nodes involved. There was no evidence of metastatic disease on abdominal exploration. The operative specimen is shown in Fig. 140.2.

Comment

In 1909, Jamieson and Dobson described *Operation for Growths in the Region of the Splenic Flexure*.[1]

> "The left colic artery is defined as it leaves the inferior mesenteric vein, and is tied at this point with the accompanying vein. The bowel is then freed by incising the peritoneum to the outer side of the descending colon and splenic flexure and separating the bowel with the growth, the peritoneum and the subperitoneal tissues containing the lymphatic glands and vessels from the posterior abdominal wall. The mesocolon is then divided from the point of ligature of the artery, upwards to a selected point on the transverse colon. The selection of this point will be determined by the extent of the transverse colon supplied by the middle colic artery; it will lie as a rule at the junction of the middle and left thirds of the transverse colon. The peritoneum is also divided in a direction downwards and outwards to the descending colon. At the selected point on the transverse colon, the bowel is divided; below, the descending colon is divided in its lower part and the operation is completed by an end-to-end anastomosis."
>
> J. Kay Jamieson, M.B.,
> Demonstrator of Anatomy in the University of Leeds
> J. F. Dobson, M.S., F.R.C.S.,
> Senior Assistant Surgeon to the Leeds General Infirmary

[1] Jamieson and Dobson [1]. This excerpt was reused with the generous permission of Wolters Kluwer Health, Inc., CCC|RightsLink®, License number 5156680911793, License date Sep 26, 2021.

An illustration of Jamieson and Dobson's operation is shown in Fig. 140.3.

Alternative operations reported for splenic flexure cancer are listed in Table 140.1.

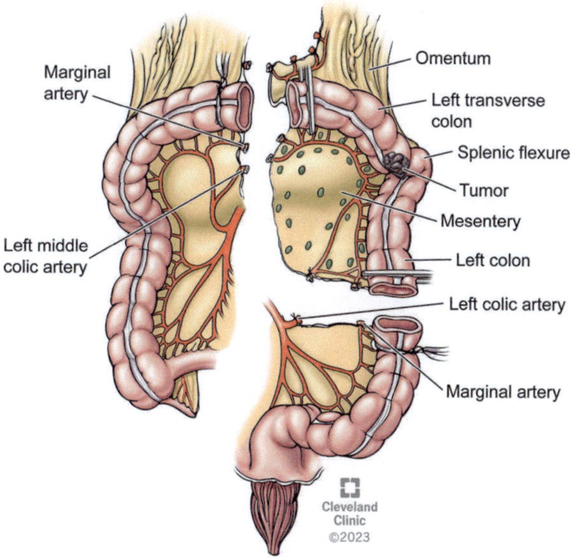

Fig. 140.3 Excision of splenic flexure cancer [1]. The cancer, the cancer bearing segment of colon extending from the left transverse colon to the lower part of the descending colon and the associated lymph node bearing mesentery were resected. The omentum attached to the left transverse colon was removed. The left middle colic artery, left colic artery, and regional marginal arteries were divided and ligated

Table 140.1 Operations for splenic flexure cancer [2, 3]

Operations
Segmental resection
Extended right hemicolectomy
Extended left hemicolectomy
Subtotal colectomy with ileosigmoid anastomosis

References

1. Jamieson JK, Dobson JF. The lymphatics of the colon. With special reference to the operative treatment of cancer of the colon. Ann Surg. 1909;50:1077–90.
2. Steffen C, Bokey EL, Chapuis PH. Carcinoma of the splenic flexure. Dis Colon Rectum. 1987;30:872–4.
3. Rega D, Pace U, Scala D, Chiodini P, Granata V, Bucci AF, et al. Treatment of splenic flexure colon cancer: a comparison of three different surgical procedures: Experience of a high volume cancer center. Sci Rep. 2019;9:10953. https://doi.org/10.1038/s41598-019-47548-z.

Transverse Colon Cancer

141

James S. Wu

Presentation A

A 65-year-old patient was referred for surgery to treat colorectal cancer situated in the mid-transverse colon. The preoperative assessment did not reveal metastatic disease.

Management

The patient underwent extended right hemicolectomy with ileocolic anastomosis (Fig. 141.1).

The cancer was located mid-way between the hepatic flexure and the splenic flexure. The terminal ileum, right colon, transverse colon and left colon along with the right colon, transverse colon and left colon mesenteries were excised. Bowel continuity was restored by ileocolic anastomosis.

J. S. Wu (✉)
Department of Colon and Rectal Surgery, Cleveland Clinic, Cleveland, OH, USA

J. S. Wu, M. D. Inkster (eds.), *Cleveland Clinic Colorectal Case Studies*,
https://doi.org/10.1007/978-3-031-39880-3_141

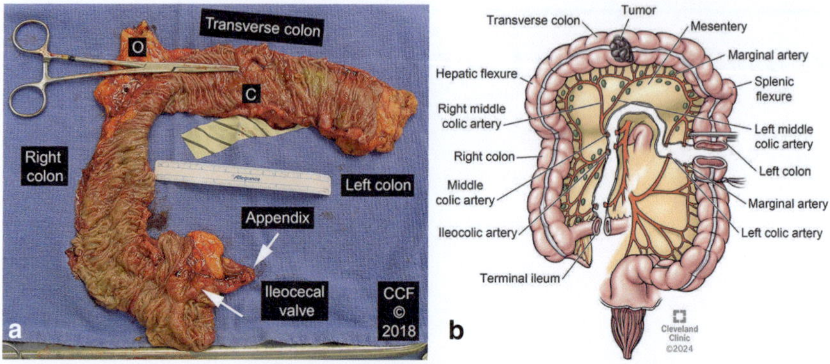

Fig. 141.1 (**a**) Extended right hemicolectomy to treat transverse colon cancer (C). The tumor site is marked by the tip of a clamp. The tumor, terminal ileum, right colon, transverse colon, and left colon with the accompanying lymph node bearing mesentery are removed. The omentum (O) marks the junction between the right and transverse colons. The ileocecal valve, appendix, right colon, transverse colon, and left colon have been labeled for reference. (**b**) Illustration of extended right colectomy for transverse colon cancer. The ileocolic, middle colic, left colic, and marginal arteries arteries are divided. The terminal ileum, right colon, transverse colon and left colon including their respective mesenteries are removed. Two methods of closing the ends of the divided colon (by clamp and by umbilical tape) to prevent bowel spillage are shown

Presentation B

A mid-transverse colon cancer was found on colonoscopy. Metastatic disease was not detected. Transverse colectomy was done (Fig. 141.2). Bowel continuity was reported by right colon to left colon anastomosis.

This cancer was located midway between the hepatic and splenic flexures. The tumor, the transverse colon and the lymph node bearing mesentery associated with the middle colic artery were removed. The omentum was removed with the colon. Bowel continuity was restored by right colon to left colon anastomosis.

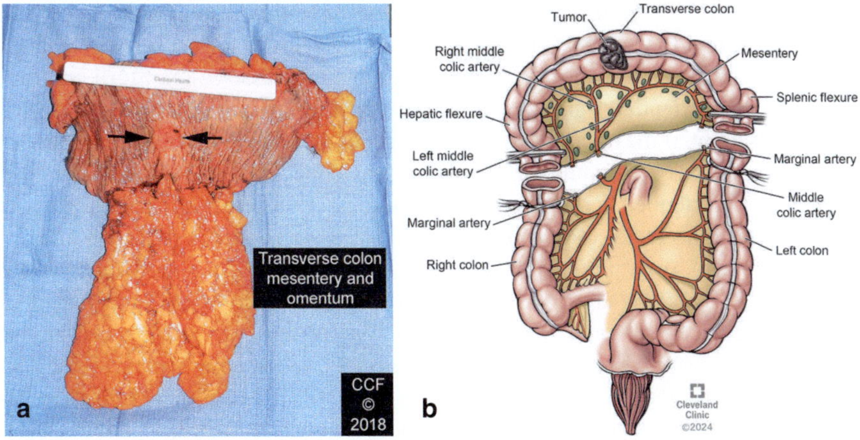

Fig. 141.2 (**a**) Transverse colectomy and omentectomy for mid-transverse colon cancer. The tumor is marked with arrows; (**b**) Illustration showing the extent of resection for transverse colectomy for cancer. The middle colic artery and marginal arteries are divided. The hepatic flexure and splenic flexures are mobilized. The tumor, distal right colon, transverse colon, and proximal left colon are excised with the lymph node bearing mesentery

Comment

Transverse colon cancers are located between the hepatic and splenic flexures. The primary arterial supply to the transverse colon is the middle colic artery with its right and left branches. Operations performed for transverse colon carcinoma include extended right colectomy, transverse colectomy, segmental colectomy, extended left colectomy, and subtotal colectomy. Cancer location guides surgical decision making. Surgery is performed with open, laparoscopic, and robotic techniques [1–4].

Kim et al. [5] performed right hemicolectomy or extended right hemicolectomy for lesions in the hepatic flexure as well as for lesions within the 10 cm distal to the hepatic flexure. Left hemicolectomy or extended left colectomy was performed for lesions in the splenic flexure as well as for lesions within the 10 cm proximal to the splenic flexure. Transverse colectomy or extended right hemicolectomy was performed for lesions in between. For Mistrangelo et al. [6], a tumor located at the hepatic flexure or within 10 cm distal to the hepatic flexure was treated by extended right hemicolectomy. A tumor at the splenic flexure or within 10 cm proximal to the splenic flexure was treated by segmental colon resection or left extended hemicolectomy. Transverse colectomy was performed for tumors located centrally in the transverse colon. Similarly, for Zeng et al. [7], a tumor located at the hepatic flexure or within 10 cm distal to the hepatic flexure was treated by extended right hemicolectomy. A tumor at the splenic flexure or within 10 cm proximal to the splenic flexure was treated by left extended hemicolectomy. Transverse colectomy was performed for tumors located centrally in the transverse colon. Storli and Eide [8] performed extended right hemicolectomy for tumors in the proximal and mid-transverse colon. If the tumor was in the left side of the transverse colon, an extended left hemicolectomy or a subtotal colectomy was done. In 2013, Van Rongen et al. [9] compared extended hemicolectomy versus transverse colectomy in patients with cancer of the transverse colon and found that 5-year survival was slightly higher for the hemicolectomy group but that this difference did not reach statistical significance. In 2016, Chong et al. [10] compared long-term oncological outcomes after transverse colectomy versus extended resection for transverse colon cancer and found that in terms of perioperative and oncological outcomes, transverse colectomy and extended colectomy did not differ. Similarly, Li et al. [11] found similar oncological and prognostic outcomes for the treatment of transverse colon cancer by transverse colectomy and extended colectomy.

References

1. Fernández-Cebrián JM, Yonte PG, Jiminez-Toscano M, Vega L, Ochando F. Laparoscopic colectomy for transverse colon carcinoma: a surgical challenge but oncologically feasible. Colorectal Dis. 2012;15:e79–83.
2. Jung KU, Park Y, Lee KY, Sohn S-K. Robotic transverse colectomy for mid-transverse colon cancer: surgical techniques and oncologic outcomes. J Robot Surg. 2015;9:131–6.
3. Kawahara H, Watanabe K, Tomoda M, Enomoto H, Akiba T, Yanaga K. Umbilical single incisional approach plus one port for partial transverse colectomy: initial operative experience. Hepato-Gastroenterol. 2014;61:1954–6.
4. de'Angelis N, Alghamdi S, Renda A, Azoulay D, Brunetti F. Initial experience of robotic versus laparoscopic colectomy for transverse colon cancer: a matched case-control study. World J Surg Oncol. 2015;13:295. https://doi.org/10.1186/s12957-015-0708-1.
5. Kim MK, Won D-Y, Lee J-K, Kang W-K, Kye B-H, Cho H-M, Kim H-J, Kim J-G. Laparoscopic surgery for transverse colon cancer: short- and long-term outcomes in comparison with conventional open surgery. J Laparoendosc Adv Surg Tech. 2015;25:982–9.
6. Mistrangelo M, Allaix ME, Cassoni P, Giraudo G, Arolfo S, Morino M. Laparoscopic versus open resection for transverse colon cancer. Surg Endosc. 2015;29:2196–202.
7. Zeng W-g, Liu M-j, Zhou Z-x, Hou H-r, Liang J-w, Wang Z, Zhang X-m, Hu J-j. Outcome of laparoscopic versus open resection for transverse colon cancer. J Gastrointest Surg. 2015;19:1869–74.
8. Storli KE, Eide GE. Laparoscopic complete mesocolic excision versus open complete mesocolic excision for transverse colon cancer: long-term survival results of a prospective single centre non-randomized study. Dig Surg. 2016;33:114–20.
9. van Rongen I, Damhuis RAM, van der Hoeven JAB, Plaisier PW. Comparison of extended hemicolectomy versus transverse colectomy in patients with cancer of the transverse colon. Acta Chir Belg. 2013;113:107–11.
10. Chong CS, Huh JW, Oh BY, Park YA, Cho YB, Yun SH, Kim HC, Lee WY. Operative method for transverse colon carcinoma: transverse colectomy versus extended colectomy. Dis Colon Rectum. 2016;59:630–9.
11. Li C, Wang Q, Jiang K-W. What is the best surgical procedure of transverse colon cancer? An evidence map and minireview. World J Gastrointestinal Oncol. 2021;13:391–9.

Right Colon Cancer (Right Hemicolectomy by the "No-Touch" Isolation Technique)

142

James S. Wu

Presentation

A 65-year-old patient was referred for surgical removal of right-sided colon cancer. Preoperative assessment did not reveal metastatic disease. The patient was deemed medically fit for surgery. Right hemicolectomy by the "no-touch" isolation technic was done. The operation and recovery were uneventful.

Comment

In 1909, Jamieson and Dobson described details for the surgical removal of cancer involving the cecum, lower part of the ascending colon, and the neighborhood of the hepatic flexure [1].

> 'THE OPERATION FOR MALIGNANT DISEASE OF THE CÆCUM, AND LOWER PART OF THE ASCENDING COLON.
>
> —In cases for radical treatment the operation necessitated by the arrangement of the lymphatics is, viz.: After exposing the field of operation the lower border of the third part of the duodenum is defined. The peritoneum over this is divided and the ileocolic vessels are found. The fatty tissue surrounding the vessels which will contain the uppermost gland of the ileocolic chain is stripped downwards with gauze, care being taken not to wound the duodenum. The artery and vein are ligatured and divided close to the superior mesenteric

J. S. Wu (✉)
Department of Colon and Rectal Surgery, Cleveland Clinic, Cleveland, OH, USA

J. S. Wu, M. D. Inkster (eds.), *Cleveland Clinic Colorectal Case Studies*,
https://doi.org/10.1007/978-3-031-39880-3_142

> artery. It is well at this stage to select the point on the transverse colon where the gut shall be divided. The transverse mesocolon is then divided up to the selected point, some branches of the middle colic artery being secured. The middle colic artery itself is carefully preserved. If the right colic artery has a separate origin from the superior mesenteric it will need ligature. The peritoneum of the mesentery is then divided in an oblique line downwards to the ileum. The ileocolic and right colic vessels, with the accompanying chain of glands, the fatty tissue and the overlying peritoneum, are then stripped downward to the ileum and cæcum and outwards to the colon. The ureter and spermatic vessels are encountered and must be avoided. The cæcum is then lifted up and the peritoneal reflection to the outer side of the colon is divided. The cæcum and appendix, the whole of the ascending colon, and the terminal portion of the ileum, with the ileocolic and right colic vessels and the lymphatic chain, can then be withdrawn from the abdomen, only remaining attached by the continuity of the intestine. The colon is divided at the previously selected point and the ileum about six inches from the valve. The operation is terminated by an ileocolostomy to the transverse colon,…
>
> OPERATION FOR GROWTHS IN THE NEIGHBORHOOD OF THE HEPATIC FLEXURE.
>
> To remove the “lymphatic area” it is necessary to tie the middle colic artery at its origin from the superior mesenteric and to remove the mesocolon from this point up to the bowel. By this step the whole of the middle colic chain of glands is secured. Ligature of the artery devitalizes so much of the ascending colon—particularly in those cases where the right colic artery has origin from the middle colic— that is necessary to remove the whole of the ascending colon, with the cæcum and terminal six inches of the ileum, the growth at the hepatic flexure, and about half of the transverse colon, completing the operation by a lateral anastomosis between the ileum and the transverse colon.”

The lines of resection for cancer according to Jamieson and Dobson in the cecum and lower part of the ascending colon are illustrated in Fig. 142.1a; those for cancer in the neighborhood of the hepatic flexure are shown in Fig. 142.1b. Their operative technique is remarkable for initial vascular ligation followed by intestinal mobilization.

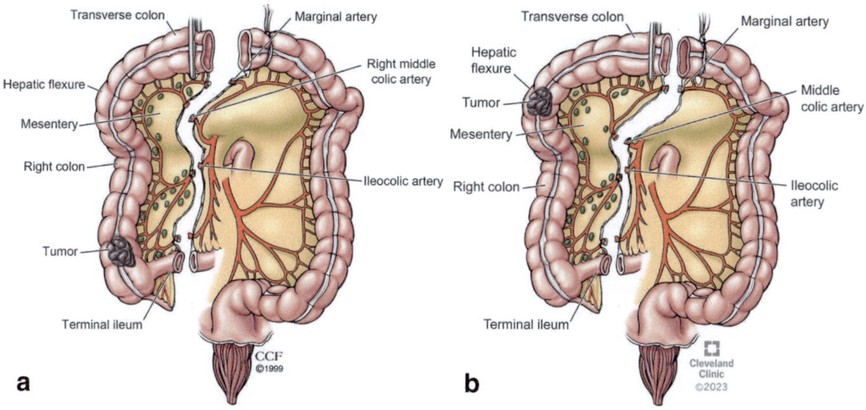

Fig. 142.1 (**a**) Right hemicolectomy for cancer of the cecum and lower part of the ascending colon. The tumor, the terminal ileum, right colon, and proximal transverse colon with the associated lymph node bearing mesentery are removed. The ileocolic artery, right branch of the middle colic artery, and marginal arteries are ligated; (**b**) Extended right hemicolectomy for cancer in the neighborhood of the hepatic flexure. The tumor, the terminal ileum, right colon, and transverse colon (where the distal resection margin includes the distal transverse colon) with the associated lymph node bearing mesentery are removed. The ileocolic artery, middle colic artery, and marginal arteries are ligated. In both of these illustrations, to prevent fecal spillage, the end of the resected colon is closed with a clamp, while the colon used for anastomosis is encircled with an umbilical tape.

(The right colic artery was not included in these illustrations because of variations in its precise arrangement including absence. See Haywood M, Molyneux C, Mahadevan V, Srinivasaih N. Right colic artery anatomy; systemic review of cadaveric studies. Tech Coloproctol 2017;21:937–943.)

"No-Touch" Isolation Right Hemicolectomy

The "no-touch" isolation technic for colon cancer resection was popularized at the Cleveland Clinic in 1953 by Dr. Rupert Turnbull [2]. Ligation of the lymphovascular pedicles before cancer manipulation was done to mitigate against intraoperative tumor spread. The rationale for the operation was based on the observations of earlier investigators. In 1938, Gordon-Watson wrote concerning venous spread in cancer of the rectum [3]:

Origin and spread of cancer of the rectum
in relation to surgical treatment
by Sir Charles Gordon-Watson, K.B.E., C.M.G.,
F.R.C.S. Eng., F.A.C.S.
Consulting surgeon, St. Bartholomew's Hospital,
St. Mark's Hospital for Diseases of the Rectum, and the
Metropolitan Hospital, London

"No doubt venous emboli can and do occasionally occur in the early stages of the disease, and this is one uncertain factor that the surgeon has to face when considering prognosis. It is possible also that manipulations during operation may be responsible sometimes for the separation of a thrombus and so cause metastasis,..."

In 1941, Dukes and Bussey described the venous spread of rectal cancer [4].

Venous Spread in Rectal Cancer
By C. E. Dukes, M.D., M.Sc., D.P.H., and H. J. R. Bussey, B.Sc.
The Pathology Department, St. Mark's Hospital, London

"In view of the severe consequences of the spread of rectal cancer by veins it is surprising that so little attention has been given to the state of the veins during routine examination of pathological specimens. Our interest in this question was first aroused by Dr. P. C. Hou of Cheeloo University, North China, who demonstrated a case of cancerous occlusion of a branch of the superior hæmorrhoidal vein. Realizing the importance of such a finding we decided to make a special study of the state of the veins in rectal cancer....

Frequency of Venous Extension

We have examined 669 operation specimens of rectal cancer... and found clumps of carcinoma cells in the hæmorrhoidal veins in 111 (16.6%)."

In 1952, Barnes described an operation that advocated vascular ligation before colon mobilization specifically in order to prevent intravascular tumor dissemination [5].

Physiologic Resection of the Right Colon.
J. Peyton Barnes, M.D., F.A.C.S
Houston, Texas

"The surgical attack on a malignant lesion, wherever located, is ordinarily carried out according to well established and thoroughly accepted principles. One such basic principle is that, whenever possible, the blood supply to and the lymphatic vessels from the lesion be severed before the lesion itself is removed or manipulated. This is to prevent forcing, by such manipulation, malignant cells into the areas beyond the site of surgery via the blood and lymph channels."

Barnes proposed the following operation that would follow these principles:

PROCEDURE

1. A transverse incision, cutting both recti about 1 inch above the umbilicus is used.
2. Resectability is decided upon.
3. The site for section of the colon is established, usually a little to the right of the main trunk of the midcolic artery.
4. The omentum is now split up to site selected for colon section.
5. The colon is cleared of all fat at the site of section and cut between clamps. A straight Ochsner clamp is used on the distal end if an end-to-end closed type of anastomosis is contemplated.

6. Beginning at the site of colon section, working from above downward, the colon and transverse mesocolon with all vessels and lymph nodes are separated from all posterior relations. As the dissection proceeds downward, all vessels are identified, doubly ligated, and cut. …in completing it one sections a branch of the mid-colic, the right colic, and the ileocolic arteries.

7. When this incision as described is complete, the site for section of the ileum is selected and cleared. The ileum is then cut between clamps….

10. Now one is ready to remove the right colon, lesion, and terminal ileum. At this point we incise the peritoneum lateral to the colon…. The colon is not mobilized from without inward.

11. Beginning medially and above, working outward and downward, the right colon, mesocolon, with all involved nodes, vessels and ileum are carefully cleaned from the underlying structures. This procedure removes the lesion *last of all.*

The technique described adheres to the principle that the blood and lymph channels of a lesion should be severed before manipulating the lesion itself."

In 1955, Fisher and Turnbull demonstrated tumor cells in the mesenteric venous blood in patients with colorectal carcinoma [6]. Tumor cells were identified histologically in seven of 25 cases (28%) and cytologically in eight (32%).

In 1967, Turnbull and colleagues compared survival rates for Stage A, B, C, and D cancers of the colon according to surgical technic (*No-Touch Isolation* versus conventional) [7, 8].

Cancer of the Colon: The Influence of the
No-Touch Isolation Technic on
Survival Rates
Rupert B. Turnbull, Jr., M.D., Kenneth Kyle, M.B., M.Ch.,
Frank R. Watson, Ph.D., John Spratt, M.D.

"In late 1953, one of us (R. B. T., Jr) adopted a technic of colon resection for cancer wherein the cancer-bearing segment was not manipulated or handled in any manner until after the lymphovascular pedicles were divided and ligated and the colon was divided at the elected sites for resection. To emphasize the type of technic, the name *no-touch isolation* was adopted. This method of resection has been applied to every cancer of the colon operated upon by the senior author since that time (1953-1964). During this time, five staff surgeons at the Cleveland Clinic Hospital continued to perform resections of the colon with the *conventional* technic, which is characterized by ligation and division of the lymphovascular pedicles *after* mobilization of the cancer-bearing segment.

Six hundred sixty-four patients were treated by one surgeon (R. B. T., Jr) who used the *no-touch isolation* technic when resection was indicated. Five other staff surgeons operated upon 232 patients using a *conventional* technic when resection was indicated."

The resectability rates were the same in both groups. The crude 5-year survival was 51% for the for the *No-Touch Isolation* technic and 35% for the *conventional* technique.

Technic

The small bowel is eviscerated to the right (Fig. 142.2). The beginning of the jejunum serves as a useful reference point. The peritoneum between the mesentery and the duodenum is divided sharply (Fig. 142.3).

The index finger of the right hand passes between the superior mesenteric artery and the duodenum (Fig. 142.4a, b).

The small intestine then is rotated to the left. The ileocolic artery is isolated from the retroperitoneal side (Fig. 142.5a, b) and divided (Fig. 142.6). The transverse colon is elevated so that the transverse colon mesentery is perpendicular to the aorta.

The right branch of the middle colic artery (RMCA) is isolated and divided (Fig. 142.7a, b, c).

Figure 142.8 shows the operation following division of the ileocolic artery and the RMCA and before right colon mobilization. Following lymphovascular isolation, the mesentery is elevated from the retroperitoneum. The terminal ileum is divided approximately 10 cm proximal to the colon. The transverse colon is divided in its midsection. The avascular lateral peritoneal attachments of the colon are divided. Finally, the specimen is removed from the operative field. The excised right colectomy specimen is shown in Fig. 142.9.

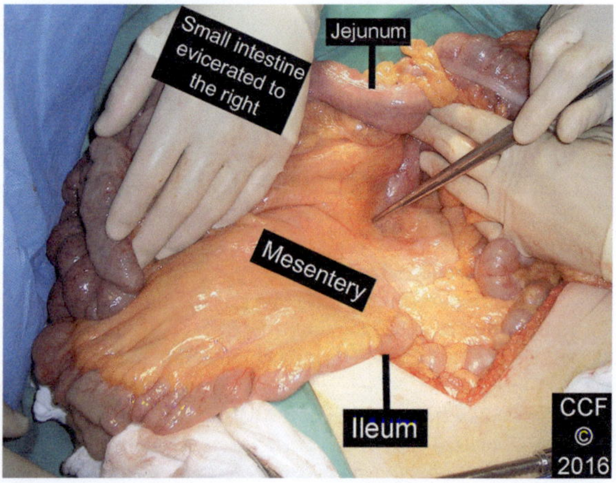

Fig. 142.2 Small intestinal evisceration to the right exposes the peritoneum located at the beginning of the jejunum (forceps)

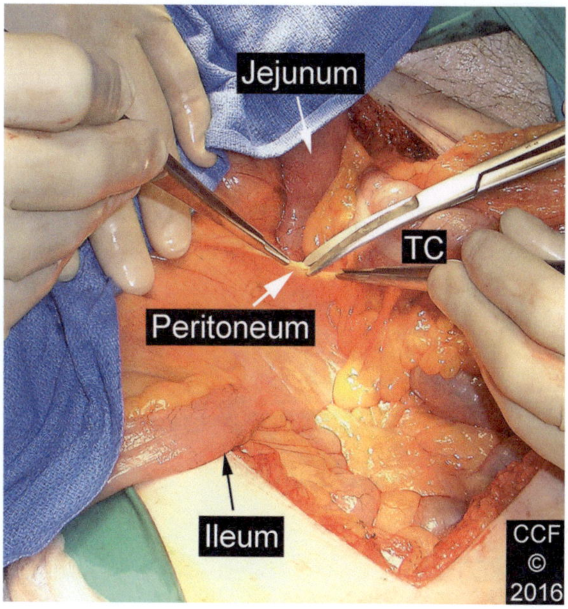

Fig. 142.3 The peritoneum covering the superior mesenteric artery (SMA) as it crosses the duodenum is divided. The jejunum, transverse colon (TC), and ileum are labeled

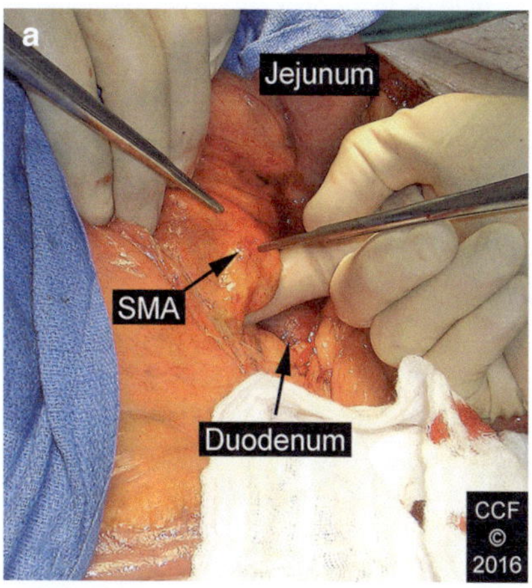

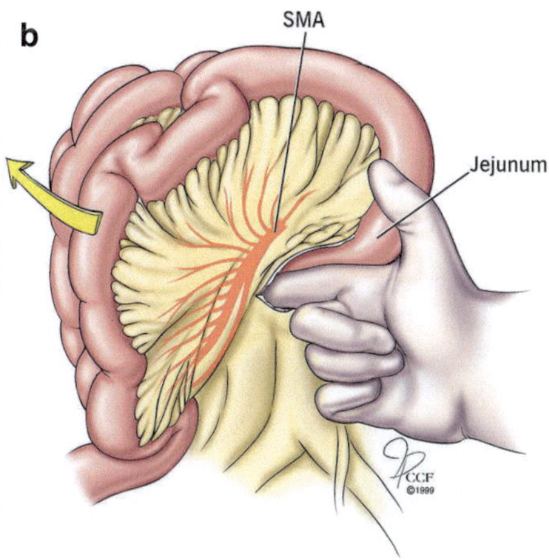

Fig. 142.4 (**a**, **b**). With the small intestine eviscerated to the right (yellow arrow), the index finger of the right hand is passed over the duodenum and under the SMA (forceps) into the retroperitoneal space

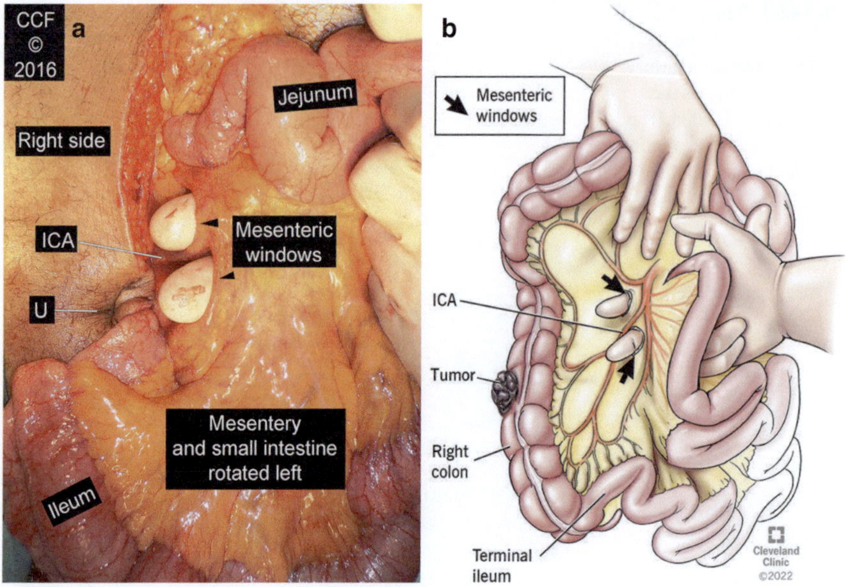

Fig. 142.5 Isolation and division of the ileocolic artery: (**a**, **b**). The ileocolic artery (ICA) is isolated retroperitoneally without mobilizing the right colon. The index and middle fingers of the right hand straddle the ileocolic artery through mesenteric windows. In the operative photo, the jejunum, small intestinal mesentery, umbilicus (U) and the right side of the abdominal wall are labeled. In the illustration, the tumor, the right colon, ileocolic artery (ICA), the terminal ileum, and the mesenteric windows (arrows) are labelled

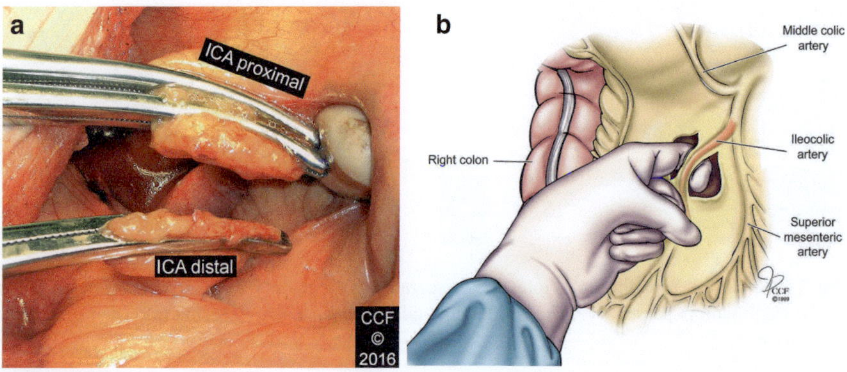

Fig. 142.6 (**a**, **b**) The ileocolic artery (ICA) is isolated and divided between clamps aligned with the tips toward the specimen. This parallel alignment allows the scissors to follow the curve of the clamps. In this case, the proximal end of the divided artery has been doubly clamped so that it may be doubly tied; # 1 or # 0 chromic suture commonly is used. The middle colic artery (MCA) and superior mesenteric artery (SMA) are labeled

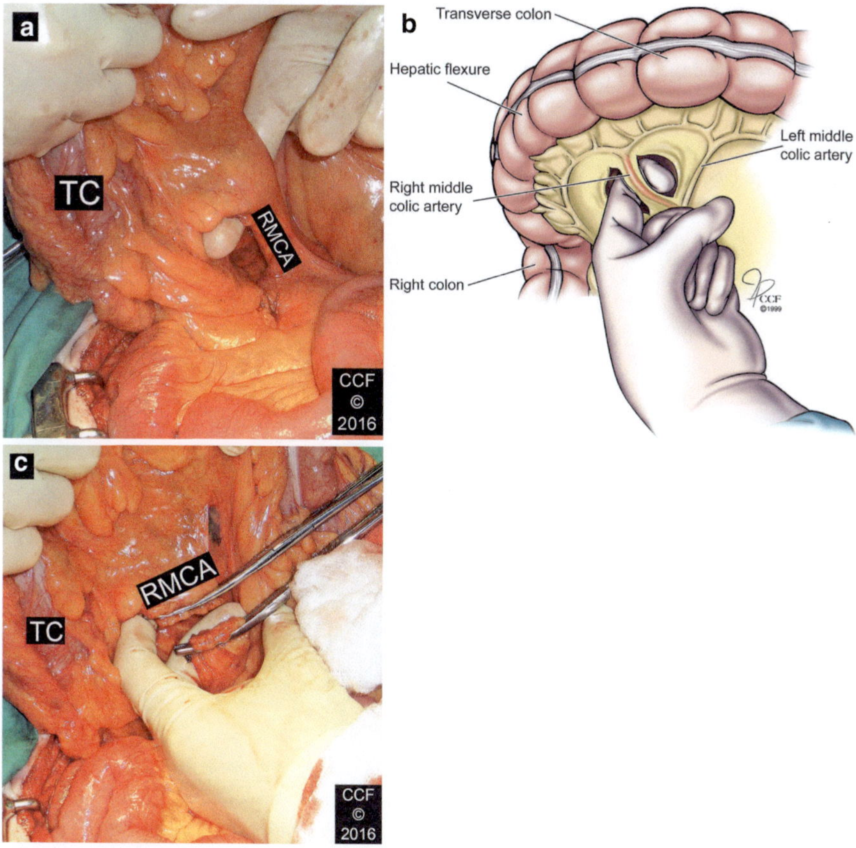

Fig. 142.7 (**a**) The transverse colon (TC) is moved perpendicularly to facilitate isolation of the RMCA; (**b**) Illustration showing isolation of the RMCA; (**c**) The RMCA is divided between curved clamps placed with tips directed toward the specimen. The right colon, right branch of the middle colic artery, hepatic flexure, transverse colon, and left branch of the middle colic artery are labelled

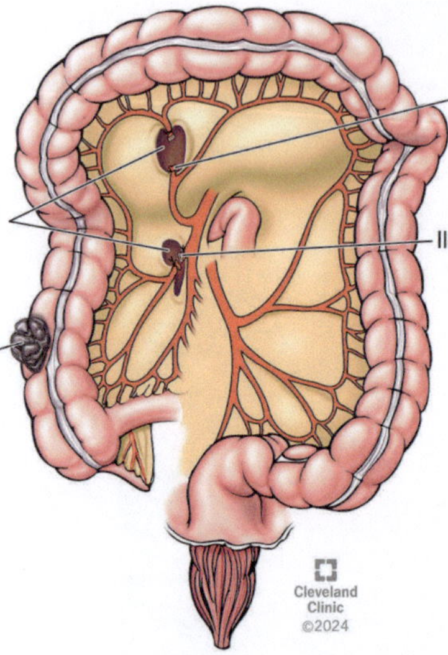

Fig. 142.8 Illustration showing ligation of the ileocolic artery and the right branch of the middle colic artery. The mesenteric windows and the tumor are labelled

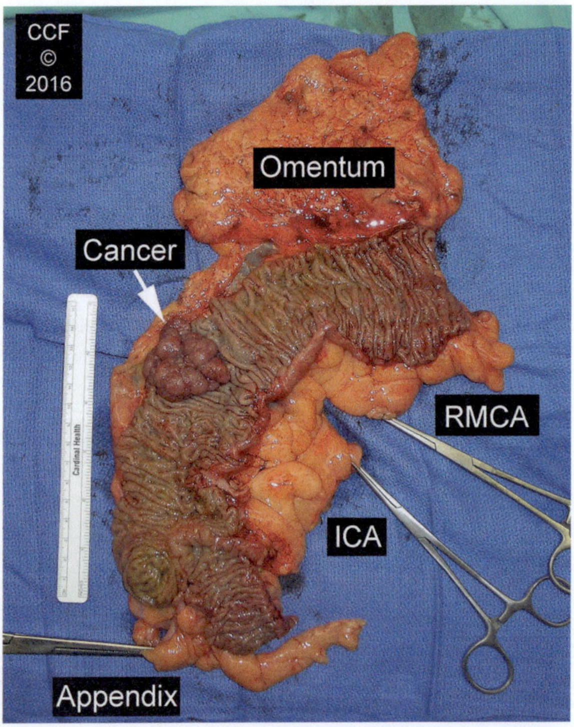

Fig. 142.9 Right hemicolectomy specimen. The mesenteric clamps identify the lymphovascular beds of the ileocolic artery (ICA) and right branch of the middle colic artery (RMCA). The proximal omentum has been removed with the specimen. The tumor is seen in the right colon. A clamp identifies the appendix

Comment

Dr. Fazio related that once the diagnosis of colon cancer had been made, Dr. Turnbull did not permit a probing abdominal examination to locate a tumor mass so as not to displace tumor cells into the portal system. Colectomy by the *no-touch isolation* technic has been investigated at other institutions. In 1988, Wiggers et al. [9] performed a controlled prospective trial of the *no-touch isolation* technique in colon cancer; the authors' data suggested a limited benefit. In 1998, Hayashi et al. [10] used mutant-allele-specific amplification (MASA) to detect occult tumor cell dissemination into the portal vein. These authors identified genetic alterations of the primary tumor in the portal blood in 8 of 11 (73%) of conventional resection technique cases, but only one of seven (14%) in the *no-touch isolation* technique had a positive result. In 1998, Slanetz [11] studied curative resections for colorectal cancer to determine the effects of the application of bowel ligatures and the sequence of mesenteric ligation on survival and recurrence as part of the *no-touch isolation* technique. Records documenting the application of bowel ligatures in 2015 consecutive curative resections for colorectal cancer and the sequence of mesenteric vessel ligation in 1663 of these cases were reviewed. The author found that bowel ligatures applied before tumor mobilization in curative resections for colorectal cancer consistently reduced cancer-related deaths and the incidence of distant, local, and suture line recurrences. In 1999, Sales et al. [12] reported on blood dissemination of colonic epithelial cells during no-touch surgery for rectosigmoid cancer. The authors concluded that the no-touch technique in colorectal surgery with primary ligation of the lymphovascular pedicle seemed to be effective in preventing blood spread of colonic cells. In 2022, Takii et al. [13] reported the results of a multicenter, open-label, randomized, phase III trial comparing the convention technique versus the *no-touch isolation* technique for primary tumor resection patient colon cancer. The study failed to confirm the superiority of the no-touch.

Biographical Note [14]

Rupert B. Turnbull, Jr. (1913–1981)

Rupert Turnbull received his medical degree from McGill University. From 1941 to 1943, he was a resident in Surgery at Gorgas Hospital, Canal Zone, Panama. During World War II, he served as a field surgeon with the First Marine Division in Okinawa, South Pacific, and Tien-Tsin, China (1943–1946). Between 1946 and 1949, he completed a Fellowship in Surgery with Dr. Thomas E. Jones, at the Cleveland Clinic Foundation. From 1950 to 1978, he served as Head, Department of Colon and Rectal Surgery, at the Cleveland Clinic. In addition to popularization of the "*no-touch isolation*" technic, Dr. Turnbull defined Stage D for metastatic colon cancer, described techniques for ostomy creation, founded the School of Enterostomal Therapy at the Cleveland Clinic, and advocated for surgery to treat the toxic megacolon phase of ulcerative colitis, and for intersphincteric proctectomy for benign disease.

References

1. Jamieson JK, Dobson JF. The lymphatics of the colon. With special reference to the operative treatment of cancer of the colon. Ann Surg. 1909;50:1077–90. This excerpt was reused with the generous permission of Wolters Kluwer Health, Inc., CCC|RightsLink®, License number 5156691277189, License date Sep 26, 2021
2. The term "No-touch" isolation technique was coined by the late Dr. Frank L. Weakley. Personal communication from Dr. Victor W. Fazio.
3. Gordon-Watson C. Origin and spread of cancer of the rectum in relation to surgical treatment. Lancet. 1938;231(5970):239–45.
4. Dukes CE, Bussey HJR. Venous spread of rectal cancer. Proc R Soc Med. 1941;34:571–3. This excerpt is reproduced with permission from SAGE Publications, CCC|RightsLink®, License Number 5134590289078, License Date Aug 23, 2021
5. Barnes JP. Physiologic resection of the right colon. Surg Gynecol Obstet. 1952;94:723–6. Reprinted with permission from Mr. Spencer Dimmick, the Journal of the American College of Surgeons, formerly Surgery Gynecology & Obstetrics, August 30, 2021
6. Fisher ER, Turnbull RB Jr. The cytologic demonstration and significance of tumor cells in the mesenteric venous blood in patients with colorectal carcinoma. Surg Gynecol Obstet. 1955;100:102–8. Reprinted with permission from Mr. Spencer Dimmick, the Journal of the American College of Surgeons, formerly Surgery Gynecology & Obstetrics, Sep 21, 2021
7. Turnbull RB, Kyle K, Watson FR, Spratt J. Cancer of the colon: The influence of the *no-touch isolation* technic on survival rates. Ann Surg. 1967;166:420–7. Permission to reproduce this excerpt was generously given by Wolters Kluwer Health, Inc, CCC|RightLinks®, License number 5134820748120, License Date Aug 23, 2021
8. Wu JS, Fazio VW. Colon cancer. Dis Colon Rectum. 2000;43:1473–86.
9. Wiggers T, Jeekel J, Arends JW, Brinkhorst AP, Kluck HM, Luyk CI, et al. No-touch isolation technique in colon cancer: a controlled prospective trial. Br J Surg. 1988;75:409–15.
10. Hayashi N, Egami H, Kai M, Kurusu Y, Takano S, Ogawa M. No-touch isolation technique reduces intraoperative shedding of tumor cells into the portal vein during resection of colorectal cancer. Surgery. 1999;125:369–74.
11. Slanetz CA Jr. Effect of no touch isolation on survival and recurrence in curative resections for colorectal cancer. Ann Surg Oncol. 1998;5:390–8.
12. Sales J-P, Wind P, Douard R, Cugnenc P-H, Loric S. Blood dissemination of colonic epithelial cells during no-touch surgery for rectosigmoid cancer. Lancet. 1999;354:392.
13. Takii Y, Mizusawa J, Kanemitsu Y, Komori K, Shiozawa M, Ohue M, et al. The conventional technique versus the no -touch isolation technique for primary tumor resection in patients with colon cancer (JCOG1006). Ann Surg. 2022;275:849–55.
14. Fazio VF. Reminiscences: Rupert Beach Turnbull, Jr., M.D., C.M., F.A.C.S., F.R.A.C.S. (H), R.S.M. (H) October 3, 1913-February 18, 1981. Dis Colon Rectum. 1982;25:219–21.

Video: Right Hemicolectomy by the "No-Touch Isolation" Technic

143

David G. Jagelman and James S. Wu

David G. Jagelman, M.B.M.S. (1939–1993) [1]

Dr. Jagelman was born in London. He graduated from the Westminster Medical School in 1963. He became a Fellow of the Royal College of Surgeons in 1970 and was awarded the prestigious Master of Surgery in 1973. In 1974, Dr. Jagelman received special training in colorectal surgery at the Cleveland Clinic with Dr. Rupert Turnbull and in 1975 was hired as a staff physician. During his career, he published nearly 200 textbook chapters, journal articles, and presentations on surgical techniques to treat inflammatory bowel disease and colorectal cancer. In 1979, he founded the Cleveland Clinic Familial Polyposis Registry. In 1988, he was appointed Chairman of the Cleveland Clinic Department of Colorectal Surgery in Fort Lauderdale, Florida.

> "His untimely death was most unfortunate not only for his family and the Cleveland Clinic, but for the thousands of patients he had helped in the past and would have helped in the future".
>
> Floyd Loop, MD
> then CEO of the Cleveland Clinic Foundation
> "Video: Right Hemicolectomy by the "no-touch isolation" Technic

Supplementary Information The online version contains supplementary material available at https://doi.org/10.1007/978-3-031-39880-3_143. The videos can be accessed individually by clicking the DOI link in the accompanying figure caption or by scanning this link with the SN More Media App.

D. G. Jagelman · J. S. Wu (✉)
Department of Colon and Rectal Surgery, Cleveland Clinic, Cleveland, OH, USA

J. S. Wu, M. D. Inkster (eds.), *Cleveland Clinic Colorectal Case Studies*,
https://doi.org/10.1007/978-3-031-39880-3_143

This video, created by Dr. Jagelman in 1986, demonstrates extirpation of a right colon cancer by the "*no-touch isolation*" technic performed by a Master surgeon.[1] The operation was popularized by Dr. Rupert Turnbull, Jr.,

Reference

1. Jagelman DG. Inherited colorectal cancer registries. ©Cleveland Clinic; 2017. (December 18, 1939-August 9, 1993). Accessed 29 Oct 2003

[1] This video is reproduced with permission from the Cleveland Clinic, Enterprise Creative Services, artphoto@ccf.org, on 05/18/22.

Appendiceal Adenocarcinoma

144

Carolyn L. Power, Michael A. Valente, Eric W. Willis, Michelle D. Inkster, and James S. Wu

Presentation

A 63-year-old man underwent a screening colonoscopy. An ulcerated cecal mass was discovered (Fig. 144.1). An arrow points to the mass on computed tomography (Fig. 144.2). Biopsy showed inflammation.

C. L. Power · M. A. Valente · J. S. Wu (✉)
Department of Colon and Rectal Surgery, Cleveland Clinic, Cleveland, OH, USA

E. W. Willis
Department of Pathology, CORPath, Columbus, OH, USA

M. D. Inkster
Department of Gastroenterology, Cleveland Clinic, Cleveland, OH, USA

J. S. Wu, M. D. Inkster (eds.), *Cleveland Clinic Colorectal Case Studies*,
https://doi.org/10.1007/978-3-031-39880-3_144

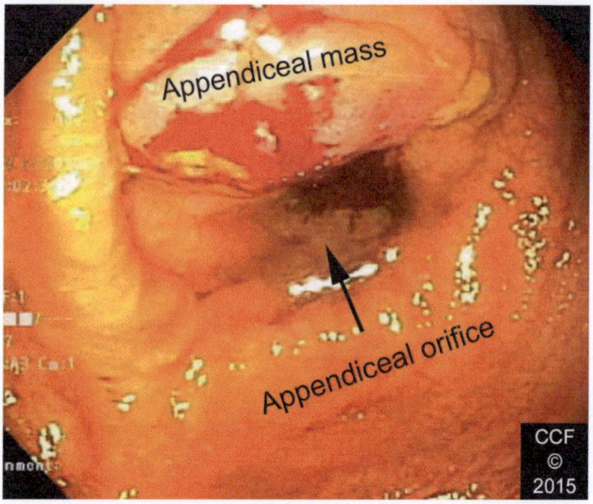

Fig. 144.1 Cecal mass (arrow), endoscopic view

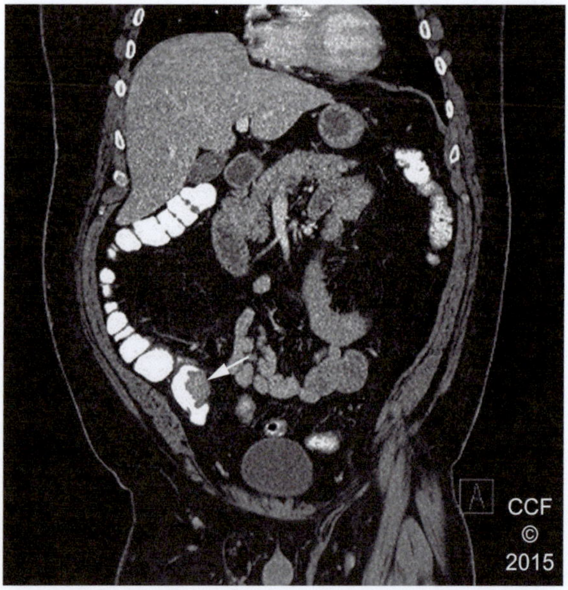

Fig. 144.2 Computed tomography of the abdomen and pelvis shows a cecal mass (arrow)

Management

At exploration, a hard cecal mass was found. Laparoscopic right hemicolectomy with ileocolic anastomosis was done. Metastatic disease was not found. Pathology showed Grade 2 (moderately differentiated) mucinous adenocarcinoma of the appendix (Fig. 144.3). The tumor invaded through the muscularis propria into the subserosa or mesoappendix, but did not extend to the serosal surface. All margins were clear of invasive carcinoma, and no lymph node involvement was found.

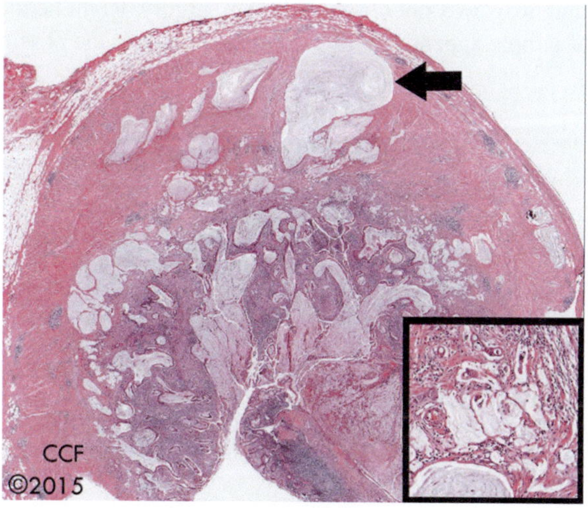

Fig. 144.3 Blue pools of mucin with floating atypical glandular cells (inset) with destructive invasion through the muscularis propria (arrow) of this appendix (Original magnification, H&E, 8×, 50×)

Comment

Primary adenocarcinoma of the appendix is rare, accounting for 0.4–1% of all gastrointestinal malignancies [1]. Diagnosis typically follows the histopathologic evaluation of surgical specimens. When symptomatic, it can present in a manner similar to acute appendicitis or with a palpable mass. A high index of suspicion is needed in order not to miss the diagnosis, especially when initial biopsy does not reveal neoplasm. Mucinous adenocarcinoma of the appendix has infrequent nodal metastases, but has a relatively high propensity for peritoneal dissemination [2]. In this case, the diagnosis was not clear until after surgery. Right hemicolectomy was done instead of simple appendectomy taking into account the possibility of malignancy [2–5].

References

1. Guraya SY, Almaramhy HH. Clinicopathological features and the outcome of surgical management for adenocarcinoma of the appendix. World J Gastrointest Surg. 2011;3:7–12.
2. Turaga KK, Pappas S, Gamblin TC. Right hemicolectomy for mucinous adenocarcinoma of the appendix: just right or too much? Ann Surg Oncol. 2013;20:1063–7.
3. Bunni J, Arnold D, Shelley-Fraser G, Shabbir J. Multidisciplinary perspective on the management of appendiceal adenocarcinoma: case review of 10 patients from a university hospital and current considerations. Clin Colorectal Cancer. 2015;14:58–62.
4. Tang LH. Epithelial neoplasms of the appendix. Arch Pathol Lab Med. 2010;134:1612–20.
5. Kawamura YJ. Management of adenocarcinoma of the appendix. J Gastroenterol. 2002;37:981.

Synchronous Colon Cancer

145

James S. Wu

Presentation

Figure 145.1 shows an example of synchronous colorectal cancers.

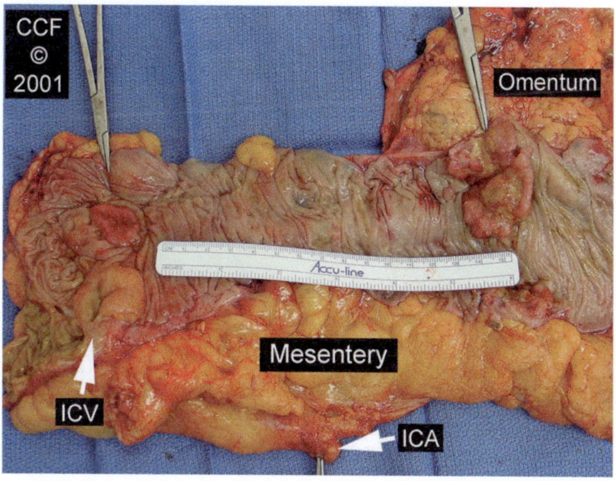

Fig. 145.1 Synchronous colon cancers in the cecum and the hepatic flexure are marked with clamps. The ileocecal valve (ICV), ileocolic artery (ICA), mesentery, and omentum are labeled

J. S. Wu (✉)
Department of Colon and Rectal Surgery, Cleveland Clinic, Cleveland, OH, USA

J. S. Wu, M. D. Inkster (eds.), *Cleveland Clinic Colorectal Case Studies*,
https://doi.org/10.1007/978-3-031-39880-3_145

Comment

More than one colorectal carcinoma occurs in a single patient in approximately 3-4% of cases in large series [1–5]. Characteristics of synchronous colorectal cancer compared to solitary colorectal cancer are listed in Table 145.1.

Following the discovery of one colon cancer, the entire colon is examined to exclude a second neoplasm. The possibility of an association with hereditary syndromes is considered. Long-term follow-up for metachronous neoplasms is indicated.

Table 145.1 Characteristics more frequently seen in synchronous colorectal cancers compared to solitary colorectal cancer

– Older
– Male
– Association with adenomatous polyps
– Proximal colon location
– Inflammatory bowel disease
– Hereditary nonpolyposis colorectal cancer
– Familial adenomatous polyposis
– Microsatellite instability-high
– Mucinous adenocarcinoma
– Precursor serrated adenomas
– Distant metastases

References

1. Hu H, Chang DT, Nikiforova MN, Kuan S-F, Pai RK. Clinicopatholologic features of synchronous colorectal carcinoma: a distinct subset arising from multiple sessile serrated adenomas and associated with high levels of microsatellite instability and favorable prognosis. Am J Surg Pathol. 2013;37:1660–70.
2. Mulder SA, Kranse R, Damhuis RA, de Wilt JHW, Ouwendijk RJT, Kuipers EJ, van Leerdam ME. Prevalence and prognosis of synchronous colorectal cancer: A Dutch population-based study. Cancer Epidemiol. 2011;35:442–7.
3. Latournerie M, Jooste V, Cottet V, Lepage C, Faivre J, Bouvier A-M. Epidemiology and prognosis of synchronous colorectal cancers. Br J Surg. 2008;95:1528–33.
4. Kaibara N, Koga S, Jinnai D. Synchronous and metachronous malignancies of the colon and rectum in Japan with special reference to a coexisting early cancer. Cancer. 1984;54:1870–4.
5. Lam AK-Y, Chan SS-Y, Leung M. Synchronous colorectal cancer: Clinical, pathological and molecular implications. World J Gastroenterol. 2014;20:6815–20.

Signet Ring Carcinoma

146

James S. Wu, Eric W. Willis, and Michelle D. Inkster

Presentation

The patient is a 55-year-old female who underwent right hemicolectomy for cancer (Fig. 146.1) found on colonoscopy. There was no evidence of metastatic disease at the time of surgery. Histopathology is shown in Fig. 146.2.

J. S. Wu (✉)
Department of Colon and Rectal Surgery, Cleveland Clinic, Cleveland, OH, USA

E. W. Willis
Department of Pathology, CORPath, Columbus, OH, USA

M. D. Inkster
Department of Gastroenterology, Cleveland Clinic, Cleveland, OH, USA

J. S. Wu, M. D. Inkster (eds.), *Cleveland Clinic Colorectal Case Studies*,
https://doi.org/10.1007/978-3-031-39880-3_146

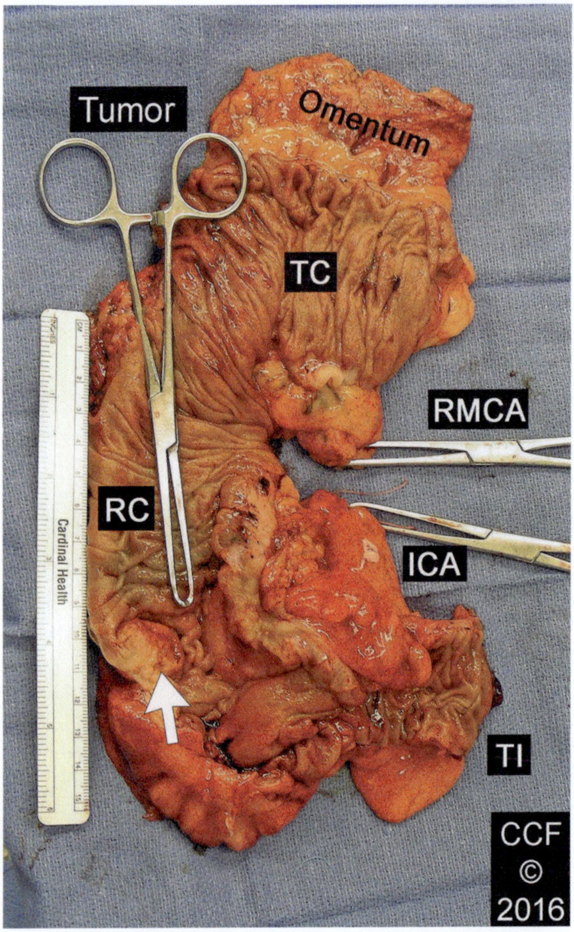

Fig. 146.1 Right hemicolectomy specimen. The tip of the vertical clamp and the white arrow point to the tumor. The horizontal clamps mark the ileocolic artery (ICA) and right branch of the middle colic artery (RMCA). The terminal ileum (TI), right colon (RC), transverse colon (TC), and omentum are labelled

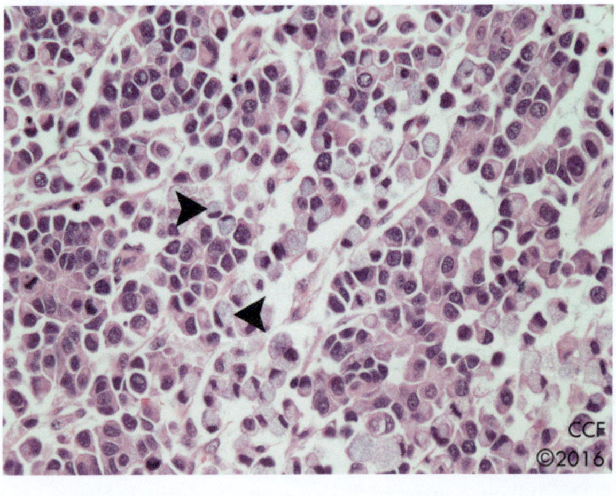

Fig. 146.2 Histopathology of the resected specimen shows mucinous adenocarcinoma, in large part signet cell type. Sections show diffuse sheets of single "signet ring" cells, consisting of an eccentrically-placed hyperchromatic nucleus, compressed by a cytoplasmic, blue–gray mucin droplet (arrowheads). Twenty-two out of 23 lymph nodes were involved with metastatic carcinoma

Comment

Primary signet ring carcinoma is encountered most commonly in the stomach. Rarer sites include gallbladder, breast, skin, and colon. In their 1951 article entitled, "Primary Linitis Plastica Type of Carcinoma of the Colon," Laufman and Saphir observed the following key features: insignificant primary site, signet ring cells, spread along the submucosa involving large portions of the affected organ, and poor prognosis [1]. Most cases of primary signet ring carcinoma of the colon are detected at an advanced stage [2–5]. Possibly, earlier detection might improve long-term prognosis. For example, in 2015, Ohnita et al. reported a case of primary signet ring carcinoma of the colon detected at an early state by magnifying endoscopy with narrow band imaging and crystal violet staining. The tumor was removed by endoscopic submucosal dissection and ileocolic resection with a favorable outcome. At 26 months after surgery, the patient was in good health with no evidence of recurrence [6].

Laufman and Safir's observation that signet ring cell carcinomas spreads along the "submucosa involving large portions of the the affected organ" returns us to the observation of Professor Sampson Handley, who in his 1910 Hunterian Lecture entitled "The Surgery of the Lymphatic System," described the pathologic findings of a case of rectal cancer treated by abdominal perineal resection. Handley's findings: "Conclusive evidence was obtained that the growth had spread by permeation along the mucous lymphatic plexus of the bowel at least as far as the point of section of the bowel 6 in. above the growth. A similar spread downward was traced as far as the region of the sphincters [7, Ch. 77, this work]". Since submucosal spread for other types of adenocarcinoma is not the norm, colorectal surgey can be done without extensive proximal and distal margins.

References

1. Laufman H, Saphir O. Primary linitis plastica type of carcinoma of the colon. Arch Surg. 1951;62:79–91.
2. Anthony T, George R, Rodriguez-Bigas M, Petrelli NJ. Primary signet-ring cell carcinoma of the colon and rectum. Ann Surg Oncol. 1996;3:344–8.
3. Tung SY, Wu CS, Chen PC. Primary signet ring cell carcinoma of the colorectum: an age- and sex-matched controlled study. Am J Gastroenterol. 1996;91:2195–9.
4. Nissan A, Guillem JG, Paty PB, Wong WD, Cohen AM. Signet-ring carcinoma of the colon and rectum: a matched control study. Dis Colon Rectum. 1999;42:1176–80.
5. Kim JH, Park SJ, Park MI, Moon W, Kim SE. Early-stage primary signet ring cell carcinoma of the colon. World J Gastroenterol. 2013;19:3895–8.
6. Ohnita K, Isomoto H, Akashi T, Hashiguchi K, Matsushima K, Minami H, et al. Early stage signet ring cell carcinoma of the colon examined by magnifying endoscopy with narrow band imaging: a case report. BMC Gastroenterol. 2015;15:86. https://doi.org/10.1186/s12876-015-0317-z.
7. Handley WS. Surgery of the lymphatic system. Br Med J 1:922–8.

Reconstruction After Left Colectomy-Transmesenteric Colorectal Anastomosis (Rombeau)

147

James S. Wu

Presentation

A patient underwent left hemicolectomy to treat a splenic flexure colon cancer. Following resection, the transverse colon would not reach the rectum (Figs. 147.1 and 147.2).

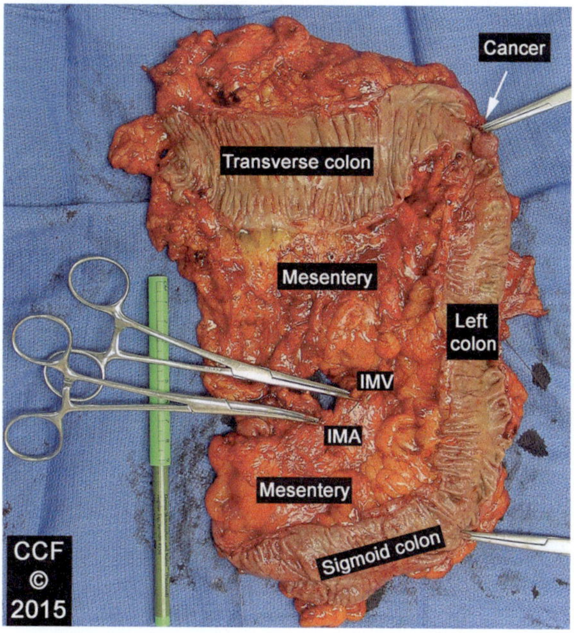

Fig. 147.1 Splenic flexure adenocarcinoma treated by left hemicolectomy. The cancer is identified by a clamp. High ligation of inferior mesenteriic artery (IMA) and the inferior mesenteric vein (IMV) was done. The transverse colon, left colon, sigmoid colon, and the mesentery are labelled

J. S. Wu (✉)
Department of Colon and Rectal Surgery, Cleveland Clinic, Cleveland, OH, USA

J. S. Wu, M. D. Inkster (eds.), *Cleveland Clinic Colorectal Case Studies*,
https://doi.org/10.1007/978-3-031-39880-3_147

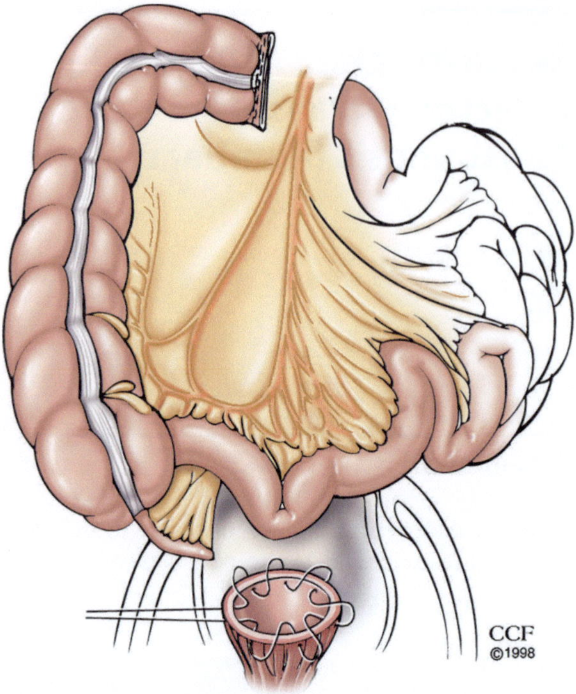

Fig. 147.2 Reconstruction is hampered because the transverse colon either crosses over the small intestine to reach the rectum or is not long enough to travel around the small intestine along the left gutter to reach the rectum

Transmesenteric Colorectal Anastomosis (Rombeau, Collins, Turnbull) [1, 2]

Following left hemicolectomy, transmesenteric colorectal anastomosis avoids compression of the terminal ileum by the transverse colon. The hepatic flexure and right colon are mobilized. The transverse colon is delivered to the rectum for anastomosis through a transmesenteric window created between the ileal and colic branches of the ileocolic artery as indicated in Figs. 147.3 and 147.4.

The positions of the colon superior and inferior to the ileal mesentery are shown in Figs. 147.4a, b.

Alternatives include right colon rotation and colorectal anastomosis (Deloyers) or ileorectal anastomosis.

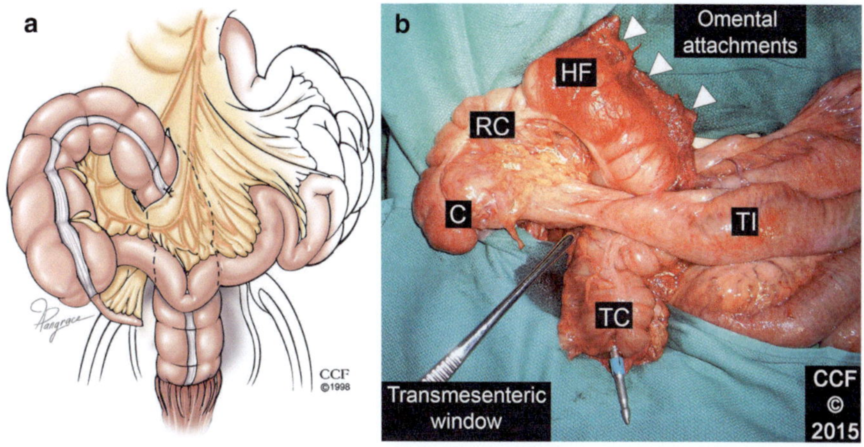

Fig. 147.3 (**a**) Illustration showing the passage of the mobilized colon through a window between the ileal and colic branches of the ileocolic artery; (**b**) Operative demonstration of this principle before anastomosis. Cecum (C), right colon (RC), hepatic flexure (HF), transverse colon (TC), terminal ileum (TI), omental attachments to the transverse colon (arrowheads)

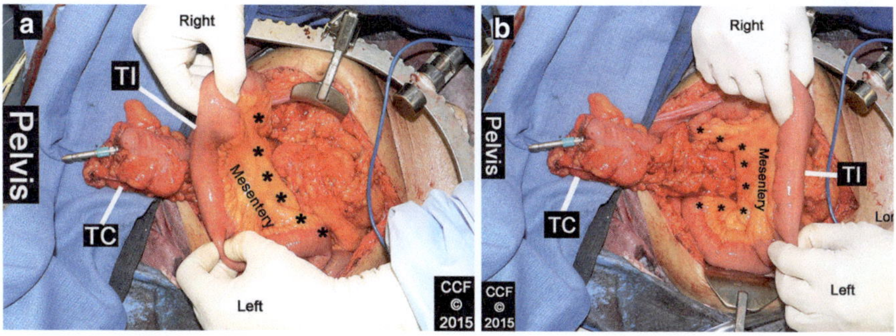

Fig. 147.4 (**a**) Superior view-relative to the mesenteric plane. The transverse colon (TC) has passed through the mesenteric window (asterisks) in the direction of the pelvis. Terminal ileum (TI); (**b**) Inferior view-relative to the mesenteric plane. The transverse colon (TC) has passed through the mesenteric window (asterisks) in the direction of the pelvis. Terminal ileum (TI)

References

1. Rombeau JL, Collins JP, Turnbull RB Jr. Left-sided colectomy with retroileal colorectal anastomosis. Arch Surg. 1978;113:1004–5.
2. Jagelman DG. Colectomy for malignant disease of the colon: the 'no touch' isolation technique. In: Fielding LP, Goldberg SM, editors. Surgery of the Colon, Rectum, and Anus. Rob and Smith's Operative Surgery. 5th ed. Oxford: Butterworth-Heinemann, Ltd.; 1993. p. 359–68.

148 Reconstruction After Left Colectomy-Right Colon to Rectum Anastomosis (Deloyers' Procedure)

Jesus Flores and James S. Wu

Introduction

Reconstruction of bowel continuity after left colectomy may be hampered because the transverse colon either crosses the small intestine to reach the rectum or is not long enough to travel around the small intestine along the left gutter to reach the rectum. In this type of situation, bowel continuity may be restored by right colon-to-rectal anastomosis (Deloyers).

Presentation

A 76-year-old female underwent sigmoid colon resection for cancer 20 years earlier. Colonoscopy revealed a large splenic flexure colon polyp that was too large to remove endoscopically.

Management

The transverse colon and left colon, including the previous colorectal anastomosis, were excised. The right colon and terminal ileum were mobilized. The appendix was removed. The right colon and its mesentery underwent a 180-degree mesoaxial rotation. Intestinal continuity was restored by right colon to rectal anastomosis (Fig. 148.1a). A contrast study demonstrated the postoperative anatomy (Fig. 148.1b).

J. Flores · J. S. Wu (✉)
Department of Colon and Rectal Surgery, Cleveland Clinic, Cleveland, OH, USA

J. S. Wu, M. D. Inkster (eds.), *Cleveland Clinic Colorectal Case Studies*,
https://doi.org/10.1007/978-3-031-39880-3_148

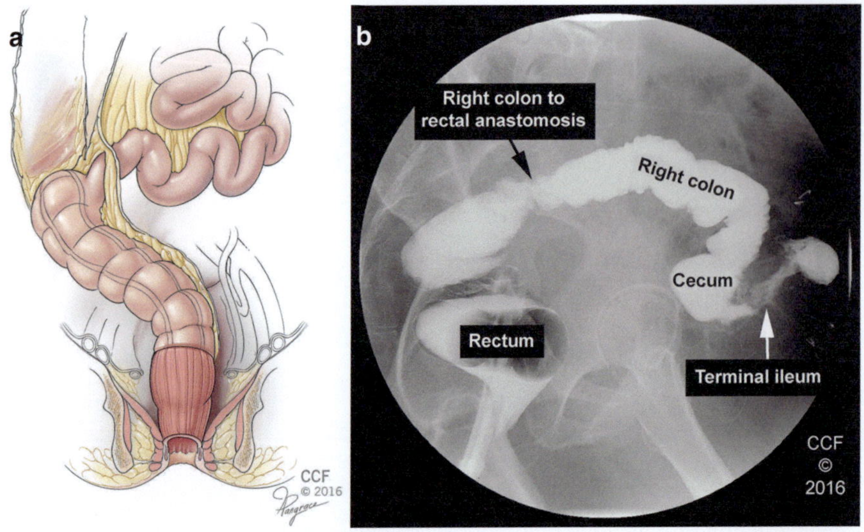

Fig. 148.1 Deloyers' procedure. (**a**) Illustration showing anastomosis of the right colon following mobilization, rotation, and anastomosis, in this illustration, to the rectum; (**b**) Contrast enema showing anatomy after intestinal reconstruction by right colon-to-rectal anastomosis. The appendix was removed to eliminate future appendicitis

Comment

In 1964, Deloyers described a technique to reconstitute large intestinal continuity [1].

La bascule du côlon droit permet sans exception de conserver le sphincter anal après les colectomies étendues du transverse et du côlon gauche (rectum y compris). Par L. Deloyers Membre d'Honneur de la Société (Bruxelles)	The rotation of the right colon allows without exception preservation of the anal sphincter after extensive colectomies of the transverse and the left colon (rectum included). By L. Deloyers Honorary Member of the Society (Brussels)

Deloyers' procedure consists of an anastomosis between the right colon and the rectum or anus after colonic mobilization with 180-degree mesoaxial rotation. Right colon perfusion is via the ileocolic artery [2–4]. Manceau [3] hypothesizes that preservation of the ileocecal junction, which acts as a sphincter, may prevent rapid inflow of ileal contents into the cecum and may improve function.

Alternatives include transmesenteric colorectal anastomosis (Rombeau) or ileorectal anastomosis.

References

1. Deloyers L. La bascule du côlon droit permet sans exception de conserver le sphincter anal après les colectomies étendues du transverse et du côlon gauche (rectum y compris). Technique-indications-Résultats immédiats et tardifs. Lyon Chir. 1964;60:404–13.
2. Shariff US, Kullar N, Dorudi S. Right colonic transposition technique: When the left colon is unavailable for achieving a pelvic anastomosis. Dis Colon Rectum. 2011;54:360–2.
3. Manceau G, Karoui M, Breton S, Blanchet A-S, Rousseau G, Savier E, et al. Right colon to rectal anastomosis (Deloyers procedure) as a salvage technique for low colorectal or coloanal anastomosis: Postoperative and long-term outcomes. Dis Colon Rectum. 2012;55:363–8.
4. Kontovounisios C, Baloyiannis Y, Kinross J, Tan E, Rasheed S, Tekkis P. Modified right colon inversion technique as a salvage procedure for colorectal or coloanal anastomosis. Colorectal Dis. 2014;16:971–5.

Intraoperative Colonic Lavage

149

James S. Wu

Presentation

A near-obstructing sigmoid colon cancer was found in a 67-year-old male by colonoscopy. The colonoscope was not able to pass proximal to the tumor. Bowel preparation before surgery was not possible. The preoperative metastatic evaluation was negative. Laparotomy and sigmoid colectomy were done. Intestinal reconstruction was carried out following intraoperative colonic lavage and colonoscopy.

Technique: Intraoperative Colonic Lavage

The appendix was removed. Warm saline was instilled into the right colon through an appendicostomy. The colonic effluent was emptied from the left colon using corrugated ventilator tubing (Figs. 149.1 and 149.2).

J. S. Wu (✉)
Department of Colon and Rectal Surgery, Cleveland Clinic, Cleveland, OH, USA

J. S. Wu, M. D. Inkster (eds.), *Cleveland Clinic Colorectal Case Studies*,
https://doi.org/10.1007/978-3-031-39880-3_149

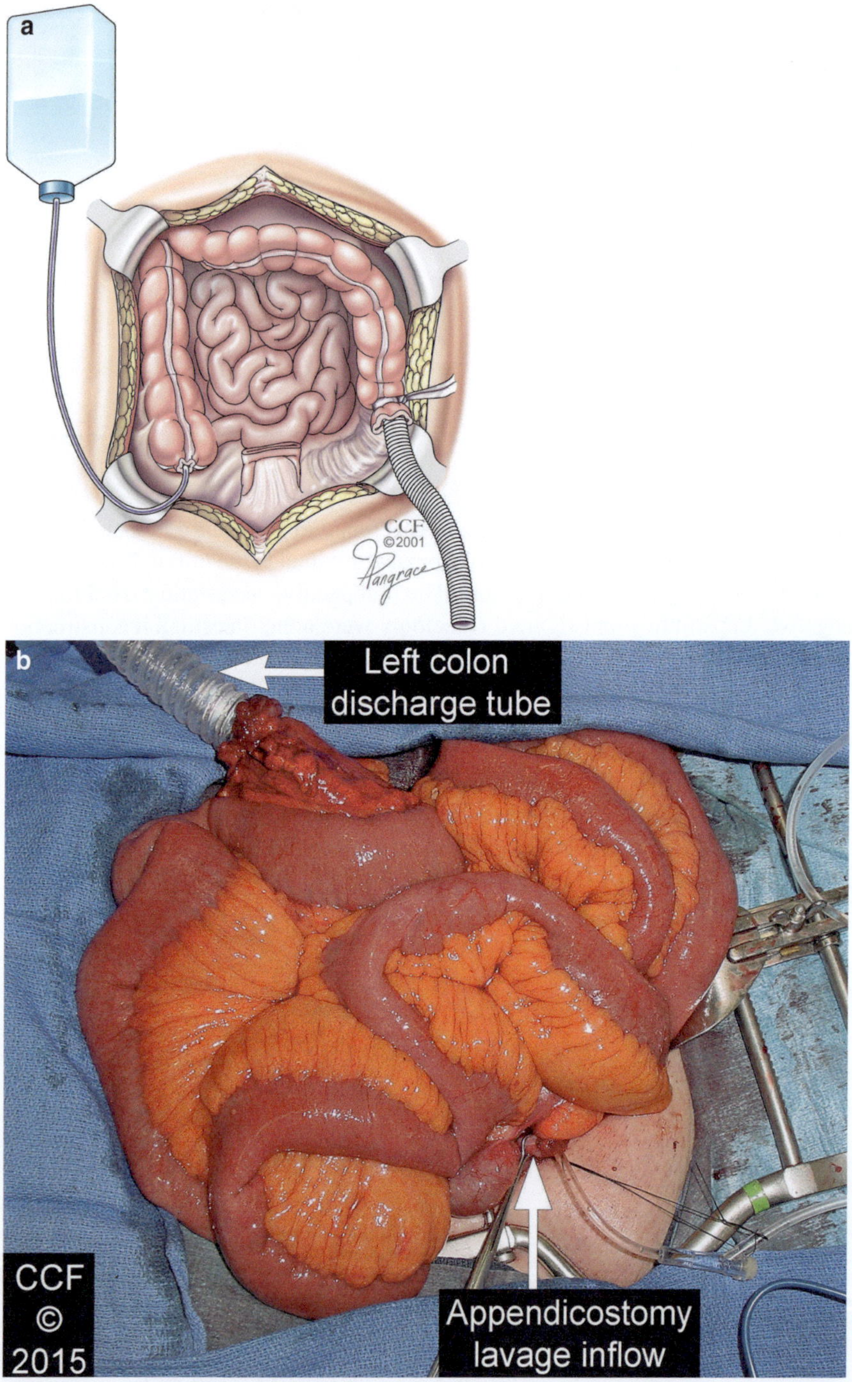

Fig. 149.1 (**a**) Intraoperative colonic lavage technique illustrated; (**b**) Intraoperative photo showing the appendicostomy inflow tube and the corrugated ventilator tubing attached to the left colon

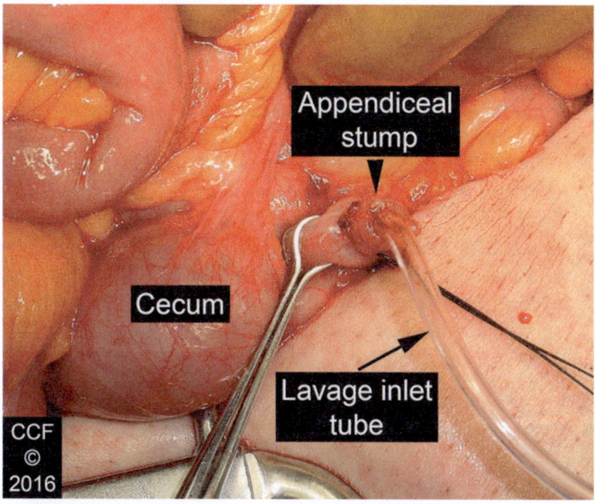

Fig. 149.2 Detail of appendicostomy. The base of the appendix in this case was grasped with a Babcock clamp. Warm saline was instilled into the colon with wide bore tubing as for cystoscopy to ensure adequate flow. Use of warm irrigation fluid prevents hypothermia

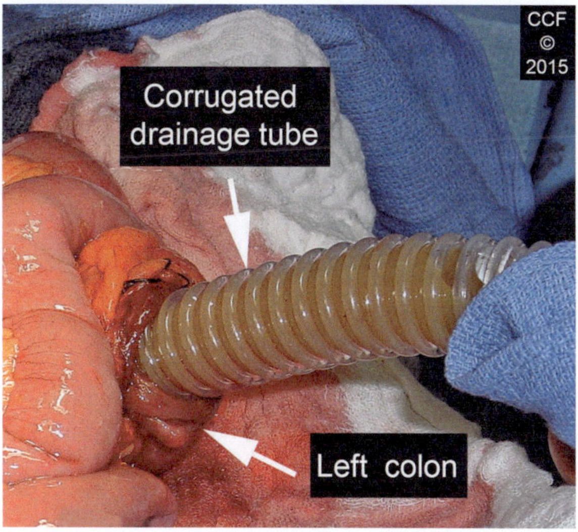

Fig. 149.3 Waste is discharged from the left colon through corrugated ventilator tubing

Comment

Because the left colon cancer was obstructing, preoperative colonoscopy was incomplete and bowel preparation was not possible. Intraoperative antegrade colonic lavage cleared the unprepared colon of feces [1–5]. Following lavage, intraoperative colonoscopy excluded synchronous lesions. Colorectal anastomosis then was done. In this case, intraoperative colonic cleansing facilitated single-stage resection and restoration of bowel continuity.

References

1. Muir EG. Safety in colonic resection. Proc R Soc Med. 1968;61:401–8.
2. Dudley HAF, Radcliffe AG, McGeehan D. Intraoperative irrigation of the colon to permit primary anastomosis. Br J Surg. 1980;67:80–1.
3. Koruth NM, Krukowski ZH, Youngson GG, Hendry WS, Logie JRC, Jones PF, et al. Intraoperative colonic irrigation in the management of left-sided large bowel emergencies. Br J Surg. 1985;72:708–11.
4. Foster ME, Johnson CD, Billings PJ, Davies PW, Leaper DJ. Intraoperative antegrade lavage and anastomotic healing in acute colonic obstruction. Dis Colon Rectum. 1986;29:255–9.
5. Pollack AV, Playforth MJ, Evans M. Peroperative lavage of the obstructed left colon to allow safe primary anastomosis. Dis Colon Rectum. 1987;30:171–3.

150 Colorectal Cancer Metastases

James S. Wu, Arthur A. Parsee, and Michelle D. Inkster

Metastatic Colon Cancer

The following computed tomographic (CT) scans and one plain radiograph show examples of colorectal cancer metastases (Figs. 150.1, 150.2, 150.3, 150.4, 150.5, 150.6, 150.7, 150.8, 150.9, and 150.10).

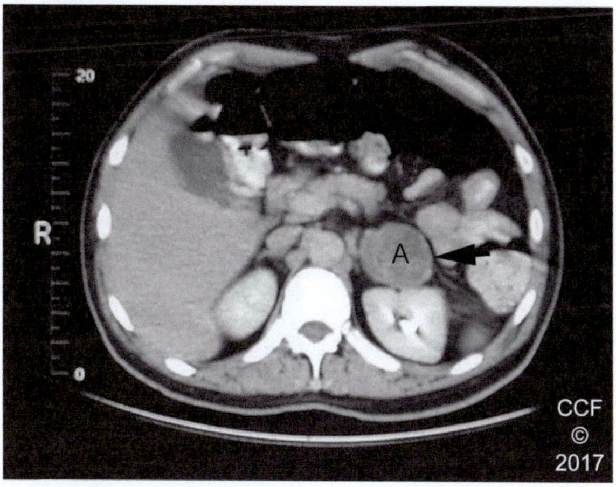

Fig. 150.1 CT scan of the abdomen (axial view) shows an adrenal metastasis (A)

J. S. Wu (✉)
Department of Colon and Rectal Surgery, Cleveland Clinic, Cleveland, OH, USA

A. A. Parsee
Department of Diagnostic Radiology, H. Lee Moffitt Cancer Center and Research Institute, Tampa, FL, USA

M. D. Inkster
Department of Gastroenterology, Cleveland Clinic, Cleveland, OH, USA

J. S. Wu, M. D. Inkster (eds.), *Cleveland Clinic Colorectal Case Studies*,
https://doi.org/10.1007/978-3-031-39880-3_150

Fig. 150.2 Plain radiograph of a patient with a colorectal cancer metastasis to the femur resulting in pathologic fracture (arrow)

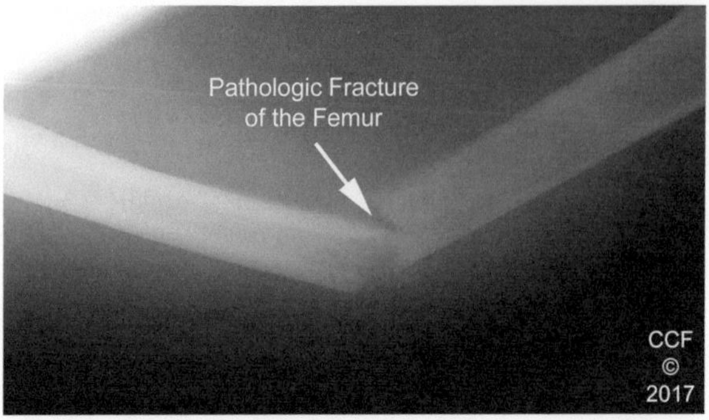

Fig. 150.3 CT scan of the abdomen (axial view) shows large liver metastases (asterisks). The stomach (S) and spleen (Sp) are labeled

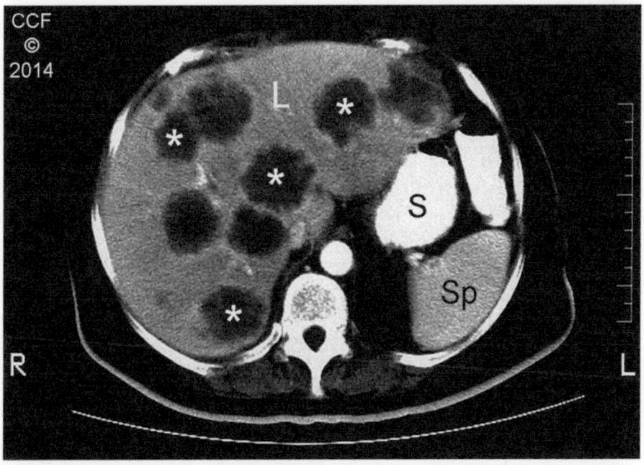

Fig. 150.4 CT scan of the abdomen (axial view) shows malignant ascites (asterisks). The borders of the border of liver and spleen are marked with arrows

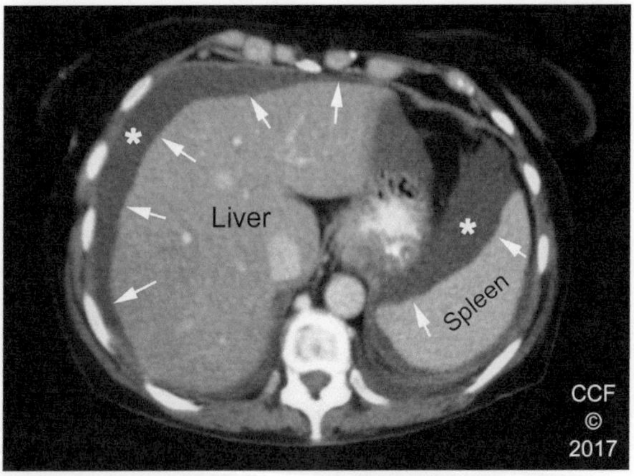

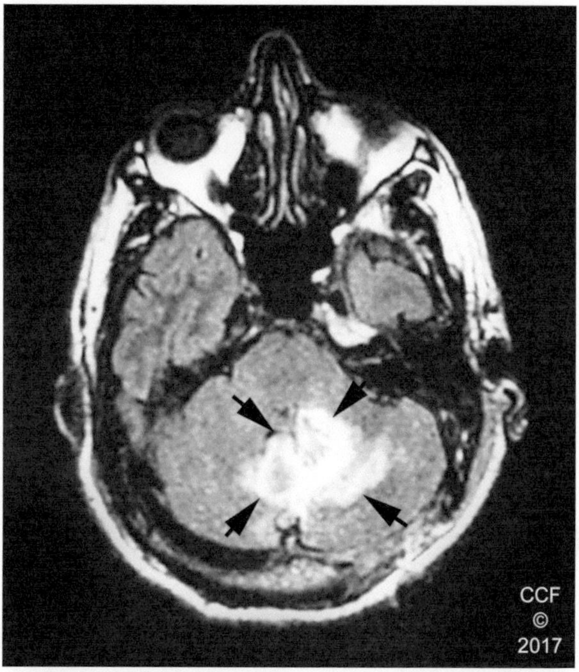

Fig. 150.5 MRI image, FLAIR sequence, shows a metastasis (arrows) to the cerebellum with effacement of the fourth ventricle

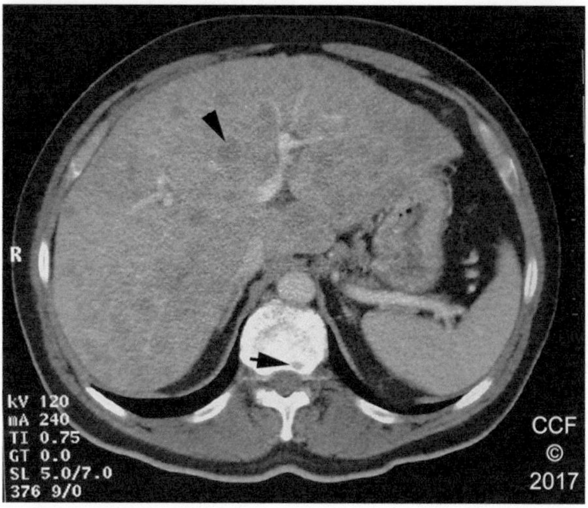

Fig. 150.6 CT scan of the abdomen (axial view) shows diffuse liver metastases (arrowhead) and a spine metastasis (arrow)

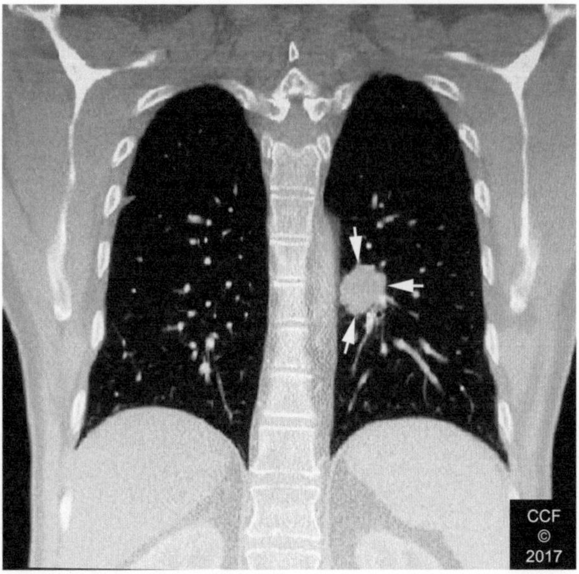

Fig. 150.7 CT scan of the chest, coronal view. A pulmonary metastasis is labeled with arrows

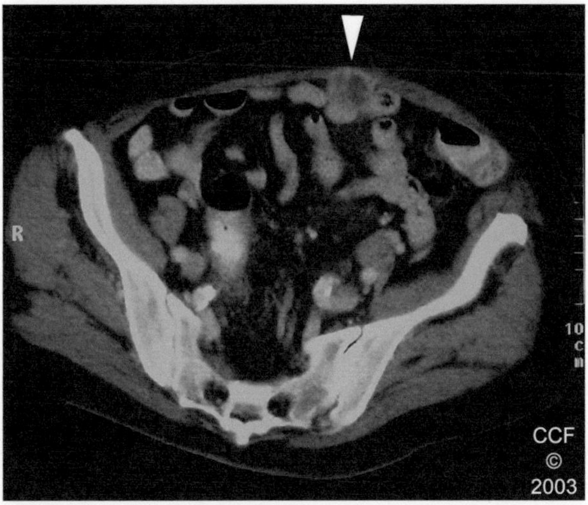

Fig. 150.8 CT scan of the abdomen, axial view. Peritoneal metastases (arrow) following colon cancer resection

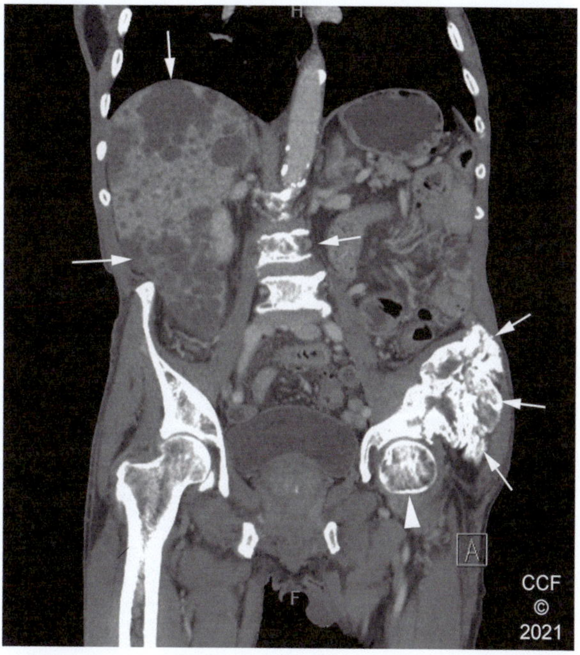

Fig. 150.9 CT scan of the abdomen, coronal view. Metastases to the liver, spine, and left pelvis are labeled with arrows. The left femoral head is labeled with an arrowhead

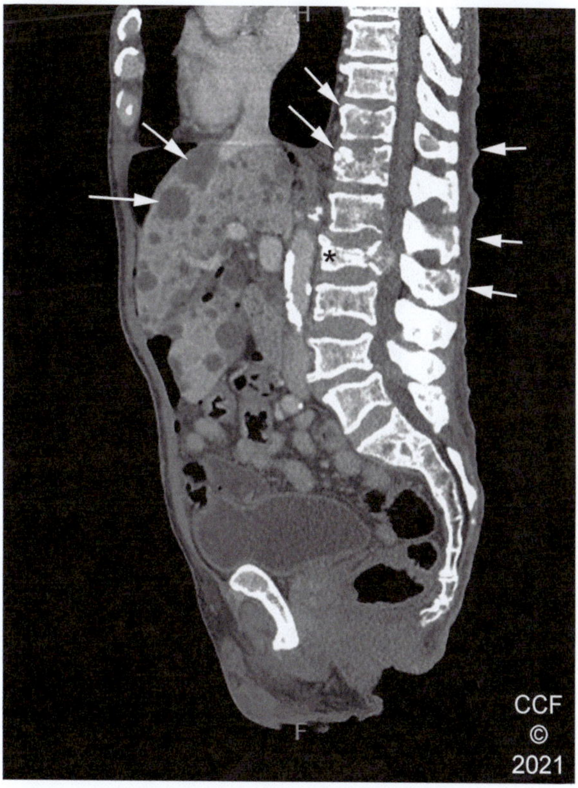

Fig. 150.10 CT scan of the abdomen, sagittal view. Metastases to the liver and spine are labeled with arrows. At L2 (asterisk), there is tumor retropulsion into the spinal canal

Comment

Approximately 20% of colorectal cancer (CRC) patients have distant metastases at the time of primary diagnosis [1].[1] In a 2015 nationwide report on colorectal cancer patients with synchronous metastases in the Netherlands, van der Geest et al. [2][2] reported the most common metastatic sites (Table 150.1).

Table 150.1 Colorectal cancer and synchronous distant metastases (2008–2011) in the Netherlands (van der Geest)

	N (%)
All patients diagnosed with CRC	47,418
Most common metastatic sites	
Liver	8123 (17)
Lung	2358 (5.0)
Peritoneum	2234 (4.7)
Bone	334 (0.7)
Brain	74 (0.2)

[1] Permission to reuse this data was generously granted by Springer Nature and Copyright Clearance Center, License number 5327240066627, License date Jun 13, 2022.

[2] Permission to reuse this data was generously granted by Springer Nature and Copyright Clearance Center, License number 5327240066627, License date Jun 13, 2022.

References

1. Riihimäki M, Hemminki A, Sundquist J, Hemminki K. Patterns of metastasis in colon and rectal cancer. Sci. Rep. 2016;6:29765. https://doi.org/10.1038/srep29765.
2. van der Geest LGM, Lam-Boer J, Koopman M, Verhoef C, Elferink MAG, de Wilt JHW. Nationwide trends in incidence, treatment and survival of colorectal cancer patients with synchronous metastases. Clin Exp Metastasis. 2015;32:457–65.

References

Intestinal Bypass for Malignant Obstruction

151

James S. Wu and Erika B. Woodrum

Presentation

An 89-year-old female underwent right hemicolectomy for colon cancer 18 months earlier. She presented with abdominal pain, nausea, vomiting, and absence of flatus. Examination revealed a hard nontender right-sided abdominal mass (Fig. 151.1). Computed tomographic (CT) scanning revealed proximal small bowel dilation, right-sided hydronephrosis, and liver metastases (Fig. 151.2a, b).

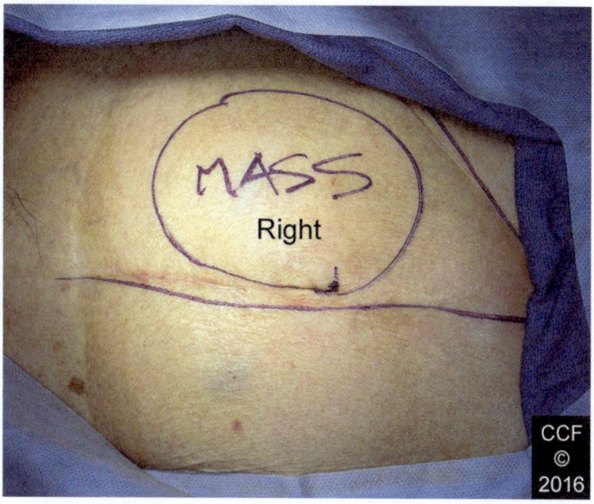

Fig. 151.1 Right-sided abdominal mass 18 months after right hemicolectomy for cancer

J. S. Wu (✉)
Department of Colon and Rectal Surgery, Cleveland Clinic, Cleveland, OH, USA

E. B. Woodrum
Medical Illustration Team, Enterprise Creative Services, Cleveland Clinic, Cleveland, OH, USA

J. S. Wu, M. D. Inkster (eds.), *Cleveland Clinic Colorectal Case Studies*,
https://doi.org/10.1007/978-3-031-39880-3_151

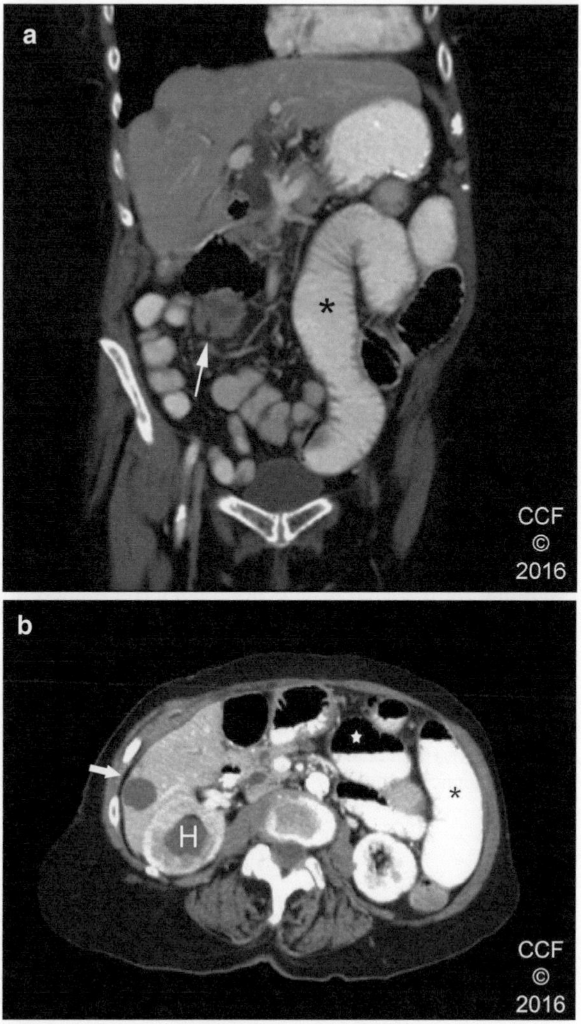

Fig. 151.2 Abdominal CT scan. (**a**) Coronal view shows a right-sided abdominal mass (arrow) and dilated proximal jejunum (asterisk); (**b**) Axial view shows right-sided hydronephrosis (H) and a liver metastasis (large arrow)

Management

Following an initial trial of nasogastric tube decompression, abdominal exploration was done. Multiple loops of small intestine were intimately associated with a right-sided retroperitoneal mass, the cause of the obstruction (Fig. 151.3). There were 100 centimeters of unobstructed jejunum from the ligament of Treitz to the mass. The obstruction was relieved by jejunum to transverse colon enterocolostomy bypass (Fig. 151.4). The bypass concept is illustrated in Fig. 151.5.

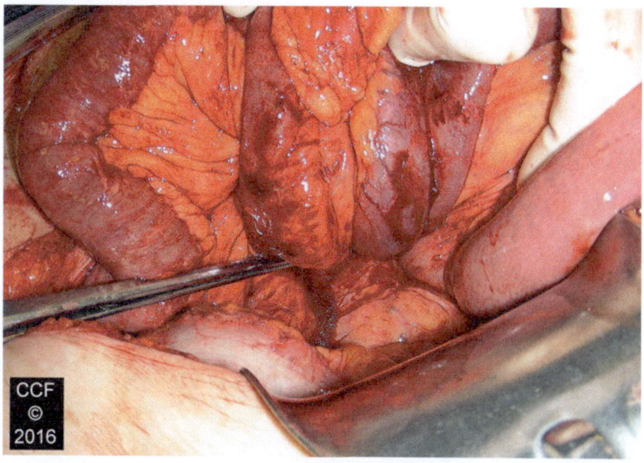

Fig. 151.3 The forceps identify the point of obstruction where multiple loops of small intestine enter a fixed mass

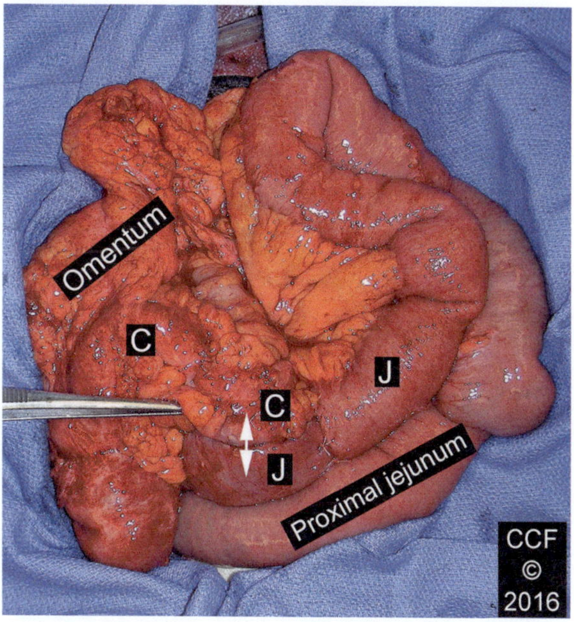

Fig. 151.4 Side-to-side anastomosis (double arrowhead, pointing scissors) between unobstructed distal jejunum (J) and distal transverse colon (C) with attached omentum

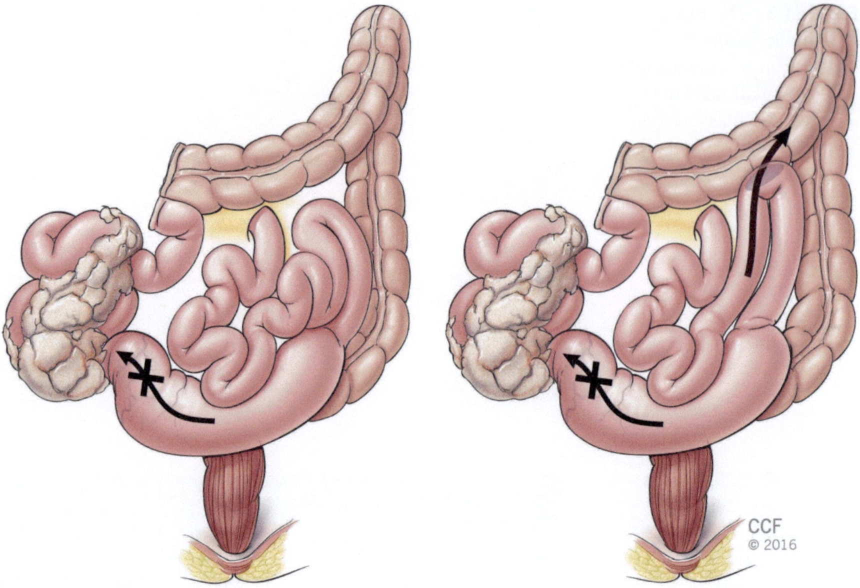

Fig. 151.5 The left-sided panel shows obstruction due to a mass following prior right colectomy. The right-sided panel shows bypass of the obstructing mass by anastomosis of the jejunum to the distal transverse colon

Comment

This patient had a firm nontender palpable mass on the right side of the abdomen following right hemicolectomy for colon cancer. The mass, arising from the retroperitoneum, caused small bowel and right ureteral obstruction. Liver metastases were present. The preoperative diagnosis was malignant obstruction. In 2004, Fazio published a treatise entitled, "Indications and Surgical Alternatives for Palliation of Rectal Cancer."[1]

> "The goals of palliation of rectal cancer are relief of disabling symptoms and maximizing quality of life. Surgical intervention is appropriate in specific situations, where the selected procedure is chosen based on likelihood of achieving these goals, balanced against the morbidity and recognition of the patient's limited life expectancy."

The principles stated are appropriate for palliation of advanced colon cancer as well.

Surgical options considered in this case included:

1. resection of the obstructed intestine,
2. proximal diversion by jejunostomy or gastrostomy,
3. intestinal bypass.

The operative was considered palliative. The patient was 89 years old. Liver metastasis was present. Because the retroperitoneal mass involved multiple loops of small intestine and the left ureter, resection was considered unfeasible. Proximal diversion would be associated with high volume postoperative fluid losses. Bypass was chosen for four reasons:

1. The unobstructed jejunum and the transverse colon were anatomically close to each other,
2. A high output stoma would be avoided,
3. The colon, with its water absorbing capacity, could be utilized,
4. The patient could eat.

Liang et al. [2] studied patients with stage IV colorectal cancers, who have unresectable primaries or extensive metastases, and found that palliative bypass or stoma creation is associated with survival for several months for a significant proportion of patients. The decision to operate in this case was made after considering prognosis and fitness for surgery. Overall care was coordinated with medical and oncology consultants [3].

References

1. Fazio VW. Indications and surgical alternatives for palliation of rectal cancer. J Gastrointest Surg. 2004;8:262–5.
2. Liang J, Church JM, Stocchi L, Fazio V, Kiran RP. Should bypass or stoma creation be undertaken for unresectable stage IV colorectal carcinoma. ANZ J Surg. 2014;84:275–9.
3. Ripamonti CI, Easson AM, Gerdes H. Management of malignant bowel obstruction. Eur J Cancer. 2008;44:1105–15.

Krukenberg Tumor

152

Kenneth D. Webster, Mark J. Melaragno, Eric W. Willis, and James S. Wu

Presentation

A 23-year-old woman presented with a left ovarian mass (Fig. 152.1). She had undergone prior colectomy for sigmoid adenocarcinoma. The serum carcinoembryonic antigen was elevated.

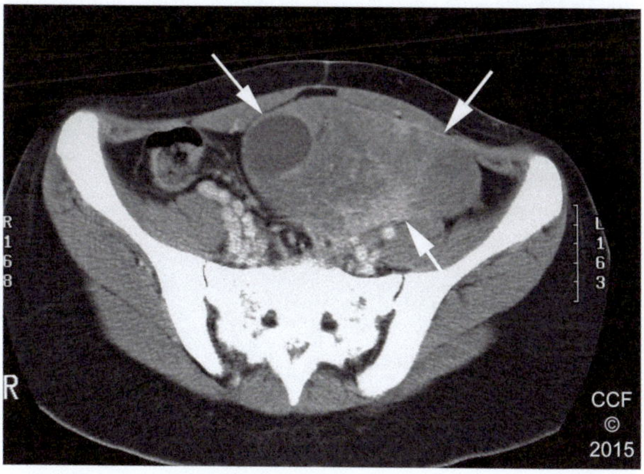

Fig. 152.1 Computed tomography (CT) shows a left ovarian mass (arrows)

K. D. Webster
Department of Obstetrics and Gynecology, Cleveland Clinic, Cleveland, OH, USA

M. J. Melaragno
Pathology & Laboratory Medicine Institute, Cleveland Clinic, Cleveland, OH, USA

E. W. Willis
Department of Pathology, CORPath, Columbus, OH, USA

J. S. Wu (✉)
Department of Colon and Rectal Surgery, Cleveland Clinic, Cleveland, OH, USA

J. S. Wu, M. D. Inkster (eds.), *Cleveland Clinic Colorectal Case Studies*,
https://doi.org/10.1007/978-3-031-39880-3_152

Management

At the time of her original colon cancer surgery, ovarian preservation had been chosen to maintain female identity and fertility. The CT scan shows a left ovarian mass (Fig. 152.1). Resection was done. The gross specimen is shown in Fig. 152.2. Histopathology of the resected specimen showed signet-ring cell carcinoma (Fig. 152.3).

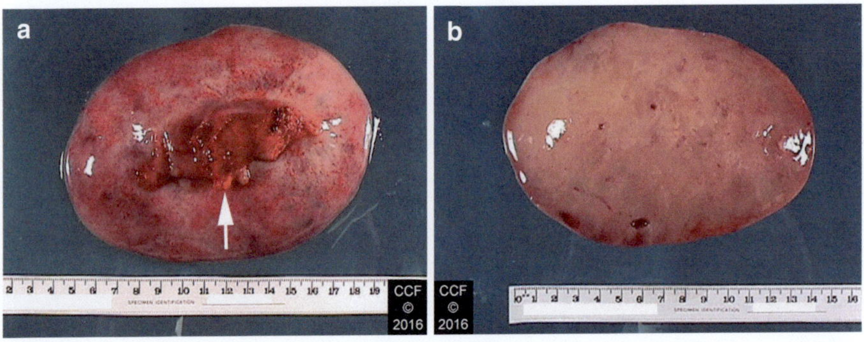

Fig. 152.2 Resected pelvic mass, (**a**) Outer surface with attached fallopian tube (arrow); (**b**) Cut surface of the bivalved ovary

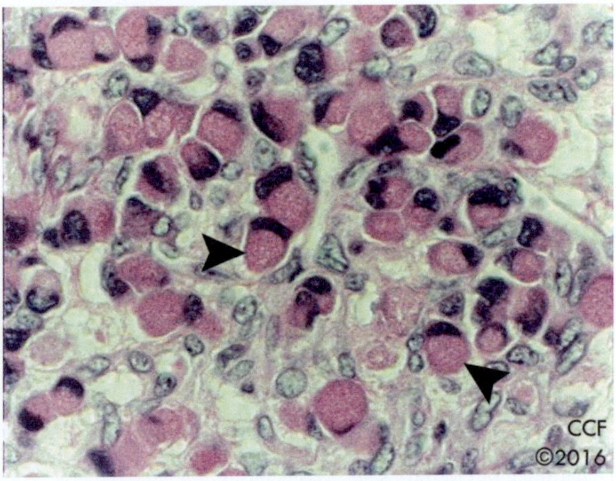

Fig. 152.3 Sections show diffuse sheets of monotonous cells with eccentric hyperchromatic nuclei compressed and indented by a mucin droplet (signet-ring cell) highlighted pink in this periodic acid-Schiff stain (arrowheads)

Comment

In his 2006 review article entitled, "From Krukenberg to Today: The Ever Present Problems Posed by Metastatic Tumors of the Ovary," Young wrote [1, 2][1]:

> "The historical timeline on the Krukenberg tumor dates back to the legendary Sir James Paget and the story is followed through the well-known, albeit flawed, contribution of Friedrich Krukenberg…."
>
> Robert H. Young,
> James Homer Wright Pathology Laboratories
> Massachusetts General Hospital
> Harvard Medical School
> Boston, MA

In 1854, Paget reported [3]:

Lectures on Surgical Pathology
Delivered at the
Royal College of Surgeons of England
By
James Paget, F.R.S.
Lately Professor of Anatomy and Surgery to the College, Assistant Surgeon and Lecturer on Physiology at St. Bartholomew's Hospital
Lecture XXX
Scirrhous or Hard Cancer

> "The most remarkable examples of hard cancers with fibrous structures that I have yet seen, have been in the ovaries of certain patients with common hard cancer of the breast or stomach."

In 1896, Krukenberg published, "Ueber das Fibrosarcoma ovarii mucocellulare (carcinomatodes)," a tumor now associated with his name [4].

Young continues:

> 'It is fitting that our knowledge of metastatic tumors goes back to one the giants of medicine, Sir James Paget whose "Lecture Notes on Surgical Pathology" contain one of the earliest mentions of what we now know to be metastasis in the ovary. As recounted by Shenoy and Scheithauer, in 1854 Paget described a distinctive form of ovarian tumor associated with breast cancer or gastric cancer of "fibrous hard" nature, almost certainly what we would now recognize as a Krukenberg tumor.
>
> The eponymous designation "Krukenberg" tumor derives from the description of 5 cases by Friedrich Ernst Krukenberg (1871-1946) in 1896 when working as a student in the laboratory of the eminent Felix Marchand, in Marburg, Germany. Marchand seems to have suggested the initial terminology "fibrosarcoma mucocellulare Carcinomatodes."'

---

[1] Permission to republish excerpts from this paper was generously granted by Wolters Kluwer Health Inc., CCC| RightsLink®, License Number 5153180051048, License Date Sep 20, 2021.

Young notes that illustrations from Krukenberg's paper show "typical signet-ring cells;" regarding the designation "Krukenberg tumor, " he writes:

> 'THE KRUKENBERG TUMOR
>
> This designation should be reserved for tumors with an appreciable component (arbitrarily defined as >10% of the tumor) of signet-ring cells and no evidence of another specific diagnosis such as clear cell carcinoma or mucinous carcinoid, or any other primary neoplasm that rarely has signet-ring cells.
>
> The designation "Krukenberg tumor" has sometimes loosely been applied to any metastatic tumor in the ovary, a practice to be avoided. Unless otherwise qualified the description implies a tumor that is metastatic to the ovary;...'

Regarding Krukenberg tumors, Kiyokawa et al. [5][2] conclude:

> "Despite Paget's priority, the eponymous designation of the tumor was based on Krukenberg's description of 6 cases 42 years later, even though he erroneously interpreted the neoplasm as a primary fibrosarcoma containing mucinous cells."

The authors note that the stomach is the most common primary malignancy that metastasizes to the ovary; other primary sites include colon and rectum, breast, small intestine, appendix, pancreas, and gall bladder/biliary tract.

McCluggage and Young [6][3] continue:

> "The occurrence of signet ring cells in primary ovarian tumors and the extent to which a proliferation of such cells can simulate the well-known metastatic signet ring cell carcinoma (Krukenberg tumor) has long been an enigmatic topic and has a checkered history. It dates back, indeed, to Krukenberg's original paper in which he presented a small series of cases which he did not recognize as being metastatic."

Ojo et al. [7] found that ovarian metastases from colorectal cancer occur in about 3% of all colorectal cancer patients. Jiang et al. [8] report a median survival of 29.6 months in patients with Krukenberg tumors of colon and rectum origin.

References

1. Young RH. From Krukenberg to today: The ever present problems posed by metastatic tumors in the ovary. Part I. Historical perspective, general principles, mucinous tumors including the Krukenberg tumor. Adv Anat Pathol. 2006;13:205–27.
2. Young RH. From Krukenberg to today: The ever present problems posed by metastatic tumors in the ovary. Part II Adv Anat Pathol. 2007;14:149–77.
3. Paget J. Lectures on Surgical Pathology. Philadelphia: Lindsay & Blakiston; 1854. p. 510.

[2]This excerpt is reproduced with the generous permission of Wolters Kluwer Health, Inc., CCC|RightsLink®, License Number 5151871098758, License date Sept 18, 2021.

[3]This excerpt is reproduced with the generous permission of Wolters Kluwer Health, Inc., CCC|RightsLink®, License Number 5151870225088, License date Sep 18, 2021.

4. Krukenberg F. Ueber das Fibrosarcoma ovarii mucocellulare (carcinomatodes). Arch Gynäkol. 1896;50:238–321.
5. Kiyokawa T, Young RH, Scully RE. Krukenberg tumors of the ovary. A clinicopathologic analysis of 120 cases with emphasis on their variable pathologic manifestations. Am J Surg Pathol. 2006;30:277–99.
6. McCluggage WG, Young RH. Primary ovarian mucinous tumors with signet ring cells. Report of 3 cases with discussion of so-called primary Krukenberg tumor. Am J Surg Pathol. 2008;32:1373–9.
7. Ojo J, De Silva S, Han E, Lin P, Wakabayashi M, Nelson R, et al. Krukenberg tumors from colorectal cancer: Presentation, treatment and outcomes. Am Surgeon. 2011;77:1381–5.
8. Jiang R, Tang J, Cheng X, Zang RY. Surgical treatment for patients with different origins of Krukenberg tumors: Outcomes and prognostic factors. EJSO. 2009;35:92–7.

Müllerian Adenocarcinoma Metastatic to the Colon

153

Michelle D. Inkster, Jacob R. Sweeney, and James S. Wu

Presentation

An 80-year-old female underwent colonoscopy because of rectal bleeding. She had a history of endometrial cancer. An ulcerated mass was found in the distal sigmoid colon (Fig. 153.1).

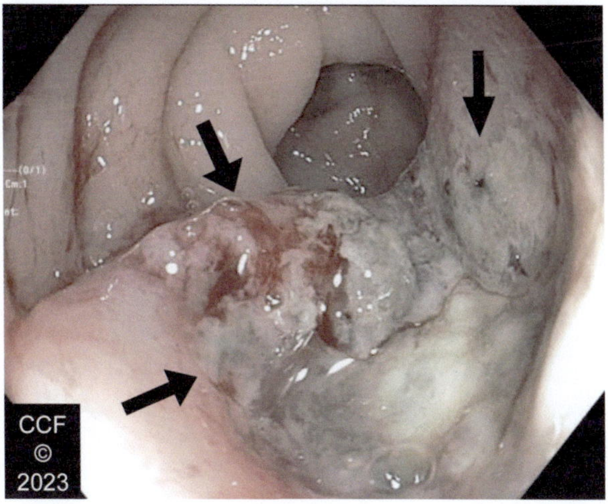

Fig. 153.1 Colonoscopic view of the ulcerated sigmoid colon mass (arrows)

M. D. Inkster
Department of Gastroenterology, Cleveland Clinic, Cleveland, OH, USA

J. R. Sweeney
Pathology & Laboratory Medicine Institute, Cleveland Clinic, Cleveland, OH, USA

J. S. Wu (✉)
Department of Colon and Rectal Surgery, Cleveland Clinic, Cleveland, OH, USA

J. S. Wu, M. D. Inkster (eds.), *Cleveland Clinic Colorectal Case Studies*,
https://doi.org/10.1007/978-3-031-39880-3_153

Pathology showed adenocarcinoma consistent with Müllerian primary (Fig. 153.2).

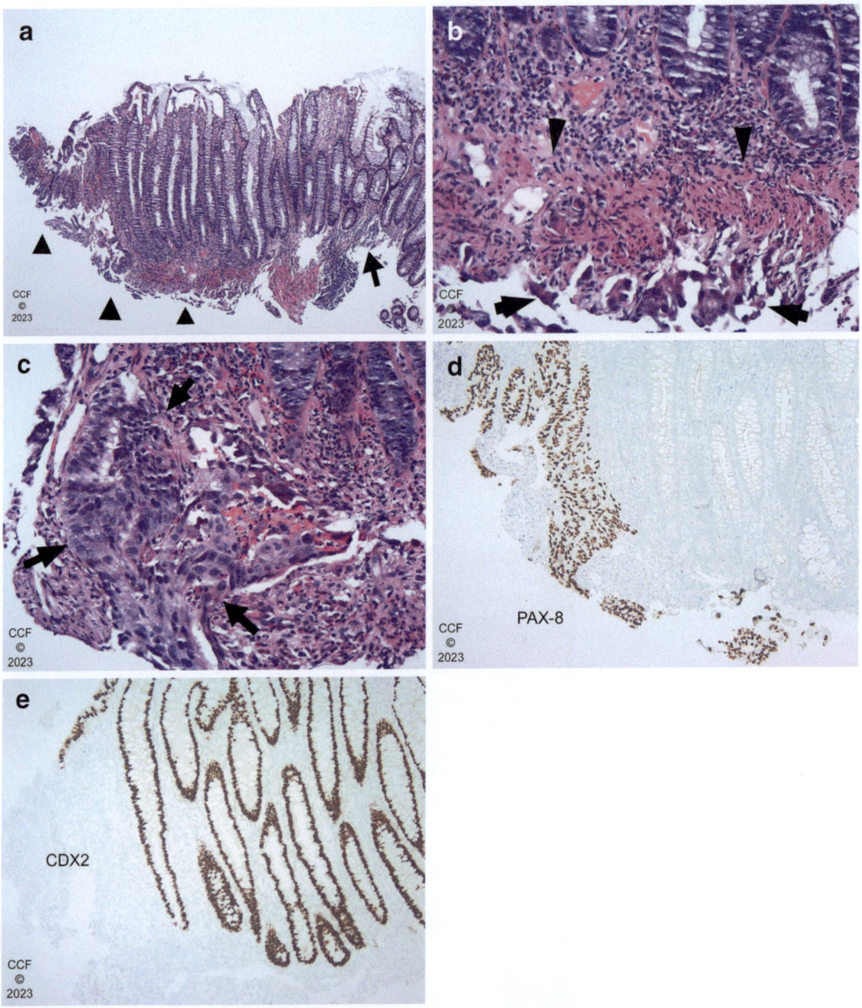

Fig. 153.2 (**a**) Low magnification (4×), adenocarcinoma as well as undermining muscularis mucosa (bottom, arrowhead), benign colonic mucosa, lower right and left, arrows. (**b**) High magnification (20×), adenocarcinoma, bottom (arrows) undermining muscularis mucosae (arrowheads). (**c**) 3-high magnification (20×), adenocarcinoma with solid growth, left, (arrowheads). (**d**) PAX-8 immunostain shows diffuse positive staining in tumor cells (left). Adjacent benign colonic epithelium (right) negative. (**e**) 5-CDX2 immunostain shows no staining in tumor cells (left) but positive staining in adjacent benign colonic epithelium (right)

Comment

This tumor easily could be mistaken for a primary colorectal adenocarcinoma. However, the patient's history of endometrial carcinoma raised the possibility of metastatic disease. The tumor's growth below the muscularis mucosa, solid growth pattern, high-grade cytology, and lack of dysplastic precursor lesions were histologic clues that suggested metastasis in this case. Positive staining for PAX8 and negative staining for CDX2 confirmed this possibility; PAX8 is positive in Müllerian primaries but negative in colorectal primaries while CDX2 is positive in colorectal primaries. Cancers of Müllerian origin metastatic to the colon are rare. In 2011, Yang et al. [1] reported 13 cases of carcinoma of Müllerian origin presenting as colorectal cancer. In 2012, Anstadt reported endometrial adenocarcinoma metastatic to the colon masquerading as a primary colon cancer [2].

A Müllerian tumor is a cancer of the uterus, ovary or fallopian tubes [3] eponymously named after Johannes Peter Müller. As outlined by Larsen [4], at about 24 days of gestation, the mesonephric ducts (Wolffian) appear [4, 5]. During the sixth week of development, the paramesonephric ducts (Müllerian) form lateral to the mesonephric ducts. Male and female genital systems are virtually identical until the end of the sixth week. In the absence of a Y chromosome, female development occurs. The paramesonephric ducts give rise to the uterus, fallopian tubes, and superior vagina [4]. In 1830, Müller reported anatomical studies on human and animal embryos that described this genital development [6].

Bildungsgeschichte der Genitalen aus anatomischen Untersuchungen an Embryonen des Menchen und der Thiere, von Dr. Johannes Müller Professor der Medicin an der Friedrich-Wilhelms-Universität zu Bonn 1830.	Educational history of the genitals from anatomical investigation of human and animal embryos by Dr. Johannes Müller Professor of Medicine at the Friedrich-Wilhelms-University in Bonn 1830.
III. Weitere Entwicklungsgeschichte der männlichen und weiblichen innern Genitalien. S. 71.	III. Further story of development of the male and female internal genitalia p.71.
Bisher waren die männlichen und weiblichen innern Genitalien nicht zu unterscheiden; alle Embryonen haben entlang dem Wolff'schen Körper einen Gang, den man für Ductus deferens eben sowohl als für Trompete halten könnte, an der entgegengesetzten inneren Seite ein keimbereitendes Genitale, das man eben so gut für Hoden als für Eierstock anzusehen berechtigt ist. Von der Gegend des Bauchringes erhebt sich eine Falte des Peritoneums nach aufwärts zum untern Ende des Wolff'schen Körpers und zu dem über diesen Körper verlaufenden Gang. Diese Falte enhält ein Bündel Fasern, noch ist die Insertionsstelle dieses Bandes, welches bei männlichen Embryonen später zum *Gubernaculum Hunteri*, bei weiblichen zum *Ligamentum uteri rotundum* wird, bei allen Embryonen gleich; es inserirt sich nämlich an den ausführenden Gang seiner Seite, am untern Ende des Wolff'schen Körpers.	Until now, the male and female inner genitalia were not distinguishable; all embryos have a duct along the Wolffian body, that one could take for ductus deferens as well as for trumpet, and on the opposite inner side a germinative genitalia, which one just as well can regard as testis or ovary. From the region of the abdominal ring a fold of peritoneum rises upwards to the inferior end of the Wolffian body and the duct running across that body. This fold contains a bundle of fibers, and the point of insertion of this ligament, which later becomes the G*ubernaculum Hunterei* in male embryos and the ligamentum uteri rotundum in females, the same in all embryos; namely, it inserts itself into the excretory duct on its side, at the lower end of the Wolffian body.
S. 74 Man sieht hieraus, dass das *Ligamentum uteri rotundum* und das *Gubernaculum Hunteri* ursprünglich ganz dieselben Dinge sind. Allein das Ligamentum uteri rotundum bleibt dem Horn des Uterus verbunden, wenn der untere Theil der ausführenden Ganges jeder Seite sich zum Horn des Uterus erweitert hat. Beim Menschen werden selbst diese Hörner zum Fundus des Uterus umgewandelt, und die Insertion des Ligamentum ist zuletzt am Uterus selbst.	p. 74 From this it can be seen that the *Ligamentum uteri rotundum* and the Gubernaculum *Hunteri* are originally exactly the same things. Only the ligamentum uteri rotundum remains connected to the horn of the uterus when the lower part of the excertory ducts of each side has widened to the horn of the uterus. In man even these horns are transformed into the fundus of the uterus, and the insertion of the ligament is finally on the uterus itself.

Biographical Note

Johannes Peter Müller (1801–1858)

Johannes Müller was a physician, physiologist, comparative anatomist, and educator. He rose to the position of Professor and Chair of Anatomy and Physiology at the University of Berlin [7, 8]. Upon Müller's death, it was one of his students, Rudolf Virchow, who gave his eulogy [9]. Virchow begins with words that express the profound grief of his colleagues.

Johannes Müller Eine Gedächtnissrede, gehalten bei der Todtenfeier am 24. Juli 1858 in der Aula der Universität zu Berlin von Rudolf Virchow Der dritte Monat ist fast vorüber seit jenem Frühlingsmorgen, an welchem die erschütternde Kunde von Johannes Müller's jähem Tode unsere Stadt durcheilte. Kein Lob bringt uns den Verlorenen zurück. Hier stehen wir, die Vertreter der grossen ärztlichen Familie, Lehrer und Lernende, Praktiker und Forscher, um es uns gegenseitig zu klagen, wie keine Sorge des Tages, keine Arbeit der Nächte unsere Bekümmerniss über einen solchen Verlust zu mildern vermag.	Johannes Müller A memorial speech given at the funeral service on July 24, 1858 in the auditorium of the University of Berlin by Rudolf Virchow The third month has almost passed since that spring morning when the shocking news of Johannes Müller's sudden death swept through our city. No praise brings back he whom we have lost. Here we stand, the representatives of the great medical family, teachers and students, practitioners and researchers, to lament to one another how no care of the day, no work of the night can lessen our Grief over such a loss.

At the end of the eulogy, Virchow notes familiar personal traits, that now gone, will be missed.

Das dunkle Auge, das so finster aussah, wenn es grübelte, das so hell aufschlagen konnte, wenn es lächeln wollte, war gebrochen. Die starke Falte des Forschers war gesunken. Die kräftige, breite Schulter lag auf immer starr. An dem mächtigen Kopf, der wie eines Kriegers des Alterthums erschien, sah man, dass ein hehrer Arbeiter des Geistes gefallen war.	The dark eye that looked so grim when it was brooding, that could open so brightly when it wanted to smile, was broken. The explorer's strong brow had fallen. The powerful, broad shoulders lay forever rigid. On the mighty head, which looked like that of an ancient warrior, one saw that a noble laborer of the spirit had fallen.

In the center of the eulogy, Virchow defines the principal tools of Müller's approach to understanding life processes, namely, *Beobachtung* (observation) and *Versuch* (experimentation). The background necessary for comprehending the observed lies in basic science and anatomy.

Die Anatomie wurde die sichere Grundlage der biologischen Anschauung; die langsam heranreifende Chemie und Physik gaben die Mittel zu einer mechanischen Erklärung der Lebensvorgänge. …dass vielmehr nur in der innigen Verbindung der durch Beobachtung und Versuch fortschreitenden Physiologie mit der Philosophie die Sicherheit vor jeder einseitigen Behandling gegeben ist.	Anatomy became the secure foundation of biology; the slowly maturing fields of chemistry and physics gave the means for a mechanical explanation of life processes. …moreover, only in the intimate combination of observation and experiment, advancing physiology with philosophy, is there security from any bias.

In the epigraph to *Bildungsgeschichte der Genitalien aus anatomischen Untersuchungen an Embryonen des Menchen und der Thiere*, Müller emphasizes that *observation (Beobachtung)* must be tireless (*unermüdete).*

Es ist nicht genug, schön und beredt die Erfahrung zu preisen, sondern die Erfahrung selbst und die unermüdete Beobachtung ist nöthig.	It is not enough, beautifully, and eloquently, to praise experience, but experience itself and tireless observation is necessary.

References

1. Yang Q, Wang H, Cho HY, Jung SJ, Kim K-R, Ro JY, et al. Carcinoma of müllerian origin presenting as colon cancer: a clinicopathologic study of 13 cases. Ann Diag Pathol. 2011;15:12–8.
2. Anstadt MJ, Lapetino SR, Defnet A, Kapur U, Shoup M. Endometrial adenocarcinoma metastatic to the colon masquerading as a primary colon cancer. J Gastroenterol Hepatol Res. 2012;1:40–3.
3. NIH-National Cancer Institute. Mullerian tumor [cited 2023 June 17] www.cancer.gov
4. Larsen WJ. Essentials of human embryology. New York: Churchill Livingstone; 1998. pages 176, 183, 188.
5. Aulie RP. Caspar Friedrich Wolff and his 'Theoria Generationis', 1759. J Hist Med Allied Sci. 1961;16:124–44. http://www.jstor.org/stable/24620814
6. Müller J. Bildungsgeschichte Der Genitalien aus anatomischen Untersuchungen an Embryonen des Menchen und der Thiere, nebst einen Anhang über die chirurgische Behandlung der Hypospadia. Düsseldorf, bei Arnz, 1830, pp. 59–61.
7. Steudel J. Johannes Müller. Encyclopaedia Britannica. Encyclopaedia Britannica, Inc., Date Published: 24 April 2023, [cited 2023 June 20]. Available from https://www.britannica.comhttps//www.britannica.com/biography/Johannes-Muller
8. Müller, Johannes Peter. [cited 2023 July 1]. Available from Encyclopedia.com
9. Virchow R. Johannes Müller. Eine Gedächtnissrede, gehalten bei der Todtenfeier am 24. Juli 1858 in der Aula der Universität zu Berlin. 1858, Berlin, Verlag von August Hirschwald, pages 3, 4, 14, 15, 19, 20, 38.

Cecal Lymphoma

154

Brian T. Hill, Eric W. Willis, and James S. Wu

Presentation

A 54-year-old male was found to have a cecal mass on colonoscopy (Fig. 154.1). Biopsies of the mass showed follicular lymphoma (Fig. 154.2a and b).

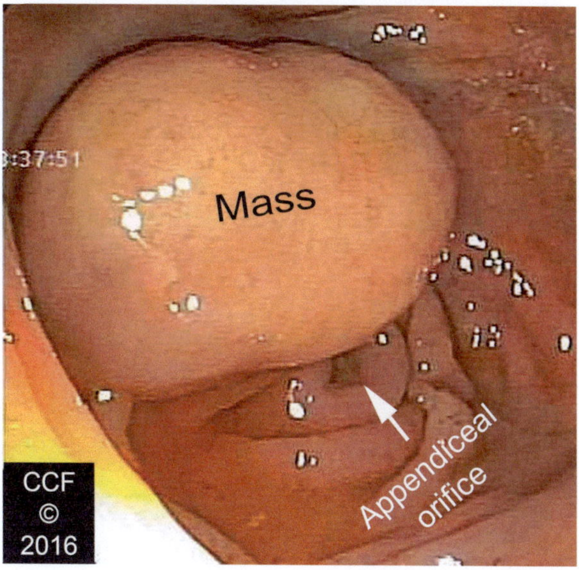

Fig. 154.1 A cecal mass adjacent to the appendiceal orifice

B. T. Hill
Cleveland Clinic Taussig Cancer Institute, Cleveland Clinic, Cleveland, OH, USA

E. W. Willis
Department of Pathology, CORPath, Columbus, OH, USA

J. S. Wu (✉)
Department of Colon and Rectal Surgery, Cleveland Clinic, Cleveland, OH, USA

J. S. Wu, M. D. Inkster (eds.), *Cleveland Clinic Colorectal Case Studies*,
https://doi.org/10.1007/978-3-031-39880-3_154

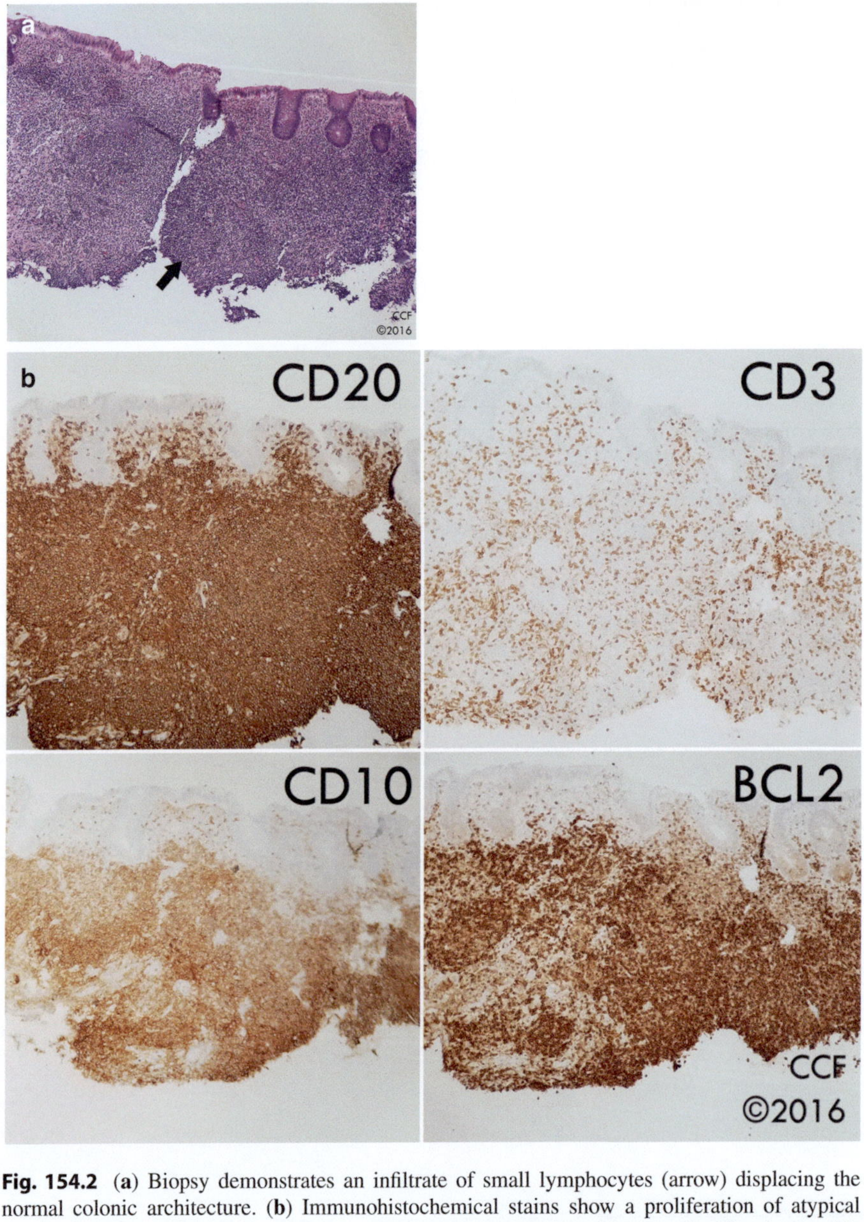

Fig. 154.2 (**a**) Biopsy demonstrates an infiltrate of small lymphocytes (arrow) displacing the normal colonic architecture. (**b**) Immunohistochemical stains show a proliferation of atypical CD20-positive B cells, which outnumber the background CD3-positive T cells. The abnormal B cells stain for CD10, BCL2, and BCL-6 (not shown). The B cells are negative for CD5, CD43, and cyclin-D1. The morphologic and immunophenotypic findings support the diagnosis of follicular lymphoma. The lymphocytes have predominantly centrocytic morphology with small, angulated nuclei. Larger centroblasts are rare, accounting for <15 cells/HPF, consistent with WHO grade 1–2 [1] (CD20 is a generic B-cell marker; CD3 is a generic T-cell marker (negative in B cells); CD10 is a germinal center marker that is also expressed in follicular lymphoma; BCL2 is an antiapoptosis protein that is expressed in follicular lymphoma. The other two markers CD5 and cyclin-D1 are meant to rule out mantle cell lymphoma)

Comment

Lymphoma is a malignancy of the lymphatic system [2, 3]. The major types of lymphoma are Hodgkin lymphoma and non-Hodgkin lymphoma. Non-Hodgkin lymphoma can arise in B-lymphocytes, T-lymphocytes, or natural killer cells. Non-Hodgkin lymphoma can be indolent or aggressive. Follicular lymphoma is the most common type of indolent non-Hodgkin lymphoma. It typically progresses slowly over months to years. Most patients are age 50 years and older. Follicular lymphoma is highly treatable but rarely enters remission without treatment. Primary colorectal lymphoma is rare representing less than 1% of colorectal malignancies. Males, in the fifth to seventh decades of life, are most commonly affected. The most common location is the cecum. The most common histology is B-cell.

Management

Management of colorectal lymphoma is done in consultation with a hematologist-oncologist. Complete resection is rarely indicated and generally reserved for cases of aggressive lymphoma (i.e., diffuse large B-cell lymphoma, Burkitt lymphoma) causing complete bowel obstruction. In the case of indolent lymphoma or nonobstructing aggressive lymphoma, biopsy is sufficient. Subsequent management involves systemic therapy tailored to the type of lymphoma with an assessment of treatment response using serial endoscopic evaluation.

References

1. Harris NL, Swerdlow SH, Jaffe ES, Ott G, Nathwani BN, De Jong D, et al. Follicular lymphoma. In: Swerdlow SH, Campo E, Harris NL, Jaffe ES, Pileri SA, et al., editors. WHO Classification of Tumours of Haematopoietic and Lymphoid Tissues. Lyon, France: IARC Press; 2008. p. 220–6.
2. NIH-National Cancer Institute. Adult non-Hodgkin lymphoma treatment (PDQ®)-Health profession version. https://www.cancer.gov/types/lymphoma/hp/adult-nhl-treatment-pdq. Accessed October 3, 2022.
3. NIH-National Cancer Institute. Adult non-Hodgkin lymphoma treatment (PDQ®)-Patient version. [cited 2002 Oct 3]. Available from https://www.cancer.gov/types/lymphoma/patient/adult-nhl-treatment-pdq

Colon Interposition for Esophageal Replacement

155

David W. Dietz, Jennifer J. Liang, Hermann Kessler, and James S. Wu

Presentation

A female patient underwent a difficult esophagectomy without reconstruction for squamous cell carcinoma of the distal esophagus. She had undergone prior antrectomy with Billroth I reconstruction for peptic ulcer disease. At presentation, she had a cervical spit esophagostomy. Colorectal surgery consultation was requested for the creation of a colonic interposition graft to act as a conduit between the proximal esophagus and the remaining stomach.

Preoperative Assessment

1. Colonoscopy was normal.
2. Three vessel mesenteric angiography showed that the circulation between the superior and inferior mesenteric arteries was intact.

Operative Strategy

The plan was to create an isoperistaltic colonic interposition graft using the transverse and splenic flexure colon.

D. W. Dietz
Department of Surgery, NYU Langone Medical Center, New York, NY, USA

J. J. Liang · H. Kessler · J. S. Wu (✉)
Department of Colon and Rectal Surgery, Cleveland Clinic, Cleveland, OH, USA

J. S. Wu, M. D. Inkster (eds.), *Cleveland Clinic Colorectal Case Studies*,
https://doi.org/10.1007/978-3-031-39880-3_155

Operative Sequence

Step 1

Through a midline incision, the lateral attachments of the colon from the cecum to the rectosigmoid junction were divided (Fig. 155.1).

Step 2

The middle colic vessels and the inferior mesenteric vein were divided (Fig. 155.2).

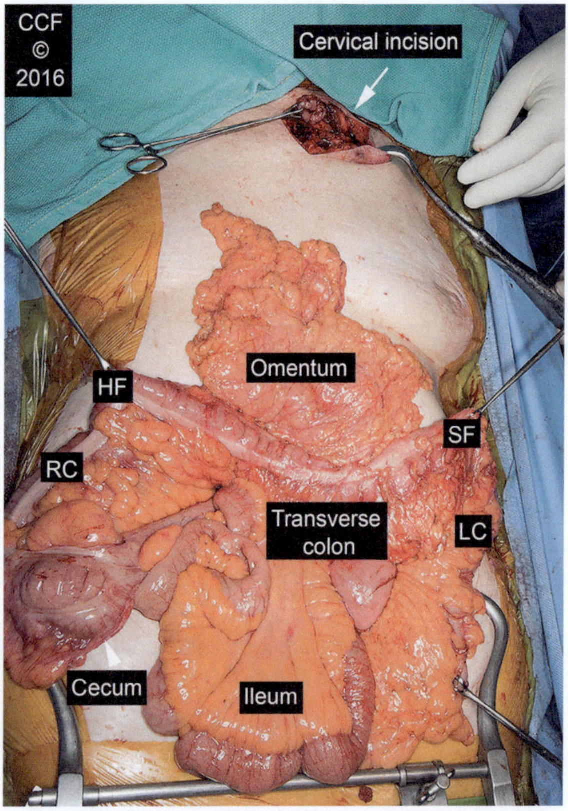

Fig. 155.1 The colon has been mobilized through a midline incision. Right colon (RC), hepatic flexure (HF), splenic flexure (SF), left colon (LC). The omentum, transverse colon, ileum, and cecum are labelled. A cervical incision is seen

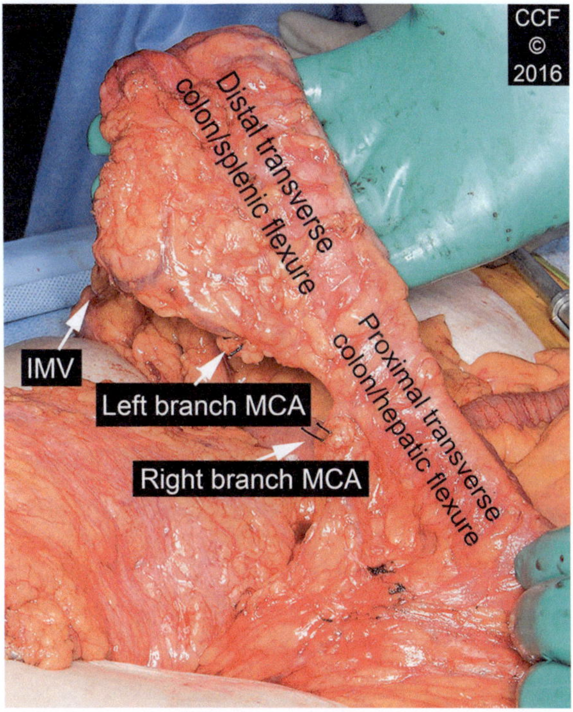

Fig. 155.2 This patient had a very short or non-existent common middle colic artery (MCA) trunk; and therefore, the individual branches had to be divided. The ligated inferior mesenteric vein (IMV), left branch of the middle colic artery (MCA), right branch of the middle colic artery (MCA) are shown. The transverse colon extending from the hepatic flexure to the splenic flexure is labelled

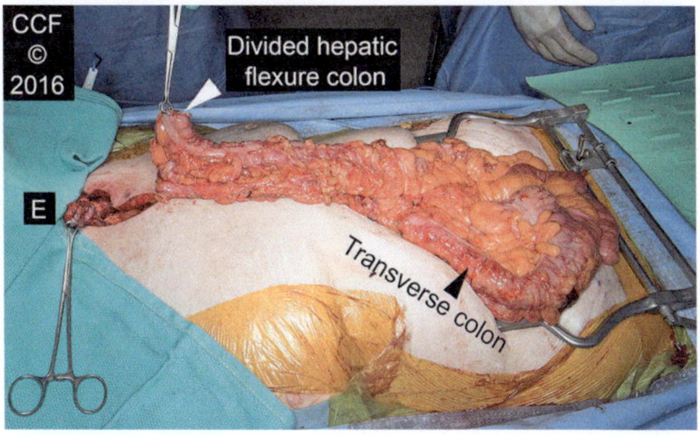

Fig. 155.3 The mobilized colon is brought up to the level of the cervical esophagostomy (E) to test for reach. The divided hepatic flexure colon and transverse colon are labelled

Step 3

After confirming sufficient length of the colon conduit, the hepatic flexure was divided with a gastrointestinal anastomosis stapler (GIA). The colon conduit was demonstrated to easily reach the neck to allow a tension-free anastomosis (Fig. 155.3). It was then passed through a tunnel in the anterior mediastinum (Figs. 155.4, 155.5).

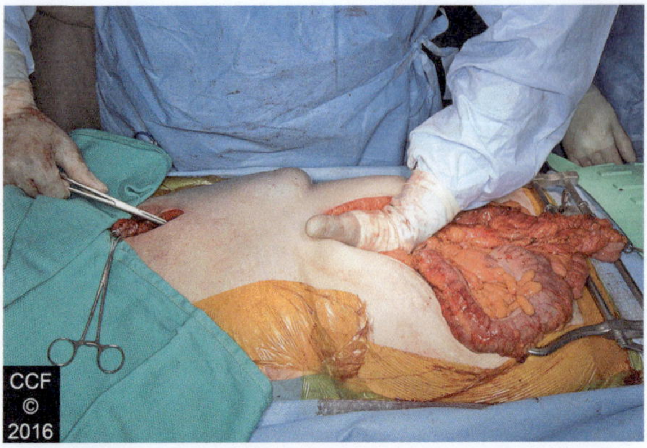

Fig. 155.4 The retrosternal space is prepared for the passage of the colon

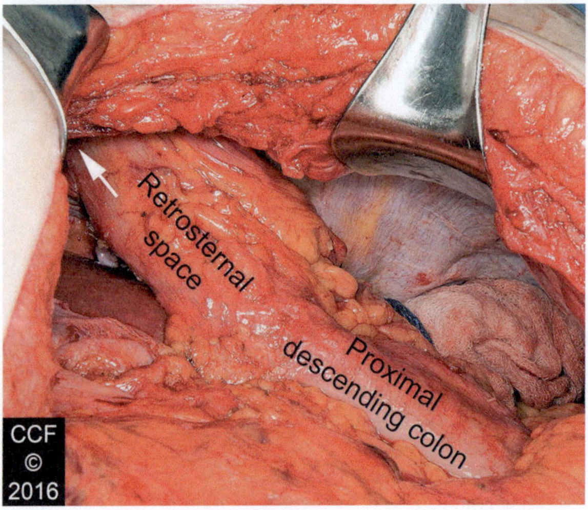

Fig. 155.5 The retrosternal space with colon interposition graft

Following preparation of a retrosternal tunnel (Fig. 155.4), the proximal end of the colon conduit was passed from the abdomen to the cervical wound. Care must be taken not to damage the mesocolon or marginal artery during this step. The esophagostomy has already been mobilized by the thoracic team (Fig. 155.5).

Step 4

Esophagocolostomy

The esophagostomy has been taken down in preparation for esophagocolic anastomosis (Fig. 155.6).

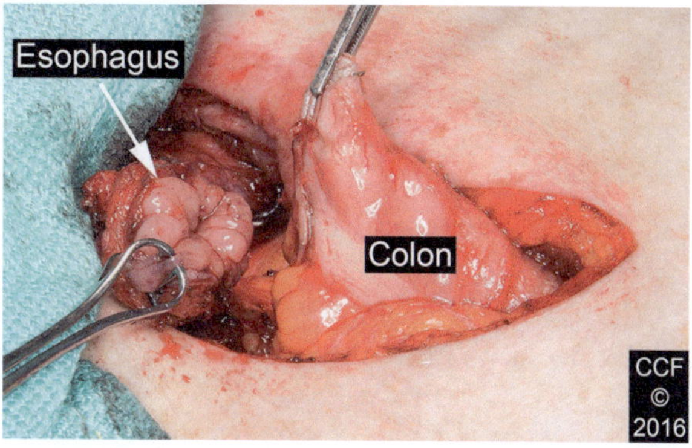

Fig. 155.6 The esophagus next to the colon in preparation for anastomosis

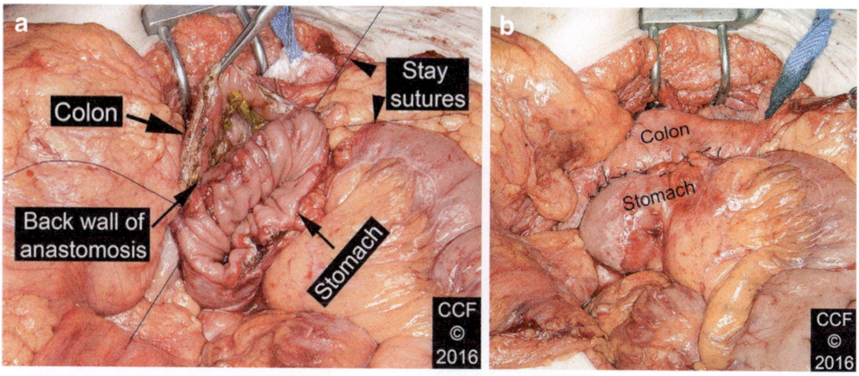

Fig. 155.7 Cologastrostomy (distal end of colon conduit to stomach). (**a**) Stay sutures identify the back wall; (**b**) Completed cologastrotomy

Step 5

The distal end of the colon graft is divided adjacent to the stomach, and an anastomosis is created (Fig. 155.7a, b). Care must be taken to divide only the colon itself. Damage to the marginal artery during this step will render the colonic conduit ischemic.

Step 6

Intestinal continuity was restored by creating a functional end-to-end colocolic stapled anastomosis (Fig. 155.8a, b).

The operative field after closure of cervical and abdominal incisions is shown in Fig. 155.9.

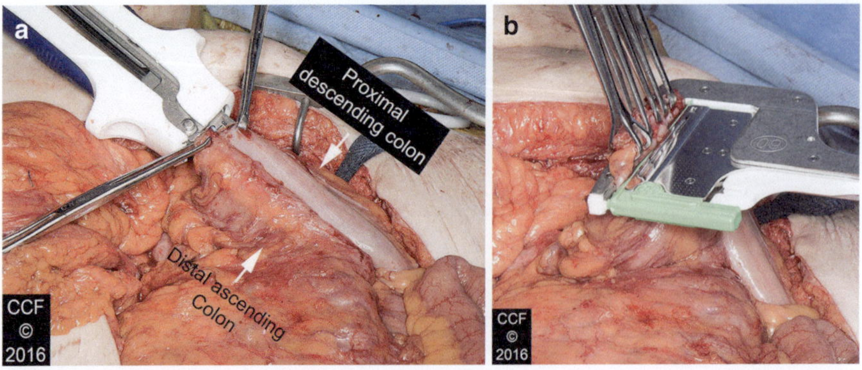

Fig. 155.8 Functional end-to-end colocolic anastomosis: (**a**) The GIA stapler divides the common wall between the two limbs; (**b**) The enterotomy is closed with a linear stapler

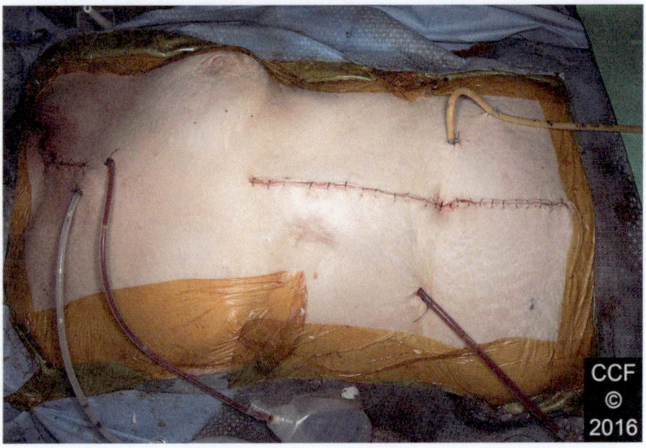

Fig. 155.9 The operative field after closure of the cervical and abdominal incisions

Comment

Colonic interposition graft can be used to reestablish gut continuity after esophagectomy for trauma or neoplasm. The first successful colon conduit was reported by Kelling in 1911 [1]. The operation involved bypass of an obstructing esophageal lesion.

Ösophagoplastik mit Hilfe des Querkolon.
Von
Prof. Dr. med. G. Kelling
in Dresden.

Es handelte sich um eine 45jährige Frau, die seit etwa ½ Jahre Schluck-beschwerden hatte und in den letzen 4 Wochen nur dünne Suppen nehmen konnte. Die Sondierung ergab ein Hindernis bei 29 cm; das Ösophagoskop zeigte ein ulzeriertes Karzinom. Pat. war damals in ziemlich gutem Ernährungszustand und wünschte dringend, wieder essen zu können.

Ein großes Stück des Querkolon wurde rechts und links abgetrennt... Die übrig gebliebenen Teile wurden durch zirkuläre Naht miteinander vernäht.

Nachdem die Naht beendet war, wurde von dem ausgeschalteten Stück des Querkolon der rechte Teil blind vernäht, der linke Teil aber in die Vorderwand des Magens eingenäht.... Das Querkolon reichte garade bis zur Mammilla. Es wurde nun ein Hautschnitt von der Höhe der Mammilla links vom Sternum senkrecht nach unten in den Laparotomieschnitt einmündend, angelegt, die Haut rechts und links ausgiebig unterminiert, das Querkolon hineingelegt und die Haut wieder zusammengenäht.

Nach 25 Tagen entschloss ich mich zur zweiten Operation. Zuerst wurde ein Schnitt am Halse an der Innerseite des linken Sternocleidomastoideus angelegt, bis etwa 1½ Querfinger breit oberhalb der Clavicula. Dann wurde der Ösophagus herauspräpariert und seine Vorderwand ringsum an die Halsfascie uneröffnet angenäht. Dann wurde der Ösophagus eröffnet.... Dann wurde zwischen der Ösophagusfistel und der Öffnung des Querkolon eine Röhre gebildet aus dem dazwischenliegenden Streifen Brusthaut.

Am 13. Tage,....
Ich liess die Pat. schlucken, und es zeigte sich, daß die Funktion der neugebildeten Speiseröhre für flüssige Kost sehr gut war.
Am 15. Tage bekam aber Pat. einen Kollaps und starb...Sektion wurde leider verweigert.

Esophagoplasty with the help of the transverse colon
by
Prof. Dr. G. Kelling
Dresden.

The case involved a 45-year-old female, who for about a half-year had difficulty swallowing and in the last 4 weeks could only eat thin soup. A sound showed a blockage at 29 cm; esophagoscopy showed an ulcerated cancer.
The patient's nutritional status was relatively good, and she desperately wished to eat again.

A large segment of the transverse colon was disconnected from the right and left sides...The remaining segments were sewn together with stitches.

After the stitching was completed, the right side of the isolated piece of transverse colon was sewn shut, the left side, however, was anastomosed to the anterior wall of the stomach...The transverse colon reached exactly to the level of the breasts...A skin incision was made from the level of the breasts to the left of the sternum which was joined perpendicularly with the laparotomy incision. The skin was undermined to the right and left; the transverse colon was then place therein and the skin was then closed.

After 25 days, I performed a second operation. First, an incision was made in the neck on the inner side of the left sternocleidomastoid about 1½ finger widths above the clavicle. Then the esophagus was dissected out and its front wall sewn unopened to the cervical fascia.
Then the esophagus was opened...Then a tunnel was constructed between the esophagus fistula and the opening in the transverse colon from the breast tissue that lay in between.
On day 13,....
I allowed the patient to drink, and it was shown that the function of the neo-digestive tube for liquid foods was good.
On day 15, the patient collapsed and died.
Autopsy unfortunately was denied.

The use of stomach as an esophageal substitute is the most commonly accepted method of esophageal reconstruction[2]. However, in patients who require a long segment of conduit for esophageal discontinuity or when a gastric conduit is unattainable, colon can be utilized. The colon has the advantage of length and reliable blood supply. Disadvantages include the longer operating time for colon mobilization and the creation of an additional anastomosis that increase the perioperative morbidity when compared to the use of gastric conduit. Complications following colonic interposition include conduit ischemia, anastomotic leak, stricture, and perioperative mortality [3–6].

Notably, the success of this operation depends on the viability of the transverse colon conduit. The blood supply starting at the aorta is: aorta to inferior mesenteric artery to left colic artery to the marginal artery of the conduit leading to the hepatic flexure.

References

1. Kelling G. Ösophagoplastik mit Hilfe des Querkolon. Zentralblatt Chir. 1911;38:1209–12.
2. Akiyama H, Miyazono H, Tsurumara M, Hashimoto C, Kawamura T. Use of the stomach as an esophageal substitute. Ann Surg. 1978;188:606–10.
3. Wain JC, Wright CD, Kuo EY, Moncure AC, Wilkins EW Jr, Grillo HC, Mathisen DJ. Long-segment colon interposition for acquired esophageal disease. Ann Thorac Surg. 1999;67:313–7.
4. Wilkins EW Jr. Long-segment colon substitution for the esophagus. Ann Surg. 1980;192:722–5.
5. Briel JW, Tamhankar AP, Hagen JA, DeMeester SR, Johansson J, Choustoulakis E, et al. Prevalence and risk-factors for ischemia, leak, and stricture of esophageal anastomosis: Gastric pull-up versus colon interposition. J Am Coll Surg. 2004;198:536–42.
6. Motoyama S, Kitamura M, Saito R, Murayama K, Sato Y, Hayashi K, et al. Surgical outcome of colon interposition by the posterior mediastinal route for thoracic esophageal cancer. Ann Thorac Surg. 2007;83:1273–8.

Small Lymphocytic Lymphoma, Mesenteric Involvement

156

Catherine L. Forse, Deepa Jagadeesh, Arthur A. Parsee, and James S. Wu

Presentation

A 75-year-old patient underwent screening colon computed tomography (CT). Colon masses or polyps >6 mm were not seen; however, the examination revealed prominent mesenteric adenopathy consistent with the patient's known history of small lymphocytic lymphoma (Fig. 156.1).

Several years before this CT colonography, the diagnosis of small lymphocytic lymphoma (SLL) was made by peripheral lymph node biopsy (Fig. 156.2a and b).

CT of the head and neck, chest, and abdomen showed lymphadenopathy throughout the neck, mediastinum, mesentery, retroperitoneum, and pelvis. Treatment included chemotherapy and supportive care.

C. L. Forse
Department of Pathology and Laboratory Medicine, Faculty of Medicine, University of Ottawa, Ottawa, ON, Canada

D. Jagadeesh
Cleveland Clinic Taussig Cancer Institute, Cleveland, OH, USA

A. A. Parsee
Department of Diagnostic Radiology, H. Lee Moffitt Cancer Center and Research Institute, Tampa, FL, USA

J. S. Wu (✉)
Department of Colon and Rectal Surgery, Cleveland Clinic, Cleveland, OH, USA

J. S. Wu, M. D. Inkster (eds.), *Cleveland Clinic Colorectal Case Studies*,
https://doi.org/10.1007/978-3-031-39880-3_156

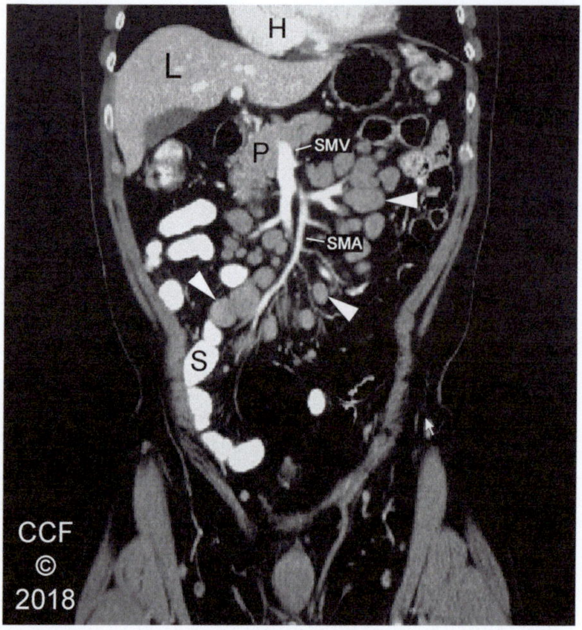

Fig. 156.1 Coronal CT image demonstrating diffuse bulky lymphadenopathy throughout the mesentery (arrowheads). The heart (H), liver (L), pancreas (P), and small intestine (S) are marked. The proximal superior mesenteric vein (SMV) is seen adjacent to the pancreas. The superior mesenteric artery is seen to the left of the SMV

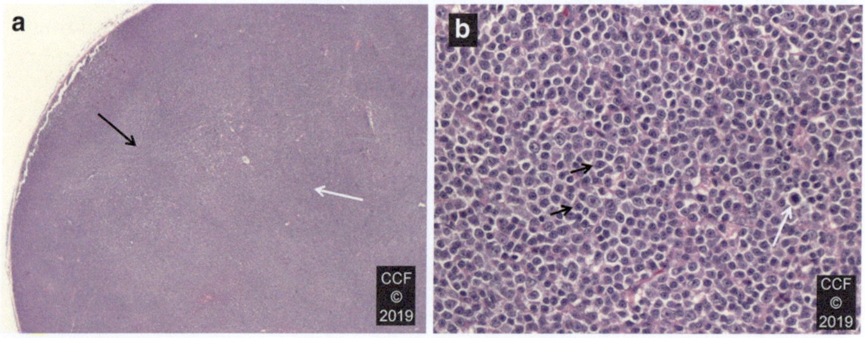

Fig. 156.2 (**a**) A supraclavicular lymph node demonstrating diffuse effacement of normal lymph node architecture. Note the alternating light (black arrow) and dark (white arrow) zones. The light zones correspond to proliferative centers which are a characteristic feature of small lymphocytic lymphoma. H&E, 20× magnification; (**b**) The lymph node is effaced by a mixed population consisting predominantly of small lymphocytes with clumped chromatin (black arrows). This is the classical histological appearance of small lymphocytic lymphoma. Mitotic activity can be identified (white arrow). H&E, 400× magnification

Comment

Chronic lymphocytic leukemia (CLL) and small lymphocytic lymphoma (SLL) are indolent B-cell malignancies that affect mature lymphocytes. They are similar diseases with different clinical presentation. CLL presents with high white cell count (leukocytosis) and lymphocyte count (lymphocytosis) and is the most common type of chronic leukemia in adults. Diagnostic criteria for CLL require $\geq 5 \times 10^9/L$ monoclonal B lymphocytes in peripheral blood [1, 2]. Peripheral blood and bone marrow are commonly involved in CLL. SLL patients present with lymphadenopathy and have $<5 \times 10^9/L$ clonal B-lymphocytes in peripheral blood [1, 2]. Common sites of involvement for SLL are lymph nodes and bone marrow. Other clinical symptoms associated with SLL include B symptoms (fever, night sweats, and unexplained weight loss), splenomegaly, and cytopenia like neutropenia, anemia, and thrombocytopenia.

Workup for SLL should include a complete blood count, complete metabolic panel, lactate dehydrogenase (LDH) and beta-2-microglobulin levels. CT scans of the neck, chest, abdomen, and pelvis can help identify lymphadenopathy and organomegaly, but are not required at the time of diagnosis. A CT scan should be done prior to initiating treatment to determine the sites of involvement. Bone marrow aspiration and biopsy are not required to establish a diagnosis. However, this should be considered prior to initiating treatment in patients with cytopenias. HIV serology should be checked in newly diagnosed patients. Hepatitis B and C virus infection status should be checked prior to initiating treatment with anti-CD20 monoclonal antibody therapy.

A diagnosis of SLL is established by lymph node biopsy. The lymph node architecture is usually effaced with small mature lymphocytes. The malignant lymphocytes are positive for surface B-cell antigens CD19, CD20, CD5, and CD23 and negative for CD10 and cyclin D1. Flow cytometry may identify monoclonal B cells that are immunophenotypically abnormal and are expressing the above B-cell markers. Fluorescence *in situ* hybridization (FISH) is helpful in identifying poor prognostic markers like 17p deletion. Other abnormalities commonly present include 13q deletion, and 11q deletion. Mutation in *TP53* gene also is a poor prognostic factor.

Asymptomatic patients at the time of diagnosis can be monitored without any treatment. Indications for treatment include the presence of B symptoms or cytopenias, massive splenomegaly, symptomatic organ involvement, or large tumor burden. Advent of novel therapies have changed the treatment landscape of CLL/SLL. Newly diagnosed CLL/SLL are treated with targeted agents like BTK (Bruton's tyrosine kinase) and BCL2 inhibitors. Ibrutinib, the first generation BTKi along with second generation BTKi, acalabrutinib and zanabrutinib, are approved to treat newly diagnosed CLL/SLL patients [3]. Ventoclax is a BCL2 inhibitor that is approved for both newly diagnosed and relapsed disease. Although rituximab, obinutuzumab and ofatumumab are approved anti-CD20 monoclonal antibodies, recent trials support the use of obinutuzumab as the preferred anti-CD20 monoclonal agent in combination with acalabrutinib and venetoclax. Other novel agents like pirtobrutinib and idelalisib also are used to manage relapsed disease. Conventional chemotherapy regimens like BR (bendamustine and rituxumab) and FCR (fludarabine, Cytoxan, and rituximab) are rarely used in the era of targeted therapy.

References

1. Zelenetz AD, Gordon LI, Wierda WG, Abramson JS, Advani RH, Andreadis CB, Bartlett N, et al. Chronic lymphocytic leukemia/small lymphocytic lymphoma, version 1.2015. J Natl Compr Cancer Netw. 2015;13:326–62.
2. Hallek M, Cheson BD, Catovsky D, Caligaris-Cappio F, Dighiero G, Döhner H, et al. iwCLL guidelines for diagnosis, indications for treatment, response assessment, and supportive management of CLL. Blood. 2018;131:2745–60.
3. Stephens DO, NCCN Guidelines Update: Chronic Lymphocytic Leukemia/Small Lymphocytic Lymphoma. J Natl Compr Canc Netw 2023;21(5.5):563–6.

Ostomy Site Selection

157

Barbara J. Hocevar, Amelia Agostinelli, and James S. Wu

Presentation

Intestinal stomas serve as the end of the gastrointestinal and urinary tracts, protect distal anastomoses, and relieve obstruction. Appropriate stoma siting is critical to postoperative stoma management. The ability to obtain a predictable seal on the pouching system decreases peristomal skin problems and helps maximize a patient's quality of life.

General Principles for the Selection of Stoma Sites [1, 2][1]

1. Select optimal stoma sites before surgery
2. As shown in Figs. 157.1 and 157.2, preferred sites are:
   - Below the umbilicus
   - Directly over the belly of the rectus abdominis muscle
   - Away from body creases, scars, and bony prominences
   - At the top of the infraumbilical fat mound
   - Visible and accessible to the patient

[1] Marking discs: Marlen Manufacturing & Development Co., 5150 Richmond Road Bedford, OH 44146, U.S.A

B. J. Hocevar
Rupert B. Turnbull, Jr., School of WOC Nursing Education, Cleveland Clinic, Cleveland, OH, USA

A. Agostinelli
WOC Nursing Department, Cleveland Clinic, Cleveland, OH, USA

J. S. Wu (✉)
Department of Colon and Rectal Surgery, Cleveland Clinic, Cleveland, OH, USA

J. S. Wu, M. D. Inkster (eds.), *Cleveland Clinic Colorectal Case Studies*,
https://doi.org/10.1007/978-3-031-39880-3_157

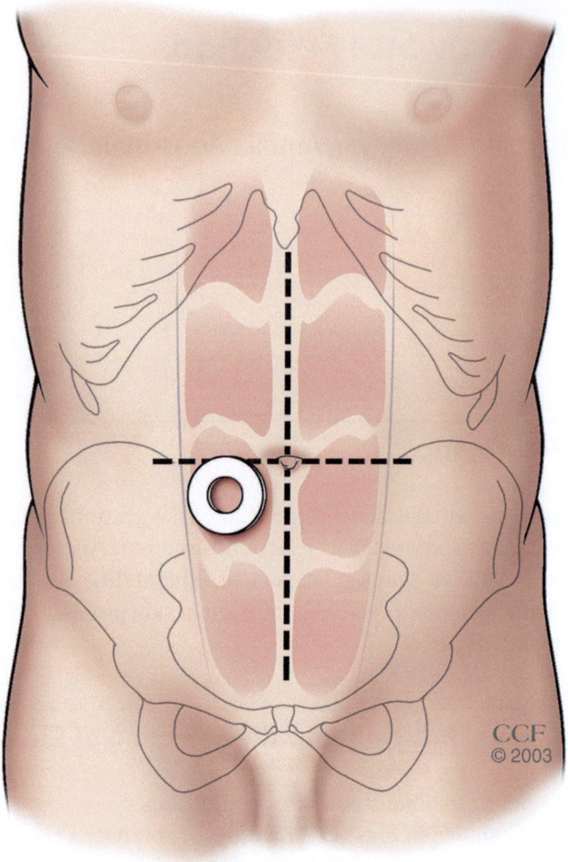

Fig. 157.1 Placement of a stoma marking disc in the optimal stoma site for a right-sided stoma

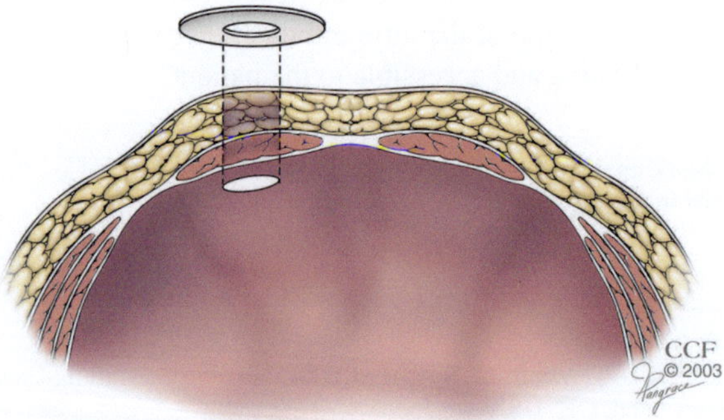

Fig. 157.2 Stoma site located over the body of the rectus abdominis muscle

3. Stoma sites are chosen with the patient supine, sitting, and standing. Selected sites are marked with indelible ink or tattooed into the dermis with India ink using a small gauge needle (Figs. 157.3, 157.4, 157.5, 157.6, 157.7, 157.8).

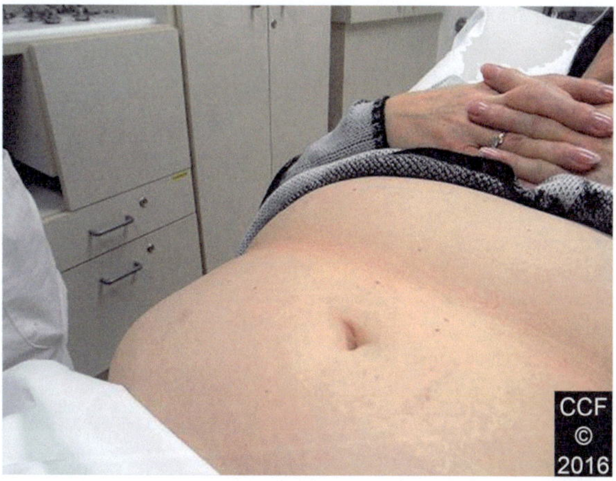

Fig. 157.3 Assessment of the abdomen lying down. Scars and creases are noted

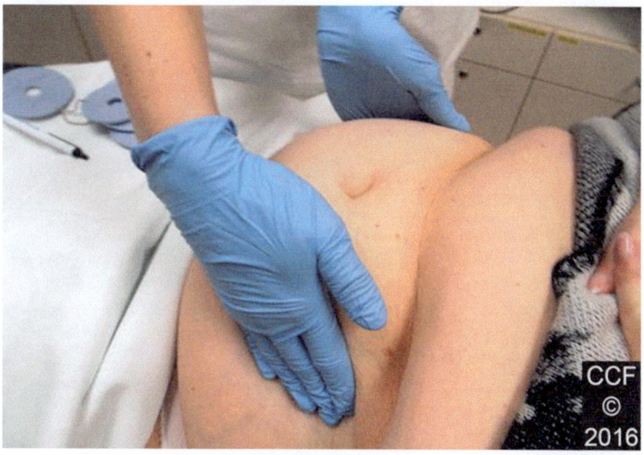

Fig. 157.4 The lateral edges of the rectus abdominis muscle are palpated

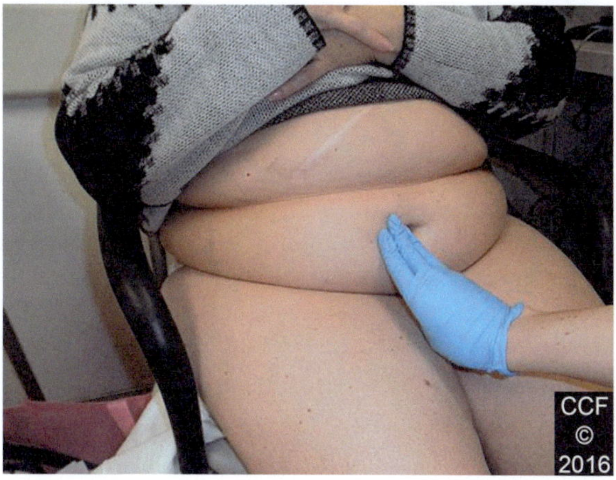

Fig. 157.5 The patient is positioned in a chair with feet on the floor. Creases and scars, not evident when the patient is supine, are sought

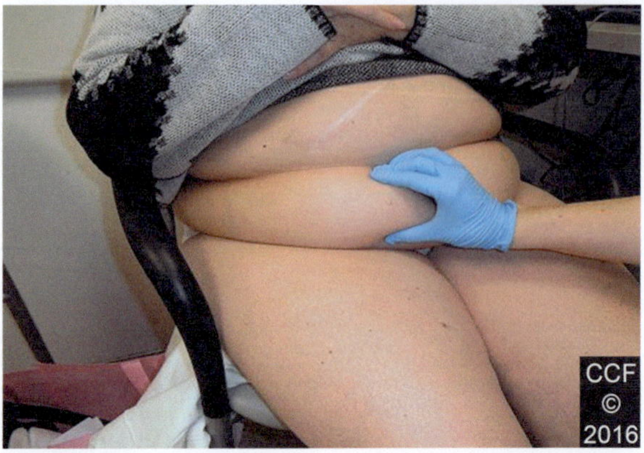

Fig. 157.6 An ostomy site is chosen on the summit of the infraumbilical fat mound. The summit is the point that protrudes out the farthest. Stoma site selection for patients who have undergone prior abdominal surgery can be challenging. The "best" ostomy sites already may have been rendered unusable. An example is shown in Fig. 157.8

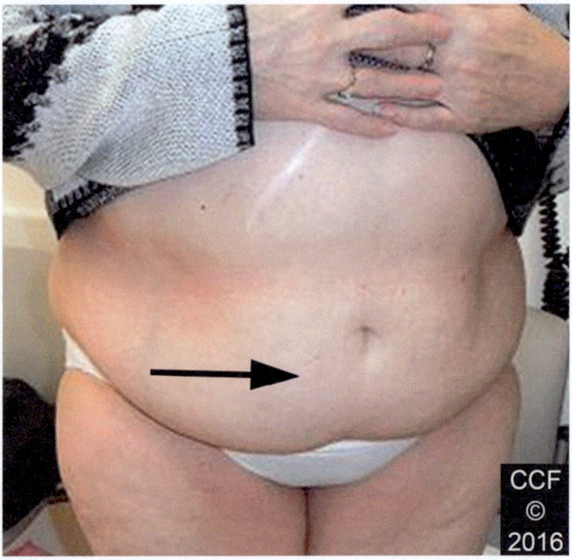

Fig. 157.7 In this case, the stoma mark is placed at the tip of the arrow: away from any skin scars, creases or folds and visible to the patient

The abdomen is assessed supine (Fig. 157.3). Skin creases and the lateral edges of the rectus are identified (Fig. 157.4). The abdomen is re-examined in the sitting position (Fig. 157.5). An ostomy site is chosen on the summit of the infraumbilical fat mound (Fig. 157.6). An example of a stoma site away from skin scars, creases, or folds that is visible to the patient is shown in Fig. 157.7. Selection of a stoma site in a patient who has had previous stoma surgery is shown in Fig. 157.8.

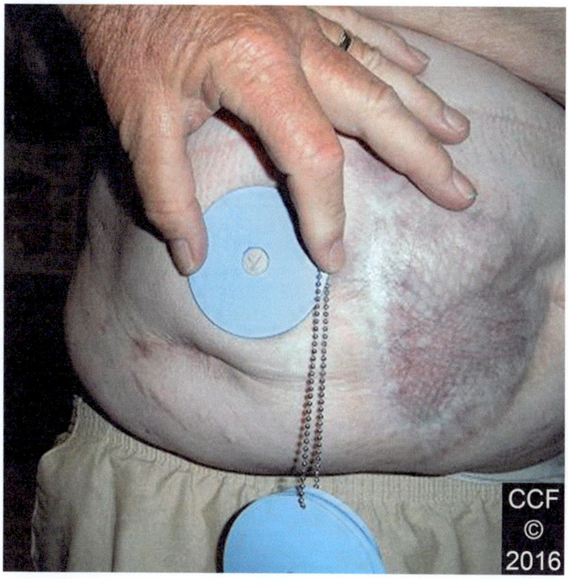

Fig. 157.8 This person has had prior surgery; one can see a prior stoma site in the patient's right lower quadrant. A healed skin graft is located on the patient's left side. The edge of the rectus was palpated. A stoma site was chosen by placing the edge of a marking disc along the midline at a site with an adjacent flat skin surface (about 2½ inches). The "x" located at the center of the marking disc identifies the surgical incision site

References

1. Turnbull RB Jr, Weakley FL. Colectomy and ileostomy for ulcerative colitis. Location of the stoma and the abdominal incision. In: Atlas of Intestinal Stomas, Chapter 1. St. Louis: The CV Mosby Company; 1967. p. 7–9.
2. Salvadalena G, Hendren S, McKenna L, Muldoon R, Netsch D, Paquette I, et al. WOCN Society and ASCRS position statement on preoperative stoma site marking for patients undergoing colostomy or ileostomy surgery. J Wound Ostomy Continence Nurs. 2015;42:249–52.

End Ileostomy Construction

158

James S. Wu and Sherief Shawki

The steps of end ileostomy creation are illustrated in Figs. 158.1, 158.2, 158.3, 158.4, 158.5, 158.6, 158.7.

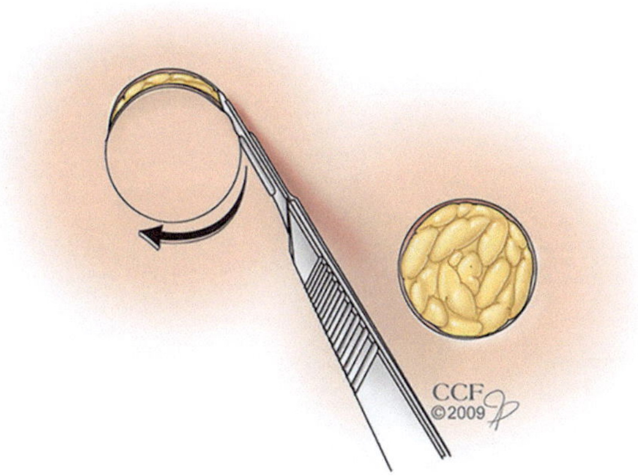

Fig. 158.1 A disc of skin approximately 1. 5 cm in diameter is excised. It is always possible to make the aperture larger. A skin opening cannot be made smaller

J. S. Wu (✉)
Department of Colon and Rectal Surgery, Cleveland Clinic, Cleveland, OH, USA

S. Shawki
Department of Colon and Rectal Surgery, Mayo Clinic, Rochester, MN, USA

J. S. Wu, M. D. Inkster (eds.), *Cleveland Clinic Colorectal Case Studies*,
https://doi.org/10.1007/978-3-031-39880-3_158

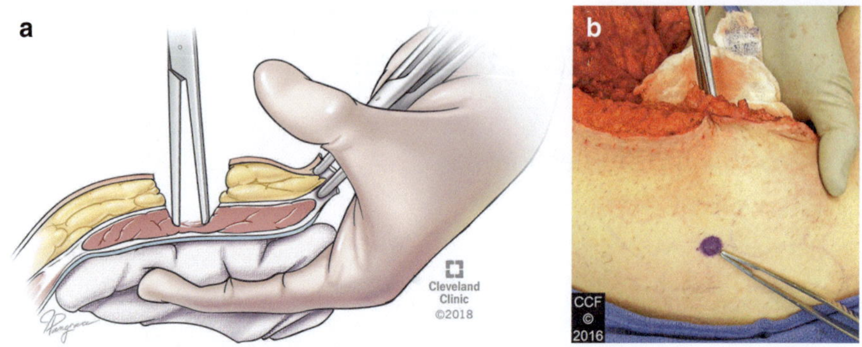

Fig. 158.2 (**a**) Illustration. Following laparotomy the abdominal wall directly beneath the ostomy aperture is suspended with a sponge first to protect the underlying small intestine and second to provide a stable platform for the ostomy aperture creation. Two clamps, one on the midline fascia and a second on the dermis, are placed. The clamps maintain the original relationship between the skin, the fascia, and the rectus muscle; (**b**) Operative photo. The skin site selected for the ostomy is marked with a tattoo (forceps). The fascial clamps and the sponge held by the operator beneath the ostomy aperture are shown

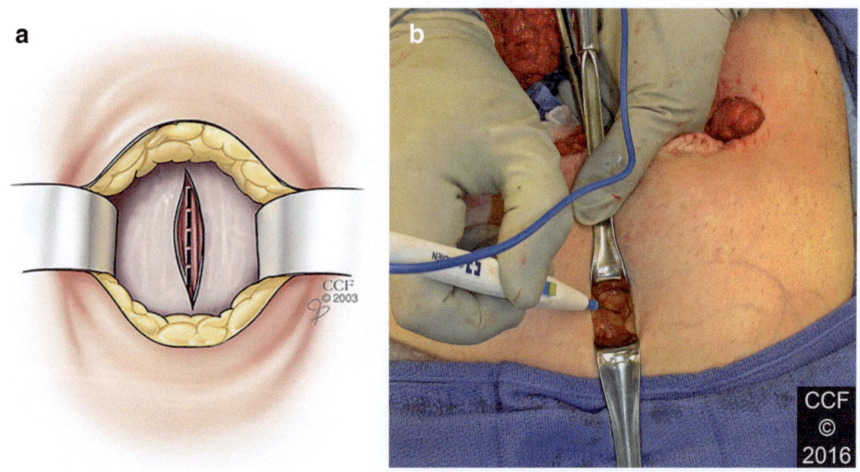

Fig. 158.3 (**a**) Illustration. The subcutaneous fat is divided with electrocautery between retractors The anterior rectus fascia is divided in a superior–inferior direction (dotted line). The fibers of the rectus muscle are separated with a blunt-tipped clamp. Muscle separation by sharp instruments is avoided in order to prevent injury to the epigastric artery; (**b**) Operative photo. The ostomy site fat is divided with electrocautery. Exposure is provided with small retractors. The fingers of the operator's left hand support the surgical site from below

Fig. 158.4 The ostomy aperture is made large enough to allow the passage of the intestine and its mesentery. For end ileostomy, this is about two fingers

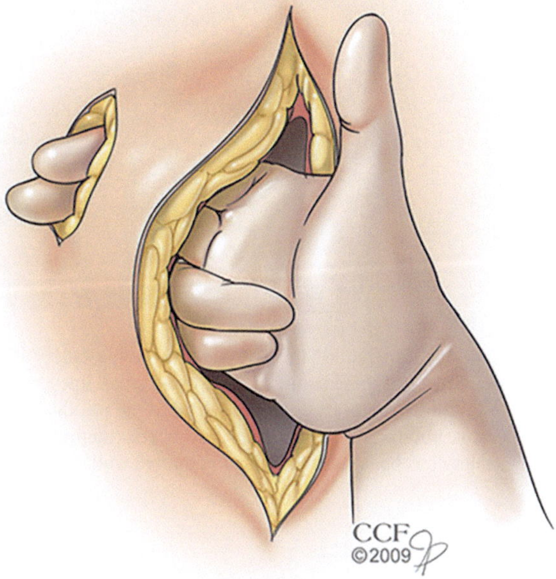

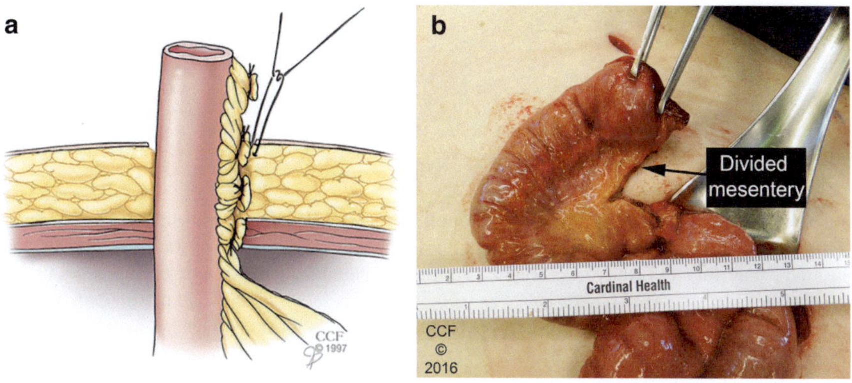

Fig. 158.5 (**a**) Illustration. The intestine is inspected to make certain there are no organoaxial twists. The distal 5 cm of mesentery is divided. The terminal ileum is brought through the ostomy aperture; (**b**) Operative photo. The distal mesentery at the end of the ileostomy is divided in order to allow the intestine to pass through the abdominal wall

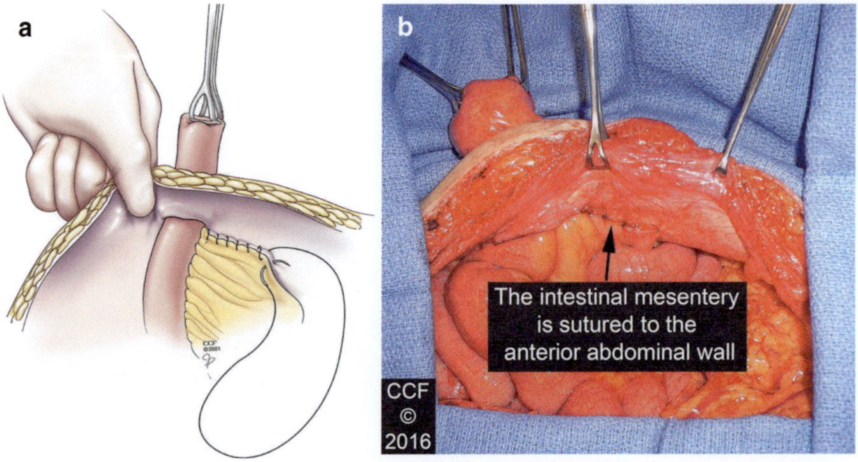

Fig. 158.6 (**a**) Illustration. The cut edge of the mesentery is sutured to the anterior abdominal wall. The purpose of these sutures is to prevent small intestinal volvulus around the fixed terminal ileum. The sutures are placed far enough from the midline to allow laparotomy incision closure; (**b**) Operative photo. The end ileostomy has been brought through the abdominal wall. The edge of the mesentery has been sutured to the abdominal wall

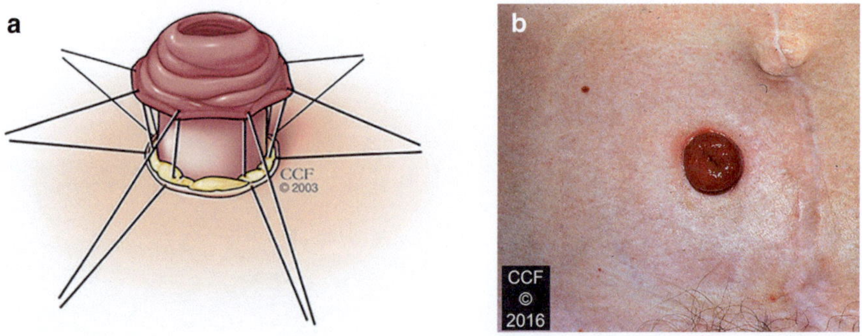

Fig. 158.7 (**a**) Illustration. Primary maturation of the end ileostomy. Full-thickness absorbable sutures (3–0 chromic) are passed first through the end of the cut edge of the intestine and then through the dermis. Full-thickness stitches through the skin are avoided in order to prevent intestinal mucosal implants (see Chap. 166, Fig. 166.3); (**b**) Operative photo. The matured stoma after healing. The stoma is located at the center of a fat mound. The skin is intact

Comment

Before primary maturation, ileostomies were exteriorized with the serosa exposed. In 1951, Warren and McKittrick described ileostomy for ulcerative colitis as follows:

"About 3 centimeters of ileum is brought beyond the skin, a glass tube or catheter is placed in the stoma to lead the discharge away, the stoma is encircled with dry gauze to which it rapidly becomes adherent and, being thus incorporated as part of the dressing, is prevented from prolapsing to the outside.
The tube is allowed to drain by gravity into the bedside bottle for a period of 5 days." [1][1]

A common complication observed for this method of ileostomy creation was *ileostomy dysfunction*.

"*Ileostomy dysfunction.* Early fixation of the ileum by the abdominal wall and later contraction of the stoma are the most harmful features resulting from ileostomy. Although complete obstruction rarely occurs at the ileostomy stoma, partial obstruction is common. It was seen in 130, or 62 percent, of our patients. It is characterized by cramp-like pain and, paradoxically, an increase in the volume of ileostomy discharge. The discharge becomes watery. In the severe cases vomiting occurs and ileostomy diarrhea becomes so severe that serious water and electrolyte deficiencies may result. The first systemic manifestation may be sudden evidence of profound fluid and electrolyte imbalance as manifested by a shock-like state."

Richard Warren, M.D., F.A.C.S.
and Leland S. McKittrick, M.D., F.A.C.S.
Massachusetts General Hospital, 1951

In 1952, Brooke described primary maturation of the ileostomy as a solution to this problem (Fig. 158.7a, b).

'An ileostomy must work perfectly if the surgical treatment of ulcerative colitis is not to fall into disrepute;....

INTESTINAL OBSTRUCTION

Intestinal obstruction is the commonest serious complication of ileostomy, but not much has been published about it. Warren and McKittrick (1951), however, have given a good account of it, using the title "ileostomy dysfunction" for the particular syndrome arising from partial obstruction which more often occurs;...

STENOSIS

Stenosis at the stoma arises, as Warren and McKittrick (1951) state, from scar tissue formed by the granulations that cover the raw serosal surface of the protruding ileum during the two postoperative weeks before the gradual evagination of the mucosa has brought that surface into continuity with the skin edge.

[1] Reprinted with permission from Mr. Spencer Dimmick, the Journal of the American College of Surgeons formerly Surgery Gynecology & Obstetrics, Oct 7, 2021

A more simple device is to evaginate the ileal end at the time of operation and suture the mucosa to the skin. "[2][2]

The Management of an Ileostomy
Including its Complications
B. N. Brooke
M.Chir. Camb., F.R.C.S.
Reader in Surgery in the University of Birmingham

Brooke's operation has remained standard since its description. Serosal fixation sutures were not part of the original operation for the following reason:

"FISTULÆ

Fistulae form for two reasons. The ileal wall may be damaged or weakened at the time of operation; a fixation suture through serosa and muscle alone without penetration of the mucosa is particularly liable to cause a subsequent breakdown of the whole thickness of the bowel wall. A suture of ligature lying close to the ileum but not penetrating it in any way can lead to the same result. In these circumstances the fistula will appear in the first ten days or so after the operation."

References

1. Warren R, McKittrick LS. Ileostomy for ulcerative colitis. Technique, complications, and management. Surg Gynecol Obstet. 1951;93:555–67.
2. Brooke BN. The management of an ileostomy including its complications. Lancet. 1952;260(6725):102–4.

[2] This excerpt is reused with the generous permission of Elsevier Science & Technology Journals, CCC | Marketplace™, Order License ID 1143931–1, Order date 28-Aug-2021

Loop Ileostomy Construction

159

James S. Wu

Presentation

In his 1958 treatise on intestinal stomas, Turnbull noted that while end ileostomy usually was performed in the course of treatment for ulcerative colitis, loop ileostomy was "rarely indicated" [1].

> "Loop ileostomy is rarely indicated but, when it is the chosen procedure, the ileum should be withdrawn through a two-finger vertical incision…. The loop is simply opened transversely so that the proximal portion is the longest. By everting the edges of the ileum and suturing them to the skin primarily, dysfunction is avoided entirely."

The loop was aligned vertically with the proximal limb superior. In 1978, Turnbull and Hewitt [2][1] spelled out details of loop-ileostomy construction.

> "CONSTRUCTION OF THE ILEOSTOMY
>
> A round disk of skin is excised at the ileostomy site. The subcutaneous fat is cut vertically until the anterior rectus is exposed. The sheath is divided caudad and cephalad for 2 inches. The rectus muscle is split vertically and the posterior sheath is exposed and also cut vertically for the same distance. The terminal loop is pulled through the abdominal wall aperture. One can easily observe when the broad fan of conduit mesentery impinges on the posterior rectus vertical slit. To gain more length, the loop is pulled back within the abdomen and the slit in the posterior rectus sheath is extended cephalad and caudad for another three inches. After several trials of pulling the loop through the aperture (with umbilical tape) with progressive enlargement of the posterior rectus slit each time, the loop of ileum will finally protrude enough. At least 1½ inches of the loop should protrude and rest easily on the skin without any tendency to withdraw into the abdomen."
>
> Rupert B. Turnbull, M.D., C.M., F.A.C.S.
> and Clarence R. Hewitt, M.D.

[1] The excerpts were reproduced with the generous permission of Elsevier Inc, CCC | RightsLink®, License Number 5156890727537, License date Sep 27, 2021

J. S. Wu (✉)
Department of Colon and Rectal Surgery, Cleveland Clinic, Cleveland, OH, USA

J. S. Wu, M. D. Inkster (eds.), *Cleveland Clinic Colorectal Case Studies*,
https://doi.org/10.1007/978-3-031-39880-3_159

The exteriorized loop of intestine is supported with a rod placed through a small opening in the mesentery. The authors instruct that the "division of the bowel on the nonfunctional side of the stoma must be four-fifths of the way across the lumen." Maturation is done with 4-0 subcuticular chromic suture.

These steps are illustrated in Figs. 159.1, 159.2, 159.3, 159.4, 159.5. A distal loop of ileum is selected that can reach the skin with the least amount of tension. A mesenteric window is made close to the intestine through which is passed an umbilical tape. The proximal and distal limbs of intestine are identified with sutures of different length or color (Fig. 159.1). The selected ileum is exteriorized taking care to avoid twists.

The umbilical tape is replaced with a 2-inch stoma rod (Fig. 159.2). The proximal ileum is marked with a blue stitch. The distal ileum is marked with a brown stitch. A transverse enterotomy is made in the distal exposed aspect of the loop (Fig. 159.3). The stoma is matured primarily (Fig. 159.4). The appearance of the matured loop ileostomy is shown in Fig. 159.5.

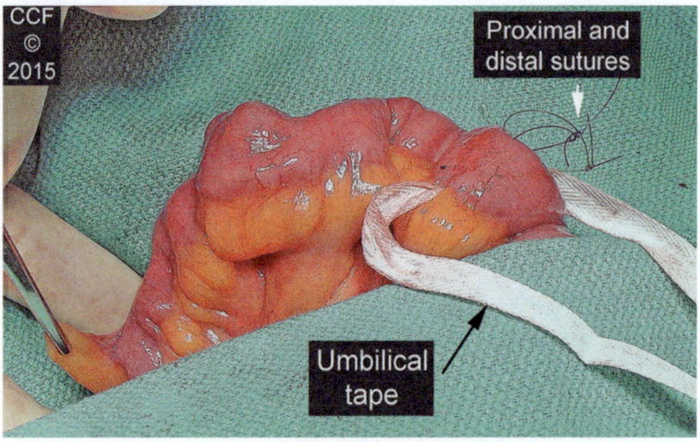

Fig. 159.1 A transmesenteric window, encircled with umbilical tape, marks the site of the future loop ileostomy. The proximal and distal limbs of ileum are identified with unique sutures. The fold of Treves (forceps) serves as a reference point that marks the distance of the ileostomy to the end of the ileum

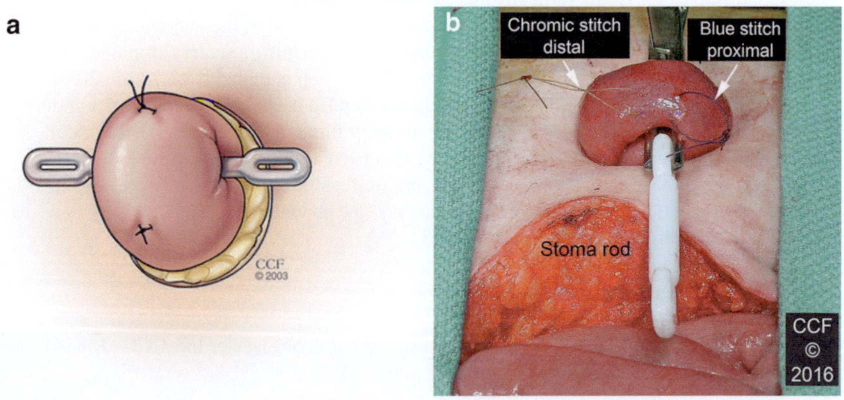

Fig. 159.2 (**a–b**) The incipient loop ileostomy is suspended over a stoma rod. The proximal and distal ends are marked with suture. In this case, "blue" (polyglycolic acid) is toward the sky, i.e., proximal, and "brown" (chromic) is down. The stoma rod is secured with a Kocher clamp

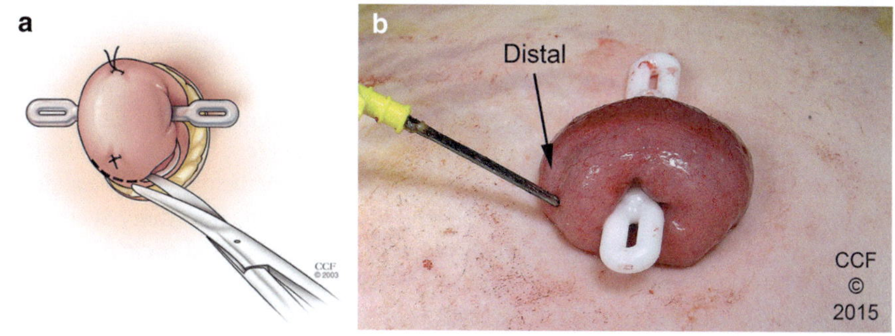

Fig. 159.3 (**a–b**) An enterotomy is made in the distal exposed aspect of the loop. The ileum is cut four-fifths of the way across (from mesentery to mesentery)

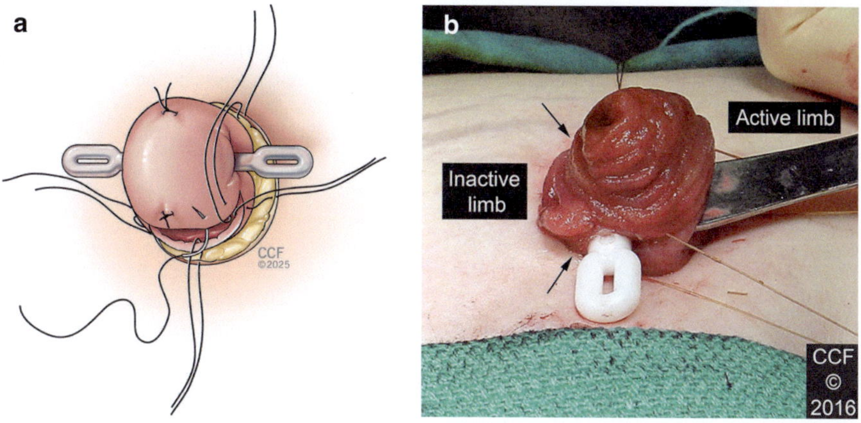

Fig. 159.4 (**a–b**) Primary maturation. The intestinal lining is everted. Maturation sutures (3-0 chromic in this case) are sewn through the full thickness of the intestine to the skin dermis. The active limb occupies about 80% of the stoma aperture circumference. The junction between the active and inactive limbs are marked with arrows

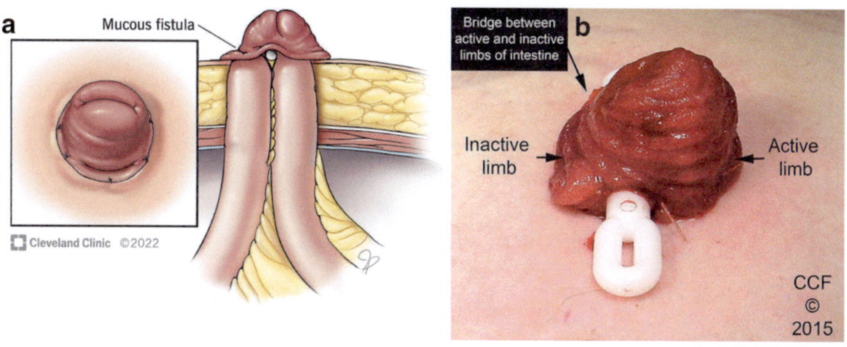

Fig. 159.5 (**a–b**) The matured loop ileostomy. The proximal matured end occupies about 80% of the stoma aperture circumference; the distal defunctionalized end occupies about 20%. The ostomy is located on a flat surface that can accommodate an appliance not too close to the midline incision. The stoma rod is removed when the intestine is secure in its position above the skin

Comment

A loop ileostomy is used to divert the fecal stream. It may serve as a temporary or permanent end of the gastrointestinal tract, protect a distal anastomosis, or prevent feces from reaching a disease process. Ileostomy site selection is made at a site that can accommodate an appliance and that can be managed by the patient. The abdominal wall stoma aperture is prepared as for end ileostomy. The ileostomy aperture is made large enough to accommodate two limbs of intestine and their mesentery. Although the indications for loop ileostomy in 1958 may have been few, advances in colon and rectal surgery have elevated loop ileostomy to a standard operative technique.

References

1. Turnbull RB Jr. Intestinal stomas. Surg Clin N Amer. 1958;38:1361–72.
2. Turnbull RB Jr, Hewitt CR. Loop-end myotomy ileostomy in the obese patient. Urol Clinc N Amer. 1978;5:423–9.

Loop-End Ileostomy Construction

160

James S. Wu

Loop-End Ileostomy

Loop-end ileostomy is an alternative to end ileostomy if the end of the ileum cannot be brought above the skin surface without tension or ischemia. Loop-end ileostomy has a mesenteric arcade that perfuses the stoma. Suspension of the loop-end ileostomy over a rod prevents stoma retraction (Fig. 160.1a–c).

In this case, two limbs of inflamed (thickened and edematous) intestine plus intervening mesentery had to be exteriorized. To achieve this, the space between the skin and the peritoneum was enlarged by dividing posterior rectus sheath, rectus muscle, anterior rectus sheath, subcutaneous fat, and skin more than usual and as much as needed (Fig. 160.2). The subsequent development of a hernia was accepted.

J. S. Wu (✉)
Department of Colon and Rectal Surgery, Cleveland Clinic, Cleveland, OH, USA

J. S. Wu, M. D. Inkster (eds.), *Cleveland Clinic Colorectal Case Studies*,
https://doi.org/10.1007/978-3-031-39880-3_160

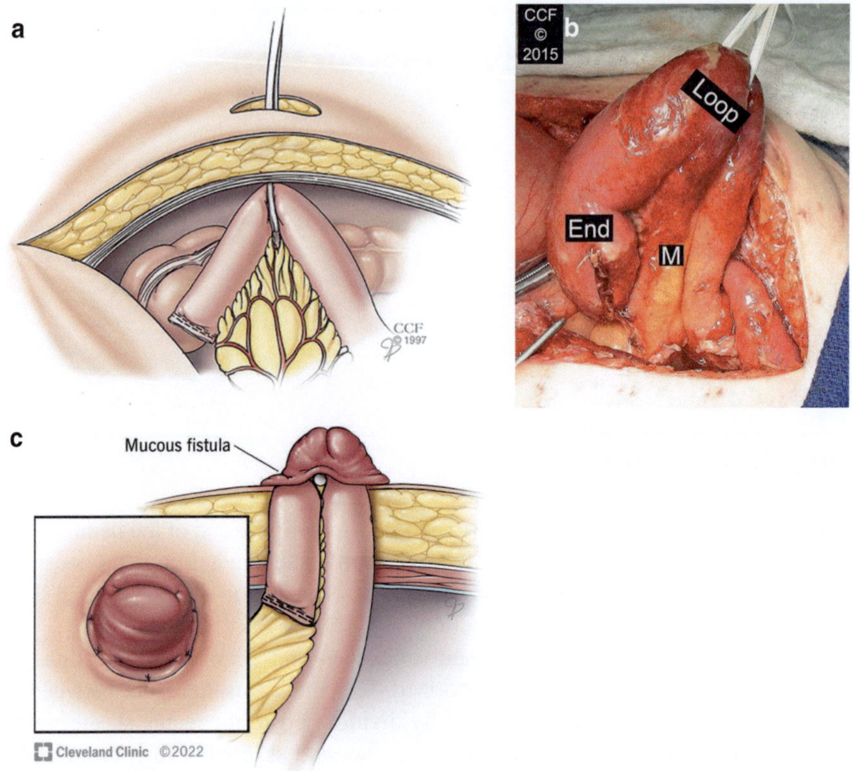

Fig. 160.1 Loop-end ileostomy. (**a**) Illustration showing the mesenteric arcade of vessels supplying the incipient loop-end ileostomy stoma; (**b**) the terminal ileum is prepared for loop-end ileostomy in a septic patient following ileocolic anastomotic leak. The anastomosis was dismantled and the ileum was exteriorized. Because the mesentery was inflamed and foreshortened, end ileostomy was not possible. In this case, the apex of the loop-end ileostomy easily reached above the skin surface (M = mesentery); (**c**) illustration of the completed loop-end ileostomy. Like loop ileostomy, the functional side of the stoma crosses over the rod so that it occupies most of the skin aperture

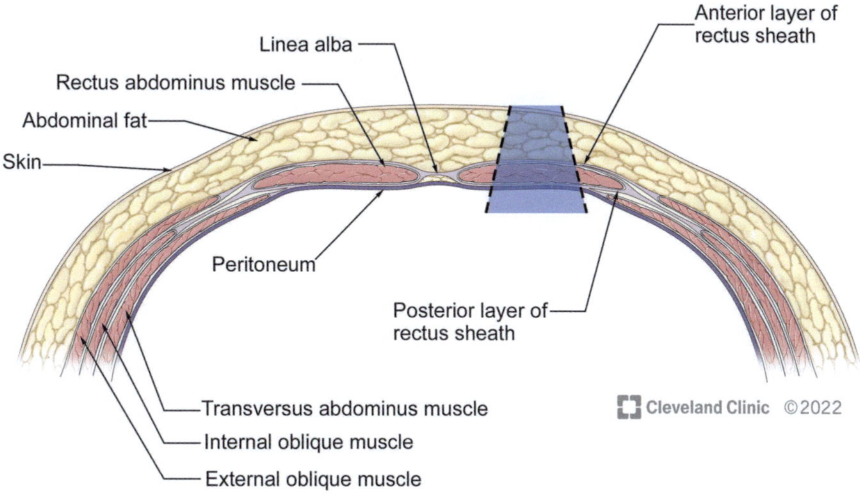

Fig. 160.2 In order to exteriorize edematous and thickened intestine/mesentery in the construction of a stoma, the space between the skin and the peritoneum is enlarged by dividing skin, fat, muscle, and fascia as much as is needed. The openings in rectus sheaths and the skin, in particular, must be enlarged. The subcutaneous space takes the form of a cone

Table 160.1 Settings appropriate for loop-end ileostomy

Obesity
Short mesentery
Irradiated ileum
Ileum affected by inflammatory bowel disease
Ileostomy in the presence of abdominal wall deformities
Jejunostomy
Supravesicular diversion with ileal conduit

Comment

In 1978, Turnbull and Hewitt [1, 2][1] described loop-end ileostomy as a solution for ileostomy creation in situations where a matured end ileostomy above the skin cannot be created. Situations where loop-end ileostomy may be indicated are shown in Table 160.1.

> "Supravesicular diversion with the ileal conduit may be difficult in obese persons because of the length of the conduit necessary to traverse the thick abdominal wall and still make a suitable projecting ileostomy. All too often the surgeon cuts into the mesentery of the ileostomy to gain length and then finds the stoma ischemic or at best retracted to the level of the skin. A collecting device cannot be worn without leakage and the patient cannot be rehabilitated."

[1]This excerpt is reproduced with the generous permission from Mr. Subash Balakruishnan, ELSEVIER | HCM – Health Content Management, reference number 210904-009370, September 4, 2021

We have used this procedure since 1961. Retraction of the stoma has never occurred. We have followed all of the patients carefully. The success rate as compared with the end stoma has been high enough to indicate that this is the most useful stoma that we have constructed in obese patients following cystectomy. If we consider loop stomas of this type done for Crohn's disease following colectomy, in excess of 600 stomas of this type have been constructed.

Obesity is the most common indication for loop-end ileostomy. Other indications include the presence of multiple abdominal scars or other abdominal deformities, and instances in which the terminal ileum is not suitable for use as an isolated segment. For example, when the terminal ileum is the site of radiation changes. When the proximal ileum or jejunum is used, the nature of the blood supply to these portions of the small intestines requires the use of the loop stoma."

Rupert B. Turnbull, Jr., M.D., C.M., F.A.C.S.,
and Clarence R. Hewitt, M.D.
Cleveland

Reference

1. Turnbull RB Jr, Hewitt CR. Loop-end myotomy ileostomy in the obese patient. Urol Clinc N Amer. 1978;5:423–9.
2. Turnbull and Hewitt's operation included ileostomy myotomies. Myotomies have been omitted from this presentation.

Loop Ileostomy Closure-Sewn

161

Douglas D. Benson, Michelle D. Inkster, and James S. Wu

Loop Ileostomy Closure: Sewn [1]

The skin around the loop ileostomy is prepared (Fig. 161.1). A peristomal skin incision is made (Fig. 161.2). The intestine is freed from attachments to subcutaneous fat and fascia (Fig. 161.3). The proximal limb is of ileum is desusscepted. The skin attached to the ileostomy is excised leaving proximal and distal limbs of intestine. The distal limb of ileum is smaller than the proximal limb (Fig. 161.4).

The smaller distal limb of intestine is widened by a Cheatle slit (Fig. 161.5). Traction stitches are placed at the mesenteric and antimesenteric borders (Fig. 161.6). The ileostomy is closed with full-thickness 3-0 polyglycolic acid (Figs. 161.6 and 161.7).

The traction sutures stretch the suture line; gaps needing additional suture are identified using the tip of a hemostat (Fig. 161.7). The intestinal lumen is considered adequate when the tips of the thumb and index finger can touch through the newly created anastomosis, as shown in Fig. 161.8.

There are many acceptable ways to close the fascia. In this case, the fascia was closed with interrupted absorbable suture. Figure 161.9 shows the surgical site after return of the intestine to the abdomen and fascial closure. The peristomal skin incision was extended superiorly in order to provide adequate exposure of the adhesive attachments between the intestine and the fascia. In this case, the superior skin incision extension was closed, and the ostomy site was loosely approximated with an absorbable purse-string suture (Fig. 161.10). Alternatively, the wound can be packed with moist gauze and healed by secondary intention.

D. D. Benson · J. S. Wu (✉)
Department of Colon and Rectal Surgery, Cleveland Clinic, Cleveland, OH, USA

M. D. Inkster
Department of Gastroenterology, Cleveland Clinic, Cleveland, OH, USA

J. S. Wu, M. D. Inkster (eds.), *Cleveland Clinic Colorectal Case Studies*,
https://doi.org/10.1007/978-3-031-39880-3_161

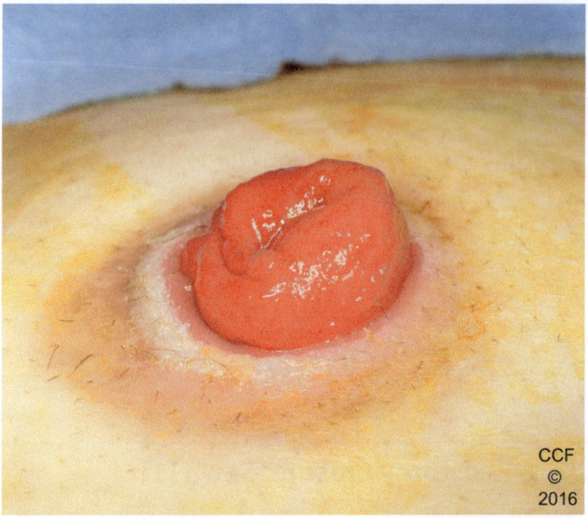

Fig. 161.1 The loop ileostomy prepared for closure

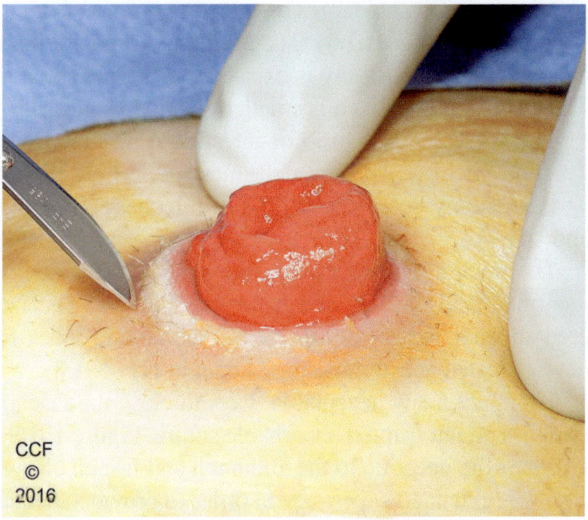

Fig. 161.2 A full-thickness peristomal skin incision is made

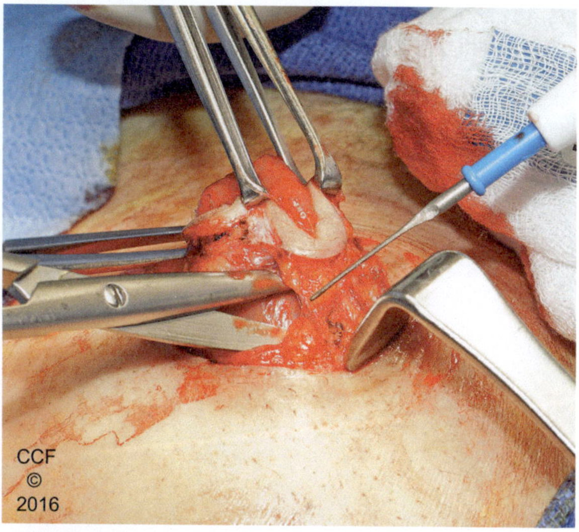

Fig. 161.3 Adhesions between the ileum and surrounding fat and fascia are divided. In this case, the scissor blades create distance between the bowel and the adhesion

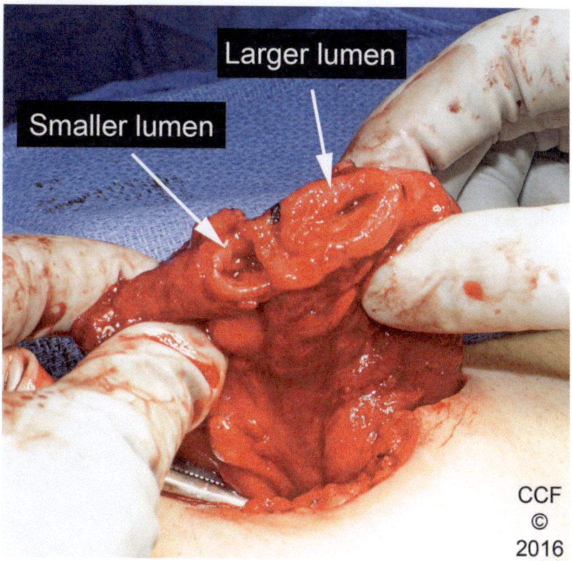

Fig. 161.4 The two intestinal limbs of the loop ileostomy are separated. A luminal size discrepancy is seen. The larger lumen corresponds to the proximal limb. The smaller lumen corresponds to the efferent defunctionalized limb

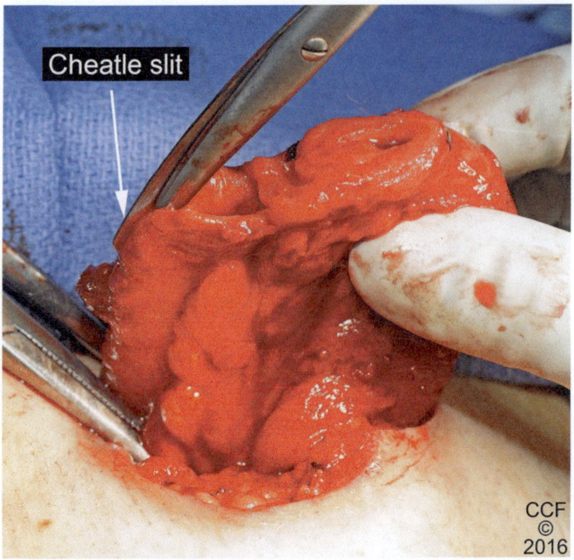

Fig. 161.5 An antimesenteric slit is made in the smaller limb of intestine to increase its luminal diameter

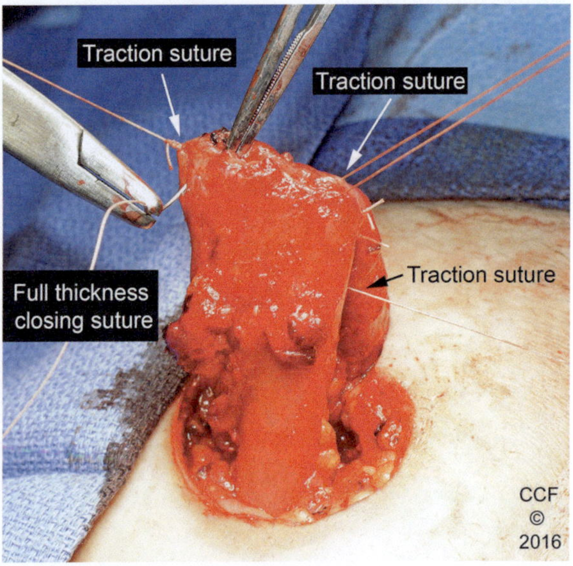

Fig. 161.6 Traction sutures are placed on the antimesenteric corners of the intestinal limbs and across the intestinal lumen to be closed in order to facilitate precise full-thickness single-layer closure. In this photograph, a closing stitch is being placed at one of the antimesenteric corners. The hemostat identifies the intestinal lumen

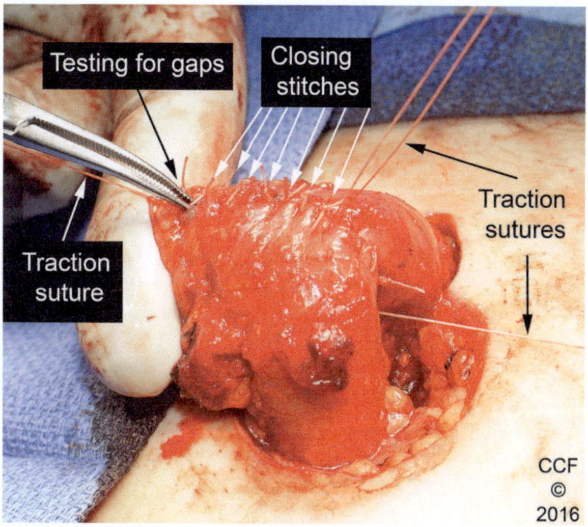

Fig. 161.7 The intestinal lumen between two traction sutures has been closed. If the tip of a hemostat can be passed between two stitches, another stitch is placed to close the gap

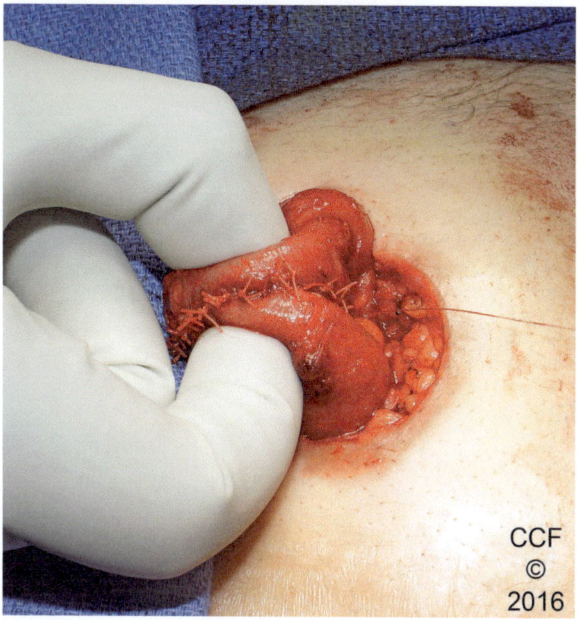

Fig. 161.8 If the thumb and forefinger can touch through the anastomosis, the luminal diameter usually is adequate

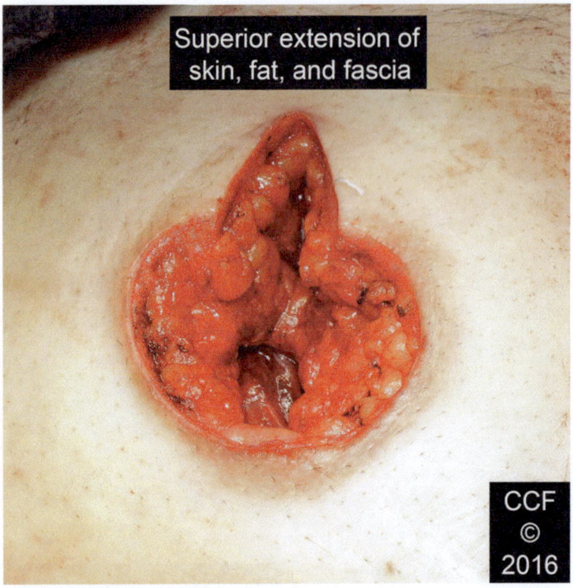

Fig. 161.9 The surgical site after return of the intestine to the abdomen and fascial closure

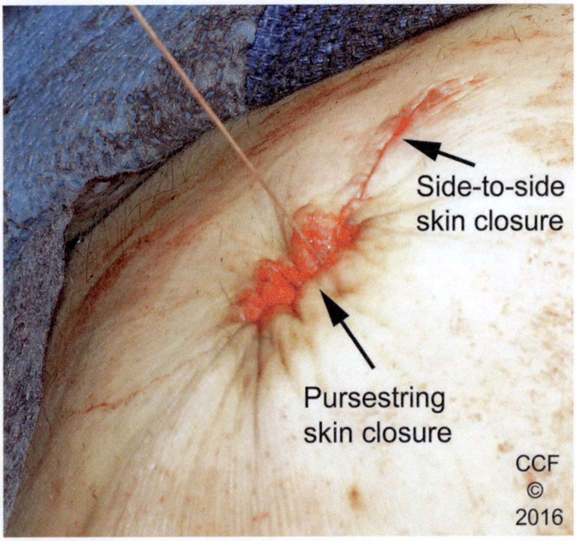

Fig. 161.10 The superior extension of the skin incision was closed with absorbable suture. The ostomy site was loosely approximated with an absorbable purse-string suture

Comment

Meticulous adhesiolysis under direct vision is required to free the intestine from the subcutaneous fat, rectus muscle, and fascia. Adequate exposure is provided by traction and countertraction. Superior or inferior extension of skin and fascial incisions may be needed to obtain adequate fascial exposure. Blind and blunt dissection is avoided. Serosal and full-thickness injuries are detected by filling the intestinal lumen with dilute iodine solution under pressure. All defects are repaired. Intestinal resection and laparotomy may be required in order to ensure safe reconstitution of intestinal continuity. The choice of stapled versus sewn anastomosis is determined by surgeon preference [2].

Biographical Note

Sir Lenthal Cheatle

George Lenthal Cheatle was born in 1865. He qualified in medicine at King's College and Hospital in 1887. As a hospital registrar he came into close association with Lister and assisted him in the last operation he performed. He served in the military during the Boer War and during the European War of 1914-1918. For his service he was made Commander of the Bath, surgeon rear-admiral and K.B.C. Early in his career, he recognized the importance of cutting and examining sections of an affected organ, and he developed a large microtome sometimes associated with this name [3].

In 1897, Cheatle described a method of uniting the intestine in which a longitudinal slit is made on the side of the intestine opposite the mesentery [4, 5].[1]

> A METHOD OF UNITING THE
> DIVIDED INTESTINE.
> By G. Lenthal Cheatle, F.R.C.S. Eng.,
> Assistant Surgeon to King's College Hospital
> and to the West London Hospital.

> "This operation has been planned upon experiments performed on the dead, and upon one in a living animal. Therefore I venture to hope that the present publication will be regarded only as a preliminary note, and not the result of matured investigations.

[1] Permission to reproduce Figs. 163.1–3 was generously provided by the LANCET PUBLISHING GROUP, Order License ID 1139329-1, Order Date 09-Aug-2021.

After the removal of the affected segment of the intestine by a section exactly transverse to the longitudinal direction of the bowel and its V-shaped piece of attached mesentery the open ends of the gut lie requiring suture. Through all the coats forming the wall of each free end a longitudinal incision is made and in each case it should be situated exactly opposite that part of the bowel to which the mesentery is attached (Fig. 161.11 [Cheatle FIG. 1.]).

The length of each incision must vary as convenience and necessity demand, but speaking generally it should at least be equal to the diameter of the tube at the seat of resection. These incisions allow the open ends of the intestine to be spread out in the shape of a fan and while in this state the separated serous surfaces can be exactly apposed as if it were back-to-back (Fig. 161.12 [Cheatle FIG. 2.]).

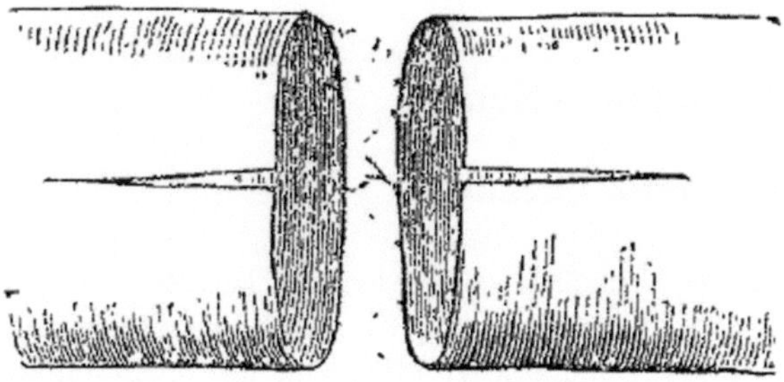

Fig. 161.11 [Cheatle FIG. 1.]. A slit is made in the anti-mesenteric walls of two segments of intestine that are to be joined

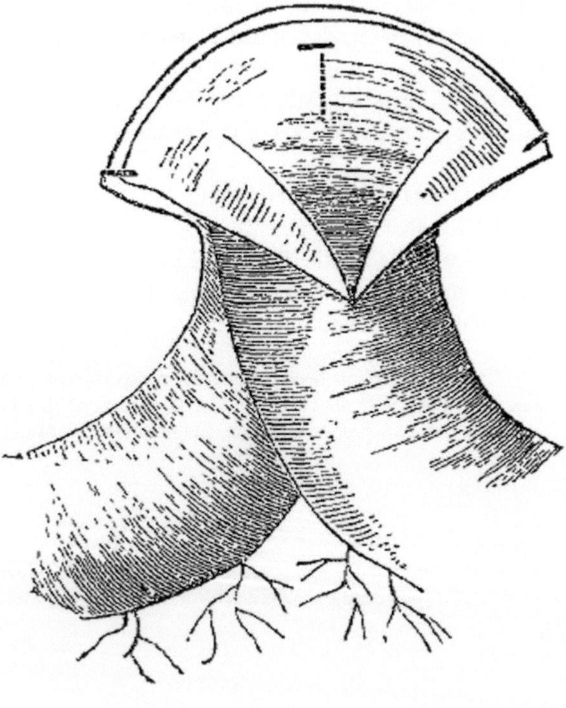

Fig. 161.12 [Cheatle FIG. 2.]. An end-to-end anastomosis is sewn. The open ends of the intestine are spread out in the shape of a fan to facilitate exact apposition

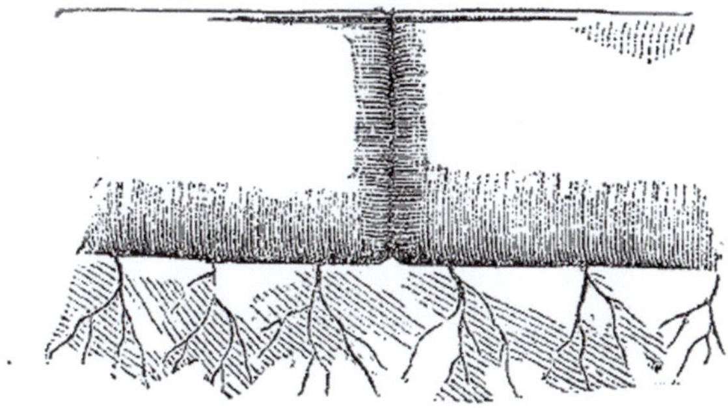

Fig. 161.13 [Cheatle FIG. 3.]. The completed intestinal anastomosis

> The ends are thus firmly joined and all that remains to be done is to suture the longitudinal incision by any of the well-known methods which the operator may prefer (Fig. 161.13 [Cheatle FIG. 3.])."

Cheatle's technique facilitates the creation of an anastomosis between two intestinal segments of unequal luminal diameter. A slit is made in the intestinal limb with the smaller diameter so that the circumference of both intestinal limbs is equal. The technique, described in 1897, remains an essential surgical skill today.

References

1. Turnbull RB Jr, Weakley FL. Closure of loop ileostomy. In: Atlas of Intestinal Stomas, Chapter 4. St. Louis: CV Mosby Co; 1967. pp. 53–7.
2. Hull TL, Kobe I, Fazio VW. Comparison of handsewn with stapled loop ileostomy closures. Dis Colon Rectum. 1996;39:1086–9.
3. Sir Lenthal Cheatle. K.C.B., C.V.O., F.R.C.S. Obituary. Br Med J. 1951;1:95–6.
4. Cheatle GL. A method of uniting the divided intestine. Lancet. 1897;149(3847);1403–4.
5. Cheatle GL. A method of uniting the divided intestine. lancet. 1897;150(3870):1113.

Loop Ileostomy Closure-Stapled

162

Emre Gorgun, H. Nail Aydin, and James S. Wu

Loop Ileostomy Closure: Stapled [1]

The operation is done in the operating room under general anesthesia in the supine position. The skin is prepared sterilely. A circumferential incision is made close to the stoma (Fig. 162.1a, b). The intestine is dissected free from the subcutaneous fat, rectus fascia, and muscle (Fig. 162.2a, b). The stoma is desuscepted. The proximal and distal limbs of intestine are separated (Fig. 162.3). The proximal and distal loops of intestine are irrigated to detect enterotomy and serosal injuries (Fig. 162.4a, b). In this stapled technique, bowel continuity is restored by functional end-to-end

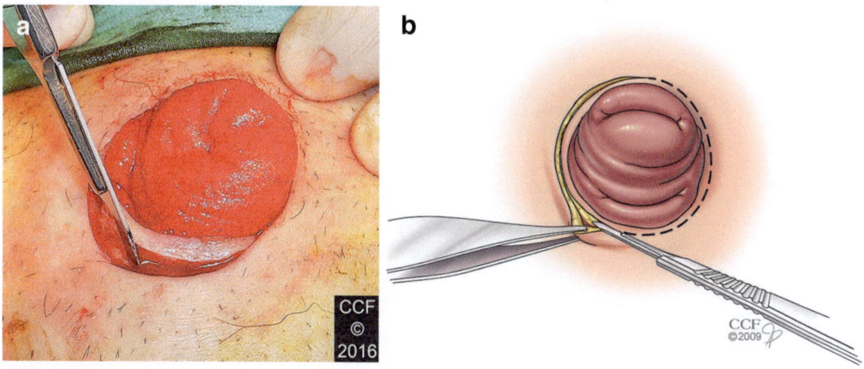

Fig. 162.1 (**a**, **b**) A circumferential full-thickness skin incision is made around the stoma

E. Gorgun · H. N. Aydin · J. S. Wu (✉)
Department of Colon and Rectal Surgery, Cleveland Clinic, Cleveland, OH, USA

J. S. Wu, M. D. Inkster (eds.), *Cleveland Clinic Colorectal Case Studies*,
https://doi.org/10.1007/978-3-031-39880-3_162

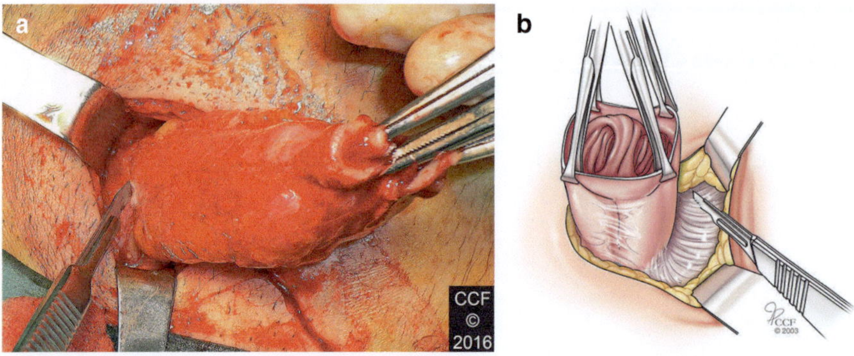

Fig. 162.2 (**a**, **b**) The two limbs of the loop ileostomy are freed from the surrounding fat and fascia by sharp dissection

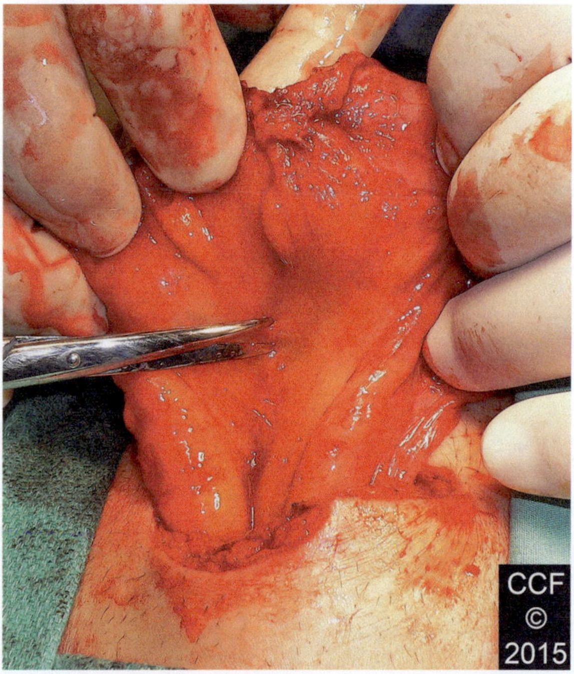

Fig. 162.3 The two limbs of ileum are separated by dividing mesenteric adhesions by sharp dissection. Adhesions are demonstrated by gentle traction

anastomosis. The antimesenteric aspects of the proximal and distal intestinal loops are divided and anastomosed using a gastrointestinal anastomosis (GIA) stapling device (Fig. 162.5a, b). The enterotomy is closed with a linear stapling device (Fig. 162.6a, b, c). The ostomy site fascia is closed (Fig. 162.7). The surgical site is allowed to heal by secondary intention.

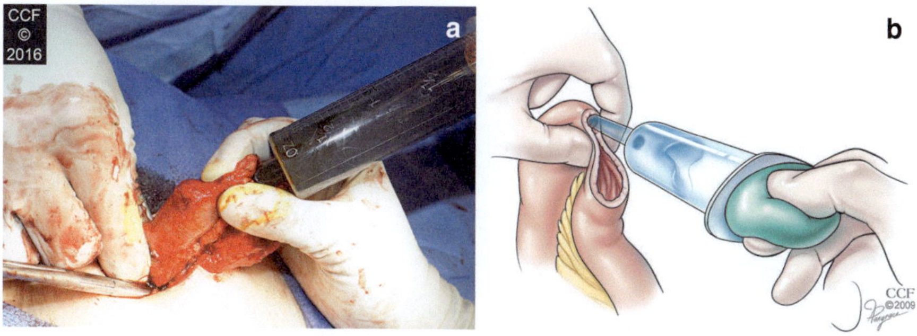

Fig. 162.4 (**a**, **b**) The proximal and distal limbs of liberated ileum are irrigated with dilute iodine solution to detect enterotomies and serosal injuries. All injuries are repaired

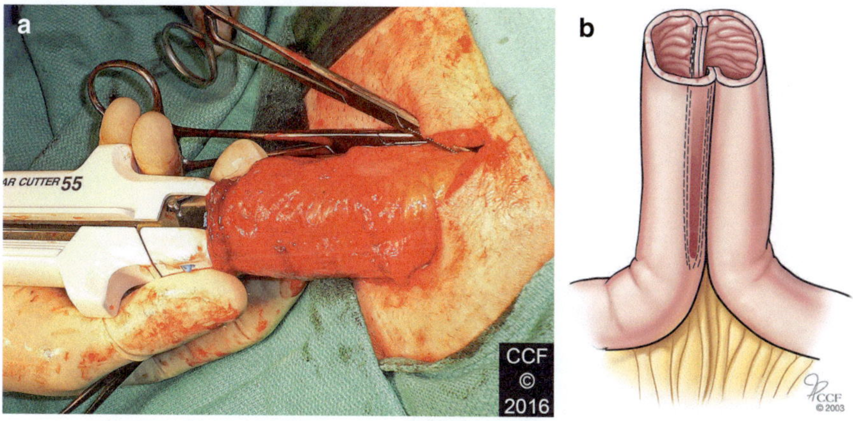

Fig. 162.5 (**a**, **b**) The antimesenteric walls of the proximal and distal limbs of intestine are simultaneously divided and anastomosed using a GIA stapler

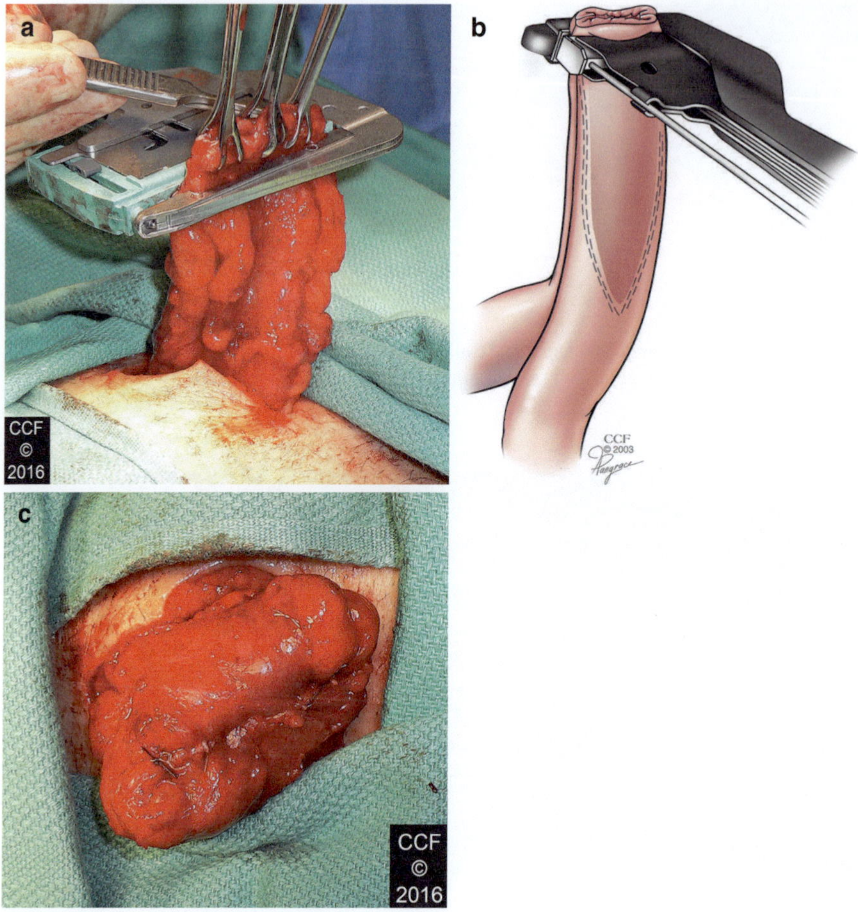

Fig. 162.6 The enterotomy is closed with a linear stapler; (**a**) operative photo showing stapled enterotomy closure. A scalpel is poised to excise the intestine excluded from the anastomosis by the staple line (**b**) medical illustration showing the same; (**c**) in this case, the staple line was buried with an additional layer of sutures

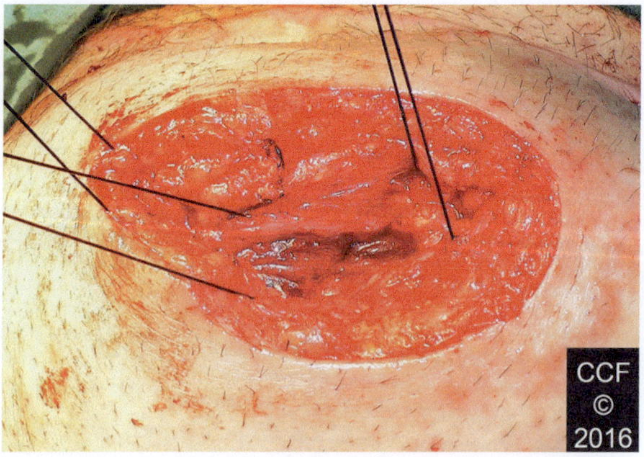

Fig. 162.7 The fascia of the ileostomy site is closed with interrupted suture. The wound was packed with moist gauze and allowed to heal by secondary intention

Reference

1. Stocchi L. Ileostomy. In: Fazio VW, Church JM, Wu JS, editors. Atlas of Intestinal Stomas, Chapter 7. Springer: New York; 2012. p. 85–95.

Philip Syng Physick

163

Michelle D. Inkster, Erika B. Woodrum, and James S. Wu

Presentation

Ostomy closure by sewn or stapled techniques now is routine. In the 1800s, this was not the case. Dr. William Gibson, then Professor of Surgery at the University of Pennsylvania, in the eighth edition of his two-volume work entitled, *Institutes and Practice of Surgery* [1] published in 1850, described in detail the pioneering method of artificial anus closure ascribed to Dr. Philip Syng Physick.

"ARTIFICIAL ANUS

When the operation for strangulated hernia has been too long delayed, and the intestine has mortified, it sometimes happens that an artificial anus is formed. In such cases the inflammation, instead of extending throughout the peritoneum, and producing the patient's death, is limited to the neighborhood of the stricture, and, terminating in the adhesive stage, glues the sound portions of the intestine to the hernia sac. This adhesion becomes firmer and firmer, in proportion as the sloughing process, going on in the protruded parts, advances, until the sloughs are thrown off, and fæces are discharged externally. By this provision of nature, effusions into the cavity of the abdomen are, in nine cases out of ten, effectually guarded against. As in every case of hernia the intestine is doubled upon itself, it follows that the two portions must lie parallel, or nearly so, with each other, and that when an artificial anus is formed, an intermediate ridge or projection will be the result. To the free admission of the fæces from the upper to the lower part of the canal, this ridge will prove in general, a serious obstacle; in most cases, indeed, there is a total cessation of fæcal discharge by the rectum; so much so that the intestine is constantly empty, or, at most, contains only a glairy mucous.

M. D. Inkster
Department of Gastroenterology, Cleveland Clinic, Cleveland, OH, USA

E. B. Woodrum
Medical Illustration Team, Enterprise Creative Services, Cleveland Clinic, Cleveland, OH, USA

J. S. Wu (✉)
Department of Colon and Rectal Surgery, Cleveland Clinic, Cleveland, OH, USA

J. S. Wu, M. D. Inkster (eds.), *Cleveland Clinic Colorectal Case Studies*,
https://doi.org/10.1007/978-3-031-39880-3_163

An artificial anus, whether induced by a wound of the abdomen, or by hernia, is a very grievous disease, not only subjecting the patient to great inconvenience, but endangering his life. Most patients, laboring under the infirmity, are troubled with colic and other derangement of the intestinal functions. Besides, they have no control, for want of a sphincter, over the fæcal discharge. A prolapsus from one or both openings of the intestine, is by no means uncommon, and is sometimes exquisitely sensible. Artificial anus, when instituted high up, or amoung the small intestines, is apt to terminate fatally—from inanition.

TREATMENT OF ARTIFICIAL ANUS

Nature will often make surprising efforts toward restoration, and is sometimes abundantly successful. If it should be found, however, after the lapse of months, that there is no prospect of amendment, an operation may be attempted for the relief of the sufferer. The indication to be fulfilled by this is to overcome the ridge-like barrier situated between the two intestines, and which prevents the direct descent of the excrement from one to the other. Desault, with this view, introduced into each orifice of the gut, plugs of lint or linen, and by these means frequently succeeded. A more expeditious, effectual, and less troublesome operation, was proposed and executed by the late Dr. Physick, between the years 1808 and 1809. A crooked needle armed with a ligature, was passed for some distance within the orifice of one gut, and brought out at the other—traversing in its passage the coats of each. The ends of the ligature were then tied at the external opening, and formed a loose loop. This being suffered to remain for a week, caused the sides of the intestines to adhere to each other. Through the consolidated ridge, thus formed, an incision was afterwards made, and a direct communication established between the upper and the lower intestine. An operation, similar to that of Dr. Physick, was afterwards performed by the late Baron Dupuytren, in Paris, and to him the merits of the proposal is generally awarded by European writers—...."

Gibson then quotes a description of a case recorded by Dr. Benjamin Horner Coates at which Dr. Physick attended.

"John Exilius, a Swedish sailor, aged nineteen years, was admitted into the Pennsylvania Hospital on the morning of 20th of October, 1808, affected with a congenital hernia. He stated that he had passed the last fourteen days without having had a stool, and that on the 29th, he had been affected with stercoraceous vomiting. These were renewed after his admission. After several other means had been employed to produce a reduction of the hernia, the operation was proceeded to at half-past three o'clock the same afternoon, by the late Professor Wistar, in the presence of Dr. Physick. The sac being opened, the intestines were found firmly adherent to the testicle, and partially so, but with equal firmness, to the abdominal ring, so as to account for the impossibility of effecting a reduction by the taxis—they appeared to be part of the ileum. A perforation existed in the side of one of them, of sufficient magnitude to permit the discharge of a considerable amount of fæces. On the 30th of October, the patient, by the regulations of the hospital, came under the care of Dr. Physick. On the 24th of December, the projecting portion of the intestine was cut off close to the ring. The two ends of the intestine were found, by a careful examination, to adhere to each other for some distance, and the form, thus presented, has been compared in this case to that of a double-barreled gun. The next method proposed by Dr. Physick, was to cut a lateral opening through the sides of the intestine where they were adherent. By introducing his finger into the intestine though one orifice, and his thumb through the other, he was enabled to satisfy himself that nothing intervened between them but the sides of the bowels. He was thus enabled, without risk, to pass a needle, armed with a ligature from one portion of the intestine into the other, through the sides which were in contact, about an inch within the orifices, which ligature was then secured with a slip-knot. This operation was performed on the 28th of January 1809. The ligature was merely drawn sufficiently tight to ensure the contact of these parts of the peritoneal tunic which were within the noose. The ligature, in this situation, gradually made its way by ulceration through the parts which it embraced, and thus loosened itself. It was at several periods again drawn to its original tightness.

After about three weeks had elapsed, concluding that the required union between the two folds of peritoneum was sufficiently ensured, Dr. Physick divided with a bistoury all the parts which now remained included within the noose of the ligature. No unfavourable symptoms occurred in consequence. On the 28th of February, the patient complained of an uneasy sensation in the lower part of the abdomen, and on the first of March he extracted with his own fingers some portions of hardened fæces from his rectum. On the 2d of March, two or three evacuations were produced in this manner. On the 3d, an enema, consisting of a solution of common salt, was directed to be given twice every day. The first of these occasioned a natural stool, about two hours after its administration. The same effect was produced on the 4th, 5th, and 6th, and the discharges from the orifices in the groin now became inconsiderable. On the 27th of July, a truss of the common construction, furnished with a very large pad, and surmounted by a large compress, was applied to the wound. By these means the discharge of fæces from the groin was completely prevented and the patient had regular evacuations per anum.... On the 10th of November, he was discharged from the hospital in good spirits, and applied himself with very good success to acquire the profession of an engraver.

Dupuytren has invented a forceps of peculiar construction called *enterotome*, for the purpose of bruising and breaking down by force the sides of the two intestines, and in this way opening a passage from one to the other."

The concept of dividing the adherent walls of proximal and distal loops of intestine attributed to Dr. Physick is illustrated in Fig. 163.1a and b.

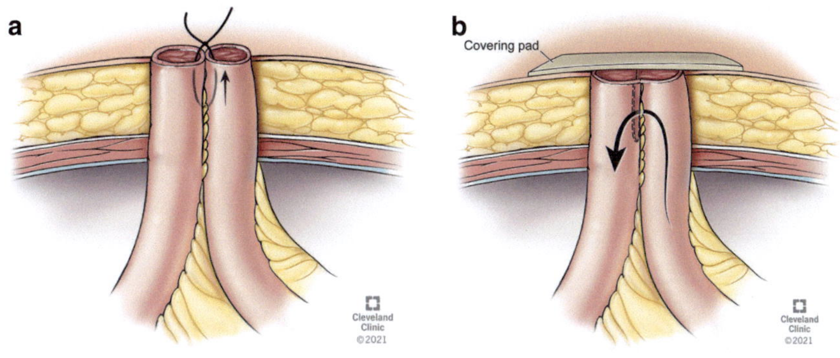

Fig. 163.1 Closure of artificial anus by cutting seton according to Physick: (**a**) A thread, passed through adherent proximal and distal limbs of intestine without entering the peritoneal cavity, is tied in a loose loop. At this stage, stool is discharged at skin level; (**b**) after the common wall is divided by the thread, stool moves from the proximal to the distal intestinal limb without exiting the skin. A surface pad catches any fecal discharge

Comment

Incarceration of a loop of ileum in a hernia resulted in a double-barreled loop ileostomy. By dividing the adherent portions of the proximal and distal limbs of intestine, stool was allowed to pass from the proximal limb to the distal limb thus re-establishing intestinal continuity. The hospitalization of the patient, John Exilius, described above was more than 1 year. In 1945, Colcock reported that this technique using a crushing clamp to divide the spur between the proximal and distal limbs of bowel was the recommended method of colostomy closure for the United States Army during World War II (Fig. 163.2) [2].[1]

Traumatic Perforation of the Colon as Seen in a General Hospital
Major Bentley P. Colcock, Medical Corps, U.S. Army

"The mortality rate following traumatic perforation of the colon in World War II has dropped to the neighborhood of 33 per cent. This represents a marked improvement over the mortality figures for World War I, which, in this type of patient, ranged from 50 to 75 per cent, and is largely due to the early replacement of blood loss by plasma, and particularly whole blood, the intraperitoneal use of the sulfonamides, and the excellent surgery being done by the well-trained abdominal surgeons in our forward field and evacuation hospitals.

(a) It is generally accepted today that the safest method of dealing with a laceration of the colon is by exteriorization of the lacerated segment of bowel.

Uniting the longitudinal bands of the colon by seromuscular sutures tied without constriction of the tissue permits the formation of a double-barreled colostomy which involves no added risk from peritonitis, and which is ideal from the point of view of the later restoration of intestinal continuity. A five- or six-inch spur not only permits the colostomy stoma to be brought well (one and one-half to two inches) above the skin level, but also insures an adequate bowel lumen after the subsequent closure. There will be no post-operative leakage of intestinal content if the spur is made of sufficient length in the first place and the bowel wall is rendered sufficiently pliable by removal of all scar tissue at the time of closure, so that it can be inverted without tension."

One of us (JSW) had the opportunity to observe the use of this "spur" crushing technique for double-barreled colostomy closure as a medical student as recently as the 1980s.

[1]Permission to reuse this excerpt was generously granted by Mr. Thomas Rexson Yesudoss, Copyrights Coordinator, ELSEVIER | HCM – Health Content Management, Unique reference number 220607-002074, on June 08, 2022

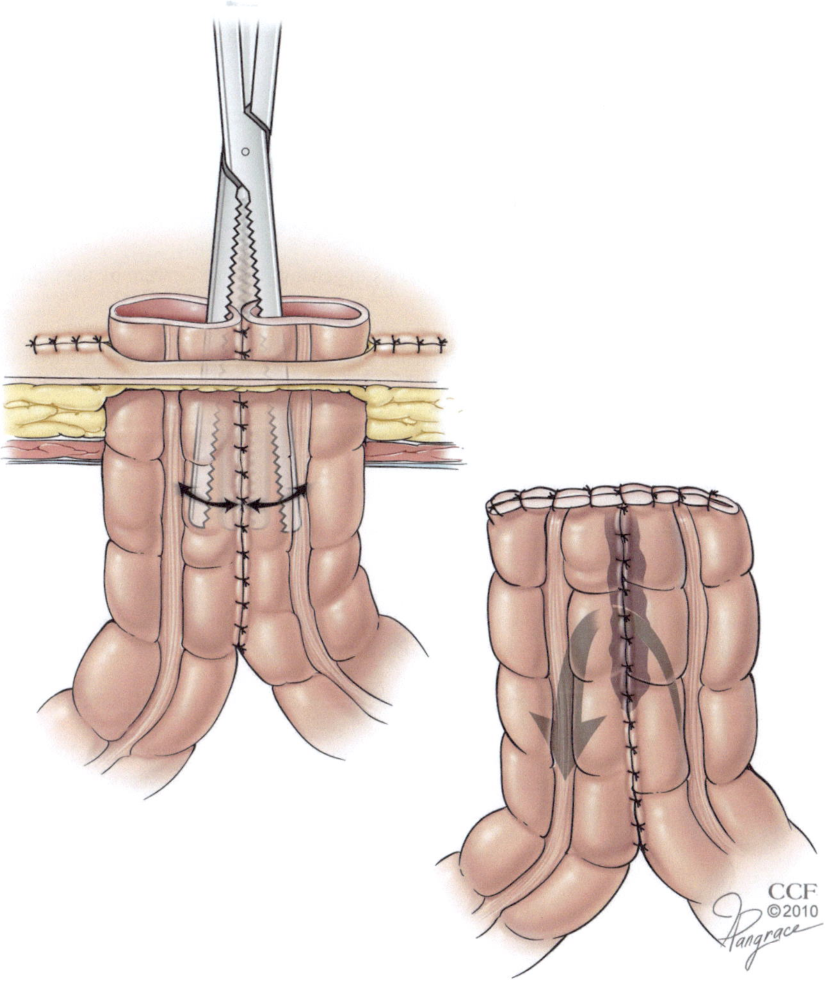

Fig. 163.2 Colostomy closure, World War II. Closure is facilitated by crushing the spur between the two limbs of colon fixed next to each other in parallel

Biographical Note

Philip Syng Physick (1768–1837)

In their work entitled, *American Medical Biographies*, Kelly and Burrage refer to Dr. Physick as the "Father of American Surgery" [3]. Following his graduation from Pennsylvania University, Physick continued his education abroad.

> 'His father was determined to give the son every opportunity of learning his profession, so sent him in 1789 to London, where he was fortunate enough to live with John Hunter and

to gain his esteem for his skillful dissections, and his influence to obtain the post of house-surgeon to St. George's Hospital, where he stayed a year. On leaving he was made a member of the Royal College of Surgeons.

Five testimonials as to "medical qualifications and correct deportment" were given young Physick when he left St. Georges and Hunter offered him a partnership. Why he refused the honor of this collaboration and the opportunity of working with Astley Cooper, Abernethy, and Home, Physick, reticent as always, does not state. He went instead to Edinburgh and took his M. D. there when twenty-four, in 1792.

Like Hunter his surgery was conservative … As to general practice he went by the light of experience of common sense….

He was professor of surgery, Pennsylvania University, 1805-19; professor of anatomy, 1819-31; president of Philadelphia Medical Society, 1824; emeritus professor of anatomy and surgery, Pennsylvania University, 1831-37; member of the Academy of Medicine of France, 1825; honorary fellow, Royal Medical and Chirurgical Society, London, 1856.'

References

1. Gibson W. Institutes and Practice of Surgery: being outlines of a course of lectures, 8E, Chapter V., Section 8. Artificial anus. Philadelphia/Pittsburgh: James Kay, Jun. and Brother/Kay and Company; 1850. p. 128–33.
2. Colcock BP. Traumatic perforation of the colon as seen in a general hospital. Surgery. 1945;17:1–10.
3. Kelly HA, Burrage WL, editors. "Physick, Philip Syng" American Medical Biographies. Baltimore: The Norman, Remington Publishing Company; 1920. pages 912-913. Google Books. [cited 2021 May 1]

Loop Transverse Colostomy 164

James S. Wu

Presentation

Consultation for fecal diversion was requested for an obese patient hospitalized in intensive care who was septic from sacral decubitus ulcers.

Management

Transverse colostomy was done. Since the transverse colon has a mobile mesentery, it easily reached the skin of the abdominal wall without tension. A stoma site was selected directly anterior to the mid-transverse colon. Preoperative preparation included a bedside plain abdominal film with a coin taped to the abdomen superior to the umbilicus. The skin beneath the coin was marked with indelible ink (Fig. 164.1).

At surgery, an incision was made that was large enough to allow the hand to enter the abdomen. The transverse colon was grasped, exteriorized, and freed from the attached omentum. The selected colon segment then was secured outside of the abdomen with a long trans-mesenteric stoma rod, opened, and primarily matured (Fig. 164.2).

J. S. Wu (✉)
Department of Colon and Rectal Surgery, Cleveland Clinic, Cleveland, OH, USA

J. S. Wu, M. D. Inkster (eds.), *Cleveland Clinic Colorectal Case Studies*,
https://doi.org/10.1007/978-3-031-39880-3_164

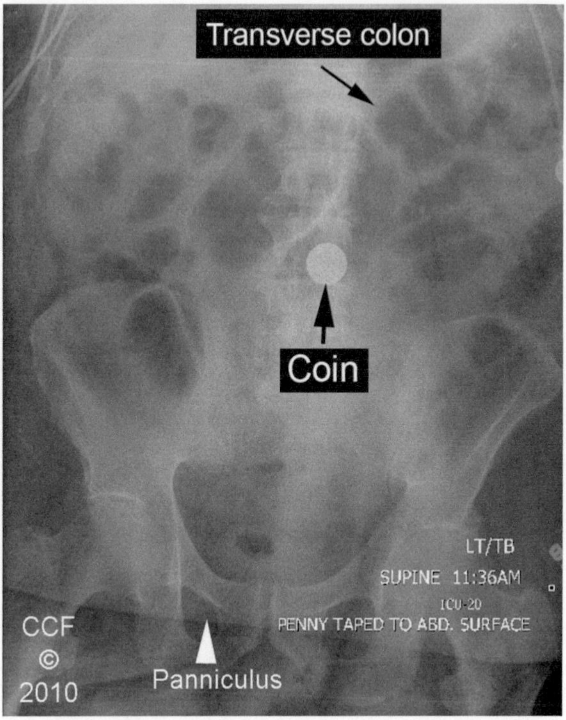

Fig. 164.1 Bedside plain abdominal film shows the relation of the transverse colon (identified by haustra) to a coin secured to the abdominal skin. This maneuver allows the operator to estimate how far superior to the coin to make an incision that will be located directly over the transverse colon. The fold of a panniculus is seen (arrowhead)

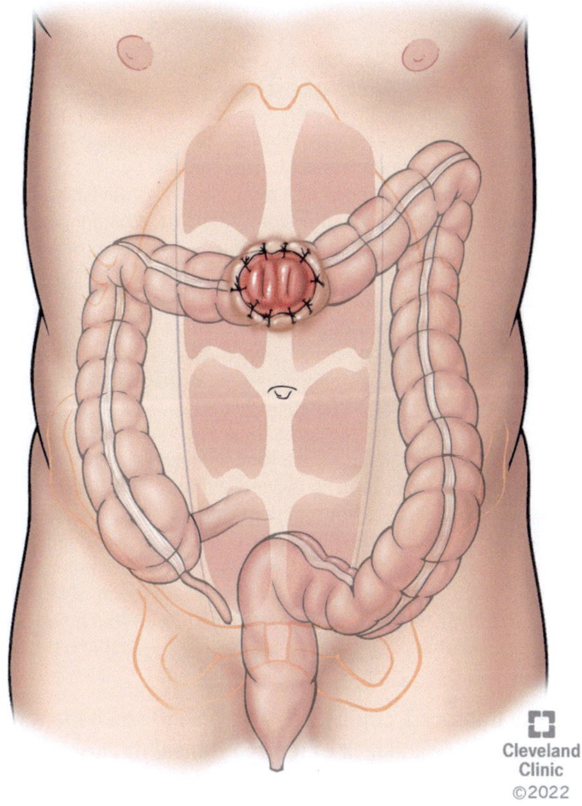

Fig. 164.2 Transverse colostomy. The mobile transverse colon and its mesentery are exteriorized. The anterior wall of the colon is opened and sutured to the dermis

Comment

Transverse colostomy was done in 1797 by M. Pierre Fine, Surgeon-in-Chief, Hospital of Geneva, and preserved for posterity by Amussat in his acclaimed *Mémoire sur la possibilité d'établir un anus artificiel dans la région lombaire sans pénétrer dans le péritoine (Memoir on the possibility of establishing an artificial anus in the lumbar region without penetrating the peritoneum)* published in 1839 [1]. Fine successfully created a diverting colostomy in a critically ill patient with obstructing rectosigmoid cancer through an incision between the navel and the pubis. His patient lived three and a half months. The position of the colostomy was determined at autopsy.

Mémoire et Observation sur L'entérotomie *Par* *M. Pierre Fine* *chirurgien en chef de l'hôpital de Genève* *Ptomatopsie*.[2] Je fis l'ouverture du cadavre le surlendemain à onze heures; je trouvai beaucoup de sérosité dans le ventre; le foie était très volumineux et très endurci, sans avoir cependent de tubérosités squirrheuses; la partie transversale du colon était celle où l'anus artificiel avait été formé; cet intestin avait conservé sa grosseur naturelle, et quoique déplacé vraisemblablement par l'expansion du gaz, il avait une position presque transversale; il avait aussi contracté des adhérences à quleques lignes autour de l'anus artificial, un peu au-dessous de cet anus; une partie d'intestin grèle en avait aussi contracté une forte, quoique peu étendue, avec les parois du ventre; enfin je trouvai à la partie tout à fait supérieure du rectum, et dans l'étendue d'un pouce et demi, une squirrhosité qui en occupait toute la circonférence, qui avait preseque oblitéré le canal intestinal, et qui était accompagnée d'une légère suppuration.	*Memoir and Observation on Enterotomy* *By* *Mr. Pierre Fine* *chief surgeon of the hospital of Geneva* *Autopsy*. I opened the body two days later at eleven o'clock; I found a lot of serous fluid in the belly; the liver was very large and very hardened, without however having scirrhous tuberosities; the transverse part of the colon was where the artificial anus had been formed; this intestine had retained its natural size, and although displaced presumably by the expansion of the gas, it had an almost transverse position; there were a few adhesions around the artificial anus. A little below that anus; a few strong but not extensive adhesions had formed between part of the small intestine and the walls of the belly; finally I found exactly superior to the rectum, measuring an inch and a half, a circumferential hard dense growth which had almost obliterated the intestinal canal, and which was accompanied by a slight suppuration.

The transverse colon likely was able to reach the lower abdomen due to its generous mesentery and lack of retroperitoneal fixation. In the current case, a coin and an abdominal plain film were used to determine the location of the transverse colon relative to the skin surface before surgery.[1]

Fine recognized the long-term effects of fecal diversion on nutrition, and recommended artificial anus creation as far away from the stomach as possible.

Second MÉMOIRE de FINE.[3] Dans mon premier Mémoire sur l'entérotomie; j'ai établi comme principe général, que l'anus artificiel doit être practiqué sur le côté gauche de l'abdomen dans la partie du tube intestinal la plus éloignée possible de l'estomac, afin que l'absorption du chyle se fasse dans une plus grande étendue et que la nutrition se ressente moins de la diminution qu'elle éprouverait, lorsque cet anus serait établi dans un endroit plus rapproché de ce viscère.	Second MEMOIR of FINE In my first memoir on enterotomy, I established as a general principle, that the artificial anus must be placed on the left side of the abdomen in the part of the intestinal tube as far as possible from the stomach, so that the absorption of the chyle is done in a large extent and that nutrition is less affected by the decrease it would experience when this anus is established in a place closer to this viscera.

[1] The inspiration for the use of a coin to determine transverse colon location in this case was a 4″ × 3″ glass slide preserved in a "lantern-slide" lecture on ulcerative colitis prepared by Dr. Frank L. Weakley at the Cleveland Clinic in the 1970s.

References

1. Amussat JZ. Mémoire sur la possibilité d'établir un anus artificiel dans la région lombaire sans pénétrer dans le péritoine. Paris: Acad R Med, Germer-Baillière; 1839. [cited 2021 Mar 3]. Available from Archive.org
2. Fine P. Memoire et observation sur l'entérotomie. In: Amussat JZ. Mémoire sur la possibilité d'établir un anus artificiel dans la région lombaire sans pénétrer dans le péritoine. Paris: Acad R Med, Germer-Baillière; 1 Oct 1839. pp. 109–114. [cited 2021 Mar 3]. Available from Archive.org
3. Amussat JZ. Mémoire sur la possibilité d'établir un anus artificiel dans la région lombaire sans pénétrer dans le péritoine. Paris: Acad R Med, Germer-Baillière; 1 Oct 1839. p. 117. [cited 2021 Mar 3]. Archive.org

"Blowhole" Colostomy

165

Ian C. Lavery, Feza H. Remzi, and James S. Wu

Presentation

An elderly male presented with large bowel obstruction from rectal cancer (Fig. 165.1).

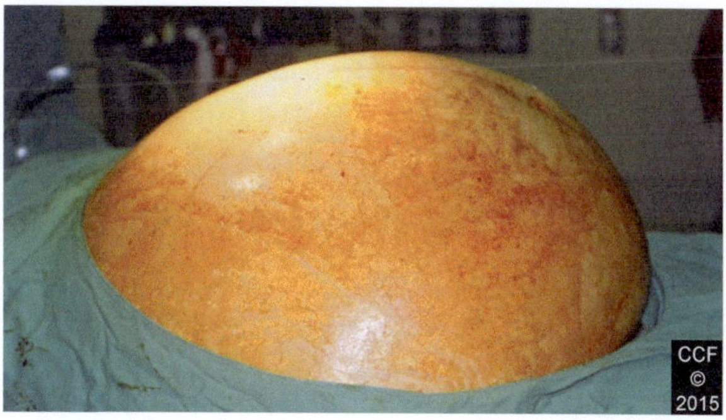

Fig. 165.1 The colon is massively distended from totally obstructing rectal cancer

I. C. Lavery · J. S. Wu (✉)
Department of Colon and Rectal Surgery, Cleveland Clinic, Cleveland, OH, USA

F. H. Remzi
Inflammatory Bowel Disease Center, NYU Langone Health, New York, NY, USA

J. S. Wu, M. D. Inkster (eds.), *Cleveland Clinic Colorectal Case Studies*,
https://doi.org/10.1007/978-3-031-39880-3_165

Management

The patient was brought to surgery. Decompression of the obstructed colon and rectum was accomplished by "blowhole" colostomy as described in Figs. 165.2, 165.3, 165.4, 165.5, and 165.6.

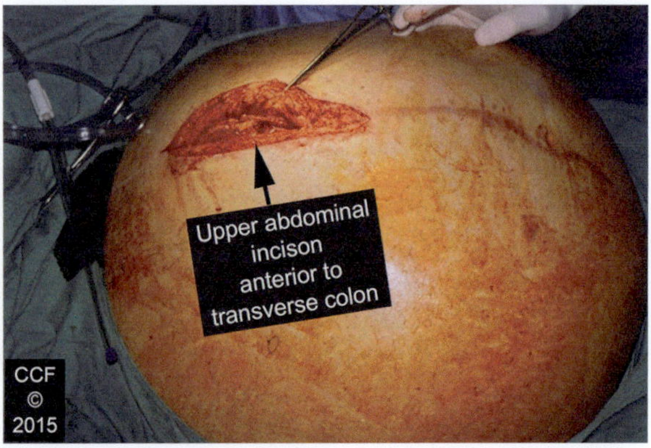

Fig. 165.2 Laparotomy incision is made anterior to the transverse colon

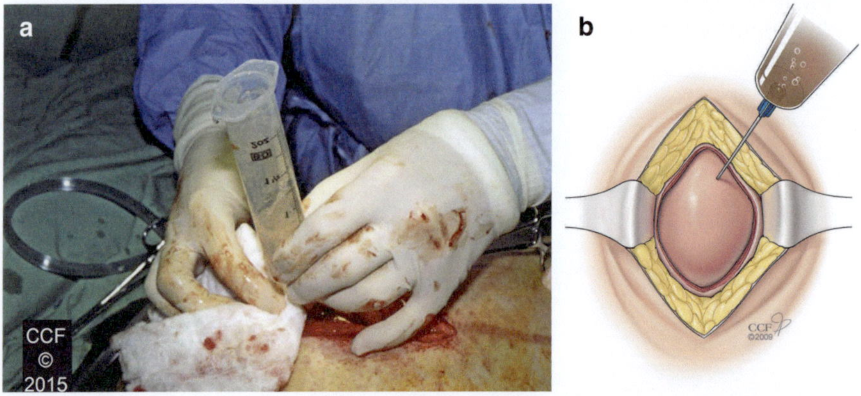

Fig. 165.3 The transverse colon is exteriorized and then decompressed with a needle attached to a syringe: (a) operative photograph; (b) illustration showing the removal of liquid stool and gas

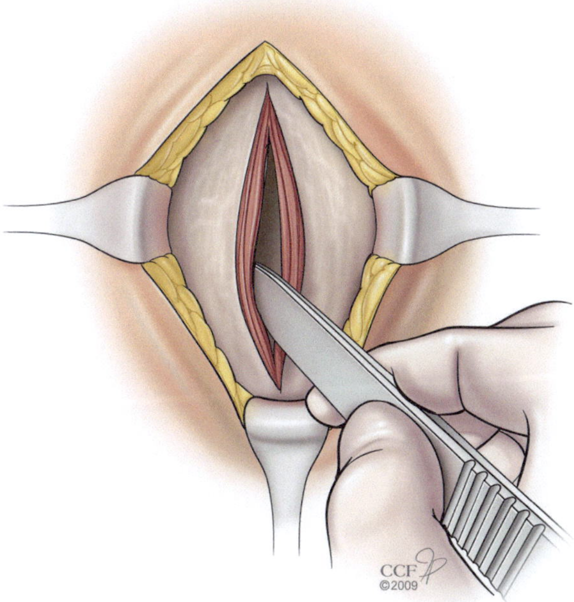

Fig. 165.4 The abdomen overlying the transverse colon is opened

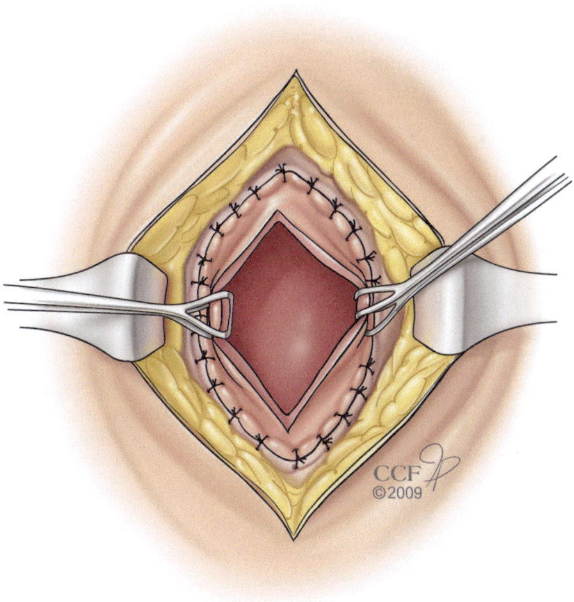

Fig. 165.5 The colonic serosa is sewn to the fascia to isolate the bowel from the peritoneal cavity. Then the colon is opened

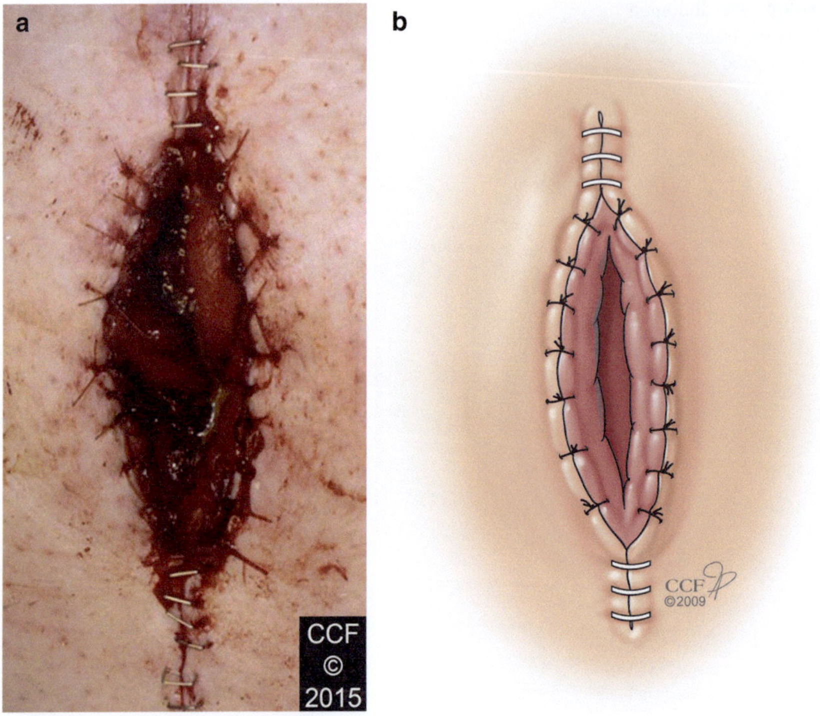

Fig. 165.6 The colostomy is matured by sewing the intestinal wall to the skin: (a) operative photograph; (b) illustration

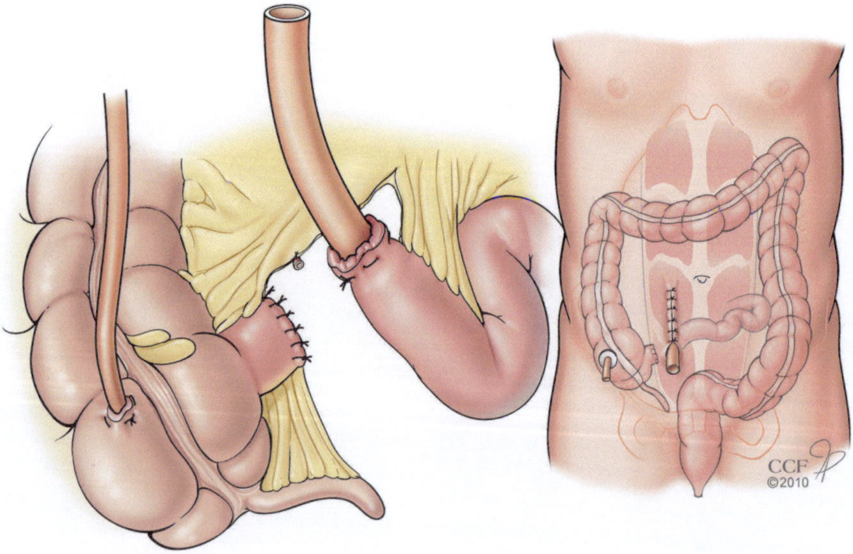

Fig. 165.7 Tube ileostomy and cecostomy to treat ulcerative colitis (Brown's operation)

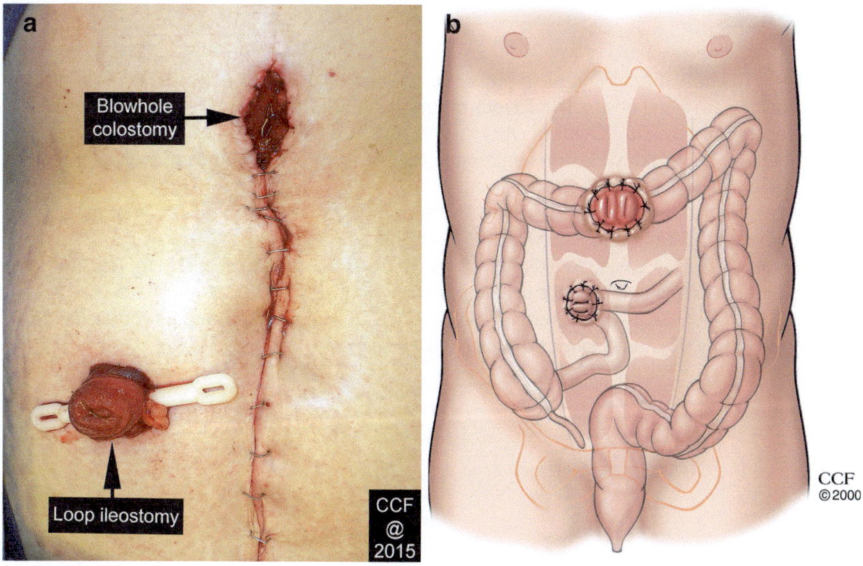

Fig. 165.8 A patient with obstructing rectal cancer was treated by loop ileostomy (suspended over a rod) and "blowhole" colostomy followed by neoadjuvant chemoradiotherapy; (**a**) intraoperative photograph; (**b**) illustration

Comment

In 1913, Brown in St. Louis returned a patient with extensive ulcerative colitis to good health by creating simultaneously tube ileostomy to divert the fecal stream and cecostomy to decompress the large intestine (Fig. 165.7) [1].

The dual concepts of Brown's operation, diversion and decompression, reappeared in "Blowhole" colostomy and ileostomy, described by Turnbull and Weakley in 1967 to decompress toxic patients with megacolon who were considered too ill to withstand abdominal colectomy [2–4]. Recent reports describe its use in toxic megacolon related to inflammatory bowel disease and pregnancy, *Clostridiodes dificile* colitis, adult Hirschprung's disease, pancreatitis with obstructing pseudocyst, and palliation for malignant bowel obstruction with metastases [5]. The procedure serves both as a bridge to definitive operation and as palliation for those with terminal illness. This chapter illustrates the use of "blowhole" colostomy alone for obstructing rectal cancer and "blowhole" colostomy plus loop ileostomy for obstructing rectal cancer prior to the administration of neoadjuvant chemoradiation (Fig. 165.8).

References

1. Brown JY. The value of complete physiological rest of the large bowel in the treatment of certain ulcerative and obstructive lesions of this organ. With description of operative technique and report of cases. Surg Gynecol Obstet 1913;16:610–3.
2. Turnbull RB Jr, Weakley FL. Decompression transverse colostomy. Atlas of Intestinal Stomas. CV Mosby: St. Louis; 1967. p. 153–9.
3. Weakley FL, Turnbull RB Jr. Exclusion and decompression for toxic dilatation of the colon in ulcerative colitis. Proc Roy Soc Med. 1970;63:73–5.
4. Turnbull RB Jr, Hawk WA, Weakley FL. Surgical treatment of toxic megacolon. Ileostomy and colostomy to prepare patients for colectomy. Am J Surg. 1971;122:325–31.
5. Remzi FH, Oncel M, Hull TL, Strong SA, Lavery IC, Fazio VW. Current indications for blow-hole colostomy. A single center experience. Int J Color Dis. 2003;18:361–4.

Five Potentially Avoidable Stoma Complications

166

Barbara J. Hocevar, Victor W. Fazio, Eric W. Willis, Sebouh Setrakian, and James S. Wu

Presentation

A common surgical aphorism states that "complications begin in the operating room." This opinion is particularly true for ostomy creation. While many postoperative problems related to intestinal stomas are unavoidable, some are preventable [1–3]. Five examples are presented.

Stoma Placement in a Skin Crease

The patient shown in Fig. 166.1a has an ileostomy that was created in a natural skin crease on the right side of the abdomen. The stoma cannot be seen with sitting or standing. The site was painful. Separation of the superior and inferior aspects of the skin crease reveals chemical destruction of the peristomal skin (Fig. 166.1b).

Comment

Preoperative selection of a flat site free from skin creases in sitting, standing, and supine positions might have prevented this complication. Ostomy relocation was needed.

B. J. Hocevar
Rupert B. Turnbull, Jr., School of WOC Nursing Education, Cleveland Clinic, Cleveland, OH, USA

V. W. Fazio · J. S. Wu (✉)
Department of Colon and Rectal Surgery, Cleveland Clinic, Cleveland, OH, USA

S. Setrakian
Pathology & Laboratory Medicine Institute, Cleveland Clinic, Cleveland, OH, USA

E. W. Willis
Department of Pathology, CORPath, Columbus, OH, USA

J. S. Wu, M. D. Inkster (eds.), *Cleveland Clinic Colorectal Case Studies*,
https://doi.org/10.1007/978-3-031-39880-3_166

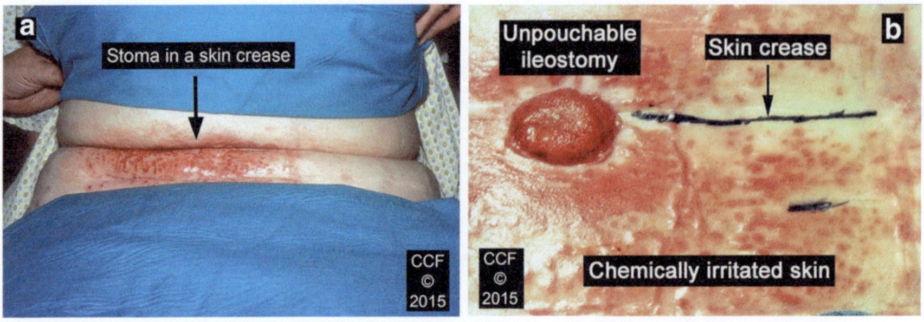

Fig. 166.1 (**a**) This stoma, located in a natural skin crease, cannot maintain an appliance; (**b**) the stoma, located at the base of the skin crease, is not pouchable. Images courtesy of Victor W. Fazio, AO, MS

Excessively Large Skin Aperture

Figure 166.2 shows separation of the mucocutaneous junction. This results in a parastomal wound that is constantly exposed to fecal effluent. In this case, the ostomy skin aperture is too large.

Comment

The skin aperture can always be enlarged; however, once created, it cannot be made smaller. This problem might have been avoided by excising a smaller skin disc initially. Other causes of mucocutaneous skin separation include poor nutritional status, stoma creation under tension, and immunosuppression.

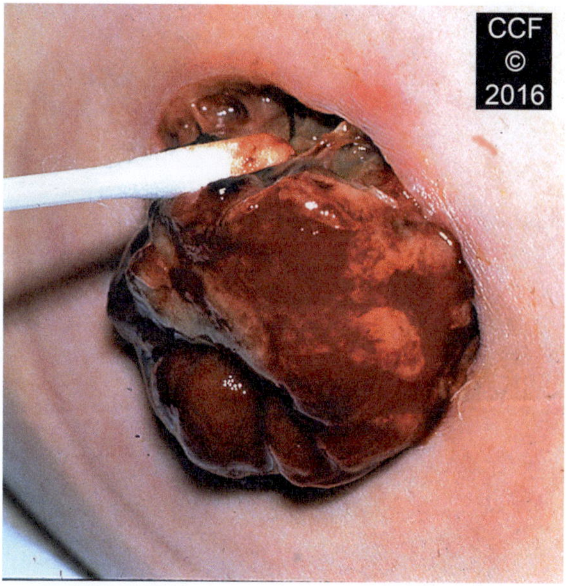

Fig. 166.2 Mucocutaneous junction separation due to an excessively large stoma skin aperture

Peri-ileostomy Mucosal Implants

A patient complained that their ileostomy appliance seal frequently leaked and that the skin barrier next to the stoma was always wet. Examination revealed circumferential peristomal mucosal implants (Fig. 166.3a). In another case (Fig. 166.3b), the appliance wafer was cut so that it did not encroach upon the implants. In both cases, mucus secretion from mucosal implants compromised the pouch seal. Figure 166.3c shows sinus tracts caused by full thickness maturation sutures placed at the time of stoma creation that later can lead to mucosal implants. Figure 166.3d shows the histologic appearance of mucosal implants.

Comment

Peristomal implants are avoided by placement of maturation sutures through the dermis. This complication occurs adjacent to both ileostomy and colostomy. Figure 166.3a-d show the macroscopic and microscopic appearance of peristomal implants adjacent to an ileostomy. Figure 166.3e shows peri-colonic implants next to a left-sided end colonoscopy. Biopsies showed colonic mucosal implants beneath the skin (Fig. 166.3f). The patient with the colostomy had lived with these implants for more than a decade without any pouching problems. The solidity of the colostomy stool compared to the liquidity of the ileostomy effluent may explain why peri-colostomy implants are better tolerated that peri-ileostomy implants.

Stoma maturation sutures are placed in the dermis (Fig. 166.3g); full thickness sutures (Fig. 166.3h) are avoided.

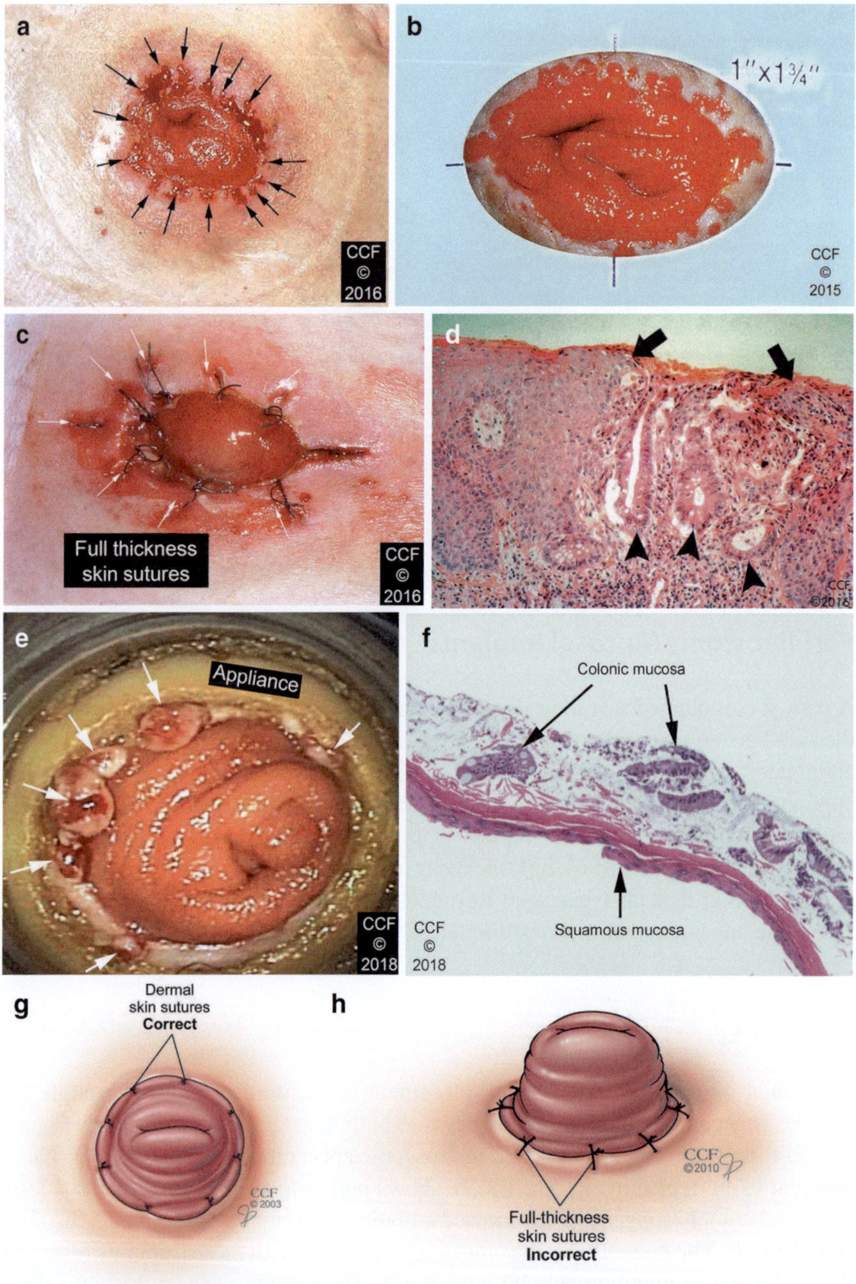

Fig. 166.3 (**a**) Peri-ileostomy mucosal implants (arrows); (**b**) Ileostomy appliance aperture cut to circumvent mucosal implants; (**c**) multiple peristomal sinus tracts caused by full thickness maturation sutures placed at the time of Ileostomy creation; (**d**) histologic sections of the excised ileostomy site following stoma relocation demonstrate squamous epithelium (arrows) interrupted by implants of intestinal-type glands (arrowheads); (**e**) peri-colostomy mucosal implants seen within the inner border of an appliance; (**f**) biopsy of the implants shows colonic mucosa embedded beneath squamous mucosa; (**g**) End view of ileostomy following correct maturation with dermal sutures (illustration); (**h**) incorrect ileostomy maturation with full thickness skin sutures (illustration)

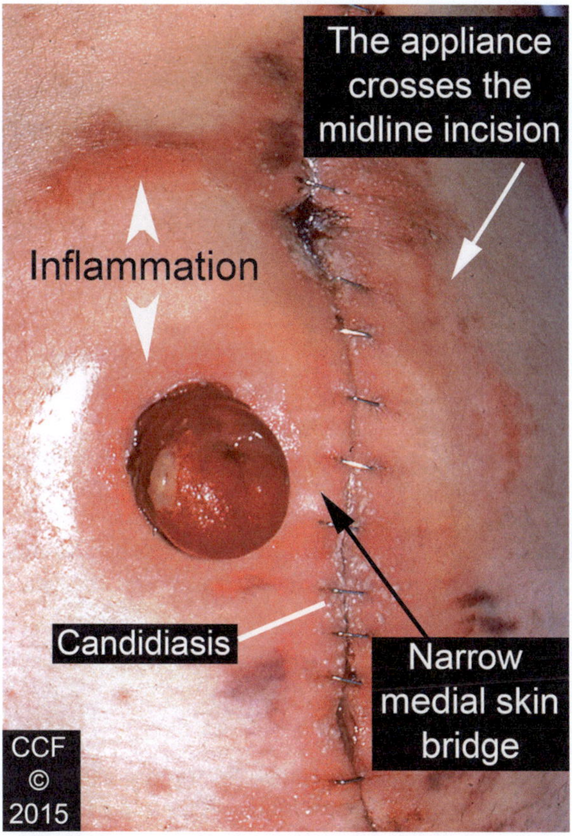

Fig. 166.4 The appliance crosses the midline incision. The medial skin bridge is narrow. The perianal skin is inflamed (arrowheads). Islands of yeast (candida) are seen along the midline incision. The ileostomy is located very close to the midline incision resulting in poor adherence of the appliance to the skin and leakage

Stoma Placement Too Close to the Midline Incision

A patient complained that their appliance could not be maintained (Fig. 166.4).

Comment

This ileostomy was placed too close to the midline. Consequently, the stoma appliance crossed over the incision. The staples raised the appliance off the skin leading to leakage and wound contamination with small intestinal fluid. Skin plasticity contributes to this problem. When the skin is stretched at the time of stoma creation, the distance between the ostomy aperture and the incision appears adequate. In the absence of stretch, the skin contracts leading to a narrow medial skin bridge. This problem can be avoided by maintaining equal traction on fascia and the skin during stoma creation and by choosing the location for the skin aperture with a sufficient skin bridge between the medial edge of the stoma and the midline incision preoperatively. The white pustules seen in the photo on both sides of the incision are islands of candidiasis resulting from excessive moisture from leakage.

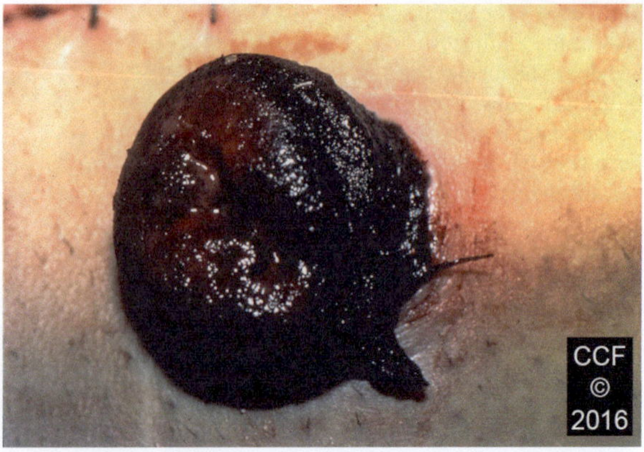

Fig. 166.5 Ischemia. Attempts to elicit bleeding from this stoma with a needle were not successful

Ischemia

The ileostomy created in this figure appeared normal at the time of its creation. Subsequent examination revealed ischemic changes (Fig. 166.5). Stomal revision was done.

Comment

Presence of the arterial supply to the end of the ileum is determined at surgery. When the mucosa at the terminus of the ileum is cut sharply, pulsatile arterial bleeding is seen. If this bleeding is not present, the intestine is trimmed proximally until definite arterial bleeding is encountered. If an end ileostomy is not possible, a loop end ileostomy is an alternative.

References

1. Stocchi L. Ileostomy. In: Fazio VW, Church JM, Wu JS, editors. Atlas of intestinal stomas. New York: Springer; 2012. p. 85–95.
2. Fazio VW, Erwin-Toth P, Church JM, Wu JS. CCF Color Photo Gallery. In: Fazio VW, Church JM, Wu JS, editors. Atlas of Intestinal Stomas. New York: Springer; 2012. p. 159–76.
3. Wound, Ostomy and Continence Nurses Society. Stoma Complications: Best Practice for Clinicians. New Jersey: Mt. Laurel; 2014.

Colonic Obstruction

167

James S. Wu and Eric W. Willis

Presentation

A 66-year-old male was seen in the emergency department for treatment of complete rectosigmoid large bowel obstruction documented by flexible endoscopy and gastrograffin enema at the referring facility. On arrival, the patient's abdomen was distended, tympanitic, and tender. Bowel sounds were absent.

Laboratory values: WBC 18,000/μl, lactate 3.2 mmol/L (0.5–2.2); Albumin 3.1 g/dl (3.5–5.0); chloride 91 mmol/L (98–110), CO_2 34 mmol/L (23–32). The patient was taken directly from the emergency department to the operating room (Fig. 167.1). Following hemodynamic resuscitation, laparotomy was done.

J. S. Wu (✉)
Department of Colon and Rectal Surgery, Cleveland Clinic, Cleveland, OH, USA

E. W. Willis
Department of Pathology, CORPath, Columbus, OH, USA

J. S. Wu, M. D. Inkster (eds.), *Cleveland Clinic Colorectal Case Studies*,
https://doi.org/10.1007/978-3-031-39880-3_167

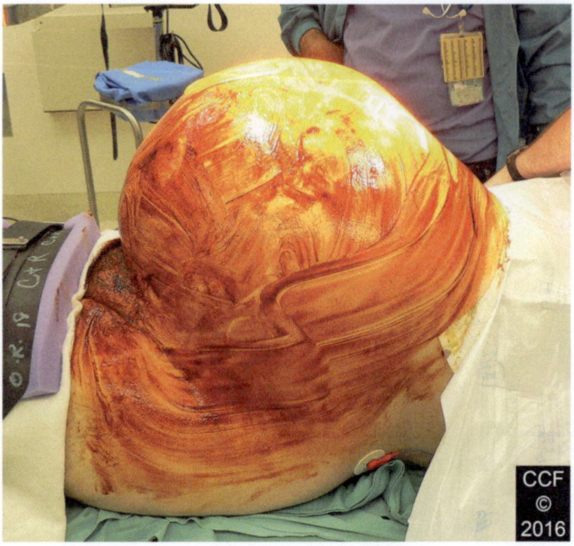

Fig. 167.1 Markedly distended abdomen just prior to laparotomy

Management

Abdominal exploration showed colonic megacolon with multiple gangrenous areas. The obstruction was caused by a rectosigmoid phlegmon. The small intestine appeared normal. Colectomy with end ileostomy was done. The gallbladder, distended and dusky, also was removed. The rectum was left in place (Fig. 167.2a, b).

Pathology showed diverticulitis with extensive pericolonic abscesses, stricture, and acute dilation of the proximal colon. Acute appendicitis also was found (Fig. 167.3a, b).

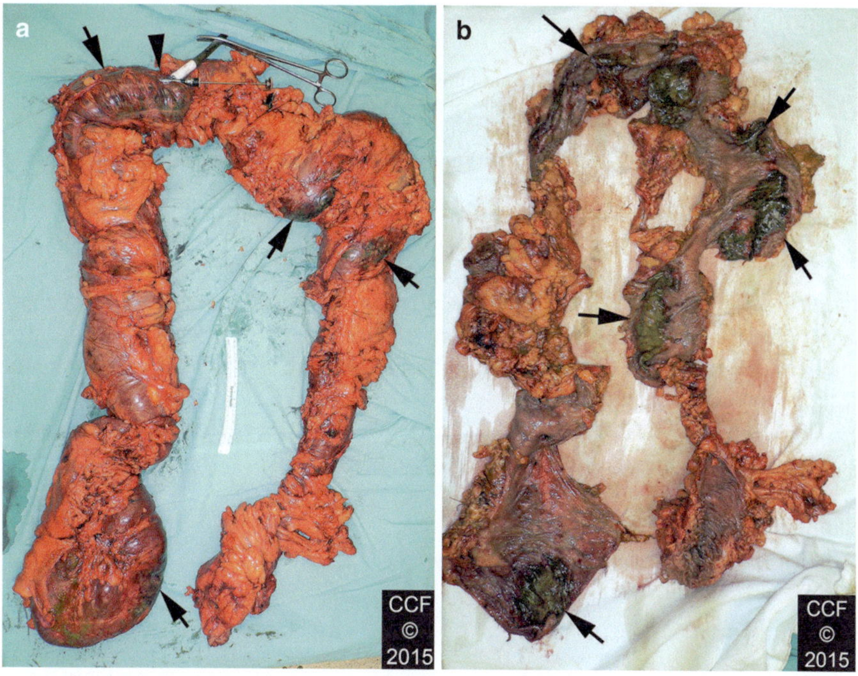

Fig. 167.2 Colectomy specimen: (**a**) external view, (**b**) intraluminal view. The cecum is located in the lower left. Gangrenous areas are identified with arrows. A venting trocar is marked with an arrowhead in (**a**)

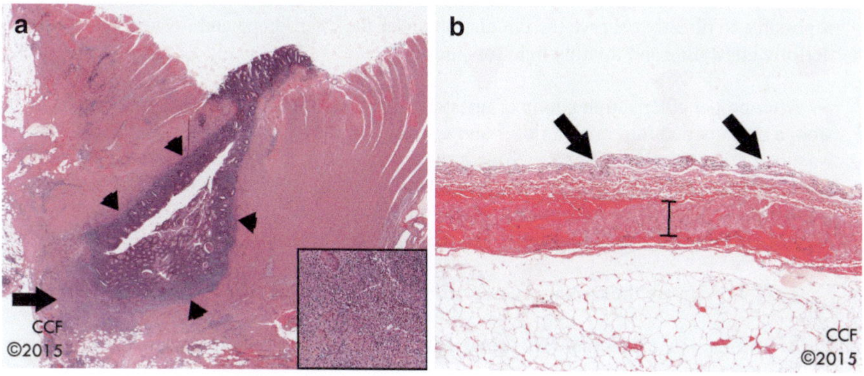

Fig. 167.3 (**a**) Diverticulitis, consisting of an outpouching of mucosa through the muscularis propria (arrowheads) with neutrophilic inflammation of the pericolonic fibroadipose tissue (arrow and inset) (Original magnification, H&E, 10×, 50×); (**b**) bowel with transmural necrosis, consisting of denuded mucosa (arrows), and muscularis propria with coagulative necrosis (brackets). The necrotic wall is significantly thinned (Original magnification, H&E, 40×)

Comment

> "It is apparent that increases in intraluminal pressure in instances of bowel obstruction may affect unfavorably the blood supply of the gut.
>
> ...the greatest stress is borne by that portion of the dilated gut which has the largest diameter."
>
> Owen H. Wangensteen,
> University of Minnesota, 1947 [1]

In this case, obstruction of the colon occurred at the rectosigmoid junction secondary to diverticular disease. The presence of a competent ileocecal valve allowed one-way traffic into the colon. Intraluminal pressure and consequent ischemia resulted in colonic gangrene.

The adverse effects of intraluminal pressure on bowel perfusion were noted in 1907 by van Zwalenburg in canine experiments [2].

Strangulation resulting from distension
of hollow viscera.
By Cornelius van Zwalenburg, M.D.,
of Riverside, Cal.

> "Several times during the past four years I have made the assertion that distension of the appendix back of an obstruction in any part of its lumen would interfere with its circulation even to the point of arresting it entirely.
>
> The following experiments upon dogs were undertaken to demonstrate this fact.
>
> The placing of an electric light bulb in the lumen of the appendix or the intestine made it possible to directly observe the circulation under the microscope and opened up a wonderfully interesting and inviting field for study.
>
> After proper etherization a loop of intestine was withdrawn through an abdominal incision, a cannula tied into one end of it and a small electric lamp into the other. The whole was then brought under the microscope and the circulation in the wall of the gut studied under different pressures by water introduced through the cannula. The degree of pressure was noted on a mercury manometer, placed in circuit with the pressure bulb. The same experiment was done on the appendix and the same results obtained.
>
> The following are the principal observations as they relate to this study.
>
> At 30 mm mercury pressure we found that some capillary streams were arrested.
>
> At 60 mm. many small veins had their currents arrested, and in most of them the stream was so slow that individual corpuscles would be seen.
>
> At 90 mm, a most interesting study presented itself. All blood streams were moving slowly and many were not moving at all."

Large intestinal obstruction is an emergency that requires timely identification and treatment. In this case, although multiple gangrenous areas of colon were present, colonic rupture, fortunately, had not occurred. The patient survived surgery and was discharged. Restoration of intestinal continuity was not done.

References

1. Wangensteen OH. Intestinal obstructions. 2nd Edition., third printing. Charles C Thomas, Springfield, Illinois, 1947, pp. 33, 39.
2. van Zwalenburg C. Strangulation resulting from distention of hollow viscera: Its bearing upon appendicitis, strangulated hernia and gall-bladder disease. Ann Surg. 1907;46:780–6.

Inflammatory Bowel Disease: An Historical Introduction

168

Michelle D. Inkster and James S. Wu

Presentation

In their discussion of the evolution of surgery for Crohn's disease, Fazio and Aufses recognize several early pioneers in the study of inflammatory bowel disease whose work often is mentioned but seldom is the center of focus: Morgagni, Coombe and Saunders, Baillie, Wilks, Dalziel, and Moschcowitz [1].

In 1762, Morgagni published *De Sedibus, Et Causis Morborum Per Anatomen Indagatis (The seats and Causes of diseases investigated by anatomy).* In volume three, "De Morbis Ventris (diseases of the belly)," he reported the case of a women who died of dysentery and whose intestines were found to be "inflammata (on fire)."

DE SEDIBUS, ET CAUSIS MORBORUM PER ANATOMEN INDAGATIS [2] De Morbis Ventris Epistola Anatomico-Medica XXXI. Art. 25 Jo. Baptiste Morgagni 25. Mulier ex dysenturia moritur. Intestina reperiuntur inflammata.	*The Seats and Causes of Diseases investigated by Anatomy* [3] Treats of Fluxes of the Belly Letter the thirty-first Articles 25 John Baptist Morgagni Chief Professor Anatomy, and President of the University at Padua 25. A woman died of a dysentery. The intestines were found to be inflam'd.

In 1793, Baillie described intestinal inflammation and sequelae including hyperemia, hemorrhage, ischemia, mucosal sloughing, perforation, and fistulization [4].

M. D. Inkster
Department of Gastroenterology, Cleveland Clinic, Cleveland, OH, USA

J. S. Wu (✉)
Department of Colon and Rectal Surgery, Cleveland Clinic, Cleveland, OH, USA

J. S. Wu, M. D. Inkster (eds.), *Cleveland Clinic Colorectal Case Studies*,
https://doi.org/10.1007/978-3-031-39880-3_168

The Morbid Anatomy of Some of the Most Important
Parts of the Human Body
Chap. VIII.
Diseased Appearances in the Intestines.
Inflammation.
Matthew Baillie, M.D., F. R.S.
Fellow of the Royal College of Physicians, and
Physician of St. George's Hospital

"The intestinal canal is subject to inflammation from a variety of causes, and therefore it is very usual to observe its effects after death. When a portion of intestine is inflamed, there is spread upon its outer surface a number of small vessels, many of which are carrying a florid blood. When the intestine is cut into, so as to exhibit its inner membrane, it appears highly vascular, from the small vessels of the villi being loaded with blood, and there are frequently to be seen a few spots of blood extravasated. In inflammation of the intestines, the peritonæum is often very little, or not at all affected. When the inflammation, however, is very great, the peritonæm is also inflamed, and covered with a layer of coagulable lymph. I have likewise seen, in violent inflammation, scattered portions of coagulable lymph thrown out upon the surface of the villous membrane. The intestine is at the same time much more thick and massy than in a healthy state, and its colour is sometimes very dark, from a large quantity of black extravasated blood. This state of an intestine has often been mistaken for mortification.

It very commonly happens that inflammation of the intestines advances to suppuration and ulceration. Ulceration, however, does not appear to be so common in the small as in the great intestines. When it takes place either in the one or the other intestine, it is attended with considerable variety in its appearance: the edges of the ulcer have sometimes considerable thickness; at other times, they are not thicker than the healthy structure of the intestine; the edges and general cavity of an ulcer are sometimes ragged, and at other times they are smooth, as if a portion had been cut out from the intestine with a knife. Sometimes, through a considerable length of the intestine (especially the great one) the inner membrane hangs in tattered shreds, occasioned by the great ravage of the ulceration. I have also seen a considerable portion of the intestine completely stripped of its inner membrane, from the extent of this process, and its muscular coat appeared as distinct as if it had been very carefully dissected.

When ulceration advances very actively, it sometimes eats through the coats of an intestine entirely. When this is the case, a portion of the contents of the intestine occasionally passes into the general cavity of the abdomen, producing there inflammation. This, however, does not very often happen; most commonly that portion of the gut where the ulcer is situated, adheres by inflammation to some other portion, or to a neighboring viscus, and a communication is formed between the one and the other. I have seen communications formed in this manner between the rectum and the bladder in a male, and between the rectum and the vagina in a female. I have even seen a communication formed between the kidney and a portion of the intestine from this cause, by which the pus produced in the kidney was evacuated through the intestine. Those communications are the means of preserving life (although in a very uncomfortable state,) for a much longer time than it could be, were the matter to pass into the general cavity of the belly. It would there produce peritonæal inflammation, which would very soon destroy."

In 1813, Combe and Saunders described a case of ileal stricture and thickening [5]:

A *Singular Case of* Stricture *and* Thickening *of the* Ileum,
by
Dr. Charles Combe.
Communicated by, Williams Saunders, M.D. F.R.S.
Fellow of the Royal College of Physicians, &c.
Read at the College, July 4, 1806.

"WILLAM PAYNE GEORGES, Esq. of a very nervous and delicate habit, had been for many years troubled with flatulency and complaints in the bowels, attended with costiveness….

This inconvenience continued to increase to the time of his death, which took place early on Sunday morning, February 9th, 1806, at which time he was more emaciated that any person we had ever witnessed.

On the next day the body was opened by Dr. Combe in the presence of Dr. Saunders, and the following appearances were observed.

The lower part of the ileum as far as the colon, was contracted, for the space of three feet, to the size of a turkey's quill. The colon had three constrictions, one about three inches long at the distance of seven inches from the cœcum, a second about one inch long at the distance of four inches from the former, and a third not quite half an inch long at the distance of three inches from the last.

Wherever the intestines were constricted, the coats were very much thickened, and exhibited an appearance of inflammation; while the blood vessels, passing though the mesentery to the intestines, were enlarged.

The time at which Mr. George perceived the great pain and uneasiness to commence after eating, corresponds with the period at which the food would naturally arrive at the beginning of the constriction of the ileum."

In 1859, Samuel Wilks reported a case of inflammatory bowel disease involving both the terminal ileum and the large intestine [6].

The Morbid Appearance of the Intestines of Miss Bankes
Letter from Dr. Wilks.
[To the Editor of the Medical Times and Gazette]

'Sir, —I beg leave to send you an account of the morbid appearances found in the intestines of Miss Bankes, together with some of the remarks which I furnished to the attorney for the prosecution several weeks before the trial. The description may be interesting to some of your readers who have not seen the appearances detailed; and the remarks will show, I hope, that a Medical witness, because of necessity employed on one side of a case, is not, therefore, an advocate on that side. This explanation appears to be needed, as the public press presumes that the Medical testimony consisted of two opposing portions—the one for the prosecution, to prove the fact of poisoning; and the other for the defence, to explain the symptoms on the supposition of natural disease.

"*Small intestine.*—On opening the intestine throughout, and beginning the examination at the upper end, nothing remarkable was observed until the lower end of the ileum was reached, when at about three feet from its termination in the cæcum, the mucous membrane commenced to exhibit an inflammatory appearance; this was evidenced by a finely granular layer of lymph in and upon the surface. It was at this part seen only on some of the more prominent folds of the mucous membrane; but on proceeding downwards, this exudation became more abundant, until it entirely covered the last foot of the ileum. This inflammatory exudation could not be scraped off, as it was firmly united to the mucous membrane, and contained in its follicles. Excepting a slight abrasion near the ileo-cæcal valve, there was no ulceration in the small intestines.

"*Large intestine.*—The mucous membrane was ulcerated from end to end; the ulcers were of all sizes, the majority being about the size of a sixpenny-piece, mostly isolated, though some had run together, and, taking them as a whole, they occupied more than half of the internal surface of the large intestine.

"Commencing with the rectum, or lower end of the large bowel, this ulceration was tolerably uniform in amount (the mucous membrane presenting these isolated patches of loss of substance) in the descending, transverse and ascending colon, until the cæcum was reached, when inflammation of the most acute and violent character was observed. In this part not only was the mucous membrane superficially ulcerated throughout, but large portions of the structure were sloughing, and almost detached from the other coats of the bowel; thus a sloughing piece of membrane, about three inches square, hung loose into the interior, and on passing the finger beneath, it was found detached even to a still greater extent the bare muscular coat was seen beneath,...

"*Remarks.*—The appearance presented by the intestines showed that the inflammation was of a most acute character, and could not have been of more than two or three weeks' duration.

"Such an acute inflammation of the large intestine, however produced, is sufficient in itself to cause death;...

"My conclusions, then are, that although this acute inflammation might be set up by an irritant poison, yet that as a primary form of disease does occasionally, though rarely, produce the same effect, I am unable to determine which was the cause in operation in the present instance." '

In 1913, Dalziel described "chronic interstitial enteritis" [7].

Chronic Interstitial Enteritis
T. K. Dalziel, M.B, C.M., F.R.F.P.S.G
Surgeon, Western Infirmary, Glasgow.

"I have the pleasure in drawing your attention to this condition, which, I think, has not yet been fully described.

Twelve years ago I saw a professional colleague, suffering from obstruction of the bowels of a fortnight's duration. previous to which he had had for several weeks numerous attacks of colic, slight attacks of diarrhoea with no tenderness over the abdomen, and very slight rise in temperature, with no appreciable alteration in the pulse-rate. When seen by me the abdomen was not distended nor were the muscles rigid, but to the hand gave a sense of putty-like resistance. As vomiting was persistent, I concluded that there might be an obstruction high up, and so opened the abdomen, to find the whole of the intestines, large and small alike, contracted, rigidly fixed, so that when a loop was lifted from the abdomen it sprang back into its sulcus. That the wall of the whole intestine was chronically inflamed there was no doubt. Nothing could be done to restore the function of the canal, and the patient died a few days afterwards."

Dalziel described additional cases in which localized disease involving the jejunum, ileum, sigmoid colon and transverse colon was found. The pathological description of these specimens were as follows:

"The earliest change in the bowel appears to be that of acute congestion. The vessels throughout are dilated, and there is much oedema of the submucosa.

With increasing infiltration the next phase arises, namely cellular and fibrinous exudation within the gut lumen (bile stained naked eye). Still later the mucous membrane is denuded of epithelium,…"

In nine cases, Dalziel boldy operated and removed the inflamed intestine.

"Treatment.

In regard to treatment, these cases which have come under observation have pursued their course uninfluenced by dietetic or medicinal treatment, and apparently only operation can afford relief, and then only if the disease be limited. Seven out of nine made a perfect recovery after the operation, and one does not hesitate in resecting large portions of intestine. The subject has been one of great interest to me for years. My friends the pathologists prefer to call it hyperplastic enteritis, and I can only regret that the etiology of the condition remains in obscurity, but I trust that ere long further consideration will clear up the difficulty."

In 1923, Moschcowitz and Wilensky [8] described, *"Non-specific granulomata of the intestine."* Cases with disease in both the large and small intestine were included.

Eli Moschcowitz, A.B., M.D.
Pathologist to Beth Israel Hospital;
Adjunct Visiting Physician, Mt. Sinai Hospital,
A.O. Wilensky, M.D.
Adjunct Visiting Surgeon to Mt. Sinai Hospital, New York

"Our purpose in this paper is to describe the pathological and some of the clinical features of a malady which, we have reason to believe is not uncommon, and yet, as far as we are aware, is not widely known in this country.

Conclusions. 1. Four cases of non-specific granulomata of the intestine are described. All involved the colon, 1 involved both colon and small intestine.

2. The histological characteristics are those of a simple granuloma. No evidence of tuberculosis, syphilis or lymphogranulomatosis are present.

3. The granulomata may involve any portion of the colon. The infiltration of the wall may be more prominent on the mucosal or the mesenteric aspect. In both instances the lumen is narrowed. Ulcerations, which are usually superficial, may be present; exceptionally, abscess formation.

4. The cause most often is unknown.

5. Clinically, these cases present signs of constriction of the intestinal lumen and a mass in some portion of the colon. Thus far, they are not diagnosticable before operation and have usually been mistaken for carcinoma and tuberculosis of the intestine."

Biographical Notes

Matthew Baillie (1761–1823)

Matthew Baillie was a Scottish pathologist. His work *Morbid Anatomy of Some of the Most Important Parts of the Human Body* (1793) was the first publication in English on pathology as a separate subject [9, 10]. The work was 314 pages and 24 chapters in length and covered diseases of the heart, thorax, lungs, mediastinum, abdominal organs including the stomach, intestines, liver, gallbladder, spleen, pancreas, kidneys, bladder, reproductive organs, and brain.

In his preface, Baillie expresses some trepidation about publishing his work recognizing his own fallibility.

> "Although I have ventured to lay this work before the Public, yet I am very sensible of its imperfections."[11]

Sir Samuel Wilks, MD, FRS (1824–1911) [12, 13]

Samuel Wilks was born in London. He received the MB degree from Guy's Hospital in 1848 and the MD in 1850. He was elected FRCP in 1856 and president of the Royal College of Physicians in 1869. In 1859 he published *Lectures on Pathological Anatomy* as Demonstrator of Morbid Anatomy at Guy's Hospital based on between 2000 and 3000 inspections standardizing pathology into the curriculum because:

> "It has always been my opinion, that every complete course of medical education should comprehend a systematic elucidation of the various morbid changes to which the human frame is subject."

References

1. Fazio VW, Aufses AH Jr. Evolution of surgery for Crohn's disease: a century of progress. Dis Colon Rectum. 1999;42:979–88.
2. Morgagni JB. De Sedibus, Et Causis Morburum Per Anatomen Indagatis Libri Quinque. Tomus Tertius, Neapoli, MDCCLXII, ex typographia Raymundiana, Sumptibus Dominici Terres; page 63. Internet. [cited 2021 April 10]. Available from Archive.org
3. Morgagni JB. The Seats and Causes of Diseases Investigated by Anatomy, in Five Books. Translated from the Latin by Benjamin Alexander, M.D., Printed for A. Millar and T. Cadell, his successor, London, 1769; 89. [cited 2021 Apr 8]. Available from Archive.org
4. Baillie M. The Morbid Anatomy of Some of the Most Important Parts of the Human Body. Printed for J. Johnson, St. Paul's Church-Yard; and G. Nicol, Pall-Mall, 1793.; chapter VIII, pp 98–101.
5. Combe C, Saunders W. A *singular* Case of Stricture *and* Thickening *of the* Ileum. Med Trans R Coll Physicians (London). 1813;4:16–21.
6. Wilks S. Morbid appearances in the intestines of Miss Bankes. Med Times Gazette (London). 1859;2:264–5.
7. Dalziel TK. Chronic interstitial enteritis. Br Med J. 1913;2:1068–70.
8. Moschcowitz E, Wilensky AO. Nonspecific granulomata of the intestine. Am J Med Sci. 1923;166:48–66.
9. Baillie M. The morbid anatomy of some of the most important parts of the human body. London: Printed for J. Johnson, St. Pauls's Church-Yard; and G. Nicol, Pall-Mall; 1793.
10. Matthew Baillie, Scottish Pathologist. The editors of Encyclopædia Brittanica. [cited 2016 Sep 13]. Available from www.brittanica.com
11. Baillie M. The Morbid Anatomy of Some of the Most Important Parts of the Human Body. London: Printed for J. Johnson, St. Pauls's Church-Yard; and G. Nicol, Pall-Mall; 1793. Preface, page X
12. Wilks S. Lectures on pathological anatomy: Delivered at Guy's Hospital during the summer sessions of 1857, 1859. Longman, Brown, Green, Longmans, and Roberts Patenoster Row 1859, p. iv.
13. Pearce JMS. Sir Samuel Wilks (1824–1911): 'The most philosophical of English Physicians.' Eur Neurol. 2009;61:119–23.

Toxic Ulcerative Colitis

169

Carolyn L. Power, David W. Dietz, Tracy L. Hull,
James M. Church, and James S. Wu

Presentation

A patient with a known history of ulcerative colitis was admitted with abdominal pain and bloody diarrhea. After three days of medical therapy, her condition had not significantly improved.

Pertinent data at that time included:

Temperature 38.5 °C
Pulse 108 bpm
WBC 13,000/μl,
Albumin 1.6 g/dL

Endoscopic and radiographic findings are shown in Figs. 169.1, 169.2, and 169.3.

C. L. Power · T. L. Hull · J. M. Church · J. S. Wu (✉)
Department of Colon and Rectal Surgery, Cleveland Clinic, Cleveland, OH, USA

D. W. Dietz (✉)
Department of Surgery, NYU Langone Medical Center, New York, NY, USA

J. S. Wu, M. D. Inkster (eds.), *Cleveland Clinic Colorectal Case Studies*,
https://doi.org/10.1007/978-3-031-39880-3_169

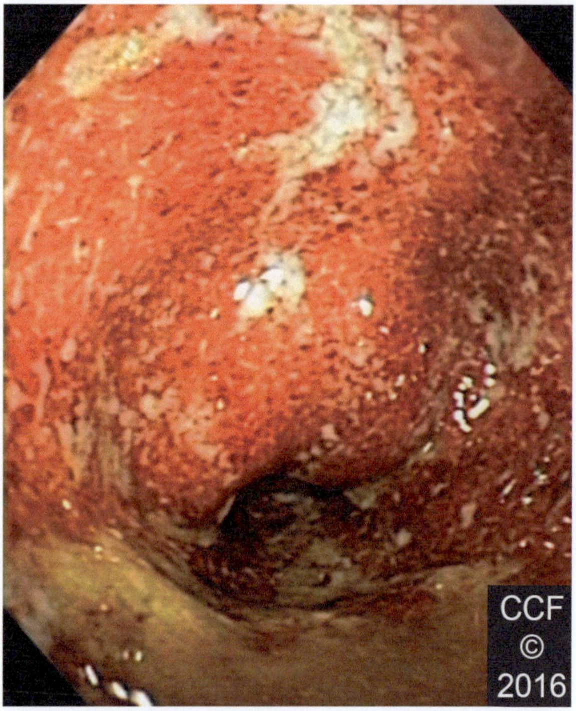

Fig. 169.1 Flexible endoscopic examination of the rectum showed moderately severe inflammation

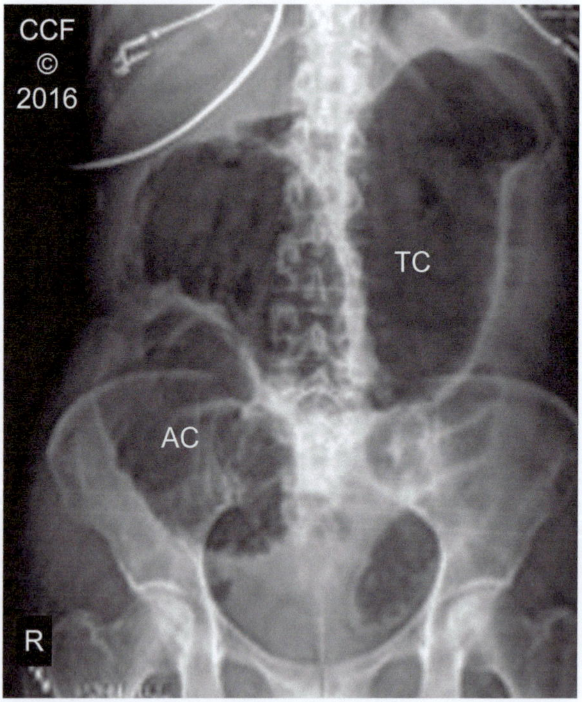

Fig. 169.2 An abdominal plain film showed marked dilation of the ascending colon (AC) and transverse colon (TC). R = right

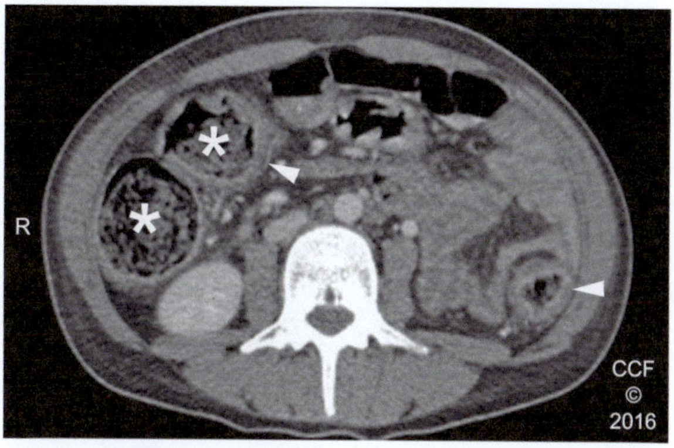

Fig. 169.3 An abdominal computed tomographic (CT) scan revealed colonic wall thickening (arrows) and retained feces (asterisks). Right (R)

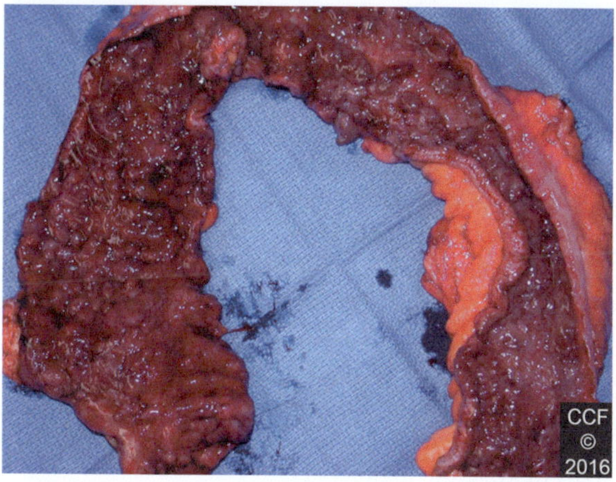

Fig. 169.4 The resected specimen showed pan-ulcerative colitis

Management

Subtotal colectomy with end ileostomy was done (Figs. 169.4 and 169.5).

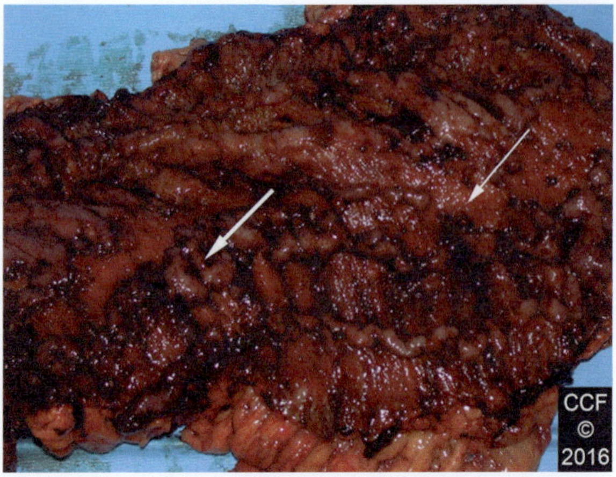

Fig. 169.5 A closer view of resected specimen shows extensive mucosal sloughing (arrows)

Comment

Indications for surgical treatment of ulcerative colitis include acute complications (toxic colitis, perforation, hemorrhage), failure of medical therapy, and the progression to dysplasia or cancer.

Toxic colitis, with or without megacolon, requires vigilance and early involvement of the surgeon. The differential diagnosis includes ulcerative colitis, Crohn's colitis, CMV colitis, *C. Difficile* colitis, drug-induced colitis, radiation induced colitis, and ischemic colitis, all of which can occur in isolation or as a complication of underlying disease.

At the Cleveland Clinic, toxic colitis is defined by the presence of two or more signs of systemic toxicity [1]:

Heart rate > 100 beats per minute
Temperature > 38.5 °C
WBC > 10,500/μL
Albumin < 3.0 g/dl

Dilation of the colon more than 5 cm is considered abnormal. Patients with colitis require multidisciplinary management including fluid resuscitation, nutritional support, and intravenous corticosteroids. Medications that can worsen the condition (notably opioids, antidiarrheal agents, anticholinergics, and NSAIDs) are stopped. Surgery is considered in the presence of toxicity, with or without megacolon. At the Cleveland Clinic, the mainstay of surgical treatment has been subtotal colectomy with end ileostomy (Fig. 169.6). Following removal of the the diseased colon, patients typically can get off chronic anti-inflammatory medications and return to a state of good health.

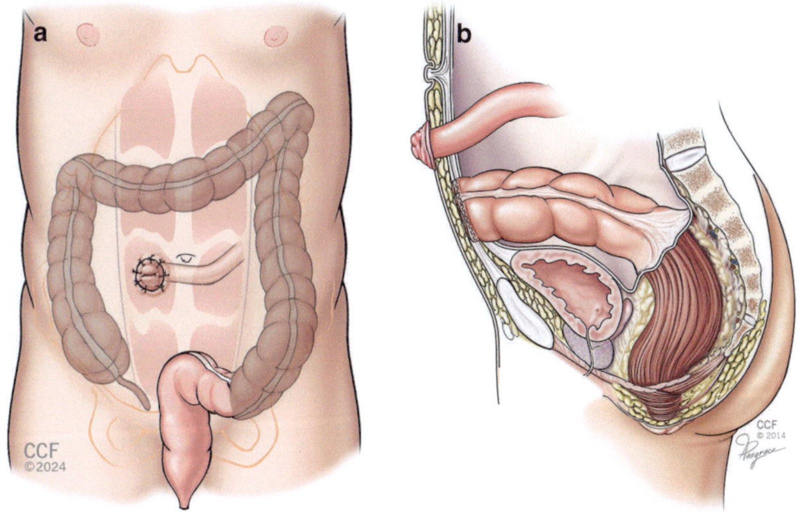

Fig. 169.6 Illustrations showing the lines for resection for subtotal colectomy. In this example, the distal sigmoid colon is secured to the distal aspect of the abdominal wound, near the pubis above the fascia but below the skin: (**a**) anterior to posterior view, (**b**) lateral view. This anatomic arrangement has three purposes: (1) in the event of rectosigmoid stump blowout, the contents of the gut will be discharged outside of the abdomen; (2) future identification of the rectosigmoid is facilitated; (3) future proctectomy is technically easier when the initial operation stops short of the pelvis

If the rectal stump is friable, it can be exteriorized to prevent rectal stump blow out (Fig. 169.7). Alternatively, the closed rectal or rectosigmoid stump is simply returned to the abdomen (Fig. 169.8). Subsequent surgery is delayed until nutritional parameters are normal and sufficient time has elapsed to allow safe reentry into the abdomen.

In 1931, Rankin, at the Mayo Clinic, described staged ileostomy followed by total colectomy for polyposis coli and for complicated chronic ulcerative colitis [3]. In 1951, Crile and Thomas described simultaneous colectomy and end ileostomy as treatment for acute toxic ulcerative colitis [4].[1]

[1] Permission to resuse these excerpts was generously provided by Elsevier and Copyright Clearance Center |RightsLink®, License number 5257221143529, License date, Feb 27, 2022

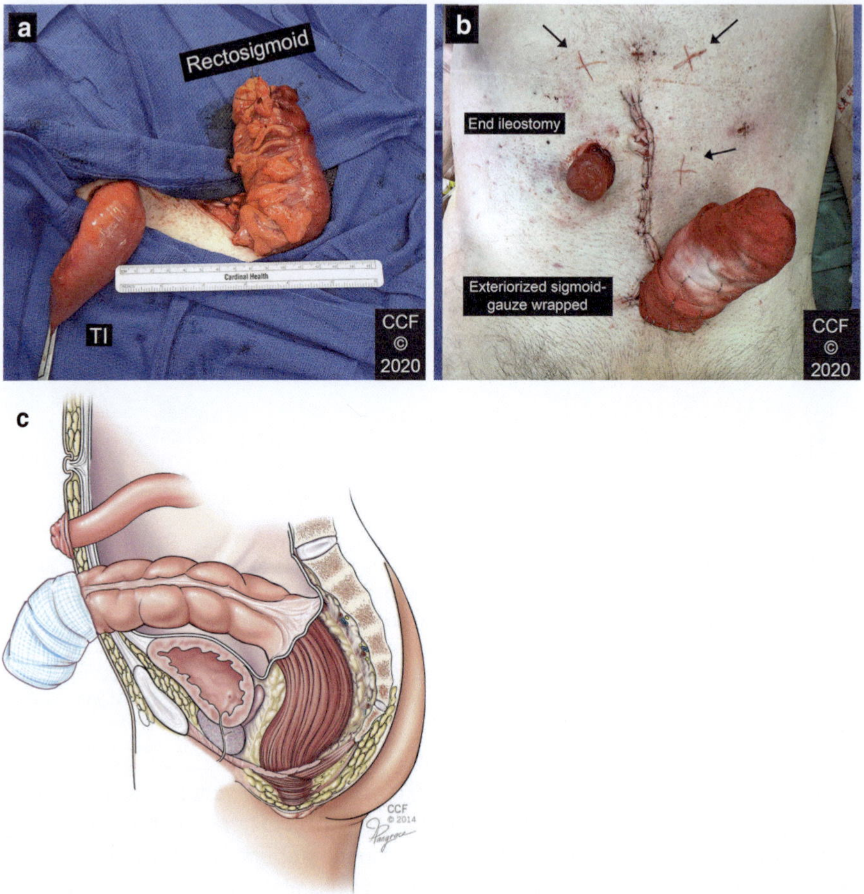

Fig. 169.7 (**a**) Following subtotal colectomy, the terminal ileum (TI) has been brought out through a premarked right lower quadrant stoma site. The rectosigmoid stump has been exteriorized though the distal end of the midline incision to avoid the adverse sequelae of rectal stump blowout. (**b**) The exteriorized rectosigmoid stump is secured in place with gauze wrapping. The end ileostomy is matured. Arrows mark alternative stoma sites (after Turnbull and Weakley's Atlas of Intestinal Stomas, 1967) [2]. (**c**) Illustration showing the end ileostomy and the exteriorized, gauze wrapped rectosigmoid colon

The Treatment of Acute Toxic Ulerative Colitis
By Ileostomy and Simultaneous Colectomy
George Crile, Jr., M.D. and C. Y. Thomas, Jr., M.D.

'In the past, ileostomy has been employed as a last resort in desperate cases in which it was apparent that medical treatment had nothing further to offer. Since the patients were often moribund, or the colon had perforated before the surgeon was asked to see the patient,

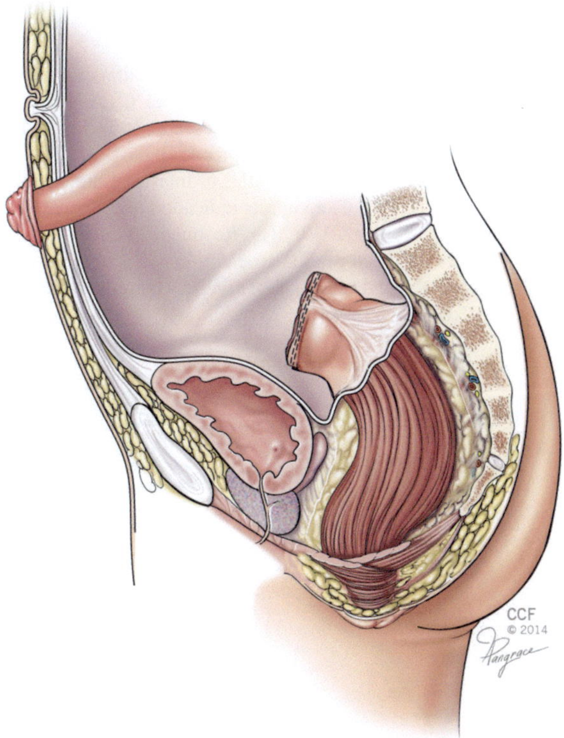

Fig. 169.8 Colectomy and end ileostomy. The distal line of resection is at the sigmoid colon proximal to the peritoneal reflexion. The rectum has been left in place

it is not surprising that the mortality rate of ileostomy performed for acute toxic ulcerative colitis was high. Perhaps if ileostomy had been done earlier in such cases, better results would have been obtained, but the fact remains that early operation was not often employed and that many patients died of ulcerative colitis either under medical treatment or after an ileostomy done late in the course of disease.

Frequently the statement has been made that a patient with acute toxic ulcerative colitis is too sick to withstand ileostomy. Often this statement is correct, because when the strain of anesthetic and operation and the inevitable disturbances of nutrition and electrolyte balance which accompany ileostomy are superimposed on the burden of anemia, sepsis and metabolic exhaustion from which the patient is already suffering, the result may be fatal. But if at the same time it is possible to remove the colon, which is the cause of the anemia and sepsis, the patient has a better chance of withstanding operation and recovering good health. Our attitude toward the patient with acute toxic ulcerative colitis, therefore has undergone an about face, and we no longer say that a patient is too sick to be operated on, but rather we agree with Ferguson[5] who said "the patients are too sick *not* to be operated on." '

References

1. Oakley JR, Fazio VW, Lavery IC. Toxic colitis and toxic megacolon: results of surgery. In: Goebell H, Malchow H, Ewe K, Koelbel Ch, editors. Falk Symposium 60. Inflammatory Bowel Disease. Progress in Basic Research and Clinical Implications. Hingham, MA: Kluwer Academic Publishers; 1991: Chapter 45. p. 361–72.
2. Turnbull RB Jr, Weakley FL. Atlas of Intestinal Stomas. St. Louis: Mosby; 1967. p. 29.
3. Rankin FW. Total colectomy; its indication and technic. Ann Surg. 1931;94:677–704.
4. Crile G Jr, Thomas CY Jr. The treatment of acute toxic ulcerative colitis by ileostomy and simultaneous colectomy. Gastroenterology. 1951;19:58–68.
5. Ferguson LK, Stevens LW. The surgery of complications of ulcerative colitis. Gastroenterology. 1948;11:640–5.

Toxic *Clostridioides difficile* Colitis

170

James S. Wu, Michelle D. Inkster,
David Hernandez Gonzalo, and Eric W. Willis

Presentation

An elderly female developed *Clostridioides difficile* colitis [1] following surgery. After an extended hospitalization, she was discharged for rehabilitation receiving an oral adjunctive agent (Vancomycin). She was re-hospitalized because of severe abdominal pain. Admitting vital signs and laboratory values are listed in Table 170.1. Computed tomographic (CT) images are shown (Fig. 170.1a-c).

Table 170.1 Vital signs and laboratory values at admission

– Temperature 35.8 °C
– Heart rate 108 bpm
– WBC 41,000/μ
– Serum albumin 2.9 g/dL

J. S. Wu (✉)
Department of Colon and Rectal Surgery, Cleveland Clinic, Cleveland, OH, USA

M. D. Inkster
Department of Gastroenterology, Cleveland Clinic, Cleveland, OH, USA

D. Hernandez Gonzalo
Department of Pathology, Immunology and Laboratory Medicine, University of Florida, Gainesville, FL, USA

E. W. Willis
Department of Pathology, CORPath, Columbus, OH, USA

J. S. Wu, M. D. Inkster (eds.), *Cleveland Clinic Colorectal Case Studies*,
https://doi.org/10.1007/978-3-031-39880-3_170

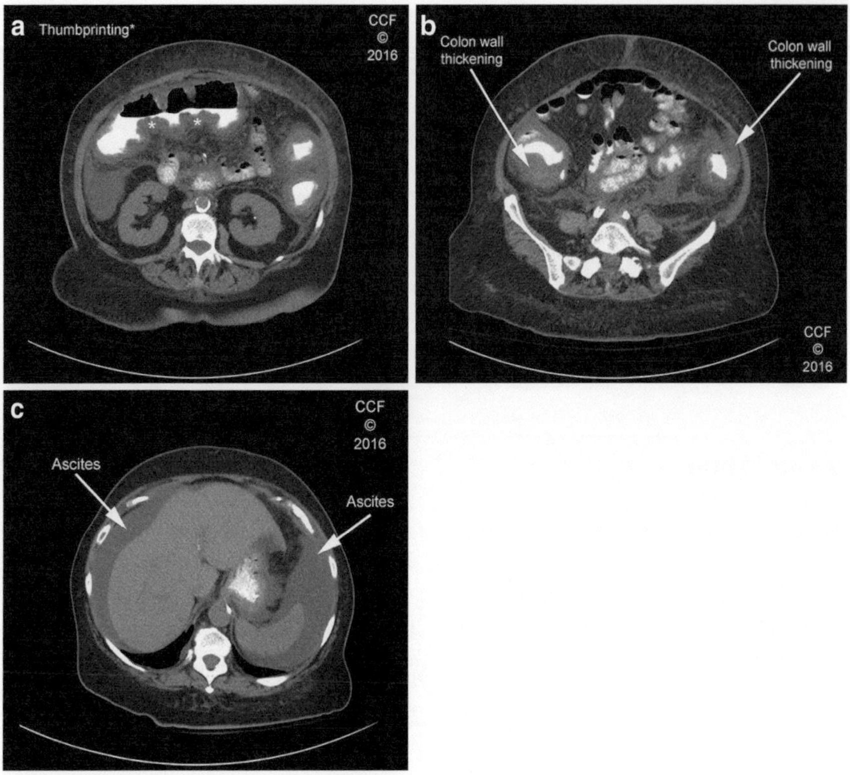

Fig. 170.1 (**a**) Mucosal thickening with "thumbprinting" (asterisks); (**b**) colon thickening (arrows); (**c**) ascites (arrows)

Management

After hemodynamic resuscitation, the patient was taken to surgery. Subtotal colectomy and end ileostomy was done. The resected specimen and histopathology are shown in Figs. 170.2 and 170.3 respectively. The patient survived surgery and was discharged from the hospital.

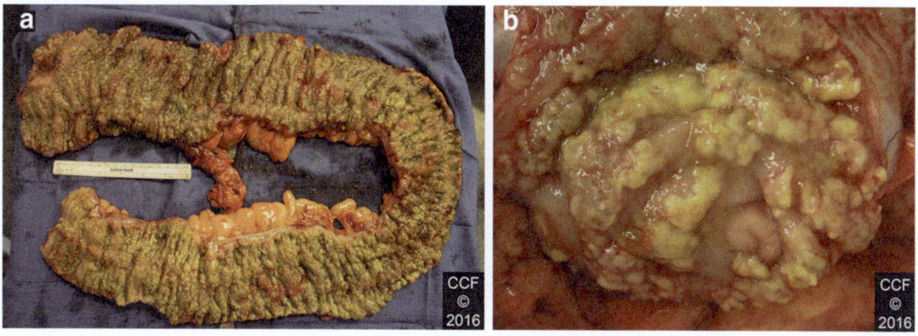

Fig. 170.2 (**a**) Subotal colectomy specimen. The entire mucosa is covered with pseudomembranes; (**b**) close-up view of pseudomembranes at the appendiceal orifice

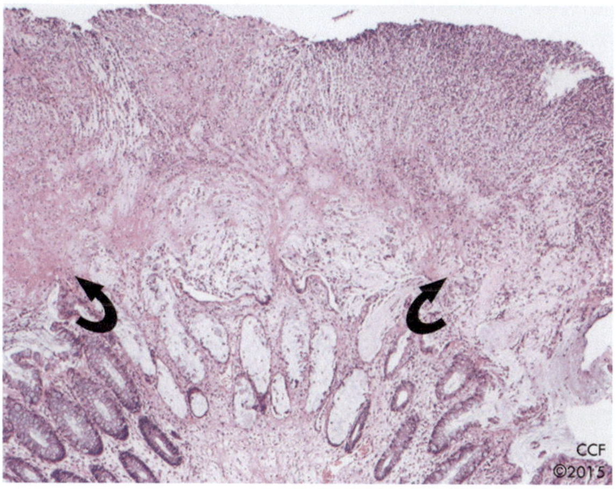

Fig. 170.3 Histopathology: "Volcano" shaped exudate with fibrin, neutrophils, and mucin. (Curved arrows indicate the edges of the volcano.) Within the crater of the volcano are dilated glands with loss of superficial epithelial cells, mimicking an ischemic pattern of injury. No chronic inflammatory infiltrate is seen in lamina propria. Nearby crypt architecture is unremarkable (hematoxylin–eosin, original magnification ×50)

Comment

In 1935, Hall and O'Toole, working at the University of Colorado School of Medicine, described a new pathogenic anaerobic bacillus that they isolated from the intestinal flora of new-born infants. Because this anaerobe was difficult to isolate, they named their new species "*Bacillus difficilis*" [2]. The authors found that the organism was associated with diarrhea and produced an exotoxin that was highly pathogenic to guinea pigs and rabbits. In 1977, Larson *et al.* described a toxin in the feces of a 12-year-old girl that developed pseudomembranous colitis after a short course of oral penicillin [3]. In 1978, Bartlett et al. [4] reported results suggesting that toxin-producing clostridia are responsible for antibiotic-associated pseudomembranous colitis. *C. difficile infection* (CDI) is a common clinical problem. Symptoms are variable and range from nuisance diarrhea to life-threatening colitis. Major risk factors for CDI are hospitalization, older age, and antibiotic exposure [5, 6]. Current methods of C. difficile detection include cell culture, toxin assays, metabolic enzyme testing, nucleic acid detection, and canine olfactory screening [7, 8].

Presentation and Management [9]

Loose watery diarrhea is a common presenting symptom. Computed tomography findings of *C. difficile* colitis include "thumb printing" [10] and colonic thickening. Ascites has been reported in cases of severe pseudomembranous colitis and is attributed to hypoalbuminemia. Hypothermia, as seen in this case, is consistent with sepsis.

Nonsurgical options for the management of *C. difficile* colitis include:

1. Stopping the offending antibiotic,
2. Treatment with adjunctive agents (vancomycin in this case),
3. Fecal transplantation.

Following resuscitation, the patient underwent urgent subtotal colectomy with end ileostomy because she had toxic colitis. As discussed in Chap. 169, toxicity is present when at least two of the four Oakley criteria are present Table 170.2 [11]. This patient had three. Following surgery, the patient survived and was discharged.

Table 170.2 Toxic colitis criteria (Oakley)

Criteria
1. Pulse > 100 beats per minute
2. Temperature > 38.5 °C
3. WBC > 10,500/μL
4. Albumin < 3.0 g/dl

References

1. Lawson PA, Citron DM, Tyrrell KL, Finegold SM. Reclassification of *Clostridium difficile* as *Clostridiodes difficile* (Hall and O'Toole 1935) Prévot 1938. Anaerobe. 2016;40:95–9.
2. Hall IC, O'Toole E. Intestinal flora in new-born infants with a description of a new pathogenic anaerobe, Bacillus difficilis. Am J Dis Child. 1935;49:390–402.
3. Larson HE, Parry JV, Price AB, Davies DR, Dolby J, Tyrrell DAJ. Undescribed toxin in pseudomembranous colitis. Br Med J. 1977;1:1246–8.
4. Barlett JG, Chang TW, Gurwith M, Gorbach SL, Onderdonk AB, Antibiotic-associated pseudomembranous colitis due to toxin-producing clostridia. N Eng J Med 1978;298:531–34.
5. Bartlett JG. Historical perspectives on studies of *Clostridium difficile* and *C. difficile* infection. Clin Infect Dis. 2008;46:S4–S11.
6. Gorbach SL, John G. Bartlett: Contributions to the discovery of *Clostridium difficile* antibiotic-associated diarrhea. Clin Infect Dis. 2014;59(S2):S66–70.
7. Carrol KC, Mizusawa M. Laboratory tests for the diagnosis of Clostridium difficile. Clin Colon Rectal Surgery. 2020;33:73–81.
8. Bomers MK, van Agtmael MA, Luik H, van Veen MC, Vandenbroucke-Grauls CMJE, Smulders YM. Using a dog's superior olfactory sensitivity to identify Clostridium difficile in stools and patients: proof of principle study. BMJ. 2012;345:e7396. https://doi.org/10.1136/bmj.e7396.
9. Poylin V, Hawkins AT, Bhama AR, Boutros M, Lightner AL, Khanna S, Paquette IM, Feingold DL. The American Society of Colon and Rectal Surgeons Clinical Practice Guidelines for the Management of Clostridioides difficile Infection. Dis Colon Rectum. 2021;64:650–68.
10. Radiology masterclass. Tutorials. Abnormal X-ray-Abnormal bowel gas pattern. Mucosal thickening-'thumbprinting'. [cited 2018 Dec 10]. Available from radiologymasterclass.co.uk.
11. Oakley JR, Fazio VW, Lavery IC. Toxic colitis and toxic megacolon: results of surgery. In: Goebell H, Malchow H, Ewe K, Koelbel Ch, editors. Falk Symposiium 60. Inflammatory Bowel Disease. Progress in Basic Research and Clinical Implications. Hingham, MA: Kluwer Academic Publishers; 1991; Chapter 45. pp. 361–72.

Cytomegalovirus Colitis

171

Michelle D. Inkster, Florian Rieder, Emre Gorgun, Catherine L. Forse, and James S. Wu

Presentation

A 52-year-old male with a past medical history of ulcerative colitis underwent colonoscopy for diarrhea and rectal bleeding (Fig. 171.1).

Biopsies were taken (Fig. 171.2a-d).

M. D. Inkster
Department of Gastroenterology, Cleveland Clinic, Cleveland, OH, USA

F. Rieder
Department of Gastroenterology, Hepatology and Nutrition, Digestive Disease Institute, Cleveland Clinic, Cleveland, OH, USA

E. Gorgun · J. S. Wu (✉)
Department of Colon and Rectal Surgery, Cleveland Clinic, Cleveland, OH, USA

C. L. Forse
Department of Pathology and Laboratory Medicine, Faculty of Medicine, University of Ottawa, Ottawa, ON, Canada

J. S. Wu, M. D. Inkster (eds.), *Cleveland Clinic Colorectal Case Studies*,
https://doi.org/10.1007/978-3-031-39880-3_171

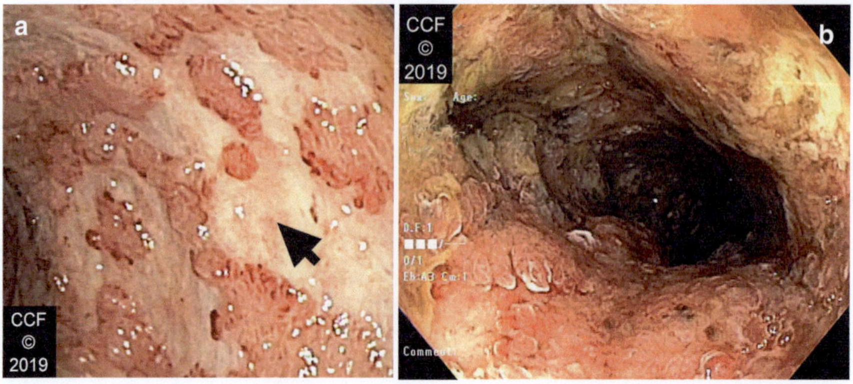

Fig. 171.1 Colonoscopy images (**a**) and (**b**) show severe inflammation with deep mucosal ulcerations exposing the underlying smooth muscle (**a**, arrow)

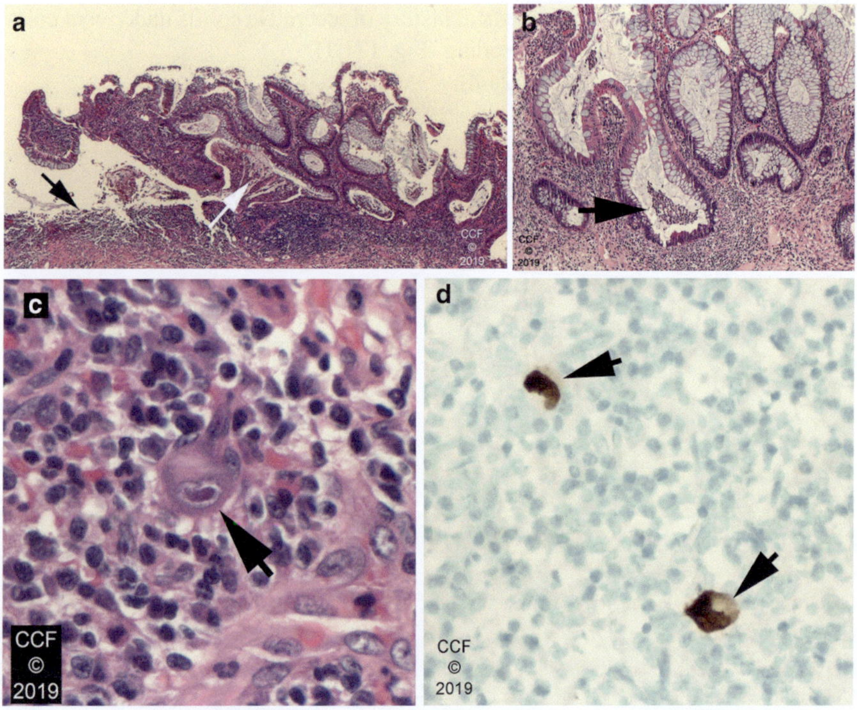

Fig. 171.2 (**a**) Colonic mucosa with ulceration (black arrow) and neutrophilic crypt abscesses (white arrow); H&E, 40× magnification; (**b**) colonic mucosa with neutrophilic crypt abscess (arrow); H&E, 100× magnification; (**c**) basophilic intranuclear inclusion (owl's eye inclusion) [arrow]; H&E, 400× magnification; (**d**) cells positive for CMV infection by immunohistochemistry (arrows); 400× magnification

Management

This patient has ulcerative colitis complicated by cytomegalovirus (CMV) infection. The enlarged cells with prominent "owl's eye" intranuclear inclusions seen in Fig. 171.2 are characteristic of CMV infection. Both an immunohistochemical stain (Fig. 171.2d) and a blood assay for CMV were positive. Because his condition was refractory to medical therapy, his colon was surgically removed (Fig. 171.3).

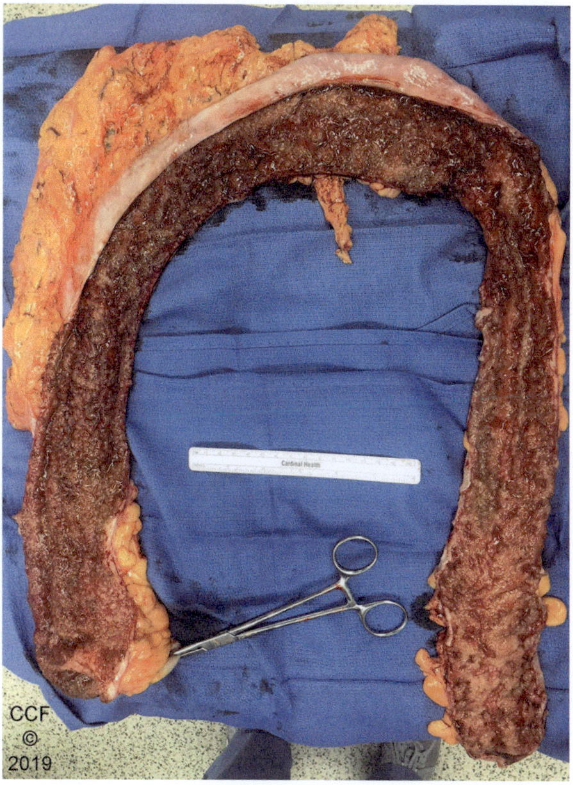

Fig. 171.3 Ulcerative colitis complicated by CMV: resected colon

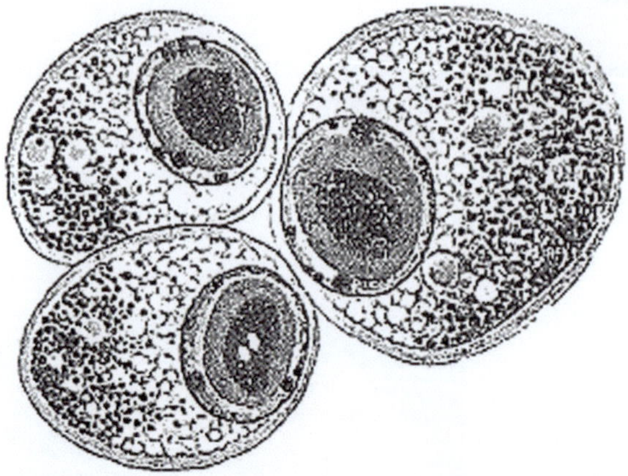

Fig. 171.4 "Protozoan-like structures" seen in the organs of a fetus with hereditary syphilis as drawn by Jesionek and Kiolemenoglou

Comment [1]

In 1904, Jesionek and Kiolemenoglou [2] described protozoan-like structures (Fig. 171.4) in the organs of a fetus afflicted with hereditary syphilis.[1]

Ueber einen Befund von protozoënartigen Gebilden in den Organen eines hereditär-luetischen Fötus. Von Dr. Jesionek und Dr. Kiolemenoglou. München Die Grösse der uns als typisch imponierenden Gebilde schwankt zwischen 20 und 30 μ. Ihre Form ist meist eine ovaläre. Sie sind von einer deutlichen, aber nicht sehr stark tingierten kutikulären Zone umrandet, welche den Eindruck einer Kapsel erregt. Innerhalb der Kapsel fällt ein stets polständiger, sehr deutlicher „Kern" auf, der seinerseits aus einem ungemein scharf prononcierten „zentralen Kernkörper" und aus zwei wohl differenzierbaren Zonen besteht, einer dunkleren Innenzone und einer helleren äusseren Zone. Der ganze Kern erscheint wie von einer Schale nach dem Zelleib hin abgegrenzt.	Concerning a discovery of a protozoan-like structure in the organs of a fetus with hereditary syphilis. By Dr. Jesionek and Dr. Kiolemenoglou Munich The size of the structures typically varied between 20 and 30 μ. Their shape is usually oval. They are surrounded by a clear, but not very strongly tinged cuticular zone, which gives the impression of a capsule. Within the capsule, there is a very distinct "core," which for its part consists of an extremely sharply pronounced "central core body" and from two differentiable zones, a darker inner zone and a brighter outer zone. The whole core appears to be separated from the cell body as if by a shell.

[1] Jesionek and Kiolemenoglou [2]. Permission to reproduce this except and figure was generously provided by Mr. Dirk Einecke, Springer Permissions, August 24, 2021.

The 1954 Nobel Prize in Physiology or Medicine was awarded jointly to John F. Enders, Thomas H. Weller, and Frederick C. Robbins "for their discovery of the ability of poliomyelitis viruses to grow in cultures of various types of tissue." [3, 4] In 1957, Weller et al. [5] described the isolation of intranuclear inclusion producing agents from infants with illnesses resembling cytomegalic inclusion disease. The name "cytomegalovirus" is credited to him [5]. The International Committee on Taxonomy of Viruses (ICTV) states that CMV is a double-stranded DNA virus and is a member of the herpes virus family [6]. In 1961, Powell and co-workers described the presence of cytomegalic inclusions in ulcerative colitis [7]. In a 2006 review, Kandiel and Lashner [8] reported a prevalence of CMV infection in acute severe colitis of 21%–34%. Active infection can be diagnosed by endoscopy, histology, serology, viral culture, antigen testing, and CMV DNA testing. The authors also reported that after antiviral therapy, colitis remission rates in inflammatory bowel diseases with CMV infection ranged from 67% to 100%.

References

1. Ho M. The history of cytomegalovirus and its diseases. Med Microbiol Immunol. 2008;197:65–73.
2. Jesionek A, Kiolemenoglou B. Ueber einen Befund von protozoënartigen Gebilden in den Organen eines hereditär-luetischen Fötus. Muenchen Med Wochenschr. 1904;51:1905–7.
3. Enders JF, Weller TH, Robbins FC. Cultivation of the Lansing strain of poliomyelitis virus in cultures of various human embryonic tissues. Science. 1949;109:85–7.
4. "The Nobel Prize in Physiology or Medicine 1954". *Nobelprizeorg* Nobel Media AB 2014. Web. 17 Feb 2018. http://www.nobelprize.org/nobel_prizes/medicine/laureates/1954/
5. Weller TH, MacAuley JC, Craig JM, Wirth P. Isolation of intranuclear inclusion producing agents from infants with illnesses resembling cytomegalic inclusion disease. Proc Soc Exp Biol Med. 1957;94:4–12.
6. International Committee on Taxonomy of Viruses (ICTV). https://ictv.global. Accessed October 3, 2022.
7. Powell RD, Warner NE, Levine RS, Kirsner JB. Cytomegalic inclusion disease and ulcerative colitis. Am J Med. 1961;30:334–40.
8. Kandiel A, Lashner B. Cytomegalovirus complicating inflammatory bowel disease. Am J Gastroenterol 2006;101:2857–65.

Ischemic Colitis with Necrosis

172

Michelle D. Inkster, Sebouh Setrakian, Eric W. Willis,
Luca Stocchi, and James S. Wu

Presentation

A 75-year-old female was found lying on the floor by a neighbor who was concerned that she had not been seen for several days. On arrival at the hospital, her vital signs were: T 36.5°C, P 152 BPM, Resp 31/min, SPB 70s mmHg. She was not responsive. Her laboratory values included: WBC 24.0 K/μl, anion gap 25, pH arterial 7.34, PaO_2, 57 mmHg; BUN 23 mg/dl, creatinine 1.1 mg/dl; electrocardiogram-atrial fibrillation with rapid ventricular response. Urinalysis showed +3 bacteria. Stool found on rectal examination was positive for occult blood. Abdominal computed tomography showed a stable 8 cm abdominal aortic aneurism. Chest radiograph showed pneumonia. Following resuscitation, upper and lower endoscopy were done. Mild gastritis was found on esophagogastroduodenoscopy. At colonoscopy, severe ulceration was noted from the rectosigmoid junction to the hepatic flexure, with areas of visible necrosis (Fig. 172.1).

M. D. Inkster
Department of Gastroenterology, Cleveland Clinic, Cleveland, OH, USA

S. Setrakian
Pathology & Laboratory Medicine Institute, Cleveland Clinic, Cleveland, OH, USA

E. W. Willis
Department of Pathology, CORPath, Columbus, OH, USA

L. Stocchi
Department of Colon and Rectal Surgery, Mayo Clinic, Jacksonville, FL, USA

J. S. Wu (✉)
Department of Colon and Rectal Surgery, Cleveland Clinic, Cleveland, OH, USA

J. S. Wu, M. D. Inkster (eds.), *Cleveland Clinic Colorectal Case Studies*,
https://doi.org/10.1007/978-3-031-39880-3_172

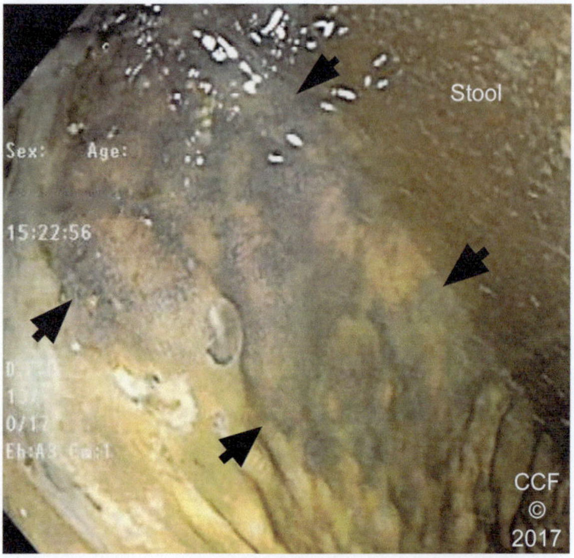

Fig. 172.1 Colonoscopy: at an area of visible necrosis, the bowel wall color was black (arrows)

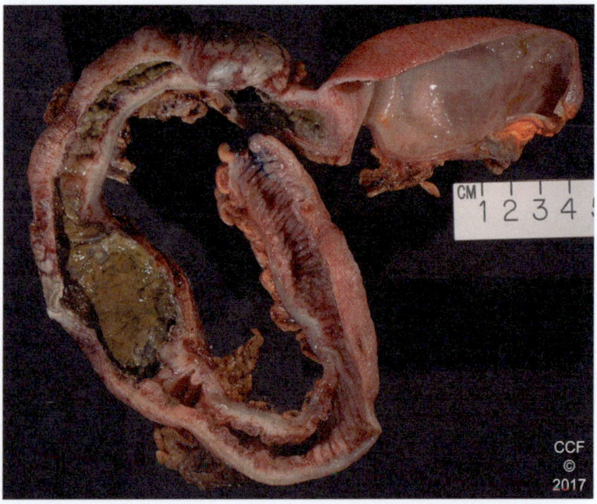

Fig. 172.2 Colectomy specimen (formalin fixed). The serosa appeared dull and fibrotic. A perforation was not present

Management

Emergent subtotal colectomy without restoration of bowel continuity was done. She was marked for a stoma preoperatively.

The serosa appeared dull and fibrotic on gross inspection (Fig. 172.2).

Histology showed transmural necrosis (Fig. 172.3).

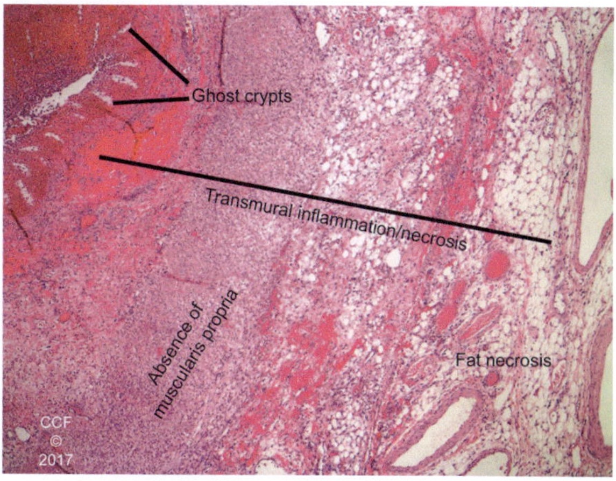

Fig. 172.3 Colon sections showed transmural necrosis with ghost crypts, absence of muscularis propria, and pericolonic fat necrosis

Table 172.1 Risk factors for ischemic colitis seen in this case

Left-sided ischemic colitis seen in advanced age
Atherosclerotic arterial disease
Hypotension
Dehydration
Atrial fibrillation
Sepsis

Comment

A possible timeline for this patient's presentation might start with urosepsis leading to diminished cognitive capacity with subsequent fall, dehydration, hypotension, atrial fibrillation, decreased organ perfusion, and colonic ischemia. She had several risk factors for ischemic colitis (Table 172.1) [1–6].

The patient's hospital course involved multiple simultaneous searches for and correction of problems. Recognition of bowel necrosis at colonoscopy led to colectomy without restitution of bowel continuity without delay.

References

1. Greenwald DA, Brandt LJ. Colonic ischemia. J Clin Gastroenterol. 1998;27:122–8.
2. Binns JC, Isaacson P. Age-related changes in the colonic blood supply: their relevance to ischaemic colitis. Gut. 1978;19:384–90.
3. Ghandi SK, Hanson MM, Vernava AM, Kaminski DL, Longo WE. Ischemic colitis. Dis Colon Rectum. 1996;39:88–100.
4. Hass DJ, Kozuch P, Brandt LJ. Pharmacologically mediated colon ischemia. Am J Gastroenterol. 2007;102:1765–80.
5. Marston A, Pheils MT, Thomas ML, Morson BC. Ischaemic colitis. Gut. 1966;7:1–15.
6. Theodoropoulou A, Koutroubakis IE. Ischemic colitis: Clinical practice in diagnosis and treatment. World J Gastoenterol. 2008;14:7302–8.

Ischemic Colitis, Reversible

173

Mark E. Baker, Catherine L. Forse, and James S. Wu

Presentation

A 60-year-old female was seen because of sudden abdominal pain, diarrhea, and bright red rectal bleeding. On examination, she was afebrile with normal vital signs. Her abdomen was soft and nontender with active bowel sounds. The white blood cell count (WBC) was 15,000/μl. The hemoglobin (Hb) was 11.0 g/dL (decreased from her baseline Hb of 12.9 g/dL). Flexible sigmoidoscopy showed diverticulosis. Computed tomography (CT) of the abdomen showed hypo-enhancing wall thickening without dilation involving the distal transverse colon to the proximal sigmoid colon (Fig. 173.1). She has a history of hypertension. Colonoscopy two years earlier showed diverticulosis.

M. E. Baker
Department of Radiology, Cleveland Clinic Lerner College of Medicine, Case Western Reserve University, Cleveland, OH, USA

C. L. Forse
Department of Pathology and Laboratory Medicine, Faculty of Medicine, University of Ottawa, Ottawa, ON, Canada

J. S. Wu (✉)
Department of Colon and Rectal Surgery, Cleveland Clinic, Cleveland, OH, USA

J. S. Wu, M. D. Inkster (eds.), *Cleveland Clinic Colorectal Case Studies*,
https://doi.org/10.1007/978-3-031-39880-3_173

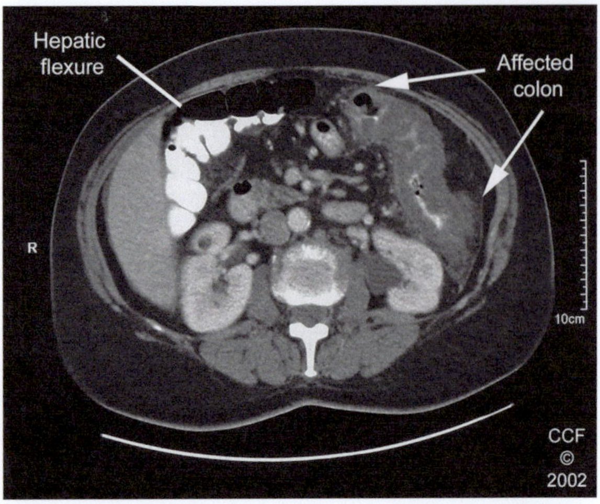

Fig. 173.1 CT scan of the abdomen shows marked colonic wall thickening and hypo-enhancement of the distal transverse colon and splenic flexure without luminal dilation. These colonic changes extended to the sigmoid colon. From an imaging standpoint, this is colitis (nonspecific) without megacolon

Management

The patient was admitted to the hospital for observation. Following the initial episode, gastrointestinal bleeding stopped spontaneously. The Hb stabilized. The WBC returned to normal. The patient was discharged 2 days after admission tolerating a diet. Follow-up colonoscopy 4 months after the bleeding event showed sigmoid diverticulosis. The mucosa, otherwise, was normal.

Comment

The patient's presentation is consistent with ischemic colitis. The word ischemia is derived from the Greek word *ischaimos,* from *ischein* to restrain (akin to Greek *echein* to hold) + *haima* blood in which there is deficient supply of blood to a body part [1]. Predisposing factors associated with IC are listed in Table 173.1 [2–4].

In 1963, Boley et al. described reversible vascular occlusion of the colon in five patients [5]. In 1966, Marston et al. [6] described a classification of ischemic colitis (Table 173.2). Gangrene involves necrosis of the entire intestinal wall resulting in spillage of feces; immediate operation is indicated. Ischemia of the mucosa and muscularis propria without perforation may recover with stricture formation. Transient ischemia affecting the mucosa alone may result in re-epithelialization of the intestine and a return to normality without specific treatment.

Table 173.1 Conditions associated with ischemic colitis [2–4]

Conditions
Cardiovascular disease
Atrial fibrillation
Peripheral vascular disease
Cerebrovascular disease
Chronic obstructive pulmonary disease
Diabetes mellitus
Hypertension
Hypotension
Medications

Table 173.2 Marston classification of ischemic colitis

Classification
– Gangrenous
– Stricturing
– Transient

In this case, the mid-section of the area of ischemic colitis was at the splenic flexure associated with a critical watershed region described by Griffiths in 1956 [7]. In 1976, Meyers reported an analysis of arteriographic studies that showed that the anastomosis at Griffith's point is present in 48%, poor or tenuous in 9%, and absent in 43% [8].

> 'This critical point is of significance in occlusive vascular impairment of the left colon, both in spontaneous instances and following surgical ligation of the inferior mesenteric artery, and in "nonocclusive" ischemic colitis.'
>
> Morton A. Meyers, MD
> The New York Hospital-
> Cornell University Medical Center
> New York

A correlation between endoscopic appearance and histopathologic findings of another case of ischemic colitis is shown in Fig. 173.2. Findings in this case included crypt atrophy, lamina propria hyalinization, and epithelial cell atrophy.

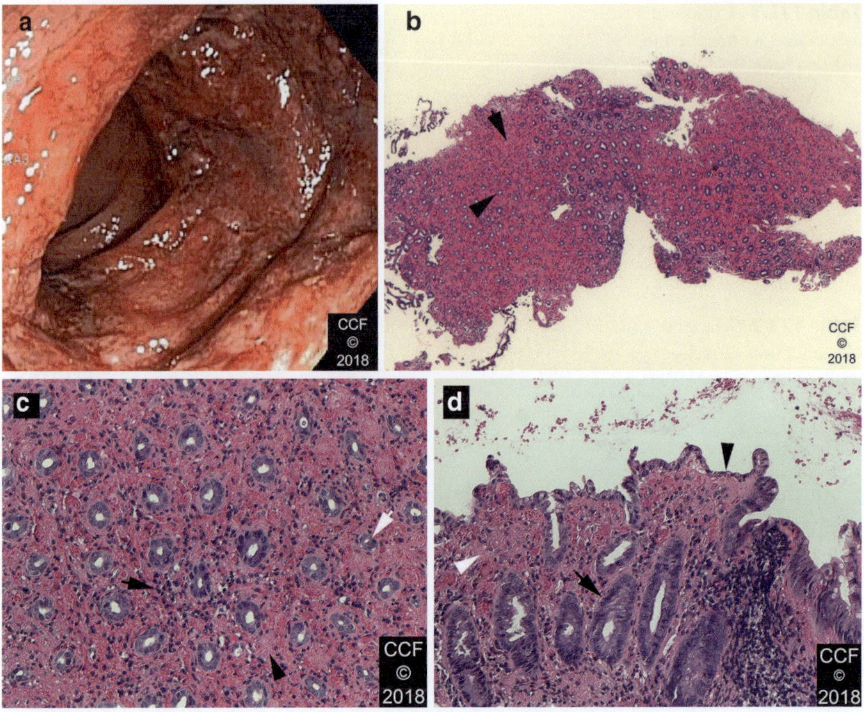

Fig. 173.2 (**a**) Ischemic colitis; (**b**) low magnification transverse section of colonic mucosa from a left colon biopsy. Note the features of chronic ischemic colitis including diffuse lamina propria hyalinization (arrow) and crypt atrophy (arrowhead) (H&E, 40× magnification). (**c**) Transverse section of colonic mucosa from a left colon biopsy demonstrating chronic ischemic colitis. There are withered, degenerating crypts (white arrow) surrounded by hyalinized lamina propria (black arrowhead) and sparse chronic inflammation (black arrow) (H&E, 200× magnification). (**d**) Longitudinal section of colonic mucosa from a sigmoid colon biopsy demonstrating chronic ischemic colitis. Note the withered crypts (arrow), surface epithelial cell atrophy (black arrowhead), and hyalinization of the lamina propria (white arrowhead) (H&E, 200× magnification)

References

1. Ischemia. Merrian-Webster dictionary. Merriam-webster.com. Accessed March 7, 2020.
2. Brandt LJ, Feuerstadt P, Longstreth GF, Boley SJ. ACG Clinical Guideline: Epidemiology, risk factors, patterns of presentation, diagnosis, and management of colonic ischemic (CI). Am J Gastroenterol. 2015;110:18–44.
3. Washington C, Carmichael JC. Management of ischemic colitis. Clin Colon Rectal Surg. 2012;25:228–35.
4. Bielefeldt K. Ischemic colitis as a complication of medication use: an analysis of the Federal Adverse Event Reporting System. Dig Dis Sci. 2016;61:2655–65.
5. Boley SJ, Schwartz S, Lash J, Sternhill V. Reversible vascular occlusion of the colon. Surg Gynecol Obstet. 1963;116:53–60.
6. Marston A, Pheils MT, Thomas ML, Morson BC. Ischaemic colitis. Gut. 1966;7:1–15.
7. Griffiths JD. Surgical anatomy of the blood supply on the distal colon. Ann Roy Coll Surg, Engl. 1956;19:241–56.
8. Meyers MA. Griffith's point: critical anastomosis at the splenic flexure. Significance in ischemia of the colon. Am J Roentgenol. 1976;126:77–94.

Immune Checkpoint Inhibitor Colitis

174

Michelle D. Inkster, Eric W. Willis, Charles M. O'Malley, Jr., and James S. Wu

Presentation

A 62-year-old female with metastatic malignancy was treated with an immune checkpoint inhibitor. Two months after starting treatment, she was admitted because of weight loss and diarrhea. She was afebrile with a pulse of 89 bpm. Admitting laboratory values included a white blood cell count of 9,600/μl (3,700–11,000/μl) and a serum albumin of 2.9 g/dl (3.9–4.9 g/dl). Stool cultures were negative for enteric pathogens. Assays were negative for *Clostridiodes difficile* and *Cytomegalovirus*. Abdominal computed tomography (CT) showed colonic dilatation (Fig. 174.1).

Colonoscopy revealed mucosal sloughing from the rectum to the transverse colon (Fig. 174.2). Biopsies showed inflammation and crypt apoptosis (Fig. 174.3a and b).

The patient was followed by surgery from the time of admission. Daily plain abdominal radiographs were taken. A week after admission, free intraperitoneal air was seen (Fig. 174.4). The patient underwent emergency subtotal colectomy and ileostomy. Pathology showed diffuse mucosal sloughing and gross perforation.

M. D. Inkster
Department of Gastroenterology, Cleveland Clinic, Cleveland, OH, USA

E. W. Willis
Department of Pathology, CORPath, Columbus, OH, USA

C. M. O'Malley, Jr.
Radiology & Diagnostic Imaging Institute, Cleveland Clinic, Cleveland, OH, USA

J. S. Wu (✉)
Department of Colon and Rectal Surgery, Cleveland Clinic, Cleveland, OH, USA

J. S. Wu, M. D. Inkster (eds.), *Cleveland Clinic Colorectal Case Studies*,
https://doi.org/10.1007/978-3-031-39880-3_174

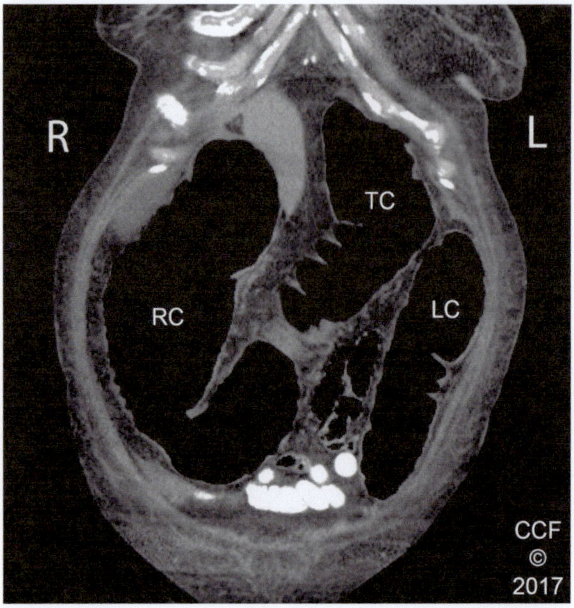

Fig. 174.1 Abdominal CT (coronal view) shows colonic dilatation. The right colon (RC), transverse colon (TC), and left colon (LC) are labeled. Right (R), left (L)

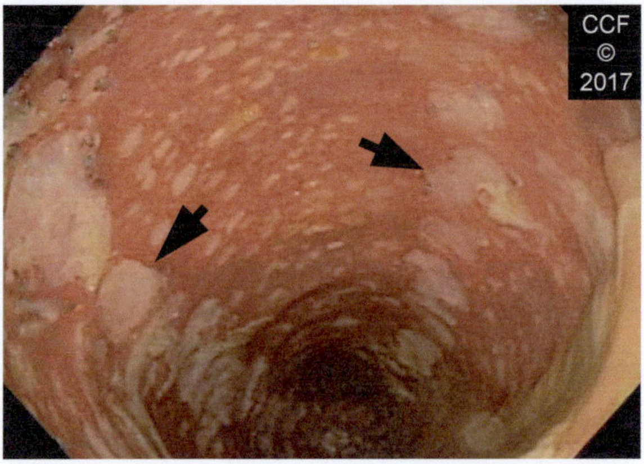

Fig. 174.2 Colonoscopy shows exposed muscularis (red colored) following diffuse mucosal sloughing. Islands of white mucosa (arrows) still remain

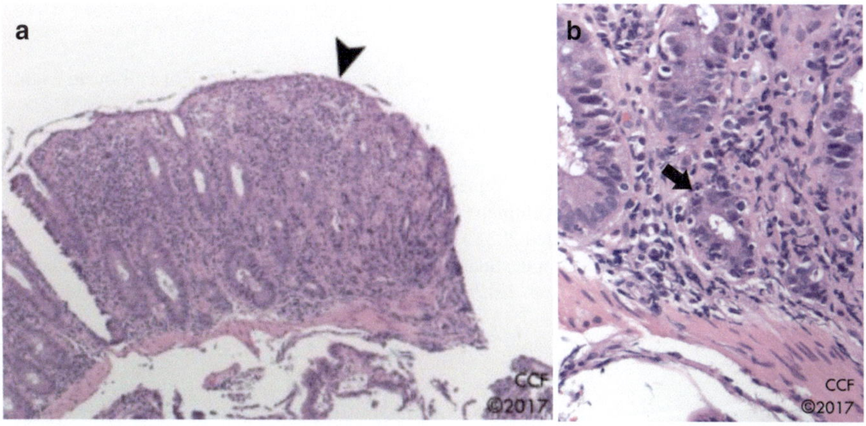

Fig. 174.3 (**a**) The colon biopsies show overall preservation of the crypt architecture with expansion of the lamina propria by lymphocytes, plasma cells, eosinophils, and neutrophils. There is neutrophil-mediated epithelial injury (arrowhead). (**b**) At higher power, increased intraepithelial lymphocytes and crypt apoptosis (arrow) are seen

Fig. 174.4 Free intraperitoneal air (arrows) is seen beneath the diaphragms on this portable upright radiograph

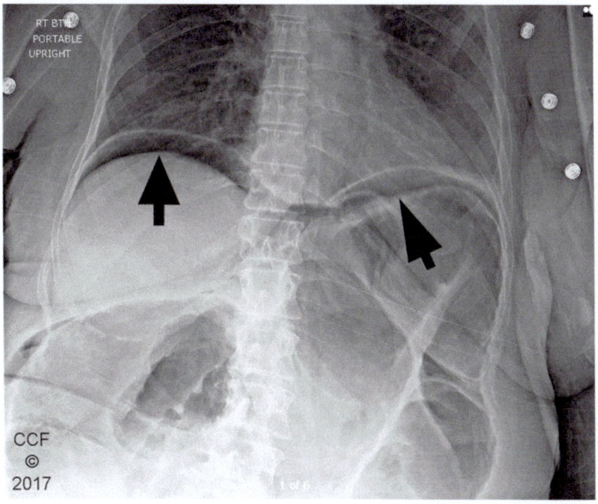

Comment

Checkpoints are controls that ensure the order of cell cycle events [1]. Immune checkpoint inhibitors (CPIs) are a class of drugs used in cancer treatment [2]. CPIs have gastrointestinal side effects, including enterocolitis [3–5]. Aware of the possible adverse consequences of CPIs, the admitting oncology team asked surgery to follow the patient from the beginning of the hospitalization. Daily plain abdominal films were ordered just in case. Sure enough, a week later, free air was detected. The patient underwent subtotal colectomy with end ileostomy without delay. Being prepared made all the difference.

References

1. Hartwell LH, Weinert TA. Checkpoints: Controls that ensure the order of cell cycle events. Science. 1989;246:629–34.
2. Benada J, Macureck L. Targeting the checkpoint to kill cancer cells. Biomolecules 2015;5:1912–37.
3. Fukomoto T, Fujiwara S, Tajima S, Tamesada Y, Sakaguchi M, Oka M, et al. Infliximab for severe colitis associated with nivolumab followed by ipilimumab. J Dermatol. 2018;45:e1–2.
4. Immunotherapy side effects. [cited 2022 Jun 11]. Available from My.clevelandclinic.org.
5. Cramer P, Bresalier RS. Gastrointestinal and hepatic complications of immune checkpoint inhibitors. Curr Gastroenterol Rep. 2017;19:3. https://doi.org/10.1007/s11894-017-0540-6.

Graft-Versus-Host Disease

175

Michelle D. Inkster, Ana E. Bennett, and James S. Wu

Presentation

A 60-year-old female with myelodysplastic syndrome underwent allogeneic bone marrow (BM) transplantation. The patient subsequently developed diarrhea and gastrointestinal bleeding. Colonoscopy was done (Fig. 175.1).

Pathology of biopsies is shown in Fig. 175.2.

M. D. Inkster
Department of Gastroenterology, Cleveland Clinic, Cleveland, OH, USA

A. E. Bennett
Pathology & Laboratory Medicine Institute, Cleveland Clinic, Cleveland, OH, USA

J. S. Wu (✉)
Department of Colon and Rectal Surgery, Cleveland Clinic, Cleveland, OH, USA

J. S. Wu, M. D. Inkster (eds.), *Cleveland Clinic Colorectal Case Studies*,
https://doi.org/10.1007/978-3-031-39880-3_175

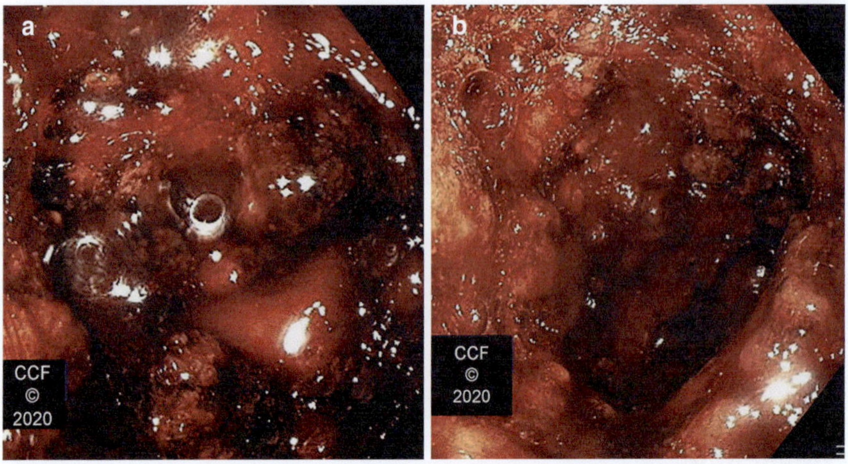

Fig. 175.1 (**a**, **b**) Colonoscopy. Blood clots and mucosal sloughing were seen from the rectosigmoid colon to the splenic flexure

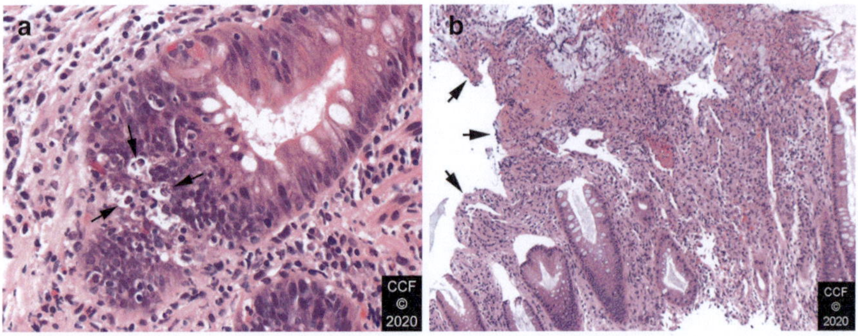

Fig. 175.2 (**a**) Epithelial apoptosis in a colonic biopsy. Large vacuoles (arrows) contain cellular debris, so called "exploding crypt cells"; (**b**) severe GVHD showing epithelial sloughing (arrows)

Comment

Vriesendorp and Heidt [1][1] summarize the discovery of graft-versus-host disease (GVHD) as follows:

> "Discovery of GvHD
>
> In 1956, Vos, Davids, Weijzen, and van Bekkem compared the survival of mice receiving supralethal TBI[2] alone with mice receiving the same dose of TBI followed by intravenously administered isologous or allogeneic BM cells.[2] Mice that received only TBI died before

[1] This excerpt was reproduced with the generous permission of Elsevier Inc., CCC | RightsLink®, License Number 5157051112642, License date Sep 27, 2021.

[2] Total body irradiation (TBI).

post-TBI day 20 from BM aplasia: the "primary" or BM syndrome. Mice treated with sufficient isologous BM cells survived. Mice treated with allogeneic BM cells died after post-TBI day 20 from a "secondary" syndrome.

Histologic studies of mice dying from the secondary syndrome confirm that these mice regenerated enough red cells, leukocytes, and platelets to survive. Instead, their cause of death was multiorgan failure in the skin, intestinal tract, liver, and lymphoid tissues,..."
Huib M. Vriesendorp and Peter J. Heidt
Leiden University Medical Center
Leiden, The Netherlands

The authors credit Barnes and co-workers [3][3] for most likely introducing the term "*graft-versus-host* reaction" in 1962.

'The "secondary disease" which afflicts mice after lethal irradiation and treatment with foreign bone marrow is now a well-known phenomenon. The clinical features of the syndrome are variable but include wasting, diarrhea, and skin lesions of varying severity. The apparent time of onset is 3 to 4 weeks after irradiation. Much evidence has accumulated from several experimental approaches suggesting that an immunological graft-*versus*-host reaction is involved in the pathogenesis of the syndrome.'
D. W. H. Barnes, J. F. Loutit, H. S. Micklem
Medical Research Council
Radiobiological Research Unit
Berkshire, England

In 1966, Billingham [4] summarized characteristics of *graft-versus-host* reaction.

"From the general principles of transplantation immunology, as they applied to conventional homograft reactions, the conditions under which a graft might be capable of initiating an immunological reaction against its host to the point of having overt consequences could easily be formulated:

1. The graft *must* contain immunologically competent cells.

2. The host must possess important transplantation isoantigens that are lacking in the graft donor, so that the host appears foreign to it and is therefore capable of stimulating it antigenically.

3. The host itself must be incapable of mounting an effective immunological reaction against the graft, at least for sufficient time for the latter to manifest its immunological capabilities—...."
R. E. Billingham
Department of Medical Genetics
University of Pennsylvania
School of Medicine
Philadelphia

Graft-versus-host reaction also referred to as graft-versus-host disease (GVHD) commonly affects the skin, liver, and the gastrointestinal tract. Gastrointestinal

---

[3]This excerpt was reproduced with the generous permission of John Wiley & Sons-Books, CCC|Marketplace™, Order License ID 1143830-1, order date 27-Aug-2021.

manifestations of GVHD include abdominal pain, diarrhea, bleeding, and malnutrition [5, 6]. The most common histological finding acute GVHD is epithelial cell apoptosis [6, 7]. Epithelial apoptotic cells are found in the regenerative areas such as the crypts. Mucosal sloughing is seen in severe cases.

References

1. Vriesendorp HM, Heidt PJ. History of graft-versus-host disease. Exp Hematol. 2016;44:674–88.
2. Vos O, Davids JAG, Weyzen WWH, van Bekkum DW. Evidence for the cellular hypothesis in radiation protection by bone marrow cells. Acta Physiol Pharmacol Neerl. 1956;4:482–6.
3. Barnes DWH, Loutit JF, Micklem HS. "Secondary disease" of radiation chimeras: A syndrome due to lymphoid aplasia. Ann N Y Acad Sci. 1962;99:374–485.
4. Billingham RE. The biology of graft-versus-host reactions. Harvey Lect 1966–67;62:21–78.
5. Sullivan KM, Mori M, Sanders J, Siadak M, Witherspoon RP, Anasetti C, et al. Late complications of allogeneic and autologous marrow transplantation. Bone Marrow Transplant. 1992;10(Suppl 1):127–34.
6. Naymagon S, Naymagon L, Wong S-Y, Ko HM, Renteria A, Levine J, et al. Acute graft-versus-host disease of the gut: considerations for the gastroenterologist. Nat Rev Gastroenterol Hepatol. 2017;14:711–26.
7. Salomao M, Dorritie K, Mapara MY, Sepulveda A. Histopathology of graft-vs-host disease of gastrointestinal tract and liver. Am J Clin Pathol. 2016;145:591–603.

Portal Hypertensive Colopathy

176

Michelle D. Inkster, Ana E. Bennett, and James S. Wu

Presentation

A 34-year-old female with Coats' syndrome (cerebral microangiopathy complicated by retinopathy, pancytopenia, and liver cirrhosis) presented for evaluation of gastrointestinal bleeding. Esophagogastroduodenopathy (EGD) showed gastric antral vascular ectasia and esophageal varices. Colonoscopy showed diffuse vascular ectasias throughout (Fig. 176.1). Biopsies were taken (Fig. 176.2).

Management

Esophageal varices seen at EGD were treated with banding. A transjugular intrahepatic portosystemic shunt (TIPS) was placed to decrease portal pressure. Following TIPS placement, bleeding decreased markedly.

On follow-up colonoscopy, vascular ectasia were still seen in the distal rectum (Fig. 176.3a); however, the endoscopic appearance of the remainder of the large intestine had returned to normal (Fig. 176.3b).

Comment

In 1991, two groups described colopathy secondary to portal hypertension one month apart.

Kozarek et al. [1] described "portal colopathy" where colonoscopy in patients with portal hypertension showed multiple vascular ectasias.

> "Twenty patients with portal hypertension related to a variety of causes prospectively underwent colonoscopy for hematochezia (n = 10), hemoccult positive stool and anemia

M. D. Inkster
Department of Gastroenterology, Cleveland Clinic, Cleveland, OH, USA

A. E. Bennett
Pathology & Laboratory Medicine Institute, Cleveland Clinic, Cleveland, OH, USA

J. S. Wu (✉)
Department of Colon and Rectal Surgery, Cleveland Clinic, Cleveland, OH, USA

J. S. Wu, M. D. Inkster (eds.), *Cleveland Clinic Colorectal Case Studies*,
https://doi.org/10.1007/978-3-031-39880-3_176

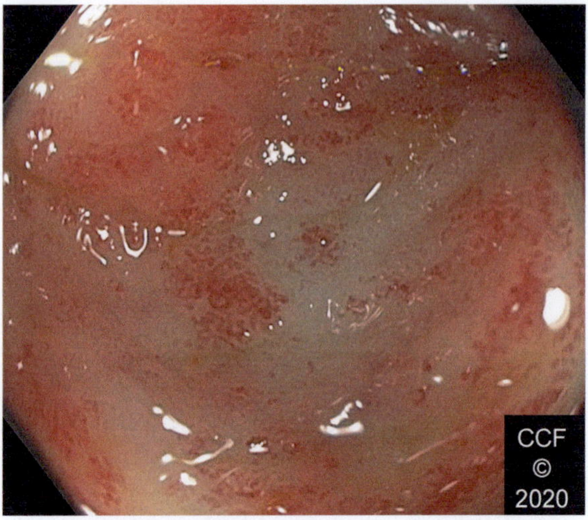

Fig. 176.1 Colonoscopy at presentation showed diffuse vascular ectasias throughout the colon and rectum

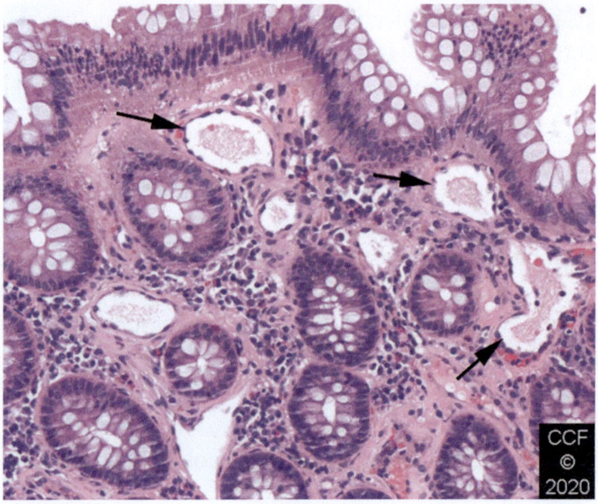

Fig. 176.2 Histology showed thickened and prominent capillaries (arrows) in the lamina propria (200×)

(n = 9), or polyp found with screening flexible sigmoidoscopy (n = 2) (includes 1 patient with anemia/heme-positive stool). Colonoscopic findings included mucosal abnormalities resembling multiple vascular ectasias in 14 (70%), 4 of whom also had endoscopic features suggesting a mild, chronic colitis[1]."
R. A. Kozarek, V. A. Botoman,
J. E. Bredfeldt, R.M. Roach, D. J. Patterson, and T. J. Ball
Virginia Mason Clinic
Seattle, Washington

Naveau and colleagues described a new entity: portal hypertensive colopathy (PHC) [2].

[1] This excerpt was reproduced with the generous permission of Elsevier, RightsLink License number 5156130896853, License date Sep 25, 2021.

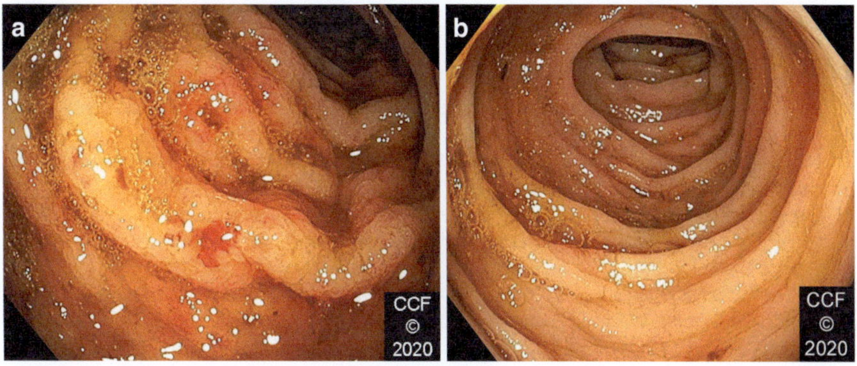

Fig. 176.3 Colonoscopy following TIPS. While the rectal mucosa showed a few residual vascular ectasias (**a**), the remainder of the colonic mucosa appeared normal (**b**)

"The aim of this paper was, first, to show in a case control study that in alcoholic cirrhotic patients colonic vascular ectasias (VE) are a complication of portal hypertension and, second, to establish in a histomorphometric study that colonic vascular ectasias and rectal varices (RV) are only endoscopic features of a new entity: portal hypertensive colopathy, the pathologic basis of which is colonic mucosal capillary ectasia[2]."
Sylvie Naveau, MD, Pierre Bedossa, MD, Thierry Poynard, MD, Benoît Mory, MD, and Jean-Claude Chaput, MD
Hôpital Antoine Béclère
Clamart Cedex, France

Portal hypertensive colopathy can cause colonic bleeding in patients with liver cirrhosis and portal hypertension. Colonoscopy and histologic examination of the colonic mucosa make the diagnosis. Lowering the portal pressure is an essential part of management [3–6].

The patient in this case had Coats disease, "*Retinal disease with massive exudation*" [7]. The association of Coats disease with liver cirrhosis and gastrointestinal bleeding was described by Bisserbe et al. in 2014 [8].

"The most characteristic features of this rare multisystem disorder are retinal telangiectasias and exsudates (Coats disease), a distinctive pattern of intracranial calcifications with leukoencephalopathy and cysts, and a high risk of gastro intestinal bleeding and portal hypertension due to the development of vascular ectasias in the stomach, small intestine and liver[3]."

Portal hypertensive colopathy is an entity that can be seen when evaluating patients with liver cirrhosis who present with gastrointestinal bleeding. Colonoscopy and histologic examination of the colonic mucosa make the diagnosis and provide direction to proper management.

---

[2]This excerpt was reproduced with the generous permission of Springer Nature BV, CCCMarketplaceTM (superscript), Order License ID 1143993-1, Order date 28-Aug-2021.

[3] Permission to reproduce this excerpt was generously provided by Elsevier Masson SAS. Tous droits réservés. Permissions France. AuthorsSupport@elsevier.com, March 3, 2024.

References

1. Kozarek RA, Botoman VA, Bredfeldt JE, Roach JM, Patterson DJ, Ball TJ. Portal colopathy: Prospective study of colonoscopy in patients with portal hypertension. Gastroenterology. 1991;101:1192–7.
2. Naveau S, Bedossa P, Poynard T, Mory B, Chaput J-C. Portal hypertensive colopathy. A new entity. Dig Dis Sci. 1991;36:1774–81.
3. Lamps LW, Hunt CM, Green A, Gray GF Jr, Washington K. Alterations in colonic mucosal vessels in patients with cirrhosis and noncirrhotic portal hypertension. Hum Pathol. 1998;29:527–35.
4. Ito K, Shiraki K, Sakai T, Yoshimura H, Nakano T. Portal hypertensive colopathy in patients with liver cirrhosis. World J Gastro. 2005;11:3127–30.
5. Rockey DC. An update. Portal hypertensive gastropathy and colopathy. Clin Liver Dis. 2019;23:643–58.
6. Balzer C, Lotterer E, Kleber G, Fleig WE. Transjugular intrahepatic portosystemic shunt for bleeding angiodysplasia-like lesions in portal-hypertensive colopathy. Gastroenterology. 1998;115:167–72.
7. Coats G. Forms of retinal disease with massive exudation. Roy Lond Ophthalmol Hosp Rep. 1908;17:440–525.
8. Bisserbe A, Tertian G, Buffet C, Turhan A, Lambotte O, Nasser G, et al. Cerebro-retinal microangiopathy with calcifications and cysts due to recessive mutations in the CTC1 gene. Rev Neurol. 2015;171:445–9.

Crohn's Colitis: Colonoscopic Appearance

177

James S. Wu

Endoscopic Features of Crohn's Colitis

In 1932, Crohn, Ginsburg, and Oppenheimer described regional enteritis [1]. In 1952, Wells described the relationship between ulcerative colitis and Crohn's disease [2]. In 1959, Brooke discussed granulomatous diseases of the intestine [3]. In 1960, Lockhart-Mummery and Morson described features of Crohn's disease confined to the colon and its distinction from ulcerative colitis [4]. Unlike ulcerative colitis, a mucosal disease that begins in the distal rectum and progresses proximally without breaks, Crohn's disease of the large bowel is a transmural granulomatous process characterized by multifocal patches of disease separated by normal segments (Table 177.1) [5].

A patient with known Crohn's colitis was referred for surveillance colonoscopy. Endoscopic findings are shown in Figs. 177.1, 177.2, 177.3, 177.4, 177.5, 177.6. "Elephant ear" perianal skin tags from another patient are shown in Fig. 177.7.

Table 177.1 Clinical features suggestive of Crohn's disease

Clinical features
Normal appearing rectum with proximal colonic disease
Perianal fistula(s) or abscesses
Indurated ("elephant ear") skin tags
Aphthous ulcers
Ileal disease
Skip lesions
Internal fistulas

J. S. Wu (✉)
Department of Colon and Rectal Surgery, Cleveland Clinic, Cleveland, OH, USA

J. S. Wu, M. D. Inkster (eds.), *Cleveland Clinic Colorectal Case Studies*,
https://doi.org/10.1007/978-3-031-39880-3_177

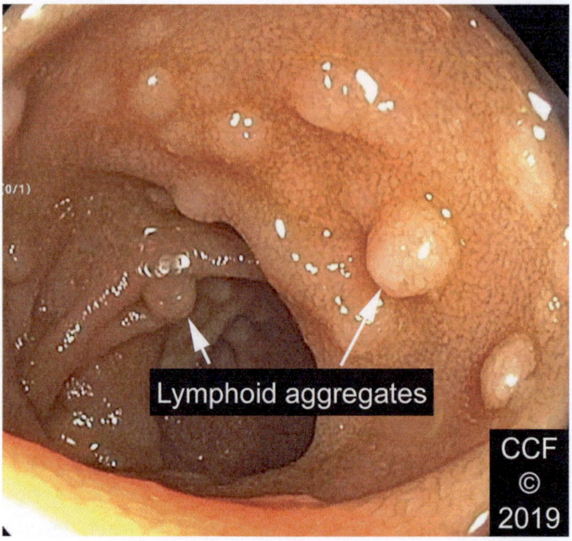

Fig. 177.1 The terminal ileum was intubated. Lymphoid aggregates (arrows) are seen [6]

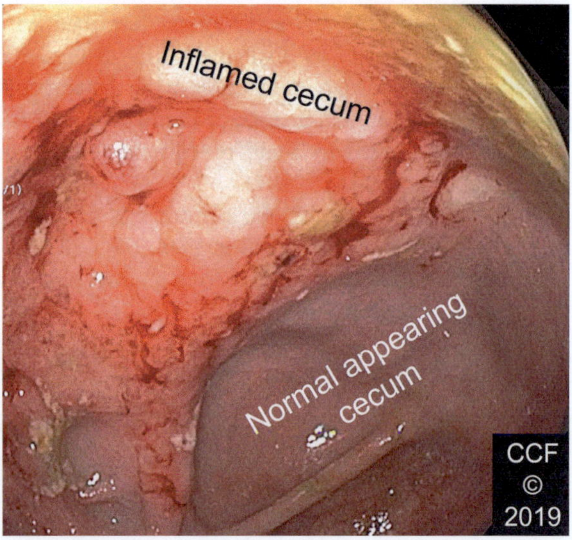

Fig. 177.2 The cecum shows inflamed mucosa adjacent to normal appearing mucosa

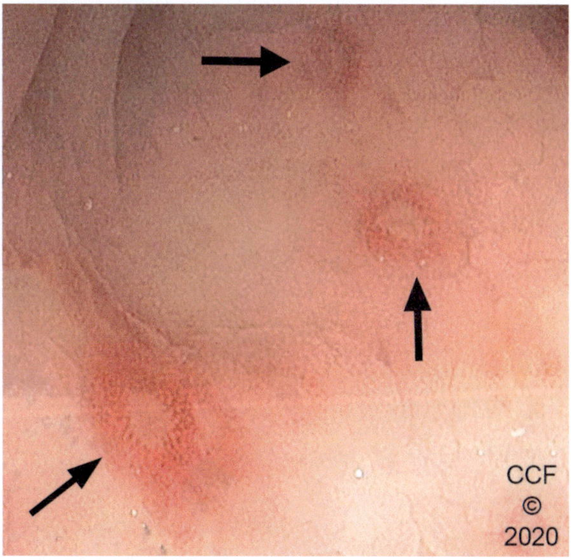

Fig. 177.3 Aphthous ulcers in the transverse colon (arrows) [7]

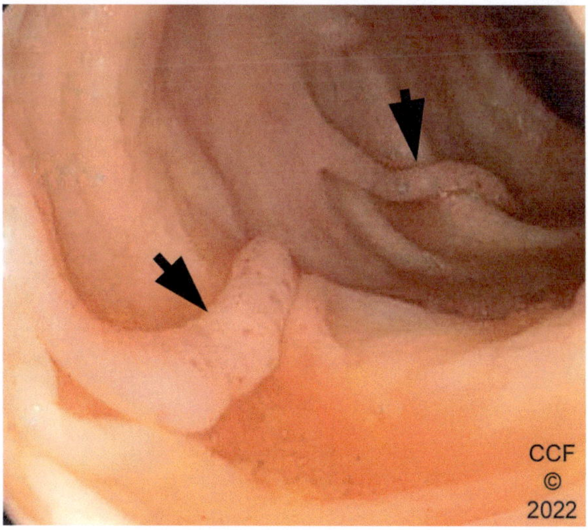

Fig. 177.4 Pseudopolyps (arrows) in a patient with inflammatory bowel disease. A pseudopolyp is defined as "a hypertrophied tab of mucous membrane resembling a polyp, but caused by ulceration surrounding intact mucosa" [8]

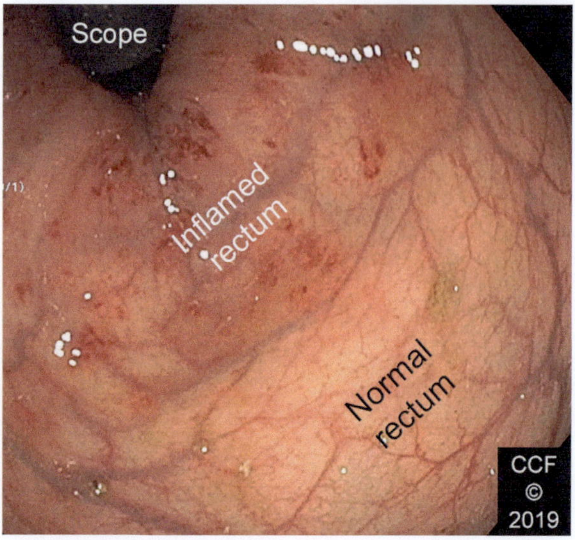

Fig. 177.5 Retroflexion in the rectum shows inflamed distal rectal mucosa adjacent to normal appearing proximal rectal mucosa

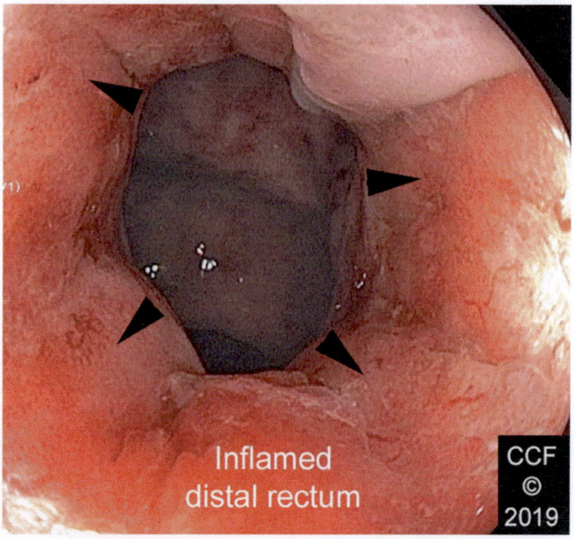

Fig. 177.6 Inflamed distal rectal mucosa seen *en face* (arrows)

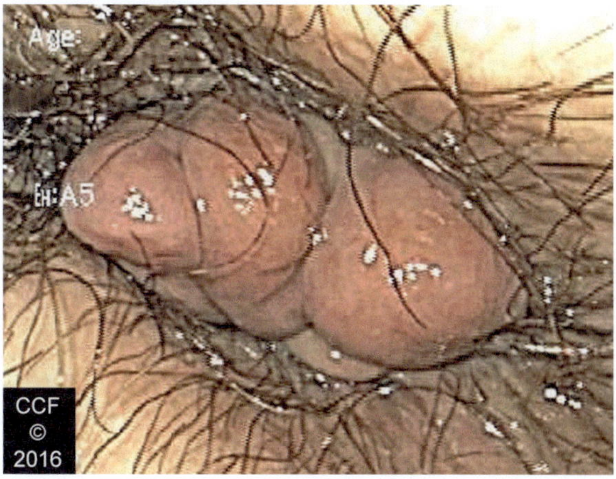

Fig. 177.7 "Elephant ear" skin tags seen on examination of the perianal skin of another patient with Crohn's disease [9]

References

1. Crohn BB, Ginzburg L, Oppenheimer GD, Regional ileitis. A pathological and clinical entity. J Am Med Assoc. 1932;99:1323–9.
2. Wells C. Ulcerative colitis and Crohn's disease. Ann R Coll Surg Engl. 1952;11:105–20.
3. Brooke BN. Granulomatous diseases of the intestine. Lancet. 1959;2(7106):745–9.
4. Lockhart-Mummery HE, Morson BC. Crohn's disease (regional enteritis) of the large intestine and its distinction from ulcerative colitis. Gut. 1960;1:87–105.
5. Fazio VF, Wu JS. Surgical therapy for Crohn's disease of the colon and rectum. Surg Clin N Am. 1997;77:197–210.
6. Moreels TG, Dewit O. Normal endoscopic appearance of the colon and the terminal ileum. In: Jouret-Mourin A, Faa G, Geboes K, editors. Colitis. Cham: Springer; 2018. p. 31–6. https://doi.org/10.1007/978-3-319-89503-1_4.
7. Laufer I, Costopoulos L. Early lesions of Crohn's disease. Am J Roentgenol. 1978;130:307–11.
8. Pseudopolyp. The Free Dictionary by Farlex. [cited 2020 Jan 18]. https://medical-dictionary.thefreedictionary.com/pseudopolyp
9. Safar B, Sands D. Perianal Crohn's disease. Clin Colon Rectal Surg. 2007;20:282–93.

Intersphincteric Proctectomy 178

James S. Wu

Presentation

A 50-year-old female with chronic ulcerative colitis underwent subtotal colectomy with end ileostomy. Following her recovery, she chose completion proctosigmoidectomy with permanent end ileostomy in order to remove the cancer risk associated with the retained inflamed rectosigmoid colon.

Intersphincteric Proctosigmoidectomy

In 1975, Turnbull and Fazio described the operation as follows [1]:

> "The Abdominopelvic Phase
>
> In the pelvic phase of proctectomy, the superior rectal artery and vein are ligated and divided at least 2 inches in front of the promontory of the sacrum. The lateral peritoneal folds are incised with scissors on each side of the rectum, and the rectum is dissected free of Waldeyer's presacral fascia all the way to the sacrococcygeal junction. The plane of dissection is between the transparent fascia that invests the posterior and lateral fat of the rectum and an alveolar space in front of the Waldeyer's fascia and laterally.
>
> The anterior dissection of the rectum is performed on the rectal side of Denonvillier's fascia, in which case the seminal vesicles of the male will not be seen and ejaculatory ganglia will be undisturbed. The anterolateral rectal stalks (through which mixed parasympathetic and sympathetic nerves course) are cut off flush with the muscular wall of the rectum. Posterior to the rectum, the presacral nerve plexes at the bifurcation of the aorta are undisturbed; the hypogastric nerve bands that approximate the rectosigmoid are visualized and gently swept laterally; and finally, the dissection is carried down to the supralevator fascia.

J. S. Wu (✉)
Department of Colon and Rectal Surgery, Cleveland Clinic, Cleveland, OH, USA

J. S. Wu, M. D. Inkster (eds.), *Cleveland Clinic Colorectal Case Studies*,
https://doi.org/10.1007/978-3-031-39880-3_178

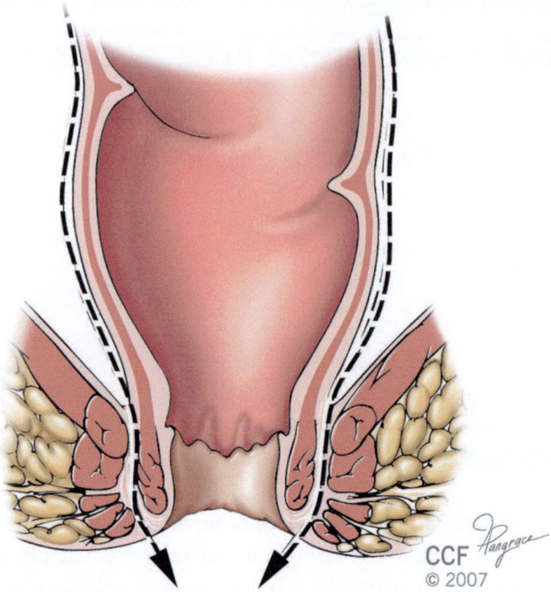

Fig. 178.1 Intersphincteric proctectomy. Incision is made in the intersphincteric groove. The rectum and internal sphincter are removed. The external sphincter and levator ani muscles are preserved

> Perineal Proctectomy
>
> The levatores ani and their dense fascial coats are preserved without injury and the subcutaneous anal muscle is removed by sharp dissection with preservation of the entire anal canal skin."

The principles of the operation are as follows:

1. Vascular division close to the rectum,
2. Pelvic mobilization close to rectum,
3. Preservation of nerve plexuses,
4. Preservation of the levatores ani,
5. Intersphincteric dissection of the anus.

The perineal portion of the operation is shown in Figs. 178.1, 178.2, 178.3, and 178.4. Figure 178.1 shows the intersphincteric lines of resection. A circumferential incision is made at the palpable intersphincteric groove (Fig. 178.2). Fig. 178.3 shows the anus dissected free of the external anal sphincter.[1]

Following removal of the specimen, the levators (Fig. 178.4) are approximated, and the skin is closed. The proctosigmoidectomy specimen is shown in Fig. 178.5.

[1] This technique of intersphincteric dissection was passed down by demonstration in the operating room to the author from Dr. Victor W. Fazio.

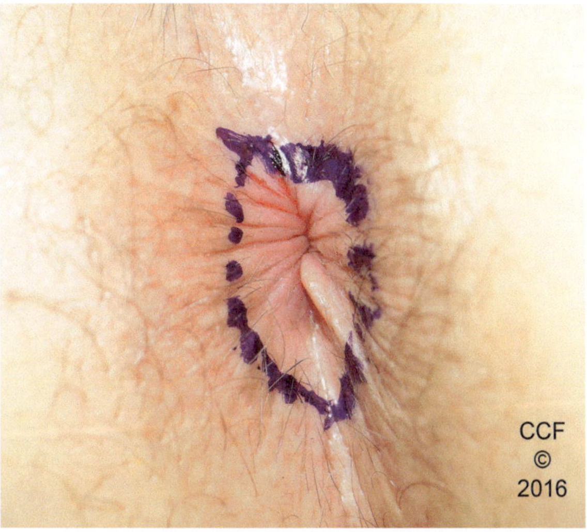

Fig. 178.2 Intersphincteric dissection. An incision is made in the intersphincteric groove, identified by palpation and here marked with ink

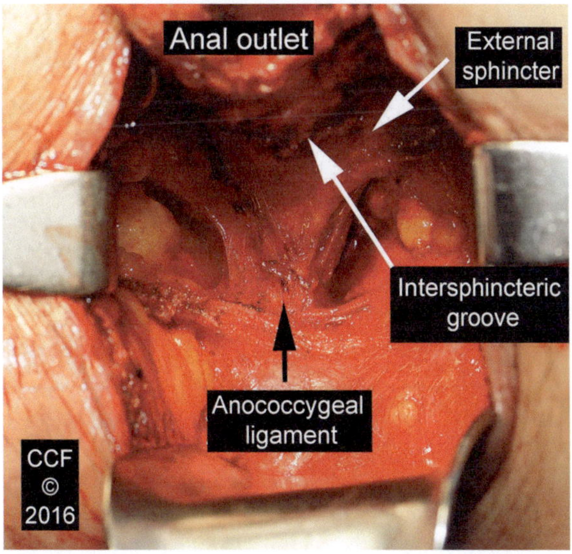

Fig. 178.3 The anus with the internal sphincter is dissected free of the external sphincter. The anococcygeal ligament is seen

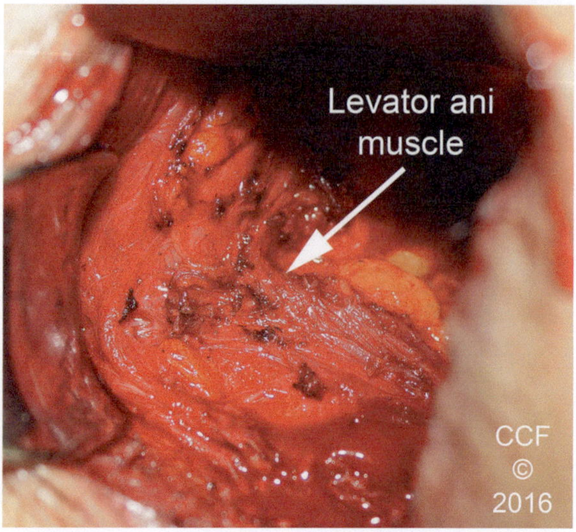

Fig. 178.4 Following removal of the anus, rectum, and sigmoid colon, the intact levator ani muscle is seen

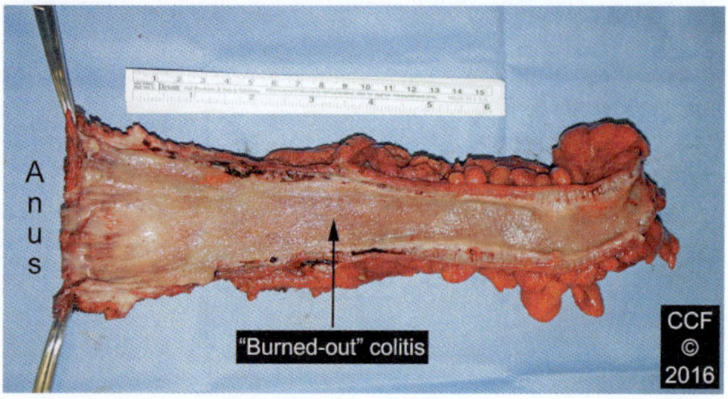

Fig. 178.5 The proctosigmoidectomy specimen. Pathology showed histologic changes consistent with "burned-out" ulcerative colitis

Comment

For benign disease, ligation of the lymphovascular supply is done close to the rectum; high ligation of the inferior mesenteric artery and vein is unnecessary. Dissection close to the rectum is done to preserve sexual function. Intersphincteric dissection with preservation and closure of the levator ani muscles helps to prevent perineal wound dehiscence and problems associated with an unhealed perineal wound [2].

References

1. Turnbull RB Jr, Fazio V. Advances in the surgical technique of ulcerative colitis surgery: Endoanal proctectomy and two-directional myotomy ileostomy. Surg Annual. 1975;7:315–29.
2. Tompkins RG, Warshaw AL. Improved management of the perineal wound after proctectomy. Ann Surg. 1985;202:760–5.

Continent Ileostomy (Kock Pouch) 179

David W. Dietz, Jean H. Ashburn, Carolyn L. Power, and James S. Wu

Presentation

A 40-year-old female with familial adenomatous polyposis underwent proctocolectomy with ileal pouch–anal anastomosis. Because of pouch complications, the pouch was excised, and she was given a conventional end ileostomy. She suffered from painful and debilitating parastomal herniation and did not like uncontrolled ileostomy function. A preoperative MRI showed that she was devoid of anal sphincter muscles. Continent ileostomy was offered.

Formation of the Continent Ileostomy

Formation of the continent ileostomy begins with marking of the stoma site. Typically, the stoma is placed through the rectus muscle in the right lower quadrant, often at the level of the anterior superior iliac spine. Situation more inferior than that usually seen for an end ileostomy is possible since a stoma appliance is not needed.

The procedure is divided into four stages:

1. Pouch construction,
2. Nipple valve formation,

D. W. Dietz
Department of Surgery, NYU Langone Medical Center, New York, NY, USA

J. H. Ashburn
Department of Colon and Rectal Surgery, Atrium Health Wake Forest Baptist, Winston-Salem, NC, USA

C. L. Power · J. S. Wu (✉)
Department of Colon and Rectal Surgery, Cleveland Clinic, Cleveland, OH, USA

J. S. Wu, M. D. Inkster (eds.), *Cleveland Clinic Colorectal Case Studies*,
https://doi.org/10.1007/978-3-031-39880-3_179

3. Valve stabilization,
4. Pouch attachment to the abdominal wall with stoma maturation.

These four stages can be further subdivided as follows:

Stage 1: S-Pouch Construction

The terminal ileum is arranged into three segments that are destined to become the pouch, the nipple valve, and the conduit to the skin (Fig. 179.1). The efferent limb of the distal-most segment is left free while the proximal aspect is sutured to the remaining two segments with serosal stitches to configure an S-shaped pouch (Fig. 179.2).

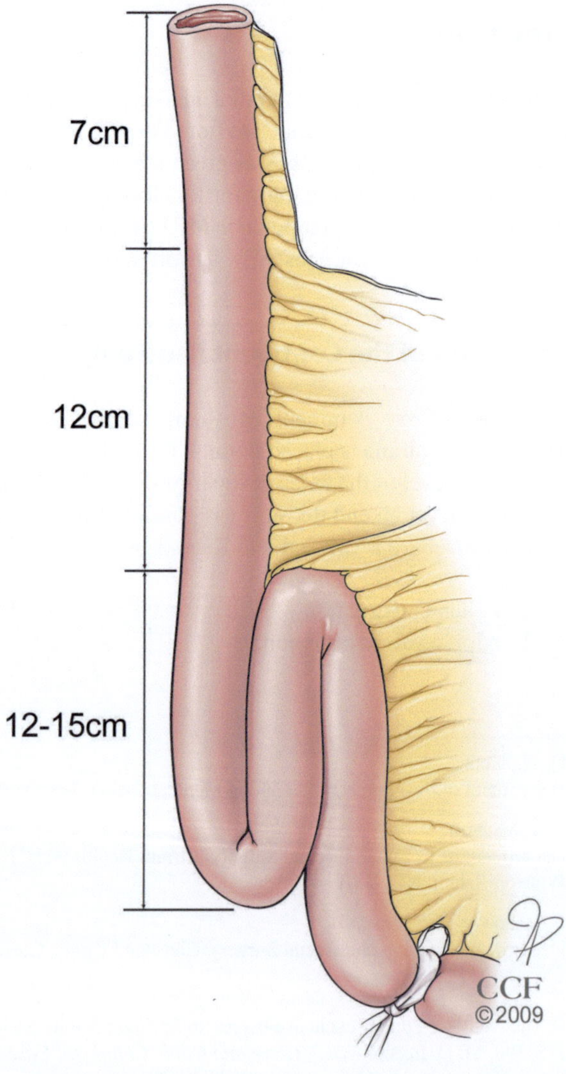

Fig. 179.1 Three 12–15 cm segments of opposed ileum are used to make the S-pouch. The 19-cm efferent limb will become the intussuscepted valve and exit conduit

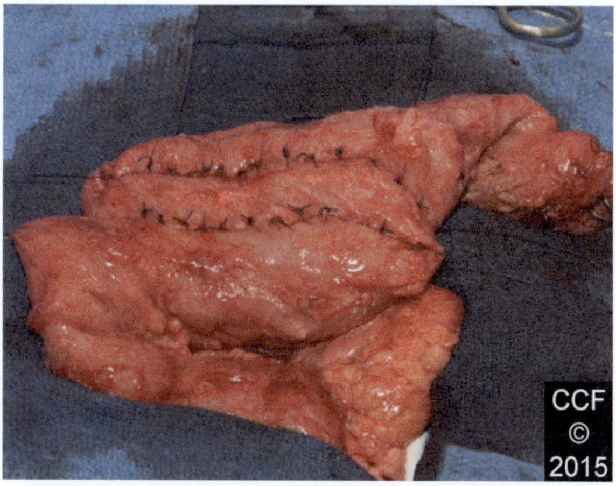

Fig. 179.2 The limbs are secured in apposition with sutures

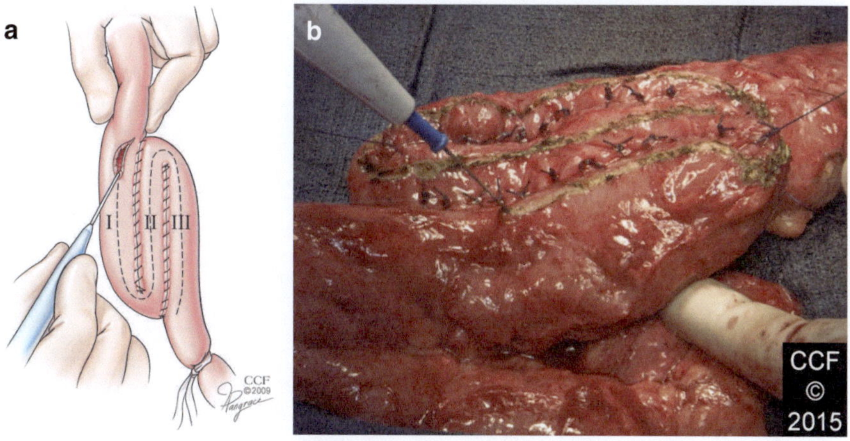

Fig. 179.3 (**a**) Illustration and (**b**) operative photo showing the creation of a long anti mesenteric incision through the three apposed limbs of ileum that will become the S-pouch

A long antimesenteric enterotomy is made in the apposed segments (Fig. 179.3a, b).

The back wall of the pouch is completed with a running full-thickness suture (Fig. 179.4a, b).

Stage 2: Nipple Valve Formation

The efferent limb of small intestine is intussuscepted to form the nipple valve (Fig. 179.5a, b).

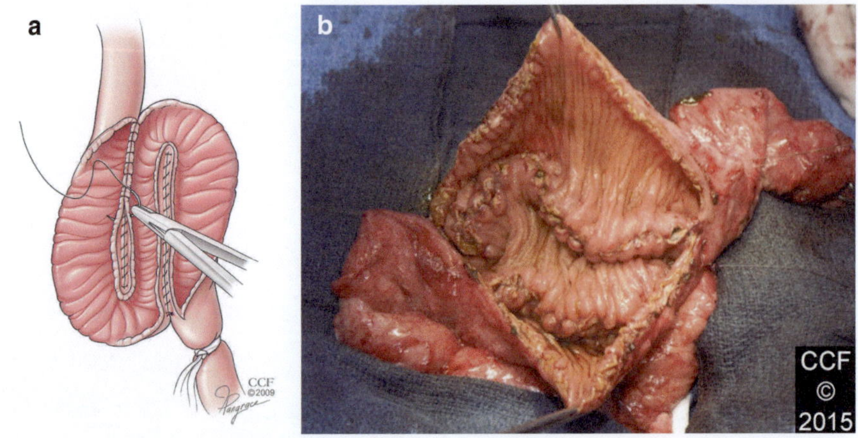

Fig. 179.4 (**a**) A running full-thickness suture is used to construct the back wall of the pouch by joining the walls of the center limb with adjacent proximal and distal limbs; (**b**) the completed back wall of the S-pouch

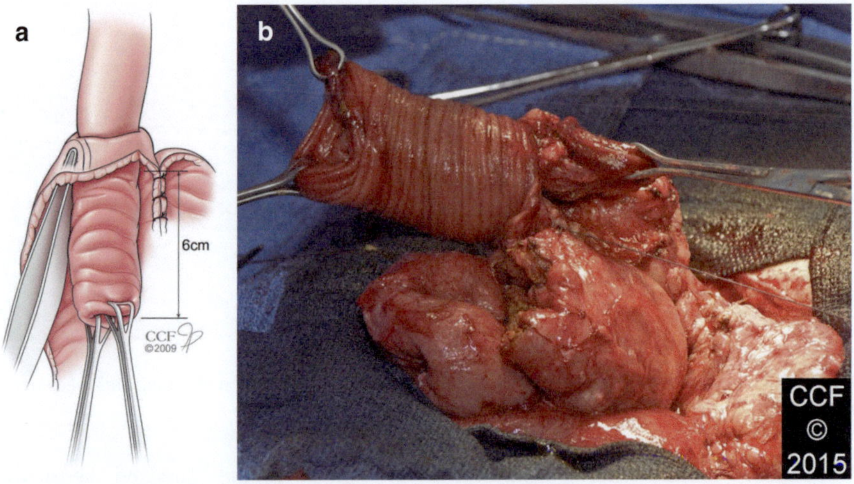

Fig. 179.5 The efferent limb is intussuscepted back into the pouch, creating a 6–7 cm valve; (**a**) two Babcock clamps stabilize the apex of the nipple valve; (**b**) a single Babcock clamp marks the most distal end of the efferent limb that will become the stoma

Stage 3. Nipple Valve Stabilization

The intussuscepted walls of the nipple valve are stapled to each other (away from the mesentery) to prevent valve desussception (Fig. 179.6a, b).

The anterior wall of the pouch is closed with suture. Closure begins where the exit conduit leaves the pouch. As the anterior pouch wall is closed over the valve,

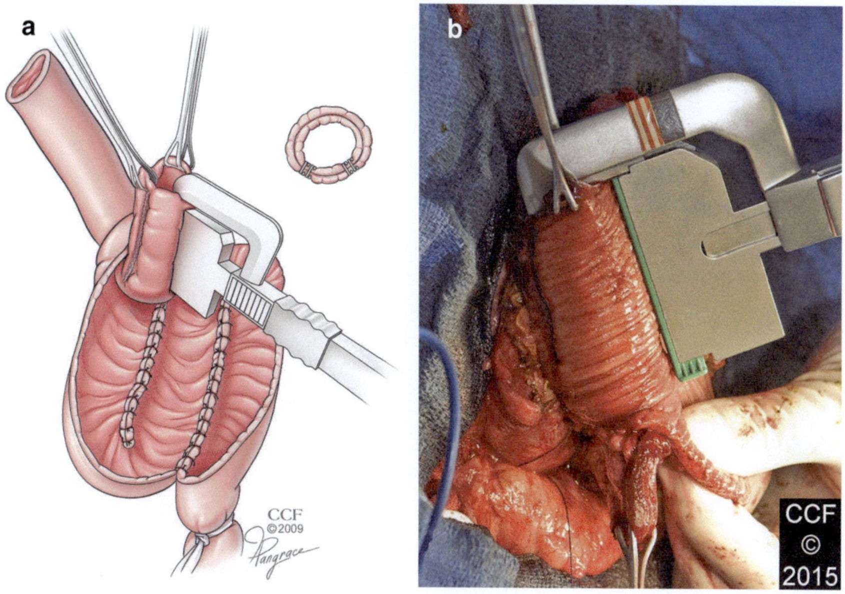

Fig. 179.6 Nipple valve intussusception is stabilized by stapling. (**a**) illustration; (**b**) operative photograph

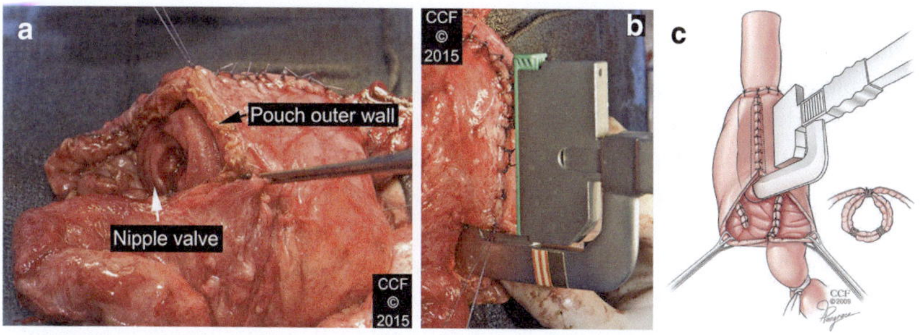

Fig. 179.7 (**a**) The nipple valve is aligned with the pouch side wall; (**b**) the nipple valve is stapled to the pouch wall; (**c**) illustration showing nipple valve-pouch stapling

sutures also incorporate the antimesenteric aspect of the valve to secure it to the pouch wall. Care is taken to avoid full-thickness bites on the valve itself to prevent fistula formation. The suture line stops at the tip of the valve. The nipple valve then is stapled to the pouch wall (Fig. 179.7). Closure of the anterior pouch wall is completed with additional sutures. Interrupted sutures placed between the serosal aspects of the pouch apex and proximal exit conduit are intended to increase valve stability.

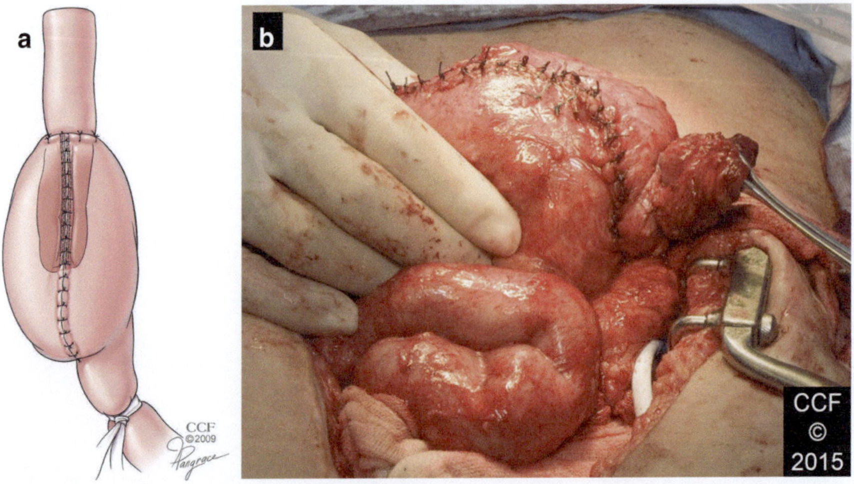

Fig. 179.8 (**a**) Illustration of the completed pouch; (**b**) In order to test the pouch for leaks and the nipple valve for continence, the afferent limb of the pouch is occluded and gentle pressure is applied to the pouch filled with saline. The clamp marks the distal end of the exit conduit that will become the stoma

Step 4: Pouch Attachment to the Abdominal Wall With Stoma Maturation

A straight continent ileostomy catheter[1] is passed through the exit conduit and into the completed pouch to confirm ease of intubation (Fig. 179.8a). With the afferent limb occluded, the pouch is filled with saline and air until tense; the catheter then is withdrawn. Suture lines are inspected for leaks, and the valve is tested for continence (Fig. 179.8b). The pouch is emptied by continent ileostomy tube reintubation. The stoma aperture is created at a previously marked site in the right lower quadrant. The pouch is placed beneath the stoma aperture, and its apex is secured to the underside of the abdominal wall at this site with permanent sutures (Fig. 179.9a). The exit conduit is brought through the abdominal wall, excess length is amputated at skin level, and the stoma is matured flush with the skin. A continent ileostomy tube is placed through the stoma into the pouch and is secured to the skin with sutures (Fig. 179.9b). A pelvic drain is placed, and the abdomen is closed (Fig. 179.10).

Demonstration of continent ileostomy intubation by a patient is shown in Fig. 179.11.

The endoscopic appearance of a continent ileostomy years after surgery is shown in Fig. 179.12.

[1] There are many commercially available straight continent ileostomy catheters. The catheter used by Dr. Fazio in the 1990's, he referred to as a "Waters tube."

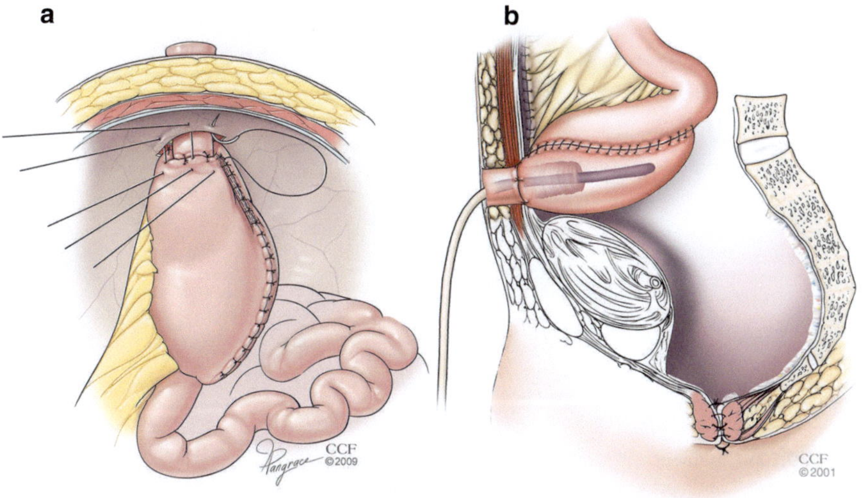

Fig. 179.9 (**a**) Securing the pouch to the fascia at the ostomy outlet; (**b**) illustration showing the pouch intubated with a drainage tube

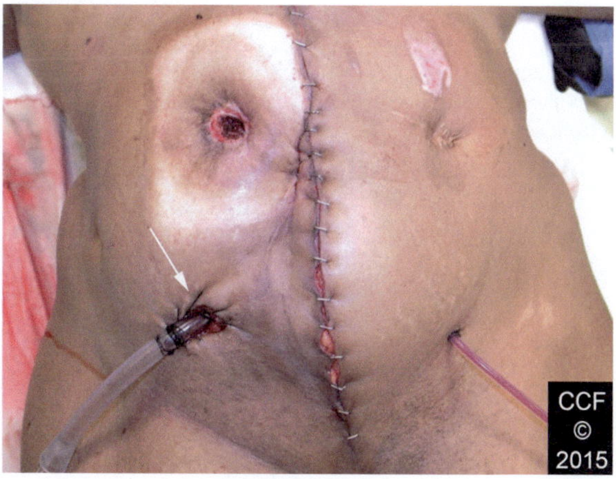

Fig. 179.10 In the immediate postoperative period, the pouch is drained continuously for four weeks (arrow). In this photograph, the site of the original conventional end ileostomy is located in the center of the appliance outline. An intra-abdominal drain is located in the left lower quadrant

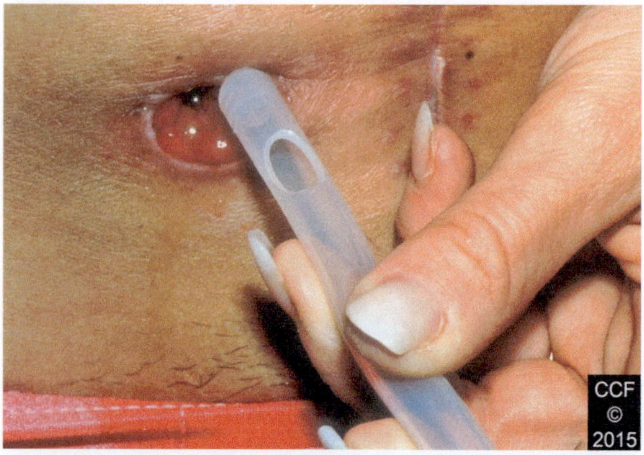

Fig. 179.11 A patient demonstrates continent ileostomy intubation during a postoperative visit 4 weeks after surgery

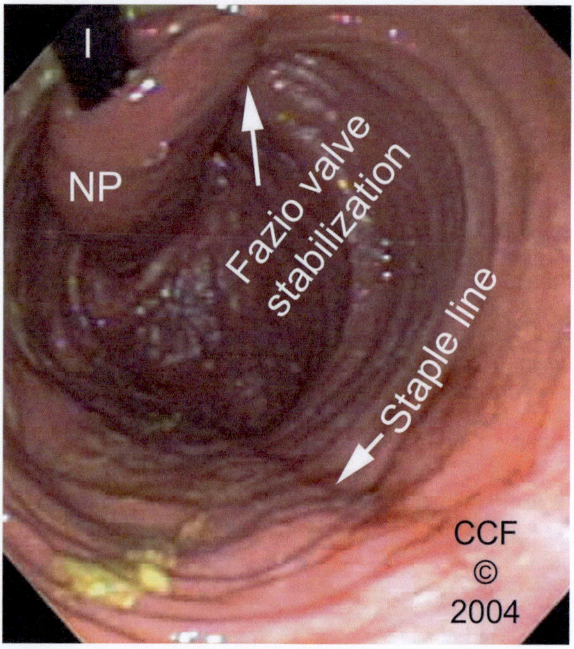

Fig. 179.12 Continent pouchoscopy. Landmarks seen include the nipple valve (NP) and a pouch staple line. In this example, the nipple was stapled to the pouch wall to prevent nipple valve slippage (Fazio valve stabilization). The examining ileoscope (I) is shown in this retroflexed view

Comments

In 1969, Kock described, "Intra-abdominal 'reservoir' in patients with permanent ileostomy," a procedure that resulted in fecal "continence" [1]. Adoption of the continent ileostomy was slow due to the complexity of the operation, high complication rates, and frequent need for reoperation. In response, continent ileostomy technique evolved [2]. Early continent ileostomies did not include a valve and relied on a long exit conduit passing through the rectus abdominis muscle to provide continence. Leakage was frequent, however, and Kock added the intussuscepted nipple valve to overcome this (Fig. 179.12). A major adverse consequence of this modification was nipple valve slippage. Fazio's stapling method, described above (Fig. 179.7), was introduced to prevent valve slippage. Other continent ileostomy designs include the "living collar" (Barnett) [3] and the "T-pouch" (Kaiser) [4]. Following the description of the restorative proctocolectomy (IPAA) for ulcerative colitis by Parks and Nicholls in 1978, use of the continent ileostomy decreased further [5]. Now, few surgeons are familiar with continent ileostomy surgery, but it still has a role in carefully selected patients who are either unsuitable for an IPAA, have a failed IPAA that cannot be salvaged, or whose conventional ileostomy is not consistent with an adequate quality of life [6].

The original continent ileostomy design by Kock was constructed from two limbs of ileum as shown in Fig. 179.13. The continent ileostomy demonstrated in this case was a three limb variant.

Continent ileostomy is associated with significant risk of complications requiring reoperation, often due to nipple valve problems. Nipple valve excision and pouch rotation can be done in some cases for pouch salvage (Fig. 179.14).

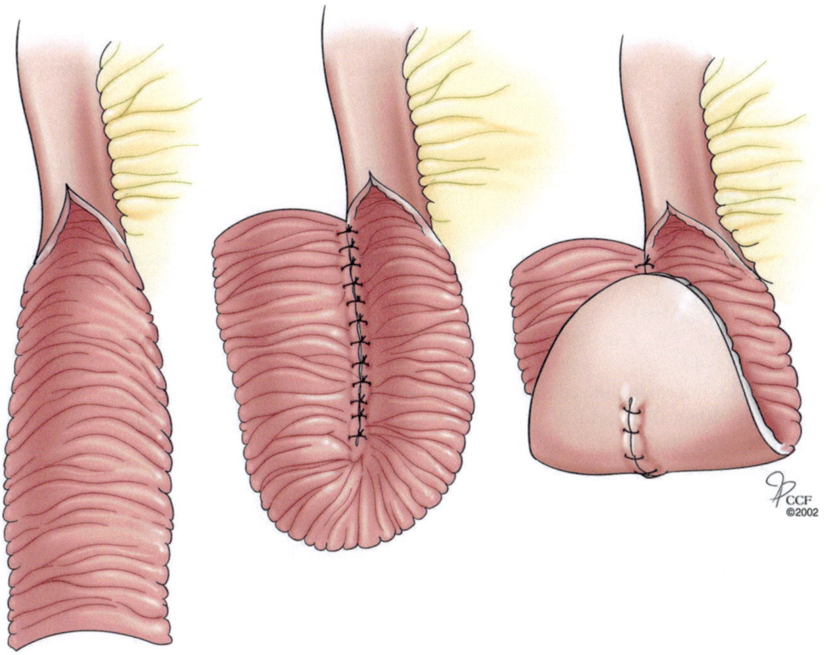

Fig. 179.13 The original continent ileostomy reported by Kock in 1969 contained two limbs with the distal ileum folded into a "U" shape. The intussuscepted nipple valve that is the hallmark of the modern continent ileostomy was a later development

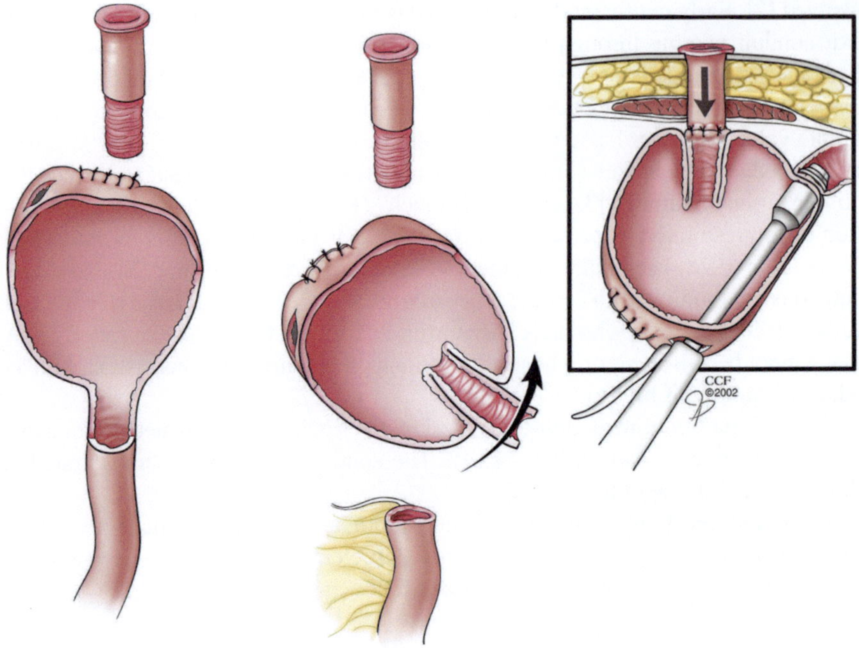

Fig. 179.14 Continent ileostomy nipple valve excision and pouch rotation: Left. The dysfunctioning nipple valve is excised; center. A new nipple valve is made from the afferent ileum. The pouch is rotated; right. the new nipple valve is attached to the abdominal wall, and intestinal continuity is restored

References

1. Kock NG. Intra-abdominal "Reservoir" in patients with permanent ileostomy. Preliminary observations on a procedure resulting in fecal "continence" in five ileostomy patients. Arch Surg. 1969;99:223–31.
2. Wu JS, Fazio VW. Continent ileostomy: Evolution of design. Clin Colon Rectal Surg. 2002;15:231–43.
3. Barnett WO. Improving the continent ileostomy. J Miss State Med Assoc. 1983;24:31–4.
4. Kaiser AM, Stein JP, Beart RW Jr. T-pouch: A new valve design for a continent ileostomy. Dis Colon Rectum. 2002;45:411–5.
5. Parks AG, Nicholls RJ. Proctocolectomy without ileostomy for ulcerative colitis. Br Med J. 1978;2(6130):85–8.
6. Aytac E, Ashburn J, Dietz DW. Is there still a role for continent ileostomy in the surgical treatment of inflammatory bowel disease? Inflamm Bowel Dis. 2014;20:2519–25.

Continent Ileostomy: Victor W. Fazio Concept Illustrations

180

Victor W. Fazio, Joyce M. Balliet, and James S. Wu

Presentation

The models for the illustrations created by Mr. Joe Pangrace were sketches drawn by Dr. Fazio on February 5, 2010. The original sketches of continent ileostomy creation were preserved by Ms. Joyce Balliet, photographer for the department of colon and rectal surgery and Dr. Fazio's assistant. Three are presented (Figs. 180.1, 180.2, and 180.3).

V. W. Fazio · J. M. Balliet · J. S. Wu (✉)
Department of Colon and Rectal Surgery, Cleveland Clinic, Cleveland, OH, USA

J. S. Wu, M. D. Inkster (eds.), *Cleveland Clinic Colorectal Case Studies*,
https://doi.org/10.1007/978-3-031-39880-3_180

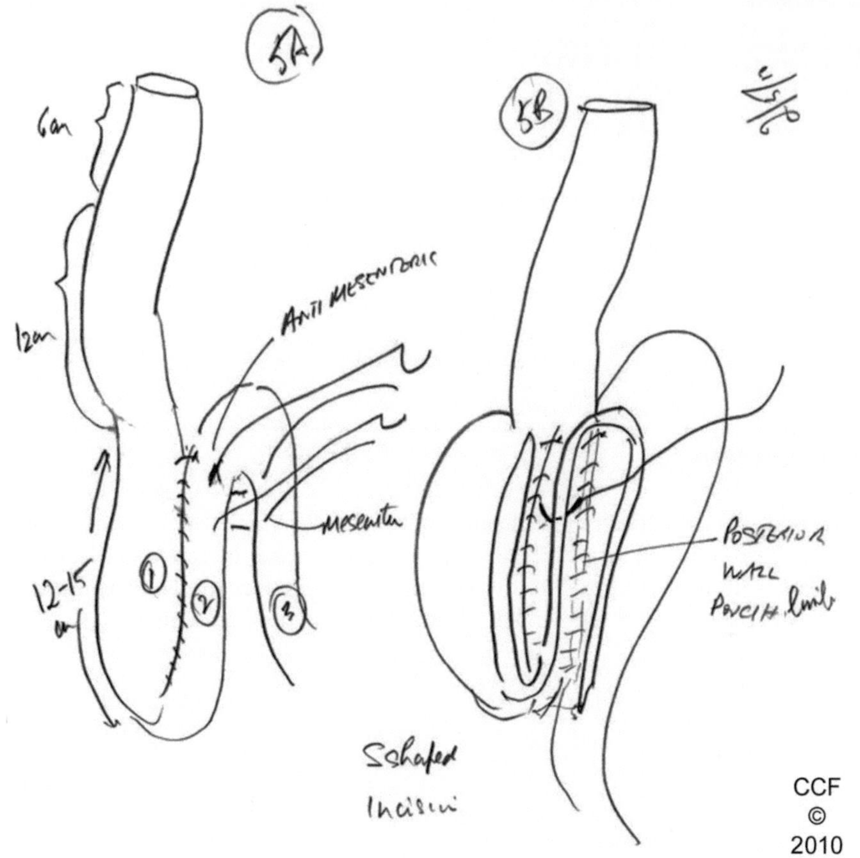

Fig. 180.1 (**a**) The terminal ileum is arranged in anticipation of "S" pouch creation. The terminal 6 cm of ileum connects the pouch to the skin. The adjacent 12 cm will be intussuscepted to create a nipple valve. The next three 12–15 cm lengths of ileum will serve as the limbs of the "S" pouch. The limbs are secured together with sutures placed at the antimesenteric border. (**b**) A "S" shaped incision is made on the antimesenteric border of the three pouch limbs. The posterior wall of the "S" pouch is created by sewing together the cut edges of the adjacent limbs of ileum

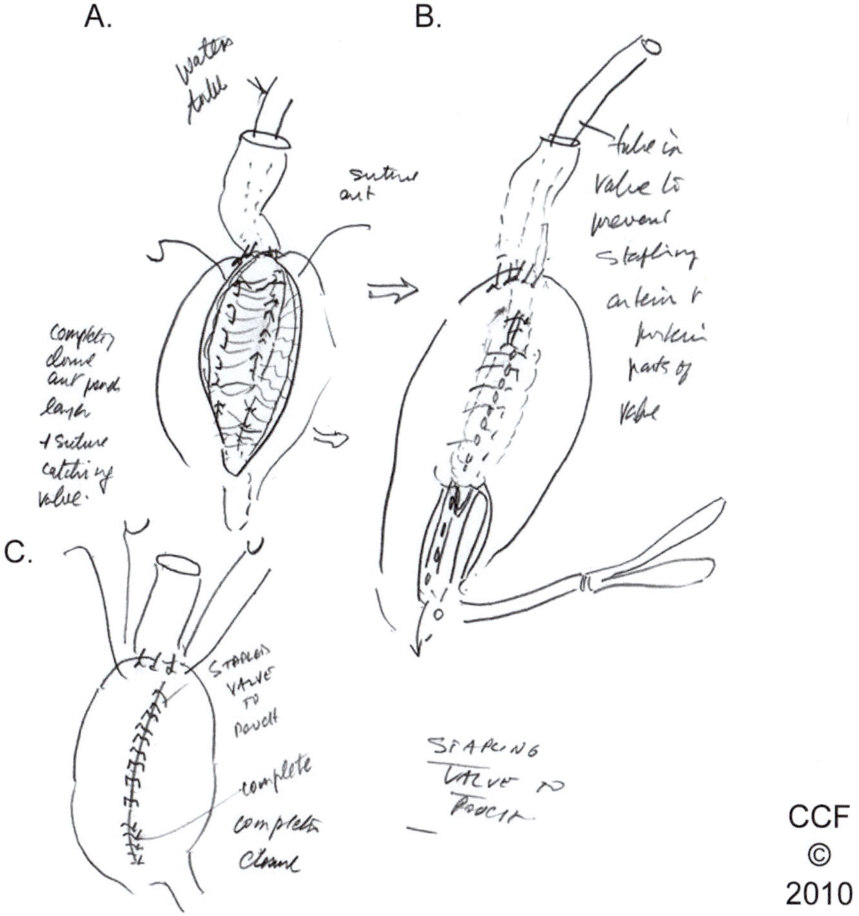

Fig. 180.2 (**a**) A straight continent ileostomy catheter (Water's tube) passes through the end of the ileum and the nipple valve into the incipient pouch. The nipple valve has been pexed bilaterally to the anterior opening of the pouch with running mattress sutures. Interrupted sutures that will close the pouch are placed; each one of these catches the nipple valve. The neck of the pouch is stitched to the ileum that connects the pouch to the skin. (**b**) Using a linear (noncutting) stapling device, the two walls of the nipple valve are stapled (1) to each other and (2) to the pouch. The straight continent ileostomy catheter prevents inadvertent stapling of the anterior and posterior parts of the valve together. (**c**) The completed continent ileostomy. The staples that secure the valve to the pouch are seen. Additional sutures complete the pouch closure

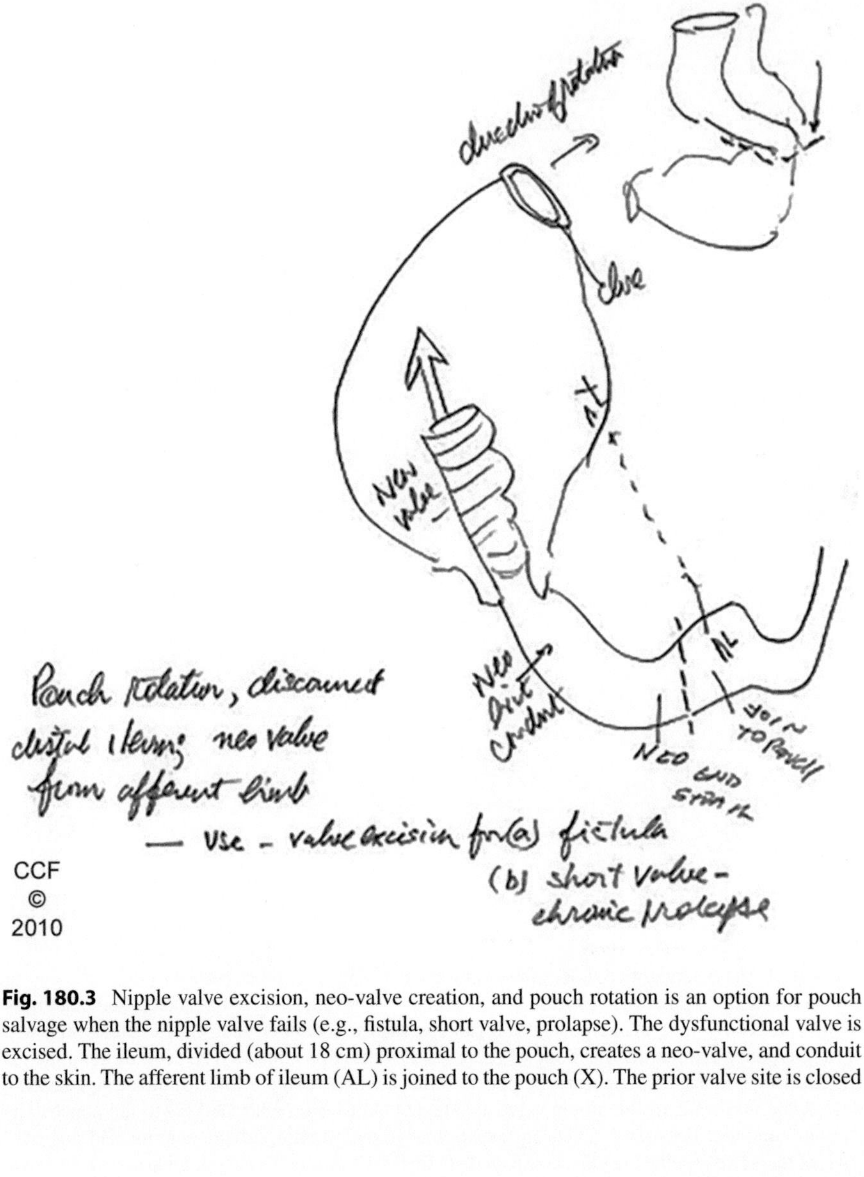

Fig. 180.3 Nipple valve excision, neo-valve creation, and pouch rotation is an option for pouch salvage when the nipple valve fails (e.g., fistula, short valve, prolapse). The dysfunctional valve is excised. The ileum, divided (about 18 cm) proximal to the pouch, creates a neo-valve, and conduit to the skin. The afferent limb of ileum (AL) is joined to the pouch (X). The prior valve site is closed

181 Continent Ileostomy Construction Video

Victor W. Fazio, Joyce M. Balliet, Apollo A. Draco, and James S. Wu

Presentation Voiceover[1]

Continent ileostomy was described by Dr. Nils Kock in 1969 as an alternative to conventional ileostomy. Kock's original design was a two-limbed reservoir.

Intussusception of the ileum at the pouch exit created a nipple valve that provided continence. Presented in this video is a variant three-limbed S-pouch with nipple valve stabilization performed by Dr. Victor Fazio in 2010 (Video 181.1).

The procedure is divided into four stages:

1. S-pouch construction;
2. Nipple valve formation;
3. Valve stabilization; and
4. Pouch attachment to the abdominal wall with stoma maturation.

[1]This video was recorded by the Cleveland Clinic Art and Photography department in 2010. The sole copy of the silent video was brought to light by Ms. Joyce Balliet, photographer for the department of Colon and Rectal Surgery and Dr. Fazio's assistant. The voice over was done by James Wu. The complete version of the video was constructed by Mr. Apollo Draco. The final version of the video was given to the Cleveland Clinic. Permission to reuse this video was granted by Cleveland Clinic, Enterprise Creative Services.

Supplementary Information The online version contains supplementary material available at https://doi.org/10.1007/978-3-031-39880-3_181.

V. W. Fazio · J. M. Balliet · J. S. Wu (✉)
Department of Colon and Rectal Surgery, Cleveland Clinic, Cleveland, OH, USA

A. A. Draco
Information Technology Institute, Cleveland Clinic, Cleveland, OH, USA

J. S. Wu, M. D. Inkster (eds.), *Cleveland Clinic Colorectal Case Studies*,
https://doi.org/10.1007/978-3-031-39880-3_181

Stage 1: S-Pouch Construction

The terminal ileum is arranged into three segments that are destined to become the pouch, the nipple valve, and the conduit to the skin. The efferent limb of the distal-most segment is left free, while the proximal aspect is sutured to the remaining two segments with serosal stitches in an S-shape. The three pouch limbs are secured in apposition with sutures. A long antimesenteric enterostomy is made through the three apposed segments. The back wall of the pouch is constructed by joining the walls of the center limb with adjacent proximal and distal limbs.

Stage 2: Nipple Valve Formation

The efferent limb is intussuscepted back into the pouch, creating a 6–7 cm nipple valve. The most distal end of the efferent limb will become the conduit to the skin.

Stage 3: Nipple Valve Stabilization

The intussuscepted walls of the nipple valve are stapled to each other (away from the mesentery) to prevent valve desussception. The anterior wall of the pouch is closed with suture. Closure begins where the exit conduit leaves the pouch. As the anterior pouch wall is closed over the valve, sutures incorporate the antimesenteric aspect of the valve to secure it to the pouch wall. Care is taken to avoid full-thickness bites on the valve itself to avoid fistula formation. The suture line is stopped at the tip of the valve.

The nipple valve then is stapled to the pouch. Closure of the anterior pouch wall is completed with additional sutures. Interrupted sutures placed between the serosal aspects of the pouch apex and proximal exit conduit are intended to increase valve stability.

Stage 4: Pouch Attachment to the Abdominal Wall With Stoma Maturation

A Waters[2] tube catheter is passed through the exit conduit and into the completed pouch to confirm ease of intubation. With the afferent limb occluded, the pouch is filled with saline and air until tense, and the catheter is withdrawn. Suture lines are inspected for leaks, and the valve is tested for continence. The pouch is emptied by Waters tube reintubation.

[2] The Waters ileostomy tube used in this case is no longer commercially available. Ileostomy catheters currently available include the Medena™ Continent Catheter (https://torbot.com) and the K-Kath Flex catheter (https://www.marlenmfg.com.) Personal communication from Ms. Barbara J. Hocevar, MSN, RN, CWOCN and Ms. Chizu Sakai-Imoto, BSN, RN, CWOCN.

The stoma aperture is created at a previously marked site in the right lower quadrant. The pouch is placed beneath the stoma aperture, and its apex is secured to the underside of the abdominal wall at this site with sutures. The exit conduit is brought through the abdominal wall. A pelvic drain is placed, and the abdomen is closed. The stoma is matured flush with the skin. A Waters tube is placed through the stoma into the pouch and is secured to the skin with sutures.

Evolution of Pelvic Pouch Surgery

182

James S. Wu

Presentation

Restorative proctocolectomy was conceived as a way of maintaining the normal route of defecation for patients with ulcerative colitis (UC) and familial polyposis coli (FAP) following proctocolectomy as an alternative to end ileostomy. Selected milestones in this journey are cited.

Ravitch and Sabiston-Anal Ileostomy With Preservation of the Sphincter [1][1]

In 1947, Ravitch and Sabiston described anal ileostomy with preservation of the sphincter, a proposed operation in patients requiring total colectomy for benign lesions.

> "Multiple polypoid adenomatosis of the colon, or multiple polyposis, has been well established to be a familial disease, beginning with the report of Cripps…. Lockhart-Mummery states that in all such patients cancer will develop if they survive. The usually recommended surgical treatment is resection of the involved bowel, which often means a total colectomy and permanent ileostomy. A number of authors recommend fulguration of polyps in the area accessible to a sigmoidoscope and resection of the remainder of the colon with ileosigmoidoscopy. Lilienthal, Soper, Erdmann, Tom Jones…, and Lockhart-Mummery all have reported successful cases by this method. Stone and Rankin have also had such cases. However, in a good number of such patients cancer has been reported to

[1] This excerpt and Figure (Ravitch and Sabiston Fig. 4, this work Fig. 182.1) are reused with the generous permission from Mr. Spencer Dimmick, the Journal of the American College of Surgeons, formerly Surgery Gynecology & Obstetrics, September 20, 2021.

J. S. Wu (✉)
Department of Colon and Rectal Surgery, Cleveland Clinic, Cleveland, OH, USA

J. S. Wu, M. D. Inkster (eds.), *Cleveland Clinic Colorectal Case Studies*,
https://doi.org/10.1007/978-3-031-39880-3_182

develop subsequently in the remaining rectal segment. We have had such an experience in this hospital.

CASE REPORT

F. K., No. 100268, a white girl of 16 years, entered the Johns Hopkins Hospital September 29, 1936, complaining of abdominal cramps and diarrhea. Her father had died of cancer of the rectum at the age of 30…. Barium enema showed countless polyps in the entire length of the colon. Sigmoidoscopy showed innumerable small bleeding polyps of the entire rectum and lower sigmoid.

Total colectomy was considered and abandoned in favor of preservation of the rectum and treatment of the distal segment with cautery. A terminal ileostomy was performed December 1, 1936, and the colon subsequently resected in stages down to the rectosigmoid. All visible polyps were fulgurated proctoscopically on 9 occasions in November and December, 1937, until no more were seen. On December 31, 1937, an ileosigmoidostomy was performed after resection of 9 cm more of the sigmoid. This specimen contained numerous polyps. She was well thereafter, in the main, and able to work. February 9, 1945, she returned obstructed by a carcinoma of the rectum. February 21, 1945, an abdominoperineal resection with permanent ileostomy was performed. There was a large adenocarcinoma in the upper end of the rectum. The remainder of the rectal mucosa was covered by innumerable benign polyps.

She died October 18, 1945, in a convalescent home of progressive cachexia presumably due to metastases – 8 years after her rectal fulgurations.

Examination of the gross specimen, with myriads of polyps carpeting the rectum, indicates the small likelihood that any considerable number of such cases will be cured if a segment of involved bowel is left behind for topical treatment. The disease is preponderantly familial, and a genetic predisposition to polyp formation should be expected to persist in this mucosa, however often it is fulgurated, with malignant degeneration constantly threatening as long as the patient lives.

In short, multiple polypoid adenomatosis of the colon is a symptomatically troublesome condition with dangerous malignant potentialities. The only safe treatment is permanent eradication of the abnormal epithelium – that is, bowel resection.

In the experiments to be described the entire colon is resected, the sphincter preserved, and the ileum mobilized and sutured to the the anus."

Mark M. Ravitch, M.D. F.A.C.S., and David C. Sabiston, Jr., From the Surgical Hunterian Laboratory of the Department of Surgery, The Johns Hopkins University Balimore, Maryland"

Operation was done on 22 dogs. Although the operation was conceived in response to FAP, the authors recognized its application to ulcerative colitis and concluded that their operation "may prove a feasible method of avoiding a permanent abdominal ileostomy in the patients requiring total colectomy for benign lesions."

Figure 182.1 shows anal ileostomy in the canine model as illustrated by Ravitch and Sabiston. In 1948, Ravitch described anal ileostomy with sphincter preservation in two patients requiring total colectomy for ulcerative colitis [2].

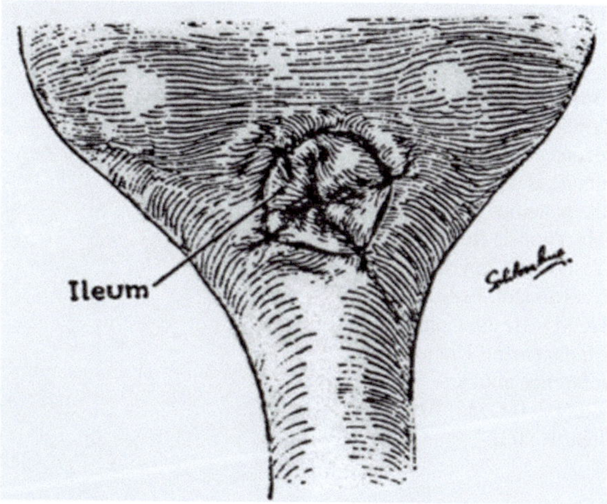

Fig. 182.1 Ravitch and Sabiston, 1947. Total colectomy with anal ileostomy and preservation of the sphincter in the canine model. The dog is positioned supine. The tail is located at 6'oclock. Reproduced with permission from the American College of Surgeons, formerly Surgery Gynecology & Obstetrics, September 20, 2021

Valiente, Rey, and Bacon–Pantaloon pouch [3][2]

In 1955, Valiente, Rey, and Bacon fashioned small intestinal reservoirs and performed pouch–anal anastomosis in dogs. They named the reservoirs, "pantaloon" pouches after small intestinal pouches made for gastric replacement [4].

> "This work deals with a proposed pull-through of the ileum through the anus with preservation of an intact sphincter mechanism, and a side-to-side ileoileostomy, the purpose of which is to establish a pouch which would serve as a reservoir for ileal contents. This pouch would obviate the almost constant need to evacuate the bowel content. The pouch is constructed in a similar manner as the technic used in the so-called "pantaloon" operation for cases of total gastrectomy. It is our belief that if an adequate pouch can be obtained and the sphincter mechanism can be preserved intact, it would be possible for these patients to retain the ileal contents enough so that only three or four bowel movements take place every day.
>
> TECHNICS APPLIED IN EXPERIMENTAL
>
> ANIMALS (DOGS)
>
> The colon and ileum are mobilized to the fullest possible extent both proximally and distally. A side-to-side ileoileostomy is performed for a total length of approximately 12 inches of the distal ileum, forming a pouch 6 inches in length after allowance for a loop long enough to reach the anus. This pouch has been constructed in three different ways; one in such a fashion that the bottom of the pouch points cephalad…, another in which the bottom of the pouch points caudad…, and the other in which a three-loop pouch is established. (Valiente Fig 5, this work Fig. 182.2).

[2]These excerpts are reused with the generous permission of Elsevier Inc., CCC | RightsLink®, License Number 5172870230644, License date Oct 20, 2021.

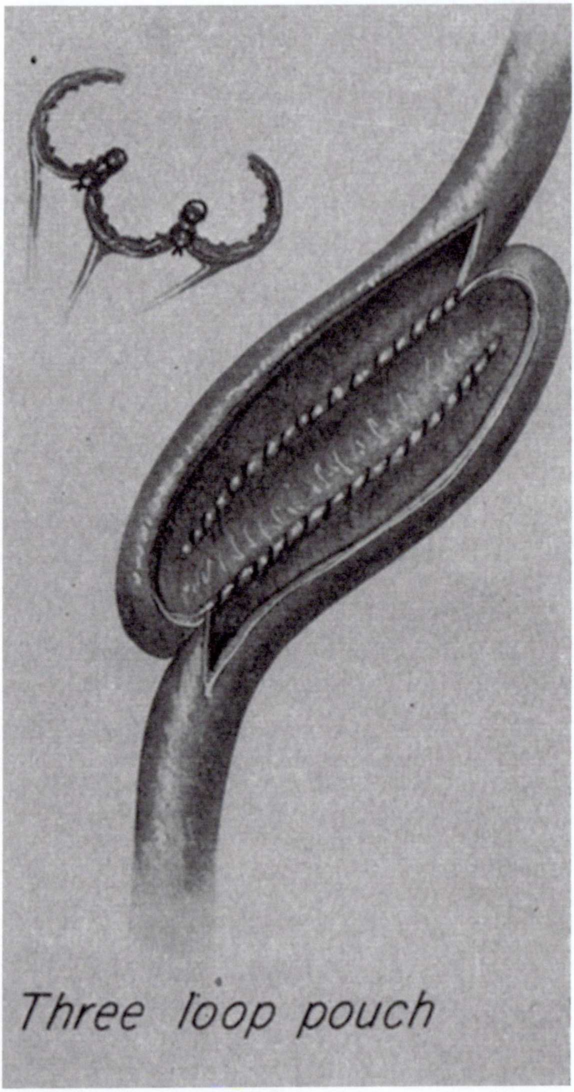

Fig. 182.2 Three loop "pantaloon" pouch devised by Valiente, Rey, and Bacon [3]. Bowel continuity was restored by ileoanal pull-through. This image is reproduced with the generous permission of Mr. Thomas Rexson Yesudoss, Copyrights Coordinator, ELSEVIER | HCM – Health Content Management, Unique reference number 220602–000635, Wed, June 1, 2022

The construction of a pouch utilizing the distal ileum has been employed experimentally in a series of seven dogs. Although five died, the results in two have been gratifying in that a satisfactory and adequate pouch was established, the sphincter control was preserved in its entirety, the number of stools decreased and their consistency became mushy to formed, while the perineal irritation was minimal. The capacity of this pouch to empty was been demonstrated by x-ray studies."

Miguel A. Valiente, M.D. (By Invitation), Hato Rey, Puerto Rico, and Harry E. Bacon, M.D. Philadelphia, Pennsylvania

In the discussion of this paper, Turnbull made the following comment:

"DISCUSSION

RUPERT B. TURNBULL (CLEVELAND, OHIO): I would like to commend the authors for trying to keep this dream of ileorectal anastomosis alive because I believe that somewhere in the future someone may perhaps solve this problem; and as the authors have stated in their work, it would be desirable to be able to remove the rectum and have intestinal continuity rather than a stoma on the abdomen. I think this is in the dream stage, however, at the present time".

Parks and Nicholls-Proctocolectomy Without Ileostomy for Ulcerative Colitis [5]

In 1978, Parks and Nicholls reported restorative proctocolectomy in patients with ulcerative colitis.

"Summary and conclusions

An operation has been developed that permits total removal of all disease-prone mucosa in ulcerative colitis but avoids the need for permanent ileostomy. The colon and upper half of the rectum are excised and the remaining inflamed mucosa is stripped from the rectal stump down to the dentate line of the anal canal. A pouch is fashioned from a triplicated loop of terminal ileum. This is drawn through the denuded rectum and an anastomosis created, via the per-anal approach, between the ileum just distal to the pouch and the mid-anal canal."

A. G. Parks, R. J. Nicholls St. Mark's Hospital and London Hospital London

In 1980, Utsunomiya et al. [6][3] described, Type B Procedure, in which a 20 cm ileal reservoir with a "J" shaped configuration, is pulled through a rectal muscular cuff denuded of mucosa. A temporary ileostomy was used (Fig. 182.3).

"Type B procedure: The point of the ileal loop which reaches the lowest level of the pelvis is selected and, at this point, usually about 20 to 30 cm from the ileal stump, a fine Nélaton catheter is placed through the mesentery for traction. The last main branches of the inferior mesenteric vessels are divided, and a slit is made in the avascular part of the mesentery. The ileocecal vessels are carefully preserved and the ileal loop extended about 10 cm. After the loop is fixed by a continuous seromuscular suture, a long side-to-side anastomosis is performed, using a GIA autosuture apparatus to create an ileal reservoir. By retracting the catheter at the apex of the loop, the reservoir is brought through the rectal cuff down to the anus.

From the perineal approach, the ileal loop is fixed to the internal sphincter by several (000) Dexon sutures, and the apex of the loop is incised by a longitudinal incision about 2 cm in length. The edge of the intestinal wall is sutured to the cut edge of the mucocutaneous junction and internal sphincter at the dentate line by interrupted sutures. The cuff is

[3]This excerpt is reused with the generous permission of Wolters Kluwer Health Inc., CCC |RightsLink®, License number 5173280499209; License date October 20, 2021.

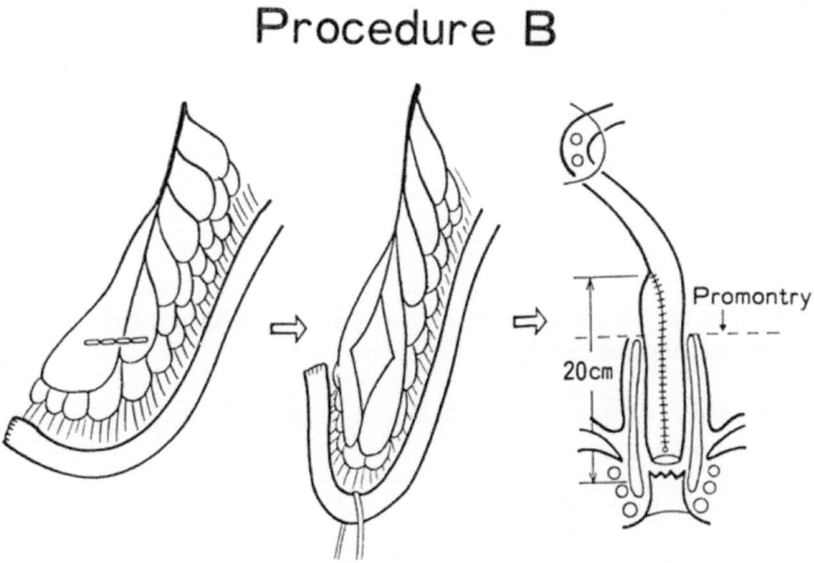

Fig. 182.3 "J-pouch" ileoanal anastomosis described by Utsunomiya in 1980. This illustration is reproduced with the generous permission of Wolters Kluwer Health, Inc., CCC | RightsLink®, License Number 5173280843258, License date October 20, 2021

> drained. From the abdomen, the rectal cuff is fixed to the pulled-through ileum by several interrupted sutures."
>
> J. Utsunomiya, M.D, T. Iwama M.D., M. Imajo, M.D., S. Matsuo, M.D., S. Sawai, M.D., K. Yaegashi, M.D., R. Hirayama, M.D.
> From the Second Department of Surgery and the Polyposis Center, Tokyo Medical and Dental University, Tokyo, Japan

Alternatively, the J-pouch is connected to the distal rectum without mucosal stripping by an end of rectum to J-pouch apex double-stapled anastomosis. This latter technique leaves a segment of inflamed columnar epithelium in place that requires surveillance for neoplasia (Fig. 182.4).

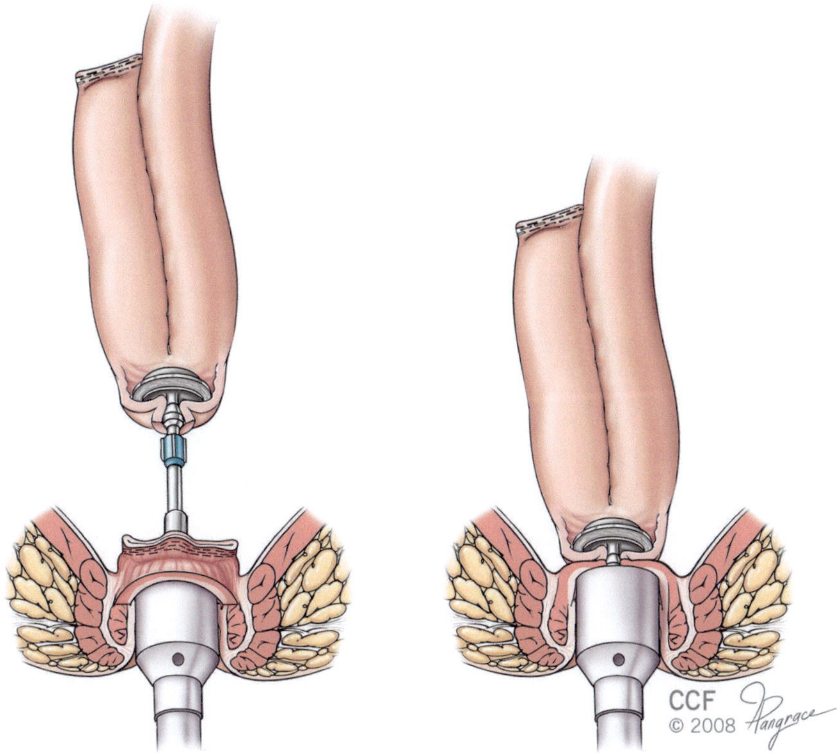

Fig. 182.4 Double-stapled end of rectum to J pouch apex anastomosis

References

1. Ravitch MM, Sabiston DC Jr. Anal ileostomy with preservation of the sphincter. Surg Gynecol Obstet. 1947;84:1095–9.
2. Ravitch MM. Anal ileostomy with sphincter preservation in patients requiring total colectomy for benign lesions. Surgery. 1948;24:170–87.
3. Valiente MA, Rey H, Bacon HE. Construction of pouch using "pantaloon" technic for pull-through of ileum following total colectomy: Report of experimental work and results. Am J Surg. 1955;90:742–50.
4. Hays RP. Anatomic and physiologic reconstruction following total gastrectomy by the use of a jejunal food pouch. Surg Forum. 1953;4:291–6.
5. Parks AG, Nicholls RJ. Proctocolectomy without ileostomy for ulcerative colitis. Br Med J. 1978;2(6130):85–8.
6. Utsunomiya J, Iwama T, Imajo M, Matsuo S, Sawai S, Yaegashi K, et al. Total colectomy mucosal proctectomy, ileoanal anastomosis. Dis Colon Rectum. 1980;23:459–66.

Ileal Pouch–Rectal Anastomosis

183

James S. Wu

Presentation

A 56-year-old female was referred for restorative proctocolectomy because of symptomatic chronic pan-ulcerative colitis with abdominal pain and colonic hemorrhage not improved by medical therapy. She had undergone prior subtotal colectomy. She was referred for completion proctosigmoidectomy and creation of a pelvic reservoir. This case shows photographs of selected steps involved in removal of the rectum for benign disease and resoration of bowel continuity by "J"-pouch to low rectal double-stapled anastomosis.

Completion Proctosigmoidectomy and Ileal Pouch Rectal Anastomosis

Step 1 Rectosigmoid Mobilization

Following mobilization, the sigmoid colon is moved anteriorly and caudally in order to expose the superior rectal artery (Fig. 183.1). The superior rectal artery is divided close to the rectum.

Step 2 Proctectomy

Following division of the superior rectal artery, gentle anterior traction is applied to the rectosigmoid in order to gain access to the presacral space. The rectum with its mesentery is separated from the sacrum by cautery dissection to the tip of the

J. S. Wu (✉)
Department of Colon and Rectal Surgery, Cleveland Clinic, Cleveland, OH, USA

J. S. Wu, M. D. Inkster (eds.), *Cleveland Clinic Colorectal Case Studies*,
https://doi.org/10.1007/978-3-031-39880-3_183

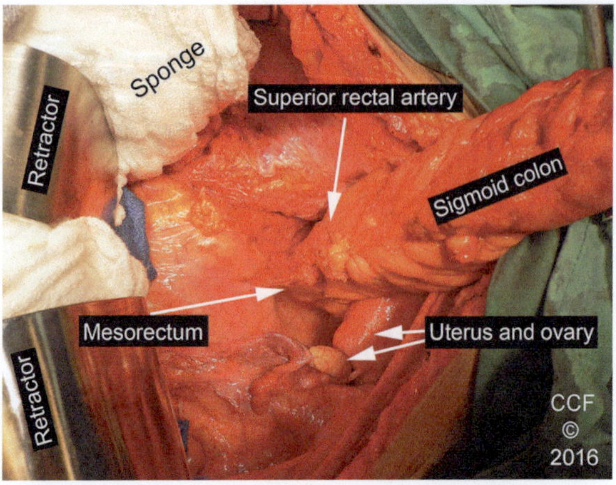

Fig. 183.1 Following mobilization, the sigmoid colon is moved anteriorly with gentle traction. The peritoneum is incised close to the rectosigmoid to expose the superior rectal artery which is divided. The uterus, ovary, mesorectum are labeled. The small intestine is kept out of the operative field by retractors and sponges

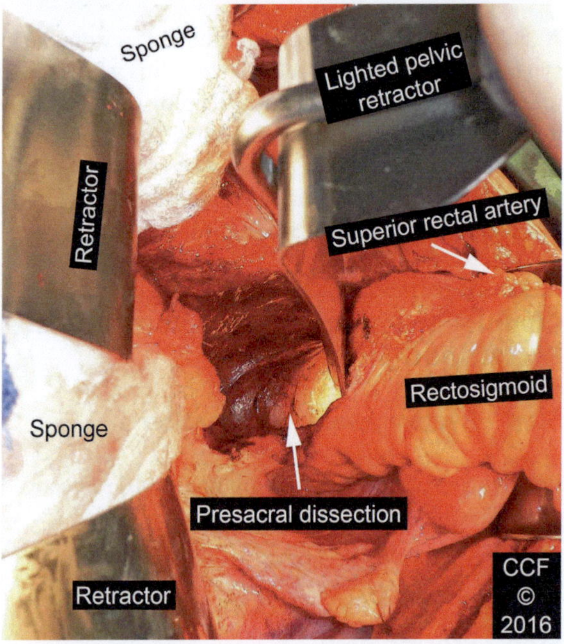

Fig. 183.2 Rectal mobilization begins posteriorly. The rectum with its mesentery is raised from the sacrum. The presacral plane of dissection is demonstrated by anterior rectosigmoid traction, in this case, aided by a straight lighted pelvic retractor. The dissection is done sharply or with cautery under direct vision to the coccyx and the levator ani muscles. The presacral fascia is not disturbed. The superior rectal artery (ligated close to the rectum), rectosigmoid colon, retractors and sponges are identified

coccyx (Fig. 183.2). Next the lateral attachments of the rectum to the pelvis (lateral stalks) are divided (Fig. 183.3 and Fig 183.4). Finally, the anterior connection of the rectum to the vagina is done sharply under direct vision, facilitated by applying posterior traction to the rectum and anterior countertraction to the vagina (Fig. 183.5). The distal rectum then is divided just above the levator ani muscles with a linear stapling device.

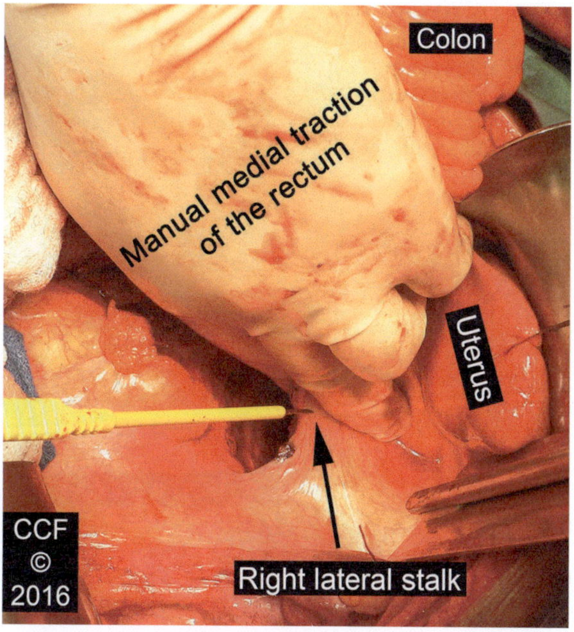

Fig. 183.3 Following posterior rectal mobilization, the lateral stalks are divided close to the rectum. In this figure, medial traction is applied to the rectosigmoid to show the line of division of the right lateral stalk. The colon and uterus are labeled

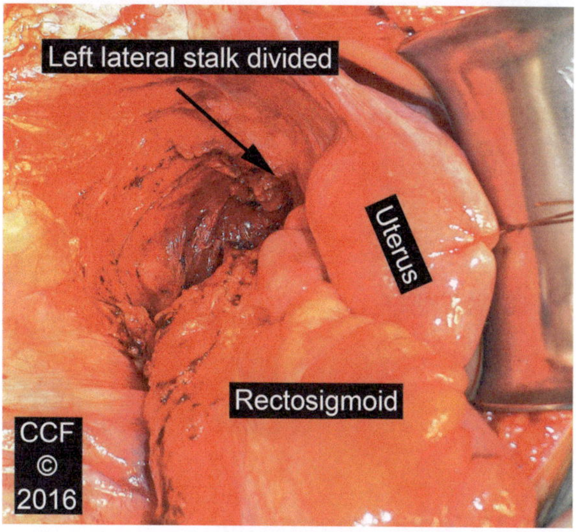

Fig. 183.4 The rectum after division of the left lateral stalk is shown

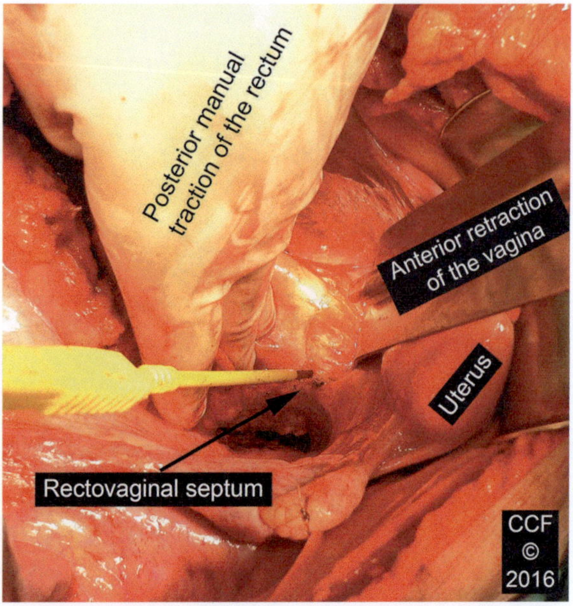

Fig. 183.5 Posterior traction is applied to the rectum while counter traction is applied to the vagina to expose the rectovaginal septum for dissection

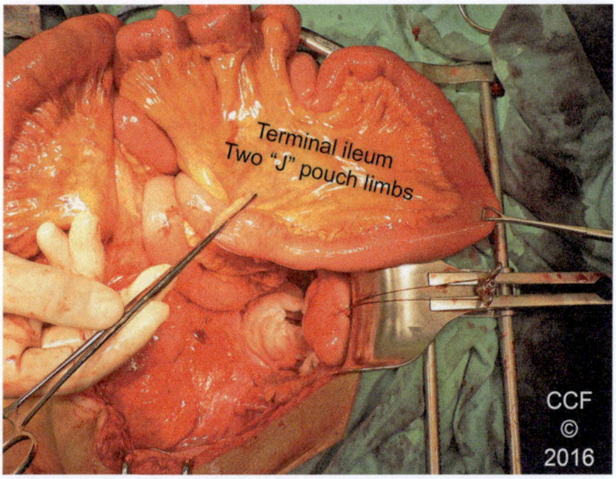

Fig. 183.6 A "J"-pouch is constructed from two 20 cm limbs of terminal ileum. The apex of the pouch is identified by a Babcock clamp. An intestinal clamp marks the end of the ileum

Step 3 "J" pouch construction

The "J" pouch is made from the distal 40 cm of ileum (Fig. 183.6). An enterotomy is made at 20 cm from the end of the ileum. A side-to-side enterostomy is made between the two 20 cm limbs of ileum using a gastrointestinal (GIA) stapler (Fig. 187.7). The pouch is then tested for leaks (Fig. 183.8). The apex of the "J"pouch is afixed with the anvil of a 31 mm end-to-anastomosis (EEA) circular stapler. The distal ileum is closed with a linear stapler (Fig. 183.9).

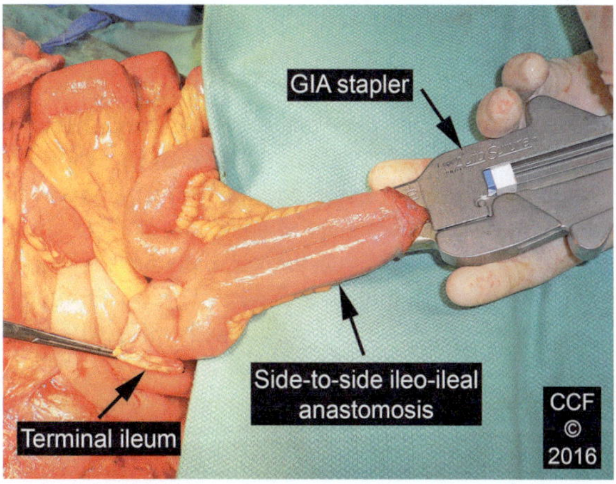

Fig. 183.7 The "J" pouch is created by side-side enteroenterostomy using two or more passes of a gastrointestinal (GIA) stapler. The mesentery is kept clear of the stapling device. The end of the ileum is marked with an intestinal clamp

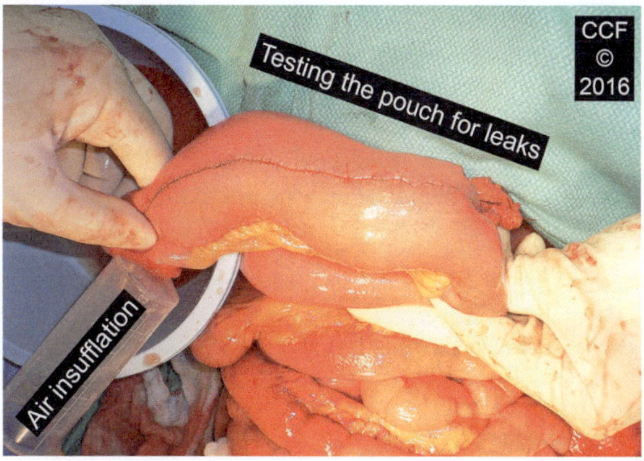

Fig. 183.8 The "J" pouch is tested for leaks. The terminal ileum proximal to the pouch and the pouch apex are closed between the thumbs and index fingers. Air is gently insufflated into the pouch through the end of the ileum

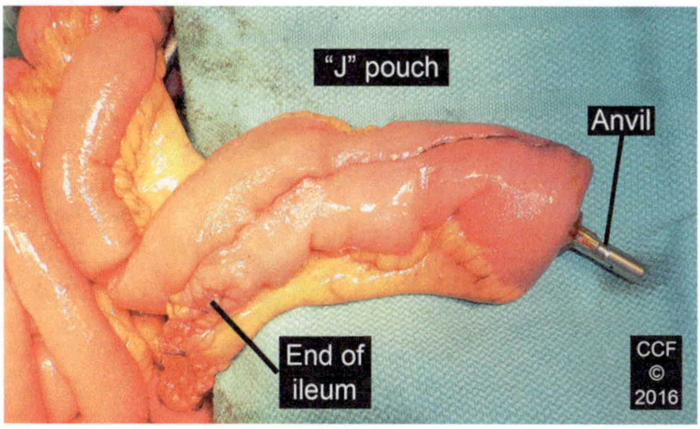

Fig. 183.9 The apex of the "J" pouch is fixed with the anvil of a circular stapling device. The end of the ileum is closed with a linear stapler

Step 4. "J" pouch to distal rectal anastomisis

The body of the circular stapler is passed into the distal rectum through the anus under direct vision. The spike of the stapler punctures the rectum posterior to the staple line (Fig. 183.10). The "J" pouch to rectal anastomosis (PRA) is made by attaching the pouch (afixed with the stapler anvil) to the body of the circular stapler and creating a double-stapled anastomosis. The anastomosis is made under direct vision making certain that the vagina is not incorporated (Fig. 183.11). Two complete anastomotic donuts are seen. The pouch-rectal anastomosis is checked for leaks by instilling air per anum with the small intestine proximal to the pouch occluded and the pelvis filled with saline.

The postoperative endoscopic images of the "J" pouch presented in this case are shown in Figs. 183.12 and 183.13.

The epithelial components of the columnar cuff, anal transitional zone, and ileal reservoir after stapled pouch-anal anastomosis was described by Thompson-Fawcett et al. [3] and Royston et al. [4]. As shown in Fig. 183.14, the ileal pouch is anastomosed to the columnar epithelium of the distal rectum. Distal to this, there is the anal transitional zone, the nonkeratinized squamous epithelium of the pecten, and the keratinized squamous epithelium of the perianal skin.

This case was entitled ileal pouch-rectal anastomosis since the pelvic pouch was anastomosed to the distal rectum, not to the anus.

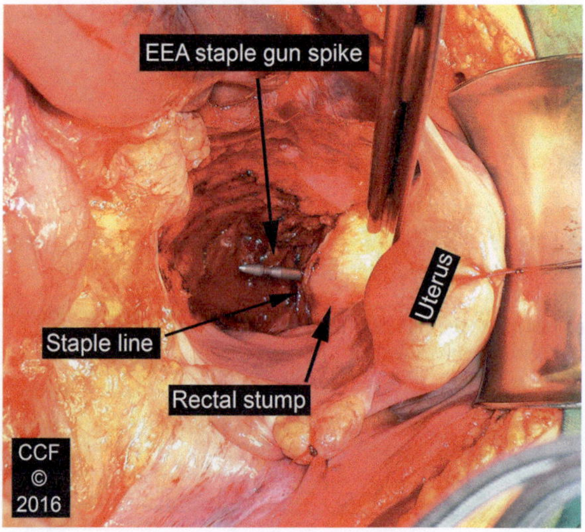

Fig. 183.10 With the body of the circular stapler inserted into the rectum, the spike of the stapler punctures the rectum posterior to the staple line at the site of rectal transection in order to keep the anastomosis away from the vagina. The uterus is labeled

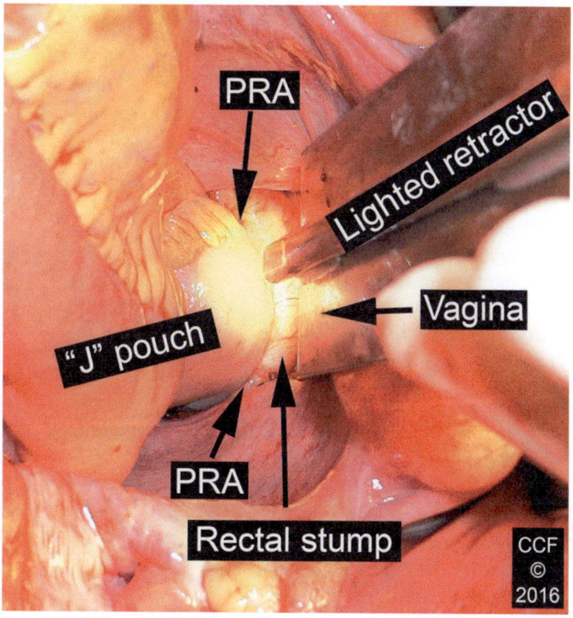

Fig. 183.11 The "J" pouch to rectal stump anastomosis (PRA) is made by the double-stapled technique. The lighted retractor keeps the vagina away from the anastomosis

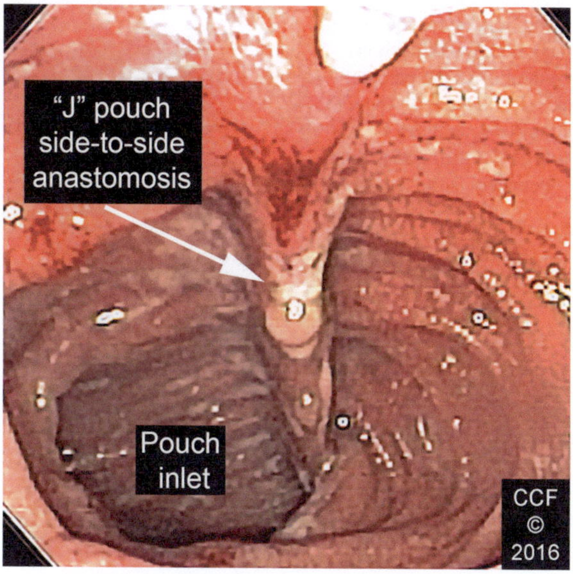

Fig. 183.12 *En face* endoscopic view of the pelvic pouch nine years after its creation. The side-to-side anastomosis within the pouch is seen in the center of the photograph. The pouch inlet is widely patent

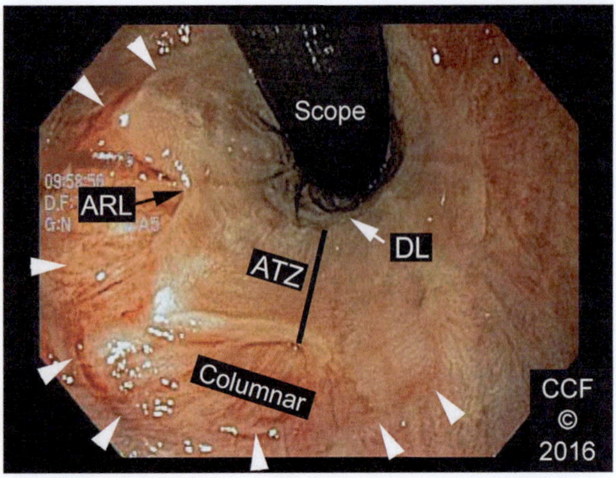

Fig. 183.13 Retroflexed view of the ileal pouch nine years after its creation. The staple line is marked by the white arrowheads. Between the staple line and the anorectal line (ARL) is columnar epithelium of the distal rectum. Between the ARL and the dentate line (DL) is the anal transitional zone (ATZ). The endoscope is labeled [1, 2]

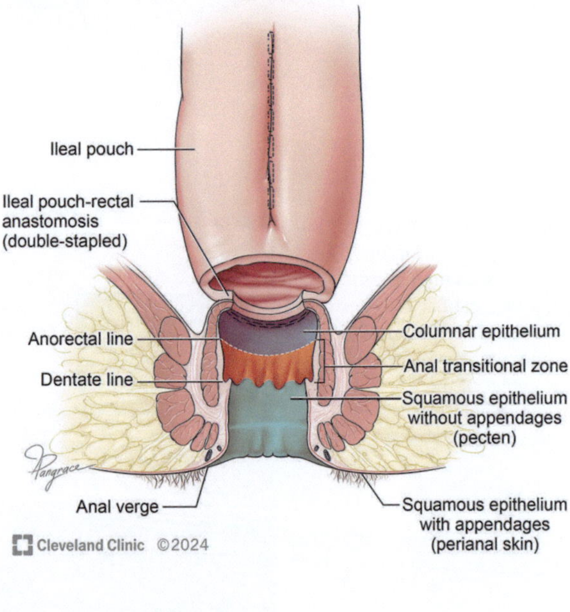

Fig. 183.14 Anatomy of the stapled ileal pouch-to-rectal anastomosis. The pouch is attached to the columnar epithelium of the rectum. The distal edge of the columnar epithelium is fused with the ATZ. Distal to the ATZ is the nonkeratinized squamous epithelium of the pecten, and the keratinized squamous epithelium of the perianal skin. The border between the stratified squamous epithelium with and without appendages is the anal verge

References

1. Herrmann G. Sur la structure et le développement de la muqueuse anale. J Anat Physiol. 1880;xvi:434–72.
2. Herrmann G, Desfosses L. Sur la muqueuse de la région cloacale de rectum. Comp Rendu Hebdo Séances Acad Sci. 1880;90:1301–2.
3. Thompson-Fawcett MW, Mortensen NJMcC, Warren BF. "Cuffitis" and inflammatory changes in the columnar cuff, anal transitional zone, and ileal reservoir after stapled pouch-anal anastomosis. Dis Colon Rectum. 1999;42:348–55.
4. Royston DJ, Warren BF. Are we reporting ileal pouch biopsies correctly? Colorectal Dis. 2011;13:1285–9.

Colorectal Cancer in Ulcerative Colitis

184

James S. Wu

Presentation

A 45 year old female who has a history of ulcerative colitis underwent colon evaluation. Barium enema showed a featureless colon with "burned-out" colitis. A persistent narrowing was seen in the region of the hepatic flexure (Fig. 184.1). At colonoscopy, the lumen was mostly devoid of mucosa (Fig. 184.2). At the hepatic flexure, a fungating carcinoma was found (Fig 184.3). The entire colon and rectum were removed (Fig. 184.4).

J. S. Wu (✉)
Department of Colon and Rectal Surgery, Cleveland Clinic, Cleveland, OH, USA

J. S. Wu, M. D. Inkster (eds.), *Cleveland Clinic Colorectal Case Studies*,
https://doi.org/10.1007/978-3-031-39880-3_184

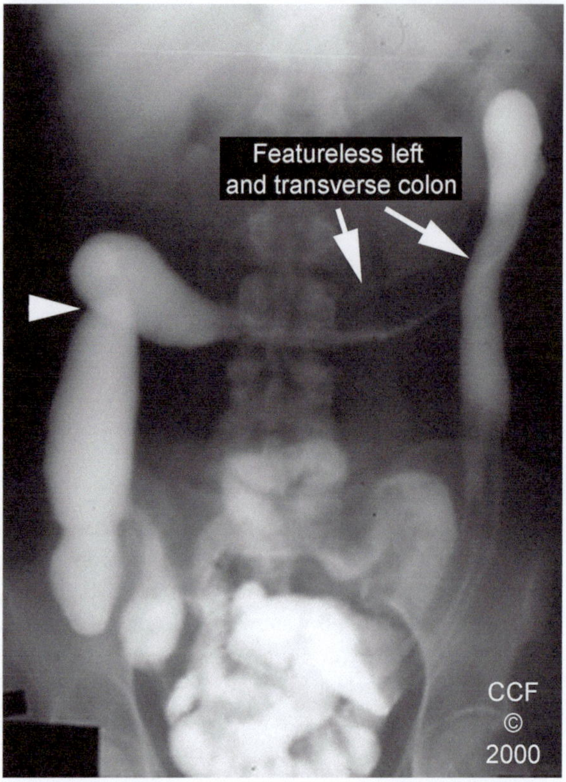

Fig. 184.1 Ulcerative colitis: barium enema shows a featureless descending and transverse colon without normal haustral markings. A fixed stricture was seen at the hepatic flexure (arrowhead)

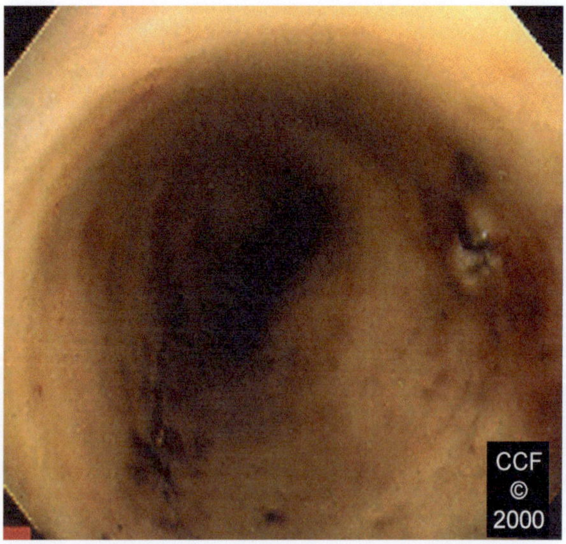

Fig. 184.2 Ulcerative colitis. The entire mucosal lining has been lost leaving exposed muscularis

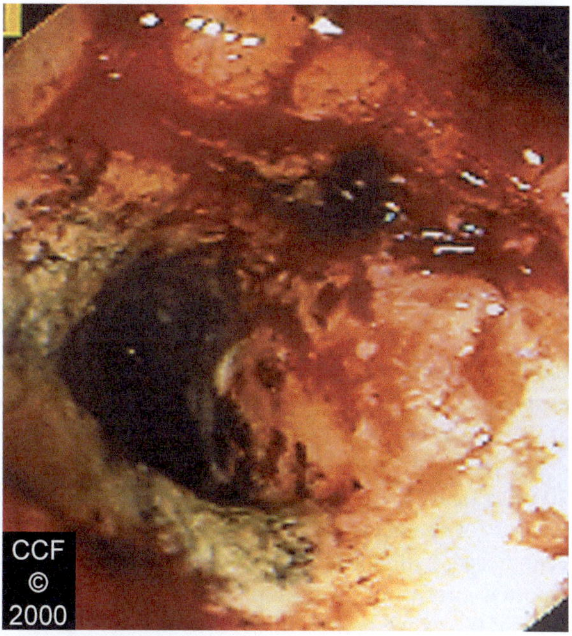

Fig. 184.3 Ulcerative colitis. Near obstructing hepatic flexure cancer

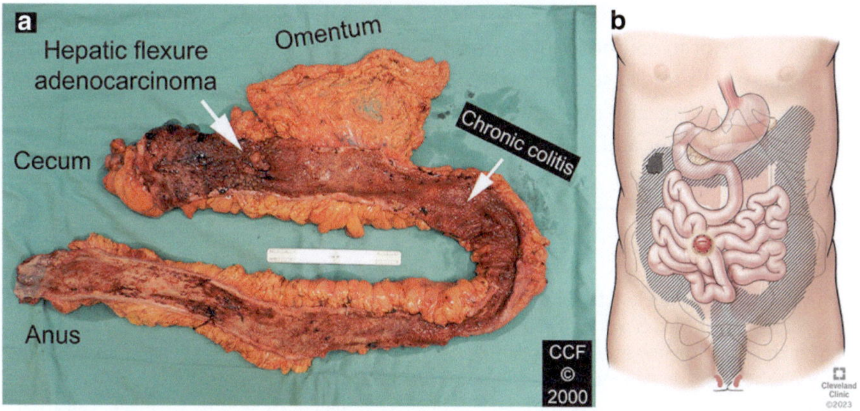

Fig. 184.4 (**a**) Proctocolectomy specimen. A hepatic flexure cancer is seen (white arrow). The entire colon and rectal mucosa was involved with chronic colitis. The cecum, omentum and anus are labelled; (**b**) Illustration showing the hepatic flexure cancer and the excised colon and rectum (total proctocolectomy with intersphincteric removal of the anus). A permanent end ileostomy is shown

Comment

Chronic Ulcerative colitis

"During the years 1921 to 1923 inclusive we have observed at the Mount Sinai Hospital a series of 29 cases.

…we have observed in 1 case a malignant degeneration of the late stage of a polypoid ulcerative colitis, with the frank occurrence of a carcinoma of the rectal wall. In brief, this was a case of a nonspecific ulcerative lesion of the colon, fourteen years or more in duration.…The sigmoidoscopic examination revealed an extensive polypoid colitis, in addition to which one observed on the left lateral wall of the rectal ampulla, growing in a mass of polyp-like excrescences, an ulcerating massive neoplasm. Sections removed for histologic examination showed the presence of adenocarcinoma."

Burrill B. Crohn, M.D. and Herman Rosenberg, M.D.
From the Medical Department
Mount Sinai Hospital
New York, 1925 [1]

Since this report, the increased risk of colorectal cancer faced by patients with ulcerative colitis has been documented [2, 3]. In a meta-analysis of 116 studies looking at the risk of colorectal cancer in ulcerative colitis, Eaden et al. [4] reported incidence rates corresponding to cumulative probabilities of 2% by 10 years, 8% by 20 years, and 18% by 30 years (irrespective of disease extent). Additional risk factors for colorectal cancer in ulcerative colitis have been recognized. Strictures, both benign and malignant, occur in ulcerative colitis. Goulston and McGovern [5] reported a series of 19 examples of benign stricture of the colon in patients with chronic ulcerative colitis. In 1992, Gumaste, Sachar, and Greenstein reported that 59 of 1156 ulcerative colitis patients (5%) developed 70 separate colorectal strictures. Seventeen of the 70 strictures (24%) proved to be malignant and the other 53 benign [6]. Prior to colonoscopy, barium enema was the primary method of examining the colon. In this case, barium enema showed a fixed narrowing at the hepatic flexure; subsequent colonoscopy revealed the cancer. Proctocolectomy was done to remove the cancer and the entire diseased large intestine.

References

1. Crohn BB, Rosenberg H. The sigmoidoscopic picture of chronic ulcerative colitis (nonspecific). Am J Med Sci. 1925;170:220–8.
2. Munkholm P. Review article: the incidence and prevalence of colorectal cancer in inflammatory bowel disease. Aliment Pharm Ther. 2003;18(Suppl. 2):1–5.
3. Lakatos PL, Lakatos L. Risk for colorectal cancer in ulcerative colitis: Changes, causes and management strategies. World J Gastroenterol. 2008;14:3937–47.
4. Eaden JA, Abrams KR, Mayberry JF. The risk of colorectal cancer in ulcerative colitis: a meta-analysis. Gut. 2001;48:526–35.
5. Goulston SMJ, McGovern VJ. The nature of benign strictures in ulcerative colitis. New Eng J Med. 1969;281:290–5.
6. Gumaste V, Sachar DB, Greenstein AJ. Benign and malignant colorectal strictures in ulcerative colitis. Gut. 1992;33:938–41.

Adenocarcinoma After Ileal Pelvic Pouch Surgery

185

Tracy L. Hull, Victor W. Fazio, Michelle D. Inkster, and James S. Wu

Presentation

A patient developed adenocarcinoma after ileal pouch surgery to treat chronic ulcerative colitis. The pouch, rectum, and anus were removed surgically. The operative specimen is shown in Fig. 185.1.

What would you call this cancer?

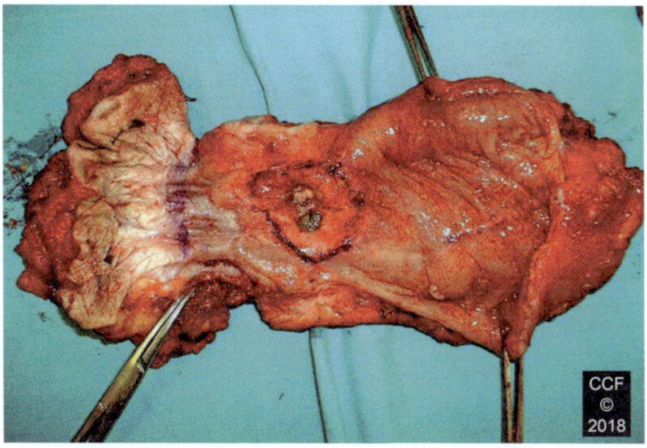

Fig. 185.1 Excised pelvic pouch. A cancer is circled with purple ink. A distal purple line marks the dentate line (courtesy Victor W. Fazio, AO, MS)

T. L. Hull · V. W. Fazio · J. S. Wu (✉)
Department of Colon and Rectal Surgery, Cleveland Clinic, Cleveland, OH, USA

M. D. Inkster
Department of Gastroenterology, Cleveland Clinic, Cleveland, OH, USA

J. S. Wu, M. D. Inkster (eds.), *Cleveland Clinic Colorectal Case Studies*,
https://doi.org/10.1007/978-3-031-39880-3_185

Comment

Dysplasia and cancer following ileal pouch–anal anastomosis (IPAA) in patients with inflammatory bowel disease was reviewed by Liu et al. in 2011 [1]. The anatomical relations of a pouch to the rectal remnant and the anoderm following stapled anastomosis are shown in Fig. 185.2.

Proximal to the ATZ is the columnar epithelium of the rectum that is derived from the hind gut [2]. In 1987, Fenger published an extensive description of the ATZ [3]. The proximal border of the ATZ is the anorectal line described by Herrmann and Desfosses in 1880 [4]. The anorectal line defines the junction between the columnar epithelium of the colorectum and the ATZ epithelium [5]. The distal border of the ATZ is the pectinate or dentate line which is continuous with the pecten described by Stroud in 1896 [6]. Distal to the dentate line is nonkeratinized squamous epithelium without skin appendages. The anal verge marks the junction between squamous epithelium with and without appendages [7]. The perianal skin is keratinized squamous epithelium with skin appendages (apocrine glands, sweat glands, and hair follicles) [8]. The relation between the columnar epithelium, ATZ, and pecten is clearly demonstrated in the retroflex view of the rectum (Fig. 185.3).

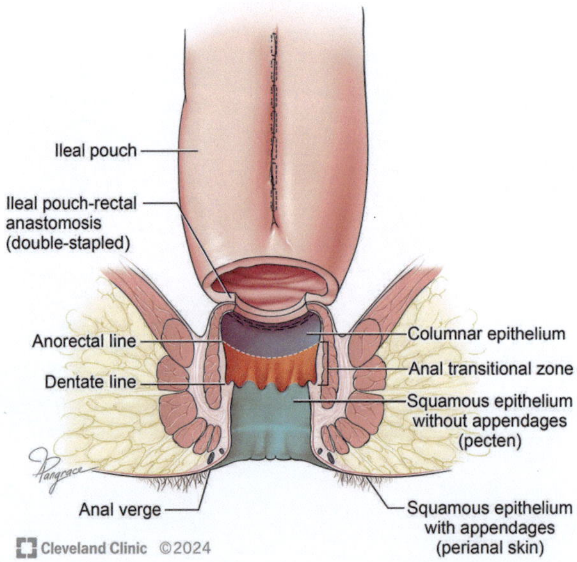

Fig. 185.2 Anatomy of an ileal pouch-rectal anastomosis (double-stapled). A two-limbed J-pouch is stapled to the rectum (columnar mucosa). The anorectal line marks the border between the columnar mucosa and the anal transitional zone. The borders of the anal transitional zone are the anorectal line proximally and the dentate line distally. Distal to the dentate line is the pecten (nonkeratinized squamous epithelium without appendages). The anal verge is the border between the pecten and the perianal skin (keratinized squamous epithelium with appendages, e.g., hair)

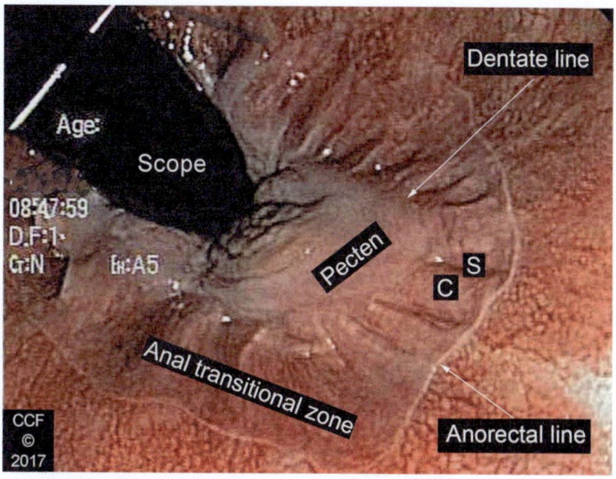

Fig. 185.3 On this colonoscopic anterior view, the anal transitional zone, pecten, and columns/sinuses of Morgagni (C/S) are seen on retroflexion with white light. Proximal to the anorectal line is columnar epithelium [9]

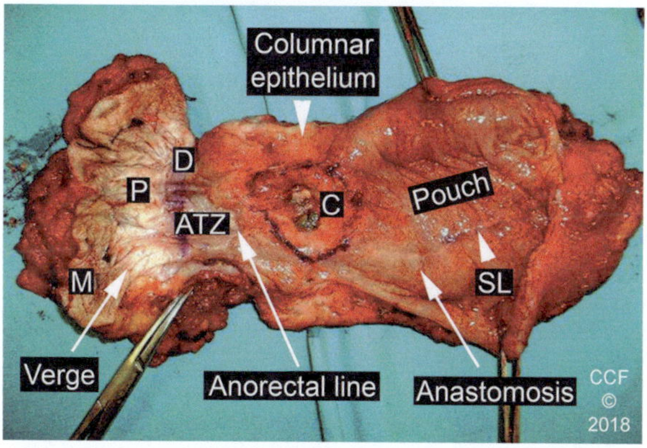

Fig. 185.4 Excised pelvic pouch with anatomic landmarks identified. The specimen consists of a pelvic pouch attached to the anorectum. The pouch is situated on the right side of the photograph; the pouch internal staple line (SL) is identified with an arrowhead. The anastomosis of the pouch to the rectum is marked with a long arrow. A cancer (C) is circled with purple ink in an area of columnar epithelium. The anal transitional zone (ATZ) is located between the anorectal line and the dentate line (D, purple line). Distal to the dentate line is the pecten (P). The pecten meets the skin of the perianal or anal margin (M) at the anal verge. This specimen was excised and marked by Dr. Victor W. Fazio

The importance of familiarity with the epithelial components of the anal canal, ATZ, columnar cuff, and ileal pouch following pelvic pouch surgery was emphasized both by Thompson-Fawcett et al. [10] and by Royston et al. [11].

In this case, the cancer in the excised specimen is located in the columnar epithelium of the rectum proximal to the ATZ and distal to the anastomosis of the rectum to the pouch. Therefore, this is a rectal cancer. It is not an ATZ cancer. It is not an ileal pouch cancer. The cancer arose in the generous amount of rectum retained at the original proctectomy. The anatomic landmarks of the excised pelvic pouch-anorectum with adenocarcinoma are shown in the labelled surgical specimen Fig. 185.4 and the accompanying medical illustration, Fig. 185.5.

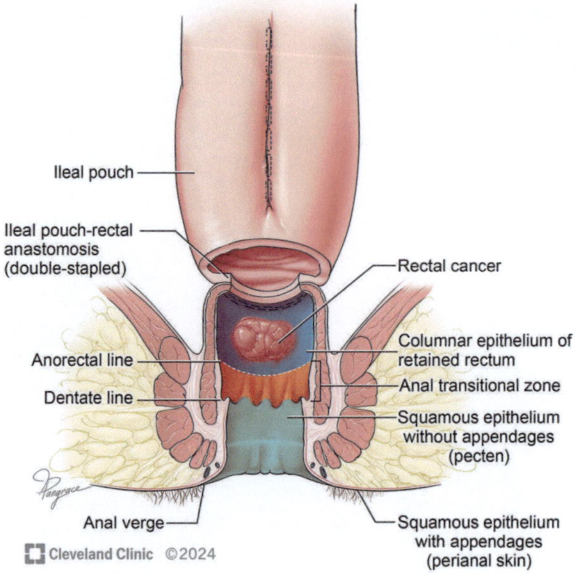

Fig. 185.5 The cancer in the excised specimen is located in the columnar epithelium of the rectum proximal to the ATZ and distal to the anastomosis of the rectum to the pouch. Pertinent anatomic landmarks (proximal to distal) include: the ileal pouch, Ileopouch-rectal anastomosis, rectal cancer, columnar epithelium of the retained rectum, anorectal line, anal transitional zone, dentate line, pecten, anal verge, and the perianal skin (a.k.a. anal margin)

References

1. Liu ZX, Kiran RP, Bennett AE, Ni RZ, Shen B. Diagnosis and management of dysplasia and cancer of the ileal pouch in patients with underlying inflammatory disease. Cancer. 2011;117:3081–92.
2. Moore KL, Persaud TVN. The anal canal. In: The Developing Human. Clinically Oriented Embryology. 8th ed. Philadelphia: Saunders Elsevier; 2008. p. 236–8.
3. Fenger C. The anal transitional zone. Acta Pathol Microbiol Immunol Scand. 1987;95(suppl 289):1–42.
4. Herrmann G, Desfosses L. Sur la muqueuse de la région cloacale du rectum. Compt Rendu Hebdo Séanc l'Acad Sci. 1880;90:1301–2.
5. Tanaka E, Noguchi T, Nagai K, Akashi Y, Kawahara K, Shimada T. Morphology of the epithelium of the lower rectum and the anal canal in the adult human. Med Mol Morphol. 2012;45:72–9.
6. Stroud BB. On the anatomy of the anus. Ann Surg. 1896;24:1–15.
7. Jabbour SK, Frassica D. Anal cancer. In: Haffty BG, Wilson LD, editors. Handbook of Radiation Oncology: Basic Principles and Clinic Protocols. Sudbury: Jones and Bartlett Publishers, LLC; 2009. p. 518.
8. American Cancer Society. What is anal cancer? [cited 2020 Feb 8]. https://www.cancer.org/cancer/anal-cancer/about/what-is-anal-cancer.html
9. Inkster MD, Wu JS. Detection of anal dysplasia by chromoendoscopy with narrow band imaging and acetic acid (NBIA) in 182 patients. Clin Surg. 2017;2:1583.
10. Thompson-Fawcett MW, Mortensen NJMcC, Warren BF. "Cuffitis" and inflammatory changes in the columnar cuff, anal transitional zone, and ileal reservoir after stapled pouch-anal anastomosis. Dis Colon Rectum. 1999;42:348–55.
11. Royston DJ, Warren BF. Are we reporting ileal pouch biopsies correctly? Colorectal Dis. 2011;13:1285–9.

Pouchoscopy: Double-Stapled J-Pouch to Rectum Anastomosis

186

James S. Wu

Presentation

A patient with ulcerative colitis underwent total proctocolectomy and reconstruction by double-stapled (DS) ileal J-pouch to rectum anastomosis. Following surgery, the patient entered a pouch surveillance program. Anatomic landmarks are illustrated in Fig. 186.1.

J. S. Wu (✉)
Department of Colon and Rectal Surgery, Cleveland Clinic, Cleveland, OH, USA

J. S. Wu, M. D. Inkster (eds.), *Cleveland Clinic Colorectal Case Studies*,
https://doi.org/10.1007/978-3-031-39880-3_186

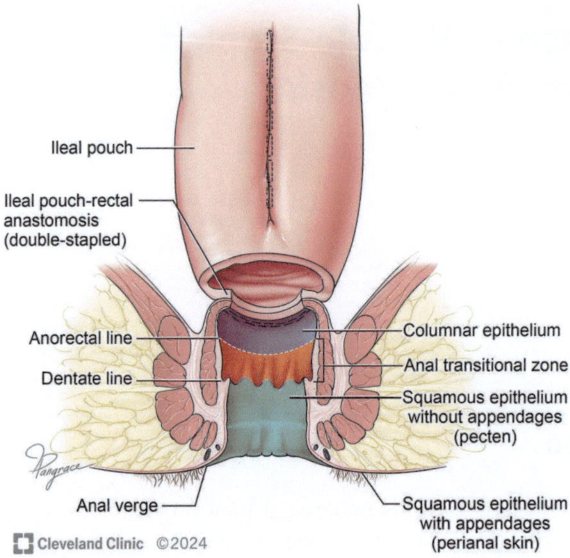

Fig. 186.1 Anatomic landmarks following DS ileal J-pouch to rectum anastomosis. The ileal J-pouch is anastomosed to the distal rectum (columnar mucosa). The anorectal line defines the proximal border of the anal transitional zone (ATZ). The distal border of the ATZ is the dentate line. Distal to the ATZ is the pecten (nonkeratinized squamous epithelium without appendages). The anal verge defines the border between the pecten and the perianal skin (keratinized squamous epithelium with appendages, e.g., hair)

Pouchoscopy

The perianal skin is inspected. The anus and the anastomosis between the rectum and the pouch is examined digitally. A fiberoptic gastroscope is introduced through the anus and advanced into the pouch. At the pouch apex, the closed end of the ileum (blind end) and the pouch communication with the proximal ileum (pouch inlet) are seen (Fig. 186.2a and b).

Mild inflammation is seen when the pouch mucosa is inspected first with white light and then with narrow band imaging (Fig. 186.3a and b).

On retroflexion, the circular shape of the anastomosis between the ileal pouch and the distal rectum is seen (Fig. 186.4).

On *en face* view, the circular shape of the anastomosis between the ileal pouch and the distal rectum is seen. The mucosa distal to the anastomosis is the columnar mucosa of the rectum (Fig. 186.5).

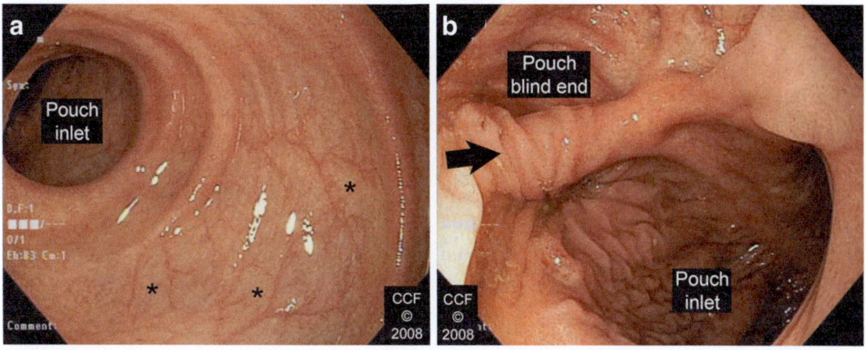

Fig. 186.2 View of the proximal end of the J-pouch. (**a**) The pouch inlet is widely patent. The ileal vascular architecture is visible (asterisks); (**b**) the closed, blind end of the pouch, and the pouch inlet (connecting the reservoir with the proximal ileum) are seen. The side-to-side entero-enterostomy is located beneath the intervening ridge (arrow)

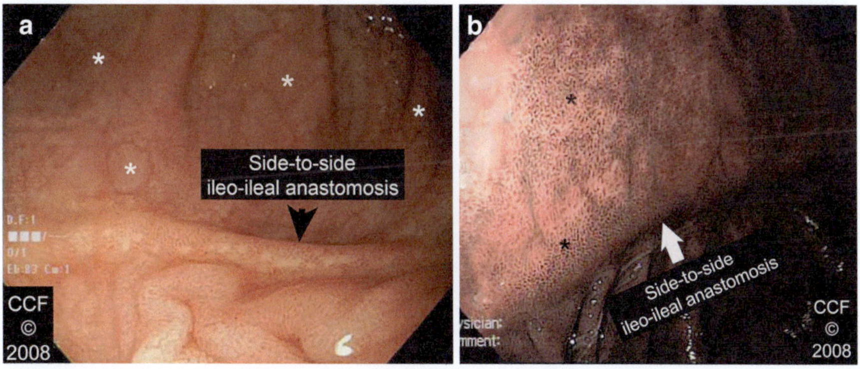

Fig. 186.3 Endoscopic view of the J-pouch body constructed by side-side ileal–ileal anastomosis (arrows). (**a**) Seen with white light, the vascular pattern of the pouch mucosa is visible (white asterisks); (**b**) seen with narrow banding imaging (where red appears black), increased vascularity (blackened mucosa, black asterisks) is seen. This appearance is consistent with mild inflammation

Distal to the rectal columnar mucosa is the ATZ, the pecten, and the perianal skin. The *en face* appearance of the pecten (nonkeratinized squamous epithelium without appendages) is shown in Fig. 186.6.

The *en face* view of the anal orifice with surrounding perianal skin is shown in Fig. 186.7.

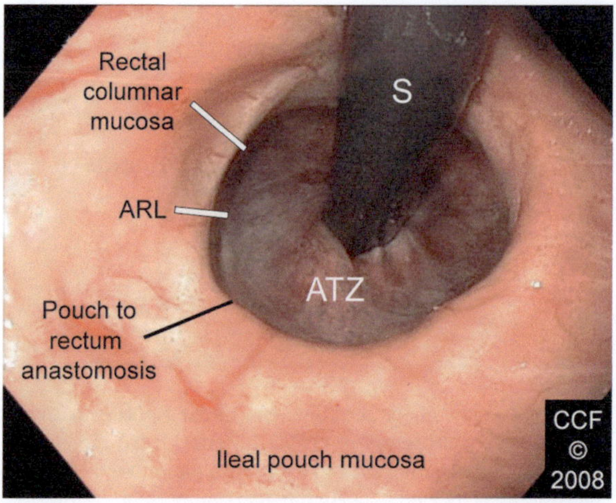

Fig. 186.4 Retroflexed view within the ileal pouch. The circular shape of the anastomosis between the ileal pouch and the distal rectum is seen (black line). Proximal to the anastomosis is the ileal pouch mucosa. Distal to the anastomosis is rectal columnar mucosa. The anorectal line (ARL) is the border between the rectal columnar mucosa and the anal transitional zone (ATZ). The endoscope is labeled with the letter S

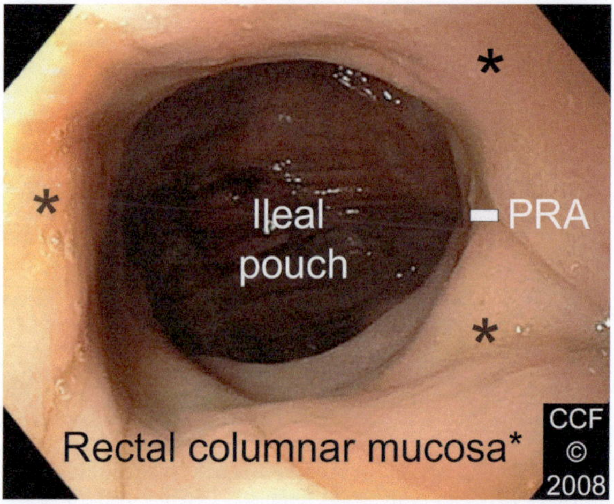

Fig. 186.5 *En face* view of the anorectum. The circular shape of the anastomosis between the ileal pouch and the distal rectum is seen (pouch to rectal anastomosis or PRA, white line). The rectal columnar mucosa distal to the anastomosis is identified with asterisks

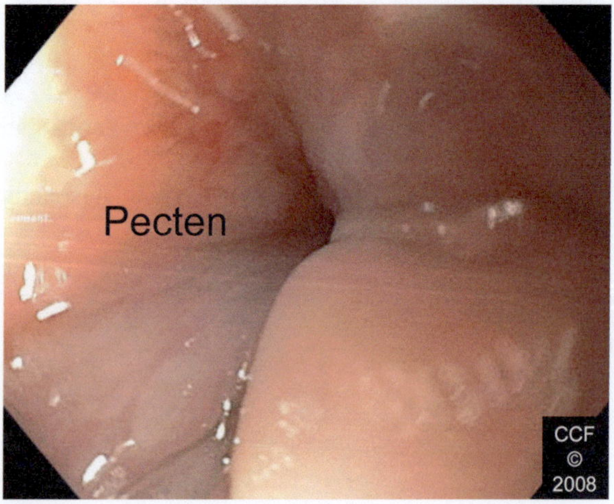

Fig. 186.6 The pecten, located distal to the ATZ, is nonkeratinized squamous mucosa without appendages (such as hair)

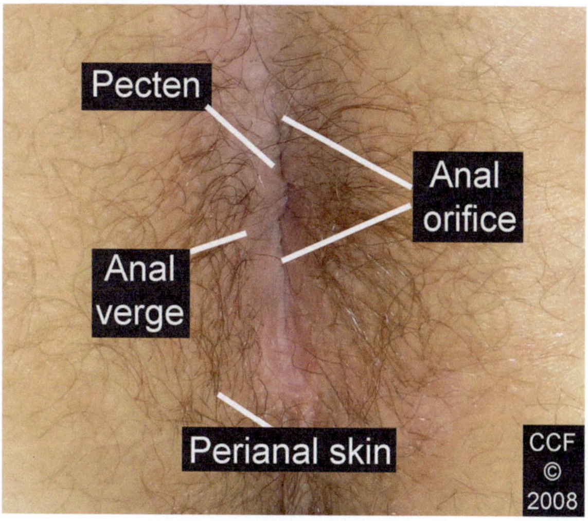

Fig. 186.7 The anal orifice is a midline slit. The perianal skin is keratinized stratified squamous epithelium with appendages (e.g. hair). The anal canal pecten is nonkeratinized stratified squamous epithelium without appendages. The anal verge is the junction between the perianal skin and the pecten

Comment

In this case, following proctocolectomy for ulcerative colitis, an ileal J-pouch was anastomosed to the distal rectum using the DS technique. Surveillance pouchoscopy provides information about anatomic structure, mucosal inflammation, anastomotic patency, and neoplastic change. Neoplasms arising in the small intestine proximal to the reservoir, the rectum, the anal transitional zone, the pecten, and the perianal skin can be seen and biopsied for histologic identification. In this case, mild inflammation was observed in the pouch. Adenomatous polyps may be found in, proximal to, and distal to the pelvic reservoirs of patients with familial adenomatous polyposis [1]. As shown in the preceding case, the rectal columnar mucosa retained after pouch to rectal anastomosis is at risk for the development of adenocarcinoma (See *Adenocarcinoma after ileal pouch surgery,* this work Chap. 185). The ATZ, pecten, and perianal squamous mucosa are at risk for the development of squamous intraepithelial lesions and anal squamous cell carcinoma [2].

References

1. New York Society of Colon and Rectal Surgeons Award at the annual meeting of the American Society of Colorectal Surgeons in Philadelphia, PA, June 26, 1997. Podium presentation. Wu JS, McGannon EA, Church JM. Ileopouch anal anastomosis does not reduce the need for endoscopic surveillance in patients with familial adenomatous polyposis. Dis Colon Rectum 1997;40(6)A4. Supervisor: James M. Church, MD. Full article: Wu JS, McGannon EA, Church JM. Incidence of neoplastic polyps in the ileal pouch of patients with familial adenomatous polyposis after restorative proctocolectomy. Dis Colon Rectum 1998;41:552–557.
2. Inkster MD, Szmulowicz UM, Wiland HO, Wu JS. Anal condyloma acuminata and anal dysplasia. In: Zutshi M, editor. Anorectal disease. Switzerland: Springer; 2016., Chapter 8. p. 189–209.

187 Anal Squamous Intraepithelial Lesion in Inflammatory Bowel Disease

James S. Wu and Eric W. Willis

Presentation

A 56-year-old man underwent subtotal colectomy with end ileostomy because of chronic large intestinal inflammatory bowel disease not responding to medical therapy. The rectum and distal sigmoid colon were left intact. Pathology showed moderate-to-severe colitis. Endoscopic examination of the rectum after surgery showed proctitis (Fig. 187.1).

Random biopsies were taken. A biopsy of the distal rectum showed squamocolumnar segment with at least high grade dysplasia, anal intraepithelial neoplasia, AIN 3, carcinoma cannot be excluded.

J. S. Wu (✉)
Department of Colon and Rectal Surgery, Cleveland Clinic, Cleveland, OH, USA

E. W. Willis
Department of Pathology, CORPath, Columbus, OH, USA

J. S. Wu, M. D. Inkster (eds.), *Cleveland Clinic Colorectal Case Studies*,
https://doi.org/10.1007/978-3-031-39880-3_187

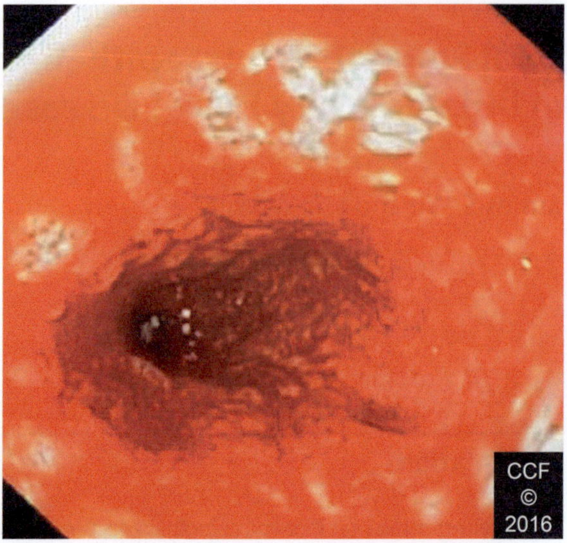

Fig. 187.1 Endoscopic appearance of the rectum after subtotal colectomy. The mucosa is inflamed

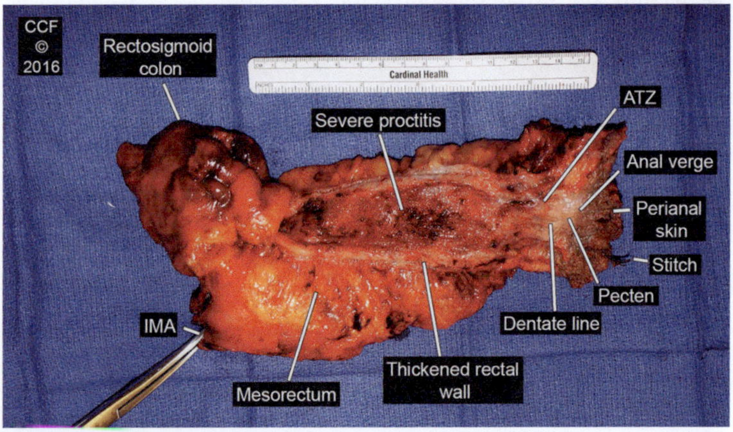

Fig. 187.2 Completion proctosigmoidectomy specimen. The inferior mesenteric artery is clamped. The rectosigmoid colon and mesorectum are labelled. Rectal wall thickening and severe proctitis are shown. Pertinent anal anatomic landmarks including the anal transitional zone (ATZ), dentate line, pecten, anal verge, and perianal skin are marked. The stitch used to close the anus at surgery is seen

Management

The patient underwent completion abdominoperineal resection (APR) with high ligation of the inferior mesenteric artery (IMA), total mesorectal excision (TME), and wide excision of the anus, levators ani and perianal skin (Fig. 187.2). The final diagnosis was anal intraepithelial neoplasia grade 3 (high-grade dysplasia/CIS); chronic active ulcerative colitis. Perirectal lymph nodes (14) were negative for malignancy (Fig. 187.3).

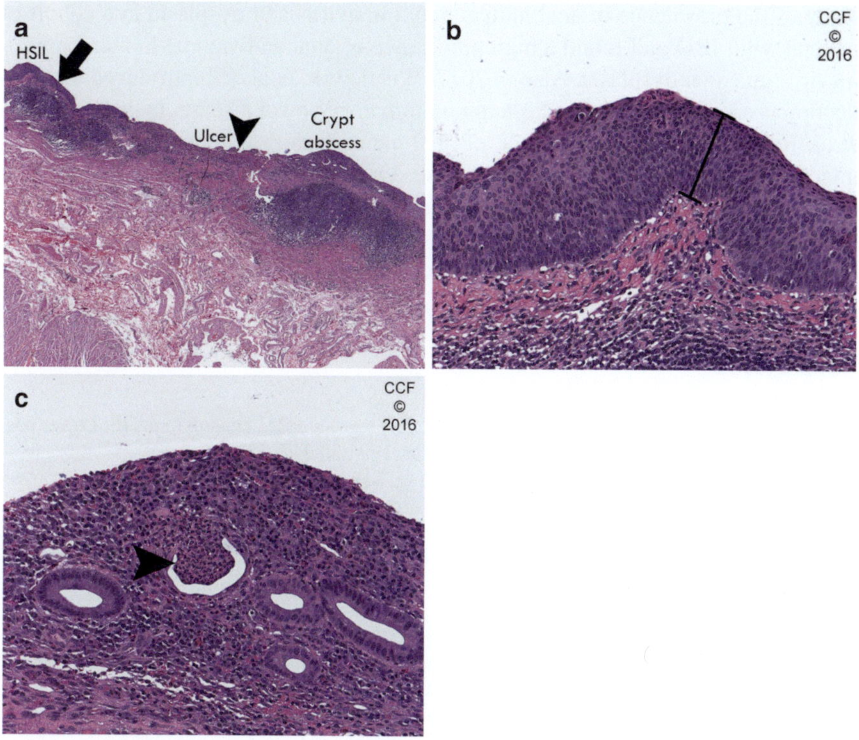

Fig. 187.3 (**a**) Low power view of the distal rectum and anus shows high-grade squamous intraepithelial lesion (HSIL) on the left (arrow), an ulcer in the middle (arrowhead), and a crypt abscess on the right, 20×; (**b**) high power view shows HSIL with hyperchromatic nuclei, increased nuclear-to-cytoplasmic ratio, and full-thickness (brackets) immaturity of the cytoplasm (200×); (**c**) active proctitis was present with cryptitis and crypt abscesses (arrowhead) [200×]

Comment

The original plan for this patient was completion proctosigmoidectomy and ileal pouch-rectal anastomosis. The plan was changed to completion proctosigmoidectomy and permanent end ileostomy because of the unexpected finding of HSIL (cannot exclude carcinoma) on anorectal biopsy. Aside from assessing the degree of columnar mucosal inflammation, endoscopic biopsies have traditionally also looked for dysplasia in the columnar epithelium [1]. Screening for anal dysplasia in patients with inflammatory bowel disease currently is not standard of care. Nevertheless, there is literature that shows an increased risk for anal SIL among inflammatory bowel disease patients. In 2010, Suneson et al. [2] found that Crohn's disease was strongly associated with increased risk for anal squamous cell carcinoma (SCC) with a standardized incidence ratio of 3.1. In 2016, Ruel et al. [3] found that SCCs, HSILs, and LSILs were identified, respectively, in six, nine, and two inflammatory bowel disease patients. In 2017, Cranston et al. [4] reported the results of a pilot study of the prevalence of anal human papillomavirus and dysplasia in a cohort of patients with IBD and found a high prevalence of anal and vaginal human papillomavirus and anal dysplasia. Also in 2017, Wisniewski et al. [5] introduced a classification proposal for anal dysplasia in inflammatory bowel disease. In 2018, Vuitton et al. [6] reported high prevalence of anal canal high-risk human papillomavirus infection in patients with Crohn's disease. One third of patients who underwent colonoscopy were found to have anal canal HPV infection. High ligation of the Inferior mesenteric artery and total mesorectal excision was done. The anus, levators and perianal skin were widely excised.

References

1. Connell WR, Sheffield JP, Kamm MA, Ritchie JK, Hawley PR, Lennard-Jones JE. Lower gastrointestinal malignancy in Crohn's disease. Gut. 1994;35:347–52.
2. Sunesen KG, Nørgaard M, Thorlacius-Ussing O, Lauerberg S. Immunosuppressive disorders and risk of anal squamous cell carcinoma: a nationwide cohort study in Denmark, 1978-2005. Int J Cancer. 2010;127:675–84.
3. Ruel J, Ko HM, Roda G, Patil N, Zhang D, Jharap B, et al. Anal neoplasia in inflammatory bowel disease is associated with HPV and perianal disease. Clin Transl Gastroenterol. 2016;7:e148.
4. Cranston RD, Regueiro M, Hashash J, Baker JR, Richardson-Harman N, Janocko L, et al. A pilot study of the prevalence of anal human papillomavirus and dysplasia in a cohort of patients with IBD. Dis Colon Rectum. 2017;60:1307–13.
5. Wisniewski A, Fléjou JF, Siproudhis L, Abramowitz L, Svrcek M, Beaugerie L. Anal neoplasia in inflammatory bowel disease: Classification proposal, epidemiology, carcinogenesis, and risk management perspectives. J Crohns Colitis. 2017;11:1011–8.
6. Vuitton L, Jacquin E, Parmentier AL, Crochet E, Fein F, Dupont-Gossat A-C, et al. High prevalence of anal canal high-risk human papillomavirus infection in patients with Crohn's disease. Clin Gastroenterol Hepatol. 2018;16:1768–76.

Terminal Ileitis

188

Michelle D. Inkster, Eric W. Willis, Andrei S. Purysko,
and James S. Wu

Presentation

A 37-year-old female presented with a 5-year history of progressively worsening abdominal pain and weight loss. The colon was endoscopically normal. A computed tomographic scan (CT) was obtained (Fig. 188.1). Treatment with steroids and mesalamine was not beneficial.

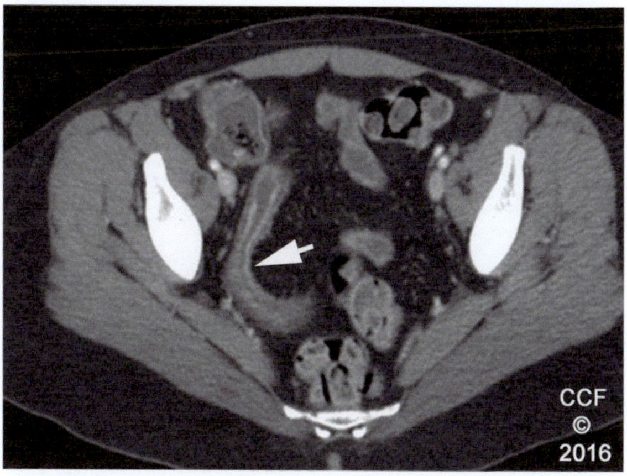

Fig. 188.1 CT enterography shows circumferential wall thickening and mucosal hyperemia of the terminal ileum. A long stricture is seen (arrow)

M. D. Inkster
Department of Gastroenterology, Cleveland Clinic, Cleveland, OH, USA

E. W. Willis
Department of Pathology, CORPath, Columbus, OH, USA

A. S. Purysko
Department of Diagnostic Radiology, Cleveland Clinic, Cleveland, OH, USA
e-mail: puryska@ccf.org

J. S. Wu (✉)
Department of Colon and Rectal Surgery, Cleveland Clinic, Cleveland, OH, USA

J. S. Wu, M. D. Inkster (eds.), *Cleveland Clinic Colorectal Case Studies*,
https://doi.org/10.1007/978-3-031-39880-3_188

Management

Ileocolic resection with neo-ileocolic anastomosis was done.

The specimen is shown in Fig. 188.2. Fat wrapping is associated with intraluminal narrowing (Fig. 188.3). Fat wrapping was consistent with terminal ileitis (Fig. 188.4).

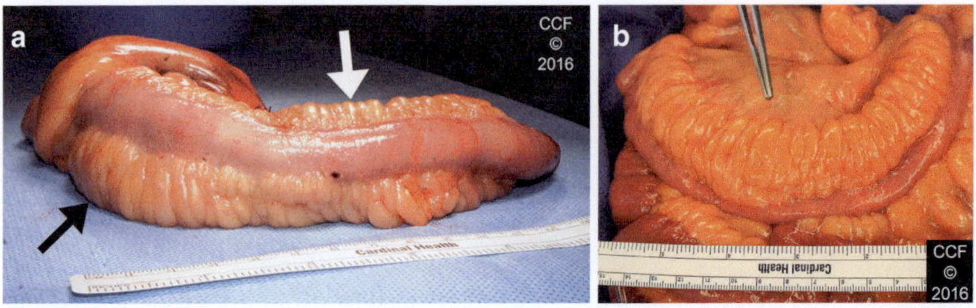

Fig. 188.2 Prominent fat wrapping is seen in the resected segment of terminal ileum indicated by an arrow in (**a**) and with forceps in (**b**)

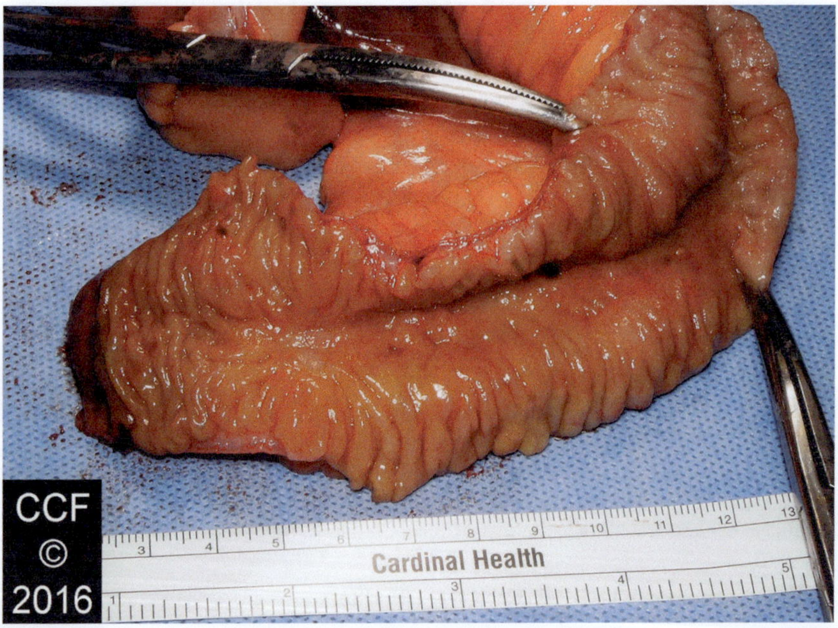

Fig. 188.3 Terminal ileitis: intraluminal stricture (clamps) associated with mesenteric fat wrapping

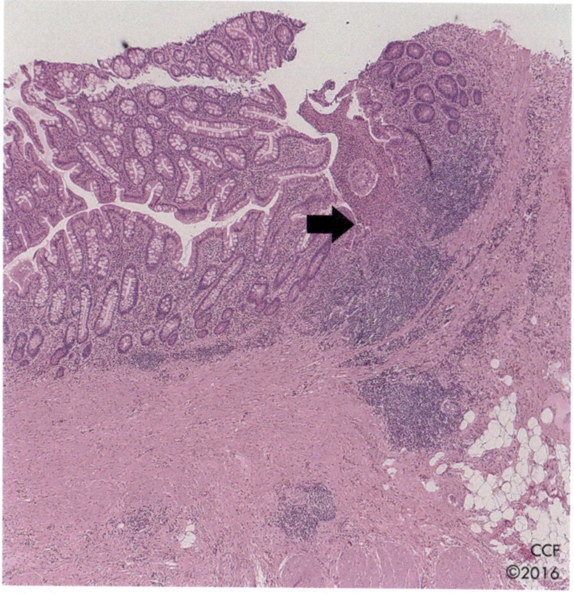

Fig. 188.4 Terminal ileitis. The mucosa shows loss of villi, crypt hyperplasia (giving the ileal mucosa a colon-like appearance), and active inflammation (arrow)

Comment

In 1932 Crohn, Ginzburg, and Oppenheimer [1] defined a disease, *Regional Enteritis*, based on the study of 14 cases. The pathologic details of the disease were based on resected specimens from thirteen of fourteen patients operated on by Dr. A. A. Berg.

Possible complications of terminal ileitis are listed in Table 188.1.

Treatment of terminal ileitis is aimed at specific complications. Generally, medical treatment is applied first. Surgery is kept in reserve until medical therapy fails or complications requiring operative intervention arise.

The surgical lines of resection recommend by the authors were as follows:

> "…in general, the proper approach to a complete cure is by surgical resection of the diseased segment of the small intestine and of the ileocecal valve with its contiguous cecum."

The optimal proximal margin of ileal resection is controversial. In a randomized controlled study, Fazio et al. [2] assigned patients undergoing ileocolic resection to two groups in which the proximal line of resection was 2 cm or 12 cm from the macroscopically involved area. The authors found that recurrence of Crohn's disease was unaffected by the width of the margin of resection from macroscopically involved bowel. Clinical assessment of the intestine is accomplished by palpating the mesentery between the thumb and forefinger as shown in Fig. 188.5.

Table 188.1 Possible complications of terminal ileitis

Thickened fibrotic mesentery
Intestinal wall thickening
Intestinal fibrostenosis
Proximal intestinal dilation
Internal fistulas
Walled off abscesses

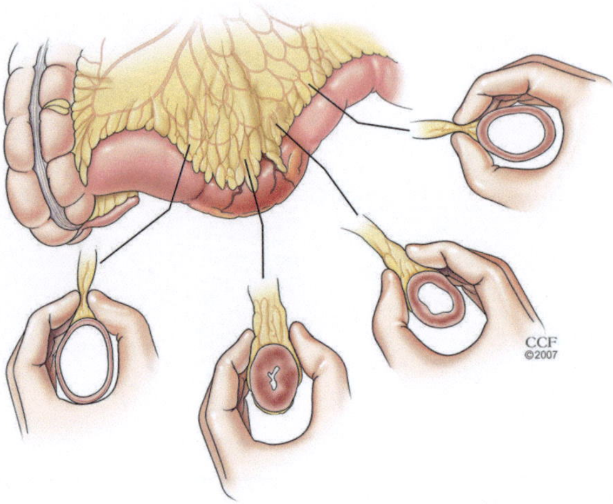

Fig. 188.5 Intestinal inflammation is associated with thickening of the adjacent mesentery. Grossly normal intestine is reached when mesenteric thickening ends (method of Dr. Victor Fazio)

References

1. Crohn BB, Ginzburg L, Oppenheimer GD. Regional ileitis: a pathologic and clinical entity. J Am Med Assoc. 1932;99:1323–9.
2. Fazio VW, Marchetti F, Church JM, Goldblum JR, Lavery IC, Hull TL, et al. Effect of resection margins on the recurrence of Crohn's disease in the small bowel. A randomized controlled trial. Ann Surg. 1996;224:563–73.

Recurrent Terminal Ileitis after Ileocolic Resection

189

James S. Wu

Presentation

A 40-year-old male patient who had a history of terminal ileitis presented with recurrent abdominal pain and intestinal obstruction. He had undergone two prior ileocolic resections, most recently 9 years earlier. Nonoperative treatment over a 6-month period had not been beneficial. A small intestinal contrast series was obtained (Fig. 189.1).

J. S. Wu (✉)
Department of Colon and Rectal Surgery, Cleveland Clinic, Cleveland, OH, USA

J. S. Wu, M. D. Inkster (eds.), *Cleveland Clinic Colorectal Case Studies*,
https://doi.org/10.1007/978-3-031-39880-3_189

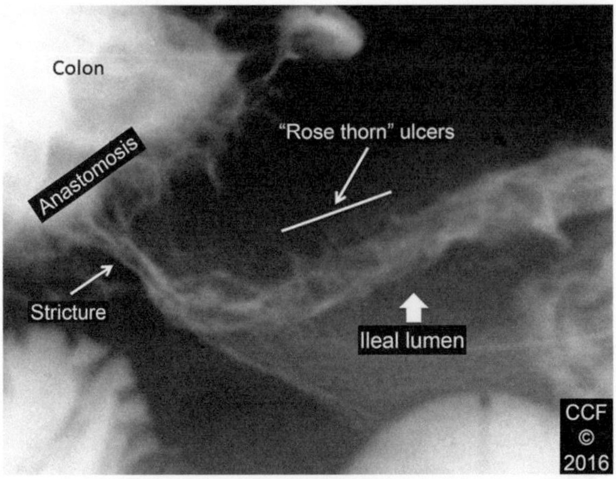

Fig. 189.1 A small bowel series shows luminal narrowing at the ileocolic anastomosis. Ileal ulcerations that arise from the intestinal lumen and penetrate the intestinal wall have the appearance of "rose thorns." The black space adjacent to the narrowed intestinal lumen is occupied by thickened bowel wall. The colon is normal

Management

The patient underwent laparotomy with ileocolic resection and neoileocolic anastomosis. Mesenteric thickening and fat wrapping for a distance of 20 cm were measured. The terminal ileum was transected 25 cm from the prior ileocolic anastomosis; 5 cm of colon were resected (Fig. 189.2). The remaining small bowel was normal and measured 350 cm from the ligament of Treitz to the neoterminal ileum.

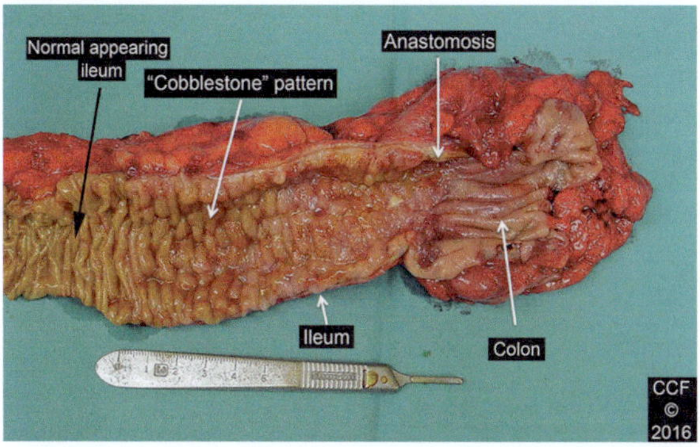

Fig. 189.2 The resected specimen shows recurrent Crohn's disease extending from the prior ileocolic anastomosis to the proximal normal ileum. Mucosal "cobblestone" changes in the diseased segment are prominent

Comment

Following initial resection for ileocolic Crohn's disease, recurrence occurs on the ileal side of the anastomosis without colonic involvement. Recurrence can be defined in symptomatic, microscopic, endoscopic, radiologic, or reoperative terms [1–6].

This was the third terminal ileal resection for this patient. Large terminal ileal loss may have long-term adverse effects on metabolic, nutritional, fluid/electrolyte, and immune functions [7, 8].

References

1. Lennard-Jones JE, Stalder GA. Prognosis after resection of chronic regional ileitis. Gut. 1967;8:332–6.
2. De Dombal FT, Burton I, Goligher JC. Recurrence of Crohn's disease after primary excisional surgery. Gut. 1971;12:519–27.
3. Greenstein AJ, Sachar DB, Pasternack BS, Janowitz HD. Reoperation and recurrence in Crohn's colitis and ileocolitits. N Engl J Med. 1975;293:685–90.
4. Rutgeerts P, Geboes K, Vantrappen G, Kerremans R, Coenegrachts JL, Coremans G. Natural history of recurrent Crohn's disease at the ileocolonic anastomosis after curative surgery. Gut. 1984;25:665–72.
5. Fazio VW, Marchetti F, Church JM, Goldblum JR, Lavery IC, Hull TL, et al. Effect of resection margins on the recurrence of Crohn's disease in the small bowel. A randomized controlled trial. Ann Surg. 1996;224:563–73.

6. D'Haens G, Baert F, Gasparaitis A, Hanauer S. Length and type of recurrent ileitis after ileal resection correlate with presurgical features in Crohn's disease. Inflamm Bowel Dis. 1997;3:249–53.
7. Silbernagl S, Despopoulos A. Color Atlas of physiology, 6E. Thieme, Stuttgart, 2009, pp. 234, 237, 251, 263.
8. Andersson H, Bosaeus I, Brummer R-J, Fasth S, Hultén L, Magnusson O, et al. Nutritional and metabolic consequences of extensive bowel resection. Dig Dis. 1986;4:193–202.

Consequences of Extensive Ileal Resection

190

Michelle D. Inkster, Gwendolyn A. Fuller, Erica C. Savage, and James S. Wu

Presentation

Sites of gastrointestinal nutrient absorption are illustrated in Fig. 190.1.

The preceding cases set the stage for a discussion about adverse sequelae that may follow extensive terminal ileal resection. The ileum constitutes about 60% of the small intestine and histologically is characterized by lymphoid tissue (Peyer's patches).

In addition to digestion and protection, functions of the ileum include absorption of vitamin B_{12} (with intrinsic factor made in the stomach), bile acids, fatty acids, fat-soluble vitamins, calcium, plus fluid and electrolytes [2]. Extensive ileal resection is associated with adverse metabolic consequences that include the following.

M. D. Inkster
Department of Gastroenterology, Cleveland Clinic, Cleveland, OH, USA

G. A. Fuller
Medical Illustration Team, Enterprise Creative Services, Cleveland Clinic, Cleveland, OH, USA

E. C. Savage
Pathology and Laboratory Medicine Institute, Cleveland Clinic, Cleveland, OH, USA

J. S. Wu (✉)
Department of Colon and Rectal Surgery, Cleveland Clinic, Cleveland, OH, USA

J. S. Wu, M. D. Inkster (eds.), *Cleveland Clinic Colorectal Case Studies*,
https://doi.org/10.1007/978-3-031-39880-3_190

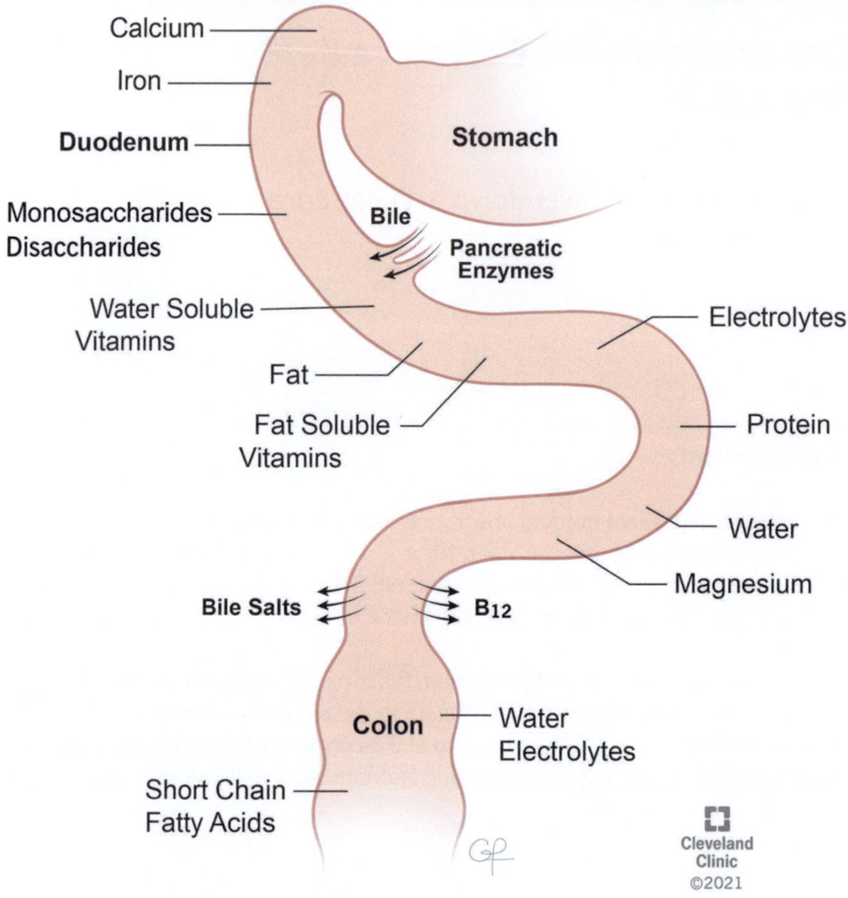

Fig. 190.1 Sites of gastrointestinal nutrient absorption (after Grant) [1]

Bile Acid Malabsorption

> "The ileum uniquely absorbs vitamin B_{12} and bile salts. Bile salts are essential for the efficient absorption of fats and fat-soluble vitamins. Normally the demand for bile salts imposed by fat absorption cannot be met by synthesis alone. The need for bile salts is met only by ileal resorption of bile salts, which are then recycled into the intestine. With ileal resection the loss of bile salts increases and is not met by an increase in synthesis. The bile salt pool is depleted and fat absorption is reduced. In addition, loss of bile salts into the colon reduces the ability of the colon to reabsorb salt and water, resulting in increased diarrhea. In the colon, bile salts are also dehydroxylated to deoxy bile salts, which induce colonic water secretion."
>
> Khursheed N. Jeejeebhoy, M.D., Ph.D., F.R.C.S.[1] [3]
> St. Michael's Hospital
> Toronto, Ontario, 2005

[1]This excerpt is reused with the generous permission of Taylor and Francis Group LLC (Books) US; CRC press, Order License ID, 156417–1, Order Date 23-Oct-2021.

Vitamin B12 Malabsorption

"The vitamin B_{12}-intrinsic factor complex is carried to its site of absorption in the ileum where it attaches to specific membrane receptors.

Any condition associated with ileal dysfunction may lead to vitamin B_{12} malabsorption and deficiency.

In Crohn's disease the absorption is dependent on the extent of the mucosal lesion and whether ileal resection has been carried out. When the resection is more than 100 cm, B_{12} malabsorption is almost invariably present. Because B_{12}-receptors are restricted to the ileum, there appears to be no adaptation of B_{12} absorption in those patients who have extensive ileal disease."

H. Schjønsby [4]
Medical Department
Aker University Hospital
Oslo, Norway, 1989

Vitamin B_{12} Deficiency

"Deficiency causes megaloblastic anemia, damage to the white matter of the spinal cord and brain, and peripheral neuropathy."

Larry E. Johnson, M.D. Ph.D.[2] [5]
University of Arkansas for Medical Sciences 2020
Merck Manual

Renal Oxalate Stones [6]

"The pathophysiology of calcium oxalate stones is related to increased urinary oxalate excretion caused by increased intestinal absorption, termed enteric hyperoxaluria (EHO) which depends on at least two mechanisms. The first is related to bile salt malabsorption in the diseased or resected distal ileum, which causes bile salt deficiency and fat malabsorption. The majority of dietary oxalate is bound to calcium and is poorly absorbed, but malabsorbed fats bind intraluminal calcium, decreasing the amount bound to oxalate and resulting in increased oxalate absorption…. The second mechanism of EHO is related to increased colonic permeability to oxalate caused by the malabsorbed fatty acids and bile salts."

Darrell S. Pardi, M.D., William J. Tremaine, M.D., William J. Sandborn, M.D., and James T. McCarthy, M.D.
Inflammatory Bowel Disease Clinic
Division of Gastroenterology, and
Division of Nephrology,
Mayo Clinic and Foundation
Rochester, Minnesota, 1998[3] [7]

[2] This excerpt is reproduced with the generous permission of Ms. Sheryl Olinsky Borg, Merck Manuals, March 11, 2022.

[3] This excerpt is reused with the generous permission of Wolters Kluwer Health, Inc., CCC | RightsLink®, License Number 5174640550033; License date Oct 23, 2021.

Malabsorption of Fat-Soluble Vitamins

"The absorption of the fat-soluble vitamins (A, D, E, and K) requires micellar solubilization by the bile salt micelles. Diseases that reduce small bowel surface area or reduce the bile salt pool, such as terminal ileal resections, are more likely to result in fat-soluble vitamin deficiencies.

Vitamin A is important in cell differentiation and proliferation. The primary clinical effects of vitamin A are related to the role of retinal as a precursor of the visual pigment, rhodopsin. Vitamin A of the 11-*cis* retinal forms is vital for night vision.

The 1, 25 form of vitamin D regulates calcium absorption from the intestine. A deficiency of vitamin D results in low serum calcium and phosphorous levels. Bone mineralization is reduced in vitamin D-deficient individuals, resulting in osteopenia in adults and rickets in children.

Vitamin E is a potent peroxyl radical scavenger… Vitamin E deficiency increases lipid peroxidation. Hemolytic anemia, ataxia and peripheral neuropathy have also been reported with vitamin E deficiency.

The predominant dietary sources of vitamin K are green leafy vegetables. Also the colonic flora produces vitamin K. Therefore, vitamin K deficiency is uncommon in patients with intact colons. Vitamin K is required for the synthesis of clotting factors in the liver, which includes factors II, VII, IX, and X. The primary symptom of vitamin K deficiency is bleeding."

James S. Scolapio, M.D.[4] [8]
Mayo Clinic
Jacksonville, Florida and
Andrew Ukleja, M.D.
Cleveland Clinic Florida
Weston, Florida

Peyer's Patches

Peyer's patches are oblong elevations of the small intestinal mucosa containing lymphoid follicles, eponymously named after the Swiss anatomist Johann Conrad Peyer (1653–1712) [9].[5] Peyer's patches are intestinal immune sensors [10] located in the terminal ileum [11].

In 1677, Peyer published *Excercitatio anatomico – medica de glandulis intestinorum* describing "intestinal glands"[12]. The 1681 edition of Peyer's work includes ICONs that illustrate his observations. ICON III is reproduced in Fig. 190.2.

[4]This excerpt is reused with the generous permission of Taylor and Francis Group LLC (Books) US, CRC PRESS, CCC | Marketplace®, License ID 1156524–1, Order Date 24-Oct-24, 2021.

[5]The endoscopic appearance of Peyer's patches is shown in the preceding chapter entitled, *Colonoscopy-Normal Landmarks,* Fig. 22.2a.

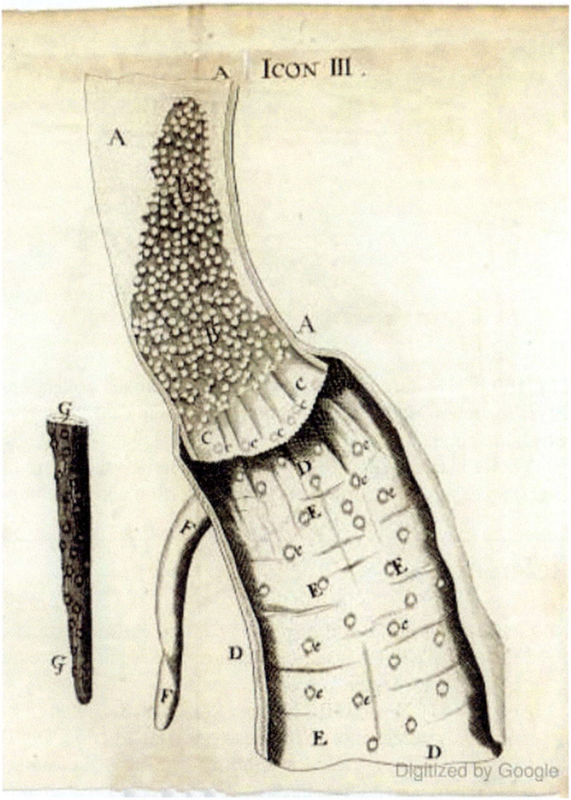

Fig. 190.2 ICON III showing the "intestinal glands" in the terminal ileum, colon, and appendix. From Peyeri, Johannis Conradi. Excercitatio anatomico medica prima de glandvlis intestinorum, 1681. Digitalized by Google; accessed from Google books, March 9, 2022

ICON TERTIA.	*IMAGE THREE.*
AAA. Extremitas ilei aperta & dilatata ut ejus interiora pateant.	AAA. Terminal ileum opened and dilated so that the interior is clearly seen.
BB. Plexus glandularum maximus totam ilei extremitatem glandulofam reddens.	BB. The largest plexus glands in the entire ileum are located at the end.
CC. Valvula Bauhini diffecta, in cujus limbo glandulae folitariæ cccc. annotantur.	CC. With Bauhin's valve dissected out, the limb of intestine cccc showing solitary glands are annotated.
DDD. Portio coli incifa & diducta ut ejus quoque glandulæ in confpectum prodeant.	DDD. Part of the colon is incised and dilated so that its glands can be inspected.
EEE, ee. Glandulæ folitariæ lenti fimiles per colum diffeminatæ.	EEE, ee. Solitary glands slowly slowly disseminated through the the colon
F.F. Inteftinum cœcum integrum.	FF. The entire cecum (appendix)
GG. Idem inverfum et ejus glandulæ appareant.	GG. The inverted appendix with its glands made apparent.

The histologic appearance of Peyer's patches is shown in Fig. 190.3.

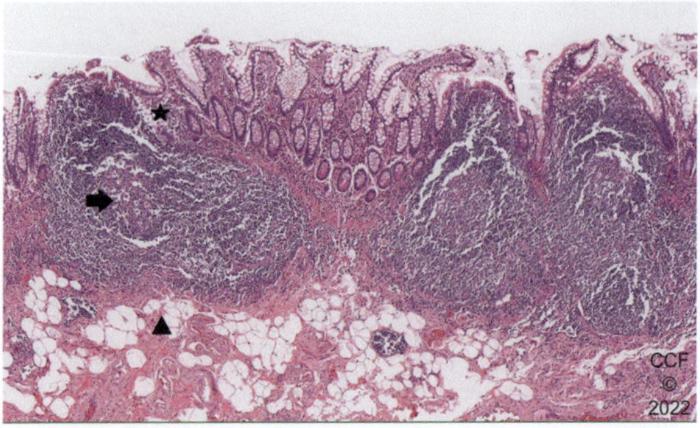

Fig. 190.3 The terminal ileum harbors specialized collections of lymphoid follicles known as Peyer's patches. Most of the lymphoid follicles in Peyer's patches contain germinal centers (arrow) which are populated by B-lymphocytes, occasional T-lymphocytes, and histiocytes known as tingible body macrophages. Peyer's patches can be seen along the interface of the lamina propria (star) and submucosa (arrowhead) with distortion and flattening of the overlying villi

References

1. Grant JP. Anatomy and physiology of the gastrointestinal tract. In: Matarese LE, Steiger E, Seidner DL, editors. Intestinal Failure and Rehabilitation. A Clinical Guide. Boca Raton: CRC press; 2005., Chapter 1. p. 5–23, Figure 1.6.
2. Andersson H, Bosaeus I, Brummer R-J, Fasth S, Hultén L, Magnusson O, et al. Nutritional and metabolic consequences of extensive bowel resection. Dig Dis. 1986;4:193–202.
3. Jeejeebhoy KN. The etiology and mechanism of intestinal failure. In: Matarese LE, Steiger E, Seidner DL (editors), Intestinal Failure and Rehabilitation. A Clinical Guide. Boca Raton: CRC press, 2005, Chapter 2, pp. 25–37.
4. Schjønsby H. Vitamin B12 absorption and malabsorption. Gut. 1989;30:1686–91.
5. Johnson LE. Vitamin B12 Deficiency. Nutritional Disorders-Manuals Professional Edition. Merck. [cited 2021 May 2]. Available from Manuals.com.
6. Corica D, Romano C. Renal involvement in inflammatory bowel diseases. J Crohns Colitis. 2016;10:226–35.
7. Pardi DS, Tremaine WJ, Sandborn WJ, McCarthy JT. Renal and urologic complications of inflammatory bowel disease. Am J Gastroenterol. 1998;93:504–14.
8. Scolapio JS, Ukleja A. Malnutrition: Vitamin and trace mineral deficiencies. In: Matarese LE, Steiger E, Seidner DL, editors. Intestinal Failure and Rehabilitation. A Clinical Guide. Boca Raton: CRC press; 2005. p. 103–13.
9. Sträuli P. Johann Conrad Peyer von Schaffhausen und seine <<Anatomisch-medizinische Methodik>>. Schweiz Med Wochen. 1959;89:825–30.
10. Jung C, Hugot J-P, Barreau F. Peyer's patches: The immune sensors of the intestine. Int J Inflam. 2010:Article 823710, 12 pages https://doi.org/10.4061/2010/823710.
11. Van Kruiningen HJ, West AB, Freda BJ, Holmes KA. Distribution of Peyer's patches in the distal ileum. Inflam Bowel Dis. 2002;8:180–5.
12. Peyeri, Johannis Conradi. Excercitatio anatomico medica prima de glandvlis intestinorum. In Parerga Anatomica et medica septem. Ratione ac experientia parentibus concepta & edita. Genevæ, Sumptibus J. Herman, Widerhold, MDCLXXXI; page 16, ICON III. [cited 2022 Mar 9]. Available from Google books.

Dividing Thickened Mesentery in Crohn's Disease 191

James S. Wu

Presentation

A patient underwent surgery to remove symptomatic stricturing terminal ileitis. A small bowel series showed a narrowed terminal ileal intestinal lumen (Fig. 191.1). Ileocolic resection was done.

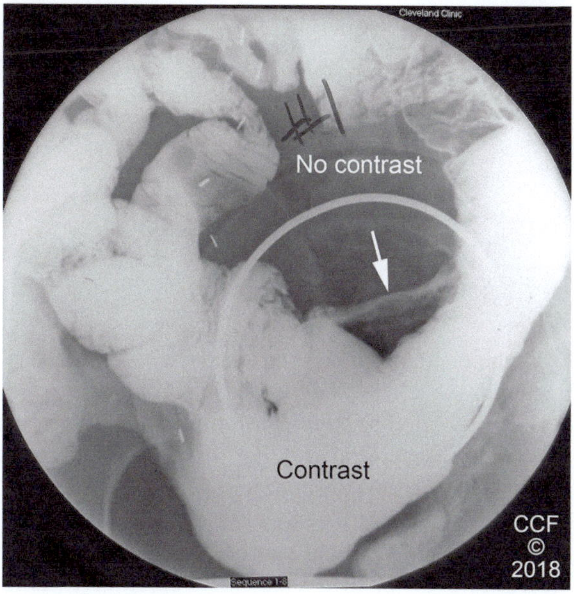

Fig. 191.1 Small bowel series shows a thin line of contrast "string sign" (arrow) that identifies the terminal ileal stricture. The absence of contrast corresponds to the space taken up by the thickened intestinal wall and its mesentery

J. S. Wu (✉)
Department of Colon and Rectal Surgery, Cleveland Clinic, Cleveland, OH, USA

J. S. Wu, M. D. Inkster (eds.), *Cleveland Clinic Colorectal Case Studies*,
https://doi.org/10.1007/978-3-031-39880-3_191

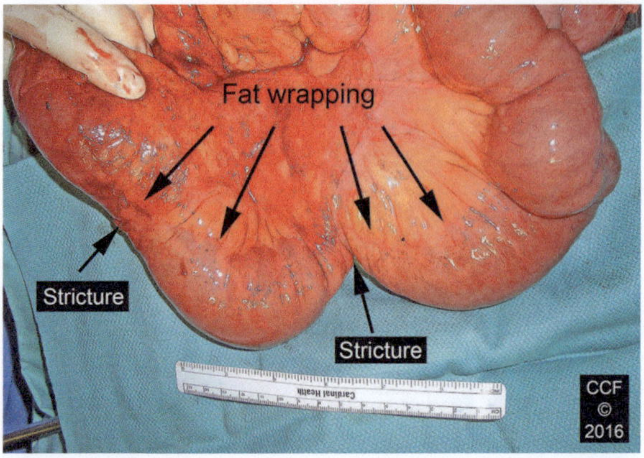

Fig. 191.2 At surgery, two strictured terminal ileal segments (short arrows) show mesenteric thickening and marked fat wrapping (long arrows)

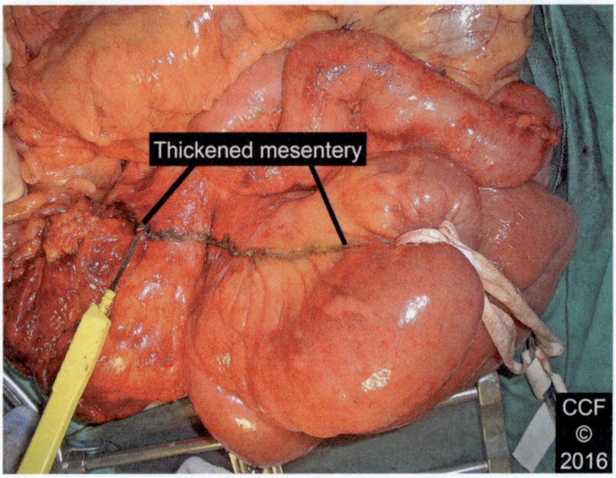

Fig. 191.3 The mesentery to be divided is marked with electrocautery. The strictured ileal segment to be resected is isolated with umbilical tapes passed through the mesentery and tied around the intestine to prevent fecal soilage

Technique: Dividing thickened ileitis mesentery using overlapping suture ligatures[1].

Two strictured segments of terminal ileum are seen in Fig. 191.2. The line of resection is demonstrated in Fig. 191.3. The mesentery is divided between clamps starting close to the intestinal wall (Fig. 191.4).

The mesentery between each pair of clamps is divided just short of the tips to avoid bleeding. A second pair of clamps is placed across the next segment of the mesentery overlapping the mesentery previously clamped but not divided. The mesentery between the second pair of clamps is then divided again just short of the end

[1] This technique was passed down from Dr. Victor W. Fazio.

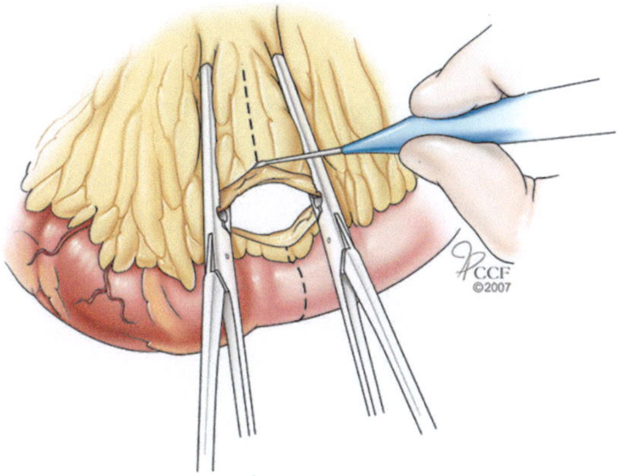

Fig. 191.4 The mesentery is divided between clamps starting at the edge of the intestine. A Kocher clamp (locking with teeth) that will not slip off of the thickened mesentery containing perfusing blood vessels is used on the side that stays with the patient. A curved Kelly clamp is applied to the side that is removed

of the clamp tips. The maneuver is repeated until the entire mesentery is divided. The technique is demonstrated in Fig. 191.5a–b. The mesenteric pedicles on the proximal side are controlled by the overlapping heavy No. 1 gauge chromic sutures (Fig. 191.6a–c). Following division of the intestine, the specimen is removed with mesenteric clamps in place (Fig. 191.7). Sites of maximum stricture in the opened specimen are marked by the clamps (Fig. 191.8).

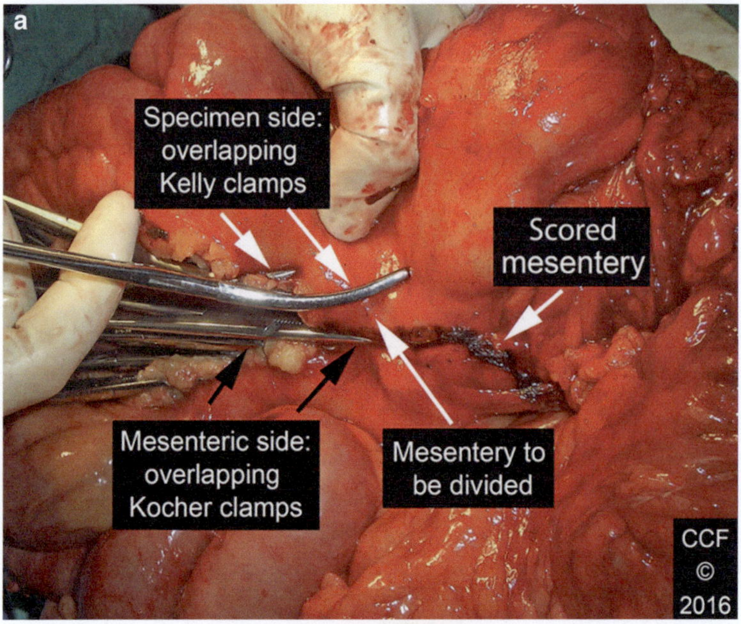

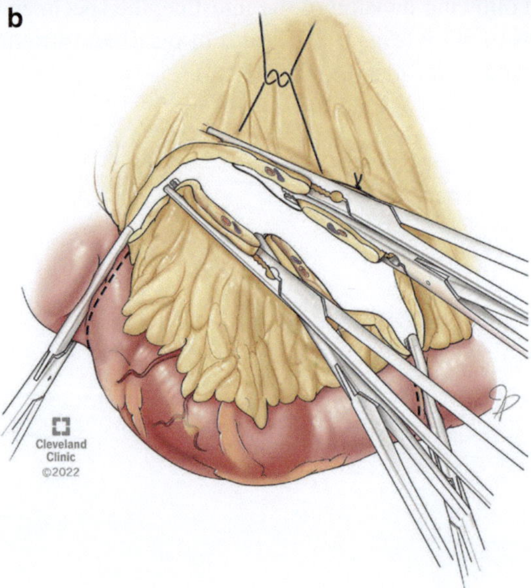

Fig. 191.5 (**a**, **b**) Starting at one end of the designated mesentery, the mesentery is divided between overlapping clamps. A Kocher clamp is used for the proximal side because it does not slip once placed. A Kelly clamp is used on the specimen side with the tips curved towards the specimen away from the line of resection. The mesentery to be divided is defined by the score on the mesentery

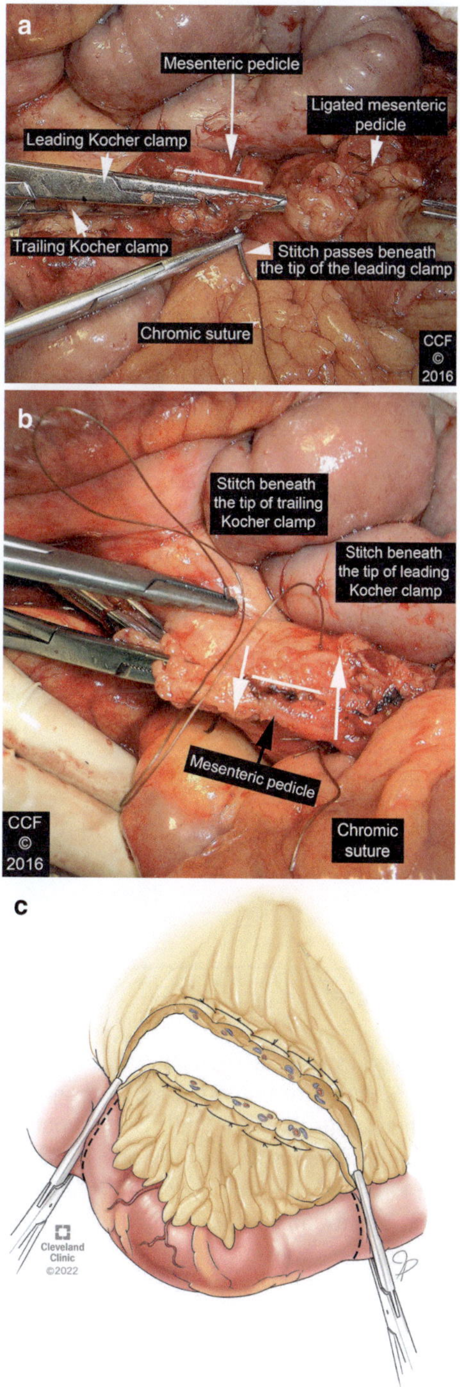

Fig. 191.6 (**a**) A No. 1 gauge chromic suture is passed beneath the tip of the leading Kocher clamp; (**b**) The mesenteric pedicles controlled by the Kocher clamps are ligated with overlapping No. 1 gauge chromic suture. The suture first passes beneath the tip of the lead clamp and then passes beneath the tip of the trailing clamp. The suture then is tied securely as the lead clamp is released slowly. Chromic suture is used because it does not slip after being tied; (**c**) Illustration showing overlying sutures tied

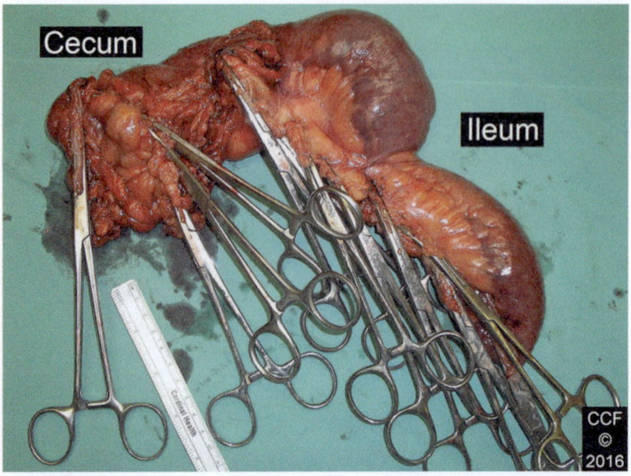

Fig. 191.7 Resected ileum and cecum with mesenteric clamps in place

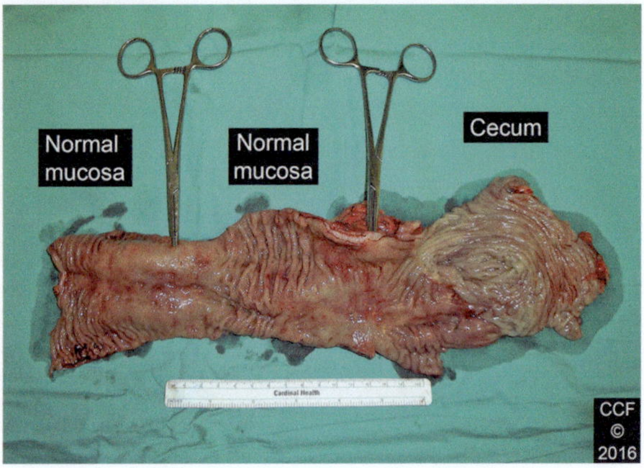

Fig. 191.8 The opened specimen shows two strictured areas with an intervening island of grossly normal appearing mucosa, two "skip" lesions. Sites of maximum stricture are marked with clamps

Comment

The blood vessels associated with ileitis can be encased in a fatty thickened mesentery. Isolation of individual arteries and veins may not be possible. The preceding method controls all blood vessels contained in the mesentery with overlapping suture ligatures. A Kocher clamp is used to secure the side of the divided mesentery that remains with the patient; this clamp crushes the mesentery within its grip and tends not to slip. Heavy No. 1 gauge chromic suture ligatures are advantageous because their knots do not untie.

Jejunoileitis-Strictureplasty

192

Victor W. Fazio and James S. Wu

Presentation

A patient with jejunoileitis developed abdominal pain and distension. Oral anti-inflammatory pills were not beneficial. A gastrointestinal contrast study was done (Fig. 192.1). At surgery, massively dilated jejunum was found followed distally by a long segment of collapsed jejunoileum (Fig. 192.2).

Closer examination of the collapsed jejunoileum revealed multiple strictures. Each stricture was located distal to a dilated segment of small intestine (Fig. 192.3). Mesenteric fat wrapping was seen on close-up view at each stricture site (Fig. 192.4).

The inflammation and subsequent luminal narrowing occurs on the mesenteric side of the bowel. The antimesenteric side of the intestine remains soft, pliable and suitable for the creation of surgical anastomoses. In this case, multiple strictureplasties were done (Fig. 192.5).

V. W. Fazio · J. S. Wu (✉)
Department of Colon and Rectal Surgery, Cleveland Clinic, Cleveland, OH, USA

J. S. Wu, M. D. Inkster (eds.), *Cleveland Clinic Colorectal Case Studies*,
https://doi.org/10.1007/978-3-031-39880-3_192

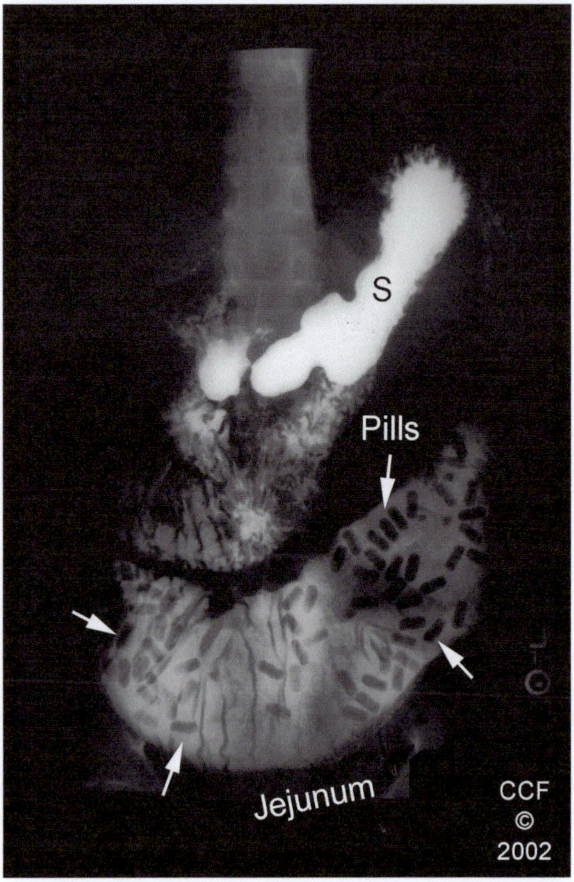

Fig. 192.1 This contrast study shows massively dilated jejunum (arrows) that contains numerous retained pills. Proximally, the stomach (S) is seen

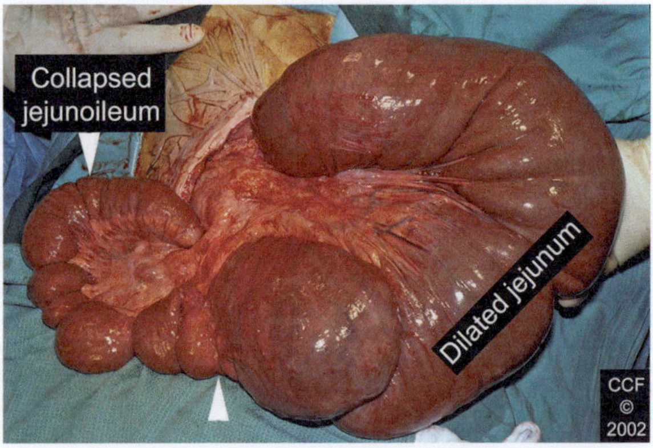

Fig. 192.2 At surgery dilated jejunum was found. Distal to this was a long segment of collapsed jejunoileum (located between arrowheads)

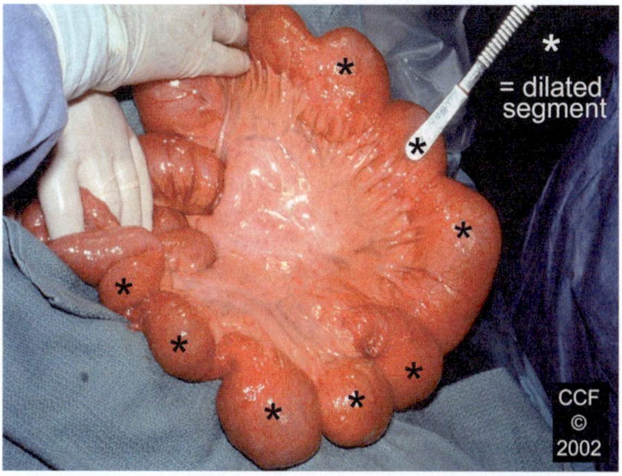

Fig. 192.3 Jejunoileitis. Alternating dilated and narrowed small intestinal segments of are seen. Multiple strictures, arising from the mesenteric side of the intestine, are seen. The dilated segments are marked with asterisks

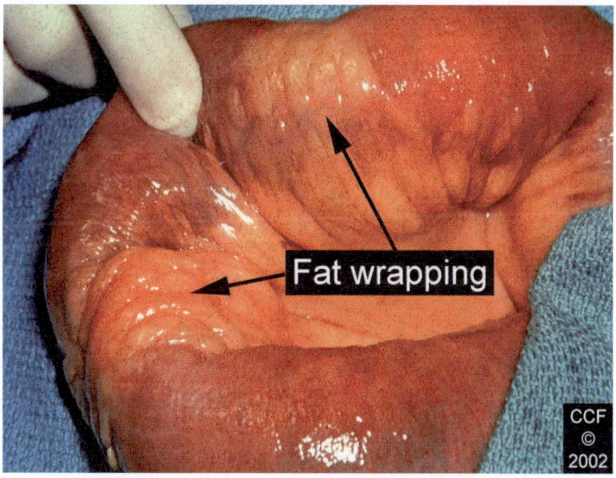

Fig. 192.4 Jejunoileal stricture. Mesenteric fat wrapping (arrows) is seen at stricture sites

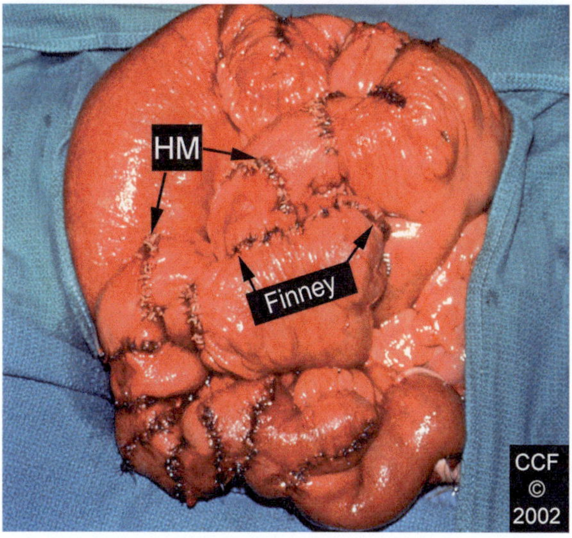

Fig. 192.5 Multiple strictureplasties. The Heineke–Mikulicz strictureplasties (HM) are identified by suture lines that run transversely across the intestine. A Finney strictureplasty, seen in the center of the photograph, has a long longitudunal suture line

Comment

Strictureplasty was described in 1977 by Katariya et al. [1] to treat intestinal strictures from tuberculosis.

> "Tubercular strictures of the small bowel, often multiple, which result from cicatricial contraction of encircling ulcers, can cause subacute or acute intestinal obstruction.
>
> In most cases surgical treatment has been either resection (treatment of choice) or enteroanastomosis…; both procedures seem drastic for a benign disease, especially for multiple strictures throughout the whole small intestine. We therefore, whenever possible, have carried out a simple procedure of stricture-plasty.
>
> The bowel is opened lengthwise by a 5-6 cm incision along the antimesenteric border and with the stricture at its mid-point. Closure is by a two-layer transverse repair (inner: continuous catgut; outer: interrupted silk)."

R. N. Katariya, S. Sood, P. G. Rao and P.L. N.G. Rao
Department of Surgery
Postgraduate Institute of Medical Education and Research
Chandigarh, India

In 1982, Lee and Papaioannou [2] used strictureplasty to treat chronic obstruction in patients with Crohn's disease of the small bowel. A distinct advantage of strictureplasty is that it preserves intestinal length to maintain adequate absorption of fluid, electrolytes, and nutrition. Intestinal preservation certainly was the reason why Dr. Fazio chose strictureplasty over resection in the case of jejunoilealitis presented above. The method was also chosen in another case involving mutiple strictures of the jejunum (Fig 192.6).

The two most commonly used strictureplasty techniques (Heineke–Mikulicz and Finney) are derived from operations originally created for pyloroplasty.

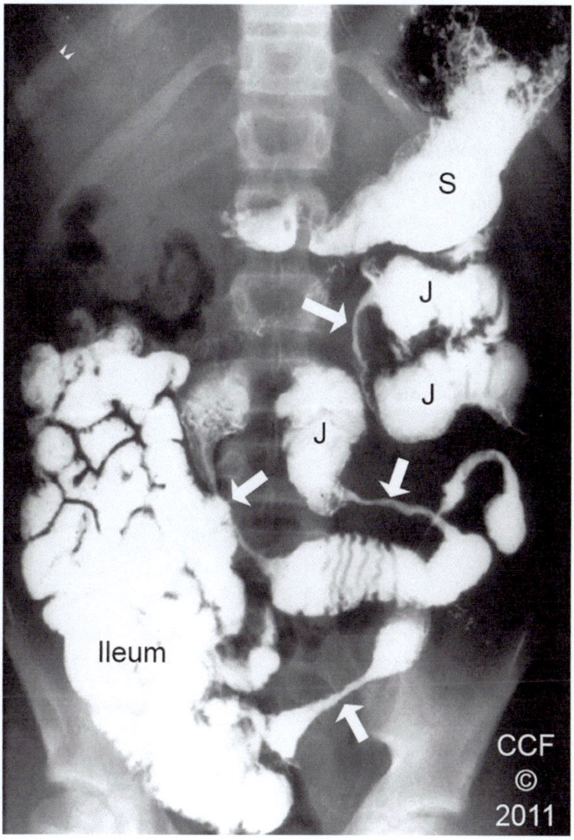

Fig. 192.6 This small bowel series shows multiple jejunal strictures (arrows). The stomach (S), jejunum (J), and ileum (I) are labeled

Heinecke–Mikulicz

In 1887, Mikulicz described the operative management of pyloric stenosis according to the method described by Heinecke [3].

Zur operativen Behandlung der Pylorusstenose. Mikulicz (Königsberg) Vor 2 Jahren hat Heinecke einen Fall von narbiger Pylorusstenose dadurch geheilt, dass er den verengerten Pylorus der Länge nach aufschnitt und die Wunde in querer Richtung vereinigte. Dieselbe Operation hat M., ohne das Verfahren von Heinecke vorher gekannt zu haben, im Februar d. J. an einer 20jährigen Frau mit hochgradiger Stenose ausgeführt.	On operative treatment of pyloric stenosis. Mikulicz (Königsberg) Two years ago, Heinecke cured a case of scarred pyloric stenosis by severing the narrowed pylorus lengthwise and uniting the wound in the transverse direction. M., without having known Heinecke method, undertook the same operation in February of this year performed on a 20-year-old woman with severe stenosis.

The concepts of this type of strictureplasty were illustrated in a woodcut published in 1887, Mikulicz (Fig. 192.7) [4].

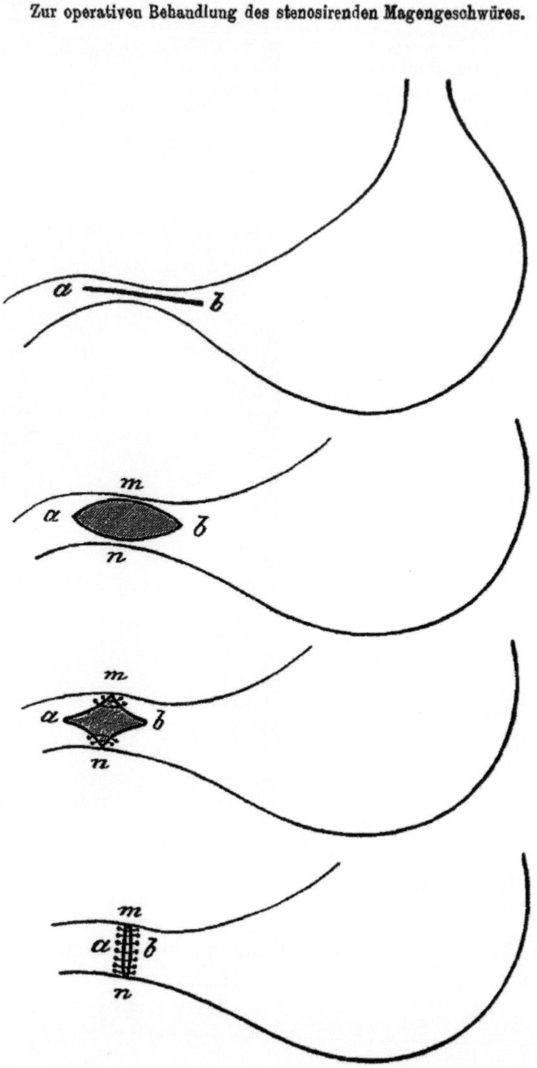

Fig. 192.7 Strictureplasty for stenosing gastric ulcer (Mikulicz 1887). A longitudinal incision is made across the pylorus (a to b). The incision is then closed in the transverse direction (m to n)

Zur operativen Behandlung des stenosirenden Magengeschwüres Von Prof. J. Mikulicz in Königsberg (mit einem Holzschnitt.) Ich habe mich schon lange mit der Idee getragen, ob es nicht möglich wäre, durch eine Art plastischer Operation am Pylorus selbst die Stenose auszugleichen und gleichzeitig dem Geschwüre selbst in entsprechenender Weise beizukommen. Nach Versuchen an der Leiche hatte ich folgendes einfache Verfahren ersonnen, dessen Plan durch die nebenstehenden Zeichnungen (Fig. 1–4) veranschaulicht ist.	Concerning the surgical treatment of stenosing gastric ulcer By Prof. J Mikulicz at Königsberg (with one woodcut.) For a long time, I have had the idea of whether it might not be possible to even out the stenosis itself by means of a kind of plastic operation on the pylorus and at the same time deal with the ulcer itself in an appropriate manner. After trials on a corpse, I devised the following simple procedure, the plan of which is illustrated by the accompanying drawings (Figs. 1–4) [this work Fig. 192.7].

The concept of luminal enlargement by longitudinal incision followed by transverse closure was extended to the small intestine a few years later by Cheatle in 1897 [5].

‘ “A method of uniting the divided intestine”

> In my most recent operations upon dogs I have brought the extremities of the longitudinal aperture into apposition, and thus fixed them and then sewed up the opening that had thereby been made transverse to, or at right angles with, the attachment of the mesentery.
>
> And hence nearly the whole length of the previously longitudinal aperture is thrown into the continuity of the lumen which must necessarily increase its size.’

By G. Lenthal Cheatle, F.R.C.S., Eng.,
Assistant Surgeon to King’s College Hospital
and to the West London Hospital

Cheatle illustrations of his longitudinal incision with transverse closure are shown in Fig. 192.8a and b.

A demonstration of what is commonly referred to as Heineke–Mikulicz strictureplasty for short intestinal strictures is shown in Fig. 192.9a–e. A longitudinal incision, made at the antimesenteric border of the bowel at the stricture site, is closed transversely.

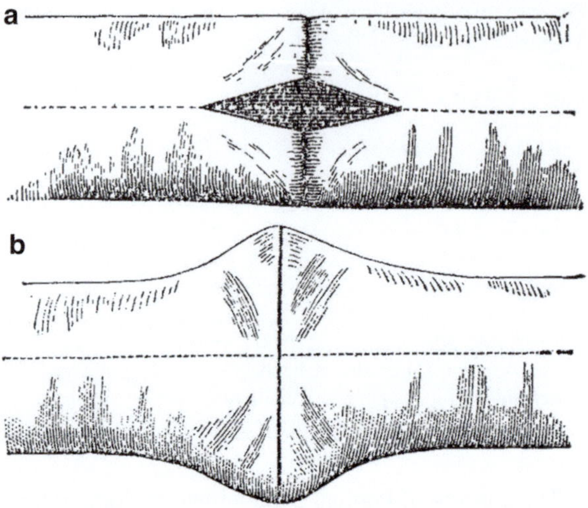

Fig. 192.8 (**a**) Concerning this illustration, Cheatle writes: "Showing the longitudinal opening into the gut after union of the cut ends. It is placed opposite to and parallel with, the mesenteric attachment. The latter is represented by a dotted line;" (**b**) Cheatle's description of this illustration is as follows: "Showing how the longitudinal opening has been made continuous with the united ends by converting it (the longitudinal opening) into a transverse one by having brought its extremities into apposition and its fixation in that direction. The mesenteric attachment is represented by the dotted line"

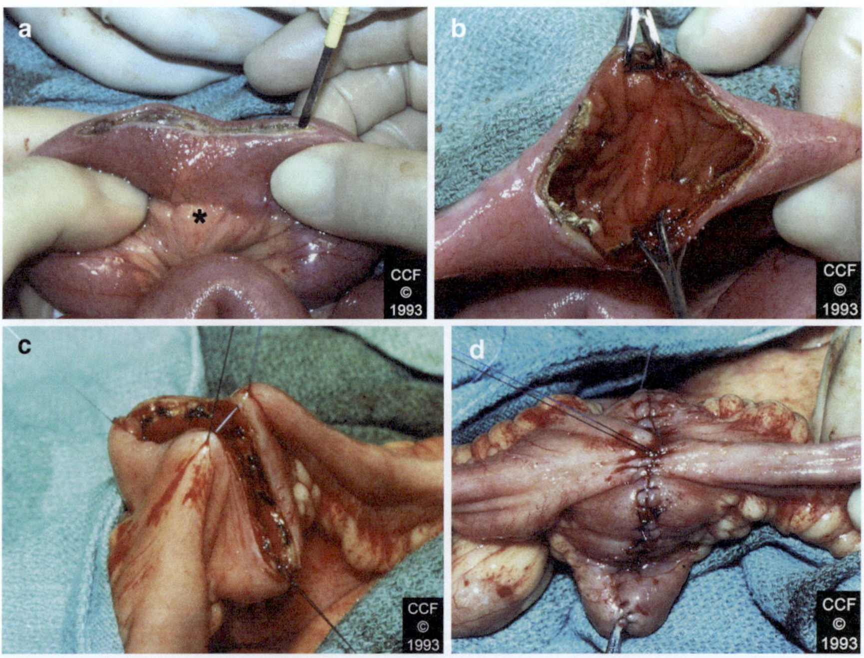

Fig. 192.9 Heineke–Mikulicz strictureplasty for small intestinal stricture: (**a**) A longitudinal incision is made along the antimesenteric border of the small intestine; (**b**) Lateral traction is applied to the mid-points of the longitudinal incision; (**c**) Traction sutures are placed in preparation for transverse incision closure; (**d**) Transverse closure of the longitudinal incision; e. Illustration showing longitudinal incision and transverse closure for Heineke–Mikulicz strictureplasty [see the following page]

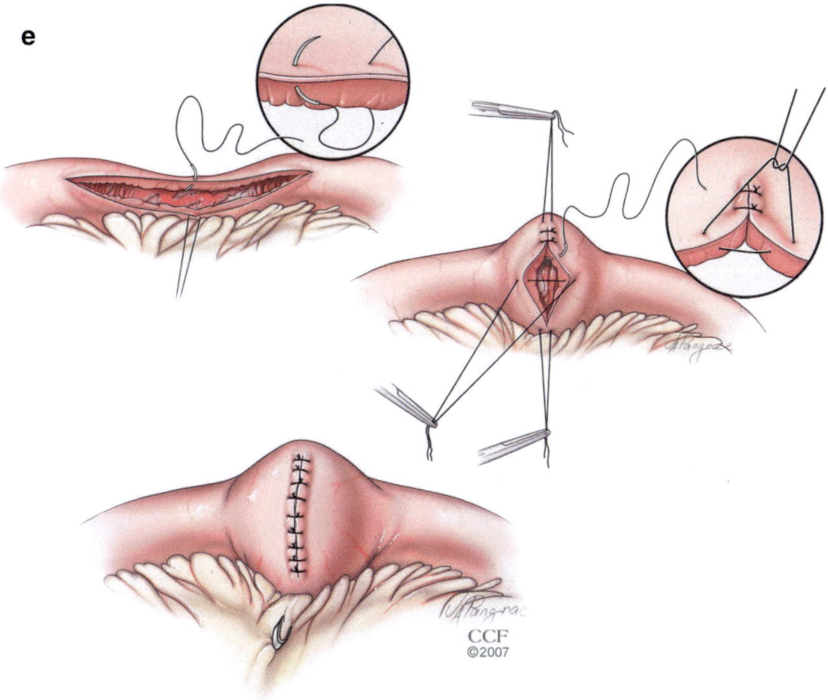

Fig. 192.9 (continued)

Finney

In 1902, Finney described *A New Method of Pyloroplasty* in which an "incision is made in the shape of a horseshoe" between the stomach and the duodenum [6]. In 1937, he described the incision in greater detail.

"Pyloroplasty and Gastroduodenostomy

> Beginning from below, on the stomach side about one-half centimeter from the lower end of the posterior suture line, and being careful to include all layers of the stomach wall, we carry the incision upward and, though the pylorus, down into the duodenum, in the shape of a narrowed inverted U, to a point opposite the start on the stomach side."[1][7]

J. M. T. Finney, Jr., M.D.
Baltimore, MD.

Finney's illustration of gastropyloroduodenostomy is shown in Fig. 192.10.

[1] The posterior suture line secures the stomach to the duodenum prior to opening the gut.

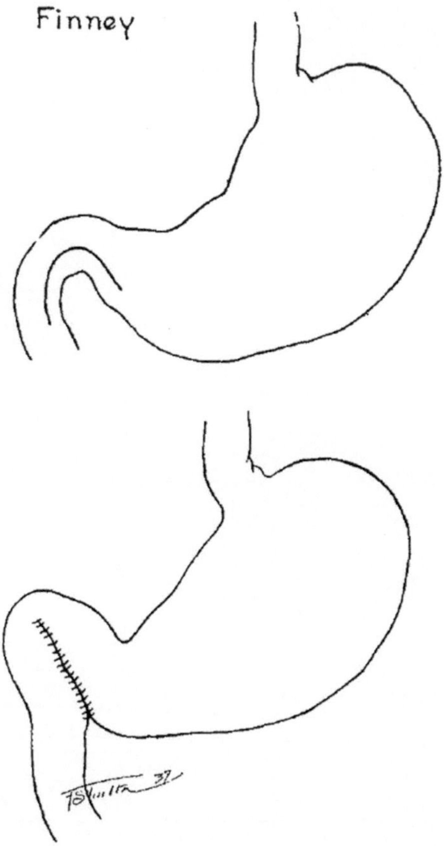

Fig. 192.10 Finney's 1937 illustrations of gastropyloroduodenostomy: Top. A "U"-shaped incision extends from the distal stomach, through the pylorus, to the proximal duodenum; Bottom. The completed gastropyloroduodenostomy. These images are reused with the generous permission of Mr. Subash Balakrishnan, Copyrights Coordinator, ELSEVIER IHCM – Health Content Management, unique reference number 211023–009364, October 23, 2021

In Crohn's disease, small intestinal strictures of up to 25 cm may be treated by side-to-side "Finney" strictureplasty (Fig. 192.11a–d). Biopsy of ulceration found during strictureplasty is done to exclude malignancy. Strictureplasty sites are marked with surgical clips for later identification. According to Tjandra and Fazio [8], situations in which strictureplasty is contraindicated include:

- overt perforation,
- fistula or inflammatory phlegmon at the intended site,
- multiple strictures in a short segment,
- excessive tension at strictureplasty closure,
- serum albumin level less than 2.0 g/dL.

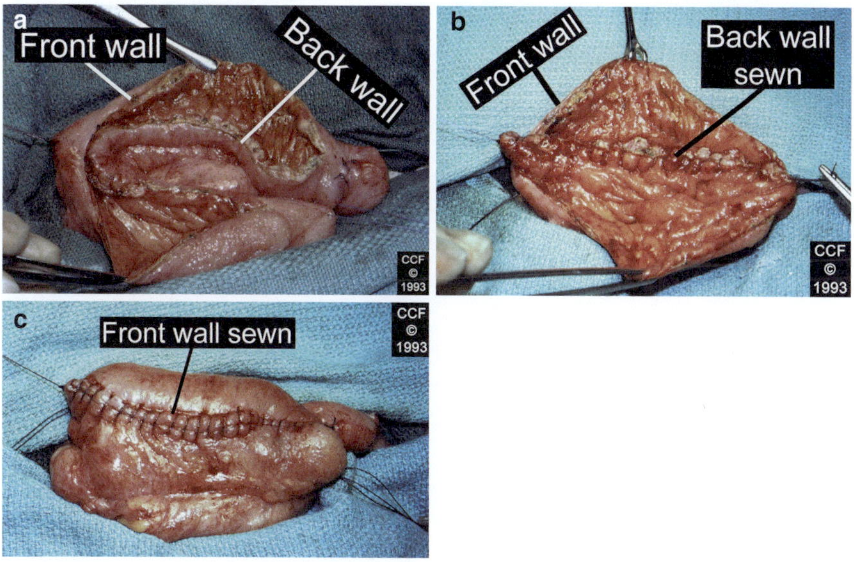

Fig. 192.11 Finney strictureplasty: (**a**) The antimesenteric border of the strictured segment of small intestine is opened. The edges of the intestine destined to become the back and front walls of the strictureplasty are labeled; (**b**) The back wall of the strictureplasty is sewn with interrupted suture; (**c**) The front wall of the anastomosis is sewn with interrupted sutures; (**d**) Illustration showing suture closure of the back (top) and front (bottom) walls of the anastomosis [see the following page]

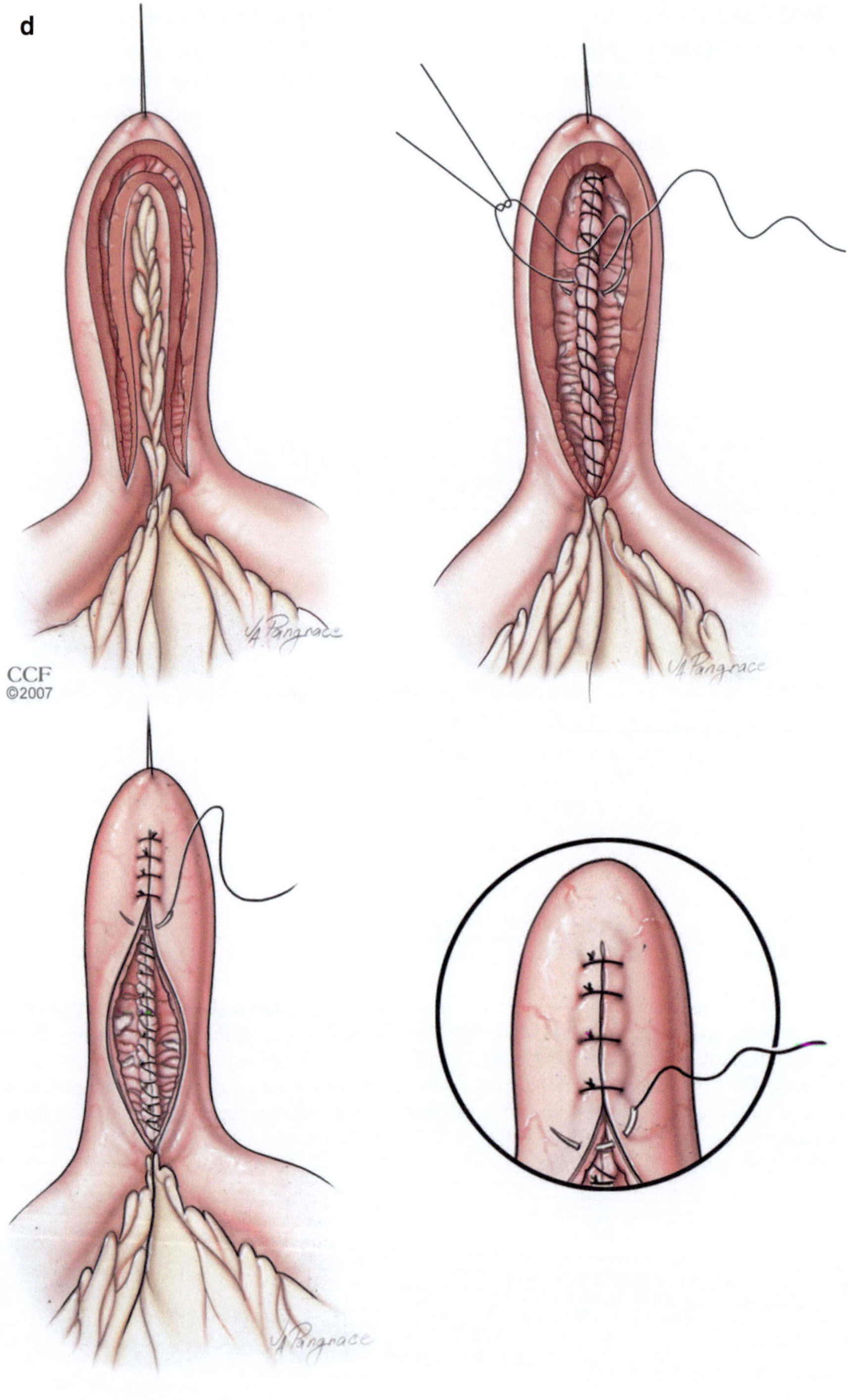

Fig. 192.11 (continued)

References

1. Katariya RN, Sood S, Rao PG, Rao PLNG. Stricture-plasty for tubercular strictures of the gastro-intestinal tract. Br J Surg. 1977;64:496–8.
2. Lee ECG, Papaioannou N. Minimal surgery for chronic obstruction in patients with extensive or universal Crohn's disease. Ann R Coll Surg Engl. 1982;64:229–33.
3. Mikulicz (Königsberg). Zur operativen Behandlung der Pylorostenose. Centralblatt Chir. 1887;25:55–6.
4. Mikulicz J. Zur operativen Behandling des stenosirenden Magengeschwüres. Arch klin Chir. 1887;34:79–90.
5. Cheatle GL. A method of uniting the divided intestine. Lancet. 1897;150(3870):1113.
6. Finney JMT. A new method of pyloroplasty. Tr Am Surg Assn. 1902;20:165–90.
7. Finney JMT. Pyloroplasty and gastroduodenostomy. Surgery. 1937;2:738–58.
8. Tjandra JJ, Fazio VW. Techniques of strictureplasty. Perspectives Colon Rectal Surg. 1992;5:189–98.

Tuberculosis 193

Michelle D. Inkster, Mark A. H. Cohen, Joseph T. Azok, Todd W. Stultz, Eric W. Willis, and James S. Wu

Presentation

A 68-year-old man was found to have severe segmental colitis at colonoscopy. Subsequently, he received anti-tumor necrosis factor therapy for two years. Despite this, his condition declined. Repeat colonoscopy showed persistent segmental colitis. He was transferred for ongoing care. At admission, the patient was febrile. He complained of weight loss, abdominal pain, and dizziness. Abdominal computed tomography (CT) findings were consistent with colitis of the proximal colon and the splenic flexure (Fig. 193.1a, b).

Chest computed tomography showed innumerable bilateral pulmonary nodules (Fig. 193.2).

Magnetic resonance imaging of the brain showed multiple contrast enhancing lesions with the largest one over the right thalamic region (Fig. 193.3).

Histology slides of biopsies from the patient's preadmission colonoscopy were obtained and stained for acid fast bacilli (AFB) (Fig. 193.4).

The patient's sputum tested positive for mycobacterium tuberculosis.

M. D. Inkster
Department of Gastroenterology, Cleveland Clinic, Cleveland, OH, USA

M. A. H. Cohen · J. T. Azok · T. W. Stultz
Radiology & Diagnostic Imaging Institute, Cleveland Clinic, Cleveland, OH, USA

E. W. Willis
Department of Pathology, CORPath, Columbus, OH, USA

J. S. Wu (✉)
Department of Colon and Rectal Surgery, Cleveland Clinic, Cleveland, OH, USA

J. S. Wu, M. D. Inkster (eds.), *Cleveland Clinic Colorectal Case Studies*,
https://doi.org/10.1007/978-3-031-39880-3_193

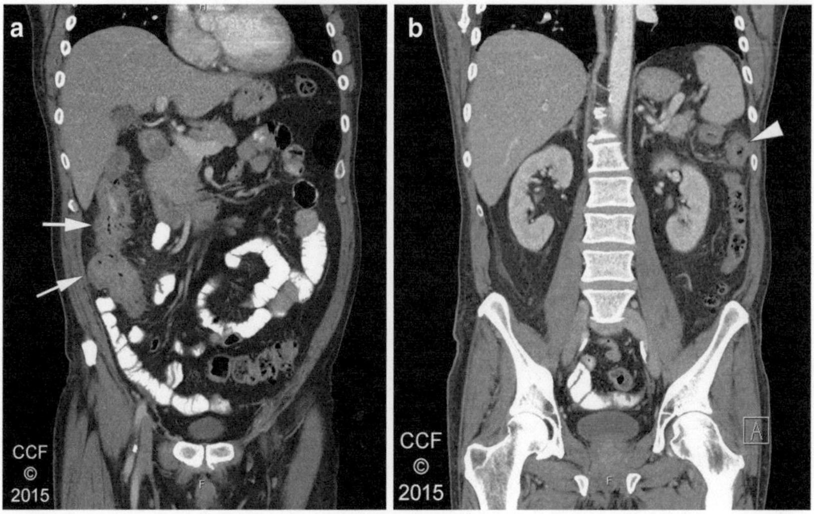

Fig. 193.1 Coronal abdominal CT images were consistent with colitis of the proximal colon (**a**, arrows) and splenic flexure (**b**, arrowhead)

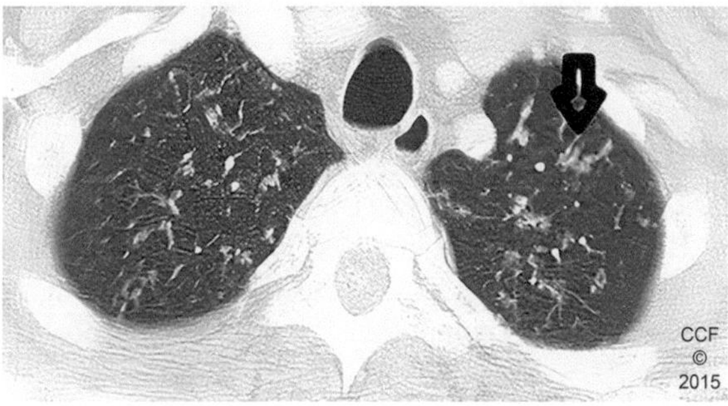

Fig. 193.2 Chest CT shows innumerable small (less than 5 mm) noncalcified bilateral diffusely scattered pulmonary nodular opacities. One prominent nodule is marked with an arrow

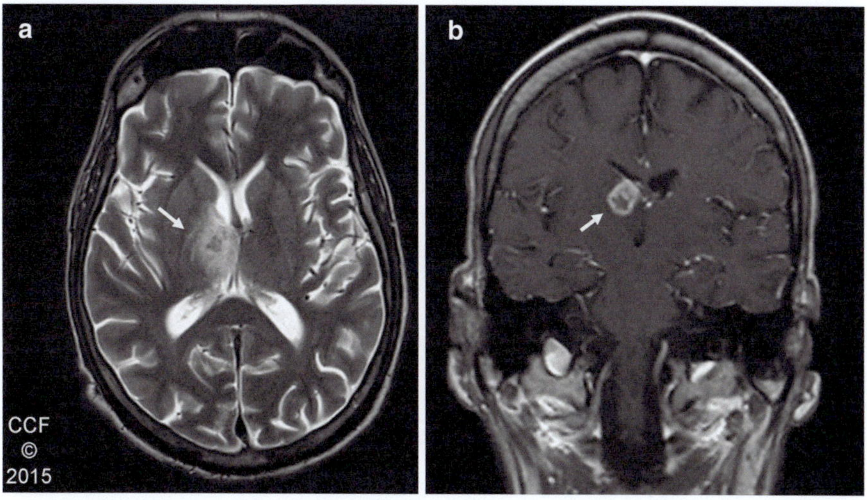

Fig. 193.3 Magnetic resonance imaging shows a large intracranial mass in the right thalamus (arrows) most suggestive of metastatic disease (**a**—axial view, **b**–coronal view)

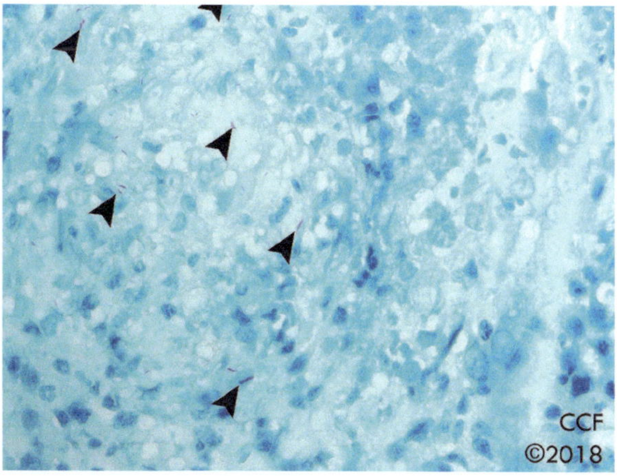

Fig. 193.4 An AFB stain highlights numerous pink-rod-shaped mycobacteria (arrowheads) within a granuloma

Management

Infectious disease consultation was obtained.

Comment

After ingestion of *M. tuberculosis,* there is an influx of macrophages and granulocytes into interstitial spaces. Tumor necrosis factor (TNF) is necessary to help dendritic cells mature so that antigen presentation can prime the immune response. Formation of granulomas represents an effort by the host to contain viable microorganisms. Administration of monoclonal anti-TNF therapy may reactivate tuberculosis [1]. Evaluation of patients for latent and active tuberculosis before initiating treatment with anti-TNF monoclonal antibody therapy is recommended [2, 3].

References

1. Ehlers S. Why does tumor necrosis factor targeted therapy reactivate tuberculosis? J Rheumatol. 2005;74:35–9.
2. Kedia S, Mouli VP, Kamat N, Sankar J, Ananthakrishnan A, Makharia G, et al. Risk of tuberculosis in patients with inflammatory bowel disease on infliximab or adalimumab is dependent on the local disease burden of tuberculosis: A systematic review and meta-analysis. Am J Gastroenterol. 2020;115:340–9.
3. Gómez-Reino JJ, Carmona L, Valverde VR, Mola EM, Montero MD, BIOBADASER Group. Treatment of rheumatoid arthritis with tumor necrosis factor inhibitors may predispose to significant increase in tuberculosis risk. Arthritis Rheum. 2003;48:2122–7.

Tuberculosis Staining

194

James S. Wu

Presentation

In 1882, Robert Koch described a method of staining that allowed the visualization of mycobacterium tuberculosis (MTB).

Die Aetiologie der Tuberculose. Von Dr. Robert Koch Regierungsrath im Kaiserl. Gesundheitsamt [1] Bei meinen Untersuchungen über die Tuberculose habe ich mich anfangs auch der bekannten Methoden bedient, ohne damit eine Aufklärung über das Wesen der Krankheit zu erlangen. Aber durch einige gelegentliche Beobachtungen wurde ich dann veranlasst, diese Methoden zu verlassen und andere Wege einzuschlagen, die schliesslich auch zu positiven Resultaten führten. Das Ziel der Untersuchung musste zunächst auf den Nachweis von irgend welchen, dem Körper fremdartigen, parasitischen Gebilden gerichtet sein, die möglicherweise als Krankheits-ursache gedeutet werden konnten. Dieser Nachweis gelang auch in der That durch ein bestimmtes Färbungsverfahren, mit Hülfe dessen in allen tuberculös veränderten Organen charactertische, bis dahin nicht bekannte Bacterien zu finden waren.	The Etiology of Tuberculosis[1] by Dr. Robert Koch Advisor to the Imperial Health Council [2] In my own studies on tuberculosis I began by using the known methods, without success. But several casual observations have induced me to forego these methods and strike out in a new direction, which has finally led me to positive results. The goal of the study must first be the demonstration of a foreign parasitic structure in the body which can possibly be indicted as the causal agent. This proof was possible through a certain staining procedure which has allowed the discovery of characteristic, although previously undescribed bacteria, in organs which have been altered by tuberculosis….

Koch documented the histologic appearance of tuberculosis stained by his method using methylene blue in meticulous color illustrations. One example of

J. S. Wu (✉)
Department of Colon and Rectal Surgery, Cleveland Clinic, Cleveland, OH, USA

J. S. Wu, M. D. Inkster (eds.), *Cleveland Clinic Colorectal Case Studies*,
https://doi.org/10.1007/978-3-031-39880-3_194

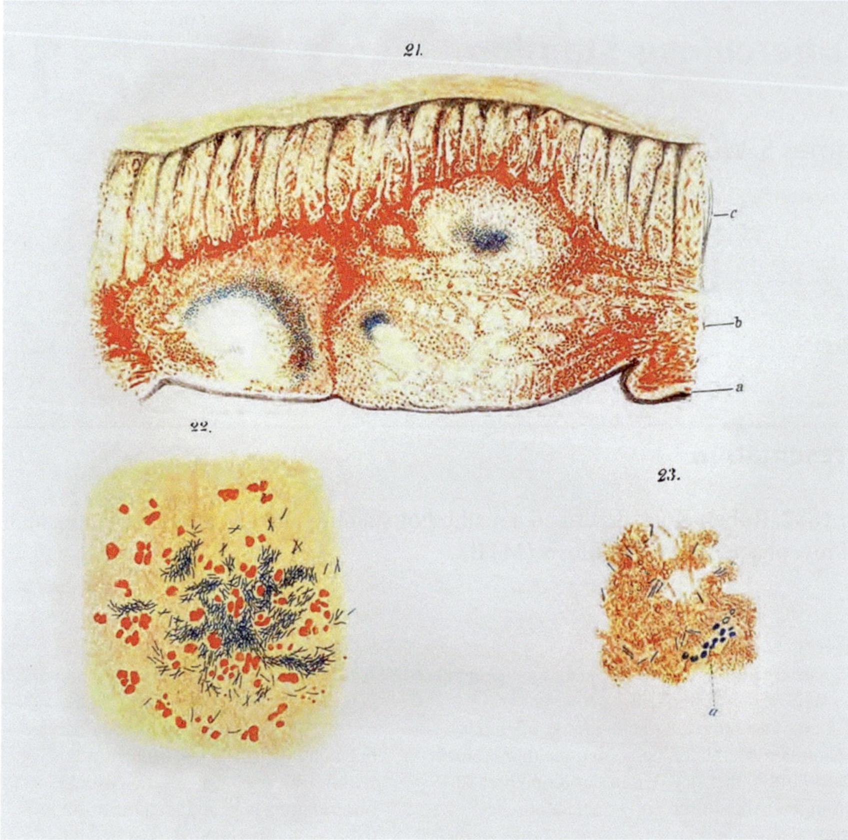

Fig. 194.1 Shown here are three illustrations by Koch, reprinted from Die Gesammelte Werke von Robert Koch, Erster Band, Tafel XXIV, Figs. 21., 22, and 23 [3]

small intestinal tuberculosis, shown in Fig. 194.1., shows slices taken through a tubercular ulcer [3].

S. 563	p. 563
Fig. 21. Schnitt in der Längsrichtung des…gezeichneten Darmes durch einige Tuberelknötchen. a Serosa. b Längmuskelschicht. c. Quermuskelschicht. 70 facher Vergrößerung.	Fig. 21. Section in the longitudinal direction… of the intestine through a few tubercle nodules. a Serosa. b. Longitudinal muscle layer. c Transverse muscle layer. 70x magnification.
Fig. 22. Eine der blau erscheinenden Stellen aus Fig. 21 bei 700 facher Vergrößerung.	Fig. 22 One of the areas appearing in blue from Fig. 21 at a magnification of 700x.
Fig. 23. Darmausleerung bei Darmphthisis. Deckglaspräparat, 700 facher Vergrößerung. Die Tuberkelbazillen blau, die übrigen Bacterien braun gefärbt. Rechts unten (a) eine Gruppe von mehr oder weniger intensiv blaugefärbten eiförmigen Bazillensporen.	Fig. 23 Evacuated bowel: intestinal tuberculosis. Coverslip preparation. 700x magnification. The tubercle bacilli are colored blue, the remaining bacteria are brown. Right below (a) a group of more or less intensely blue-colored egg-shaped bacillus spores.

Later in 1882, Paul Ehrlich described an improved method that involved using of aniline, fuchsin, and mineral acid [4]. Ehrlich here is describing the characteristic of acid fastness, the property that gives a bacterium the ability to resist decolorization by acids during staining. Bacterium of the genus Mycobacterium including *M. tuberculosis* and *M. leprae* have this property [5].

"Modification der von Koch angegebenen Methode der Färbung von Tuberkelbacillen
Paul Ehrlich
Wie bekannt, besteht die von Herrn Reg.-Rath Koch angegebene Methode darin, dass er Trockenpräparate in einter schwach alkalischen Lösung von Methylenblau färbt. Nach 24 Stunden setz er sie der Erwirkung einer Versuvin-Lösung aus. Dann wird das Präparat braun, und es zeigt sich, dass sämmtliche Elemente intensive braun sind und nur der Bacillus rein und intensiv blau bleibt.

Für die Färbung verwende ich ein mit Anilinöl gesättigtes Wasser, das sich durch Schütteln von Wasser mit überschüssigem Anilinöl und Filtriren durch ein angefeuchtetes Filter binnen wenigen Minuten herstellen lässt. Der so gewonnenen wasserklaren Flüssigkeit fügt man tropfenweise von einer gesättigten alkoholischen Fuchsin- oder Methylviolettlösung so lange hinzu, bis eine deutliche Opalescenz der Flüssigkeit eintritt, die die Sättigung mit Farbstoff anzeigt. Auf dieser Flüssigkeit lässt man die Präparate schwimmen und sieht sie binnen ¼ bis ½ Stunde intensiv in dem betreffenden Farbton sich anfärben. Die isolirte Tinction der Tuberculosebacillen gelingt nun unter dem Einfluss des Vesuvin gar nicht oder nur sehr langsam, es ist erforderlich, Säuren anzuwenden und bin ich bald zur Anwendung starker, ich möchte sagen, heroischer übergegangen. Am meisten empfiehlt sich Säuergemisch, das aus 1 Volumen officineller Saltpetersäuer und 2 Voluminibus Wasser besteht. Man sieht unter seinem Einfluss in wenig Secunden das Präparat erblassen, es heben sich gelbe Wolken hervor, und das Präparat wird weiss. Untersucht man in diesem Stadium das Präparat, so ergiebt sich, dass Alless entfärbt ist, und nur der Bacillus die intensive Färbung beibehalten hat. Man könnte jetz schon ein derartiges Präparat untersuchen, doch sind die technischen Schwierigkeiten ausserordentlich gross, den Bacillus enzustellen. Es empfiehlt sich, den Untergrund anzufärben und zwar, wenn das Präparat violett ist, gelb, wenn es roth ist, blau."

"A method for staining the tubercle bacillus
Paul Ehrlich [6][1]
As it is known, the method of Herr Reg.-Rath Koch consists of staining dried preparations in a weakly alkaline solution of methylene blue. After 24 hours, they are then treated with a solution of vesuvin. Then the preparation becomes brown, and under the microscope all of the substances are strongly brown, while the bacillus alone remains intense blue.

For the staining I use water-saturated aniline oil. This is prepared by shaking water with an excess of aniline oil and filtering through a moist filter. To the water-clear liquid obtained is added dropwise an alcoholic-saturated solution of fuchsin or methyl violet until a distinct opalescence develops which indicates that the dye is saturated. The preparations are immersed in this liquid and within one-fourth to one-half hour they have become intensely colored. The differentiation of the tubercle bacilli proceeds only very slowly with vesuvin, so that it is necessary to use acid. I have used strong, even heroic, concentrations of acid. The most effective is to mix one volume officinal nitric acid and two volumes of water. Within a few seconds one can see the preparation fade under the acid treatment, yellow clouds are given off, and the preparation becomes white. If one would examine the preparation at this stage, one would see that everything had been decolorized except the bacteria, and they had remained intensely colored. Such a preparation could be examined at this stage, but the technical difficulties are considerable, since it is difficult to focus on the bacilli. It is better to stain the background in a contrasting color, such as yellow, if the preparation is violet, or blue, if the preparation is red."

[1] Permission to reuse excerpts from references 2 and 5 were generously given by the American Society for Microbiology Press, Copyright Limited License Agreement Invoice No.: P2022.2, July 13, 2022.

In addition to his work on the visualization of tuberculosis, Ehrlich is recognized as the founder of chemotherapy [7]. In 1910, Ehrlich and Hata published Die experimentelle Chemotherapie der Spirillosen [8].

"Die experimentelle Chemotherapie der Spirillosen (Syphilis, Rückfallfieber, Hühnerspirillose, Frambösie)	"The experimental chemotherapie of spirilloses (syphilis, relapsing fever, chicken spirillosis, yeast infections)
Von	By
Paul Ehrlich und S. Hata	Paul Ehrlich and S. Hata
Schlußbemerkung	Closing remarks
Von	By
Paul Ehrlich	Paul Ehrlich
Beherrscht wird das ganze Gebiet von einem ganz einfachen, ich möchte sagen selbstverständliche Grundsatz. Wenn für die Chemie das Gesetz gilt: corpora non agunt nisi liquida, so is für die Chemotherapie maßgebend: corpora non agunt nisi fixata!"	The entire area is governed by a very simple, I would like to say, self-evident principle. If for chemistry, the law applies: bodies do not act except through liquid; then for chemotherapy, the law applies: bodies do not act without fixation!"

The 1908 Nobel Prize in Physiology or Medicine was awarded jointly to Ilya Ilyich Mechnikov and Paul Ehrlich "in recognition of their work on immunity" [9].

References

1. Die KR. Aetiologie der Tuberculose. Berliner Klin Wochenschr. 1882;No. 15:221–30.
2. Koch R. The etiology of tuberculosis. In: Milestones in Microbiology 1545-1940., translated and edited by Thomas D. Brock. Washington, DC: ASM Press; 1999. p. 109–15.
3. Koch R. Die Ätiologie der Tuberkulose. (Mitteilungen aus dem Kaiserl. Gesundheitsamte, Bd. II. Berline 1884.) In: Koch, R, Gaffky G, Pfuhl E. Gassammelte Werke von Robert Koch, Erster Band, herausgegeben von Schwalbe J, Verlag von Georg Thieme, Leipzig, 1912; Hierzu Tafel XXIV, Figs., 21-23, Erklärung der Abbildungen, p.563. [cited 2022 Aug 27]. Accessed from Google Books.
4. Ehrlich P. Modification der von Koch angegebenen Methode der Färbung von Tuberkelbacillen. Dtsch med Wschr. 1882;8:269–70. in Himmelweit F. (ed), The collected Papers of Paul Ehrlich, Vol 1, Pergamon Press, London, 1960; pp 311–313.
5. Bayot ML, Mirza TM, Sharma S. Acid Fast Bacteria. 2023 Aug 7. In: StatPearls [Internet]. Treasure Island (FL): StatPearls Publishing; 2024 PMID: 30725806.
6. Ehrlich P. A method for staining the tubercle bacillus. In: Milestones in Microbiology 1545-1940., translated and edited by Thomas D. Brock. Washington, DC: ASM Press; 1999. p. 118–20.
7. Kaufmann SHE. Paul Ehrlich: founder of chemotherapy. Nature Rev. 2008;7:373.
8. Ehrlich P, Hata S. Die experimentelle Chemotherapie der Spirillosen. (Syphilis, Rückfallfieber, Hühnerspirillose, Frambösie). Verlag von Julius Springer, Berlin, 1910;114. Accessed from Archive.org July 30, 2021.
9. The Nobel Prize in Physiology or Medicine 1908. NobelPrize.org. Nobel Media AB 2020. Sat. 20 Jun 2020. <https://www.nobelprize.org/prizes/medicine/1908/summary/.

Extraintestinal Manifestations of Inflammatory Bowel Disease

195

Aaron Brzezinski, Careen Y. Lowder, Michelle D. Inkster, Catherine L. Forse, Arthur A. Parsee, and James S. Wu

Extraintestinal Manifestations of Inflammatory Bowel Disease

The extra-intestinal complications of Crohn's disease and ulcerative colitis: A study of 700 patients

"The separation of extra-intestinal manifestations of inflammatory bowel disease into the two main groups which we have proposed seems reasonably consistent with the data and with current ways of thinking about these disorders.

One group ("B") is clearly related to disturbed small bowel function: *malabsorption* of fat, carbohydrates, and vitamin B_{12}, clearly representing loss of small bowel absorption function especially in the ileum; *gallstones,* secondary to diminished ileal reabsorption of bile salts; *kidney stones*, due to fluid and electrolyte losses plus the recently described increased absorption of oxalate; *ureteral obstruction* and *enterovesical fistulae*, secondary to direct extension of ileal disease. This group of disorders occurs most often in patients with Crohn's disease involving the ileum.

The other group ("A") appears to be more closely related to the inflammatory activity of the underlying bowel disease and to be associated with the involvement of the colon more

A. Brzezinski · M. D. Inkster
Department of Gastroenterology, Cleveland Clinic, Cleveland, OH, USA

C. Y. Lowder
Cole Cye Institute, Cleveland Clinic, Cleveland, OH, USA

C. L. Forse
Department of Pathology and Laboratory Medicine, Faculty of Medicine, University of Ottawa, Ottawa, ON, Canada

A. A. Parsee
Department of Diagnostic Radiology, H. Lee Moffitt Cancer Center and Research Institute, Tampa, FL, USA

J. S. Wu (✉)
Pathology & Laboratory Medicine Institute, Cleveland Clinic, Cleveland, OH, USA

Department of Colon and Rectal Surgery, Cleveland Clinic, Cleveland, OH, USA

J. S. Wu, M. D. Inkster (eds.), *Cleveland Clinic Colorectal Case Studies*,
https://doi.org/10.1007/978-3-031-39880-3_195

than of the small bowel. By analogy with the arthritis of viral hepatitis, and in keeping with some evidence regarding circulating antigen-antibody complexes, these extra-intestinal manifestations may have an immunologic basis possibly by the deposition of antigen-antibody complexes in the synovium, skin, and choroid apparatus of the eye."

Adrian J. Greenstein, M.B., B.Ch., F.A.C.S., F.R.C.S. (Eng., Ed.), Henry D. Janowitz, M.D., M.S., F.A.C.P., and David B. Sachar, M.D., F.A.C.P., F.A.C.G. Mount Sinai School of Medicine, New York, 1976 [1][1]

Extraintestinal manifestations in Crohn's disease and ulcerative colitis: results from a prospective population-based European inception cohort

"EIM (Extraintestinal manifestations) can be classified conceptually into two distinct pathogenetic categories: immune-mediated conditions, which in common with the bowel disease have an immunological pathogenesis, and non-immune-mediated conditions, which are caused by metabolic and other processes that are secondary to the bowel disease. To the first group belong the arthropathies, skin disorders, eye disorders, and sclerosing cholangitis; to the second group can be counted cholelithiasis, nephrolithiasis, and anemia."

Rune Isene, Tomm Bernklev, Ole Høie, Pia Munkholm, Epameonondas Tsianos, Reinhold Stockbrücker, et al. behalf of the EC-IBD Study Group, 2015 [2][2]

Renal involvement in inflammatory bowel diseases

"The most frequently involved organs are the joints (peripheral arthritis, sacroileitis, anky losing spondylitis), the skin (erythema nodosum, pyoderma gangrenosum), the eyes (episcleritis, uveitis), the liver and the biliary tract (primary sclerosing cholangitis, gallstones).

Renal involvement has been considered as an EIM and has been described both in Crohn's disease (CD) and in ulcerative colitis (UC). The most frequent renal diseases in patients with IBD are: nephrolithiasis, tubulointerstitial nephritis, glomerulonephritis and amyloidosis."

Domenico Corica, Claudio Romano,

Department of Pediatrics,
University of Messina,
Messina, Italy, 2016[3][3]

Examples of EIMs of inflammatory bowel disease follow.

[1]This excerpt is reused with the generous permission of Wolters Kluwer Health, Inc., CCC | RightsLink® License Number 5174811074308, License date Oct 23, 2021.

[2]This excerpt is reused with the generous permission of Ms. Lee-Ann Anderson | Senior Permissions Executive, Journals, Taylor & Francis Group: permissionrequest@tandf.co.uk; 4 Park Square, Milton Park, Abingdon, OX14 4RN, Ref: LA/IGAS/P21/1687, 15 December 2021.

[3]This excerpt is reused with the generous permission of Oxford University Press, CCC | RightsLink®, License number 5174921343749, License date Oct 23, 2021.

Pyoderma Gangrenosum

Pyoderma gangrenosum (PG) is a chronic noninfectious condition marked by the formation of purplish nodules and pustules that tend to coalesce and form ulcers [4]. Examples of PG of the leg and peristomal skin are shown in Fig. 195.1a-b. The histologic appearance of PG from a left leg biopsy is shown in Fig. 195.1c-d.

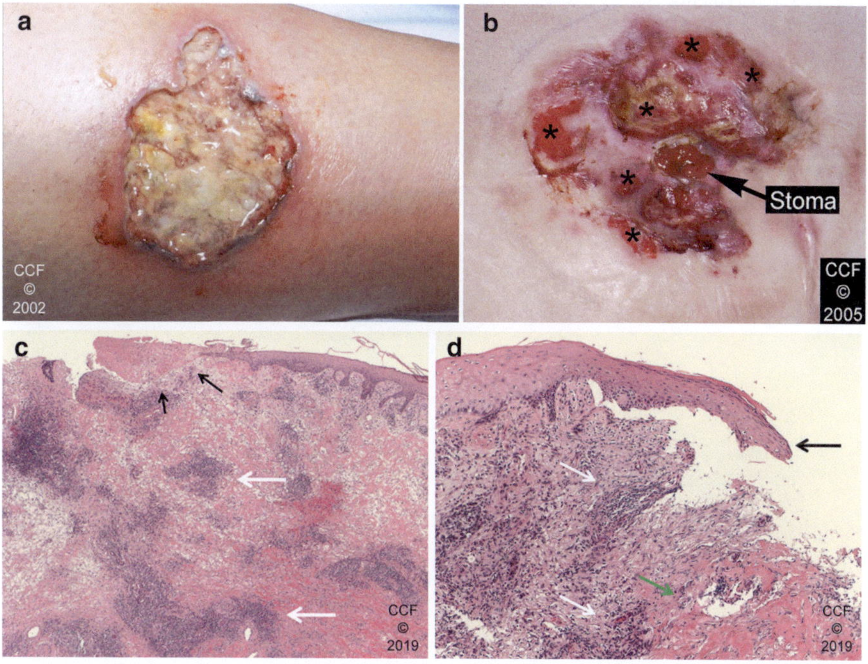

Fig. 195.1 (**a**) Pyoderma gangrenosum of the leg; (**b**) Peristomal pyoderma gangrenosum (asterisks) surrounding a stoma. (**c**) Skin biopsy from an ulcer on the left leg of a patient presenting clinically with pyoderma gangrenosum. There is a pronounced necroinflammatory infiltrate with loss of the overlying epidermis, consistent with an ulcer (black arrows). Note the superficial and deep perivascular acute and chronic inflammatory infiltrates in the dermis adjacent to the ulcer (white arrows). H&E, 40× magnification; (**d**) Skin biopsy from a left leg ulcer in a patient presenting clinically with pyoderma gangrenosum. The overhanging epidermis adjacent to the ulcer (see black arrow) can sometimes be seen as rolled edges by the treating clinician. Acute and chronic inflammation (white arrows) mixed with fibrin (green arrow) are noted within the dermis. H&E, 100× magnification

Erythema Nodosum

Pellicer et al. [5] describe erythema nodosum as a panniculitis that presents as multiple deep-red tender, painful nodules, distributed usually over the shins. An example of erythema nodosum of the leg is shown in Fig. 195.2.

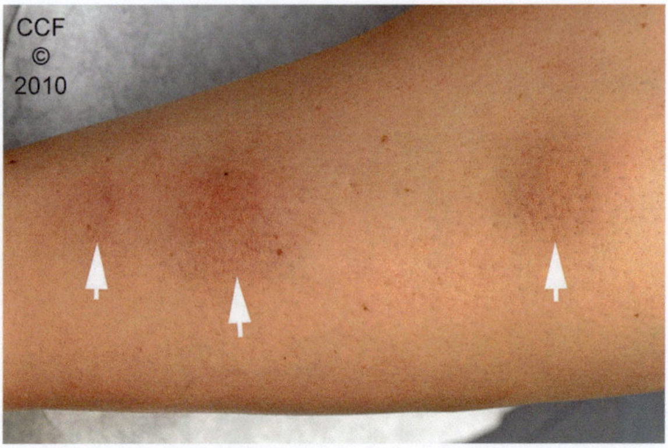

Fig. 195.2 Erythema nodosum of the leg (arrows)

Primary Sclerosing Cholangitis

PSC-IBD: a unique form of inflammatory bowel disease disease associated with primary sclerosing cholangitis

> "Primary sclerosing cholangitis (PSC) is a chronic cholestatic disease of unknown aetiology, characterized by inflammation and fibrosis of the biliary tree. PSC may eventually progress to hepatic cirrhosis and subsequent liver failure, and is accompanied by an increased risk of cholangiocarcinoma. PSC may occur in the presence or absence of inflammatory bowel disease (IBD). The prevalence of IBD (typically chronic ulcerative colitis (CUC)) among PSC patients is approximately 70-80% while only 2-7.5% of patients with CUC will develop PSC."

EV Loftus, Jr, GC Harewood, CG Loftus,
WJ Tremaine, WS Harmsen, AR Zinsmeister, DA Jewell, WJ Sandborn,
Division of Gastroenterology and Hepatology,
Mayo Clinic,
Rochester, MN, 2005 [6][4]

A cholangiogram showing multiple biliary tree strictures is shown in Fig. 195.3.

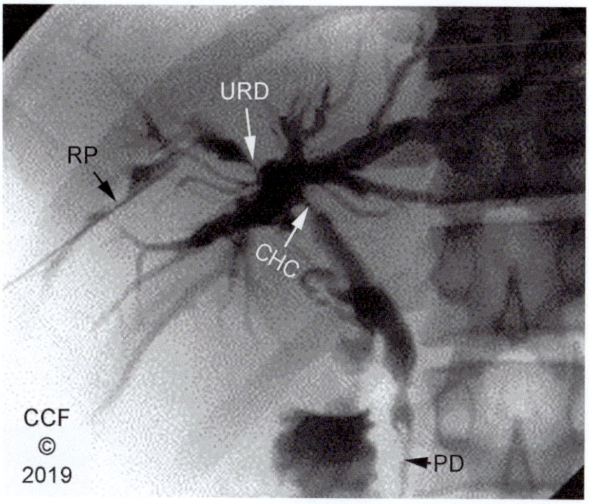

Fig. 195.3 Cholangiogram showing biliary strictures. The upward arrow shows a stricture at the common hepatic confluence (CHC). The downward arrow shows a stricture in the upper right duct, presumably draining segments VIII and VII (URD = upper right duct). There are smaller strictures towards the periphery as well, mostly on the right (right periphery, RP). There is also a physiologic narrowing of the common bile duct as it enters the pancreatic head (pancreatic duct, PD)

[4] Reuse of this excerpt was covered by Fair Use per British Medical Journal permissions.

As the strictures are isolated primarily to the intrahepatic branches, PSC would be the leading diagnosis.

Ophthalmologic Extraintestinal Manifestations of Inflammatory Disease

Presentation

A 65-year-old woman with Crohn's disease presented with severe scleritis, keratitis, and episcleritis (Fig. 195.4a–c) while being treated with Imuran (azathioprine). Treatment with prednisone controlled the pain but did not clear up the scleritis. She had an excellent response to Humira® (adalimumab) (Fig. 195.4d–e).

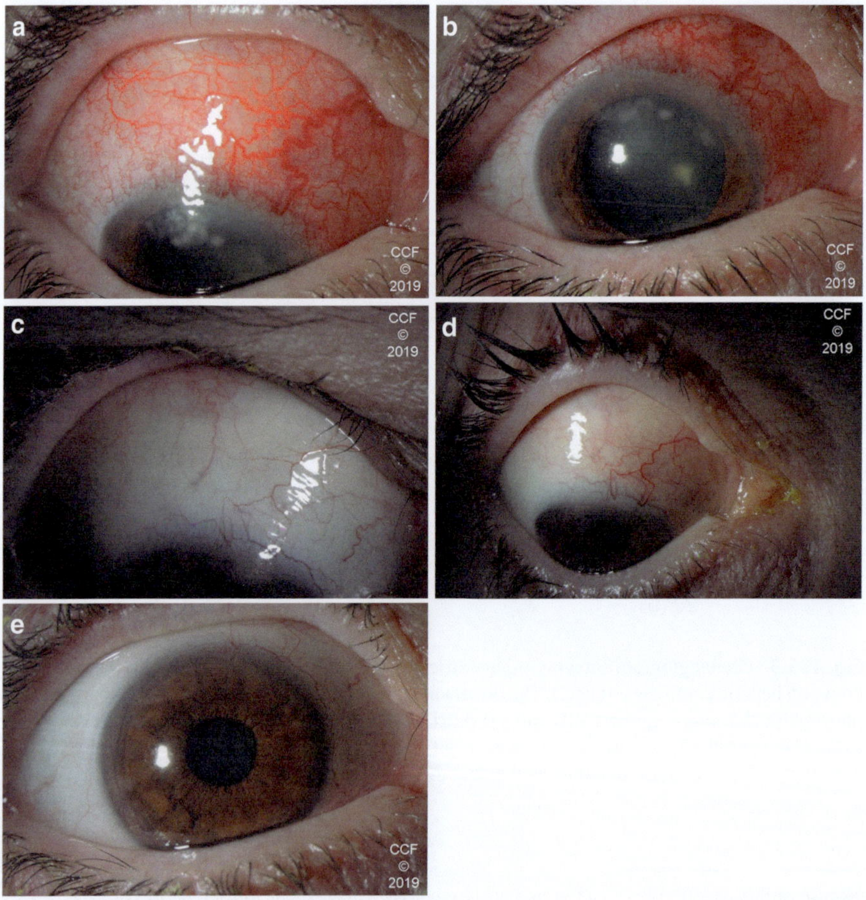

Fig. 195.4 (**a** and **b**) Severe scleritis and keratitis; (**c**) Episcleritis; (**d**) Scleritis that is responding to HUMIRA® (adalimumab); (**e**) Resolved sclerokeratitis

Nephrolithiasis

Renal calcium oxalate calculi may be seen in patients who have undergone extensive terminal ileal resection.[5]

References

1. Greenstein AJ, Janowitz HD, Sachar DB. The extra-intestinal complications of Crohn's disease and ulcerative colitis: A study of 700 patients. Medicine. 1976;55:401–12.
2. Isene R, Bernklev T, Høie O, Munkholm P, Tsianos E, Stockbrügger R, et al. Extraintestinal manifestations in Crohn's disease and ulcerative colitis: results from a prospective, population-based European inception cohort. Scand J Gastroenterol. 2015;50:300–5.
3. Corica D, Romano C. Renal involvement inflammatory bowel diseases. J Crohns Colitis. 2016;10:226–35.
4. "Pyoderma gangrenosum." *Merriam-Webster.com Medical Dictionary*, Merriam-Webster. [cited 2020 Jun 23]. Available from https://www.merriam-webster.com/medical/pyoderma%20gangrenosum
5. Pellicer Z, Santiago JM, Rodriguez A, Alonso V, Antón R, Bosca MM. Management of cutaneous disorders related to inflammatory bowel disease. Ann Gastroenterol. 2012;25:21–36.
6. Loftus EV Jr, Harewood GC, Loftus CG, Tremaine WJ, Harmsen WS, Zinsmeister AR, et al. PSC-IBD: a unique form of inflammatory bowel disease associated with primary sclerosing cholangitis. Gut. 2005;54:91–6.

[5] See Chap. 190, *Consequences of extensive ileal resection.*

Meckel's Diverticulum

196

Michelle D. Inkster, Leonard A. Kahn, James E. Lapinski, Luca Stocchi, and James S. Wu

Presentation

A 42-year-old male presented with abdominal pain accompanied first by discharge of melena and then by bright red blood per rectum. Esophagogastroduodenoscopy was unremarkable. Colonoscopy did not reveal a bleeding source. A tagged red cell scan showed active bleeding in the pelvic small bowel (Fig. 196.1a, b). Angiography, however, did not identify an active bleeding site. Because of continued acute blood loss anemia (Hb 6.7 g/dL), he was transfused with a total of seven units of packed red blood cells. Next, a nuclear medicine gastric ectopic Meckel's scan was done (Fig. 196.2).

M. D. Inkster
Department of Gastroenterology, Cleveland Clinic, Cleveland, OH, USA

L. A. Kahn
Radiology & Diagnostic Imaging Institute, Cleveland Clinic, Cleveland, OH, USA

J. E. Lapinski
Pathology & Laboratory Medicine Institute, Cleveland Clinic, Cleveland, OH, USA

L. Stocchi
Department of Colon and Rectal Surgery, Mayo Clinic, Jacksonville, FL, USA

J. S. Wu (✉)
Department of Colon and Rectal Surgery, Cleveland Clinic, Cleveland, OH, USA

J. S. Wu, M. D. Inkster (eds.), *Cleveland Clinic Colorectal Case Studies*,
https://doi.org/10.1007/978-3-031-39880-3_196

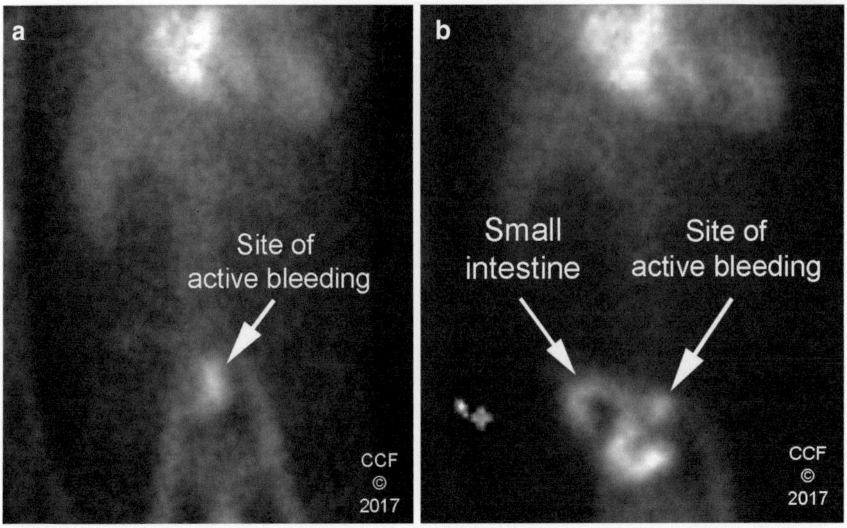

Fig. 196.1 Tagged red blood scan. (**a**) Immediate active bleeding is seen in the right pelvis; (**b**) A subsequent image shows activity at the site of active bleeding and in the adjacent small intestine

Fig. 196.2 A nuclear medicine ectopic Meckel's scan with 10.3 MCi Tc 99m pertechnetate given intravenously. Dynamic imaging of the abdomen was obtained for 30 min. The abnormal focus of activity in the mid-abdomen (arrow) suggests ectopic gastric mucosa. Activity in the gastric area (G) and the bladder (B) also is seen

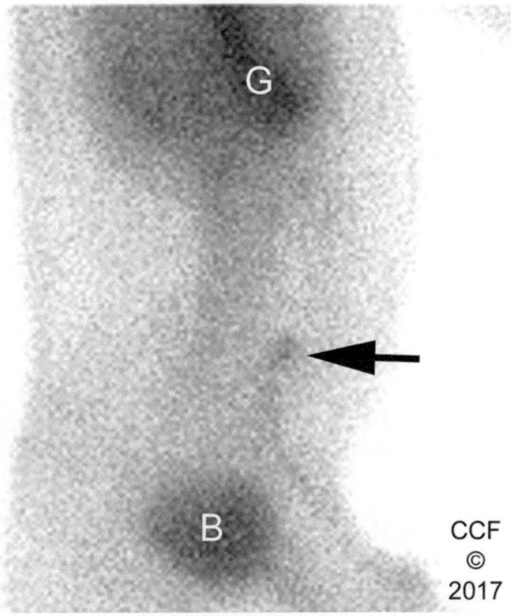

Management

A Meckel's diverticulum, found approximately 40 cm from the ileocecal valve, was excised surgically. Pathology confirmed the presence of a Meckel's diverticulum with gastric heterotopia, focal mucosal ulceration, and pyloric gland metaplasia (Fig. 196.3a–d).

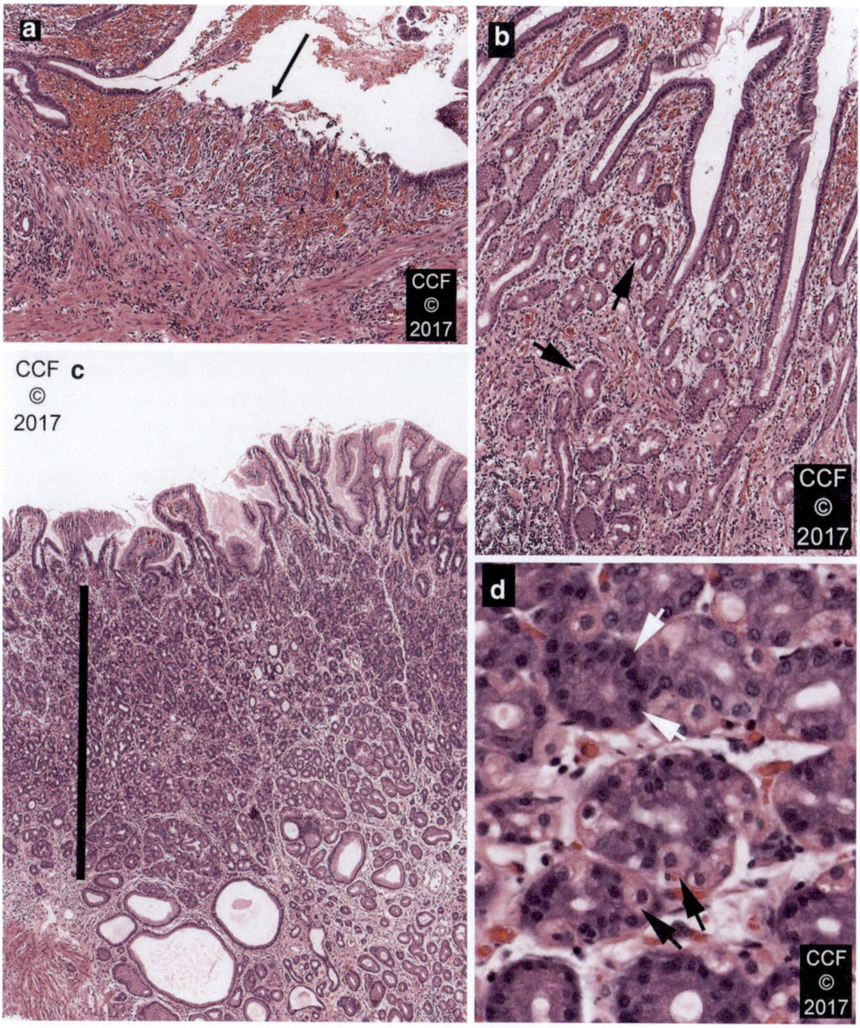

Fig. 196.3 Gastric heterotopia. (**a**) Nonspecific mucosal ulceration possibly due to mucosal prolapse or peptic injury in the setting of gastric heterotopia (arrow); (**b**) pyloric gland metaplasia (arrows); (**c**) Gastric heterotopia (boundary defined by the black line); (**d**) Gastric heterotopia (high magnification). Oxyntic-type glands are present with chief cells characterized by basophilic cytoplasm (white arrows) and parietal cells with eosinophilic cytoplasm (black arrows)

Comment

An example of a Meckel's diverticulum is shown in Fig. 196.4.

In 1809, Johann Friedrich Meckel, the younger, published a treatise entitled "Divertikel am Darmkanal" (Intestinal divertula) [1].

Ueber die Divertikel am Darmkanal, vom Prof. Meckel S. 422. Dies ist die, welche den Namen des Divertikels, Darmanhanges oder Darmfortsatzes führt, gewiss jedem nur etwas beschäftigen Zergliederer mehrmals vorgekommen,... S. 423. Mit dem allgemeinen Namen des Darmanhanges or Darmfortsatzes, belegt man alle diejenigen blind geendigten hohlen Erhabenheiten, welche über den Umfang des Darmkanals hervorspringen, und deren Höhle mit der seinigen zusammenhängt. S. 424. Man findet nemlich I) Darmanhänge, die eine rundliche, kugelförmige Gestalt haben, und mit einer etwas zusammengezogen Grundfläche auf dem Darmkanal sitzen. S. 428. Meiner Meinung nach, die ich auch schon früher, wiewohl nur beyläufig.., geäussert habe, haben sie in der anfänglich Statt findenden Communication zwischen der Nabelblase und dem Darmkanale ihren Grund,… S. 452–453. Ist es mir gelungen, auf dem vorigen Seiten das wahre Wesen Darmanhanges zu schildern, so fällt damit zugleich die…als bestimmte Wahrheit aufstellte Behauptung, dass der Blinddarm und der Wurmfortsatz der ductus umbilico - intestinalis sey,...	On diverticula of the intestinal canal by Professor Meckel This is that, which is called diverticulum, intestinal appendix or intestinal appendage, certainly now is encountered frequently only by busy dissectors, … Concerning the generally named intestinal appendix or intestinal appendage, it can be proved that all of those blindly ending hollow raised structures and their lumens which arise from their association with the intestinal canal are related. One can find namely I) intestinal appendages, which have a rounded spherical shape, and sit on the intestinal canal with a slightly contracted base. It is my opinion, which I stated previously, if only casually, that initially they have a communication with the umbilical vesicle and the intestinal canal as their origin,… If I succeeded in the preceding pages in describing the true nature of the intestinal appendix, then at the same it follows, the presented assertion as certain truth, that the appendix or worm appendage are the ductus umbilicointestinalis….

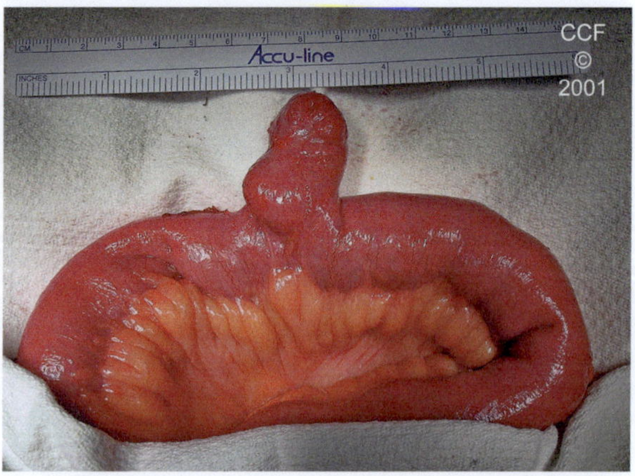

Fig. 196.4 A Meckel's diverticulum located in the terminal ileum and found incidentally at another surgery

A year earlier, in his comprehensive work entitled *Beyträge zur vergleichenden Anatomy*[2] *(A Contribution to Comparative Anatomy)*, Meckel notes that these *angebornes* (innate) diverticula arise from the small not the large intestine.

Beyträge zur vergleichenden Anatomie JF Meckel Professor der Anatomie und Chirurgie zu Halle, 1808 S. 93. Folgende Gründe scheinen mir zu beweisen, dass Divertikel Ueberreste dieser Verbinding des Darmkanals mit der Nabelblase sind: 2) Finden sie sich, wie es scheint, immer nur am dünnen Darme, denn unter einer beträchlichen Menge, die ich besitze, findet sich kein einziges am dicken und noch habe ich bey keinem Schriftsteller ein bestimmt beschreibenes, angebornes Divertikel anderswo als am dünnen Darme erwähnt gefunden.	Contributions to Comparative Anatomy JF Meckel Professor der Anatomie and Surgery, at Halle, 1808 The following reasons appear to prove to me, that Diverticula are the remains of a connection of the intestinal tract with the umbilical vesicle: 2) These are found, it appears, only on the small intestine. Among the considerable quantity which I possess, there is not a single large intestinal one. And yet I have not found a certain description mentioned by any writer of an innate diverticulum elsewhere other than on the small intestine.

Meckel concludes that the diverticula arising from the small intestine are of umbilical origin. It is now recognized that Meckel's diverticulium is a vestigial remnant of the omphalomesenteric duct. It is a true diverticulum as it contains all three layers of the small intestine. In 1905, Kelly and Hurdon described four types of Meckel's diverticulum (Kelly and Hurdon, Figs. 309–312, this work, Figs. 196.5, 196.6, 196.7, and 196.8) [3].

> "**Embryology of Meckel's Diverticulum.**—In the very young embryo the short and straight intestinal tube is still in open communication with the yolksac, which is situated directly in front of it. As the structures forming the body wall grow from the sides toward the front, they gradually narrow down the communicating portion between the intestinal tube and yolk-sac until it is but a narrow channel. This is the vitello-intestinal or omphalo-mesenteric duct, which normally becomes obliterated and absorbed as soon as the body wall of the embryo is closed. It if fails to disappear, it may persist in the adult as Meckel's diverticulum, of which we distinguish four different types.

By
Howard A. Kelly, A.B., M.D.
Professor of Gynecology
in the Johns Hopkins University
and
E. Hurdon, M.D.
Assistant in Gynecology
In the Johns Hopkins University,
Baltimore.

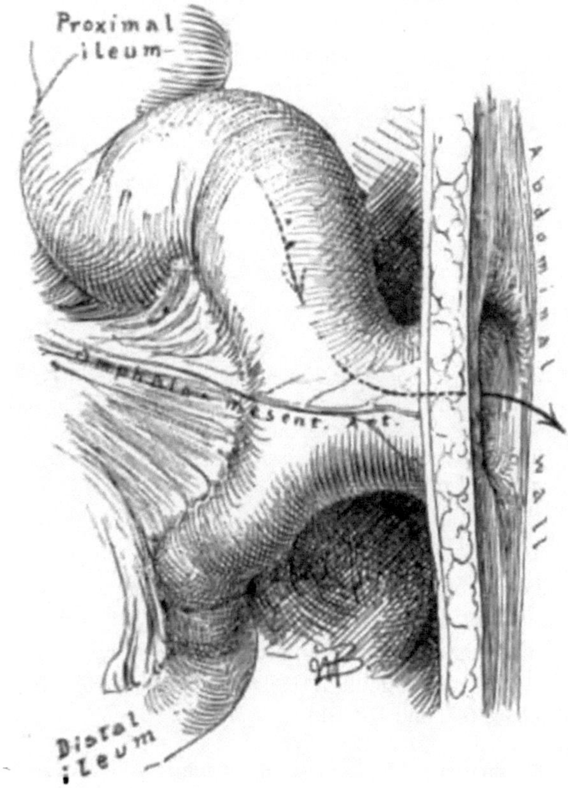

Fig. 196.5 Type I. Diagram of the most primitive form of Meckel's diverticulum, resembling the Original Vitelline Duct. It appears as a short canal which connects the ileum with a ventral fissure, the extent of which may be considerable. The canal is accompanied by the remains of the omphalo-mesenteric vessels

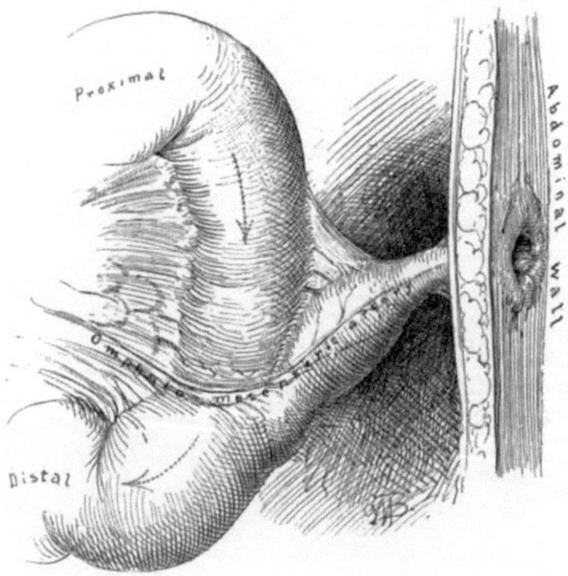

Fig. 196.6 Type II. Diagram of a more advanced form of the diverticulum. The fissure persists, but is narrower, the canal longer and more slender, and, owing to an intact anal orifice, the intestinal contents pass in the usual manner. The omphalo-mesenteric vessels accompany the canal

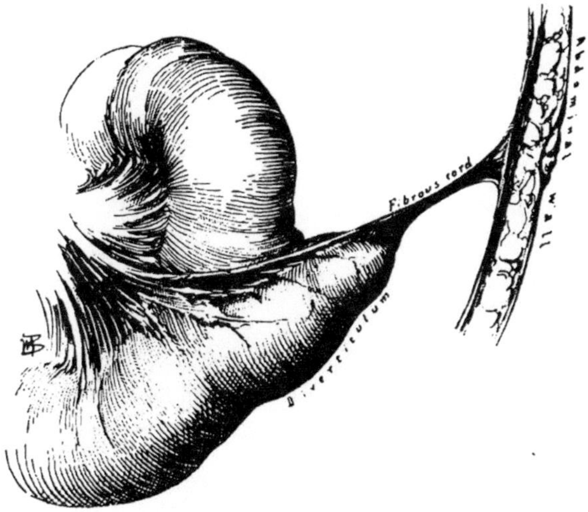

Fig. 196.7 Type III. Diagram of a still further advanced form of diverticulum. The ventral fissure is closed and the distal portion of the canal has become transformed into a fibrous cord, which may or may not contain remains of the omphalo-mesenteric vessels. The proximal portion has retained its lumen and appears as a sac attached to the free border of the ileum

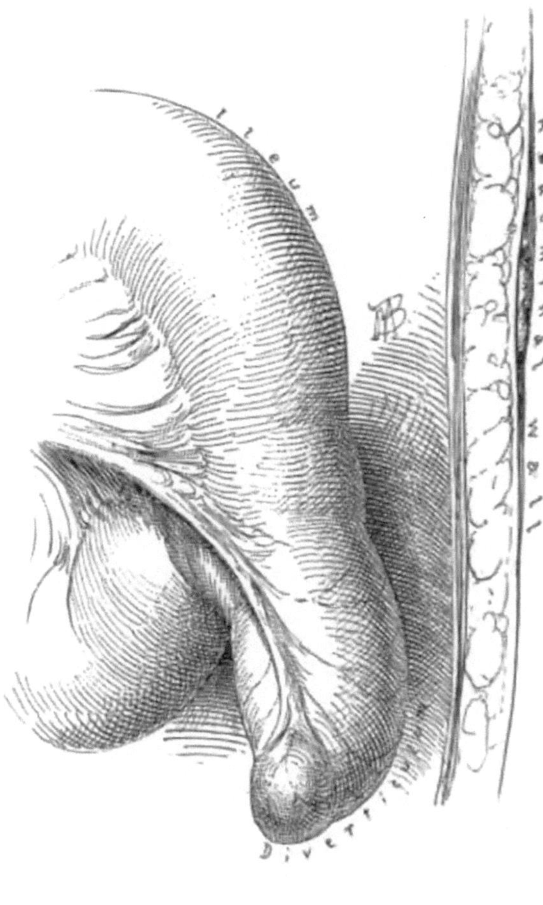

Fig. 196.8 Type IV. The usual form of Meckel's diverticulum. The proximal portion of the original vitelline duct persists, but having become closed at its end and detached from the umbilical region, it appears as a pouch hanging free from the convex border of the ileum. The omphalo-mesenteric vessels run up to its tip

Table 196.1 Meckel's diverticulum: rule of 2's

2% of the population
2 feet from the ileocecal valve
2 inches in length
2 types of heterotopic tissue (gastric and pancreatic)
Presentation before the age of 2

A memory aid regarding Meckel's diverticulum is the rule of 2's (Table 196.1) [4].

References

1. Meckel JF. Ueber die Divertikel am Darmkanal. Archiv für die Physiologie. 1809;9:421–53.
2. Meckel JF. Beyträge zur vergleichenden Anatomy, Erster Band, Erstes Heft, Leipzig, 1808, Bey Carl Heinrich Reclam; pp. 92–93. [cited 2019 Oct 02]. Available from Google Books. Books.google.com.
3. Kelly HA, Hurdon E. Meckel's Diverticulum. in: The Veriform Appendix and its Diseases. WB Saunders and Company, Philadelphia, 1905:594–602. Accessed 28 Sep 2022.
4. Stallion A, Shuck JM. Meckel's diverticulum. In: Holzheimer RG, Mannick JA, editors. Surgical Treatment: Evidence-Based and Problem-Oriented. Munich: Zuckschwerdt; 2001.

Jejunal Carcinoma

197

James S. Wu and Eric W. Willis

Presentation

A 57-year-old female was admitted with nausea and vomiting. Computed tomography shows dilated jejunum (Fig. 197.1).

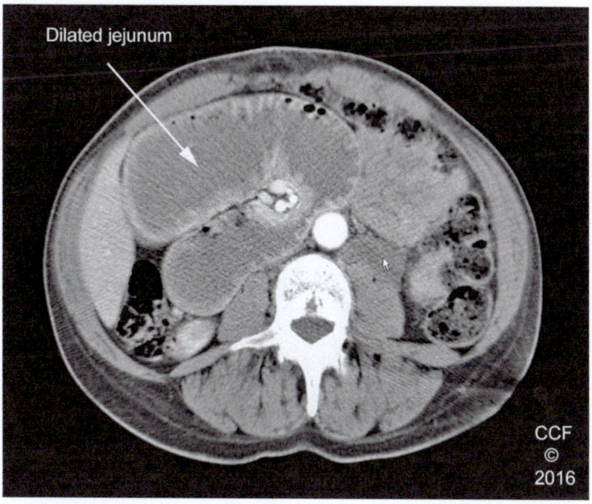

Fig. 197.1 Computed tomography shows small bowel obstruction with marked dilation of the jejunum (arrow)

J. S. Wu (✉)
Department of Colon and Rectal Surgery, Cleveland Clinic, Cleveland, OH, USA

E. W. Willis
Department of Pathology, CORPath, Columbus, OH, USA

J. S. Wu, M. D. Inkster (eds.), *Cleveland Clinic Colorectal Case Studies*,
https://doi.org/10.1007/978-3-031-39880-3_197

Management

At surgery, an obstructing jejunal tumor was found and resected (Fig. 197.2). The difference in the diameter between the obstructed and nonobstructed jejunum is demonstrated in Fig. 197.3. The opened resected specimen, Fig. 197.4, showed near circumferential luminal narrowing.

Pathology showed jejunal adenocarcinoma (Fig. 197.5). The pathologic stage was T3N0. Metastatic disease was not found.

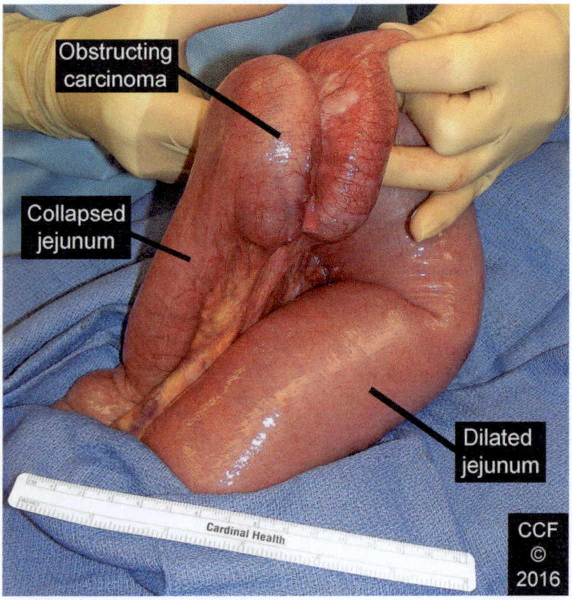

Fig. 197.2 The obstructing jejunal mass marks a site of transition between dilated and collapsed intestine

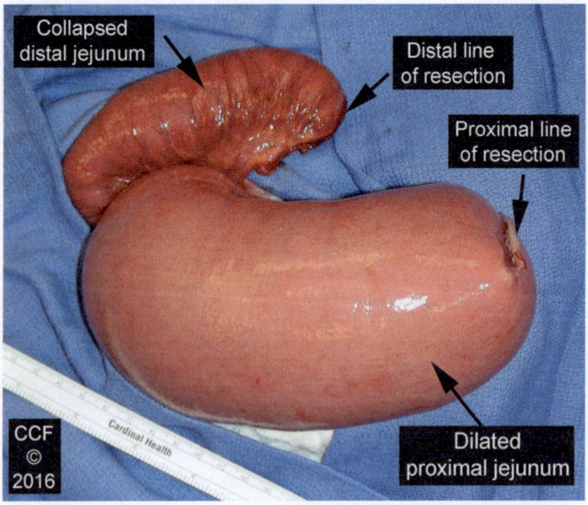

Fig. 197.3 Following resection of the tumor, the difference in luminal diameter between the proximal obstructed jejunum and the distal collapsed jejunum easily is seen

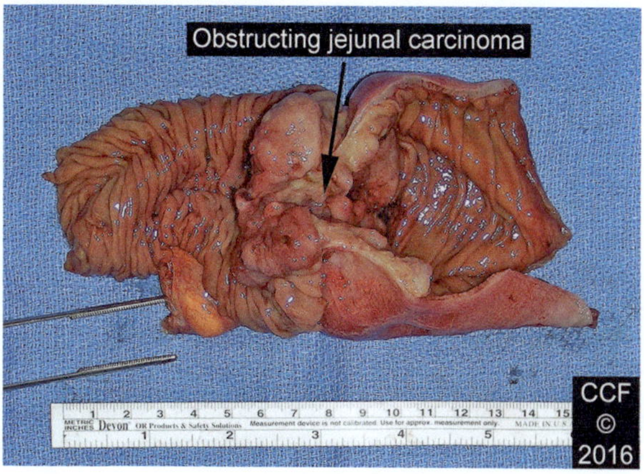

Fig. 197.4 The resected specimen shows near circumferential luminal narrowing

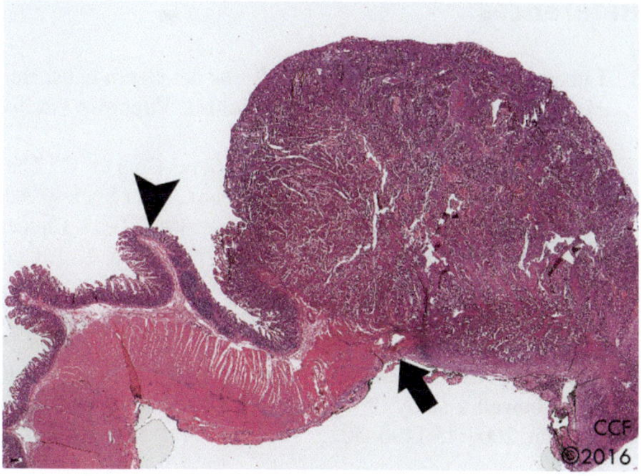

Fig. 197.5 Jejunal adenocarcinoma. An exophytic mass penetrates through the muscularis propria (arrow). The arrowhead shows uninvolved jejunum

Comment

In 1888, Lubarsch reported two cases of primary cancer of the ileum in which he established a link between adenomatous polyps of the small intestine and cancer [1].

Ueber den primären Krebs des Ileum nebst Bemerkungen über das gleichzeitige Vorkommen von Krebs und Tuberculose. Von Dr. Otto Lubarsch früherem Assistenten am pathologischen Institut zu Breslau, 1888 Zwei Fälle von primären Krebs des Ileum, welche ich im letzen Jahre zu untersuchen Gelegenheit hatte, veranlassten mich zu einem genaueren Studium der Krebse und adenomatösen Polypen des Dünndarms.	On the primary cancer of the ileum and remarks on the simultaneous occurrence of cancer and tuberculosis. By Dr. Otto Lubarsch former assistant at the Pathological Institute of Breslau, 1888 Two cases of primary cancer of the ileum, which I had occasion to examine in the last year, led me to a detailed study of the cancers and adenomatous polyps of the small intestine.

In 1999, Howe et al. [2] described 4995 cases of small bowel adenocarcinoma found in the National Cancer Data Base between 1885 and 1995. Of these, 55% occurred in the duodenum, 18% in the jejunum, and 13% in the ileum. The overall 5-year disease-specific survival was 30.5% with a median survival of 19.7 months. In 2004, Dabaja et al. [3] reported 217 patients with adenocarcinoma of the small bowel. The tumor was located in the jejunum in 25% of cases; of these, the 5-year survival rate was 30%. In 2011, Kushwaha et al. [4] warn that in India the diagnosis of jejunal adenocarcinoma is illusive because its presentation is similar to that of tuberculosis. In 2002, Abrahams et al. [5] reported 37 cases of adenocarcinoma of the small bowel. There were 10 cases of resected jejunal adenocarcinoma for which the 5-year survival was 33%. Pathologic features, including positive surgical margins, extramural venous spread, positive lymph nodes, poor tumor differentiation, depth of invasion, and history of Crohn's disease, were major prognostic indicators.

References

1. Lubarsch O. Ueber den primären Krebs des Ileum nebst Bemerkungen über das gleichzeitige Vorkommen von Krebs und Tuberculose. Virchows Archiv f Path Anat Physiol kiln Med. 1888;111:280–317.
2. Howe JR, Karnell LH, Menck HR, Scott-Conner C. The American College of Surgeons Commission on Cancer and the American Cancer Society. Adenocarcinoma of the small bowel: review of the National Cancer Data Base, 1985-1995. Cancer. 1999;86:2693–706.
3. Dabaja BS, Suki D, Pro B, Bonnen M, Ajani J. Adenocarcinoma of the small bowel. Presentation, prognostic factors, and outcome of 217 patients. Cancer. 2004;101:518–26.
4. Kushwaha JK, Sonkar AA, Saraf A, Singh D, Gupta R. Jejunal adenocarcinoma: An elusive diagnosis. Indian J Surg Oncol. 2011;2:197–201.
5. Abrahams NA, Halverson A, Fazio VW, Rybicki LA, Goldblum JR. Adenocarcinoma of the small bowel: a study of 37 cases with emphasis on histologic prognostic factors. Dis Colon Rectum. 2002;45:1496–502.

Jejunal Gastrointestinal Stromal Tumor 198

Michelle D. Inkster, Eric W. Willis, Matthew D. Kroh, and James S. Wu

Presentation

A 52-year-old female was referred for an opinion about recurrent gastrointestinal (GI) bleeding. She had three prior episodes of GI bleeding requiring transfusion of four units of blood each time. Colonoscopy, esophagogastroduodenoscopy, small bowel capsule studies, and routine computed tomography (CT) of the abdomen/pelvis did not reveal a source of bleeding. CT enterography (Fig. 198.1a, b), however, showed a jejunal lesion (arrow). Resection was done. The gross specimen (Fig. 198.2a, b) and the histopathology (Fig. 198.3) are shown.

M. D. Inkster
Department of Gastroenterology, Cleveland Clinic, Cleveland, OH, USA

E. W. Willis
Department of Pathology, CORPath, Columbus, OH, USA

M. D. Kroh
Department of General Surgery, Digestive Diseases Institute, Cleveland Clinic, Cleveland, OH, USA

J. S. Wu (✉)
Department of Colon and Rectal Surgery, Cleveland Clinic, Cleveland, OH, USA

J. S. Wu, M. D. Inkster (eds.), *Cleveland Clinic Colorectal Case Studies*,
https://doi.org/10.1007/978-3-031-39880-3_198

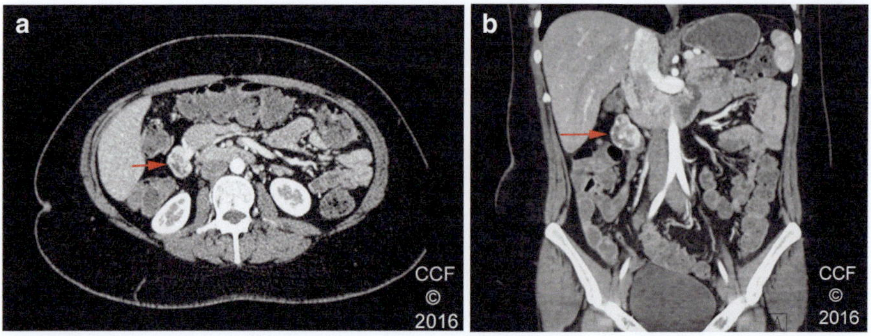

Fig. 198.1 CT enterography reveals a jejunal lesion (arrow); (**a**) Axial view; (**b**) Coronal view

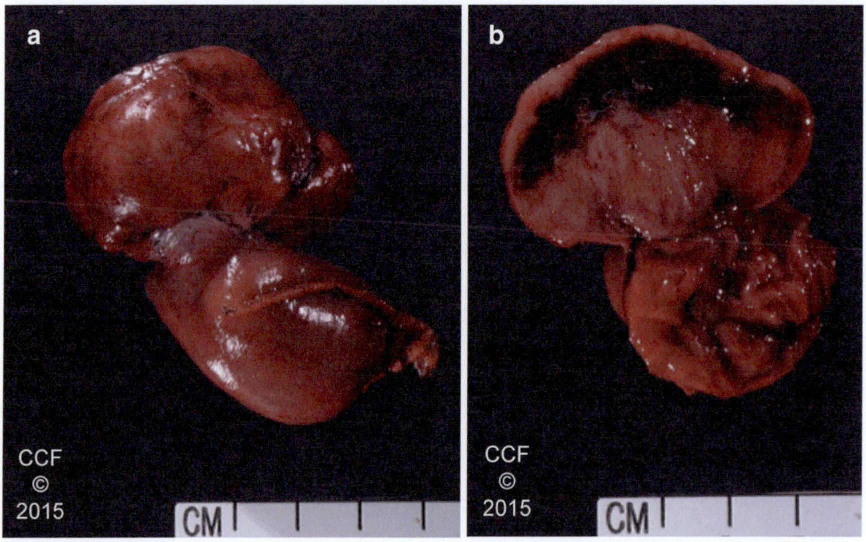

Fig. 198.2 The resected specimen; (**a**) Outer surface; (**b**) Inner surface

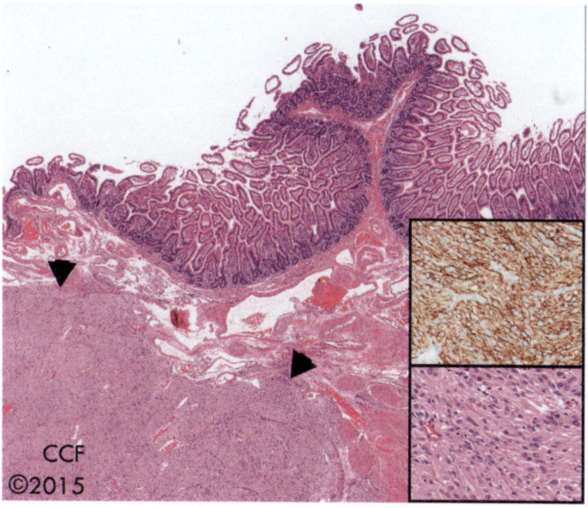

Fig. 198.3 Well-circumscribed submucosal spindle cell neoplasm with a pushing border (arrowheads) and bland cytology with 1 mitosis per 5 mm^2 (Lower inset). The tumor cells stain positive for DOG-1 and CD117 (cKit) (Upper inset)

Comments

This is a rare case of gastrointestinal bleeding from a jejunal gastrointestinal stromal tumor (GIST). Gastrointestinal GISTS are spindle cell tumors that are generally centered in the muscularis propria. GISTs occur in the esophagus, stomach, small intestine and colorectum. Bleeding is a common symptom. Immunostaining with a combination of DOG1 and CD117 antibodies favor the diagnosis of GISTS [1, 2].

References

1. Voltaggio L, Montgomery EA. Gastrointestinal tract spindle cell lesions—just like real estate, it's all about location. Mod Pathol. 2015;28:S47–S66.
2. Novelli M, Rossi S, Rodriguez-Justo M, Taniere P, Seddon B, Toffolatti L, et al. DOG1 and CD117 are the antibodies of choice in the diagnosis of gastrointestinal stromal tumours. Histopathol. 2010;57:259–70.

Pseudomyxoma Peritonei (Low-Grade Appendiceal Mucinous Neoplasm) 199

Michael A. Valente, Paresh Mahajan, Scott A. Robertson, Michelle D. Inkster, and James S. Wu

Presentation

A 56-year-old male presented with right lower quadrant pain and slowly increasing abdominal distension. Abdominal computed tomography was done (Fig. 199.1).

M. A. Valente · J. S. Wu (✉)
Department of Colon and Rectal Surgery, Cleveland Clinic, Cleveland, OH, USA

P. Mahajan
Radiology & Diagnostic Imaging Institute, Cleveland Clinic, Cleveland, OH, USA

S. A. Robertson
Pathology & Laboratory Medicine Institute, Cleveland Clinic, Cleveland, OH, USA

M. D. Inkster
Department of Gastroenterology, Cleveland Clinic, Cleveland, OH, USA

J. S. Wu, M. D. Inkster (eds.), *Cleveland Clinic Colorectal Case Studies*,
https://doi.org/10.1007/978-3-031-39880-3_199

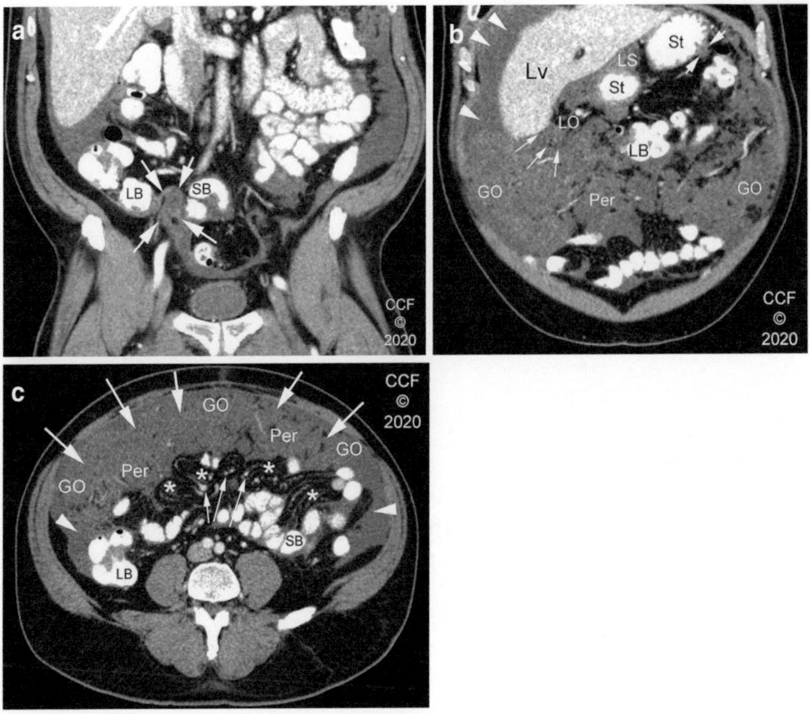

Fig. 199.1 (**a**) Right lower quadrant 1.5 cm diameter, dilated, mucin-filled appendix (arrows), proximally inseparable from a diffuse peritoneal infiltrative process; (**b**) Extensive peritoneal metastases—numerous coalescent nodules in the greater omentum (GO) often referred to as "omental caking," the lesser omentum (LO), extending into the lesser sac (LS) via the epiploic foramen (long arrows). Serosal implants (short arrows). Small volume perihepatic ascites (arrow heads); (**c**) Extensive peritoneal carcinomatosis—numerous coalescent nodules (arrows) in the greater omentum (GO), and small volume ascites (arrow heads). Mesenteric micronodules and fluid (asterisks), mesenteric vessels (small arrows); At surgery, a perforated appendix with intra-abdominal mucous was found. Pathology showed high- and low-grade mucinous cancer. LB = large bowel, Lv = liver, Per = peritoneal cavity, SB = small bowel, St = stomach

Management

At surgery, gelatinous ascites was found and removed. The intra-abdominal portion of the liver, mesentery, omentum, peritoneum, intestine, and spleen was covered with tumor nodules. Appendectomy, splenectomy, peritonectomy, and intraoperative abdominal irrigation with hyperthermic chemotherapy were done (Fig. 199.2a–f).

Pathology showed low-grade appendiceal mucinous neoplasm (LAMN) (Fig. 199.3a–d).

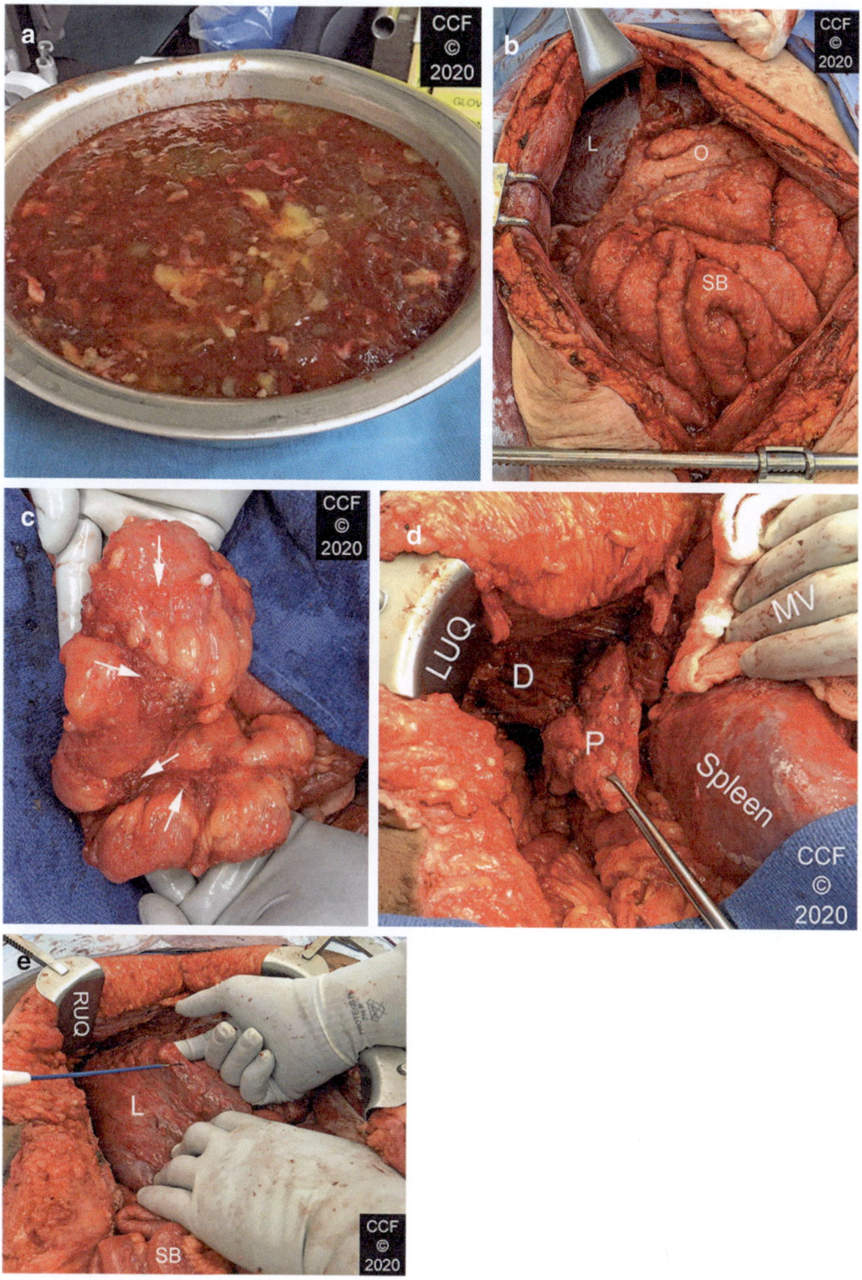

Fig. 199.2 (**a**) Gelatinous ascites removed from the abdomen; (**b**) Tumor nodules covering the liver (L), omentum (O), and small bowel (SB); (**c**) Tumor nodules covering the surface of the mesentery [arrows]; (**d**) Peritoneal (P) stripping of the left hemidiaphragm (D). The spleen SP has been labeled; (**e**) Removing Glission's capsule with tumor (Bovie tip) from the liver (L). The small bowel (SB) is labeled

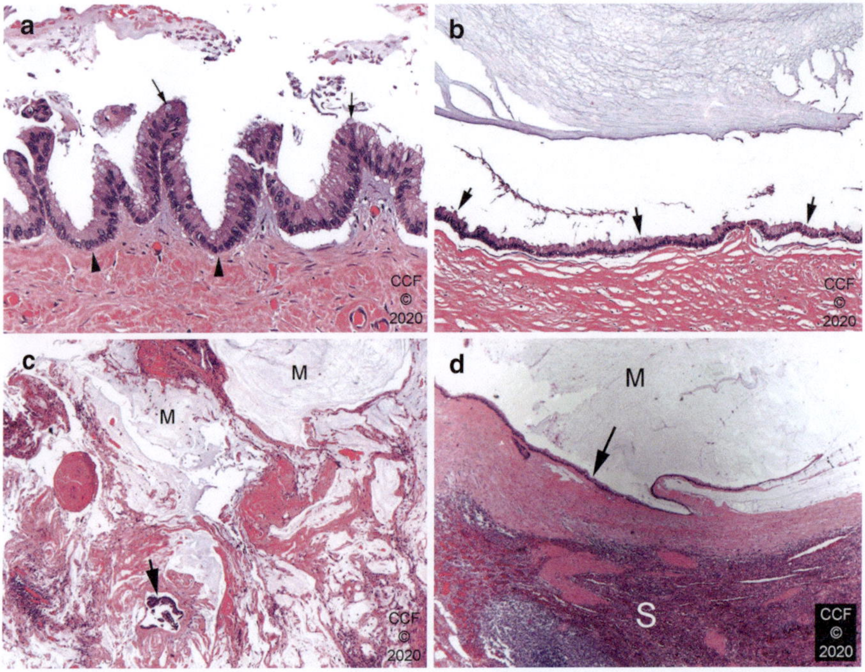

Fig. 199.3 (**a**) LAMN epithelium often demonstrates villous projections composed of hypermucinous (arrows) columnar cells. Also, there is a characteristic absence of lamina propria underneath the neoplasm (arrowheads); (**b**) LAMN mucinous epithelium may have a flattened configuration (arrows); (**c**) Large areas of the tissue show dissecting pools of mucin (M), with only scattered islands of neoplastic cells (arrow); (**d**) The neoplasm spreads in a "pushing" pattern, and lacks the infiltrative growth of conventional adenocarcinoma. Here, LAMN (arrow) pushes against the spleen (S), but does not invade it

Comment

Ballentine et al. [1] write that pseudomyxoma peritonei (PMP) is "a clinical syndrome characterized by intraperitoneal mucinous implants and progressive accumulation of mucinous ascites, most of which are now thought to arise from peritoneal dissemination of LAMNs." In 2017, Carr et al. [2] note that low-grade appendiceal mucinous neoplasms are "mucinous neoplasms without infiltrative invasion."

The word "pseudomyxoma" is derived from "pseudo" (factitious) and "myxoma." The term "myxoma" was introduced by Virchow in 1857 in his description of a malignant fatty tumor that he referred to as a "Schleimgeschwulst" [3].

Ein fall von bösartigen, zum Theil in der Form des Neuroms auftretenden Fettgeschwülsten Von Rud. Virchow Auf der Höhe ihrer Entwickelung stellten sie, wie ich schon bemerkte, eine art von Lipom dar; im Anfange der Bildung konnte man sie als Schleimgeschwulst (Tumor mucosus, Myxoma) bezeichen.	A case of malignant fatty tumors, some of which appear in the form of a neuroma By Rud. Virchow At the height of their development they represent, as I already have remarked, a type of lipoma; at the beginning of their formation, one could describe them as a mucous tumor (tumor mucosus, Myxoma).

In Rokitansky's *Handbuch der allgemeinen pathologischen Anatomie* (Handbook of general pathologic anatomy) [1842–1846], he applied the word "colloid" to describe a pathologic texture.

Das Colloid [4 p. 304] Das colloid ist eine im Allgemeinen halbflüssige, einer saturirten Gummi- oder Leimlösing, einem Obstgelée vergleichbare klebende Substanz,...	Colloid [5 p. 116] Colloid is a semi-fluid adhesive substance, resembling a saturated solution of gum or glue, or a fruit jelly.

Colloid was one of several terms that Rokitansky used to describe cancers that had gelatinous character: *cancer colloide, gallertkrebs, alveolarkrebs (colloid cancer, genlatinous cancer, alveolar cancer)*. He found these cancers located on the peritoneum and the ovary and concluded that they are more "gutartigste (good-natured)" compared with other cancers.

Gallertkrebs, Cancer colloide, — Alveolarkrebs, C. aréolaire, gélatiniforme [4].

Auch in der Reihe der Krebse finden wir ein gallerthaltiges, colloides Aftergebilde, den Gallertkrebs, noch bekannter unter dem name Alveolarkrebs — ein Name, welcher durch die so gewöhnliche alveolare Textur des Gebildes veranlasst wurde.

Der Gallertkrebs kömmt in zwei Formen vor:

1. Er stellt eine graulich-gelbliche, gelbröthliche, auch wohl hie und da farblose, einer stockenden Gallerte ähnliche durchscheinende, zitternde, kleistrige,[1]bei einigem Volumen höckerig-unebene, gelappte Masse dar,…
2. Als sog. Alveolarkrebs—von Otto 1816 als eine besondere Art des Magenskirrhus aufgeführt, Cancer gélatiniforme, aréolaire Cruveilhier's.

Das Aftergebilde besteht im Allgemeinen der charakteristischen Hauptmasse nach aus Follikeln (Alveolis) von bald sehr zartem durchsichtigen, bald dichterem massenreicheren weissen atlasartig-glänzenden Fasergefüge, welche eine farblose oder blass-gelbliche, grauliche, durchsichtige Gallerte enthalten.

Von den einzelnen Formen ist es auf der Peritonäum besonders die erste form, aber auch die alveolare; die vereinzelten Knötchen haben die Bedeutung discreter Alveoli. Im Ovarium ist es ganz besonders der zu Cysten sich entwickelnde Alveolarkrebs; er stellt hier einen sehr gewöhnlichen Hydrops cysticus areolarkrebsiger Natur dar.

Der reine Gallertkrebs ist unter den Krebsen der gutartigste; eine ihm zur Seite gehende Cachexie ist, wenn er nicht durch excedirende Massenwucherung einen Erschöpfungszustand nach sich gezogen hat, minder palpabel als bei andern Krebsen;…

Zudem ist er sehr gewöhnlich solitär, dabei aber andererseits durch seine Ausbreitung und namentlich durch das Übergreifen von seinem ursprünglichen Sitze auf contigue Gewebe, unter diesen vor Allen auf seröse Häute unter die diffuse Wucherung auf diesen ausgezeichnet.

Colloid, Gelatinous Cancer Alveolar Cancer (C. Aréolaire) [5].

In the array of cancers, we again encounter a gelatinous, colloid new-growth, namely, *gelatinous cancer*, better known under the epithet *alveolar*, derived from its very frequent *alveolar fabric*.

This species occurs under two forms:

1. It presents a yellow-gray, yellowish-red, here and there colorless, firm, jelly-like, transparent, tremulous, sizy, and when voluminous, irregularly clavate, lobulated mass.
2. So-called alveolar cancer—Cited by Otho, in 1816, as a peculiar kind of stomach-scirrhus—cancer gélatiniforme, aréolaire of Cruveilhier.

The growth consists mainly and characteristically of follicles (alveoli) of either very delicate, pellucid, or of more compact and massive, white satin-like, shining fiber-texture, containing a colorless or a pale yellow, grayish, diaphanous gelatine.

Upon the peritoneum the first form is predominant, but not to the exclusion of the alveolar, the scattered tubercula having the character of isolated alveoli. In the ovary the cyst-like alveolar cancer is prevalent, very often as encysted dropsy of the areolar cancer-form.

Pure gelatinous cancer is the least malignant of any, and, unless it prove exhausting by dint of surpassing volume, a dependent cachexia is less pronounced than in other cancers. It is for the most part solitary, although somewhat prone to extend to continuous organs, and to scatter to itself over serous surfaces,…

[1] A translation of the word *kleistrige* is *sticky*. Dr. Swaine's translation employs the word *sizy*.

In 1884, Werth published "Pseudomyxoma Peritonei" (PMP), a complication of ovarian cysts [6].

Klinische und anatomische Untersuchungen zur Lehre von den Bauchgeschülsten und der Laparotomie. Von Prof. Werth In Kiel II. Pseudomyxoma Peritoneum Mit dieser Bezeichnung möchte ich eine Veränderung des Peritoneum belegen, die zuweilen als Complication von Eierstockscysten beobachtet, im Ganzen bisher wenig beachtet und, so weit dies geschehen, irrig gedeutet worden ist. Die fragliche Veränderung beruht auf einer eigenthümlichen Reaction des Peritoneum gegen den auf dem Wege spontaner Cystenperforation in die Bauchhöhle gelangten geleeartigen Inhalt, wie ihn manche Kystome führen, die sich durch Dünnwandigkeit und Neigung zu spontaner Eröffnung, sowie meist durch rasches Wachsthum auszuzeichnen pflegen. Bei der Operation resp. Autopsie findet man in solchen Fällen die Bauchhöhle in Allen ihren Abschnitten mit dieser gelatinösen Masse erfüllt, diese aber nur zum Theil frei in derselben gelegen, zum Theil in form dicker halbdurchsichtiger Schwarten der Innenfläche der Bauchwand und den Eingeweiden aufgelagert und fest anhaftend.	Clinical and anatomical investigations for teaching about abdominal tumors and laparotomy Von Prof. Werth in Kiel II. Pseudomyxoma Peritonei With this name, I would like to document a change in the peritoneum, which sometimes is seen as a complication of ovarian cysts, that as a whole has received little attention, and as far as this has happened, has been misinterpreted. The change in question is based on a peculiar reaction of the peritoneum to the jelly-like substance that fills the abdominal cavity after spontaneous perforation of cysts which are thin-walled, undergo rapid growth, and tend to open spontaneously. At operation or autopsy one finds in such cases that the abdominal cavity is filled in all of its sections with a gelatinous mass, that is partially free and partially firmly adherent as thick semitransparent rinds to the inner surface of the abdominal wall and the guts.

In 1901, Fraenkel [7] reported a case of PMP associated with appendiceal rupture discovered at autopsy.

Ueber das sogennante Pseudomyxoma peritonei. Von Eug. Fraenkel Aus dem pathologischen Institut des allgemeinen Krankenhauses Hamburg-Eppendorf. Die Beobachtung betrifft einen unter dem Bilde des Encephalomalacie verstorbenden 79 jährigen Mann, bei dessen Sektion ausser multiplen encephalomalacischen, durch Sklerose der Hirnarterien bedingten Herden…, das ganze kleine Becken anfüllender, sich aufwärts in beide Region. Iliacae fortsetzender Gallertmassen festgestellt wurde. Bei der weiteren Untersuchung gelang es unschwer, als Ausgangspunkt für die namentlich in der Beckenhöhle angesammelten Gallertmassen den mit dem gleichen Inhalt erfüllten, an einer Stelle geborstenen Wurmfortsatz ausfindig zu machen.	Concerning the so-called pseudomyxoma peritonei By Eug. Fraenkel From the Pathological Institute of the General Hospitals Hamburg-Eppendorf This observation concerns a 79-year old man who appeared to have died from encephalomalacia, during whose autopsy, apart from multiple encephalomalacic foci caused by sclerosis of the cerebral artery…., filling the whole small pelvis, spreading upwards into both iliac regions, continuous gelatinous masses were detected. On further investigation, it was not difficult to locate the appendix, that had ruptured at one point, as the starting point of the gelatinous masses that had collected in the pelvic cavity.

In 1987, Sugarbaker et al. presented a curative approach to treatment of malignant PMP [8].[2]

> Malignant Pseudomyxoma Peritonei of Colonic Origin.
> Natural History and Presentation of a Curative Approach to Treatment.
>
> "Pseudomyxoma peritonei is an unusual malignancy arising from the goblet cells of the large bowel or appendix. Its characteristic clinical features are low histologic grade of malignancy and widespread dissemination throughout the abdominal cavity. In a clinical study of 14 patients, the most common initial symptoms were abdominal distension or right lower quadrant pain suggestive of appendicitis. All patients underwent radical procedures in an attempt to surgically removal all gross disease from the abdomen.
>
> Six cycles of intraperitoneal 5-FU and three doses of mitomycin C were used following cytoreductive surgery in seven patients. Five of these seven patients are disease free following staging by celiotomy with two- to four-year follow-up. This new treatment strategy, designed to cure some patients with pseudomyxoma peritonei, has given favorable results in a disease that previously had a uniformly lethal outcome."
>
> Paul H. Sugarbaker, M.D., Kenneth Kern, M.D., Ernest Lack, M.D. From the Emory Cancer Center, Atlanta Georgia, Surgery Branch, NCI, DCT, and the Anatomic Branch, NIH, Bethesda, Maryland

Secondary delayed re-entry of the abdomen in patients with cancer of the colon and rectum was described in 1949 by Wangensteen [9].

> Cancer of the Colon and Rectum.
> With special reference to... secondary delayed re-entry of the abdomen in patients exhibiting lymph node involvement
>
> "I have been proposing to my colleagues that we should reenter the abdomen of patients with gross lymph node involvement (Dukes' group C) three to four months after the initial operation, to do a "wiping-up" operation."
>
> Owen H. Wangensteen, M.D.
> University of Minnesota
> Minneapolis

In 1995, Sugarbaker reported that the cytoreductive approach for PMP may require six peritonectomy procedures to resect or strip cancer from all intra abdominal surfaces. [10].

---

[2] Permission to reproduce this excerpt was generously provided by Wolter's Kluwer Health, Inc., CCC|RightsLink®, License number 5133450260151, License date Aug 21, 2021.

Biographical Note

Karl Freiherr von Rokitansky (1804–1878)

In the Editor's Preface to his 1855 English translation of Rokitansky's *Manual of Pathologic Anatomy*, Swaine provides the following biography [5 p. viii].

> '"Charles Rokitansky, the founder of the German [it should rather have been called Austrian] medico-anatomical school, was born at Königsgraetz, in Bohemia, was educated at the Gymnasium of Leitneritz, and graduated, at Vienna, in 1828. Shortly afterwards he was appointed Assistant in the pathologico-anatomical department of the University, and, in 1834, Professor of Pathological Anatomy. At the same time he was instituted Prosector at the General [united Civil and Military] Hospital at Vienna, and also sole medico-legal Anatomist for the examination of all doubtful cases of death throughout that metropolis.
>
> "The immense fund of materials thus placed at his disposal [the number of corpses dissected by him is summed up at 30,000] was almost entirely reserved for the elaboration of that grand work on pathological anatomy, which, in the consciousness of having thoroughly mastered the subject, he gave to the world between the years 1842 and 1846; which has passed, *unaltered*, through three reimpressions; and which, under the auspices of the Sydenham Society, has been translated into the English language."
>
> "In 1849, Rokitansky was appointed Dean of the Medical Faculty, and, in 1850, Rector of the University, of Vienna."'

References

1. Ballentine SJ, Carr J, Bekhor EY, Sarpel U, Polydorides AD. Updating staging and patient outcomes in low-grade appendiceal mucinous neoplasms. Mod Pathol. 2021;34:104–15.
2. Carr NJ, Bibeau F, Bradley RF, Dartigues P, Feakins RM, Geisinger KR, et al. The histological classification, diagnosis and differential diagnosis of mucinous appendiceal neoplasms, appendiceal adenocarcinomas and pseudomyxoma peritonei. Histopathology. 2017;71:847–58.
3. Virchow R. Ein Fall von bösartigen, zum Theil in der Form des Neuroms auftretenden Fettgeschwülsten. Arch Pathol Anat Phys Klin Med. 1857;11:281–288.
4. Rokitansky C. Handbuch der allgemeinen pathologischen Anatomie. Wien: Braumüller & Seidel; 1846, pp. 353, 354, 357, 358. Digitized by the Internet Archive in 2015. https://archive.org. Accessed 07 Dec 2020.
5. Rokitansky C. A Manual of Pathologic Anatomy, Vol I. Translated from the German by Swaine WE, Philadelphia: Blanchard & Lea; 1855, pp. Editor's preface p. viii, 202, 204. Digitalized in Google Play. Accessed 07 Dec 2020.
6. Werth R. Klinische und anatomische Untersuchungen zur Lehre von den Bauchgeschülsten und der Laparotomie. Arch Gynecol Obstet. 1884;24:100–118.
7. Fraenkel E. Ueber das sogenannte Pseudomyxoma peritonei. Muench Med Wochenschr. 1901;48:965–70. HathiTrust, http://www.hathitrust.org.
8. Sugarbaker PH, Kern K, Lack E. Malignant pseudomyxoma peritonei of colonic origin: natural history and presentation of a curative approach to treatment. Dis Colon Rectum. 1987;30:772–9.
9. Wangensteen OH. Cancer of the colon and rectum. With special reference to (1) earlier recognition of alimentary tract malignancy; (2) secondary delayed re-entry of the abdomen in patients exhibiting lymph node involvement; (3) subtotal primary excision of the colon; (4) operation in obstruction. Wis Med J. 1949;48:591–7.
10. Sugarbaker PH. Peritonectomy procedures. Ann Surg. 1995;221:29–42.

Intestinal Foreign Bodies

200

Michelle D. Inkster, Christian G. Massier, Christopher R. Daigle, and James S. Wu

Presentations

Foreign bodies can enter the gastrointestinal tract accidentally or purposefully. Some will pass spontaneously while others require an intervention to remove them. Foreign bodies may be removed manually, endoscopically, or surgically. Illustrative examples follow.

Figure 200.1a, b shows a small intestinal endoscopy capsule that has become stuck at a terminal ileal stricture.

Figures 200.2, 200.3, and 200.4 are plain films that show ingested foreign bodies.

Figure 200.5a, b shows a rectal vibrator that had to be removed in the operating room.

Figure 200.6a, b shows a rectal foreign body that removed endoscopically with a snare.

Figure 200.7 is an abdominal radiograph that shows the internal workings and the outline of the outer shell of a foreign body at presentation in the rectum.

M. D. Inkster
Department of Gastroenterology, Cleveland Clinic, Cleveland, OH, USA

C. G. Massier
Department of General Surgery, Cleveland Clinic, Cleveland, OH, USA

C. R. Daigle
Department of Surgery, Cleveland Clinic Akron General Hospital, Akron, OH, USA

J. S. Wu (✉)
Department of Colon and Rectal Surgery, Cleveland Clinic, Cleveland, OH, USA

J. S. Wu, M. D. Inkster (eds.), *Cleveland Clinic Colorectal Case Studies*,
https://doi.org/10.1007/978-3-031-39880-3_200

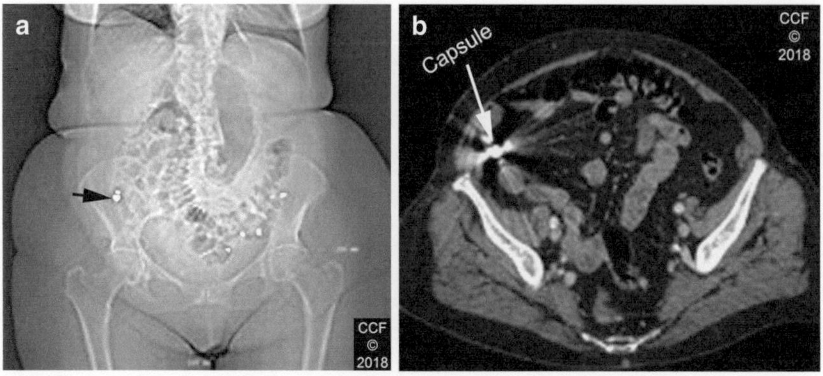

Fig. 200.1 Small intestinal capsule endoscopy was done as part of the evaluation for abdominal pain. The examination revealed a terminal ileal stricture at which point the capsule became entrapped. (**a**) Abdominal plain film shows the capsule in the right lower quadrant (arrow); (**b**) Computed tomography (CT) shows the capsule in the terminal ileum

Fig. 200.2 This patient ingested pins (arrow) and a nail (arrowhead). The items were removed surgically

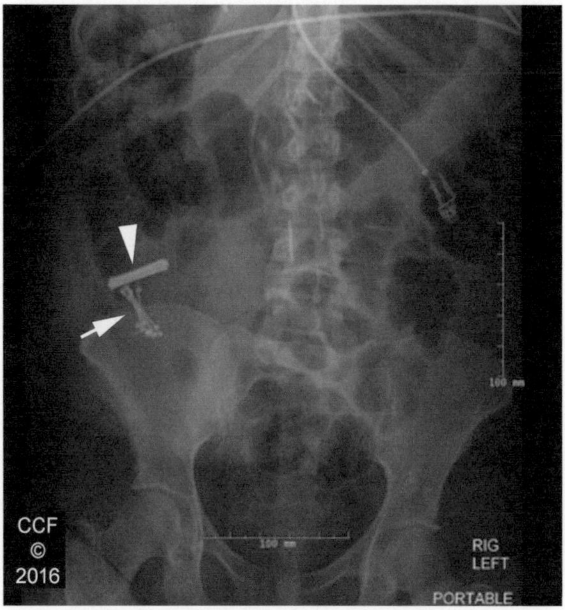

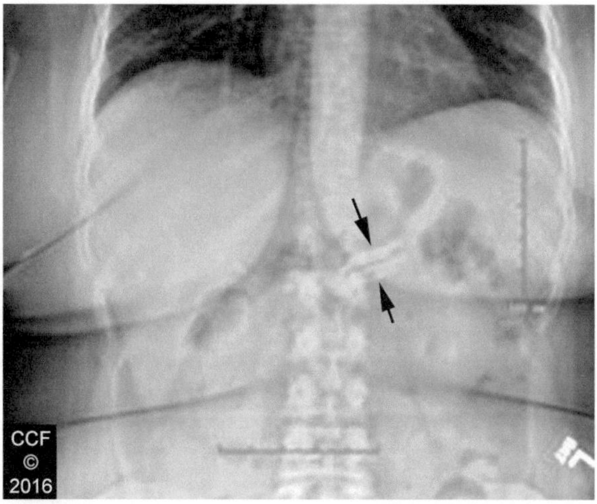

Fig. 200.3 A swallowed double-edged razor blade (arrows) is seen on this abdominal film. Surgery was required to remove it

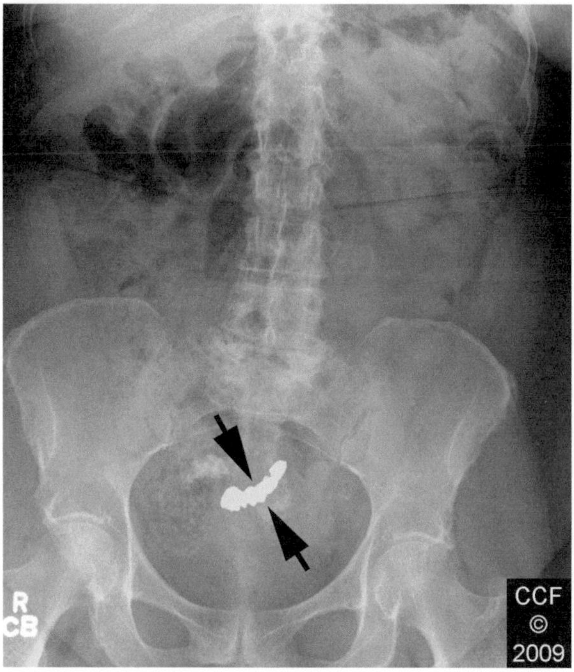

Fig. 200.4 Dentures were swallowed by accident. The patient was seen at a routine office visit. The patient did not complain of abdominal pain. Examination did not show tenderness. Plain abdominal films showed the dentures (arrows). The dentures eventually passed by natural means. An intervention. was not required

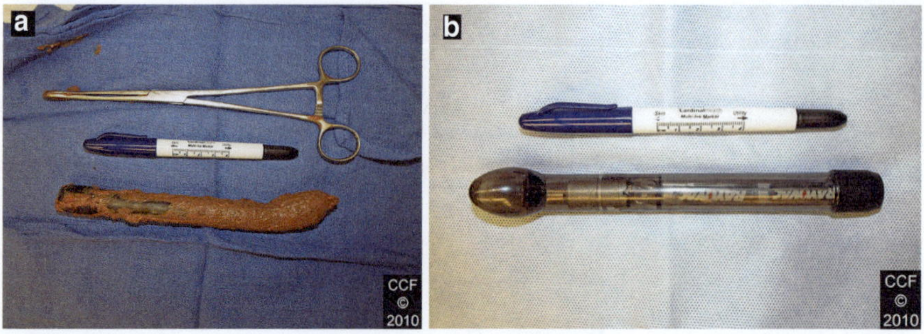

Fig. 200.5 Rectal vibrator. A male patient was seen complaining that he was not able to recover a vibrator that he had inserted into his rectum. Examination did not reveal peritoneal signs. Endoscopic attempts at removal were unsuccessful. The patient was brought to the operating room. Under general anesthesia, the anal sphincters relaxed. Proctoscopy through an operating anoscope facilitated removal of the vibrator. The patient was admitted for observation. Follow-up abdominal films and examination were normal. The patient was discharged. (**a**) Vibrator immediately after removal; (**b**) Vibrator-cleaned

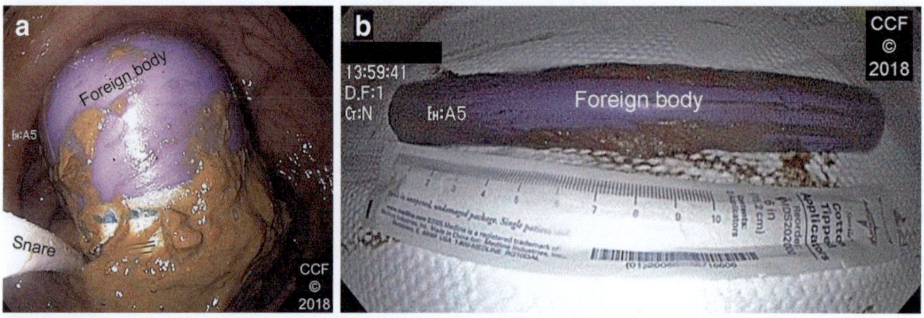

Fig. 200.6 This patient presented with a "toy" that could not be manually removed from the rectum. (**a**) Endoscopic snare removal of the foreign body, (**b**) Foreign body after removal. The patient was discharged after serial normal abdominal examinations and abdominal films were obtained

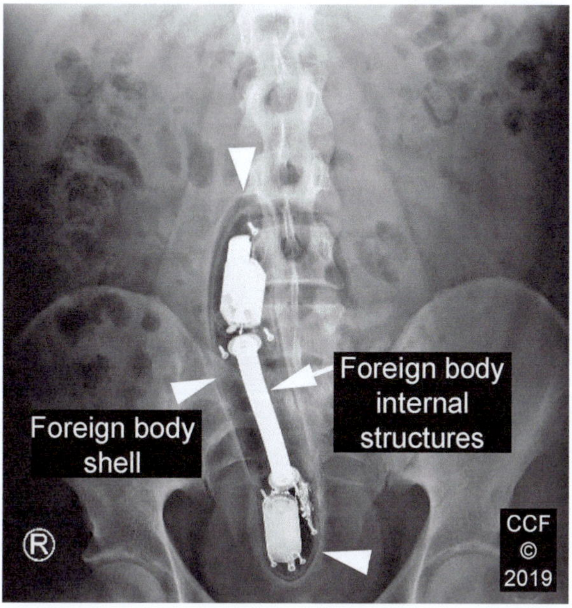

Fig. 200.7 Abdominal radiograph shows the internal structure (arrows) and the outer shell (arrowheads) of a rectal foreign body. Removal in the operating rooms under anesthesia was required

Comment

Foreign bodies can enter the gastrointestinal tract accidentally or purposefully. Ingestion of foreign bodies occurs commonly. Consultation with otorhinolaryngology is suggested for foreign bodies at or above the level of the cricopharyngeus. Management of foreign bodies or ingested food in the esophagus involves caregivers skilled in esophagogastroduodenoscopy. The majority of ingested foreign bodies will pass spontaneously. Impaction, perforation, or obstruction tend to occur at points of angulation or narrowing. Sharp and pointed objects are more likely to cause perforation [1]. Rectal foreign bodies are challenging because of the possibilities of perforation (acute and delayed), bleeding, and anatomic barriers that hinder removal [2, 3]. Removal may be accomplished manually, endoscopically, or surgically. Relaxation of the anal sphincter with an anal block may assist with removal [4].

References

1. Ikenberry SO, Jue TL, Anderson MA, Appalaneni V, Banerjee S, Ben-Menachem T, et al. Management of ingested foreign bodies and food impactions. Gastrointest Endosc. 2011;73:1085–91.
2. Goldberg JE, Steele SR. Rectal foreign bodies. Surg Clin N Am. 2010;90:173–84.
3. Cologne KG, Ault GT. Rectal foreign bodies: what is the current standard? Clin Colon Rectal Surg. 2012;25:214–8.
4. Coskun A, Erkan N, Yakan S, Yildirim M, Cengiz F. Management of rectal foreign bodies. World J Emerg Surg. 2013;8:11. http://www.wjes.org/content/8/1/11

Intestinal Intussusception

201

Michelle D. Inkster, Bradley L. Cole, Patrick J. O'Keefe, and James S. Wu

Presentation A

An 18-year-old male presented with small bowel obstruction. Computed tomography (CT) of the abdomen was obtained (Fig. 201.1).

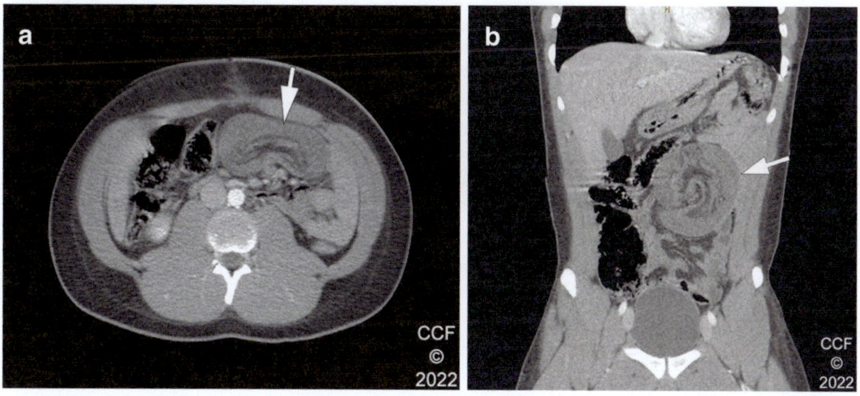

Fig. 201.1 Small bowel intussusception seen on CT scanning. Two walls of an inner limb of intestine are seen within two walls of an outer limb of intestine. (**a**) Axial view showing longitudinal intestinal orientation (arrow); (**b**) Coronal view showing cross-sectional orientation (arrow)

M. D. Inkster
Department of Gastroenterology, Cleveland Clinic, Cleveland, OH, USA

B. L. Cole · P. J. O'Keefe
Radiology & Diagnostic Imaging Institute, Cleveland Clinic, Cleveland, OH, USA

J. S. Wu (✉)
Department of Colon and Rectal Surgery, Cleveland Clinic, Cleveland, OH, USA

J. S. Wu, M. D. Inkster (eds.), *Cleveland Clinic Colorectal Case Studies*,
https://doi.org/10.1007/978-3-031-39880-3_201

Management

Surgical resection was done. Pathology showed hemorrhagic ischemic mucosa.

Presentation B

A 50-year-old female presented with cyclic colicky abdominal pain. A CT scan of the abdomen was obtained (Fig. 201.2).

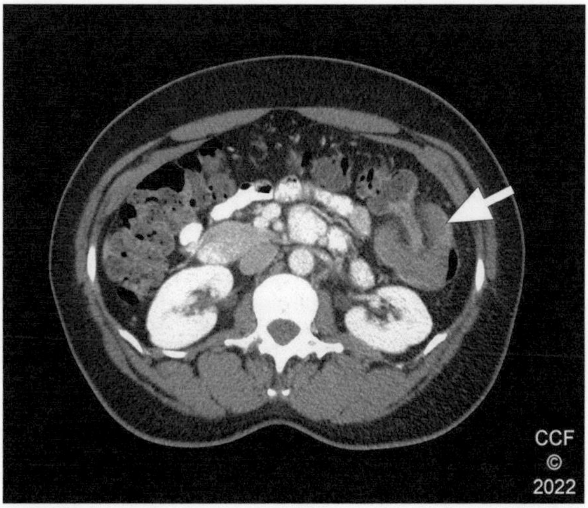

Fig. 201.2 CT scan shows a proximal colonic lipoma (arrow) likely acting as a lead point for of colocolonic intussusception

Management

Surgical resection was done. Pathology showed a submucosal lipoma, transmural ischemic injury, and reactive lymph nodes.

Comment

Intussusception is a disorder where one part of the intestine slides into another in a telescoping manner and causes inflammation and obstruction. The condition commonly is seen in young children at the junction of the small and large intestine.

In his 1884 book entitled, *Intestinal Obstruction and its Varieties*, Treves named intussusception as a cause of intestinal obstruction [1].

> "INTUSSUSCEPTION: PATHOLOGY
>
> By the term intussusception is understood the prolapse of one part of the intestine into the lumen of an immediately adjoining part.
>
> '**Pathological anatomy**. —If an intussusception be viewed in vertical section it will be seen to be composed of six layers of intestine, three on either side of the central canal, all more or less parallel to one another. It will be noticed also that the arrangement of the layers is such that mucous membrane lies in contact with mucous membrane, and peritoneum with peritoneum. On horizontal section the invaginated mass will show three concentric rings of bowel, with of course the same mutual relations with regard to the mucous and serous surfaces. All parts of the intussusception are named, and the nomenclature has suffered somewhat from an exuberance of terms. The external of the three layers is known as the intussuscipiens, the sheath, or the receiving layer (*la gaîne* of the French). The innermost cylinder is known as the entering layer, and the middle one as the returning layer. Taken together, these two layers form the intussusceptum (*le boudin* of the French). The "neck" of the intussusception is at its upper part, where the returning layer joins the sheath. The ridge formed by the junction of these two layers is known as le bourrelet. The "apex" of the intussusception is at the lower part of the intussusceptum, where the entering and returning layers join.'
>
> Frederick Treves, F.R.C.S.
> Hunterian Professor of Anatomy at
> The Royal College of Surgeons of England

Treve's illustration of the pathological anatomy of intussusception is shown in Fig. 201.3.

Concerning adult intestinal intussusception, Valentini et al. [2] [1] state that:

> "Intestinal intussusception in adults is considered uncommon, accounting for an estimated 5% of all intussusceptions and representing only 1% of intestinal obstructions. Unlike pediatric intussusception, which is usually idiopathic, adult intussusception is most often secondary to an identifiable cause. Many pathological conditions, such as malignant or benign

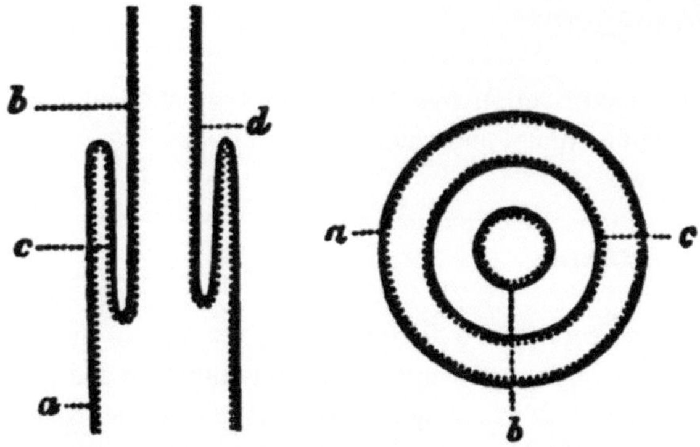

Fig. 201.3 Vertical and Transverse Sections of an Intussusception. (**a**) the sheath or intussuscepiens; (**b**) the entering or inner layer; (**c**) the returning or middle layer. From Treves. *Intestinal Obstruction and its Varieties* (Treves, Fig. 30)

neoplasms, polyps, Meckel's diverticulum, and postoperative adhesions, may act as leading points by altering bowel peristalsis. Association with malignant tumors is more common in large bowel intussusception (65–70% of cases), while small bowel intussusceptions are secondary to a malignancy in 30–35% of cases only.

The image pattern varies according to location, axis of section, bowel wall thickness, and lumen patency. The appearance of an intussusception on CT images is similar to that of a "target" mass when the CT beam is perpendicular to the longitudinal axis of the intussusception and to that of a "sausage" mass when the CT beam is parallel or oblique to the longitudinal axis."

References

1. Treves F. Chapter VIII. Intussusception: Pathology. Intestinal Obstruction: Its Varieties, with their Pathology, Diagnosis, and Treatment. Philadelphia: Henry C. Lea's Son & CO., 1884. p. 166–8. Accessed from Google books May 30, 2022
2. Valentini V, Buquicchio GL, Galluzzo M, Ianniello S, Di Grezia G, Ambrosio R, et al. Review article. Intussusception in adults: The role of MDCT in the identification of the site and cause of obstruction. Gastroenterol Res Pract. 2016; Article ID 5623718, 10 pages. https://doi.org/10.1155/2016/5623718

On Complications

202

James S. Wu and Michelle D. Inkster

De Ente et Essentia Quia parvus error in principio, magnus est in fine S. Thomae Aqvinatis [1]	On Being and Essence A small mistake in the beginning is a big one in the end St. Thomas Aquinas [2]

Common Surgical Aphorism

Complications begin in the operating room.

La philosophie de la chirurgie, René Leriche, Professeur au Collège de France, 1951 [3] L'echec est pour nous toujours cruel, même s'il n'est que relatif. Tout chirurgien porte en lui un petit cimetière, dans lequel il va de temps en temps faire oraison, cimetière d'amertume et d'hysope [4], auquel il demande la raison de certains de ses insuccès.	*The philosophy of surgery* René Leriche, Professor, College of France, 1951 Failure is always cruel to us, even if it is only relative. All surgeons carry with them a little cemetery in which they go time to time to pray, a cemetery of bitterness and hyssop, in which the reasons for certain of these failures is demanded.

> "The challenges of avoidance and treatment of complications toll heavily on every surgeon's energies."
>
> Bernard T. Ferrari, John E. Ray, Byron J. Gathright, 1985 [5]

James S. Wu
Department of Colon and Rectal Surgery, Cleveland Clinic, Cleveland, OH, USA

M. D. Inkster
Department of Gastroenterology, Cleveland Clinic, Cleveland, OH, USA

J. S. Wu, M. D. Inkster (eds.), *Cleveland Clinic Colorectal Case Studies*,
https://doi.org/10.1007/978-3-031-39880-3_202

Mea Maxima Culpa: Dealing with Surgical Complications

"In whatever way we choose to address our complications, either in our clinical practice or on the basis of consultation, we must challenge ourselves to be responsive in identifying sentinel causality."

JaBaris D. Swain, MD, MPH, 2014 [6]

Omnes enim peccaverunt et egent gloriam Dei Epistula ad Romanos 3:23 [7]	For all have sinned, and come short of the glory of God. Letter of St. Paul to the Romans, 3:23 [8]

Et cognoscetis veritatem et veritas liberabit vos Evangelium Secundum Ioannem 8:32 [9]	And you shall know the truth: and the truth shall make you free. The Gospel According to John 8:32

Good judgment comes from experience
Experience comes from bad judgment[1]

"A good workman always tries to leave the place better than when they found it;
A poor workman always blames his tools."
Old Australian saying[2]

"If you make errors (and, if you operate, you will), it is incumbent upon you to get your patient to safety."

Victor W. Fazio, AO, MS

References

1. S. Thomae Aqvinatis. Angelici Doctoris. De ente, & effentia. Apud Ioannem Baptiftam Bertonum, MDCVI. Accessed from Archiv.org December 15, 2023.
2. Aquinus T. De Ente et Essentia, On Being and Essence, a translation and interpretation by Joseph Kenny, O.P., 1965. https://Isadore.co>aquinas>DeEnte&Essentia.htm.
3. Leriche R. La philosophie de la chirurgie. Paris: Flammarion; 1951. Deuxième partie, chapitre premier. p. 176–7.
4. Hyssop is a plant cited in the Passover (Exodus 12: 22) used for ceremonial cleansing. Bible plants. Old Dominion University. ww2.odu.edu. Accessed 08 Mar 2021.
5. Ferrari BT, Ray JE, Gathright BJ (editors). Complication of Colon and Rectal Surgery. Prevention and Management. Preface. Philadelphia: W.B. Saunders Company, 1985.
6. Swain JD. Mea maxima culpa—dealing with surgical complications. Bull Am Coll Surg. 2014;99:14. bulletin.facs.org, published January 3, 2014.
7. St. Paul. Epistula Ad Romanos. Chapter 3: Verse 23. The Latin Vulgate New Testament Bible. Vulgate.Org. Accessed 14 Jun 2021.
8. Paul S. In: Chamberlin RB, Feldman H, editors. the Epistle of Paul to the Romans, 3:23. The Dartmouth Bible. Boston: Houghton Mifflin Company; 1950. The Riverside Press Cambridge, Page 1091.
9. John. Evangelium Secundum Ioannem-Chapter 8:Verse 32. The Latin Vulgate New Testament Bible. Vulgate.org. Accessed 3 Oct 2021.

[1] This quote has been attributed to many. Who said it first, we don't know.

[2] Work ethic passed to Dr. Inkster from her father, Mr. Henry George Inkster.

Superior Mesenteric Vein Transection 203

James S. Wu

Presentation

A 77-year-old female was undergoing a right hemicolectomy for colon cancer. During mobilization of the hepatic flexure, the superior mesenteric vein (SMV) was completely transected (Fig. 203.1). One thousand milliliters of blood was lost quickly. The SMV ends were ligated to control bleeding. The colectomy

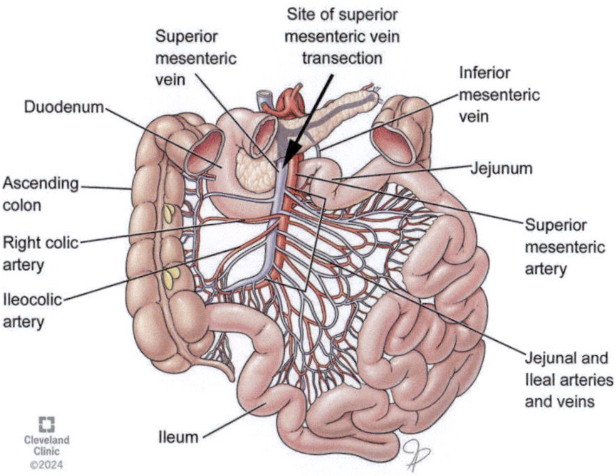

Fig. 203.1 The superior artery perfuses the jejunum, ileum, right colon, and transverse colon (not shown). Transsection of the SMV near the pancreas results in the extravasation of venous return these organs and prevents their venous return from reaching the portal system

J. S. Wu (✉)
Department of Colon and Rectal Surgery, Cleveland Clinic, Cleveland, OH, USA

J. S. Wu, M. D. Inkster (eds.), *Cleveland Clinic Colorectal Case Studies*,
https://doi.org/10.1007/978-3-031-39880-3_203

was completed. Intraoperative hypotension was corrected by the transfusion of four units of packed red blood cells. The small intestine became markedly edematous due to venous obstruction.

Management

Intraoperative consultation with the solid organ transplantation service was requested. The ends of the SMV were freshened. After obtaining vascular control, a human cadaveric iliac vein interposition graft was sewn in between the proximal superior mesenteric vein to the splenic vein (Fig. 203.2). Flow was excellent. The small intestine edema steadily decreased and the intestine returned to a normal appearance except for the terminal ileum. The distal 10 cm was ischemic and was resected. An end ileostomy was created. Colon pathology returned the diagnosis of moderately differentiated adenocarcinoma. There was no evidence of malignancy in 25 lymph nodes. Restoration of intestinal continuity was done six months later.

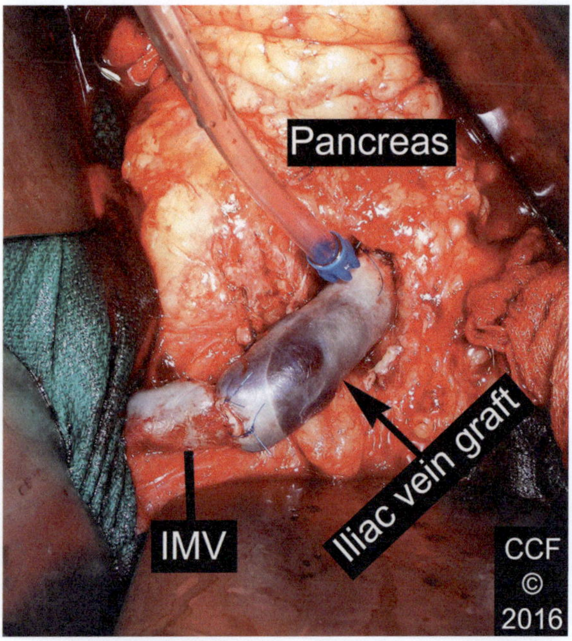

Fig. 203.2 Reconstruction following complete superior mesenteric vein disruption during right colon mobilization. Reconstruction was accomplished using a cadaveric human iliac vein interposition graft (arrow). The native SMV anastomosed to the iliac vein graft is labeled. The transection occurred at the lower border of the pancreas

Comment

In this case, injury was caused by excessive traction on the superior mesenteric vein and its middle colic venous branches during hepatic flexure mobilization. Without immediate restoration of venous outflow, small and large intestinal infarction would have followed. This potentially life-threatening problem would have been avoided by gentler handling of the colon and its mesentery. The surgeon in this case (JSW) and his patient were fortunate to have an expert in venous reconstruction available. This case stresses the importance of gentleness in tissue handling, the potential disastrous consequences of not heeding this universal rule, and the blessing of colleagues to whom one can turn for help.

Abdominal Compartment Syndrome

204

James S. Wu

Presentation

A 64-year-old female presented with a complete small bowel obstruction two years after subtotal colectomy with end ileostomy (left-sided) for ulcerative colitis. Laparotomy with extensive lysis of adhesions and stoma translocation was done to relieve the obstruction. The fascial bridge between the original left-sided ileostomy site and the midline incision had disintegrated. The ileostomy was translocated to the right side. The fascia and skin were closed. On the first postoperative day, the patient complained of severe abdominal pain. Serum electrolytes included: Na 143 mEq/L, K 4.1 mEq/L, Cl 110 mEq/L, and HCO_3^- 17 mEq/L. The bladder pressure was elevated at 37 mm Hg. The patient was returned to the operating room. The abdomen was opened. Doppler pulses along the intestinal mesentery were present. Examination of the intestine with a Wood's lamp after injection of intravenous fluorescein showed that the intestine was perfused (Fig. 204.1).

At the end of the re-exploration, complete fascial closure could not be done without tension.

J. S. Wu (✉)
Department of Colon and Rectal Surgery, Cleveland Clinic, Cleveland, OH, USA

J. S. Wu, M. D. Inkster (eds.), *Cleveland Clinic Colorectal Case Studies*,
https://doi.org/10.1007/978-3-031-39880-3_204

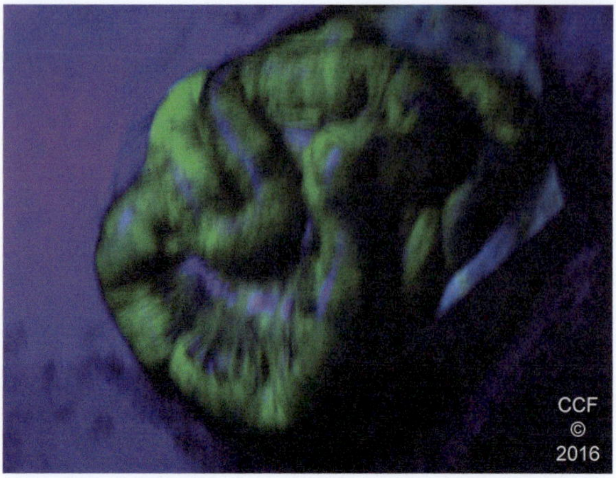

Fig. 204.1 The small intestine was viewed with a Wood's ultraviolet lamp after intravenous injection of fluorescein. The entire small bowel was perfused

Management

Fascial closure at the previous left-sided ileostomy site could not be done because the fascial bridge between the previous stoma and the midline involving the upper half of the laparotomy incision had disintegrated. The lower half of the laparotomy incision was closed with midline stitches reinforced with retention sutures. Coverage of the intestine protruding from the upper half of the incision was accomplished by suturing porcine mesh to the facscia (Fig. 204.2). The skin over the upper incision and the original left-sided ostomy was approximated using a combination of staples and dental rolls (Fig. 204.3). Healing was uneventful (Fig. 204.4).

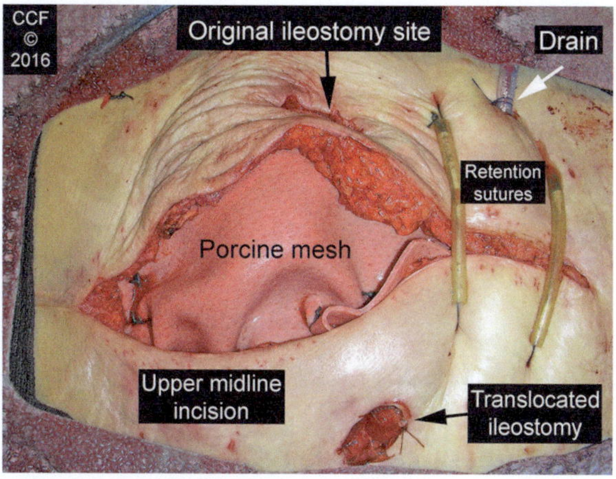

Fig. 204.2 The fascia in the upper half of the incision could not be closed primarily without tension. Porcine mesh, sewn to the fascia, provided intestinal coverage. The fascia of the lower incision was closed successfully; retention sutures were placed to prevent dehiscence. The ileostomy was translocated from the left to the right side. A temporary drain is located in the left lower quadrant

Fig. 204.3 The skin overlying the porcine mesh including the original stoma site was closed using dental rolls and staples

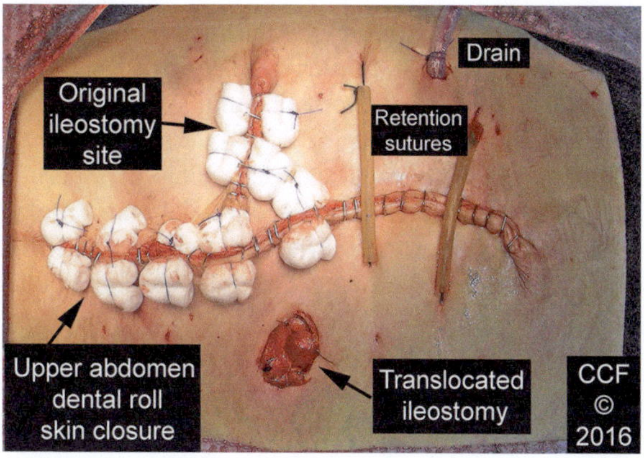

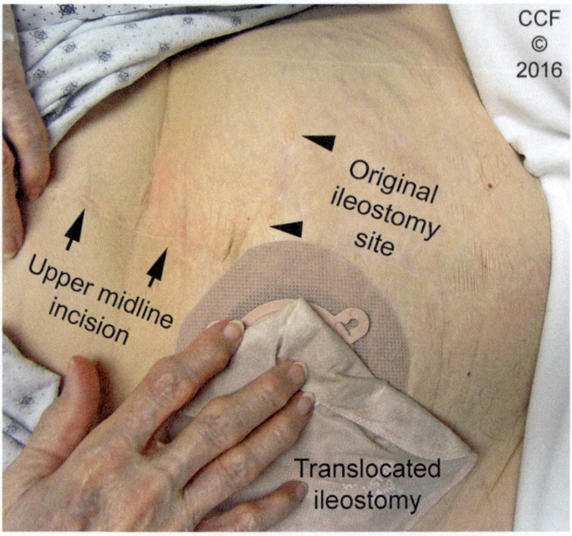

Fig. 204.4 Healing at six months following removal of staples, retention sutures, and dental rolls

Comment

In 1911, Emerson demonstrated by animal experiments that elevated intra-abdominal pressure decreases internal perfusion and can result in death [1]. In 1984, Kron identified elevated intra-abdominal compartment pressure as an indication for abdominal re-exploration [2]. An International Conference of Experts on Intra-abdominal Hypertension and Abdominal Compartment Syndrome defined intra-abdominal hypertension as an intra-abdominal pressure at or above 12 mmHg. Abdominal compartment syndrome was defined as an intra-abdominal pressure above 20 mmHg with evidence of organ dysfunction/failure requiring invasive measures [3]. Elevated intra-abdominal pressure may be determined by direct or indirect methods [4]. Monitoring by measuring bladder pressures via Foley catheter is comparable to intraperitoneal pressure measurement but is noninvasive. Abdominal decompression is indicated for abdominal compartment syndrome [5, 6]. If the abdomen cannot be closed after decompression, the intestines can be covered with prosthetic material.

Following surgery, this patient developed abdominal compartment syndrome characterized by abdominal pain, elevated abdominal compartment pressures (>20 mmHg), and metabolic acidosis (high chloride, low bicarbonate). The patient was returned to the operating room. The abdomen was opened. Intestinal viability was confirmed by the assessment of mesenteric pulses and inspection of the small intestine with intravenous fluorescein. After the abdomen was opened to relieve the pressure, the patient's own fascia could not be closed without tension in the area of the original stoma where the midline fascia had been lost. Three maneuvers were

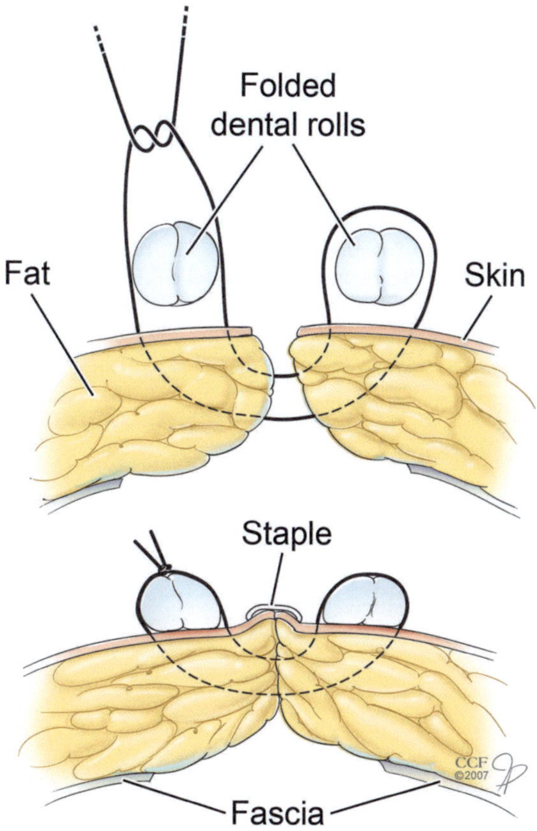

Fig. 204.5 Dental roll closure of the abdomen. The skin and subcutaneous fat are closed using vertical mattress sutures sewn over dental rolls that have been folded in a "U" shape. The dental rolls distribute even pressure on the skin and maintain wound edge approximation. The top illustration shows the passage of a mattress suture through the skin, fat, and dental rolls. The bottom illustration shows the tied suture and a skin staple. The abdominal wall fascia, shown in both the top and the bottom illustrations is not closed. If the dental rolls are kept dry, they can stay in place for several weeks

used to close the abdomen. Abdominal closure at the distal midline incision was reinforced with retention sutures. The fascia at the upper part of the incision was bridged with porcine mesh. The entire skin closure was done using cotton dental rolls as shown in Fig. 204.3 and illustrated in Fig. 204.5.[1]

References

1. Emerson H. Intra-abdominal pressures. Arch Intern Med. 1911;7:754–84.
2. Kron IL, Harman PK, Nolan SP. The measurement of intra-abdominal pressure as a criterion for abdominal re-exploration. Ann Surg. 1984;199:28–30.

[1] Dental roll skin closure: Technique passed down from Dr. Victor W. Fazio.

3. Kirkpatrick AW, Roberts DJ, Jaeschke R, De Waele J, De Keulenaer B, Duchesne J, et al. Methodological background and strategy for the 2012-2013 updated consensus definitions and clinical practice guidelines from the abdominal compartment society. Anaesthesiol Intensive Ther. 2015;47:s63–s78.
4. Schein M, Wittmann DH, Aprahamian CC, Condon RE. The abdominal compartment syndrome: The physiological and clinical consequences of elevated intra-abdominal pressure. J Am Coll Surg. 1995;180:745–53.
5. Burch JM, Moore EE, Moore FA, Franciose R. The abdominal compartment syndrome. Surg Clin North Am. 1996;76:833–42.
6. Saggi BH, Sugerman HJ, Ivatury RR, Bloomfield GL. Abdominal compartment syndrome. J Trauma: Injury, Infect, Crit Care. 1998;45:597–609.

Anastomotic Stricture-Balloon Dilation 205

James S. Wu

Presentation

A patient underwent low anterior resection of the rectum with colorectal anastomosis and temporary loop ileostomy. Endoscopic examination of the anastomosis six weeks after surgery showed a stricture (Fig. 205.1).

Endoscopic balloon stricture dilation was done (Figs. 205.2 and 205.3).

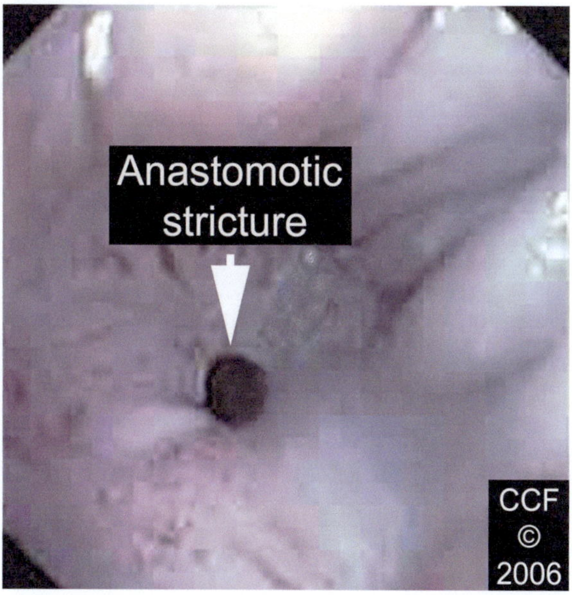

Fig. 205.1 A colorectal anastomotic stricture detected 6 weeks after low anterior resection of the rectum with stapled colorectal anastomosis

J. S. Wu (✉)
Department of Colon and Rectal Surgery, Cleveland Clinic, Cleveland, OH, USA

J. S. Wu, M. D. Inkster (eds.), *Cleveland Clinic Colorectal Case Studies*,
https://doi.org/10.1007/978-3-031-39880-3_205

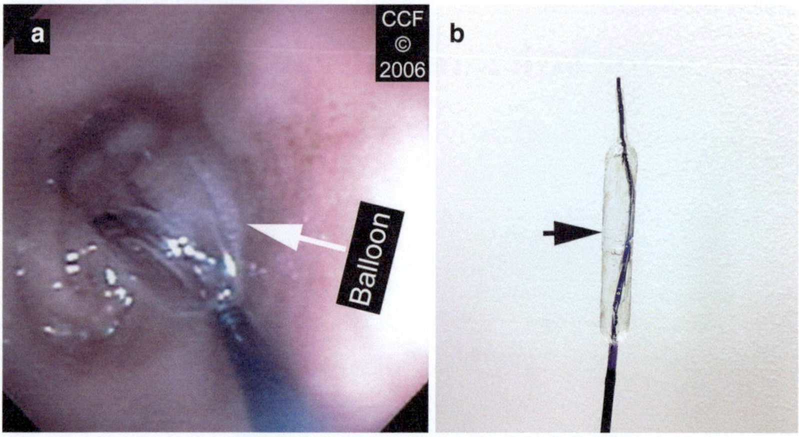

Fig. 205.2 (**a**) Endoscopic balloon dilation of the colorectal anastomotic stricture; (**b**) Balloon dilator (arrow) (The balloon dilators used in this case were made by the Boston Scientific, Company, www.bostonscientific.com)

Fig. 205.3 The appearance of the colorectal anastomosis (arrows) following serial balloon dilations (8 mm × 1 min, 10 mm × 1 min, and 15 mm × 1 min)

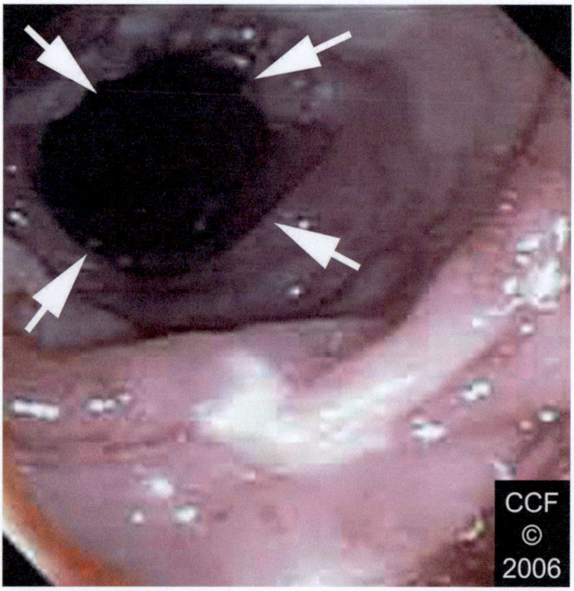

Comment

Ideally, following colorectal anastomosis, a widely patent colorectal anastomosis will be seen as shown in Fig. 205.4.

An anastomotic stricture seen at postsurgical examination (six weeks in this case), often can be enlarged by serial balloon dilation [1].

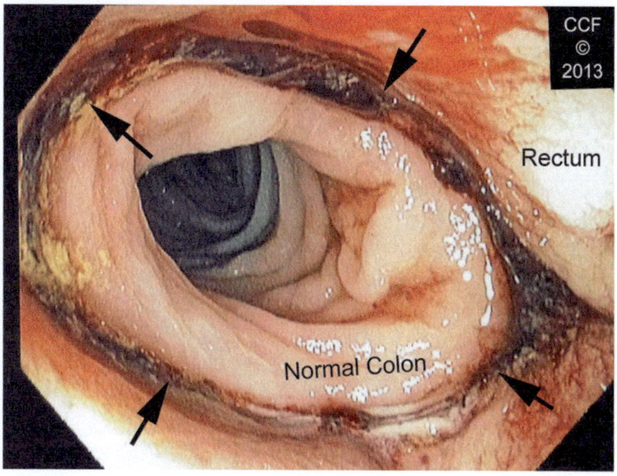

Fig. 205.4 End-to-end colorectal anastomosis seen 6 weeks after surgery. The anastomosis is widely patent with a continuous staple line (arrows). The intestine on each side of the anastomosis is normal. Dilation was not required in this case

Reference

1. Siddiqui UD, Banerjee S, Barth B, Chauhan SS, Gottlieb KT, Konda V, et al. Tools for endoscopic stricture dilation. Gastrointest Endosc. 2013;78:391–404.

Anastomotic Leak

206

James S. Wu and Sherief Shawki

Presentation

A 56-year-old male underwent right hemicolectomy with end of terminal ileum to side of transverse colon stapled anastomosis to treat a large cecal adenoma. On postoperative day five, bilious drainage was noted at the incision. The patient was returned to the operating room. Anastomotic dehiscence was found (Fig. 206.1).

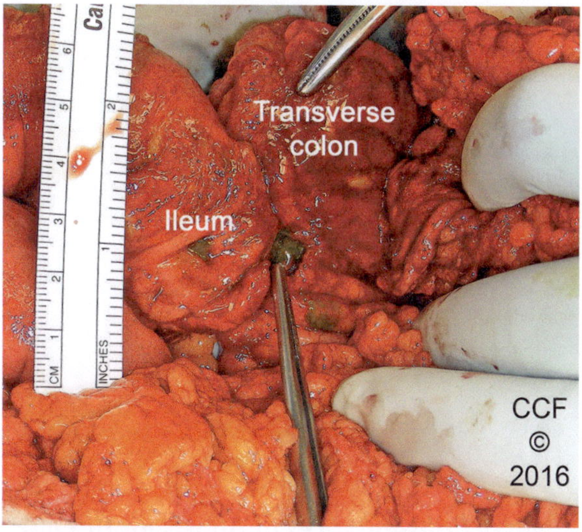

Fig. 206.1 The end of the terminal ileum has been anastomosed to the side of the transverse colon. The forceps point to the anastomotic dehiscence

J. S. Wu (✉)
Department of Colon and Rectal Surgery, Cleveland Clinic, Cleveland, OH, USA

S. Shawki
Department of Colon and Rectal Surgery, Mayo Clinic, Rochester, MN, USA

J. S. Wu, M. D. Inkster (eds.), *Cleveland Clinic Colorectal Case Studies*,
https://doi.org/10.1007/978-3-031-39880-3_206

Management

Feces were removed by suction and irrigation. The anastomosis was disassembled. The transverse colon was secured to the fascia at the superior aspect of the midline incision. A loop-end ileostomy was created at a preselected right lower quadrant stoma site. A negative pressure sponge dressing was applied to the incision.

Comment [1–7]

Factors That Favor a Successful Intestinal Anastomosis

Healthy intestine
Good blood supply
No tension
Adequate nutrition

Factors That May Contribute to Anastomotic Leakage

Technical errors
Inadequate blood supply
Inadequate intestinal approximation
Tension
Distal obstruction
Malnutrition
Immunosuppression
(a) Steroids
(b) anti-inflammatory agents
(c) chemotherapeutic agents
Infection
Irradiation
Prolonged operative time
Anastomosis below the peritoneal reflection
Tobacco abuse
Hypothermia
Collagen vascular disease
Diabetes
Hypertension
Atherosclerosis

Adverse Consequences of Anastomotic Leak

Increased mortality
Increased length of hospital stay
Reoperation
Unexpected ostomy
Sepsis

Multisystem organ failure
Coagulopathy
Enterocutaneous fistula
Delayed return to work
Negative impact on quality of life

Recognition

High index of suspicion
Deviation from the normal postoperative course
Fever
Tachycardia
Leukocytosis
Ileus
Oliguria
Mental status change
Circulatory collapse
Radiographic diagnosis

Anastomotic leak-General Management Principles

Stop the contamination
(a) Fecal stream diversion
(b) Leak closure
(c) Washout
(d) Drainage
Antibiotics
Nutritional support

Intestinal anastomotic leak leads to significant morbidity and mortality. It is always on our minds.

References

1. Schrock TR, Deveney CW, Dunphy JE. Factors contributing to leakage of colonic anastomosis. Ann Surg. 1973;177:513–8.
2. Bielecki K, Gajda A. The causes and prevention of anastomotic leak after colorectal surgery. Klin Onkol. 1999;12:25–30.
3. Gibbs J, Cull W, Henderson W, Daley J, Hur K, Khuri SF. Preoperative serum albumin level as a predictor of operative mortality and morbidity. Arch Surg. 1999;134:36–42.
4. Hyman N, Manchester TL, Osler T, Burns B, Cataldo PA. Anastomotic leaks after intestinal anastomosis. Ann Surg. 2007;245:254–8.
5. Suding P, Jensen E, Abramson MA, Itani K, Wilson ER. Definitive risk factors for anastomotic leaks in elective open colorectal resection. Arch Surg. 2008;143:907–12.
6. Wild T, Rahbarnia A, Kellner M, Sobotka L, Eberlein T. Basics in nutrition and wound healing. Nutrition. 2010;26:862–6.
7. Trencheva K, Morrissey KP, Wells M, Mancuso CA, Lee SW, Sonoda T, Michelassi F, et al. Identifying important predictors for anastomotic leak after colon and rectum resection. Ann Surg. 2013;257:108–13.

Small Bowel Obstruction, Adhesive

207

James S. Wu

Presentation

A 52-year-old female underwent abdominal colectomy and ileorectal anastomosis. Six months later, she presented with nausea and vomiting. Endoscopic examination of the anastomosis was normal. An upright abdominal plain film showed gaseous distention of mid-abdominal small bowel (Fig. 207.1). Nasogastric decompression and intravenous fluid resuscitation were started. Although the patient subsequently passed small amounts of flatus, she felt nauseated each time the nasogastric tube was clamped. A water-soluble contrast study showed dilated proximal and collapsed distal small bowel (Fig. 207.2).

J. S. Wu (✉)
Department of Colon and Rectal Surgery, Cleveland Clinic, Cleveland, OH, USA

J. S. Wu, M. D. Inkster (eds.), *Cleveland Clinic Colorectal Case Studies*,
https://doi.org/10.1007/978-3-031-39880-3_207

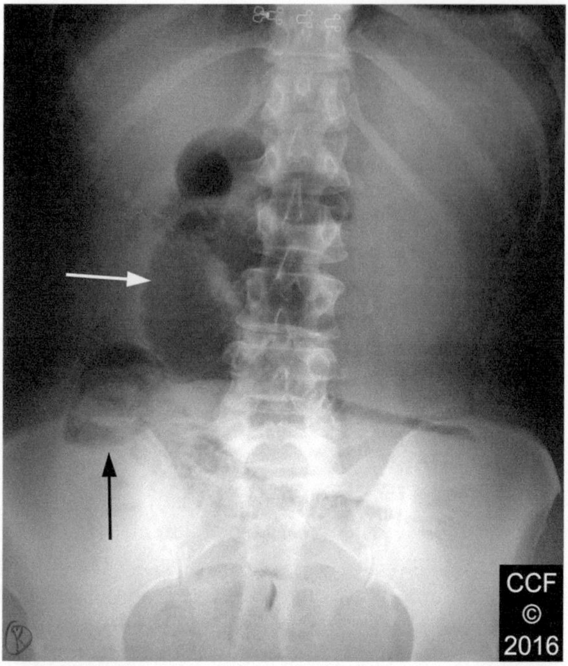

Fig. 207.1 An abdominal plain film shows gaseous distension of several loops of small bowel within the mid-abdomen (white arrow). An air fluid level is marked (black arrow)

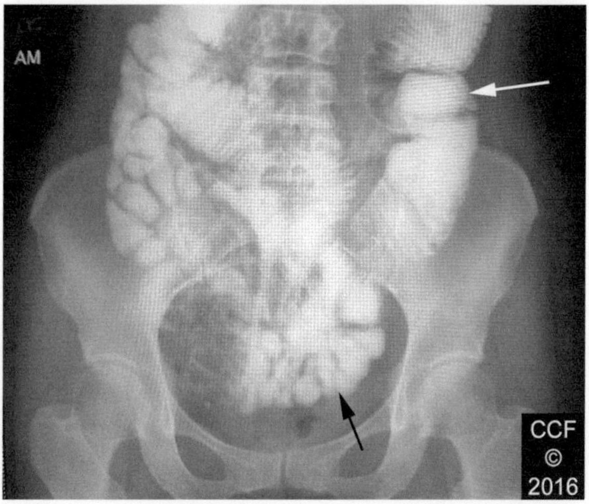

Fig. 207.2 Small bowel series with water-soluble contrast shows dilation of the proximal jejunum (white arrow). Contrast reaches collapsed distal small bowel (black arrow)

Management

Three days after admission, surgery was done. Laparotomy revealed dilated proximal and collapsed distal small intestine (Fig. 207.3). The small bowel was obstructed partially by a single adhesive band (Fig. 207.4). Band division relieved the obstruction.

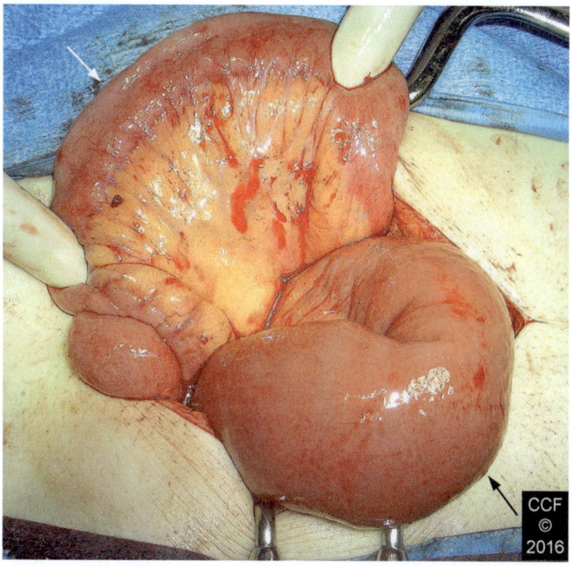

Fig. 207.3 Small bowel obstruction. Dilated proximal small bowel (black arrow) and collapsed distal small bowel (white arrow) are shown

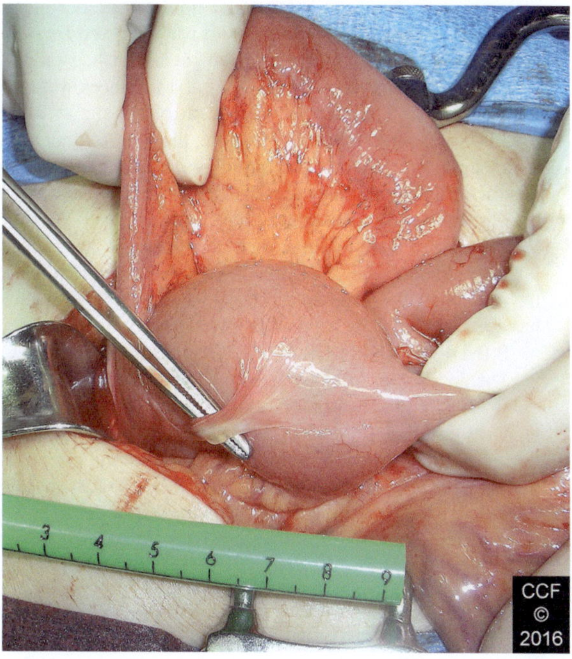

Fig. 207.4 The cause of the obstruction was a single adhesive band (forceps)

Comment

Small bowel obstruction (SBO) is caused by tumors, hernias, adhesions, neurogenic paralysis, intussusception, volvulus, and foreign body effects. Initial treatment includes intravenous fluid and electrolyte resuscitation plus intestinal decompression by nasogastric suction drainage.

Indications for operation include obstruction with strangulation and failure of conservative management. The absence of intestinal activity in the early postoperative period due to paralytic ileus commonly is seen.

Biographical Note

Owen Wangensteen (1898–1981)

In his groundbreaking work, *Intestinal Obstructions*, Wangensteen proposed the use of conservative decompression to treat intestinal obstruction [1].

> "DECOMPRESSION BY APPLICATION OF SUCTION TO DUODENAL.
> TUBES IN OBSTRUCTION
> A FACTORS SUGGESTING USE OF CONSERVATIVE DECOMPRESSION
> From determinations made upon fluid escape occurring through an enterotomy tube from a gut obstructed by adhesions, it was observed frequently that, after an initial escape of small amounts of gas and fluid, the gut established again its own continuity with little or no subsequent drainage. On the contrary, instances were observed in which the drainage was profuse and continued independent of the site at which the drainage vent had been established. It was reasoned, therefore, that the continuance of profuse drainage following high jejunostomy or low enterostomy was dependent on the persistence of a high degree of obstruction, that minimal escape of gas or fluid through an enterostomy tube indicated that the obstructive mechanism must have relented.
> These observations suggested the possibility of decompressing the gut in certain instances of mechanical obstruction without operation. The observations with relation to the fluid lost through an enterostomy have been extended since the employment of suction has been applied to an inlying duodenal tube, to include gas escape as well.
> B INDICATIONS FOR THE EMPLOYMENT OF DECOMPRESSION BY SUCTION
> The decision as to what agency is to be selected in securing relief of the obstruction is obvious when the obstruction is strangulating in nature or an obstruction of the colon with great distention is present. In either instance, early operation is *urgently* indicated. When, however, the obstruction is simple in character and concerns the small intestine, the determination of the best remedial measure may be no easy task. In the main, it may be said, that a trial with suction applied to an inlying duodenal tube is permissible in those cases in which clear indication for immediate operation does not exist."

Owen H. Wangensteen, BA, MD, PhD
Professor of Surgery of the University of Minnesota and
Surgeon in Chief of the University of Minnesota Hospital

Wangensteen's experimental conclusions challenged surgical dogma that favored early operation for small bowel obstruction. In 2021, Diaz et al. [2] reexamined a rule that previously had been ingrained in the surgical mindset.

> 'Traditionally, surgeons have been taught: "Never let the sun set or rise on a bowel obstruction," and that operating early was best. However, with advances in imaging and a better understanding of the natural history of SBO, urgent operations are becoming less common with more than 70% of patients successfully treated non-operatively.'[1]

Following nasogastric gastric tube placement, timing of tube removal may be guided by a poem taught to me when I was a medical student by Dr. Kenneth J. Bennett.

"Bile is green,
Obstruction is seen.
Bile is yellow,
Feed the fellow."

Biographical Note Owen H. Wangensteen (1898–1981) A remembrance from the Archives of the American College of Surgeons reads:

> 'Owen H. Wangensteen, MD, PhD, FACS, was a renowned surgeon from Minnesota who had a deep influence in the areas of research, teaching, and the practice of surgery.
> In his capacity as a teacher, Dr. Wangensteen employed the Socratic method, which he used to foster independent thought and research amongst his students. Beyond the classroom, he believed that surgeons were split into two distinct groups, "those who see what they believe and those who believe what they see." He was passionate in trying to produce the latter,…
>
> Dr. Wangensteen's passion for surgery did not stop when he retired from the profession. He went on to write a book with his wife entitled *The Rise of Surgery: From Empiric Craft to Scientific Discipline*.' [3, 4]

A book review by Dr. David Sabiston of "*The Rise of Surgery: From Empiric Craft to Scientific Discipline*," reads as follows:

> 'A SCHOLARLY WORK occasionally appears which justifies extraordinary praise. Such is clearly true of this outstanding contribution by Owen and Sarah Wangensteen. In the opening sentence of the preface, they penetrate directly to the mark in stating: "If all of Medicine from anatomy to zoology were taught with a view to the historic background of each discipline privileged to carry a badge of its own, our students would be taught better." It is from this viewpoint that the authors present a carefully edited and thoughtfully selected complication of the history of surgery.
>
> The impact of this outstanding work is clearly stated in the dedication. "May the spirit of inquiry, the love of leaning, and the appreciation of the history of medicine create in our medical schools an intellectual atmosphere that will heighten greater commitment and accountability in its service to mankind.'
>
> David C. Sabiston, Jr., M.D., 1980 [5][2]

---

[1] This excerpt is reused with the generous permission of Elsevier, CCC|RightsLink, License Number 5897260335306; License date Oct 27, 2024.

[2] Permission to reproduce this excerpt was generously provided by Wolters Kluwer Health, Inc, CCC|RightsLink®, License number 5136861089653, License Date Aug 27, 2021.

References

1. Wangensteen OH. Intestinal Obstructions. 2nd ed. Springfield, Illinois: Fourth printing, Charles C. Thomas; 1949. pp. 138 and 149.
2. Diaz A, Ricci KB, Rushing AP, Ingraham AM, Daniel VT, Paredes AZ, et al. Re-examining "never letting the sun rise or set on a bowel obstruction" in the era of acute care surgery. J Gastrointest Surg. 2021;25:512–22.
3. Wangensteen OH, Wangensteen SD. The Rise of Surgery from Empiric Craft to Scientific Discipline. Minneapolis: University of Minnesota Press; 1978.
4. Owen H. Wangensteen, 1898–1981. Reproduced with permission from the Archives of the American College of Surgeons, August 23, 2021.
5. Sabiston DC, Jr. The Rise of Surgery: From Empiric Craft to Scientific Discipline. Ann Surg. 1980;191:117.

Small Bowel Obstruction-Internal Hernia 208

James S. Wu

Presentation A

A 45-year-old patient underwent laparoscopic-assisted abdominal colectomy with end ileostomy for toxic ulcerative colitis. The operation was performed through an 8-cm midline abdominal incision centered around the umbilicus. The rectosigmoid stump was closed with staples and secured above the fascia at the distal aspect of the incision. Four months after surgery, the patient complained of nausea, vomiting, and severe abdominal pain. She was seen without delay and taken to surgery. The main operative finding is shown in Fig. 208.1.

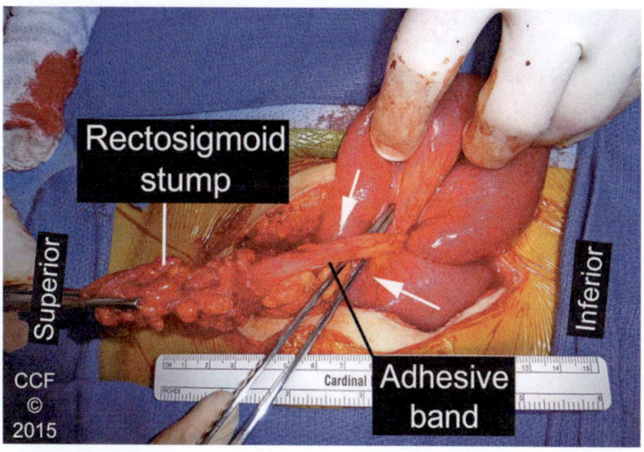

Fig. 208.1 The rectosigmoid stump (white line) has been freed from the abdominal wall. Small intestine (arrows) has been trapped by an adhesive band (black line) attached to the rectosigmoid stump on its inferior surface. The adhesion has been elevated by forceps

J. S. Wu (✉)
Department of Colon and Rectal Surgery, Cleveland Clinic, Cleveland, OH, USA

J. S. Wu, M. D. Inkster (eds.), *Cleveland Clinic Colorectal Case Studies*,
https://doi.org/10.1007/978-3-031-39880-3_208

A loop of small intestine had become trapped in the space between the rectosigmoid stump and the anterior abdominal wall/pelvis. Division of the adhesion relieved the obstruction. The intestine was viable; resection was not needed. The rectosigmoid was returned to the abdomen, unattached to the abdominal wall.

Comment

Following subtotal colectomy for toxic colitis through a long midline incision, the rectosigmoid stump may be secured above the fascia adjacent to the pubis symphysis. The benefits of this maneuver are twofold. First, the rectosigmoid stump is easy to locate at future operations. Second, in the event of a rectosigmoid stump blowout, the contents of the rectosigmoid are discharged above the fascia, thus avoiding peritonitis. In this case, the rectosigmoid stump was secured above the fascia close to the umbilicus following minimally invasive colectomy. This left a space between the rectosigmoid stump and the anterior abdominal wall/pelvis through which the small intestine herniated (Fig. 208.2).

Internal herniation of small intestine through this space caused small intestinal obstruction. Had the condition been neglected, small intestinal ischemia or infarction might have occurred.

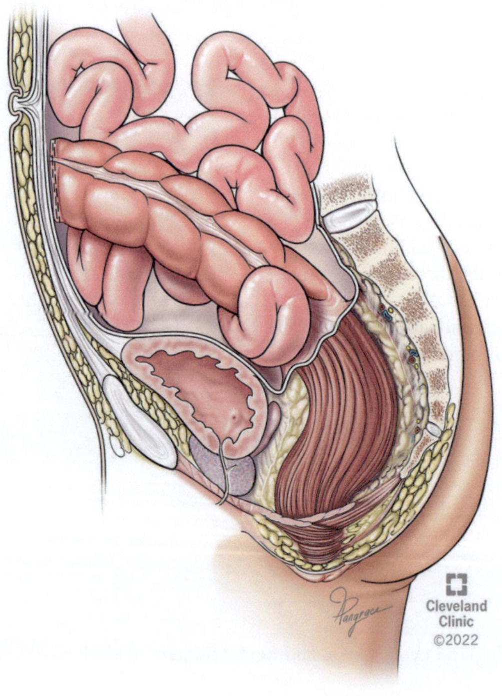

Fig. 208.2 Following subtotal colectomy, the rectosigmoid stump has been secured to the anterior abdominal wall. The small intestine has herniated between the rectosigmoid and the anterior abdominal wall/pelvis

Martin et al. [1][1] summarize hernias as follows:

> "Hernias are of two main types, external and internal. External hernias refer to prolapse of intestinal loops through a defect in the wall of the abdomen or pelvis, and internal hernias are defined by the protrusion of a viscus through a normal or abnormal peritoneal or mesenteric aperture within the confines of the peritoneal cavity.
>
> Although internal hernias have an overall incidence of less than 1%, they constitute up to 5.8% of all small bowel obstructions, which, if left untreated, have been reported to have an overall mortality exceeding 50% if strangulation is present".

Presentation B

A 62-year-old female was admitted to the hospital for observation because of abdominal pain, nausea, and vomiting. She had undergone several abdominal operations previously. At the time of admission, her vital signs were within the normal range except for a slight elevation in her heart rate. The pain was intermittent; it came in waves, gradually increasing in severity then abating. At the time of admission, her abdominal examination was described as soft and nontender. Radiographs showed features consistent with small bowel obstruction. Intravenous fluid resuscitation was started. A nasogastric tube was placed. Over the following 20 hours, the patient's pain became more severe (10/10) and constant. She was transferred to the intensive care unit following abrupt hemodynamic collapse and then emergently rushed to surgery. The appearance of the terminal ileum on opening the abdomen is shown in Fig. 208.3.

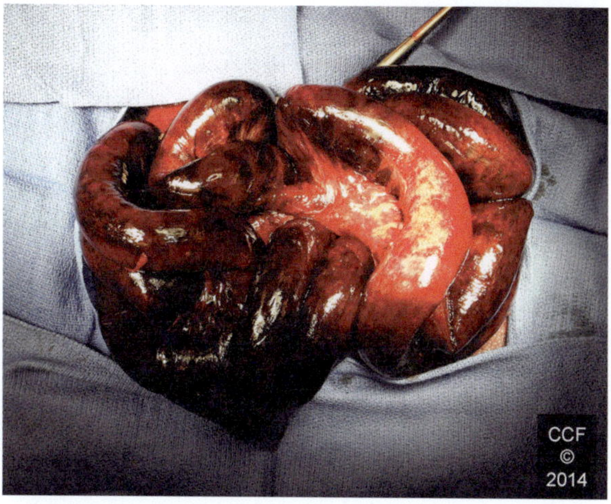

Fig. 208.3 Infarcted terminal ileum

[1] Permission to reuse these excerpts was requested from the Radiological Society of North America. I was notified that a formal permission was not needed on October 27, 2021. Proper APA/MLA citation format was requested.

Comment

The patient's small bowel obstruction was caused by an internal hernia. The trapped intestine became ischemic; and, eventually, it infarcted. This catastrophic end might have been avoided had surgery been done earlier. A major factor that allowed the right course of therapy not to be followed in this case may have been what Martin and Stephen call a "lack of situational awareness" on the part of the care-giving team [2]. These authors specifically discuss *pain out of proportion to examination findings* associated with bowel ischemia and other "time-dependent and life-threatening" emergencies. Bala et al. [3] cite a mortality in the range of 50% for untreated acute mesenteric ischemia and stress the importance of early diagnosis and surgery.

References

1. Martin LC, Merkle EM, Thompson WM. Review of internal hernias: Radiographic and clinical findings. AJR Am J Roentgenol. 2006;186:703–17. https://doi.org/10.2214/AJR.05.0644.
2. Martin S-J, Stephen VS. Pitfalls in medicine: pain out of proportion to examination findings. Br J Hosp Med. 2022. https://doi.org/10.12968/hmed.2021.0599.
3. Bala M, Kashuk J, Moore EE, Kluger Y, Biffl W, Gomes CA, et al. Acute mesenteric ischemia: guidelines of the World Society of Emergency Surgery. World J Emerg Surg. 2017;12:38. https://doi.org/10.1186/s13017-017-0150-5.

209 Food Bolus Obstruction

Barbara J. Hocevar and James S. Wu

Presentation

A 69-year-old female underwent proctocolectomy with end ileostomy to treat ulcerative colitis. Many years later, after eating coleslaw (finely chopped cabbage), she presented to the emergency room with abdominal pain and bloating. Ileostomy function had ceased. Plain abdominal radiographs (Fig. 209.1) and computed tomographic images of the abdomen (Fig. 209.2a, b, and c) were obtained.

B. J. Hocevar
Rupert B. Turnbull, Jr., School of WOC Nursing Education, Cleveland Clinic, Cleveland, OH, USA

J. S. Wu (✉)
Department of Colon and Rectal Surgery, Cleveland Clinic, Cleveland, OH, USA

J. S. Wu, M. D. Inkster (eds.), *Cleveland Clinic Colorectal Case Studies*,
https://doi.org/10.1007/978-3-031-39880-3_209

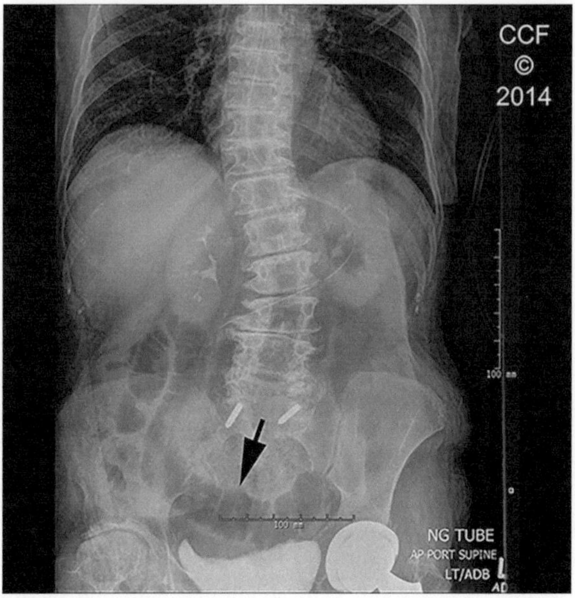

Fig. 209.1 A plain abdominal radiograph shows a dilated air-filled loop of intestine (arrow). Scoliosis and a left hip prosthesis also are seen

Management

The working diagnosis was "food bolus obstruction." The ileostomy was intubated with a lubricated Foley catheter and gently lavaged with normal saline. Catheter withdrawal resulted in the discharge of undigested vegetable matter and flatus (Fig. 209.3). Subsequent plain abdominal radiography showed disappearance of the dilated small bowel (Fig. 209.4).

Comment

Food bolus obstruction is a clinical syndrome that occurs when incompletely digested food, usually vegetable matter, forms an obstructing phytobezoar proximal to the abdominal wall fascia [1–3]. The mechanism of obstruction is similar to blockage of a kitchen sink (Fig. 209.5).

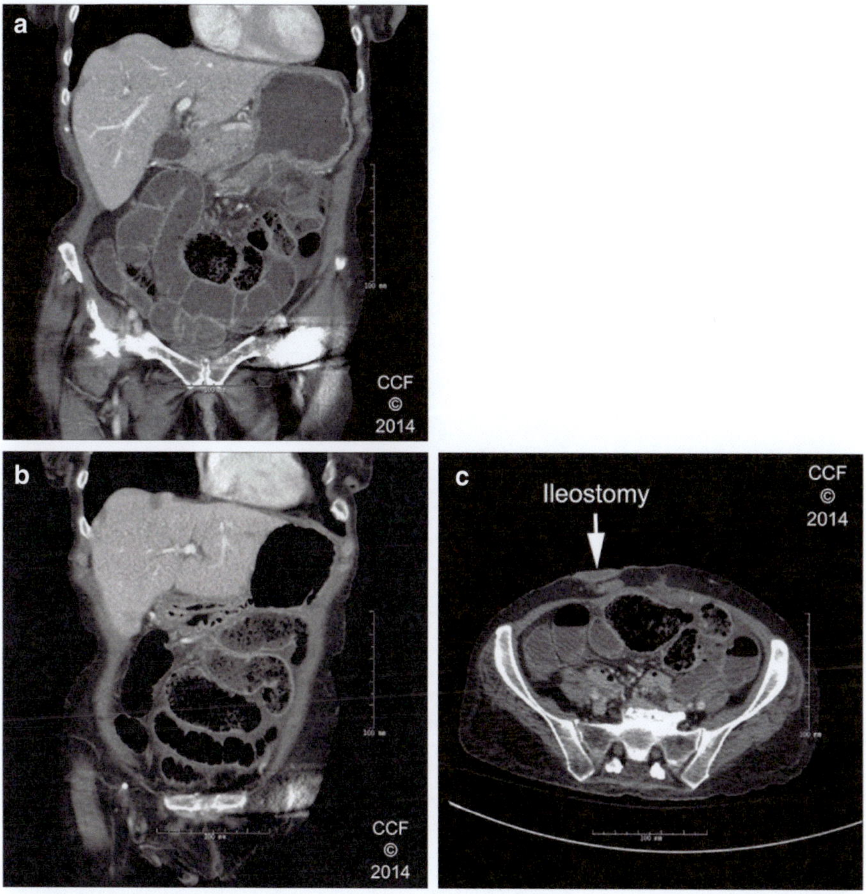

Fig. 209.2 Computed tomography of the abdomen. (**a**) A coronal view of the abdomen shows dilated fluid-filled loops of small intestine; (**b**) A second coronal view anterior to (Fig. 209.2a) shows dilated air filled loops of small intestine; (**c**) Axial view shows an ileostomy (arrow) located in the right lower quadrant

Management of Food Bolus Obstruction

The following is adapted from the R. B. Turnbull, Jr., MD, School of WOC Nursing Education, (2015) lesson on Ileal Lavage [4].

Conservative management of suspected food bolus obstruction can be done at home. Signs of a food bolus obstruction include thin, liquid, foul smelling output or lack of output for four to six hours; crampy abdominal pain particularly near the stoma; stomal and/or abdominal distension; and nausea or vomiting. If there is no vomiting, measures can be undertaken at home to relax the abdominal muscles and stimulate peristalsis. These measures would include:

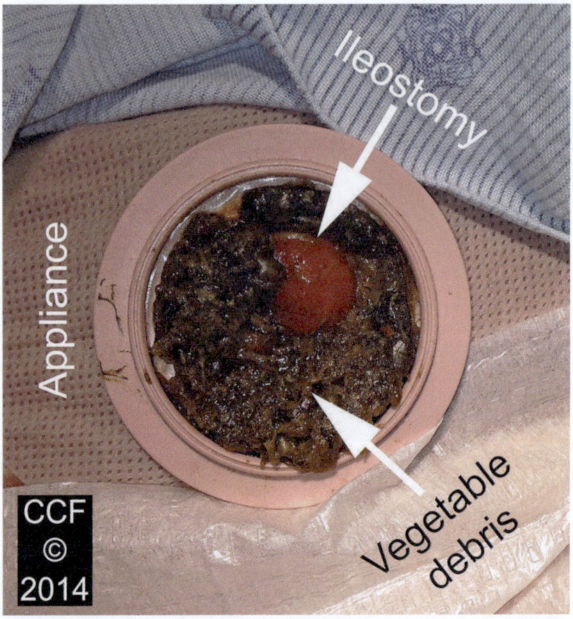

Fig. 209.3 Stoma irrigation resulted in the efflux of flatus and partially digested vegetable matter

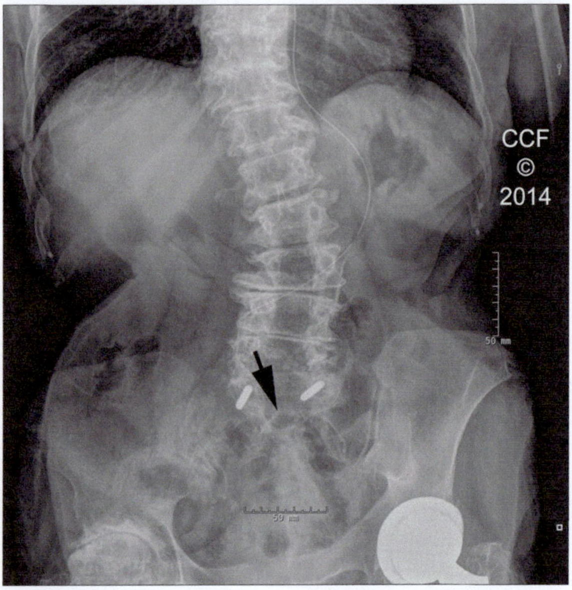

Fig. 209.4 The dilated small intestine previously seen in Fig. 209.1 has disappeared following catheter lavage of the ileostomy. The approximate location of the dilated small bowel previously seen is marked with an arrow

- Walking.
- Avoiding solid foods.
- Drinking warm fluids.
- If no output, no eating or drinking.
- Peristomal massage.

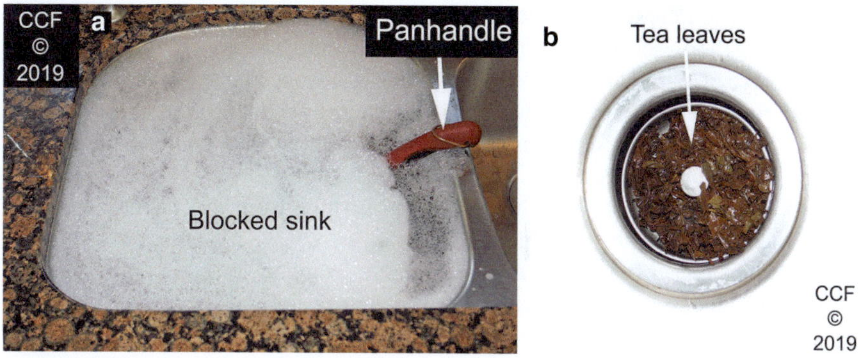

Fig. 209.5 (**a**) Water and bubbles in a blocked kitchen sink; (**b**) Tea leaves, matted together at the sink outlet, were the cause of the sink blockage

- Knee-chest position to see if the bolus can be dislodged.
- Warm tub bath to relax abdominal muscles.

If vomiting occurs or symptoms worsen, the individual is advised to seek medical attention. They should be advised to bring all of their pouching supplies with them.

A complete history and physical exam, IV fluid resuscitation, blood work, and a flat plate or CT of the abdomen are usual first steps in the medical work-up. If a food bolus is confirmed or suspected, an ileal lavage may be required. Steps in this procedure are listed below:

1. Assemble equipment: Foley catheter, 18-20Fr., irrigation set, ostomy pouching system and irrigation sleeve, water soluble lubricant, non-sterile gloves, drainage receptacle, 1000 cc of normal saline, bed protection pads, personal protective equipment including gown and face shield (when the food bolus breaks up, it can come out of the stoma under force!).
2. If needed, medicate the patient. This helps to relax the rectus abdominus muscle, which can make the lavage more effective.
3. Position the patient supine and protect the bed with bed protection pads.
4. If available, apply ostomy irrigation sleeve per guidelines with the spout placed into a drainage receptacle. If an irrigation sleeve is not available, direct the drainage spout of the pouch into the receptacle and cut a small "x" at the top of the pouch.
5. Lubricate your pinkie finger, insert into stoma, and notice the direction of the intestine. If the food bolus is encountered, gently attempt to break it up with your finger.
6. Lubricate the end of the indwelling catheter with water-soluble lubricant and connect to the irrigation syringe that is filled with 60 cc of normal saline.

7. Slowly insert the catheter into the lumen of the stoma (either through the top of the irrigation sleeve or through the "x" cut into the pouch). Slowly instill 40–60 cc of saline into the catheter while it is advanced into the bowel.
   (a) You will notice that saline/intestinal contents will come around the catheter.
   (b) If no resistance is met, slowly advance the catheter using an in-and-out" motion.
   (c) Periodically disconnect the irrigation syringe from the catheter to allow luminal contents to drain out.
   (d) The catheter may be advanced its entire length as long as no resistance is encountered. If this occurs, the problem is not caused by a food bolus obstruction.
   (e) Remove the catheter from the bowel intermittently to assess catheter patency.
8. Repeat the above steps until there is relief or a negative response.
9. A positive response = progressive discoloration of the returned solution or effluent containing fiber or food particles. A maximum of 1000 cc of saline in increments of 40–60 cc can be used.
10. Negative response = clear return of the solution after 500 cc of solution has been used.
11. When the procedure is discontinued, remove irrigation sleeve/old pouch. Before repouching, measure the size of the stoma as it can become swollen. Repouch with appropriately sized pouching system.
12. Review with the patient foods that cause food bolus obstruction as well as the need to chew foods thoroughly.

References

1. Verstandig AG, Klin B, Bloom RA, Hadas I, Libson E. Small bowel phytobezoars: detection with radiography. Radiology. 1989;172:705–7.
2. George AJ, Fallaize RC, Bennett J, Shabbir J. Ileostomy obstruction by ingested apricot stone with clinical-radiological-pathological correlation. BMJ Case Rep. 2015. https://doi.org/10.1136/bcr-2015-210594.
3. Jain M, Pielage P, De-Ryke R. Plum stones: an unusual cause of ileostomy obstruction demonstrated by sonography. J Clin Ultrasound. 1988;26:416–7.
4. Turnbull RB Jr, School of WOC Nursing Education. Lesson on ileal lavage (with permission); 2015.

210 Postpolypectomy Colon Coagulation Syndrome

James S. Wu, Sean W. Carlson, and Michelle D. Inkster

Presentation

A 67-year-old female patient underwent colonoscopy with hot snare removal of a 15 mm sessile sigmoid colon polyp (Fig. 210.1). Eight hours later, she was seen in the emergency department because of severe left lower quadrant pain (T 38.0°C, serum white blood cell count (WBC) 13 K/μL). Physical examination showed focal left lower quadrant tenderness. Computed tomography (CT) of the abdomen and pelvis showed pericolonic fat stranding along a short segment of sigmoid colon, but no free air (Fig. 210.2).

J. S. Wu (✉)
Department of Colon and Rectal Surgery, Cleveland Clinic, Cleveland, OH, USA

S. W. Carlson
Department of Radiology, UPMC Children's Hospital of Pittsburgh, Pittsburgh, PA, USA

M. D. Inkster
Department of Gastroenterology, Cleveland Clinic, Cleveland, OH, USA

J. S. Wu, M. D. Inkster (eds.), *Cleveland Clinic Colorectal Case Studies*,
https://doi.org/10.1007/978-3-031-39880-3_210

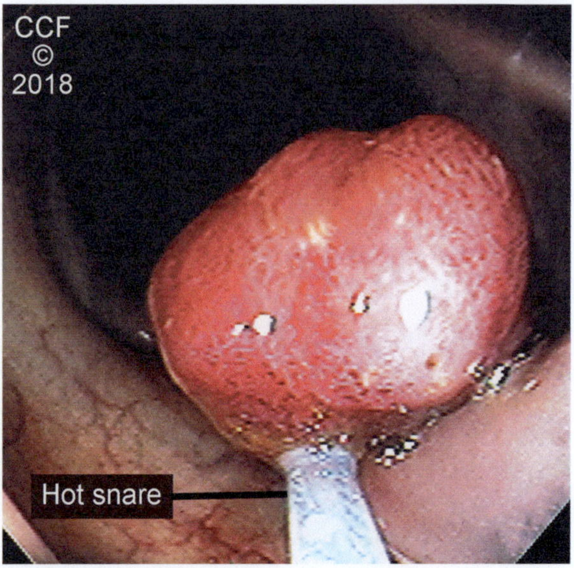

Fig. 210.1 Sigmoid colon polyp removed by hot snare

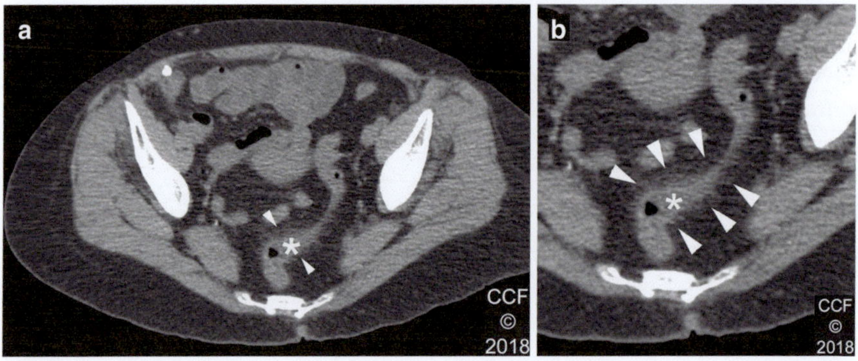

Fig. 210.2 CT shows areas of pericolonic fat stranding (arrow heads) adjacent to the sigmoid colon (asterisk) [(**a**) Axial view; (**b**) Magnified and cropped axial image]

Management

The patient was admitted to the hospital. Intravenous fluid and antibiotics were administered. Food was withheld. Physical findings, vital signs, and serum WBC were monitored closely. She passed flatus on the day after admission. Leukocytosis gradually resolved. Abdominal pain and tenderness decreased on serial examinations. A diet gradually was reintroduced. She was discharged on hospital day four.

Comment

In 1980 at the Second International Congress on Colonoscopy and Diseases of the Large Bowel, Waye described "The postpolypectomy coagulation syndrome":

> 'The major complications of colonoscopic polypectomy are perforation and bleeding, but there is another complication which I have called the "postpolypectomy coagulation syndrome." So far, this has not appeared in the medical literature, but it is a very real problem for those who remove colon polyps. The "coagulation syndrome" occurs after polypectomy and consists of localized abdominal pain, signs of peritoneal irritation, and fever. This syndrome is caused by thermal injury to tissue during electrocautery. Tissue necrosis extends into the submucosa, causing a variable amount of symptomatic reaction.'
>
> Jerome D. Waye, MD [1][1]
>
> Mount Sinai School of Medicine, New York

Postpolypectomy coagulation syndrome (PPCS) mimics colonic perforation [2]. Patients present with abdominal pain and tenderness. Fever, tachycardia, and leukocytosis may be seen [3]. Radiologic studies help to ensure no underlying free air. As seen in this case, CT may reveal wall thickening and/or pericolonic fat stranding involving the affected segment of bowel. In the absence of perforation, treatment is nonoperative and includes intravenous fluids, bowel rest, antibiotics, and close clinical monitoring. With improvement, diet and activity gradually are advanced [4].

Biographical Note

Jerome D. Waye, MD [5][2].

Dr. Jerome D. Waye was born in Shanghai, China, and emigrated to Kankakee, Illinois, at the age of 5 years. He received his undergraduate education at the Massachusetts Institute of Technology and his medical degree from Boston University Medical School.

> "… where he was on scholarship and worked 3 jobs, 1 of which was drawing blood on the Third Surgical Service at Boston City Hospital, where he rose at 4:30 each morning to draw blood from 60 surgical patients. In exchange for this service, the hospital provided clothing (white uniforms found in the hospital laundry discard bins) and food and lodging (in the old tuberculosis wards)."

Dr. Waye did his internship, residency, and gastroenterology fellowship at Mount Sinai Hospital in New York. A pioneer in the field of colonoscopy and Master Clinician, Dr. Waye is currently Professor of Medicine and Director of the Center for Advanced Colonoscopy and Therapeutic Endoscopy-Sinai.

---

[1] This excerpt was reproduced with the generous permission of Elsevier, CCC|RightsLink®, License Number 5162141076022, License date Oct 04, 2021.

[2] This excerpt is reused with the generous permission of Elsevier Science & Technology Journals, CCC|Marketplace™, Order License ID: 1156716-1, Order Date: 25 Oct 2021.

References

1. Waye JD. The postpolypectomy coagulation syndrome. Gastrointest Endosc. 1981;27:184.
2. Benson BC, Myers JJ, Laczek JT. Postpolypectomy electrocoagulation syndrome: a mimicker of colonic perforation. Case Rep Emerg Med. 2013. Article ID 687931, 3 pages. https://dx.doi.org/10.1155/2013/687931.
3. Kedia P, Waye JD. Colon polypectomy: A review of routine and advanced techniques. J Clin Gastroenterol. 2013;47:657–65.
4. Jehangir A, Bennett KM, Rettew AC, Fadahunsi O, Shaikh B, Donato A. Post-polypectomy electrocoagulation syndrome: a rare case of acute abdominal pain. J Comm Hosp Intern Med Perspect. 2015;5:29147. http://dx.doi.org/10:3402/jchimp.v5.29147.
5. Jerome D. Waye, MD. VideoGIE. 2019;4:99–101. https://doi.org/10.1016/j.vgie.2019.01.007.

Iatrogenic Colon Perforation-Laparotomy

211

James S. Wu and David M. Einstein

Presentation

A 50-year-old female underwent colonoscopy with sigmoid colon polypectomy. In recovery, she complained of severe abdominal pain and bloating. She was not able to pass flatus. An abdominal plain film was obtained (Fig. 211.1).

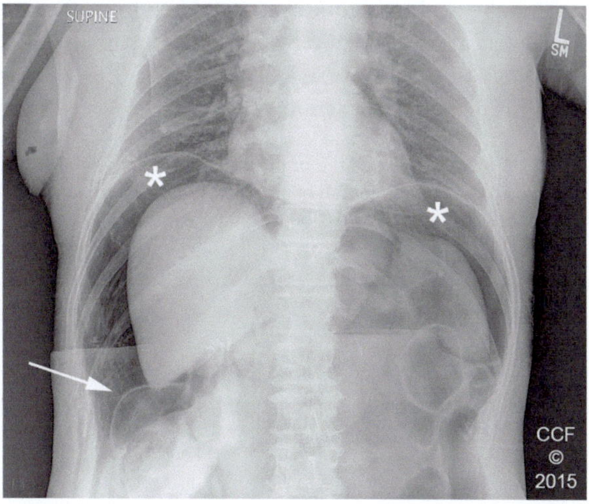

Fig. 211.1 Plain film of the abdomen shows free subdiaphragmatic air (asterisks). The arrow points to an intestinal wall flanked by air on both sides (Rigler's sign)

J. S. Wu (✉)
Department of Colon and Rectal Surgery, Cleveland Clinic, Cleveland, OH, USA

D. M. Einstein
Radiology & Diagnostic Imaging Institute, Cleveland Clinic, Cleveland, OH, USA

J. S. Wu, M. D. Inkster (eds.), *Cleveland Clinic Colorectal Case Studies*,
https://doi.org/10.1007/978-3-031-39880-3_211

Management

This patient was taken to surgery. Laparotomy revealed perforation at the sigmoid colon polypectomy site. The colon edges at the perforation were debrided to normal, well-vascularized tissue. Suture closure of the perforation and abdominal washout was done. The patient recovered uneventfully.

Comment

This is an example of a low energy, small colonic wound diagnosed and treated without delay after mechanical bowel preparation. Primary repair was appropriate therapy. Colostomy or proximal diversion were not indicated. Repair in this case was done by laparotomy.

Biographical Note

Leo George Rigler (1896–1979) [1]

Leo George Rigler was born in Minneapolis, Minnesota. He received his undergraduate and medical degrees from the University of Minnesota. His internship was done at the St. Louis City Hospital. He ultimately rose to the positions of Chair of the Department of Radiology at the University of Minnesota and Professor of Radiology at the University of California, Los Angeles. Concerning the sign that bears his name, Rigler wrote:

> "A roentgenologic sign of pneumoperitoneum hitherto not reported or clearly defined is described. It consists of the demonstration of the outer as well as the inner bowel wall due to the accumulation of gas between the loops of bowel [2]."[1]

References

1. Lewicki AM. The Rigler sign and Leo G. Rigler. Radiology. 2004;233:7–12.
2. Rigler LG. Spontaneous pneumoperitoneum: A roentgenologic sign found in the supine position. Radiology. 1941;37:604–7.

[1] Permission to reproduce this excerpt was generously provided by Ms. LaShundra Carson, permisions@rsna.org, 24 Aug 2021.

Iatrogenic Colon Perforation-Endoscopic Repair

212

John A. Dumot and James S. Wu

Presentation

An elderly female underwent polypectomy of a left colon polyp. The patient immediately developed abdominal pain and distension. The polypectomy defect was closed immediately using two endoluminal clips. Computed tomography showed massive free air and colonic intraluminal clips (Fig. 212.1). The patient was

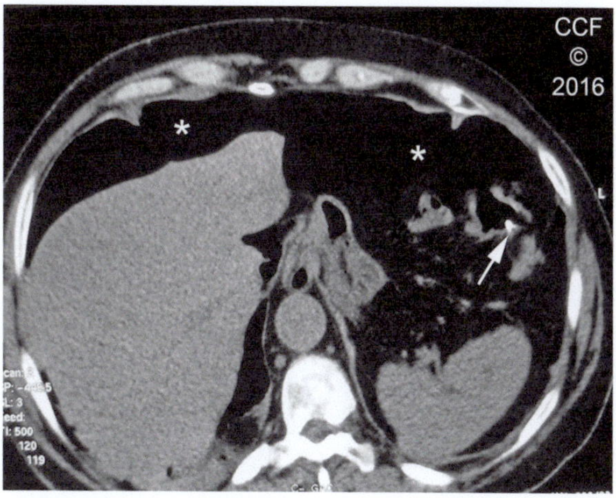

Fig. 212.1 Computed tomography shows free intra-abdominal air (asterisks) following colonoscopic left colon polypectomy. The hole was closed at the time of endoscopy with metal clips (arrow)

J. A. Dumot
Department of Gastroenterology, University Hospitals of Cleveland, Cleveland, OH, USA

J. S. Wu (✉)
Department of Colon and Rectal Surgery, Cleveland Clinic, Cleveland, OH, USA

J. S. Wu, M. D. Inkster (eds.), *Cleveland Clinic Colorectal Case Studies*,
https://doi.org/10.1007/978-3-031-39880-3_212

admitted to the hospital. Oral intake was withheld. Intravenous fluid and antibiotics were administered. Sepsis did not occur. Bowel functioned returned. The patient was discharged after several days without further adverse event.

Comment

This is an example of a iatrogenic perforation created during endoscopic polypectomy. The perforation was recognized immediately, and the defect was closed with endoluminal clips. Factors that contributed to a successful outcome in this case included small defect, immediate recognition and treatment, admission for observation, antibiotics, and a prepared colon [1, 2].

References

1. Sileri P, Del Vecchio Blanco G, Benavoli D, Gastpari AL. Iatrogenic rectal perforation during operative colonoscopy: closure with endoluminal clips. J Soc Laparoendoscop Surg. 2009;13:69–72.
2. Pohl J. Endoluminal repair of iatrogenic colonic perforation. Video J Encycloped GI Endosc. 2013;1:325. https://doi.org/10.1016/S2212-0971(13)70142-0.

Postpolypectomy Hemorrhage

213

Michelle D. Inkster, Ihab S. Haddadin, and James S. Wu

Presentation

A patient presented for a routine colonoscopy. A large polyp was removed from the ascending colon during the colonoscopy. The patient presented to the Emergency Department later that day with rectal bleeding. Her hemoglobin had decreased from a baseline of 10 g/dL to 3 g/dL. The patient refused blood products. Repeat colonoscopy showed a large amount of blood in the colon. Angiography showed active bleeding in the ascending colon (Fig. 213.1). This vessel was treated with transcatheter arterial coil embolization (Fig. 213.2). Hemostasis was achieved, and the patient was discharged from the hospital several days later without further bleeding.

M. D. Inkster
Department of Gastroenterology, Cleveland Clinic, Cleveland, OH, USA

I. S. Haddadin
Radiology & Diagnostic Imaging Institute, Cleveland Clinic, Cleveland, OH, USA

J. S. Wu (✉)
Department of Colon and Rectal Surgery, Cleveland Clinic, Cleveland, OH, USA

J. S. Wu, M. D. Inkster (eds.), *Cleveland Clinic Colorectal Case Studies*,
https://doi.org/10.1007/978-3-031-39880-3_213

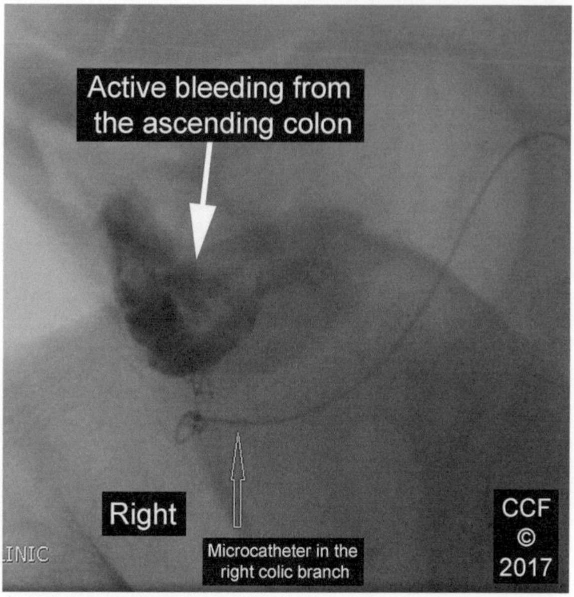

Fig. 213.1 Angiogram showing active bleeding (arrow) in the ascending colon. A microcatheter is located in a branch of the right colic artery

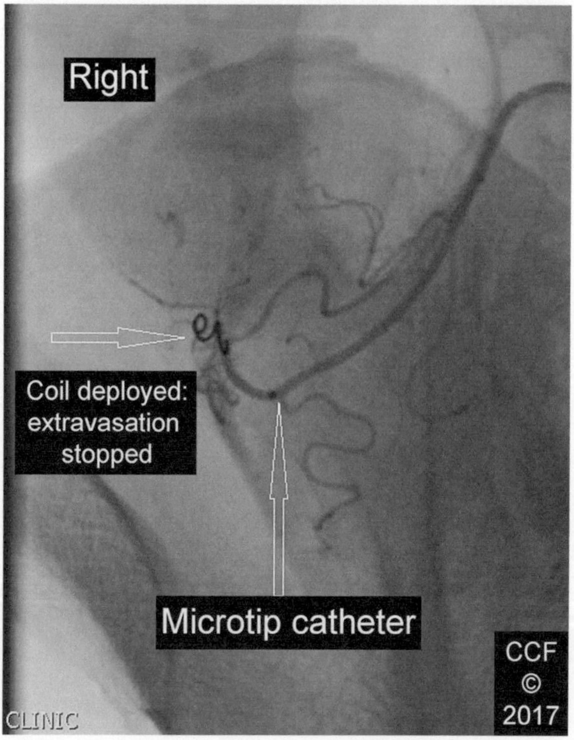

Fig. 213.2 Successful treatment of polypectomy site bleeding by transcatheter arterial coil embolization. The microcatheter tip is marked with a long arrow. The coil is marked with a short arrow

Comment [1–8]

Delayed hemorrhage after colonic polypectomy is a complication that can be life-threatening. Initially, steps are taken to establish hemodynamic stability and normalize clotting parameters. When active hemorrhage is ongoing, therapeutic measures include repeat endoscopy, angiography, and surgery. Endoscopic techniques used to stop active hemorrhage include adrenaline injection, clipping, and snare. For this patient, who refused blood products, embolization was an acceptable alternative that, fortunately, was successful.

References

1. Rex DK, Lewis BS, Waye JD. Colonoscopy and endoscopic therapy for delayed post-polypectomy hemorrhage. Gastrointest Endosc. 1992;38:127–9.
2. Waye JD, Kahn O, Auerbach ME. Complications of colonoscopy and flexible sigmoidoscopy. Gastrointest Endosc Clin N Am. 1996;6:343–77.
3. Gibbs DH, Opelka FG, Beck DE, Hicks TC, Timmcke AE, Gathright JB Jr. Postpolypectomy colonic hemorrhage. Dis Colon Rectum. 1996;39:806–10.
4. Paspatis GA, Paraskeva K, Theodoropoulou A, Mathou N, Vardas E, Oustamanolakis P, et al. A prospective, randomized comparison of adrenaline injection in combination with detachable snare versus adrenaline injection alone in the prevention of postpolypectomy bleeding in large colonic polyps. Am J Gastroenterol. 2006;101:2805–9.
5. Uno Y, Satoh K, Tuji K, Wada T, Fukuda S, Saito H, Munakata A. Endoscopic ligation by means of clip and detachable snare for management of colonic postpolypectomy hemorrhage. Gastrointest Endosc. 1999;49:113–5.
6. Church JM. Experience in the endoscopic management of large colonic polyps. ANZ J Surg. 2003;73:988–95.
7. Gravante G, Delogu D, Venditti D. Post-endoscopic polypectomy delayed bleeding concomitant with an abdominoperineal resection: a case report. Eur Rev Med Pharmacol Sci. 2007;11:355–7.
8. Rosetti A, Buchs NC, Breguet R, Bucher P, Terraz S, Morel P. Transarterial embolization in acute colonic bleeding: review of 11 years of experience and long-term results. Int J Color Dis. 2013;28:777–82.

Colonoscope Caught in an Inguinal Hernia

214

David C. Baringer, Arthur A. Parsee, and James S. Wu

Presentation

A 60-year-old male was referred for colonoscopy. Under conscious sedation, the endoscope was passed into the cecum and withdrawn. Upon withdrawal, however, the colonoscope became trapped in a left-sided inguinal hernia (Fig. 214.1).

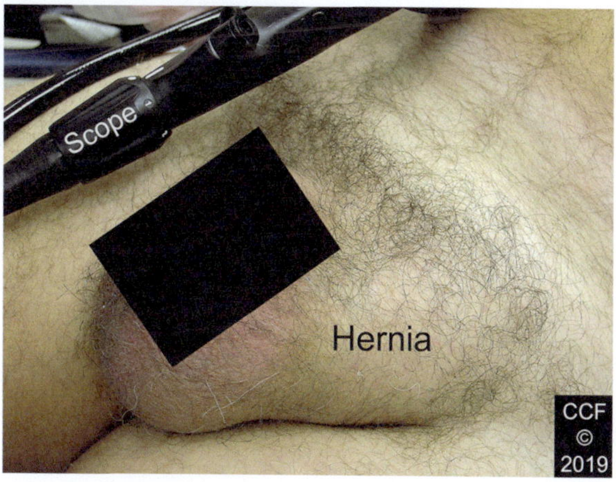

Fig. 214.1 The colonoscope and a loop of sigmoid colon are trapped in a left inguinal hernia

D. C. Baringer
Department of General Surgery, Cleveland Clinic, Cleveland, OH, USA

A. A. Parsee
Department of Diagnostic Radiology, H. Lee Moffitt Cancer Center and Research Institute, Tampa, FL, USA

J. S. Wu (✉)
Department of Colon and Rectal Surgery, Cleveland Clinic, Cleveland, OH, USA

J. S. Wu, M. D. Inkster (eds.), *Cleveland Clinic Colorectal Case Studies*,
https://doi.org/10.1007/978-3-031-39880-3_214

Management

General anesthesia was administered. Fluoroscopy showed that the colonoscope and a loop of sigmoid colon had become trapped in a left inguinal hernia (Fig. 214.2).

With fluoroscopy, the colonoscope was removed successfully. The patient subsequently underwent elective left inguinal hernia repair.

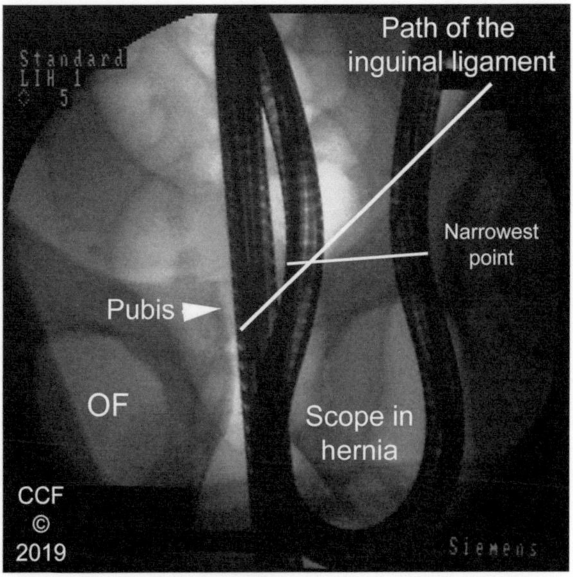

Fig. 214.2 Fluoroscopic image of the colonoscope in a loop of redundant sigmoid colon trapped in a left-sided inguinal hernia. The point of greatest narrowing is where the hernia passes beneath the inguinal ligament, OF = obturator foramen

Comment

Colonoscope incarceration in inguinal hernias has been reported infrequently [1–4]. This complication occurred because the sigmoid colon was not attached to the retroperitoneum, was redundant, had a long mesentery, and was located adjacent to a left inguinal hernia. A barium enema of another patient (Fig. 214.3) shows a redundant sigmoid colon and its relation to other parts of the large intestine.

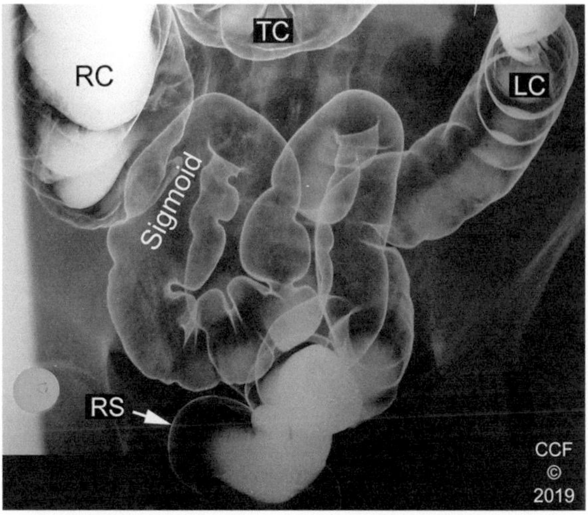

Fig. 214.3 Unlike the rectum and the left colon, the mesentery of the sigmoid colon is not fixed to the pelvis or to the retroperitoneum. In some cases, the sigmoid colon can move within the abdominal cavity accompanied by its mesentery. As shown in this double-contrast enema, the sigmoid is particularly redundant, LC = left colon, RC = right colon, RS = rectosigmoid, TC = transverse colon

References

1. Rees BI, Williams LA. Incarceration of hernia after colonoscopy (letter). Lancet. 1977;1:371.
2. Kolton WA, Coller JA. Incarceration of a colonoscope in an inguinal hernia: "pulley" technique of removal. Dis Colon Rectum. 1991;34:191–3.
3. Tan VP-Y, Lee YT, Poon JTC. Incarceration of a colonoscope in an inguinal hernia: Case report and literature review. World J Gastrointest Endosc. 2013;5:304–7.
4. Wang X, Zhang Y. Incarceration of a colonoscope within an inguinal hernia. An unusual complication. Biomed Res. 2017;28:9822–4.

Caput Medusa

215

James S. Wu

Presentation

The ileostomy appearance of a patient who had undergone total proctocolectomy with end ileostomy for ulcerative colitis is shown in Fig. 215.1.

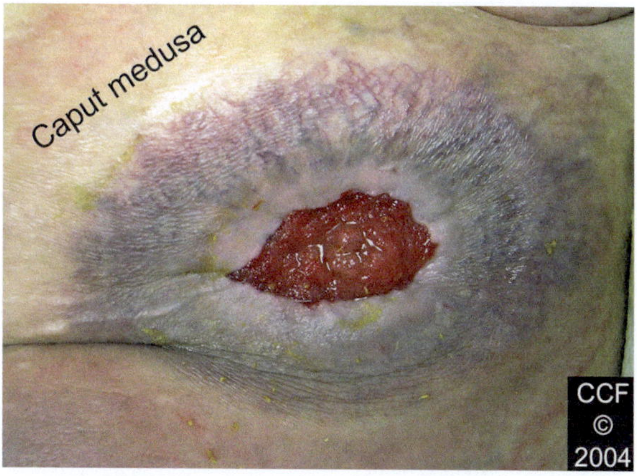

Fig. 215.1 Engorged blood vessels (a.k.a. caput Medusa) surround the ileostomy

J. S. Wu (✉)
Department of Colon and Rectal Surgery, Cleveland Clinic, Cleveland, OH, USA

J. S. Wu, M. D. Inkster (eds.), *Cleveland Clinic Colorectal Case Studies*,
https://doi.org/10.1007/978-3-031-39880-3_215

Comment

The peristomal blood vessels (Fig. 215.1) are varices seen in an ulcerative colitis patient who after proctocolectomy and end ileostomy developed primary portal hypertension complicated by cirrhosis and peristomal variceal bleeding. Islam and Morris-Stiff [1] describe a similar presentation and advise that cirrhosis and portal hypertension be kept in mind as a possible cause of peristomal hemorrhage.

> "A 44-year-old man presented with acute onset painless haemorrhage from his ileostomy. He had undergone panproctocolectomy for ulcerative colitis 17 years previously. Immediately following admission, he experienced further massive hemorrhage, developing hypovolaemic shock. Active resuscitation including suturing of a bleeding stomal varix was successful.
>
> However he reattended 8 days later with further significant hemorrhage. Investigation with CT revealed portal hypertension and cirrhosis. The patient is currently awaiting a transjugular intrahepatic portosystemic shunt (TIPS) procedure… to alleviate his portal hypertension.…"

Management options for bleeding peristomal varices are listed in Table 215.1 [2–5].

Farmer et al. [6] refer to peristomal varices as "The bleeding grapes of wrath" because of their purplish coloration and their association with massive peristomal hemorrhage. The term "grapes of wrath" harkens back to the Battle Hymn of the Republic published in 1862 [7].

> "Battle Hymn of the Republic
> Mine eyes have seen the glory of the coming of the Lord:
> He is trampling out the vintage where the grapes of wrath are stored;
> He hath loosed the fateful lightening of His terrible swift sword:
> His truth is marching on."
>
> Julia Ward Howe (Mrs. Dr. S. G. Howe)

Run afoul of the grapes of wrath and prepare to meet the lightening of His terrible swift sword.

Table 215.1 Management of bleeding peristomal varices

Recumbent position
Pressure
Sclerotherapy
Suture ligation
Cautery
Epinephrine
β-Blockade
Coil embolization
Portosystemic shunt
Mucocutaneous disconnection
Liver transplantation

Because of their serpentine appearance, the term Caput Medusa (Medusa's head) has been attached to peristomal varices. In their translation of the fourth book of Ovid's *Metamorphoses* describing the origin of Medusa, Sir Samuel Garth, John Dryden et al. write [8]:[1]

Metamorphoses
Book 4

"Medusa once had charms; to gain her love
A rival crowd of envious lovers strove.
They, who have seen her, own, they ne'er did trace
More moving features in a sweeter face.
Yet above all, her length of hair, they own,
In golden ringlets wav'd, and graceful shone.
Her Neptune saw, and with such beauties fir'd,
Resolv'd to compass, what his soul desir'd.
In chaste Minerva's fane, he, lustful, stay'd,
And seiz'd, and rifled the young, blushing maid.
The bashful Goddess turn'd her eyes away,
Nor durst such bold impurity survey;
But on the ravish'd virgin vengeance takes,
Her shining hair is chang'd to hissing snakes.
These in her Aegis Pallas joys to bear,
The hissing snakes her foes more sure ensnare,
Than they did lovers once, when shining hair."

Ovid
Publius Ovidius Naso (43 BCE-17 CE) [9]
Roman Empire

Gaze upon the Gorgon's face and be turned to stone. This myth is particularly disturbing because it tells the story of an innocent woman who is raped by a powerful male figure and then, as a victim, is punished with disfigurement, ostracized from society, and, ultimately, hunted down and murdered.

References

1. Islam KA, Morris-Stiff G. Bleeding stomal varices: a marker of chronic liver disease. BMJ Case Rep. 2009;2009:bcr02.2009.1568.
2. Farquharson AL, Bannister JJ, Yates SP. Peristomal varices life threatening or luminal? Ann R Coll Surg Engl. 2006;88:W6–8.
3. Pennick MO, Artioukh DY. Management of parastomal varices: who re-bleeds and who does not? A systemic review of the literature. Tech Coloproctol. 2013;17:163–70.

[1] I received notification from classics.mit.edu that the works on site are in the public domain.

4. Spier BJ, Fayyad AA, Lucey MR, Johnson EA, Wojtowycz M, Rikkers L, et al. Bleeding stomal varices: case studies and systematic review of the literature. Clin Gastroenterol Hepatol. 2008;6:346–52.
5. Wu JS, Fazio VF. Difficult Stomas. Perspec Colon Rectal Surg. 1998;10:33–60.
6. Farmer AD, Sadler GJ, Swarbrick ET. The bleeding grapes of wrath. Gut. 2009;58:1459. https://doi.org/10.1007/978-3-031-39880-3_21510.1136/gut.2008.173161.
7. Howe JW. Battle hymn of the republic. Atlantic Monthly, Oliver, Ditson & Co., Boston, 1862. 9(52):10.
8. Garth S, Dryden J, et al. 2019. Ovid. Metamorphoses. http://classics.mit.edu//Ovid/metam.html
9. Ovid. www.Brittanica.com; Accessed October 28, 2024.

Ileostomy Fistula

216

Alexander G. Heriot, Lewis A. Diulus III, and James S. Wu

Presentation

A 22-year-old female underwent total proctocolectomy with end ileostomy for Crohn's disease. She developed an enterocutaneous fistula at the skin level on the medial aspect that led to problems with pouching and with skin irritation at the fistula site.

Management

At surgery, the fistula was identified with a curved clamp (Fig. 216.1). A circumferential incision was made around the stoma close to the intestine. The stoma was mobilized from the skin, soft tissue, and fascia (Fig. 216.2). The fistula-bearing segment was amputated distal to the fistula. A new stoma was then matured primarily at the original stoma site (Fig. 216.3).

A. G. Heriot
Department Colorectal Surgery, Peter MacCallum Cancer Centre, Melbourne, Australia

L. A. Diulus III
Crystal Plastic Surgeons, Akron, OH, USA

J. S. Wu (✉)
Department of Colon and Rectal Surgery, Cleveland Clinic, Cleveland, OH, USA

J. S. Wu, M. D. Inkster (eds.), *Cleveland Clinic Colorectal Case Studies*,
https://doi.org/10.1007/978-3-031-39880-3_216

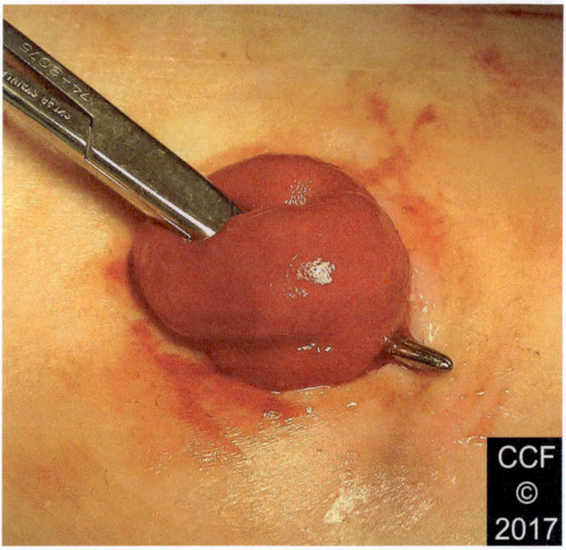

Fig. 216.1 A clamp passes through the stoma opening and exits at the skin level

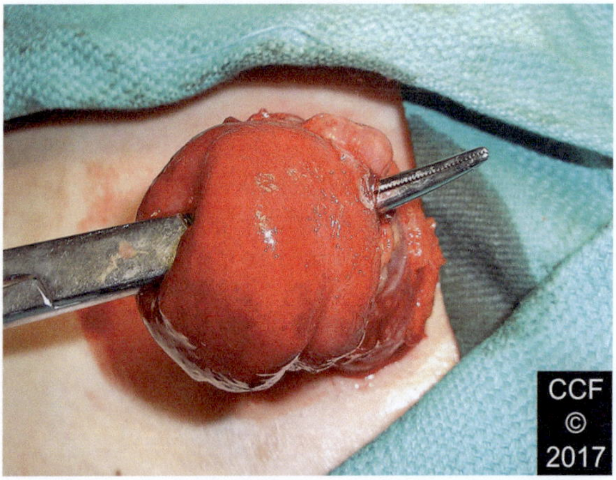

Fig. 216.2 The stoma has been mobilized by dissecting the distal end of the ileum free of surrounding skin, soft tissue, and fascia

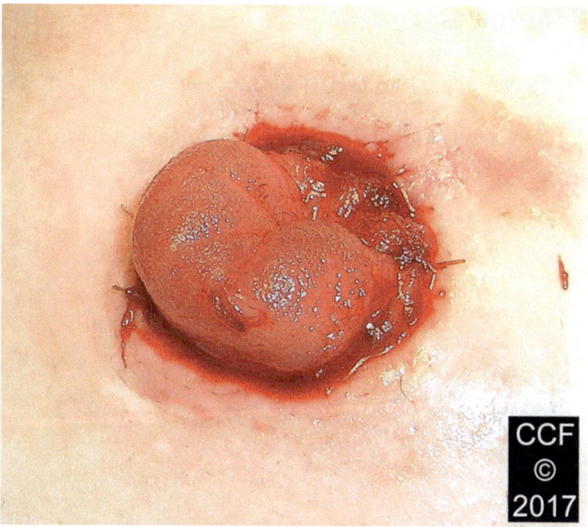

Fig. 216.3 Following amputation of the previous stoma with the fistula, the mobilized ileum was rematured at the same site

Comment

In his 1952 description of the primarily matured ileostomy, Brooke [1][1] wrote:

> "FISTULÆ
>
> Fistulæ form for two reasons. The ileal wall may be damaged or weakened at the time of operation; a fixation suture through serosa and muscle alone without penetration of the mucosa is particularly liable to cause a subsequent breakdown of the whole thickness of the bowel wall. A suture or ligature lying close to the ileum but not penetrating it in any way can lead to the same result. In these circumstances the fistula will appear in the first ten days or so after the operation. A fistula at the skin level develops at any time after the operation through chafing of the stoma against the flange of the bag.
>
> Fistulae are avoided therefore by the elimination of fixation sutures, by suturing without tension the structures round the ileum, and by the proper siting of the stoma;…. The formation of a new ileostomy by further operation is the only cure for either type of fistula,…"
>
> B. N. Brooke,
> M.Chir. Camb., F.R.C.S.
> Reader in Surgery in the University of Birmingham

Recurrent transmural intestinal inflammation and local trauma may also result in fistulae.

The operation performed here was stoma mobilization, excision, and rematuration. Alternatives include loop-end ileostomy and stoma relocation [2].

[1] The is excerpt was reproduced with the generous permission of the Lancet publishing group, CCC|Marketplace™, Order License ID 1143931-1, Order Date 28 Aug 2021.

References

1. Brooke BN. The management of an ileostomy, including its complications. Lancet. 1952;260(6725):102–4.
2. Steel MCA, Wu JS. Late stomal complications. Clin Colon Rectal Surg. 2002;15:199–207.

Colostomy Prolapse

217

John P. Cullen and James S. Wu

Presentation

A patient who had received an end colostomy to divert the fecal stream away from sacral pressure ulcers presented with colostomy complications that included prolapse, bleeding, mucosal ulceration, and difficulty with stoma pouching (Fig. 217.1a, b).

J. P. Cullen · J. S. Wu (✉)
Department of Colon and Rectal Surgery, Cleveland Clinic, Cleveland, OH, USA

J. S. Wu, M. D. Inkster (eds.), *Cleveland Clinic Colorectal Case Studies*,
https://doi.org/10.1007/978-3-031-39880-3_217

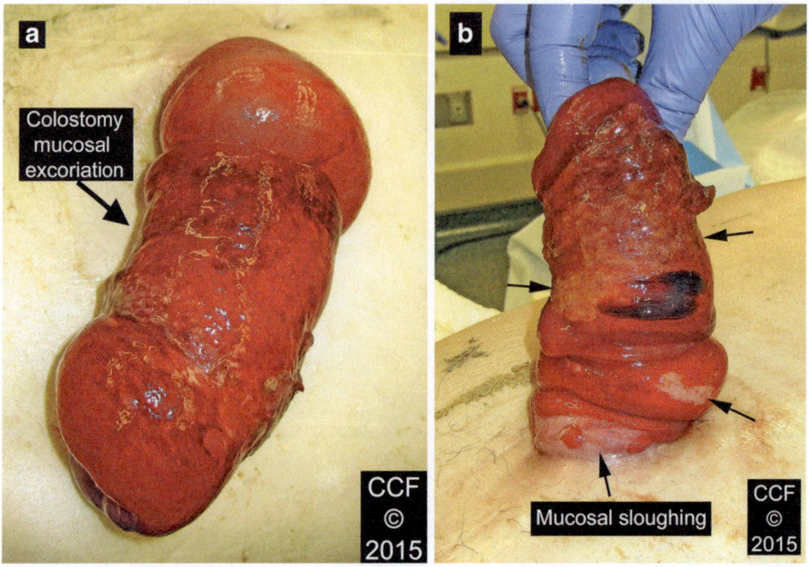

Fig. 217.1 (**a**) Superior view of prolapsed colostomy shows mucosal excoriation (arrow); (**b**) Inferior view of the same colostomy shows areas of mucosal sloughing (arrows) with exposed muscularis (white areas)

Management

Local colostomy revision was done. A circumferential incision was made at the mucocutaneous junction (Fig. 217.2). The outer tube of prolapsed colostomy was peeled away from the underlying inner tube. (Fig. 217.3). The redundant large intestine and its mesentery were divided (Fig. 217.4). The colostomy was rematured primarily (Fig. 217.5).

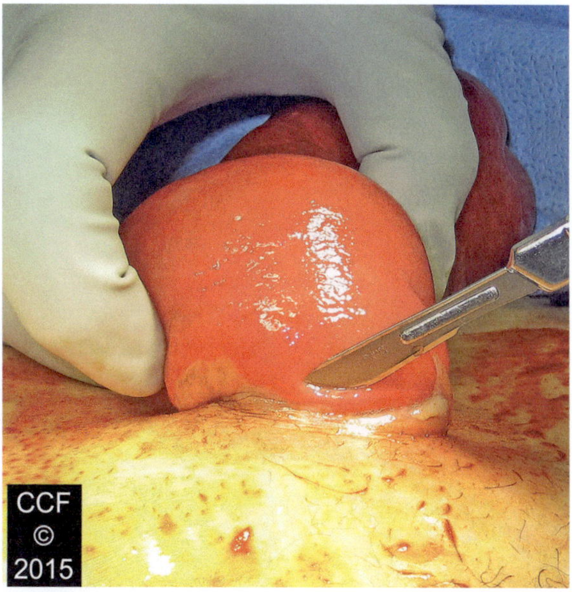

Fig. 217.2 The mucocutaneous junction is divided

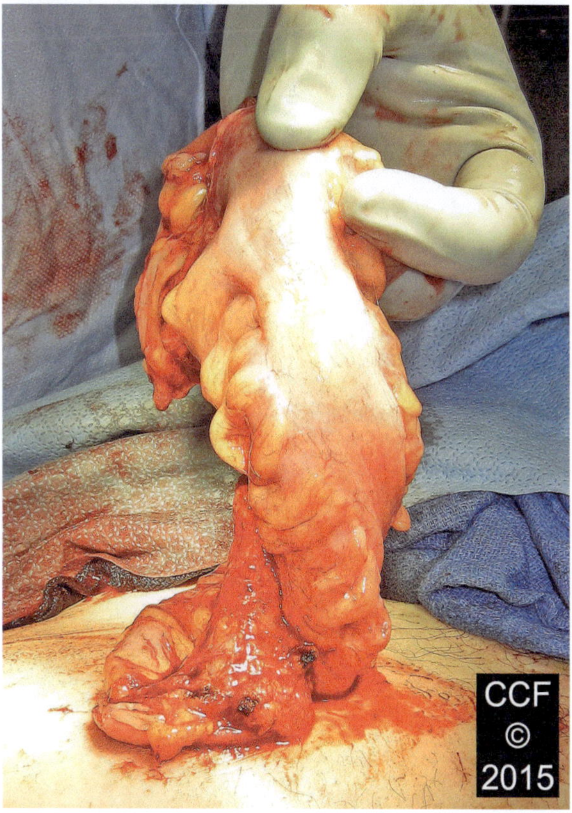

Fig. 217.3 The outer tube of the colostomy prolapse has been peeled away from thinner tube leaving a single tube of protruding colon

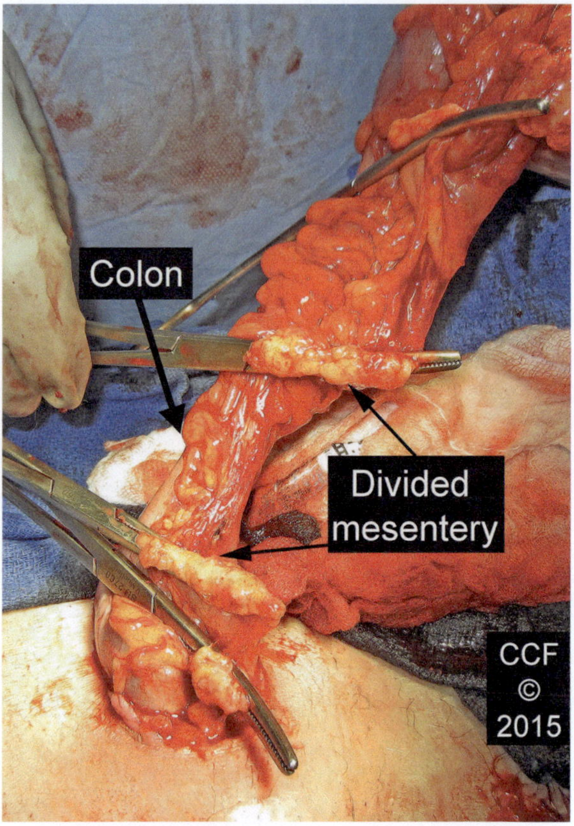

Fig. 217.4 The mesocolon and colon are divided

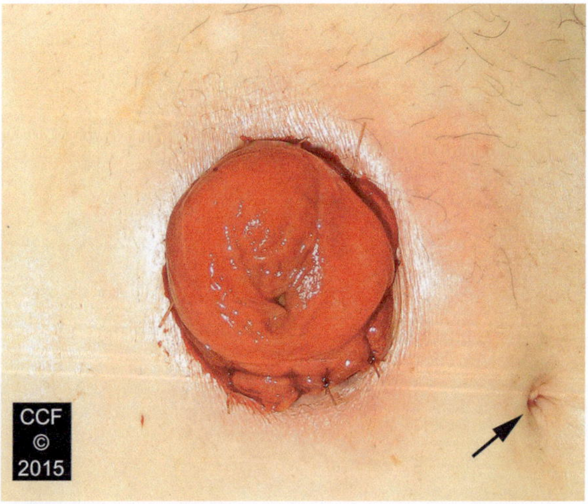

Fig. 217.5 The primarily matured colostomy following transection of the redundant prolapsed colon. The arrow shows the relationship of the colostomy to the umbilicus

Comment

Colostomy prolapse occurs when the everted full thickness of the bowel wall protrudes from the ostomy site. Predisposing factors include increased intra-abdominal pressure and mesocolon redundancy. Indications for repair include pouch leakage, incarceration, recurrent trauma, bleeding, and unacceptable body image [1]. Surgical options include colostomy closure, stoma translocation, and excision of redundant colon (as was done in this case) [2].

References

1. Steel MCA, Wu JS. Late stomal complications. Clin Colon Rectal Surg. 2002;15:199–207.
2. Szmulowicz UM, Hull TL. Stoma prolapse. In: Fazio VW, Church JM, Wu JS, editors. Atlas of Intestinal Stomas. NY: Springer; 2012., ch. 22,. p. 249–72.

Stitch Abscess

218

James S. Wu

Presentation

A 56-year-old patient underwent a laparoscopic procedure using a supraumbilical port.

At follow-up, persistent purulent drainage from the port-site incision was seen (Fig. 218.1).

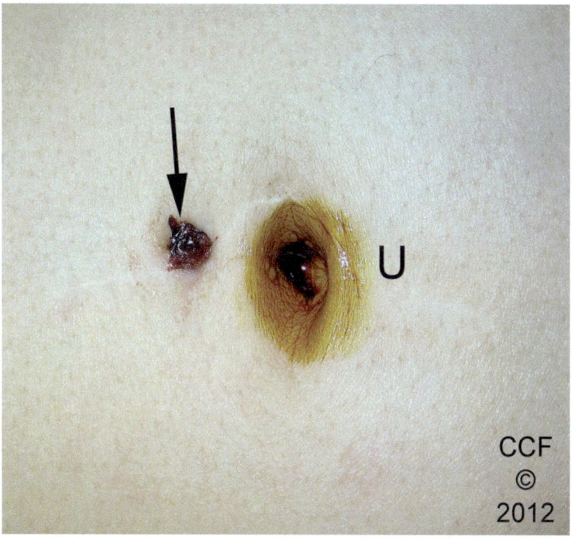

Fig. 218.1 Purulent drainage from a laparoscopic port site (arrow) adjacent to the umbilicus (U) is seen

J. S. Wu (✉)
Department of Colon and Rectal Surgery, Cleveland Clinic, Cleveland, OH, USA

J. S. Wu, M. D. Inkster (eds.), *Cleveland Clinic Colorectal Case Studies*,
https://doi.org/10.1007/978-3-031-39880-3_218

Management

Wound probing with a blunt-tipped clamp revealed a loose fascial stitch (Fig. 218.2). The stitch was removed with gentle traction (Fig. 218.3).

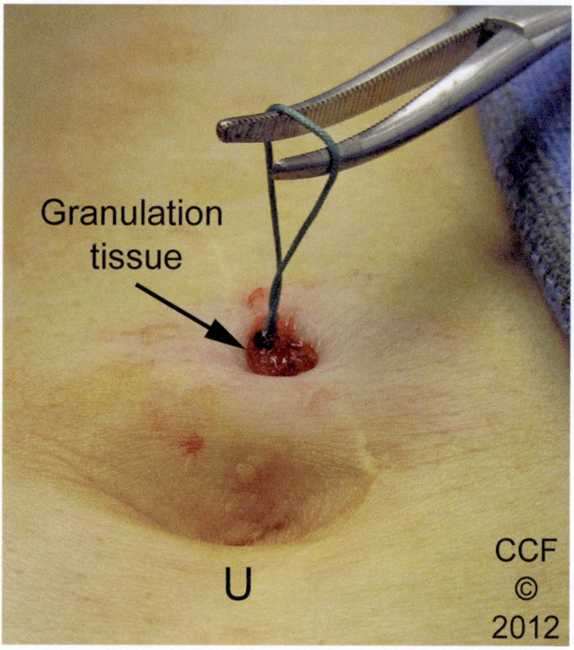

Fig. 218.2 A fascial closure stitch is elevated with a blunt-tipped clamp. Granulation tissue and the umbilicus (U) are labeled

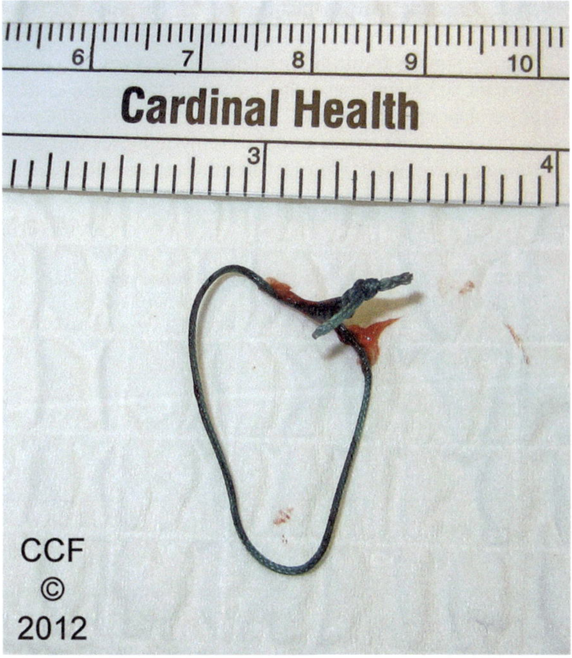

Fig. 218.3 The fascial stitch, made of braided nylon, following removal

Comment

In 1912, Crandon and Ehrenfried described causes of stitch abscess [1].

> "STITCH ABSCESS
>
> Stitch abscesses are most apt to occur after abdominal operations. Surface suture holes may become infected from unclean suture material, from bacteria in or on the skin or on the surgeon's hands, from strangulation of the tissues by tying the sutures too tightly, or from tension resulting under the swelling incident on normal repair. Abscess in the incision develops secondarily from the infection of coagulated blood or serum collected between poorly approximated planes of tissue, from an untied vessel, or a vessel pierced unwittingly in sewing up the skin, or as a result of bruising of the edges of the incision by stretching or rough retraction. An abscess may develop either in the incision or in the suture tract from contact with the drainage in infected cases. The liability to these occurrences is greater in the presence of a thick, fatty, abdominal wall. If it arises from an infected hematoma, the first discharges have the chocolate color of decomposed blood.
>
> Ordinarily, if the pus forms in the loose subcutaneous tissues, it either finds its way to the skin surface along a suture track, or else it burrows its way to the incision line and discharges thorough this."
>
> L. R. G. Crandon, A.M, M.D.
> Albert Ehrenfried, A.B., M.D.,
> Harvard Medical School
> Boston

In 2002, concerning suture sinuses, Simon and Brenner wrote that [2]:[1]

"**Suture sinuses** form when a suture site becomes infected. A suture sinus is a tract leading from the suture material within the wound to the skin surface that continually drains serous or purulent material. A small abscess called a *stitch abscess* often forms beneath the sinus. A suture sinus or suture abscess usually indicates that a foreign body, which may be the suture material itself, is present and has become infected in the wound. As long as the suture remains in place the sinus will persist. These infections occur most commonly with silk and other multifilament sutures and are least often seen with monofilament synthetics. Explore the sinus tract gently with a probe, and remove the suture with a skin hook when possible; if this is not possible; wait a few weeks for spontaneous ejection to occur".

Robert R. Simon, M.D.
Rush Medical College
Chicago
Barry E. Brenner, M.D., Ph.D.
University of Arkansas
Little Rock

References

1. Crandon RG, Ehrenfried A. Surgical After-treatment. A manual of the conduct of surgical convalescence. 2nd ed. Philadelphia: W.B. Saunders Company; 1912. pp. 253–4. Accessed from Google Books, 26 Sep 2022.
2. Simon RR, Brenner BE. Suture sinuses. In: Emergency procedures and techniques. 4th ed. Philadelphia: Lippincott Williams & Wilkins|Wolters Kluwer; 2002. p. 416.

[1] The excerpt is reproduced with the generous permission of Ms. Caren Erlichman, Wolters Kluwer permissions, 23 Aug 2021.

Fascial Dehiscence

219

James S. Wu and Michelle D. Inkster

Presentation

A 45-year-old man underwent anterior resection of the rectosigmoid colon for cancer. He was discharged on the seventh postoperative day. Twenty days after discharge, a clear pink-tinged drainage from the incision was seen when staples were removed. Probing revealed fascial separation.

Management

Wound exploration in the operating room showed inferior fascial dehiscence (Fig. 219.1). Fascial reclosure could not be done without tension. The intestines were covered with omentum, and negative pressure wound therapy (vacuum-assisted closure) was initiated (Fig. 219.2).

Serial images of the wound over time are shown in Fig. 219.3a–c.

J. S. Wu (✉)
Department of Colon and Rectal Surgery, Cleveland Clinic, Cleveland, OH, USA

M. D. Inkster
Department of Gastroenterology, Cleveland Clinic, Cleveland, OH, USA

J. S. Wu, M. D. Inkster (eds.), *Cleveland Clinic Colorectal Case Studies*,
https://doi.org/10.1007/978-3-031-39880-3_219

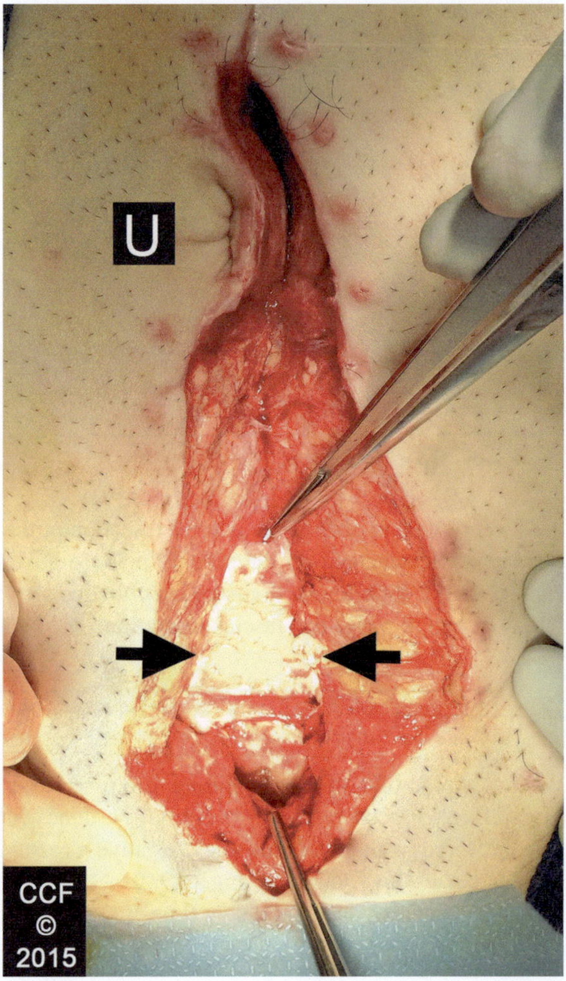

Fig. 219.1 Wound exploration showed separation of the inferior one-third of the fascia indicated by forceps and arrows. The wound base showed a necrotic yellow eschar overlying healthy omentum. The umbilicus (U) is identified

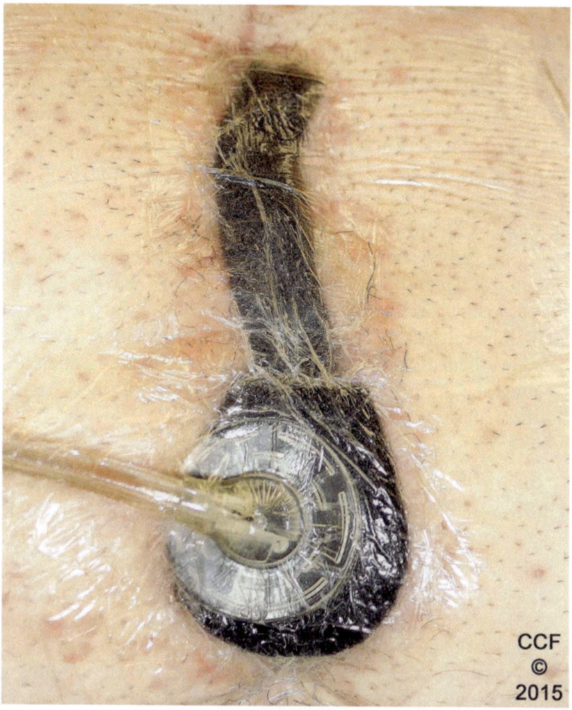

Fig. 219.2 A sponge was cut to fit the wound. The wound was covered with a clear adhesive covering. Suction (60 mm Hg) is applied to the sponge through a cut in adhesive covering

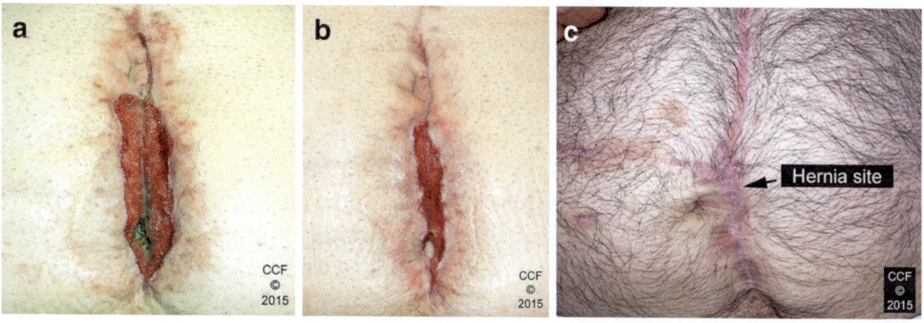

Fig. 219.3 (**a**) The wound 3 weeks after vacuum dressing application. (**b**) Wound appearance 5 weeks after vacuum dressing application. At this point, the negative pressure dressing was discontinued and replaced with a wet to dry gauze dressing. (**c**). The wound appearance 1 year after surgery. An incisional hernia was found at the site of the fascial dehiscence

Comment

Risk factors for acute abdominal fascial dehiscence include technical problems with wound closure, increased intra-abdominal pressure, infection, malnutrition, anemia, chronic lung disease, emergency surgery, wound tension, prior surgery, obesity, smoking, steroids, and cancer [1–5]. In this particular case, wound closure was achieved using negative pressure wound therapy. Although the process was complicated by incisional hernia, the worse complication of enterocutaneous fistula was avoided. The omentum was used to prevent intestinal exposure to the atmosphere or dressing material.

In volume II of *The Genuine Works of Hippocrates*, translated from the Greek by the surgeon, Frances Adams, and published in 1886, treatment of ulcers by the application of negative pressure by "cupping" is described [6].

> "ON ULCERS
>
> 17. When in cupping, the blood continues to flow after the cupping-instrument has been removed, and if the flow of blood, or serum be copious, the instrument is be applied again before the part is healed up, so as to abstract what is left behind. Otherwise coagula of blood will be retained in the incisions, and inflammatory ulcers will arise from them. In all such cases the parts are to be bathed with vinegar, after which they are not to be wetted; neither must the person lie upon the scarifications, but they are to be anointed with some of the medicines for bloody wounds."

In 1908, Meyer and Schmieden published a book entitled, *Bier's Hyperemic Treatment,* focusing on the teachings of the German surgeon, August Bier [7].

> "BIER'S HYPEREMIC TREATMENT
>
> Obstructive Hyperemia by Means of Suction Apparatus.
>
> For some years Bier has been employing suction apparatus (also called vacuum apparatus, suction cups, cupping glasses) for the induction of artificial hyperemia.
>
> In making use of these vacuum apparatus we not only rely on the artificial hyperemia they produce, but also, and by no means least, on their mechanical effect.
>
> If we place such a glass over a diseased area which presents a sinus in its middle, the pus and with its bacteria are aspirated from the depth, slowly and painlessly; often necrotic tissue, or even sequestra of small size, are brought to the surface. This suction is particularly valuable, for the granulations lining the fistulous tract or the abscess cavity are in this manner also brought under hyperemia, and the current of secretion thus directed outwardly, bathes and cleanses them gently but thoroughly."

Examples of Bier's cupping glasses are shown in Fig. 219.4.

In 1993, Fleischmann et al. [8] described vacuum sealing as treatment of soft tissue damage in open fractures in 15 patients. Drainage tubes were placed into a polyvinyl foam that filled in a wound or tissue defect. The authors reported efficient cleaning and conditioning of the wound, marked proliferation of granulation tissue, and no bone infection. More recently, negative pressure wound therapy (NPWT) technology also known as VAC (vacuum-assisted closure) applies negative pressure to a sealed wound dressed with a porous sponge. This technology was described by Morykwas and Argenta [9, 10].

Benefits of VAC therapy shown in Table 219.1.

Wound dehiscence is one application of this technology [11].

Table 219.1 Benefits of VAC therapy

- increased local blood flow,
- active promotion of granulation tissue,
- adaptation to the contours of deep and irregularly shaped wounds,
- decrease in bacterial colonization,
- decreased edema.

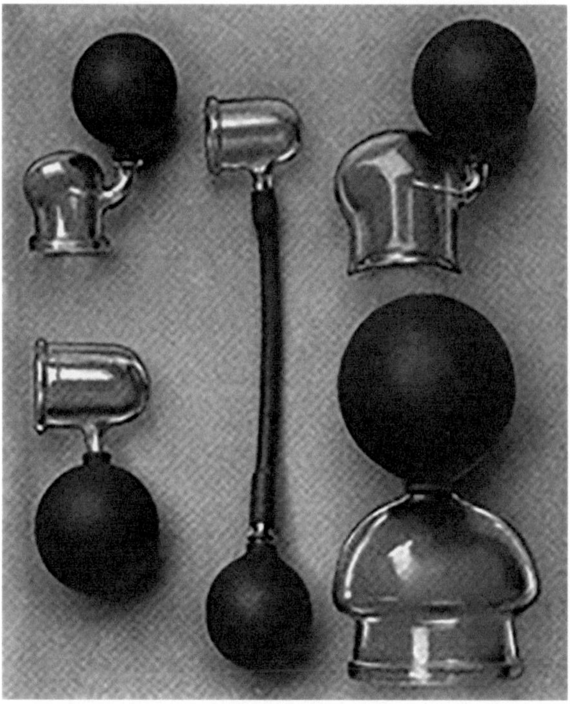

Fig. 219.4 These figures represent vacuum glasses for the collection of wound secretions (Meyer and Schmieden [7])

References

1. Webster C, Neumayer L, Smout R, Horn S, Daley J, Henderson W, Khuri S, et al. Prognostic models of abdominal wound dehiscence after laparotomy. J Surg Res. 2003;109:130–7.
2. Khan MN, Naqvi AH, Irshad K, Chaudhary AR. Frequency and risk factor of abdominal wound dehiscence. J Coll Physicians Surg Pak. 2004;14:355–7.
3. Mäkelä JT, Kiviniemi H, Juvonen T, Laitinen S. Factors influencing wound dehiscence after midline laparotomy. Am J Surg. 1995;170:387–90.
4. Wahl W, Menke H, Schnütgen M, Junginger Th. Die Fasciendehiscenz-Ursache und Prognose. Chirurg. 1992;63:666–71.
5. Rodriguez-Hermosa JI, Codina-Cazador A, Ruiz B, Roig J, Gironès J, Pujadas M, et al. Risk factors for acute abdominal wall dehiscence after laparotomy in adults. Cir Esp. 2005;77:280–6.
6. Adams F. On ulcers. In: The genuine works of Hippocrates, vol. II. New York: William Wood and Company; 1886. p. 293–306. Accessed from Google Books, 06 Feb 2022.
7. Meyer W, Schmieden V. Bier's Hyperemic Treatment in Surgery, Medicine, and the Specialties. A manual of its practical application. Philadelphia: Saunders; 1908. p. 44, 47, 49, 50. Accessed from Google Books, 6 Feb 2022.
8. Fleischmann W, Strecker W, Bombelli M, Kinzl L. Vakuumversigelung zur Behandlung des Weichteilschadens bei offenen Frakturen. Unfallchirurg. 1993;96:488–92.
9. Morykwas MJ, Argenta LC, Shelton-Brown EI, McGuirt W. Vacuum-assisted closure: A new method for wound control and treatment: Animal studies and basic foundation. Ann Plast Surg. 1997;38:553–62.
10. Argenta LC, Morykwas MJ. Vacuum-assisted closure: A new method for wound control and treatment: Clinical experience. Ann Plast Surg. 1997;38:563–77.
11. Schoemann MB, Lentz CW. Treating surgical wound dehiscence with negative pressure dressings. Ostomy Wound Manage. 2005;51(2A Suppl):15S–20S.

Incisional Hernia Repair with Mesh

220

Douglas D. Benson and James S. Wu

Presentation

A patient developed a ventral hernia after prior surgery when a left lower quadrant colostomy was created. Repair with mesh was done after mechanical bowel preparation.

Procedure

Step 1. The abdomen was prepared sterilely, and the colostomy was isolated from the hernia repair site (Fig. 220.1). After the fascia was freed from the overlying fat and skin, repair was done with synthetic mesh (Fig. 220.2).

The appearance of the mesh after circumferential mattress suture placement is shown in Fig. 220.3. The incision was closed with a combination of staples and dental rolls (Fig. 220.4).

The surgical incision site was covered with a sterile dressing before the colostomy was exposed (Fig. 220.5). An appliance then was applied to the colostomy (Fig. 220.6).

D. D. Benson
Rocky Mountain Colon and Rectal Surgeons, Lone Tree, CO, USA

J. S. Wu (✉)
Department of Colon and Rectal Surgery, Cleveland Clinic, Cleveland, OH, USA

J. S. Wu, M. D. Inkster (eds.), *Cleveland Clinic Colorectal Case Studies*,
https://doi.org/10.1007/978-3-031-39880-3_220

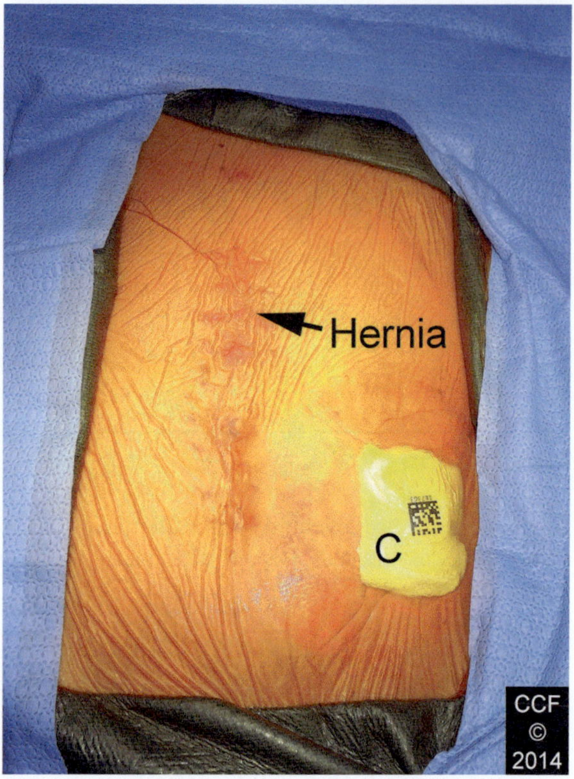

Fig. 220.1 The colostomy (C) was isolated from the hernia repair site with absorbent gauze and Iodine impregnated adhesive barrier

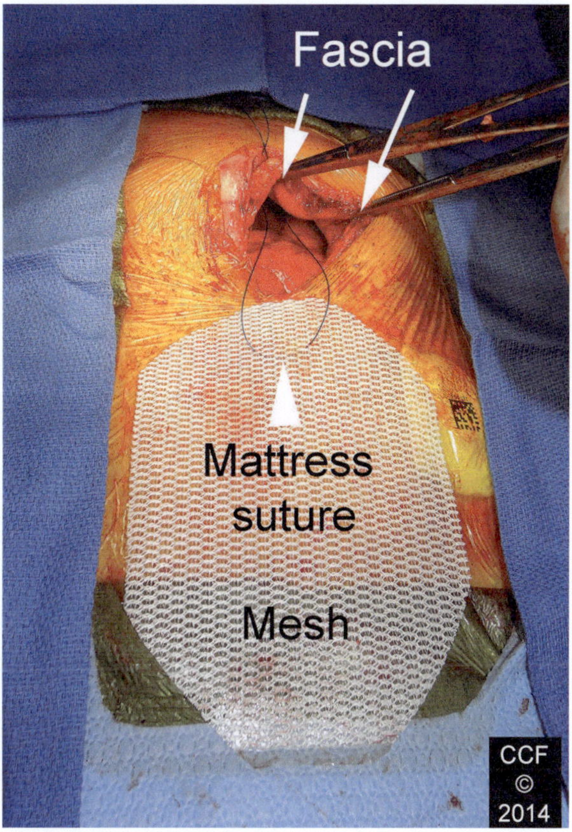

Fig. 220.2 After the fascia was freed from the overlying fat and skin, repair was done with synthetic mesh. The mesh was secured to the abdominal wall fascia with mattress sutures (fascia-mesh-mesh-fascia)

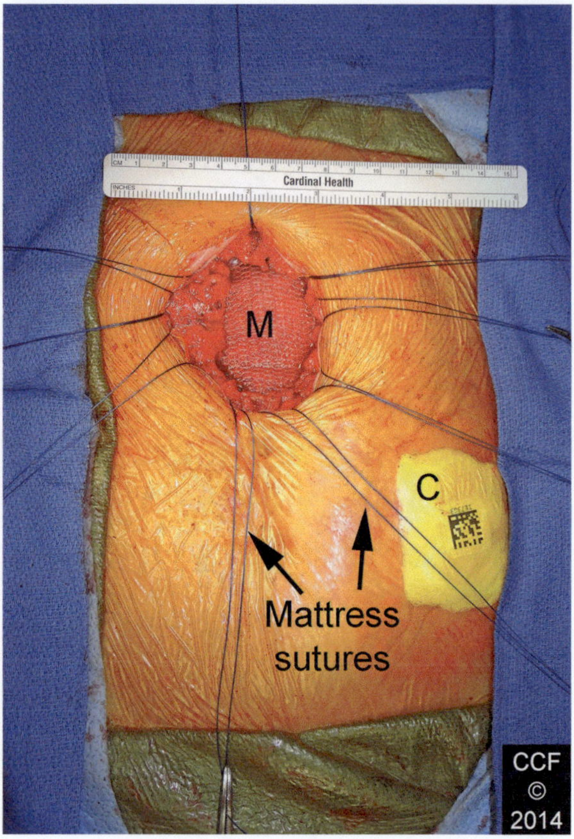

Fig. 220.3 The mesh (M) was secured to the fascia with circumferential mattress sutures. The colostomy (C) remains isolated from the mesh

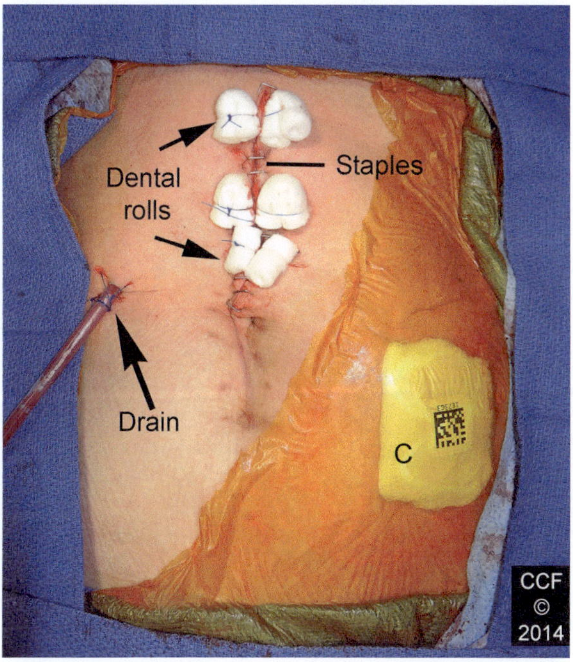

Fig. 220.4 The incision was closed with a combination of staples and dental rolls. A temporary drain was placed. The colostomy (C) remains isolated

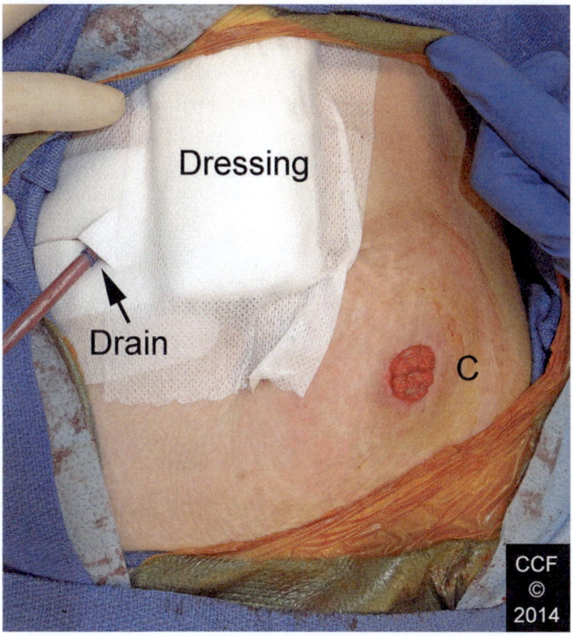

Fig. 220.5 The surgical site and drain were dressed before the colostomy (C) was exposed

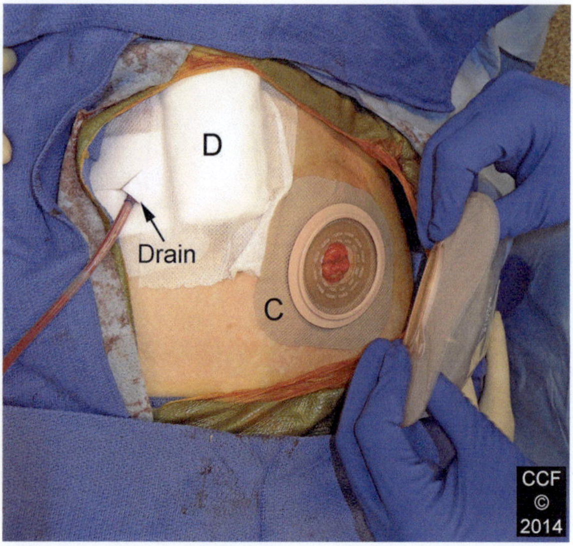

Fig. 220.6 An appliance was applied to the colostomy (C). The hernia repair dressing is identified by the letter "D." A temporary bulb-suction wound drain has been placed

Comment

Hernia repair using prosthetic mesh in the presence of a colostomy requires complete isolation of the surgical site from the ostomy. The mesh was secured to the fascia with circumferential mattress sutures that prevented intestine from herniating anterior to the mesh. The skin covering the mesh repair was closed with staples plus buttressing dental rolls. The dental rolls and staples were kept dry and left in place for several weeks until the skin closure was secure[1].

[1] The dental roll skin closure technique was passed down to us from Dr. Victor W. Fazio. See Chap. 204, Abdominal Compartment Syndrome, this work.

Paracolostomy Hernia Repair

221

James S. Wu

Presentation

A 56-year-old male underwent proctectomy with permanent end colostomy. He developed a paracolostomy hernia that became increasingly uncomfortable. He requested hernia repair. The patient stated that he is able to maintain a colostomy appliance for 4 days without leak. The skin around the colostomy was well preserved.

Management

The patient underwent paracolostomy hernia repair. Three incisions were considered: midline, keyhole, and lateral as shown in Fig. 221.1.

J. S. Wu (✉)
Department of Colon and Rectal Surgery, Cleveland Clinic, Cleveland, OH, USA

J. S. Wu, M. D. Inkster (eds.), *Cleveland Clinic Colorectal Case Studies*,
https://doi.org/10.1007/978-3-031-39880-3_221

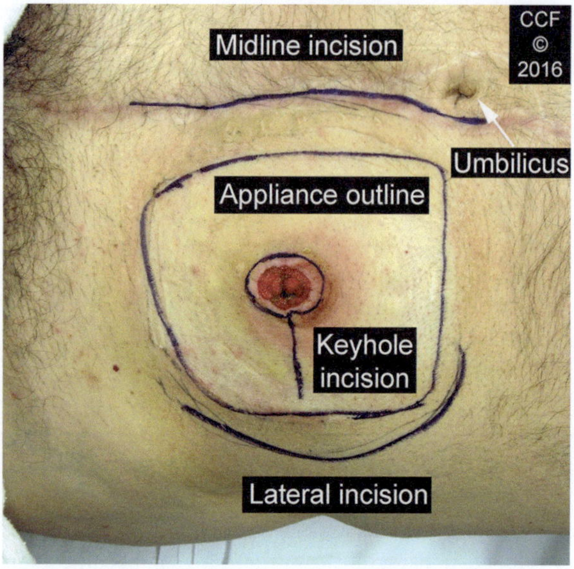

Fig. 221.1 Three approaches to parastomal hernia repair: medially through a midline incision; laterally from outside of the appliance outline; and directly adjacent to the ostomy through a "keyhole" incision

Step 1

The operative site was prepared sterilely, and the colostomy was isolated from the operative field with a skin adherent barrier dressing (Fig. 221.2).

In this case, paracolostomy hernia repair was done through a lateral incision (Fig. 221.3).

The hernia was exposed as seen in Fig. 221.4.

The hernia sac was opened exposing the hernia contents (Fig. 221.5).

A piece of mesh was prepared for repair of the fascial defect (Fig. 221.6).

The mesh was positioned around the colon at the level of the fascia (Fig. 221.7).

The mesh is secured to the fascia with nonabsorbable suture (Fig. 221.8).

The soft tissue was approximated over the mesh repair (Fig. 221.9).

The surgical site was irrigated and closed over temporary drain (Fig. 221.10).

The wound was inspected 2 weeks after discharge following staple removal (Fig. 221.11).

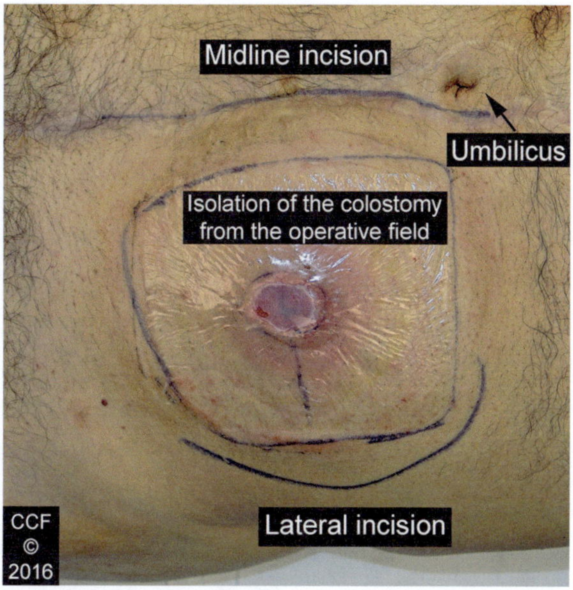

Fig. 221.2 The colostomy has been isolated from the midline and lateral incision sites to prevent enteric contamination

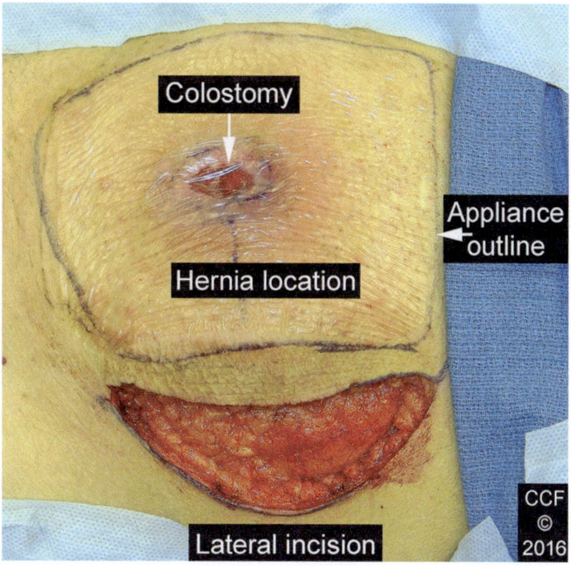

Fig. 221.3 A curved incision was made lateral to the boundaries of a colostomy appliance faceplate. The colostomy is isolated from the surgical site

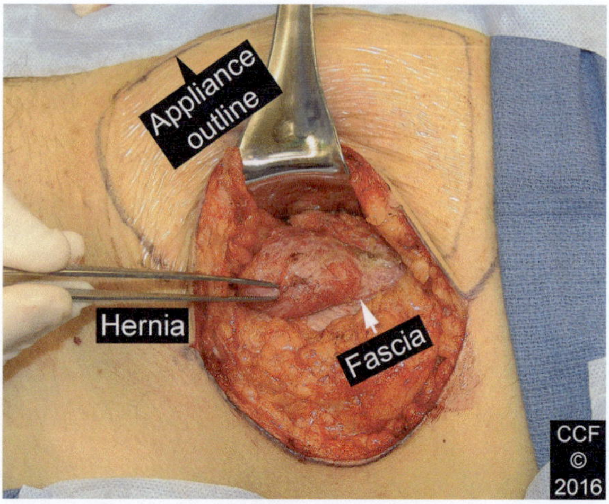

Fig. 221.4 The hernia sac with underlying intestine is seen adjacent to the fascia

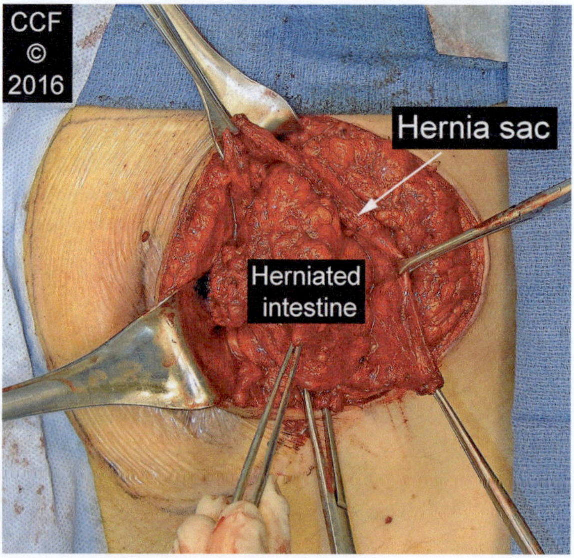

Fig. 221.5 The hernia contents were exposed after the hernia sac is opened

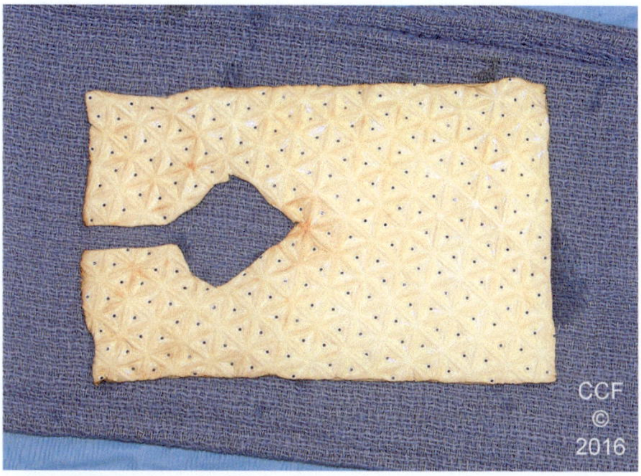

Fig. 221.6 A piece of Gortex™ mesh was prepared for implantation. A "keyhole" was created that will encircle the colon

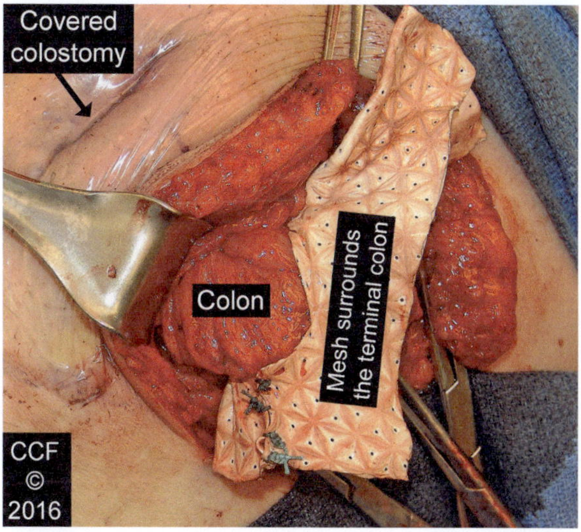

Fig. 221.7 The mesh was wrapped around the colon leading to the colostomy (arrow). The colostomy remains completely isolated from the mesh by the skin adherent barrier. The opening in the mesh was sutured closed

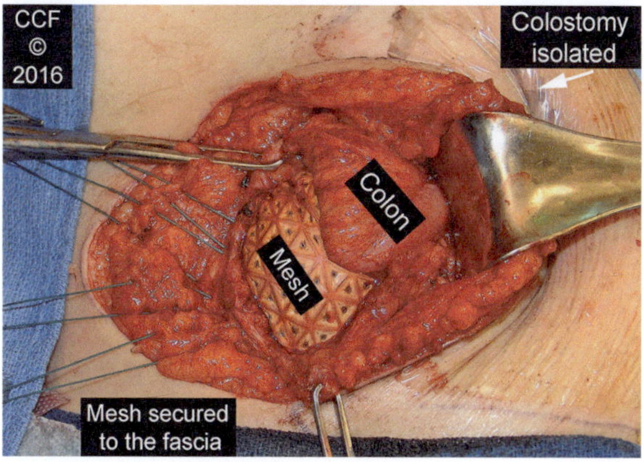

Fig. 221.8 The mesh was secured to the fascia circumferentially with nonabsorbable suture. The mesh remains isolated from the colostomy to avoid contamination

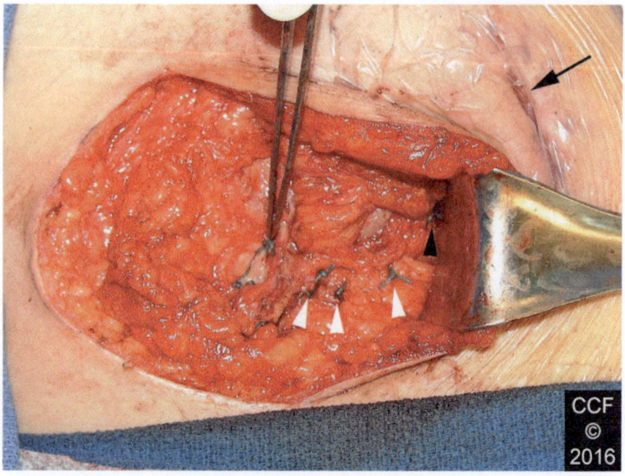

Fig. 221.9 The mesh repair was covered with soft tissue secured with suture (white arrows). The colostomy site remained isolated from the operative field (black arrow)

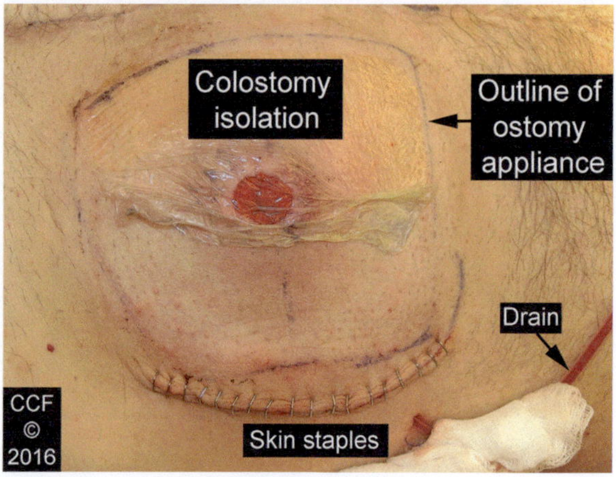

Fig. 221.10 The skin was closed with staples over a drain

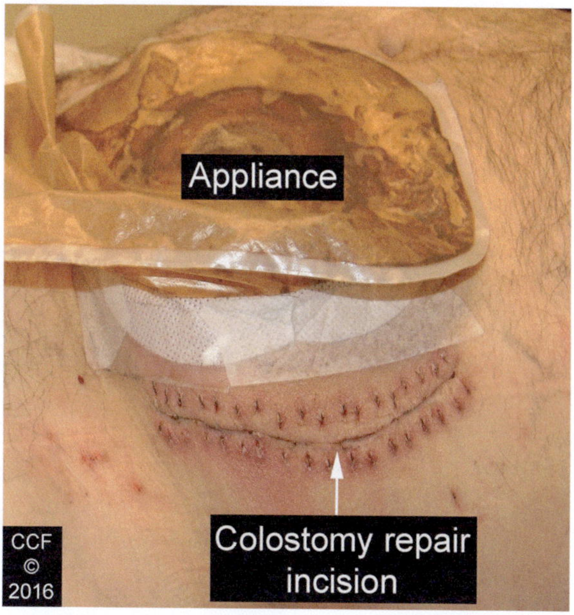

Fig. 221.11 The healed surgical incision at 2 weeks. The colostomy appliance does not touch the wound

Comment

Complications Related to Colostomy Herniation

> "Some degree of herniation around the colostomy is so common that this complication may be regarded as virtually inevitable".
> John Goligher
> Emeritus Professor Surgery,
> University of Leeds
> Consulting Surgeon,
> St. Mark's Hospital for
> Diseases of the Rectum and Colon, 1984 [1]

Peristomal hernia is common because the stoma has created an unnatural defect in the abdominal wall. Protrusion of abdominal contents through the stoma fascial aperture is a consequence of the pressure differential between the intra-abdominal cavity and the atmosphere. Asymptomatic hernias do not require repair [2]. Surgical options for peristomal hernia repair are listed in Table 221.1.

In this case, hernia repair was accomplished using Thorlakson's lateral approach (Fig. 221.12) [3].

Table 221.1 Surgical options for peristomal hernia repair

Local repair
Stoma relocation
Stoma closure

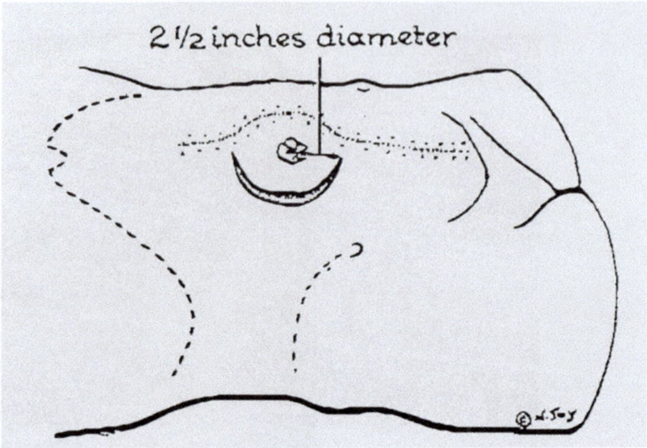

Fig. 221.12 Thorlakson's technique for parastomal hernia. Reprinted with permission from Ms. Andrea Musolf, the Journal of the American College of Surgeons, formerly Surgery Gynecology & Obstetrics, July 28, 2021

References

1. Goligher J. Surgery of the Anus, Rectum, and Colon. 5th ed. London: Ballière Tindall; 1984. p. 703.
2. Steel MCA, Wu JS. Late stomal complications. Clin Colon Rectal Surg. 2002;15:199–207.
3. Thorlakson RH. Technique of repair of herniations associated with colonic stomas. Surg Gynecol Obstet. 1965;120:347–50.

Marjolin's Ulcer

222

Victor W. Fazio and James S. Wu

Presentation

A patient presented with a 10 cm painful skin lesion adjacent to an ileostomy that had been created 44 years earlier (Fig. 222.1). A parastomal ulcer first appeared 6 years earlier and gradually increased in size. Biopsy revealed squamous cell carcinoma.

Management

The patient underwent wide excision of the ileostomy, the cancer, and the surrounding abdominal wall soft tissue. Margins were free of tumor. A new ileostomy was made on the opposite side of the abdomen (Fig. 222.1, site marked by the letter "X") [1].

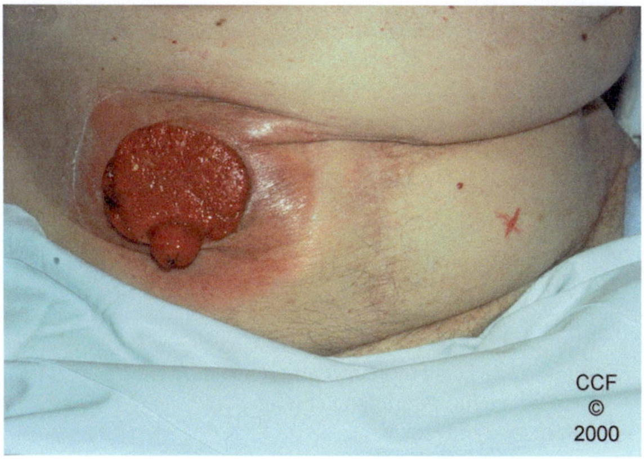

Fig. 222.1 A squamous cell carcinoma surrounds the right lower quadrant ileostomy. A new ileostomy site has been marked with the letter "X" on the patient's left

V. W. Fazio · J. S. Wu (✉)
Department of Colon and Rectal Surgery, Cleveland Clinic, Cleveland, OH, USA

J. S. Wu, M. D. Inkster (eds.), *Cleveland Clinic Colorectal Case Studies*,
https://doi.org/10.1007/978-3-031-39880-3_222

Comment

The development of squamous cell carcinoma in an unhealed wound is eponymously associated with Jean-Nicholas Marjolin. In 1846, Marjolin published a treatise entitled *Ulcère* in the *Dictionaire de Médicine, Tome Trentième* (Paris, 1846) [2][1].

Marjolin's section entitled *Ulcères cancroïdes* in the *Dictionnaire* reads as follows:

Ulcères cancroïdes [2].—On donne ce nom à des ulcères qui offrent la plupart des caractères des ulcères cancéreux, et qui sont cependent d'une autre nature. La peau et les origines des membranes muqueuses en sont le siége le plus fréquent; ils se développent plus souvent sur le visage que sur les autres régions du corps. Les bords et la base de ces ulcères sont durs, inégaux; leur surface est rouge ou livide, grisâtre ou gangréneuse, tantôt lisse, tantôt rugueuse, inégale; ils fournissent un pus ichoreux, àcre, fétide; quelquefois ils sont aride; ces ulcères sont douloureux et quelquefois rongeans. Les ganglions lymphatiques situés dans leur voisinage sont souvent engorgés.	Cancroid ulcers.—This name is given to ulcers which offer most of the characteristics of cancerous ulcers, and which are of another nature. The skin and origins of the mucous membranes are the most frequent sites; they develop more commonly on the face than on other parts of the body. The edges and base of these ulcers are hard, uneven; their surface is red or livid, greyish of gangrenous, sometimes smooth, sometimes rough, uneven; these ulcers are painful and sometimes gnawing. Lymph nodes in their vicinity often are engorged.

Marjolin's *Ulcère Cancroïdes* is consistent with the eponymous definition attributed to him.

In 1903, Da Costa described two cases of "chronic ulcers of the cutaneous surface which became carcinomatous." Da Costa concluded:

> "The characterization of this condition as Marjolin's ulcer I think to be proper, because it was first carefully studied and accurately described by Professor Marjolin, of Paris, over fifty years ago.
>
> It is a very ancient and well-demonstrated belief that cancer may arise, and, in fact, is rather apt to arise, in an area of chronic inflammation [3];…"
>
> John Chalmers Da Costa, M.D.
> Professor of Principles of Surgery and of
> Clinical Surgery
> in the Jefferson Medical College
> Philadelphia

Fordyce, writing in *Keen's Surgery* (1911), defined Marjolin's ulcer [4].

> "**Malignant Disease of Scars and Ulcers.—Marjolin's ulcer**, described by Marjolin over fifty years ago, and more recently revived by Da Costa, is the designation applied to chronic ulcers which have undergone malignancy."
>
> John A. Fordyce, M.D.
> New York

[1] This citation is on page 26. Accessed from Google Books August 29, 2022.

References

1. Wu JS, Sebek BA, Fazio VW. Parastomal squamous cell carcinoma in an ileostomy 44 years after proctocolectomy. J Am Coll Surg. 2000;191:107.
2. Marjolin. Ulcère. Dictionaire de Médicine ou Repertoire Général des Sciences Médicales. Deuxième Edition, Tome trentième et dernier. ULC-WIS., Paris, LABÉ, Libraire de la faculté de médecine; Place de L'école de Médicine, 4. 1846. p. 10–29.
3. Da Costa JC. Carcinomatous changes in an area of chronic ulceration, or Marjolin's ulcer. Ann Surg. 1903;37:496–502.
4. Fordyce JA. In: Keen WW, editor. Malignant Disease of Scars and Ulcers.—Marjolin's ulcer. In: Surgery: Its Principles and Practice, vol. 2. Philadelphia: WB Saunders Co.; 1911. p. 631. Accessed from Internet Archive July 19, 2021.

References

223 Enterocutaneous Fistula

James S. Wu

Presentation

A 30-year-old female underwent ileocolic resection for terminal ileitis with abscess. The operation was complicated by three enterocutaneous fistulae. The patient was referred for management.

Examination of the abdomen at presentation is shown in Fig. 223.1. Computed tomography showed contrast extravasation but no undrained fluid collections (Fig. 223.2).

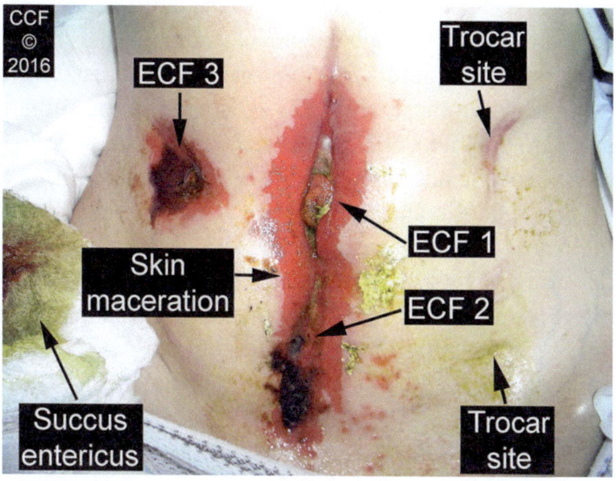

Fig. 223.1 Two enterocutaneous fistulas (ECF 1-2) are located in the midline incision. A third fistula (ECF3) is seen on the right side of the abdomen. The skin adjacent to the ECFs is macerated due to constant exposure to succus entericus. Two laparoscopic trocar sites are labelled

J. S. Wu (✉)
Department of Colon and Rectal Surgery, Cleveland Clinic, Cleveland, OH, USA

J. S. Wu, M. D. Inkster (eds.), *Cleveland Clinic Colorectal Case Studies*,
https://doi.org/10.1007/978-3-031-39880-3_223

Fig. 223.2 Computed tomography shows contrast extravasation but no undrained fluid collections

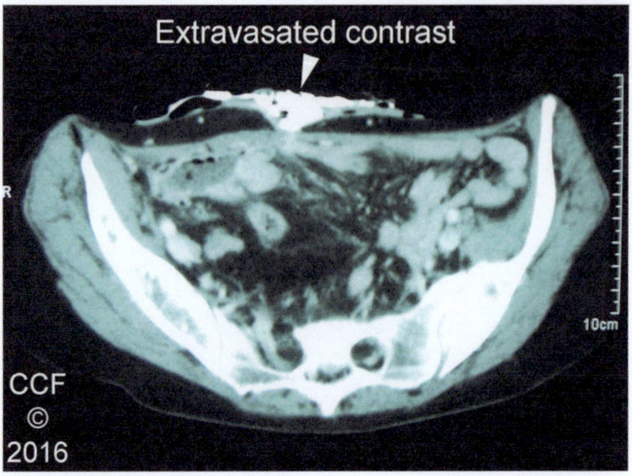

Management

The patient was seen by the wound and ostomy service who pouched the fistulae to protect the adjacent skin. Home hyperalimentation was administered for a period of 6 months. Oral intake, initially withheld, was resumed as the appearance of the skin improved (Fig. 223.3).

Surgery to takedown the enterocutaneous fistulae was done. The case was scheduled as the first case and the only case of the day. Ureteral catheters were placed. The abdomen was entered through the previous midline incision. Extensive lysis of the adhesions was done. The entire small intestine was mobilized from the ligament of Treitz to an ileocolic anastomosis (Fig. 223.4). Three fistulous origins were found. Fistula 1 originated from an ileocolic anastomosis. Fistula number 2 came from ileum located close to the ileocolic anastomosis. Fistula 3 was located distant from the other two.

The ileocolic anastomosis was disassembled. The segment of intestine containing fistulas 1 and 2 was excised. The neo-terminal ileum was used to create an end ileostomy. The colon was closed and returned to the abdomen. The segment of intestine containing fistula 3 was excised even though the fistula had closed following hyperalimentation; Intestinal continuity was restored by sewn end-to-end anastomosis. The length of small intestine from the ligament of Treitz to the neo-terminal ileum was 330 cm. A gastrostomy tube was placed. The midline wound could not be completely closed. The upper two-thirds of the incision were covered with a sheet of prosthetic mesh (Fig. 223.5).

The appearance of the wound 6 weeks after surgery is shown in Fig. 223.6. Intestinal function had returned, and a diet was resumed.

The prosthetic mesh was kept in place until a healthy bed of granulation tissue covered the midline wound. Replacement with skin ultimately followed (Fig. 223.7).

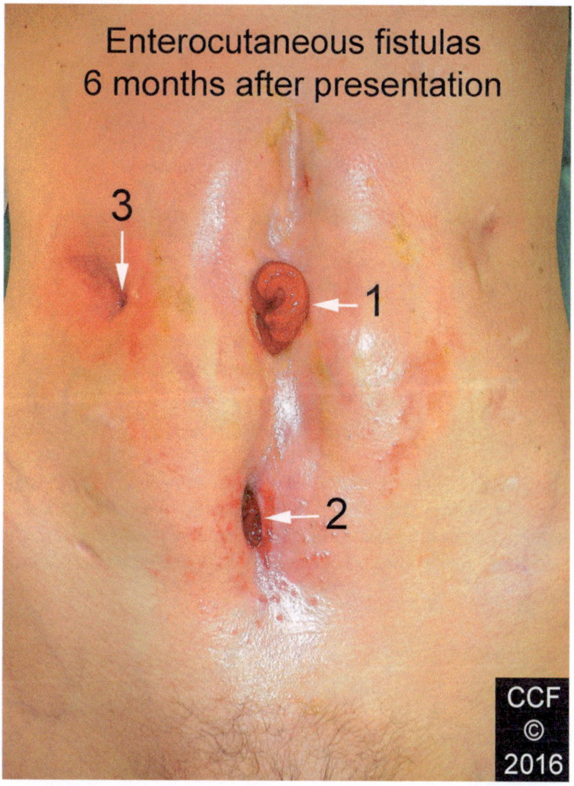

Fig. 223.3 The appearance of the abdominal skin following 6 months of hyperalimentation and dedicated wound and ostomy nursing care. Midline fistulae 1 and 2 were still active. Fistula number 3 had closed. Skin maceration had markedly improved

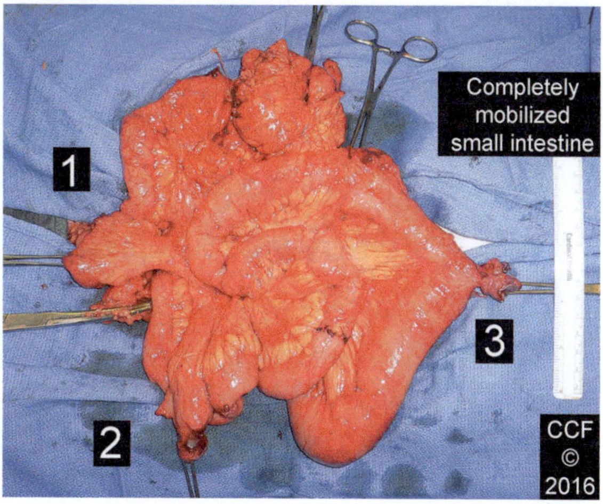

Fig. 223.4 The origins of the three enterocutaneous fistulae are labelled 1, 2, and 3. Other clamps identify sites of small bowel injury (e.g. serosal tears) that required repair

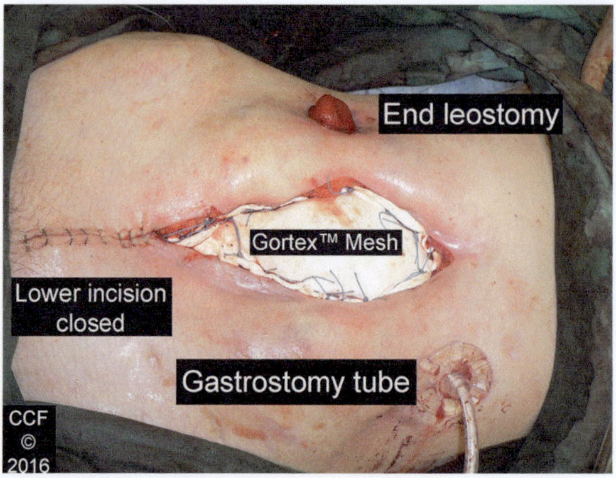

Fig. 223.5 Following take down of enterocutaneous fistulae, small intestinal continuity was restored. An end ileostomy was created. A percutaneous gastrostomy tube was placed in left upper quadrant for intestinal decompression and for tube feeding. The fascia of the upper portion of the abdominal incision could not be closed. The intestine was covered with a piece of Gortex™ sewn to the fascia

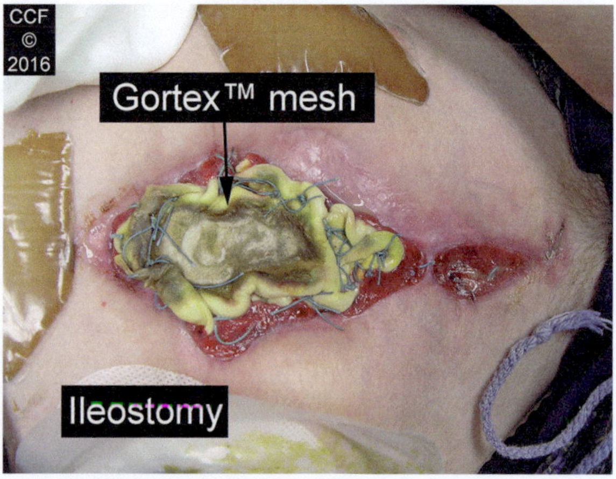

Fig. 223.6 The appearance of the Gortex™ mesh 6 weeks after surgery. The edge of the ileostomy appliance is seen at lower left

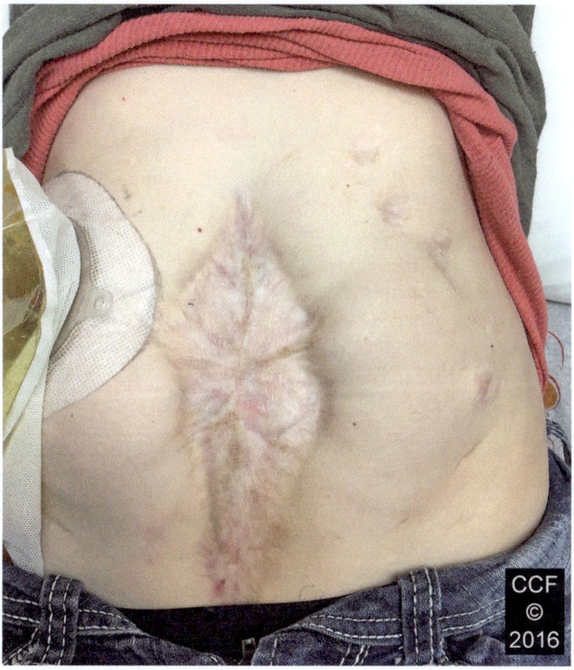

Fig. 223.7 The final appearance of the midline wound 10 years after surgery

Comment [1–6]

Enterocutaneous fistulae are abnormal connections between the intestine and the skin. Causes are shown in Table 223.1.

Principles of non-operative management are listed in Table 223.2. Treatment of patients with enterocutaneous fistulae is a multidisciplinary team effort involving committed specialists in surgery, gastroenterology, medicine, nutrition, enterostomal therapy, radiology, and mental health.

Some enterocutaneous fistulae will close spontaneously obviating the need for surgery. Some are almost asymptomatic; surgery may not be indicated in this group either. Definitive surgery is considered for enterocutaneous fistulae that persist despite optimal non-operative support. Principles of surgery for enterocutaneous fistula are listed in Table 223.3. Reoperation is delayed until: 1. sufficient time has elapsed to allow for regression of intra-abdominal inflammatory processes and 2. patient medical fitness for surgery is optimized. It is prudent to schedule the surgery as the first and the only case of the day. The aims of surgery are to resect the fistulae and restore intestinal continuity. Having an exit strategy in reserve is helpful in situations where continuation of an operation may make things worse.

In this case, coverage of the intestine was accomplished using Gortex™ mesh. The mesh was kept in place until a bed of granulation tissue had formed.

Table 223.1 Causes of enterocutaneous fistula

Malignancy
Inflammatory bowel disease
Anastomotic leak
Radiation
Infection
Foreign body
Iatrogenic
Trauma

Table 223.2 Principles of nonoperative management of enterocutaneous fistula

Correction of fluid and electrolyte imbalance
Drainage of fluid collections
Treatment of sepsis
Control of fistula output
Provision of nutrition

Table 223.3 Principles of surgery for enterocutaneous fistula

Delay until intra-abdominal conditions are optimal
Delay until systemic conditions are optimized
Resect the fistula and reconstitute intestinal continuity
Provide coverage for the intestine

This operation eliminated the enterocutaneous fistulae and allowed the patient to resume oral nutrition free of hyperalimentation. In this particular case, it was the surgeon's choice to stop the operation at this point and not connect the small intestine to the colon. Voltaire's poem *La Bégueule (conte moral)* [7][The prude, (moral tale)] begins with two lines:

Dans ses écrits[1] un sage Italien	In his writing a sage Italian
Dit que *le mieux est l'ennemi du bien*	States that *the best is the enemy of good.*

The Italian proverb to which Voltaire refers is stated in the final sentence of *Art dramatique* in *Questions sur L'Encyclopédie par des Amateurs, seconde Partie* (1770) [8].

Il meglio e l'inimico del bene	*The best is the enemy of good*

[1] The original letter "f" has been changed to the modern letter "s." for example, the original "Dans fes écrit," has been change to "Dans ses écrit."

References

1. Joyce MR, Dietz DW. Management of complex gastrointestinal fistula. Curr Probl Surg. 2009;46:384–430.
2. Schechter WP, Hirshberg A, Chang DS, Harris HW, Napolitano LM, Wexner SD, Dudrick SJ. Enteric fistulas: Principles of management. J Am Coll Surg. 2009;209:484–91.
3. Lloyd DAJ, Gabe SM, Windsor ACJ. Nutrition and management of enterocutaneous fistula. Br J Surg. 2006;93:1045–55.
4. Lee S-H. Surgical management of enterocutaneous fistula. Korean J Radiol. 2012;13(S1):S17–20.
5. Truong A, Hanna MH, Moghadamyeghaneh Z, Stamos MJ. Implications of preoperative hypoalbuminemia in colorectal surgery. World J Gastrointest Surg. 2016;8:353–62.
6. Gribovskaja-Rupp I, Melton GB. Enterocutaneous fistula: Proven strategies and updates. Clin Colon Rectal Surg. 2016;29:130–7.
7. Voltaire. La Bégueule, conte moral. A Geneve, MDCCLXXII. Accessed from Google Books, 29 Aug 2022.
8. Voltaire. Art dramatique. In: Questions sur L'Encyclopédie par des amateurs, seconde Partie, M. DCC. LXX; p. 250. Accessed from Internet Archive, October 29, 2024.

224 Enterocutaneous Fistula-Pouching

Chizu Sakai-Imoto, Barbara J. Hocevar, and James S. Wu

Presentation

A 60-year-old female presented with three enterocutaneous fistulae (Fig. 224.1). The fistulae are scattered in a wound that has little granulation tissue and a small amount of slough tissue along the periphery. An ileostomy is seen in the right lower quadrant. The fistulas produced over 1200 cc/24 h of liquid effluent that led to skin irritation. Wound, ostomy, and continence (WOC) nurses were consulted to devise a pouching system that ideally would contain the fistula output and protect the skin with reasonable wear time and cost.

The supplies needed to successfully pouch these enterocutaneous fistulae and the large wound are shown in Fig. 224.2 At the initial assessment, the abdominal skin was examined specifically for skin creases (Fig. 224.3). The skin creases are leveled out using wedges of skin barrier (Fig. 224.4). A ring of skin barrier "petals" is then applied circumferentially around the wound to act as a platform for the application of the pouching system (Fig. 224.5). The pouching system is applied to the ring of skin barrier petals (Fig. 224.6). The completed pouch is seen in Fig. 224.7 with the lid applied.

C. Sakai-Imoto
WOC Nursing Department, Cleveland Clinic, Cleveland, OH, USA

B. J. Hocevar
Rupert B. Turnbull, Jr., School of WOC Nursing Education, Cleveland Clinic, Cleveland, OH, USA

J. S. Wu (✉)
Department of Colon and Rectal Surgery, Cleveland Clinic, Cleveland, OH, USA

J. S. Wu, M. D. Inkster (eds.), *Cleveland Clinic Colorectal Case Studies*,
https://doi.org/10.1007/978-3-031-39880-3_224

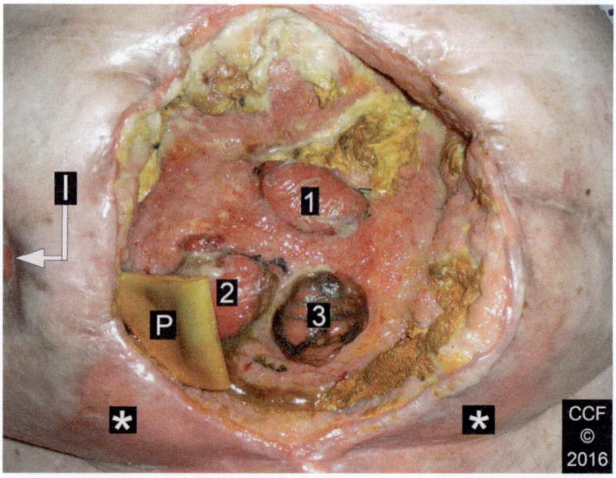

Fig. 224.1 Fascial dehiscence resulted in exposure of multiple loops of small intestine. Three enterocutaneous fistula (labelled 1, 2, and 3) are seen in the wound. The small intestinal effluent caused significant skin irritation (asterisks). A penrose drain (P), draining an abscess, is seen at the right side of the wound. An arrow points to the edge of an ileostomy appliance

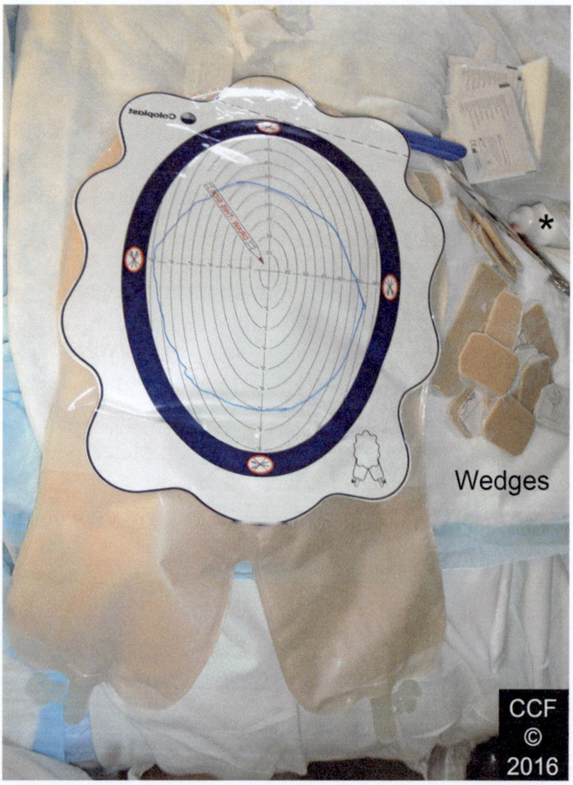

Fig. 224.2 An array of products are needed for pouching the enterocutaneous fistulae, among them: a large pouching system with skin barrier attached, wedges of skin barrier, adhesive remover, skin barrier powder (asterisk), and paste

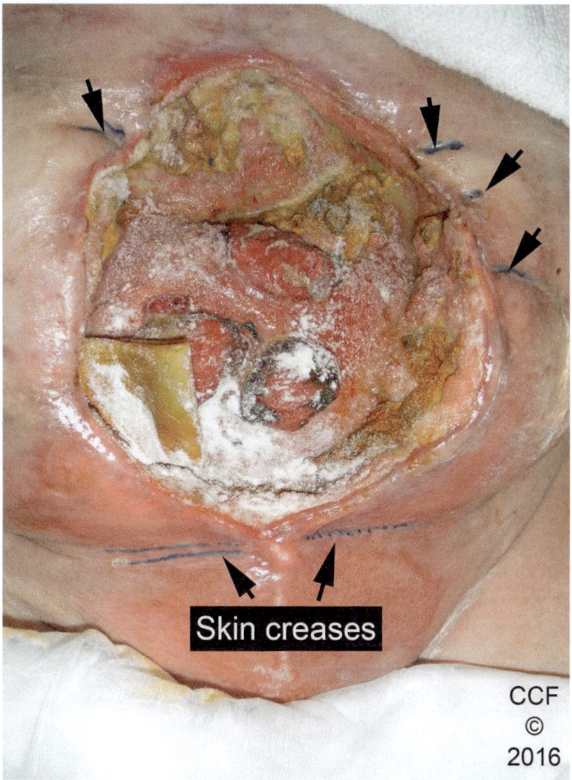

Fig. 224.3 The abdomen was assessed in the sitting position, and areas of creasing were identified. These areas were marked with indelible marker (arrows); the patient's abdomen looked flat in the supine position, so it was necessary to identify areas of dips and creases to assist with appropriate wedge placement

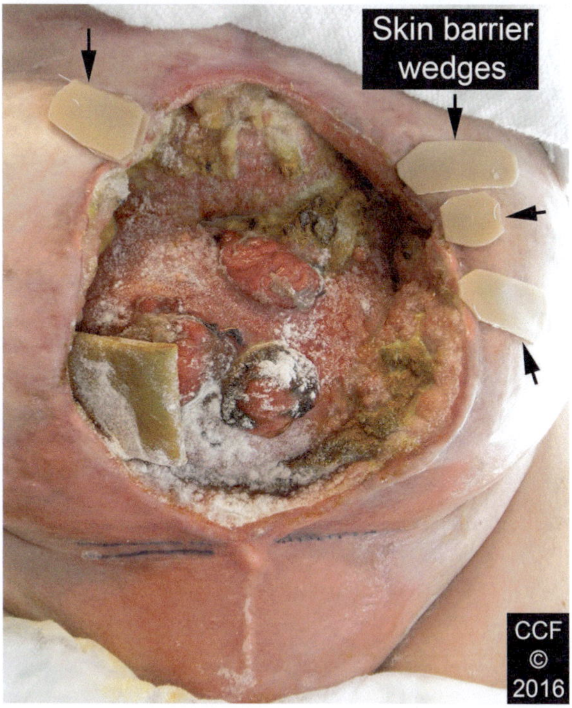

Fig. 224.4 Wedges of skin barrier (arrows) are applied to creases to level out these areas. This process facilitates pouch adherence

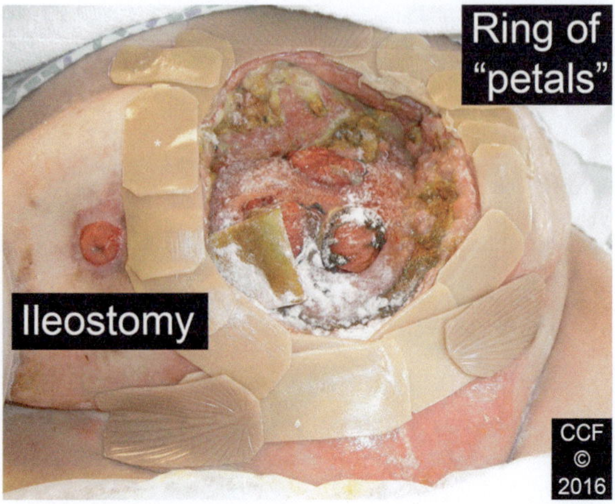

Fig. 224.5 Petaling, that is, placing pieces of skin barrier around a large opening, protects exposed skin. These petals also provide support to soft abdominal tissues, creating a platform that provides for improved pouch adhesion. Caulking with a small amount of skin barrier paste helps seal the wedges and fill in any small open areas. The ring of skin barrier petals surrounds multiple enterocutaneous fistulas. A non-functioning ileostomy is labelled

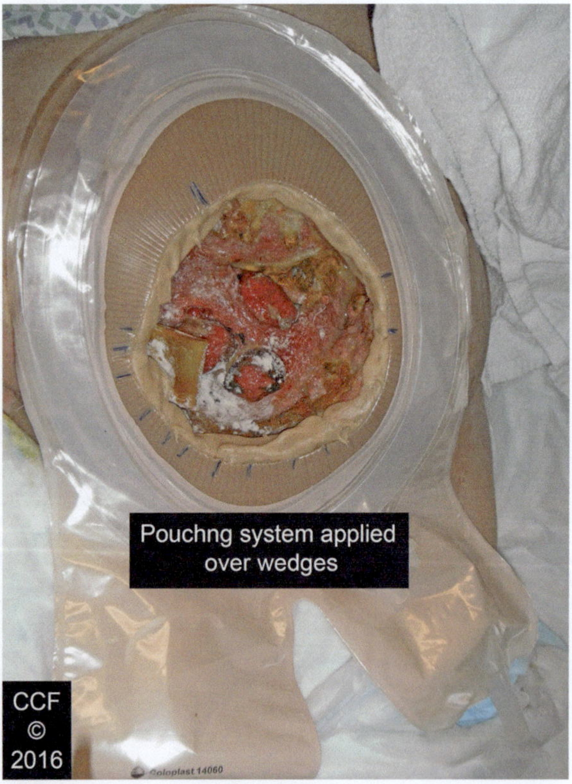

Fig. 224.6 Note the blue lines along the inner diameter of the pouch. These are areas where radial slits were made in the pouch to help it conform to uneven contours around the wound. Skin barrier paste is applied on top of the inner pouch edge to serve as a caulk. This particular appliance was made by the Coloplast Company

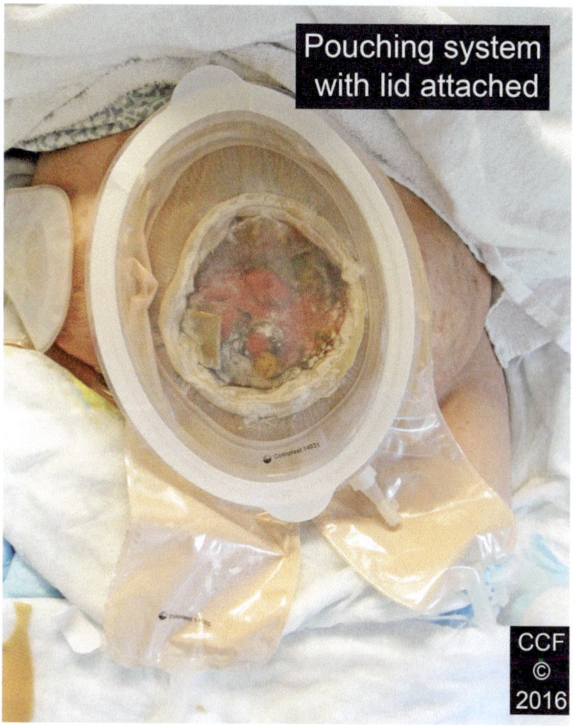

Fig. 224.7 The fistula pouch was placed vertically in order to accommodate the size of the wound and facilitate emptying. Skin barrier powder was applied inside the pouch to prevent skin barrier paste from adhering to the pouch

Comment [1]

Management goals in this case include fistula effluent collection and skin protection with a pouching system that will allow patient mobility and control odor at reasonable cost. A pouching system with a large circumference that encompassed the entire wound was required. Denuded skin was dusted with skin barrier powder. Wedges of solid sheet skin barrier leveled skin creases and provided a flat surface for pouching. Skin barrier paste was applied to caulk seams. The pouch was then applied vertically in order to accommodate the size of the wound and facilitate pouch emptying. The fistula pouch was attached to a gravity drainage bag in order to prevent the weight of the effluent from weakening the pouch seal. This system took approximately 45 min to 1 h to apply and had a wear time of 5–7 days for this bedridden patient [2].

Editor's Comment

This case demonstrates the invaluable contribution that WOC-trained nurses provide to the care of patients with enterocutaneous fistulae. The ostomy/wound care of these patients requires expertise, commitment, and, above all, compassion.

References

1. Erwin-Toth P, Hocevar B, Stricker LJ. Wound, ostomy, and continence/enterostomal therapy (WOC/ET) nursing. In: Fazio VW, Church JM, Wu JS, editors. Atlas of Intestinal Stomas. New York: Springer; 2012. p. 75–84.
2. The appliances shown in this case were made by the Coloplast Company, https://products.coloplast.us.

Portal Venous Gas and Pneumatosis Intestinalis

225

Alexander G. Heriot, Ajay Bhardwaj, Arthur A. Parsee, Michelle D. Inkster, and James S. Wu

Presentation A

Two weeks after complicated surgery, an elderly man developed fever and leukocytosis. A CT scan was obtained that showed gas in the wall of the jejunum (Fig. 225.1) and in the portal vein (Fig. 225.2).

A. G. Heriot
Department Colorectal Surgery, Peter MacCallum Cancer Centre, Melbourne, Australia

A. Bhardwaj
Radiology and Diagnostic Imaging Institute, Cleveland Clinic, Cleveland, OH, USA

A. A. Parsee
Department of Diagnostic Radiology, H. Lee Moffitt Cancer Center and Research Institute, Tampa, FL, USA

M. D. Inkster
Department of Gastroenterology, Cleveland Clinic, Cleveland, OH, USA

J. S. Wu (✉)
Department of Colon and Rectal Surgery, Cleveland Clinic, Cleveland, OH, USA

J. S. Wu, M. D. Inkster (eds.), *Cleveland Clinic Colorectal Case Studies*,
https://doi.org/10.1007/978-3-031-39880-3_225

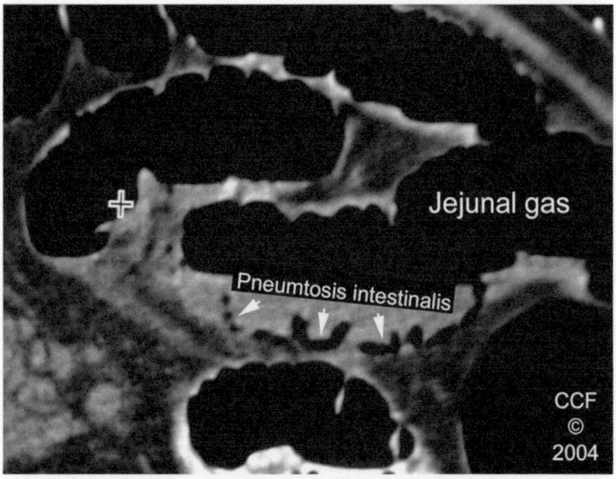

Fig. 225.1 Abdominal CT scan shows pneumatosis intestinalis (PI). Gas is seen in the intestinal lumen and in the intestinal wall (arrows)

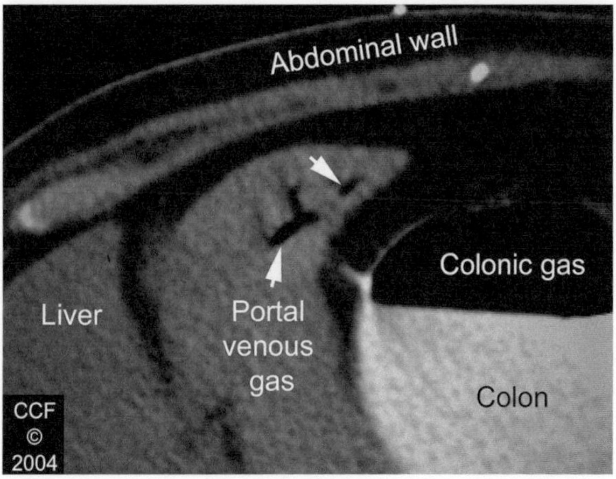

Fig. 225.2 Abdominal CT scan shows portal venous gas. Gas is seen in the colonic lumen and in the portal venous vessels in the liver (arrows). The abdominal wall is labelled

Management

Findings at laparotomy included gangrene of the gall bladder and of the jejunum. The gall bladder (Fig. 225.3) and the ischemic jejunum (Fig. 225.4) were resected.

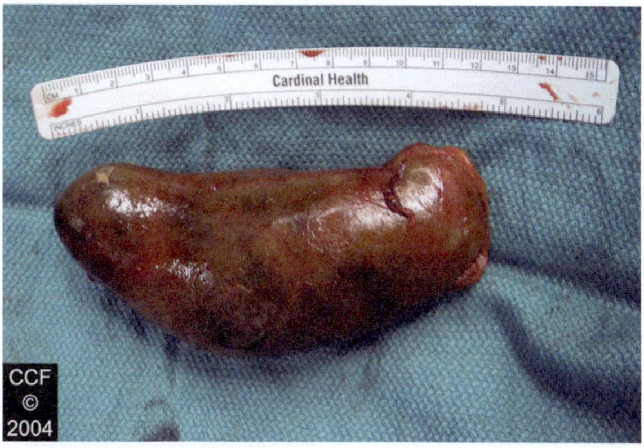

Fig. 225.3 Operative cholecystectomy specimen showing gangrenous cholecystitis

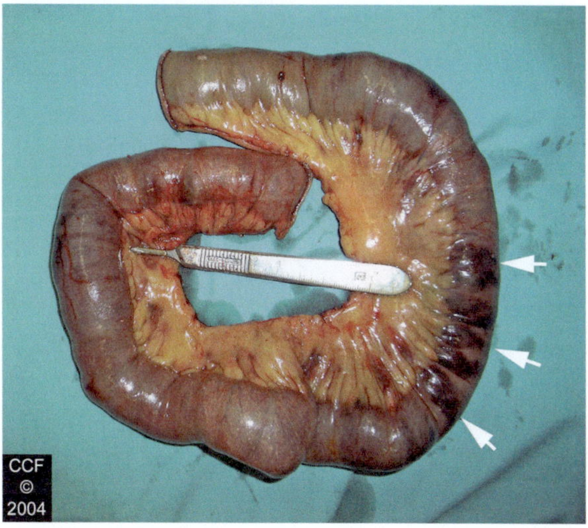

Fig. 225.4 Resected specimen showing ischemic jejunum with gangrenous segment (arrows)

Presentation B

A 50-year-old female underwent colonoscopy because of foul-smelling stool. She was otherwise healthy. Diffuse bullous lesions were seen (Fig. 225.5).

Management

Non-operative treatment consisting of antibiotics and hyperbaric oxygen was offered [1].

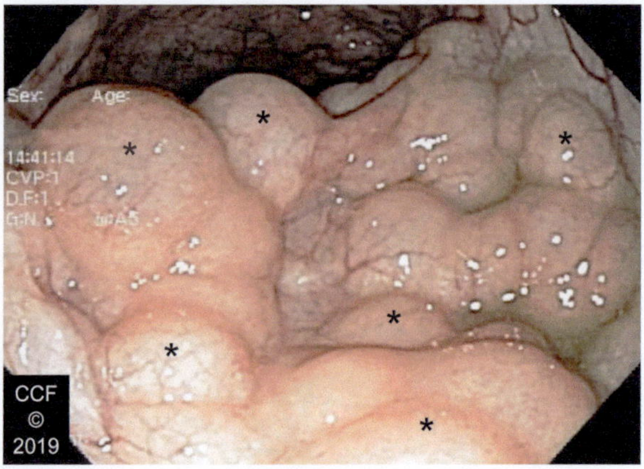

Fig. 225.5 Multiple gas-filled blebs (asterisks) seen at colonoscopy

Presentation C

A male with alcoholic cirrhosis underwent banding of esophageal varices. Following the procedure, he developed abdominal pain. An abdominal CT scan was obtained (Fig. 225.6) that showed pneumtosis intestinalis (PI).

Management

Signs of sepsis were not seen. Management consisted of observation only.

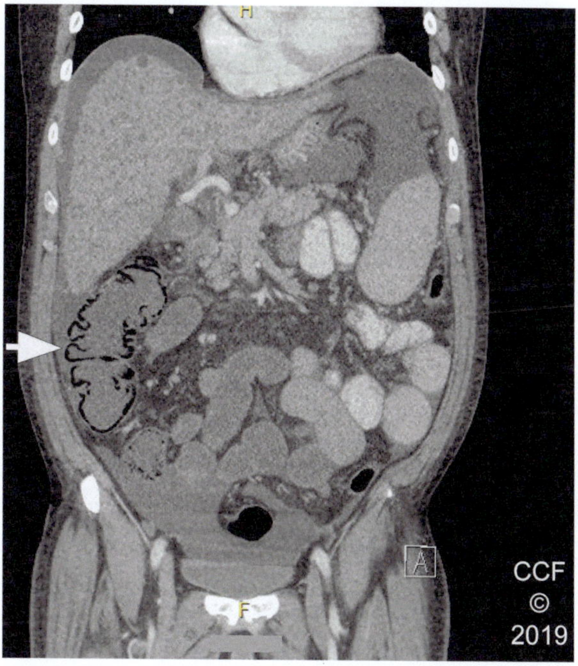

Fig. 225.6 This abdominal CT was obtained after esophageal banding. Pneumatosis is seen in the right colon (arrow). There is fluid between the diaphragm and the liver consistent with cirrhosis associated ascites

Comment

Hepatic Portal Venous Gas (HPVG)

In 1955, Wolfe and Evans described postmortem gas in the portal veins of the liver in six infants who died with marked distension of the bowel. Postmortem blood cultures grew *E. coli* [2]. The authors concluded:

> "Thus, it is reasonable to suppose that gas under increased tension in the lumen of the bowel enters the mesenteric veins and collects in the portal system of the liver. This concept is supported by the demonstration of pneumatosis of the bowel in 3 cases."

John N. Wolfe, M.D., and William A. Evans, M.D.
Department of Radiology of the Children's Hospital of Michigan
Detroit, Michigan

In the majority of cases, the radiologic finding of HPVG is associated with potentially life threatening conditions in which gas enters the portal system usually from a gastrointestinal source such as necrotic bowel, gastric ulcer, or enterocolitis. Prompt surgical intervention is considered up front. However, HPVG also occurs after endoscopic procedures, and these may follow a benign course. In general, HPVG is approached as if it were caused by serious pathology first. Conservative treatment is considered only after the exclusion of intra-abdominal catastrophe [3–5].

Pneumatosis Intestinalis (PI)

PI is air trapped in the walls of the intestine. In 1783, du Vernoi [6] described PI as air trapped under the external and internal skins of the intestines.

Joh. Georf du Vernoi anatomische Beobachtungen der unter der äussern und inner Haut der Gedärme und eingeschlossen Luft.

Ich kann nicht mit Gewissheit sagen, ob schon irgendwo Beobachtungen von solchen Geschwülsten der Gedärme aufgezeichnet sind. Ich fand nemlich auf der äussern Fläche des Darmes eine beträchtliche Länge hindurch sehr viel Stellen, in welchen die äussere Haut zu einem blasenartigen Geschwulste erhaben war. Von diesen Erhabenheiten waren einige breiter, andere enger, und mehr oder weinger hervorstehend. Einige umfassten die ganzen Peripherie des Darmes als ein Ring, so dass der Darm in dieser Stelle merklich dicker war. Alle hatten sie die eigene Farbe der Gedärme. Dem äussern Ansehen nach schienen sie mit einer durchsichtigen weissen Materie a efüllt zu sehn, wenn man sie aber aufschnitt, so fand man inwendig weisse dem Scheibenhonig ähnliche Fächer, die trocken waren in keine Feuchtigkeit enthielten.

Joh. Georg du Vernoi anatomic observations of air trapped under the outer and inner skin of the intestines.

I cannot say with certainty whether observations of such tumors of the intestines have been recorded anywhere. I found many places on the outer surface of the intestine over a considerable length, in which the outer skin was raised to form a blister-like tumor. Of these elevations some were broader, others narrower, and more or less prominent. Some encompassed the entire periphery of the bowel as a ring, so that the bowel was noticeably thicker in that area. They all had their normal intestinal color. From the outside they seemed to be filled with a transparent white matter, but when they were cut open one found inside white compartments, like honeycomb, which were dry and contained no moisture.

Causation, Diagnosis, and Management of PI

"Two basic mechanical features characterize the majority of cases of PI: mucosal injury, the most important and prevalent feature, and increased intraluminal pressure. Increased intraluminal pressure may be produced by bowel obstruction, ileus, or iatrogenically by upper or lower GI endoscopy.

Patients manifesting symptoms or signs of abdominal distress merit an aggressive surgical approach. Associated acidosis and hyperamylasemia suggest necrotic bowel and portend a grave prognosis. The finding of PI radiographically without associated clinical evidence of intra-abdominal pathology does not necessitate operative exploration. These patients may be followed expectantly."

Stuart J. Knechtle, M.D., Andrew M. Davidoff, M.D., and Reed P. Rice, M.D.
From the Departments of Surgery and Radiology
Duke University Medical Center
Durham, North Carolina [7]

"Pneumatosis intestinals is most often secondary to another medical condition. The diagnosis is most often made radiologically with a computed tomography scan. The disease severity ranges from benign to life-threatening. Predictors of poor outcomes include pH less than 7.3, bicarbonate level of less than 20 mEq/L, lactate level of more than 2 mmol/L, amylase level of more than 200 U/L, and portal venous gas on imaging. Early recognition of life threatening signs and symptoms is critical. Treatment options include bowel rest, antibiotics, surgery and more recently, the use of hyperbaric oxygen therapy."

Joseph D. Feuerstein, MD, Nicole White, MD, and Tyler M. Berzin, MD, MS
Division of Gastroenterology,
Department of Medicine,
Beth Israel Deaconess Medical Center, and
Harvard Medical School,
Boston, MA [8]

References

1. Masterson JST, Fratkin LB, Osler TR, Trapp WG. Treatment of pneumatosis cystoides intestinalis with hyperbaric oxygen. Ann Surg. 1978;187:245–7.
2. Wolf JN, Evans WA. Gas in the portal veins of the liver in infants: A Roentgenographic demonstration with postmortem anatomical correlation. Am J Roentgenol Rad Ther Nuc Med. 1955;74:486–9; This excerpt is reused with the generous permission of the American Roentgen Ray Society, Date Oct 5, 2021.
3. Liebman PR, Patten MT, Manny J, Benfield JR, Hechtman HB. Hepatic — portal venous gas in adults: Etiology, pathophysiology and clinical significance. Ann Surg. 1978;187:281–7.
4. Abboud B, El Hachem J, Yazbeck T, Doumit C. Hepatic portal venous gas: Physiology, etiology, prognosis and treatment. World J Gastroenterol. 2009;15:3585–90.
5. Hussain A, Mahmood H, El-Hasani S. Portal vein gas in emergency surgery. World J Emerg Surg. 2008;3:21.
6. du Vernoi JG. Anatomische Beobachtungen der unter der äussern und innern Haut der Gedärme eingeschlossen Luft. Physikal Med Abhandl Kayser Akad Wiss Petersb. 1783;2:182–8; aus dem Lateinischen übersetzt von J.L.C. Mümler; 2:1783. Accessed from Deutsche Digitale Bibliotek. Kultur und Wissen online. September 25, 2022.

7. Knechtle SJ, Davidoff AM, Rice RP. Pneumatosis intestinalis. Surgical management and clinical outcome. Ann Surg. 1990;212:160–5; These excerpts are reused with the generous permissionof Wolters Kluwer Health, Inc., CCC | RightsLink®, License Number 5901460726136, License date Nov 03, 2024.
8. Feuerstein JD, White N, Berzin TM. Pneumatosis intestinalis with a focus on hyperbaric oxygen therapy. Mayo Clinc Proc. 2014;89:697–703. This excerpt is reused with the generous permission of Elsevier, CCC|RightsLink; License Number 590147048246; License date Nov 03, 2024.

Abdominal Pain-Neutropenia

226

James S. Wu and Michael O. Christian

Presentation

A 59-year-old female, receiving radiation and chemotherapy to treat anal squamous cell carcinoma, was admitted to the hospital with severe abdominal pain and nausea.

Physical Findings

VS: T97.9°C, BP 93/56 mm Hg, P 76 bpm, RR 19/min

Examination

Complaint: severe left lower abdominal pain

Abdomen: focal severe left lower quadrant tenderness

Laboratory

White blood cell count 0.7 × K/μL (absolute neutrophil count 500/μL); Hemoglobin 9.2 g/dl; Platelet count 86 K/μL

Computed tomography (CT) shows diverticulitis of the left colon (Fig. 226.1).

J. S. Wu (✉)
Department of Colon and Rectal Surgery, Cleveland Clinic, Cleveland, OH, USA

M. O. Christian
Radiology & Diagnostic Imaging Institute, Cleveland Clinic, Cleveland, OH, USA

J. S. Wu, M. D. Inkster (eds.), *Cleveland Clinic Colorectal Case Studies*,
https://doi.org/10.1007/978-3-031-39880-3_226

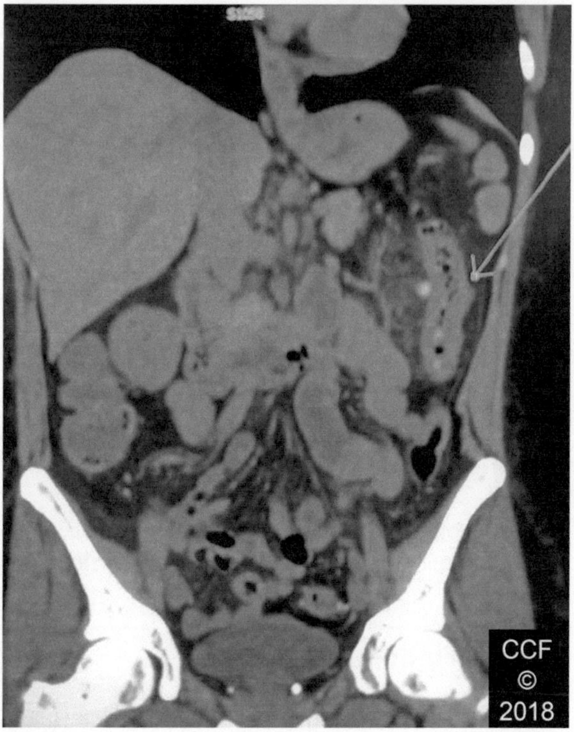

Fig. 226.1 CT scan shows diverticulitis of the descending colon (arrow) with pericolonic infiltration

Management

The patient was admitted to the hospital. Food was withheld. Intravenous fluids, antibiotics, and colony-stimulating factor were administered. The patient's abdominal pain gradually diminished, and her white cell count improved over several days. Food was reintroduced, and she was discharged.

Comment

This patient presented with abdominal pain and neutropenia (white blood cell count 0.7 K/μL, absolute neutrophil count 500/μL) during the course of chemotherapy and radiation. CT indicated a colonic source. Treatment focused on improving neutrophil counts with colony-stimulating factor and treatment of possible infection with antibiotics. Normally, there are at least 1500 neutrophils per microliter of blood. For granulocyte (neutrophil) counts between 100/μL and 1500/μL of blood, the term "granulocytopenia" or "neutropenia" is used. This means that too few neutrophils are present. The lower the neutrophil count and the longer it remains low, the higher

Table 226.1 Causes of abdominal pain in the neutropenic patient (after Badgwell)

Enterocolitis
Small bowel obstruction
Clostridium difficile colitis
Diverticulitis
Appendicitis
Cholecystitis
Colonic pseudo-obstruction
Splenic rupture

Table 226.2 Management of abdominal pain in the neutropenic cancer patient

Rapid and accurate diagnosis
Improvement of neutrophil count
Supportive care – Intravenous fluid and electrolyte resuscitation – Antibiotics – Hemodynamic support – Nutrition – Gastrointestinal tract decompression – Restriction of oral intake
Timely surgical intervention

the risk of developing a dangerous infection.[1] Neutropenia is a side effect associated with chemotherapy. Badgwell et al. reported the causes of abdominal pain in the neutropenic cancer patient listed in Table 226.1 [1].

General principles of management of abdominal pain in the neutropenic cancer patient are shown in Table 226.2.

Timely Surgical Intervention

> "More than 60% of our patients with neutropenic enteropathy had their symptoms resolve with conservative therapy alone. All of these patients had prolonged neutropenia, but when normal levels of circulating granulocytes returned, their symptoms resolved in all cases.
>
> Our approach to the neutropenic cancer patient with abdominal pain is based on the concept that surgical intervention should be avoided in patients with neutropenic enteropathy."
>
> H. Fletcher Starnes Jr, MD, Francis D. Moore Jr, MD,
> Steven Mentzer, MD, Robert T. Osteen, MD,
> Glenn D. Steele Jr, MD, and Richard E. Wilson, MD,
> Department of Surgery, Brigham and Women's Hospital,
> Harvard Medical School,
> Boston, Massachusetts 1986 [2][2]

[1] Cleveland Clinic. Agranulocytosis. https://my.clevelandclinic.org/health/diseases/15262-agranulocytosis. Date published: November 27, 2017.

[2] This excerpt is reproduced with the generous permission of John Wiley and Sons, CCC|Rightslink®; License number 5140121002121, License date 01 Sep 2021.

"The decision to operate in the treatment of abdominal pain in neutropenic patients can be exceedingly difficult. It is recognized that surgical morbidity and mortality are increased in this subset of patients. Traditional surgical teaching would advise operative intervention in patients with physical findings suggestive of peritonitis. Such an approach in this patient population would result in most of the patients being treated surgically. One must be very thorough in the evaluation of these patients to ensure that needless operations are avoided and yet safeguard that surgically treated disease is not left untended."

LCDR David S. Wade, MC, USN,
Harold Douglass, Jr, MD,
Hector R. Nava, MD, Marion Piedmonte, MA
Departments of Surgical Oncology and Biomathematics, Roswell Park Memorial Institute, Buffalo, NY and,
Department of Surgery, Uniformed Services University of the Health Sciences, Bethesda, Md
1990 [3][3]

"The clinical course of patients with hematological disease, especially after treatment, is often complicated by gastrointestinal infections. Between 1986 and 1990 a total of 18 patients affected with hematologic disease and presenting with an acute abdomen were admitted to the surgery department at the University of Rome "La Sapienza". Most patients were affected with acute or chronic myeloid leukemia (61%) and lymphoma. Five patients with acute appendicitis, three with necrotizing enterocolitis, three with spontaneous hemoperitoneum, three with cholecystitis, two splenic infarctions and two intestinal occlusions were diagnosed.

Symptoms were often vague and non-specific and blood counts revealed neutropenia in all but two patients,… All patients underwent surgical procedures within 48 hours of admission to the department. In all cases of necrotizing enterocolitis, intestinal resections, either ileal or colonic, were followed by an immediate anastomosis in two layers. Intensive hematological and antibiotic post surgical care was performed in all patients. Seven patients presented minor complications (38.8%), and only one died (5.5%).

Emergency surgical treatment may be safely carried out in patients with hematological diseases presenting with an acute abdomen. Intensive postsurgical care is mandatory for the recovery of patients and the patient's critical condition should not be a deterrent to surgical intervention."

Piero Chirletti, Paolo Barillari, Paolo Sammartino,
Maurizio Cardi, Roberto Caronna, William Arcese,
Concetta Petti, and V. Stipa,
Universita' di Roma "La Sapienza", Patologia Chirurgica IX, Cattedra di Ematologia, Roma, Italy [4][4]
1993

"Neutropenic patients with abdominal pain present a particular challenge because of their increased susceptibility to infection and the rapidity with which such sepsis can become overwhelming. Indeed, infection remains the leading cause of death in patients with haematological malignancy and frequently the causative organisms are Gram-negative bacilli of autogenous gastrointestinal origin. The situation is further compounded for the attending surgeon because many of the accepted criteria for surgical intervention, e.g., fever and leukocytosis, may not necessarily be present or, if present, may be of limited clinical value. The

[3] Permission to reuse this excerpt was generously granted by Terri S. Carter, managing editor, JAMA surgery, jamasurg@jamanetwork.org, 30 Aug 2021.

[4] Permission to reuse this excerpt was generously granted by Taylor & Francis, Publisher, http://www.tandfonline.com, CCC | RightsLink®, 30 Aug 2021.

knowledge that surgery is followed by greater morbidity and mortality rates in these patients because of co-existing medical problems further complicates decision making."

N. Williams and A. D. N. Scott
Glenfield General Hospital
Leicester, UK
1997 [5][5]

"Abdominal infections are an important cause of morbidity and mortality in neutropenic patients. We present a retrospective series of 16 patients, mostly with acute leukemia, who developed severe abdominal infections during chemotherapy-induced neutropenia between 1991 and 1997. Thirteen patients presented with enterocolitits and 3 patients presented with cholecystitis. Eight patients died. Bacteremia was present in 6 patients, 4 patients suffered from proven or strongly suspected fungal infections, and 1 patient suffered from cytomegalovirus infection. Early surgical management was required in a patient with intestinal obstruction, whereas other patients could be managed conservatively. Two patients with acute cholecystitis were treated with antibiotics until the end of neutropenia and then were resected. Severe abdominal infections in neutropenic patients, which are often fatal, were caused by nonbacterial micororganisms in one-fourth of the cases and could be managed conservatively in most instances."

Marcus Gorschlüter, M.D., Axel Glasmacher, M.D., Corinna Hahn, Ph.D.,
Claudia Leutner, M.D., Günter Marklein, M.D., Jürgen Remig, M.D.,
Ingo G. H. Schmidt-Wolf, M.D., Tilman Sauerbruch, M.D.,
Departments of Internal Medicine, Radiology, Medical Microbiology and Immunology, and Surgery
University of Bonn, Germany
2001 [6][6]

In 2018, Saillard et al. [7][7] reported a review and meta-analysis aimed to determine the prognostic impact of abdominal surgery in cancer patients with neutropenic enterocolitis (NE).

"This meta-analysis included studies analyzing cancer patients presenting with NE, treated with surgical or medical treatment,… The endpoint was hospital mortality. Surgery was not associated with an excess risk of mortality compared to medical treatment. Defining the optimal indications of surgical treatment is needed."

Groupe de Recherche en Réanimation Respiratoire du patient d'Onco-Hématologie

References

1. Badgwell BD, Cormier JN, Wray CJ, Borthakur G, Qiao W, Rolston KV, et al. Challenges in surgical management of abdominal pain in the neutropenic cancer patient. Ann Surg. 2008;248:104–9.

[5] This excerpt is reused with the generous permission of John Wiley and Sons, CCC | RightsLink®, License Number 51622400924531, License date 5 Oct 2021.

[6] This article abstract excerpt is reused with the generous permission of Taylor & Francis, permissionrequest@tandf.co.uk, CCC | RightsLink®, Date: 30 Aug 2021.

[7] Under the terms of creative commons CC by license, permission to reuse this excerpt is not required provided the original work is properly cited, SpringerNature, CCC | RightsLink®, Date: Sept 8, 2021.

2. Starnes HF Jr, Moore FD Jr, Mentzer S, Osteen RT, Steele GD Jr, Wilson RE. Abdominal pain in neutropenic cancer patients. Cancer. 1986;57:616–21.
3. Wade DS, Douglass H, Nava HR, Piedmonte M. Abdominal pain in neutropenic patients. Arch Surg. 1990;125:1119–27.
4. Chirletti P, Barillari P, Sammartino P, Cardi M, Caronna R, Arcese W, Petti C, Stipa V. The surgical choice in neutropenic patients with hematological disorders and acute abdominal complications. Leuk Lymphoma. 1993;9:237–41. https://doi.org/10.3109/10428199309147376.
5. Williams N, Scott ADN. Neutropenic colitis: a continuing surgical challenge. Br J Surg. 1997;84:1200–5.
6. Gorschlüter M, Glasmacher A, Hahn C, Leutner C, Marklein G, Remig J, Schmidt-Wolf IGH, Sauerbruch T. Severe abdominal infections in neutropenic patients. Cancer Investig. 2001;19:669–77. https://doi.org/10.1081/CNV-100106141.
7. Saillard C, Zafrani L, Darmon M, Bisbal M, Chow-Chine L, Sannini A, Brun J-P, et al. The prognostic impact of abdominal surgery in cancer patients with neutropenic enterocolitis: a systematic review and meta-analysis, on behalf the Groupe de Recherche en Réanimation Respiratoire du patient d'Onco-Hématologie (GRRR-OH). Ann Intensive Care. 2018;8:47. https://doi.org/10.1186/s13613-018-0394-6.

Operative Injury to Irradiated Small Intestine

227

Susan L. Gearhart, Erika B. Woodrum, and James S. Wu

Presentation

A 60-year-old female with a history of cervical cancer was treated by hysterectomy and external beam radiation. Subsequently, she developed symptoms from radiation injury to the bladder. Laparoscopic bladder augmentation was scheduled. During surgery, an extensive lysis of adhesions was done. This part of the operation was complicated by enterotomies. Intraoperative consultation was requested. The abdomen was opened. Examination showed three enterotomies which transected more than 50% of the luminal diameter. The three sites were located 175 cm, 180 cm, and 190 cm from the ligament of Treitz. The injured ileum showed bowel wall and mesenteric thickening (Fig. 227.1).

S. L. Gearhart
Department of General and Colon & Rectal Surgery, Johns Hopkins Bayview Medical Center, Baltimore, MD, USA

E. B. Woodrum
Medical Illustration Team, Enterprise Creative Services, Cleveland Clinic, Cleveland, OH, USA

J. S. Wu (✉)
Department of Colon and Rectal Surgery, Cleveland Clinic, Cleveland, OH, USA

J. S. Wu, M. D. Inkster (eds.), *Cleveland Clinic Colorectal Case Studies*,
https://doi.org/10.1007/978-3-031-39880-3_227

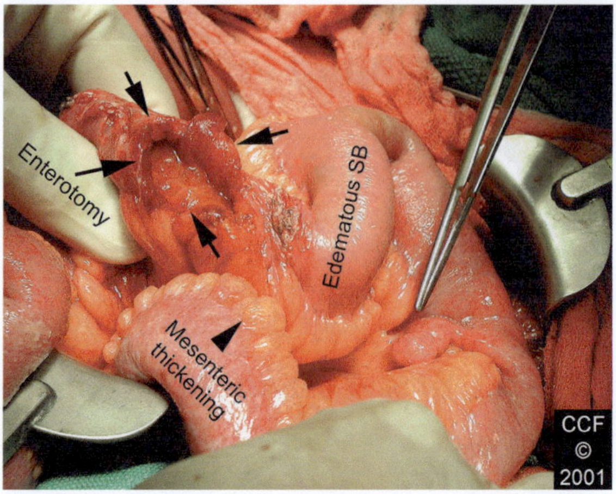

Fig. 227.1 An enterotomy (arrows) to edematous small intestine with thickened mesentery (arrowhead) consistent with radiation injury is shown

Management

The three enterotomies were repaired with interrupted suture. The small intestine was divided 170 cm from the ligament of Treitz, proximal to the repaired enterotomies. The proximal end of the divided intestine was anastomosed to normal appearing transverse colon (Fig. 227.2). An illustration of the operation is shown in Fig. 227.3. The repaired distal terminal ileum was returned to the abdomen. Additional adhesiolysis to liberate small intestine located in the pelvis was not done.

Pressure was applied to the right colon. Retrograde movement of air into the terminal ileum was not seen.

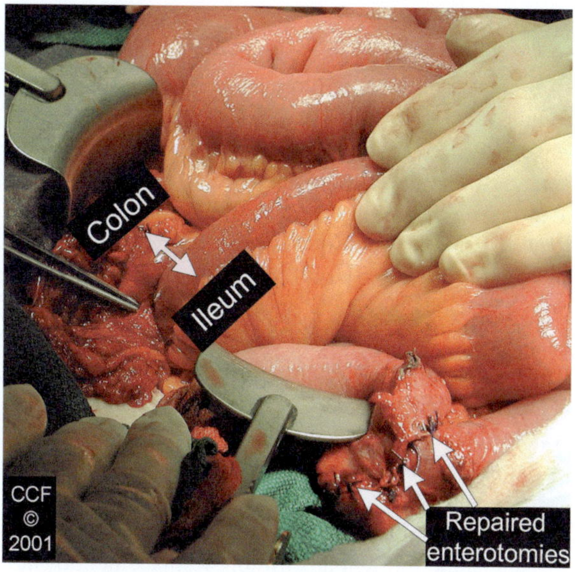

Fig. 227.2 Repaired injured irradiated terminal ileum is marked with arrows. The ileum was divided proximal to the repairs. The proximal end of the divided intestine was anastomosed to the transverse colon

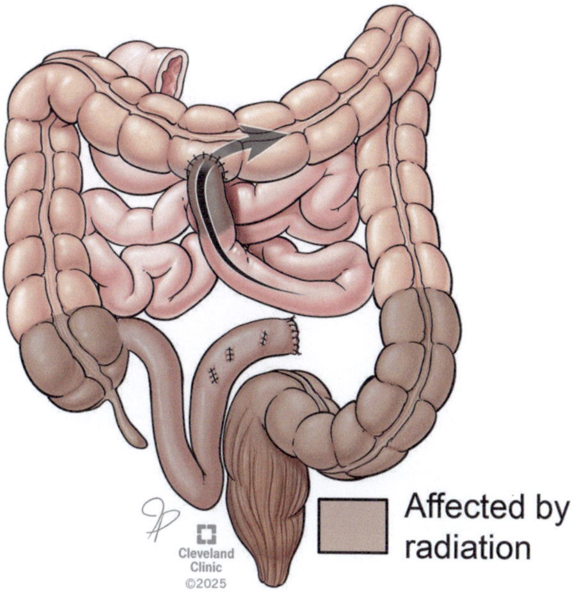

Fig. 227.3 Enterotomies in irradiated terminal ileum were repaired (stitches). The small intestine proximal to the injured segment was anastomosed to the transverse colon. Intestine affected by radiation is shaded in brown

Comment

In this case, three enterotomies were made during adhesiolysis. Each of the three injured ileal sites showed signs of radiation injury. The three enterotomies were repaired. Although the enterotomy repairs seemed watertight at surgery, postoperative anastomotic leak was of concern since both sides of each repair involved irradiated bowel. Therefore, the small intestine was divided proximal to the enterotomy repairs. Bowel continuity was restored by anastomosing the proximal limb of divided small intestine to the transverse colon. The rationale for this choice was as follows.

(a) The distal ileum containing the repairs drains antegrade into the colon.
(b) The competent ileocecal valve prevents retrograde pressure on the three enterotomy repairs.
(c) An anastomosis involving the transverse colon ensures that one side of the anastomosis (colon) had a good blood supply as advised by Galland and Spencer [1].
(d) The length of small intestine (170 cm) plus colon would be adequate for water and some nutrient absorption. Replacement of nutrients absorbed by the terminal ileum would be required.
(e) Extensive pelvic lysis of adhesions to liberate all of the ileum fixed in the pelvis was avoided.
(f) Intestine was not removed unnecessarily.

Dr. Fazio once recounted to the one of the authors (JSW) that he had to operate on a former patient of Dr. Frank Weakley. The patient had already lost a large length of small intestine, and short bowel syndrome was a concern. Something that Dr. Weakley had done gave him confidence that all would be fine. Dr. Weakley had left a segment of small intestine out of continuity. Rather than excise it, he left it in the abdomen, and exteriorized one end as an enterocutaneous fistula as described by Thiry [2] in 1865 (Fig. 227.4), in case, at another operation in the future, it might be needed. It was.

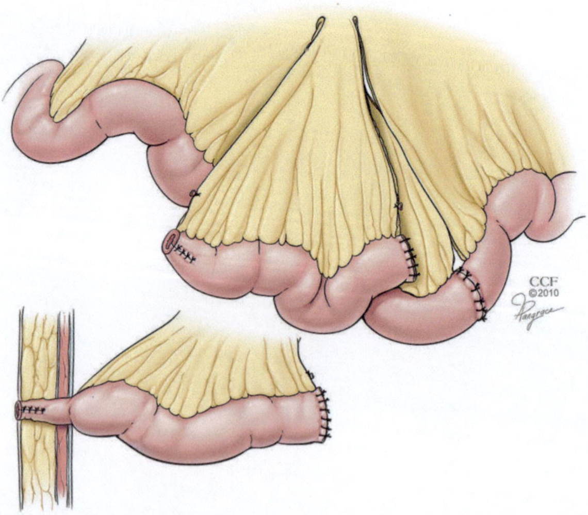

Fig. 227.4 Thiry fistula. One end of an isolated segment of small intestine is exteriorized to vent intestinal secretions. the other end is closed. Continuity of the remaining small intestine is restored

References

1. Galland RB, Spencer J. Surgical management of radiation enteritis. Surgery. 1986;99:133–9.
2. Thiry L. Über eine neue Methode, den Dünndarm zu isoliren. Sitzungsberichte der Kaiserlichen Akademie der Wissenschaften. Mathematisch-Naturwissenschaftliche Classe. Abt. 1, Mineralogie, Botanik, Zoologie, Anatomie, Geologie und Paläontologie. 1865;50:77–96.

Radiation Enteritis with Stricture

228

James S. Wu and Daniela Allende

Presentation

A 50-year-old female presented with nausea, vomiting, and abdominal pain.

She had a history of anal cancer treated with chemotherapy and radiation. Computed tomographic (CT) images of the abdomen are shown in Figs. 228.1 and 228.2.

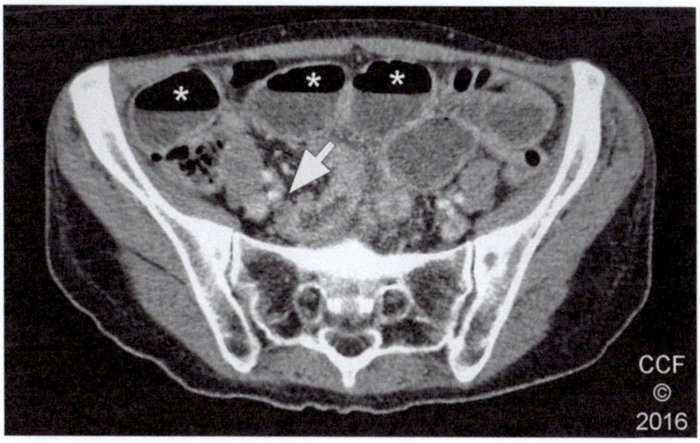

Fig. 228.1 Axial CT of the pelvis shows dilated small intestine with air-fluid levels (asterisks) and a stricture in the distal ileum located in the pelvis (arrow)

J. S. Wu (✉)
Department of Colon and Rectal Surgery, Cleveland Clinic, Cleveland, OH, USA

D. Allende
Pathology & Laboratory Medicine Institute, Cleveland Clinic, Cleveland, OH, USA

J. S. Wu, M. D. Inkster (eds.), *Cleveland Clinic Colorectal Case Studies*,
https://doi.org/10.1007/978-3-031-39880-3_228

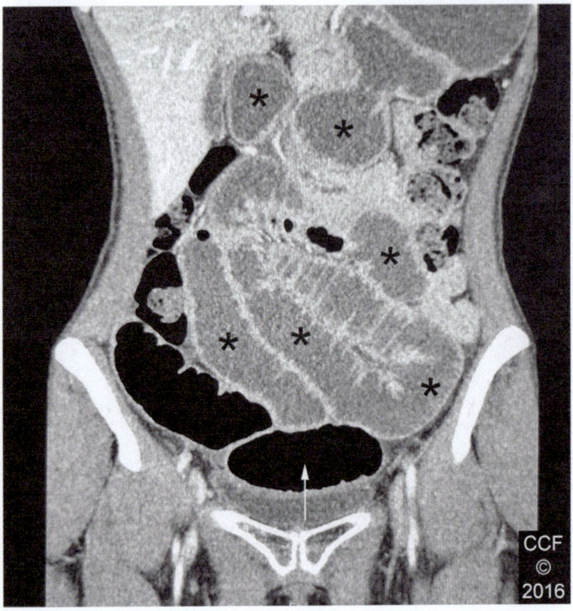

Fig. 228.2 A coronal CT slice shows multiple loops of air (arrow) and fluid (asterisks) filled dilated small intestine

Management

At surgery, an inflamed strictured segment of terminal ileum was found in the pelvis (Fig. 228.3). The adjacent terminal ileum was not strictured but was inflamed (Fig. 228.4).

The terminal ileum and right colon were mobilized (Fig. 228.5). The terminal ileum containing the stricture, right colon, and proximal transverse colon were resected (Fig. 228.6). Intestinal continuity was restored by ileocolic anastomosis.

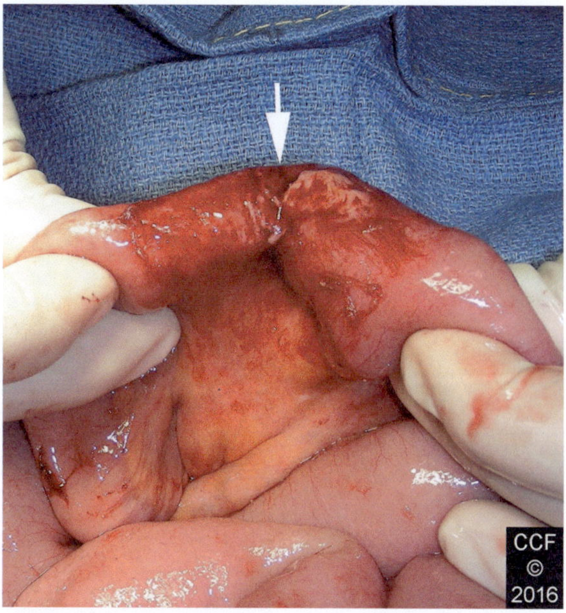

Fig. 228.3 Strictured and obstructed segment (arrow) of irradiated distal ileum

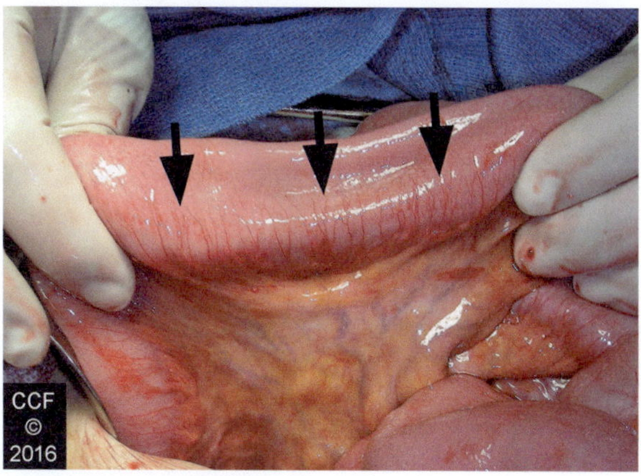

Fig. 228.4 This segment of distal ileum was located in the pelvis and showed hyperemic vessels on the mesenteric side of the intestine (arrow) consistent with radiation injury

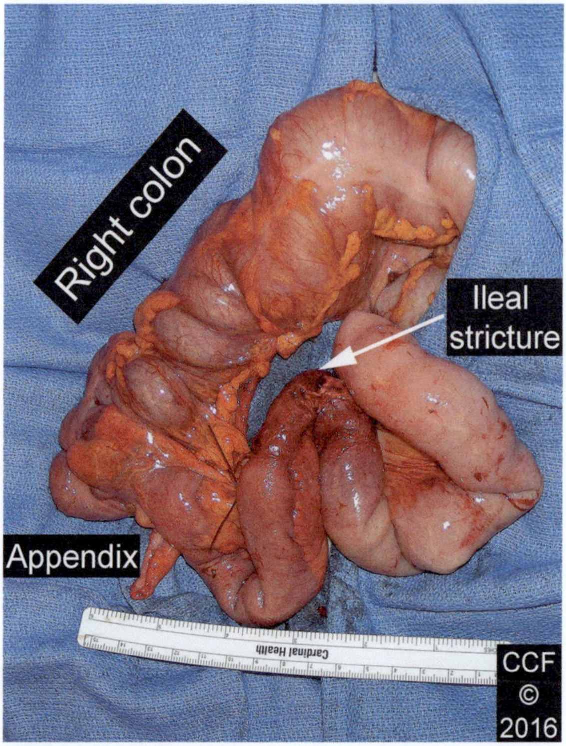

Fig. 228.5 Mobilized terminal ileum and right colon. The stricture is located about 20 cm proximal to the colon. Hyperemia of the distal terminal ileum, cecum, and proximal right colon is seen. The appendix is labelled

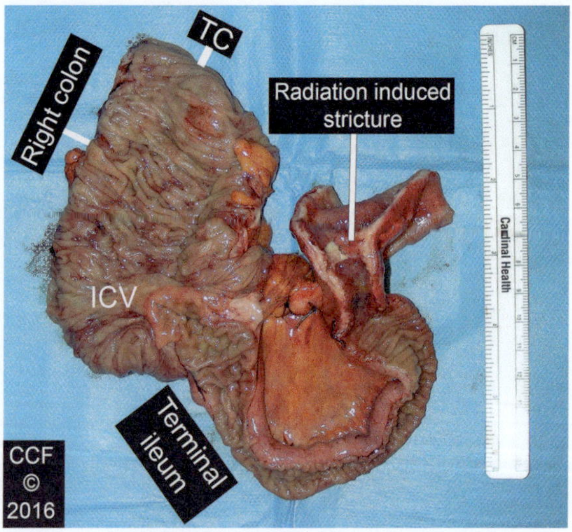

Fig. 228.6 Proximal transverse colon (TC), right colon, and terminal ileum specimen (opened). A radiation induced fibrotic stricture is noted 20 cm from the ileocecal valve (ICV)

Comment

> "The delivery of therapeutic radiation doses often is limited by the tolerance of the most sensitive normal tissues in the radiated field."
>
> Gerald Marks, M.D.
> and Mohammed Mohiuddin, M.D.
> Thomas Jefferson University.
> Philadelphia [1].

Structures neighboring the target of radiation therapy are subject to unintended injury. For the small bowel, the minimal tolerance dose (TD/5/5), the dose that leads to ulceration or stricture in 1% to 5% of patients within 5 years, is 4500 cGy. The maximal tolerance dose (TD/50/5), the dose that produces damage in 25% to 50% of patients in 5 years, is 6500 cGy. For patients who receive pelvic radiation, intestinal injury occurs most commonly to the rectum, terminal ileum, cecum, and sigmoid colon. Common radiation-induced intestinal injuries are shown in Table 228.1 [2]. The terminal ileum, about 20 cm from the colon, naturally lies in the pelvis and is the segment of small intestine most likely to be injured by radiation.

The histopathologic finding associated with radiation intestinal injury is endarteritis obliterans, defined by Merriam-Webster's Dictionary as "endarteritis in which the intimal tissue proliferates and ultimately plugs the lumen of an affected artery" (Fig. 228.7) [3, 4].

The operation performed in this case involved resection not only of the strictured segment by also of the adjacent right colon. Anastomosis was made between the neoterminal ileum and the transverse colon following the 1986 recommendation of Galland and Spencer that in the surgical management of radiation enteritis, nonirradiated bowel is used for at least one end of an anastomosis. The indications for radiotherapy in their study were mostly cancers anatomically located in the pelvis.

Table 228.1 Common radiation-induced intestinal injuries

Proctitis
Enteritis
Colitis
Stricture
Fistula
Obstruction
Hemorrhage
Pain
Malignancy

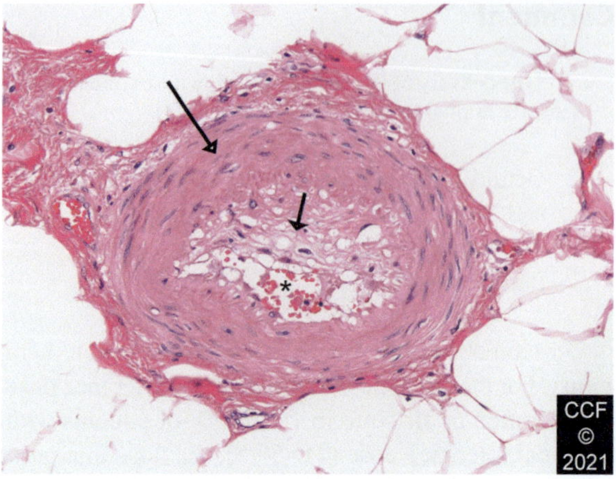

Fig. 228.7 The image shows a cross-section of an arteriole with thickened muscularis layer (long arrow) and intimal hyperplasia (short arrow) obliterating the lumen. Note the prominent endothelial cells in the luminal surface (asterisk) (H&E stain, 20×)

Surgical management of radiation enteritis

"Patients who develop intestinal problems after pelvic or abdominal radiotherapy for malignant disease should be assumed to be suffering from radiation-damaged bowel until proven otherwise.

Early reports of patients with radiation enteritis who were treated by primary resection and anastomosis showed a high anastomotic leakage rate with correspondingly high operative mortality rates. In our earlier report we noted that the ascending, transverse, and descending colon were usually free of radiation-induced lesions. Since then, whenever possible, we have used this part of the bowel for one end of an anastomosis."

R. B. Galland, M.D., F.R.C S. and J. Spencer, M.S., F.R.C.S.
Hammersmith Hospital,
London [5][1]

References

1. Marks G, Mohiuddin M. Radiation enteritis and colitis. In: Fazio VW, editor. Current Therapy in Colon and Rectal Surgery. Toronto: B.C. Decker; 1990. p. 377–83.
2. DeCosse JJ, Rhodes RS, Wentz WB, Reagan JW, Dworken HJ, Holden WD. The natural history and management of radiation induced injury of the gastrointestinal tract. Ann Surg. 1969;170:369–84.
3. "Endarteritis obliterans."Merriam Webster.com Medical Dictionary. Merriam-Webster, https://www.merriam-webster.com/medical /endarteritis%20obliterans. Accessed 10 Oct. 2021.
4. Sheaff M, Baithun S. Pathological effects of ionizing radiation. Curr Diagn Pathol. 1997;4:106–15.
5. Galland RB, Spencer J. Surgical management of radiation enteritis. Surgery. 1986;99:133–9.

[1]This excerpt was reproduced with generous permission from Mr. Subash Balakrishnan, ELSEVIER|HCM-Health Content Management, Reference number 210906-016600, September 7, 2021.

Colovaginal Anastomosis

229

Victor W. Fazio and James S. Wu

Presentation

A female patient underwent low anterior resection of the rectum with reconstruction. On the fourth postoperative day, she noted the passage of flatus and stool from her vagina. She was referred to the colon and rectal surgery service. A vaginogram was ordered (Fig. 229.1).

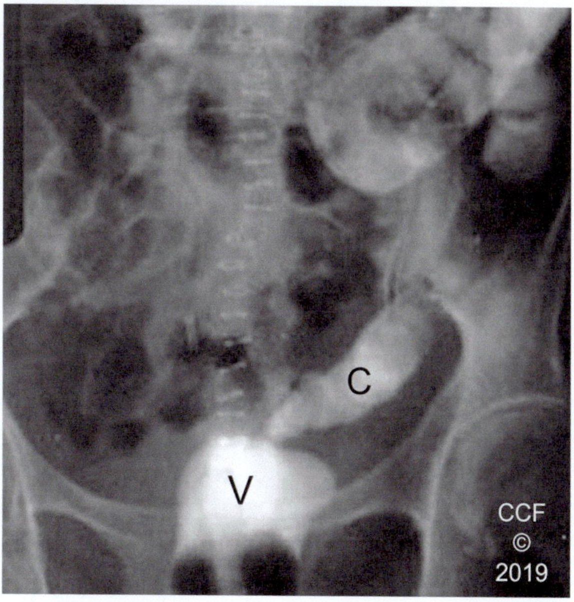

Fig. 229.1 Water-soluble contrast instilled into the vagina (V) immediately appears in the colon (C)

V. W. Fazio · J. S. Wu (✉)
Department of Colon and Rectal Surgery, Cleveland Clinic, Cleveland, OH, USA

J. S. Wu, M. D. Inkster (eds.), *Cleveland Clinic Colorectal Case Studies*,
https://doi.org/10.1007/978-3-031-39880-3_229

Management

The patient was taken to surgery. The colovaginal anastomosis was taken down, and anastomosis of the colon to the rectum was done.

Comment

Colovaginal anastomosis is an unusual complication associated with the stapling technique. It can occur either by placement of the stapling gun into the vagina or by including the vagina in a colorectal anastomosis [1–4]. Direct visual identification of anatomic landmarks including the anus, the vagina, and the proximal rectum may help to prevent this problem (Figs. 229.2 and 229.3).

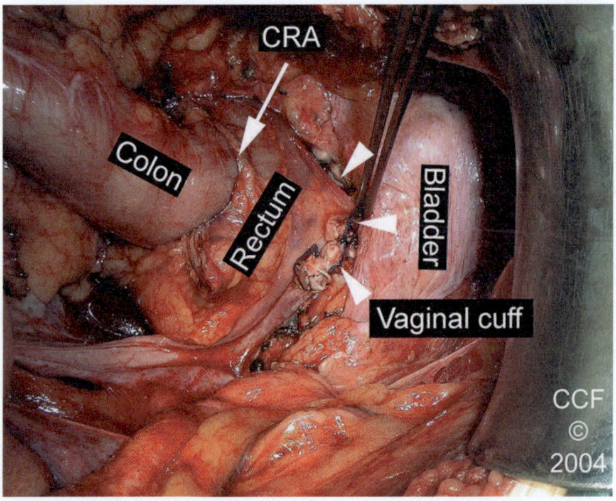

Fig. 229.2 Anatomic landmarks seen during anterior resection of the rectosigmoid colon with colorectal anastomosis (CRA). The patient has undergone prior hysterectomy. The vaginal cuff is seen in between the rectum and the bladder, clear of the CRA

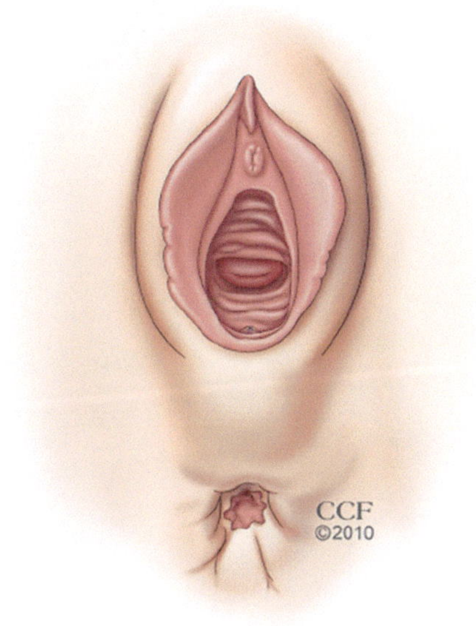

Fig. 229.3 The relation of the vagina and the anus in the lithotomy position. The vaginal opening is much larger than the anus. In addition, the internal anal sphincter is closed and must be dilated in order to pass a stapling instrument into the rectum

References

1. Yan Z, Liao G. Colovaginal anastomosis: an unusual complication of stapler use in restorative procedure after Hartmann operation. World J Surg Oncol. 2005;3:74. https://doi.org/10.1186/1477-7819-3-74.
2. Yodonawa S, Ogawa I, Yoshida S, Ito H, Kobayashi K, Kubokawa R. Rectovaginal fistula after low anterior resection for rectal cancer using a double stapling technique. Case Rep Gastroenterol. 2010;4:224–8. https://doi.org/10.1159/000318745.
3. Panovski M, Sazdovska IR, Fildisevski I, Dzambaz D, Spirov V. Colovaginal anastomosis: A totally unacceptable surgical error. Int J Surg Case Rep. 2015;7:66–9.
4. Emoto S, Nozawa H, Yoneyama S, Murono K, Kaneko M, Sasaki K, et al. Rectovaginal fistula after low anterior resection for rectal cancer healed by non-operative treatment. Int J Surg Case Rep. 2017;41:121–3.

Deep Venous Thrombosis, Pulmonary Embolus-Rudolf Virchow

230

Leonard A. Kahn and James S. Wu

Presentation

Deep venous thrombosis and pulmonary embolus are complications seen after colon and rectal surgery (Figs. 230.1 and 230.2).

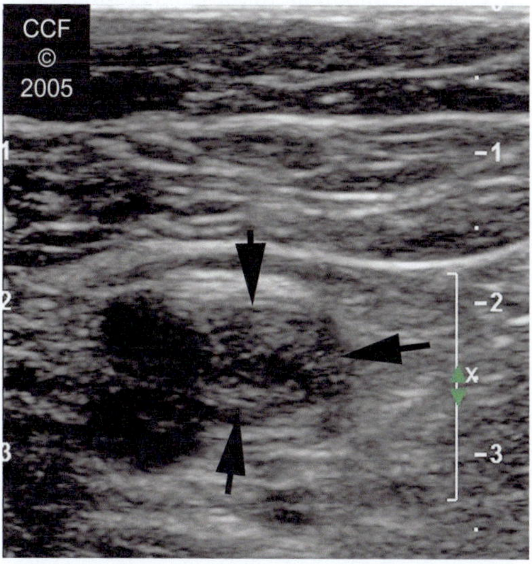

Fig. 230.1 Lower extremity duplex Doppler ultrasound shows deep venous thrombosis (arrows)

L. A. Kahn
Radiology & Diagnostic Imaging Institute, Cleveland Clinic, Cleveland, OH, USA

J. S. Wu (✉)
Department of Colon and Rectal Surgery, Cleveland Clinic, Cleveland, OH, USA

J. S. Wu, M. D. Inkster (eds.), *Cleveland Clinic Colorectal Case Studies*,
https://doi.org/10.1007/978-3-031-39880-3_230

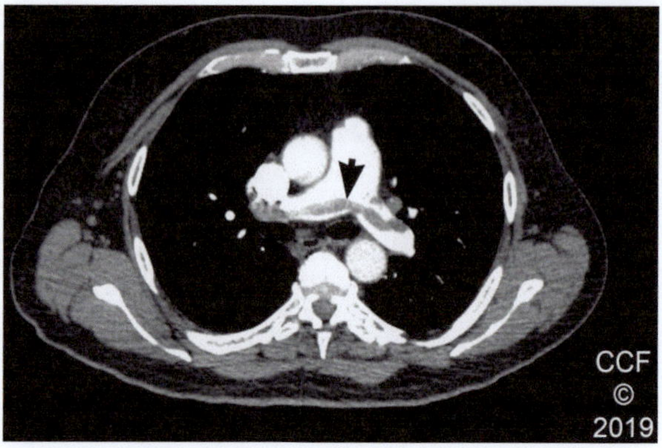

Fig. 230.2 Computed tomography pulmonary angiogram shows a saddle pulmonary embolus (arrowhead)

Comment

In 1862, Virchow described *Phlogose und Thrombose in Gefässsystem* (Inflammation and Thrombosis in the Vascular System) in which he identified three factors important to thrombus formation.

Phlogose und Thrombose in Gefässsystem. Gesammelte Abhandlungen zur Wissenschaftlichen Medicin von Rudolf Virchow Professor an der Universität zu Berlin [1] Seite 524–526 Unter diesen sind es aber namentlich drei, welche gefunden zu haben ich als einen wesentlichen Erfolg meiner Arbeiten betrachte und ohne welche die Geschichte der Thrombusbildung ihren räthselhaften Charakter noch lange nicht verloren haben würde. Ich stelle sie hier nochmals zusammen, weil sie für die Beurtheilung meiner Auffassung durchaus wesentlich sind: 1. *Die Unterscheidung von ursprünglichem und fortgesetztem Pfropf* 2. *Die Bedeutung der Klappensinus und der partiellen Ausbuchtungen der Gefässwand* 3. *Die Unterbrechung der Continuität des Blutstromes.*	Inflammation and thrombosis in the vascular system Collected Treatises on Scientific Medicine By Rudolf Virchow Professor, the University of Berlin Among these, there are three, in particular, which I have found to be essential to the success of my work, and without which the history of thrombus formation would by no means have lost its enigmatic character. I put them together again here, because they are essential to the judgment of my opinion: 1. The distinction between *the original and the continued clot* 2. *The importance of the valve sinus and the partial bulges of the vessel wall* 3. *Interruption of the continuity of the bloodstream.*

In 1858, Virchow delivered a series of 20 lectures at the Pathological Institute of Berlin based on cellular pathology. His tenth lecture, entitled, "Die metastasirende Dyscrasie," described thrombosis, emboli, and pulmonary embolism (Lungenmetastasen).

DIE CELLULARPATHOLOGIE
In ihrer Begründing auf physiologische und pathologische Gewebelehre.
Zwanzig Vorlesungen, gehalten während der Monate Februar, März und April 1858 im pathologischen Institute zu Berlin
von
Rudolph Virchow
Arzte a. d. Charité
Zehnte Vorlesung [2]
Die metastasirende Dyscrasie
Seite 178

Lassen wir also die Entzündung bei Seite and halten wir uns einfach an die Gerinnung des Blutes, an die Bildung des Gerinnsels (Thrombus), so scheint es am bequemsten, diesen ganzen Vorgang in dem Ausdrucke der Thrombose zusammen zu fassen.

Seite 183–5

Denn natürlich ensteht die Frage, in wie weit durch die Erweichung der Thromben besondere Störungen im Körper hervorgerufen werden können, welche man mit dem Namen Pyämie bezeichnen könnte. Hierauf ist zunächst zu erwidern, dass allerdings sehr häufig secundäre Störungen veranlasst werden, aber nicht so sehr dadurch, dass die Erweichungsmassen unmittelbar in das Blut kommen, als vielmehr dadurch, dass grössere oder kleinere Massen von dem Ende des erweichenden Thrombus abgelöst, mit dem Blutstrom fortgeführt und in entfernte Gefässe eingetrieben werden. Dies gibt den sehr häufigen Vorgang der von mir sogenannten Embolie.

Est ist dies ein Ereigniss, welches wir hier nur kurz berühren können. An den peripherischen Venen geht die Gefahr hauptsächlich von den kleinen Aesten aus. Gar nicht selten werden diese mit Gerinnselmasse ganz erfüllt. So Lange indess der Thrombus sich nur in dem Aste selbst befindet, so lange ist für den Körper keine besondere Gefahr vorhanden; das Schlimmste ist, dass sich ein Abcess bildet, in Folge einer Peri- oder Mesophlebitis, der sich nach Aussen öffnet. Allein die meisten Thromben der kleinen Aeste beschränken sich nicht darauf, bis an den Stamm vorzudringen; ziemlich constant lagert sich an das Ende des Thrombus neue Gerinselmasse Schicht um Schicht vom Blute ab, der Thrombus setzt sich über das Ostium hinaus in den Stamm in der Richtung des Blutstromes fort, wächst in Form eines dicken Cylinders weiter und wird immer grösser und grösser. Bald steht dieser fortgesetzte Thrombus in gar keinem Verhältniss mehr zu dem ursprünglichen (autochthonen) Thrombus, von dem er ausgegangen ist. Der fortgesetzte Thrombus kann die Dicke eines Daumens haben, der ursprüngliche die einer Stricknadel. Aus einer Vena lumbalis kann z. B. en Pfropf so dick, wie die letzte Phalanx des Daumens, sich in die Cava fortsetzen.

Diese fortgesetzten Pfröpfe bringen die eigentliche Gefahr mit sich; an ihnen erfolgt die Abbröckelung, welche zu secundären Verschliessungen entfernter Gefässe führt. Hier ist der ort, wo durch das vorüberströmende Blut grössere und kleinere Partikeln abgerissen werden. Durch das ursprünglich verstopfte Gefäss strömt überhaupt kein Blut, da ist die Circulation gänzlich unterbrochen; aber in dem grösseren Stamme, durch welchen das Blut immer noch fortgeht, und in welchen nur von Strecke zu Strecke Thrombuszapfen hineinragen, kann der Blutstrom kleinere Partikelchen lostrennen, mitschleppen und in das nächste Arterien- oder Capillarsystem festkeilen.

CELLULAR PATHOLOGY
as based upon physiological and pathological histology.
Twenty lectures delivered in the Pathological Institute of Berlin during the months of February, March and April, 1858
by
Rudolph Virchow
Physician to the Charité Hospital
Lecture X [3]
Metastatical dyscrasiæ
Page 199

If we therefore leave inflammation on one side and confine our attention simply to the coagulation of the blood, to the formation of the clot (thrombus), it seems most convenient to comprehend the whole of this process under the term *Thrombosis.*

Pages 204–207

For the question naturally arises how far particular disturbances that can be designated by the name of the pyæmia may, in consequence of the softening of the thrombi, be evoked in the body. To this in the first place we may answer that secondary disturbances certainly are very frequently occasioned, but not so much by the immediate introduction of the softened masses as fast as they become liquid into the blood, as by the detachment of larger or smaller fragments from the end of the softening thrombus which are carried along by the current of blood and driven into remote vessels. This gives rise to the very frequent process upon which I have bestowed the name of *Embolia.*

This is an occurrence which we can here only briefly touch upon. In the peripheral veins the danger proceeds chiefly from the small branches. By no means rarely do these become quite filled with masses of coagulum. As long however as the thrombus is confined to the branch itself, so long as the body is not exposed to any particular danger; the worst that can happen is that, in consequence of a peri- or meso-phlebitis, an abscess may form and open externally. Only the greater number of the thrombi in the small branches do not content themselves with advancing up to the level of the main trunk, but pretty constantly new masses of coagulum deposit themselves from the blood upon the end of the thrombus layer after layer, the thrombus is prolonged beyond the mouth of the branch into the trunk in the direction of the current of the blood, shoots out in the form of a thick cylinder farther and farther, and becomes continually larger and larger. Soon this *prolonged* thrombus no longer bears any proportion to the original (*autochthonous*) thrombus, from which it proceeded. The prolonged thrombus may have a thickness of a thumb, the original one that of a knitting needle. From a lumbar vein, for example, a plug may extend into the vena cava as thick as the last phalanx of the thumb

It is these prolonged plugs that constitute the source of real danger; it is in them that ensues the crumbling away which leads to secondary occlusions in remote vessels. They are the parts from which larger or smaller particles are torn away by the blood as it streams by.

Through the vessel originally occluded no blood at all flows; in it the circulation is entirely interrupted; but in the larger trunk through which the blood still continues its course, and into which only at intervals the thrombus-plugs project, the stream of blood may detach minute particles, hurry them away with it, and wedge them tightly into the nearest system of arteries or capillaries.

So sehen wir, dass in der Regel alle Thromben aus der Peripherie des Körpers secundäre Verstopfungen und Metastasen in der Lunge erzeugen. I habe lange Zweifel getragen, die metastatischen Entzündungen der Lunge sämmtlich als embolische zu betrachten, weil es sehr schwer ist, die Gefässe in den kleinen metastatischen Heerden zu untersuchen, aber ich überzeuge mich immer mehr von der Nothwendigkeit, diese Art der Entstehung als die Regel zu betrachten. Wenn man eine grössere Reihe von Fällen statistisch vergleicht, so zeigt sich, dass jedesmal, wo Metastasen vorkommen, auch Thrombose gewisser Gefässe besteht. Wir haben z. B. eben jetz eine ziemlich grosse Puerperalfieber-Epidemie gehabt. Dabei stellte sich heraus, dass, so mannigfaltig die Formen der Erkrankung auch waren, doch alle diejenigen Fälle, welche mit Metastasen in den Lungen verbunden waren, auch mit Thrombose im Bereiche des Beckens oder der unteren Extremitäten verlaufen waren, während bei den Lymphgefäss-Entzündungen die Lungenmetastasen felhten. Solche statistische Resultate haben eine gewisse zwingende Nothwendigtkeit, selbst wo der strenge anatomische Nachweis felht. In die Lungen-Arterie dringen die eingeführten Thrombus-stücke natürlich je nach ihrer Grösse verschieden weit ein. Gewöhnlich setz sich ein solches Stück da fest, wo eine Theilung des Gefässes stattfindet, weil die abgehenden Gefässe zu klein sind, um das Stück noch einzulassen. Bei sehr grossen Stücken werden schon die Hauptstämme der Lungenarterie verstopft, und es tritt augenblickliche Asphyxie ein;…	Thus we see, that as a rule all the thrombi from the periphery of the body produce secondary obstructions and metastatic deposits in the lungs. I long entertained doubts whether I ought to consider the metastatic inflammations of the lungs one and all as embolical, because it is very difficult to examine the vessels in the small metastatic deposits, but I am continually becoming more and more convinced of the necessity of regarding this mode of origin as the rule. When a considerable number of cases are compared statistically, the result obtained is that every time metastatic deposits occur, thrombosis is also present in certain vessels. Quite recently, for example, we have had a tolerably severe epidemic of puerperal fever, and in this it was found that, however, manifold the forms of the disease assumed, yet all those cases which were accompanied by metastases in the lungs, were also attended with thrombosis in the region of the pelvis or in the lower extremities, whilst in the inflammations of lymphatic vessels the pulmonary metastases were wanting. Such statistical results carry with them a certain amount of compulsory conviction, even where strict anatomical proof is wanting. Into the pulmonary artery the introduced fragments of thrombus of course penetrate to different depths according to their size. Usually a fragment of the kind sticks fast where a division of the vessel takes place, because the diverging vessels are too small to admit it. In the case of very large fragments even the principal trunks of the pulmonary artery are blocked up, and instantaneous asphyxia ensues;…

Virchow's woodcut (Holzschnitt) engraving of a saddle pulmonary embolus (Fig. 230.3) is shown below.

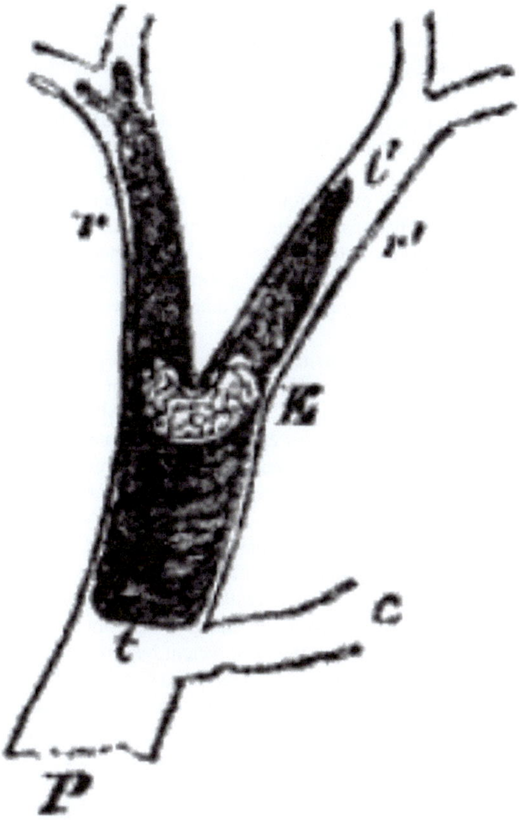

Fig. 230.3 Embolie der Lungenarterie. *P.* Mittelstarker Ast der Lungenarterie. *E.* der embolus, auf dem Sporn der sich theilenden Arterie reitend. *t, t'* der einkapselnde (secundäre) Thrombus: *t*, das Stück vor dem Embolus, bis zu dem nächst höheren Collateralgefäss *c* reichend; *t'* das Stück hinter dem Embolus, die abgehenden Aeste *r; r'* grossentheils füllend und zuletzt konisch endigend. [2, S. 185].

Embolia of the pulmonary artery. *P.* Moderately large branch of the pulmonary artery. *E.* The embolus astride upon the angle (spur—Sporn), formed by the division of the artery. *t, t'*. The capsulating (secondary) thrombus: *t*, the portion in front of the embolus reaching to the next highest collateral vessel, *c: t'*, the portion behind the embolus, in a great measure filling up the diverging branches, *r, r'*, and ultimately terminating in the form of a cone. [3, pp. 206–207]

Biographical Note

Rudolf Virchow died in 1902. His life was reviewed in an Obituary published in the British Medical Journal from which a few lines here are reproduced [4].

Obituary,
Rudolf Virchow, M.D.,
Professor of Pathological Anatomy,
University of Berlin

'Rudolf Ludwig Karl Virchow was born on October 13, 1821, at Schivelbein, a small town in Pomerania. He was the son of a shopkeeper,... In 1835 he entered the gymnasium of Cöslin, the chief town of the district. He passed out of the gymnasium first on the list of the *Abiturienten* in 1839. Among the subjects in which he presented himself for examination was Hebrew, which he had taken up merely from a love for the study of languages.

Virchow entered the Friedrich Wilhelm Institute, founded for the education of medical officers for the Prussian Army.

Almost immediately after graduation, Virchow was appointed Assistant to the Prosector of the Charité Hospital. That post was then held by Robert Froriep, and on his resignation in 1846 Virchow was chosen as his successor. In the following year, Virchow qualified as *Privat - docent*. About the same time, in conjunction with his friend Benno Reinhardt, he founded the famous *Archiv* which bears his name, and which he continued to edit until his death.

In 1856 Virchow received an invitation to become Professor of Pathology at Berlin. He accepted it on the condition that an institute for practical work was founded. When he entered on his career as professor at Berlin the museum of Morbid Anatomy contained only some 1,500 preparations. When, on his eightieth birthday, he received the congratulations of the scientific world in the new Pathological Museum which is the outcome of his own indefatigable exertions, the number of preparations in it was stated to be nearly 23,000.

THE "CELLULARPATHOLOGIE."

In 1858 appeared the *Cellularpathologie*, in which he laid the foundations of scientific pathology. The conception on which the whole structure rests is formulated by the author in the famous proposition, *Omnis cellula a cellula*. The work is one of the classics of medical literature, one of the great landmarks in the road leading from the darkness of ignorance to the light of knowledge. Of this monument of patient research and brilliant generalization, Lord Lister said that it "had swept away the false and barren theory of a structureless blastema, and established the true and fertile doctrine that every morbid structure consists of cells which have been derived from pre-exiting cells as a progeny .... Even those morbid structures which deviate most from the normal structure are known to be derived as a progeny from normal tissue—from normal cells, driven to abnormal development by injurious agencies." The principles set forth in the *Cellularpathologie* were applied by Virchow to the elucidation of the genesis and development of tumours in his other great work, *Die krankhaften Geschwülste*, which was published between 1863 and 1867.'

References

1. Virchow R. Phlogose und Thrombose im Gefässsystem. Gesammelte Abhandlungen zur Wissenschaftlichen Medicin. Zweite unveränderte Ausgabe, HAMM, G. GROTE'sche Buchhandlung (C. Müller), 1862;458, 524–526. Google Books www.books google.com. Accessed 15 Jun 2020.
2. Virchow R. Die Cellularpathologie in ihrer Begründing auf physiologische und pathologische Gewebelehre. Zwanzig Vorlesungen, gehalten während der Monate Februar, März und April 1858 im pathologischen Institute zu Berlin. Berlin 1858, Verlag von August Hirschwald.. Google Books. www.books.google.com. Accessed 31 Mar 2019.
3. Virchow R. Cellular Pathology as based upon Physiological and Pathological Histology. Twenty lectures delivered in the Pathological Institute of Berlin during the months of February, March and April, 1858. Translated from the second edition of the original by Frank Chance, London, John Churchill, MDCCCLX, Lexture X. Metastatical Dyscrasiæ, pages 196–219. Google Books. www.books.google.com. Accessed 31 Mar 2019.
4. Rudolf Virchow MD. Obituary. Br Med J. 1902;2:795–802.

Superior Mesenteric Artery Syndrome 231

James S. Wu, Arthur A. Parsee, and Michelle D. Inkster

Presentation

A 40-year-old patient was readmitted to the hospital after colectomy because of abdominal pain, nausea, and vomiting. An abdominal computed tomographic (CT) scan was obtained (Fig. 231.1).

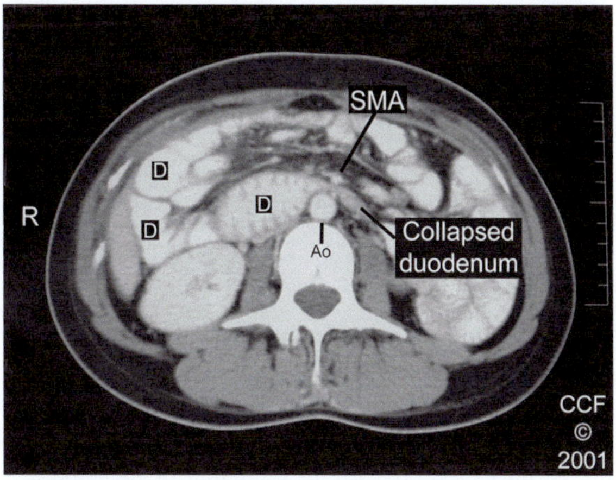

Fig. 231.1 Abdominal computed tomography (CT) shows compression of the third portion of the duodenum between the superior mesenteric artery (SMA) and the aorta (AO). The duodenum proximal to the point of compression is dilated (D). Distal to this point, the intestine is collapsed

J. S. Wu (✉)
Department of Colon and Rectal Surgery, Cleveland Clinic, Cleveland, OH, USA

A. A. Parsee
Department of Diagnostic Radiology, H. Lee Moffitt Cancer Center and Research Institute, Tampa, FL, USA

M. D. Inkster
Department of Gastroenterology, Cleveland Clinic, Cleveland, OH, USA

J. S. Wu, M. D. Inkster (eds.), *Cleveland Clinic Colorectal Case Studies*,
https://doi.org/10.1007/978-3-031-39880-3_231

Management

The upper gastrointestinal tract was decompressed with a nasogastric tube (NGT) attached to suction. Oral intake was withheld, and hyperalimentation was started. Bowel function gradually returned. The NGT was removed, and oral nutrition was resumed.

Comment

In 1861, Rokitansky [1] described incarceration of the lower duodenum by the superior mesenteric artery.

Lehrbuch der Pathologischen Anatomie von Carl Rokitansky Professor an der Universität zu Wien, 1861 "a) Incarceration. Die inneren Incarcerationen lassen sich auf folgende Arten zurückführen: 1. Die incarceration ist durch den Druck bedingt, welchen eine Darmportion und ihr Gekröse auf ein Darmstück ausübt, indem sie auf diesen lastet und dasselbe von vorne nach der hinteren starren Bauchwand hin comprimirt. Hieher gehört die Compression des unteren Querstücks des Duodenums durch das Dünndarmgekröse und zwar durch die in die Gekrösewurzel eintretende A. mesent. sup. …"	Textbook of Pathological Anatomy By Carl Rokitansky Professor, University of Vienna, 1861 "a) Incarceration Internal incarcerations can be traced back in the following ways: 1. Incarceration is caused by pressure which a portion of the intestine and its mesentery exert on a segment of bowel, by bearing on it and compressing it from the front towards the rigid posterior abdominal wall. Here the compression of the lower transverse part of the duodenum is caused by the small intestinal mesentery, and indeed by the superior mesenteric artery in the mesenteric root."

The superior mesenteric artery syndrome is obstruction caused by compression of the third portion of the duodenum by the superior mesenteric artery. In 1921, Wilkie used the phrase "chronic duodenal ileus" to describe *post-mortem* cases "where a greatly dilated and congested duodenum was found, the dilatation extending as far as the crossing of the superior mesenteric vessels." [2] In 1927, Wilkie proposed the pathogenesis of this condition. [3][1]

CHRONIC DUODENAL ILEUS.
By D. P. D. Wilkie, M.Ch., F.R.C.S.,
Professor of Surgery, University of Edinburgh.

[1] This excerpt is reused with the generous permission of Oxford University press, CCC|RightsLink®, license number 5175950900400, license date Oct 25, 2021.

"During the past six years considerable interest and not a little controversy have been aroused over the significance of the dilated duodenum and the question as to whether in the condition designated, "chronic duodenal ileus" we have a true pathologic and clinical entity. We are all familiar with the importance of the duodenal segment of the gut, with the toxicity of its content when obstructed, and the grave and often fatal constitutional disturbances which follow a complete blockage of its lumen. In cases of so-called gastromesenteric ileus we have both clinical and postmortem evidence that an organic obstruction of the third part of the duodenum by the root of the mesentery is the active factor in producing the ileus."

In 2010, concerning the etiopathogenesis of the superior mesenteric artery (SMA) syndrome, Mandarry and colleagues wrote [4]:

"Any factor decreasing the intervening space around the duodenum or altering its relation to the surrounding anatomical structures will *result in external compression or occlusion of the duodenum, by decreasing the aortomesenteric angle*."

In 2025, the National Organization of Rare Diseases (NORD) summarized SMA syndorme as follows:

"Superior mesenteric artery (SMA) syndrome is a rare condition that involves compression of the third portion of the duodenum which is the upper part of the small intestines just past the stomach. This condition occurs when the third part of the duodenum is compressed between two arteries – the main artery of the body called the abdominal aorta (AA) and one of its branches called the SMA. The SMA provides blood supply to the small intestines and the first part of the colon. Compression of the SMA against the AA can prevent duodenal contents from draining into the jejunum (upper small intestine) hence the inability to get proper nutrition leading to weight loss and malnutrition. Pain from the compression can be debilitating, causing "food fear" and aggravating the condition. Nausea and vomiting are manifestations of the compression of the duodenum. When weight loss is persistent, the mesenteric fat pad decreases and causes a decrease in the angle between the SMA and AA hence aggravating the compression and obstruction. Prompt diagnosis and early treatment are essential to avoid significant complications or death." [5]

The mechanism of this compression is illustrated in Fig. 231.2.

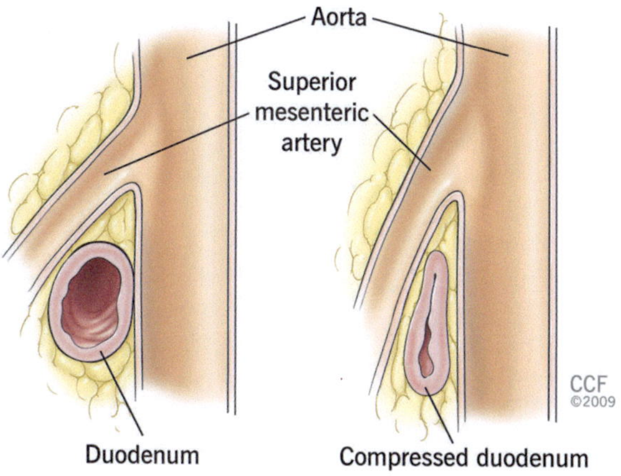

Fig. 231.2 (Left) The normal relationship between the aorta, superior mesenteric artery, and the duodenum; (right) the duodenum is compressed between the superior mesenteric artery and aorta resulting in obstruction

In this particular case, the cause of the patient's condition was attributed to significant weight loss following surgery. Treatment was supportive and included gastrointestinal decompression and hyperalimentation followed by restoration of an oral diet. In general, surgery is chosen as a treatment option only if nonoperative therapy fails.

References

1. Rokitansky C. Lehrbuch der Pathologischen Anatomie, Dritte umgearbeitete Auflage, Dritter Band. Wien: Wilhelm Braumüller; 1861, p. 187. Internet Archive. www.archiv.org. Accessed 13 Oct 2019.
2. Wilkie DPD. Chronic duodenal ileus. Br Med J. 1921;2(3176):793–95.
3. Wilkie DPD. Chronic duodenal ileus. Am J Med Sci 1927;173:643–9.
4. Mandarry M, Zhao L, Zhang C, Wei ZQ. A comprehensive review of superior mesenteric artery syndrome. Eur Surg. 2010;42:229–36.
5. National Organization for Rare Disorders (NORD). Superior mesenteric artery syndrome. In: Rare disease database. National Organization for Rare Disorders (NORD); 2022. Available at: https://rarediseases.org/rare-diseases/superior-mesenteric-artery-syndrome/#complete-report.

Gallstone Pancreatitis

232

Michael O. Christian, Michelle D. Inkster, and James S. Wu

Presentation

A patient who had a history of colorectal cancer reported severe abdominal pain. He was admitted to the colorectal service. Examination showed tenderness in the mid-upper abdomen. Computed tomography of the abdomen was obtained (Fig. 232.1).

M. O. Christian
Radiology & Diagnostic Imaging Institute, Cleveland Clinic, Cleveland, OH, USA

M. D. Inkster
Department of Gastroenterology, Cleveland Clinic, Cleveland, OH, USA

J. S. Wu (✉)
Department of Colon and Rectal Surgery, Cleveland Clinic, Cleveland, OH, USA

J. S. Wu, M. D. Inkster (eds.), *Cleveland Clinic Colorectal Case Studies*,
https://doi.org/10.1007/978-3-031-39880-3_232

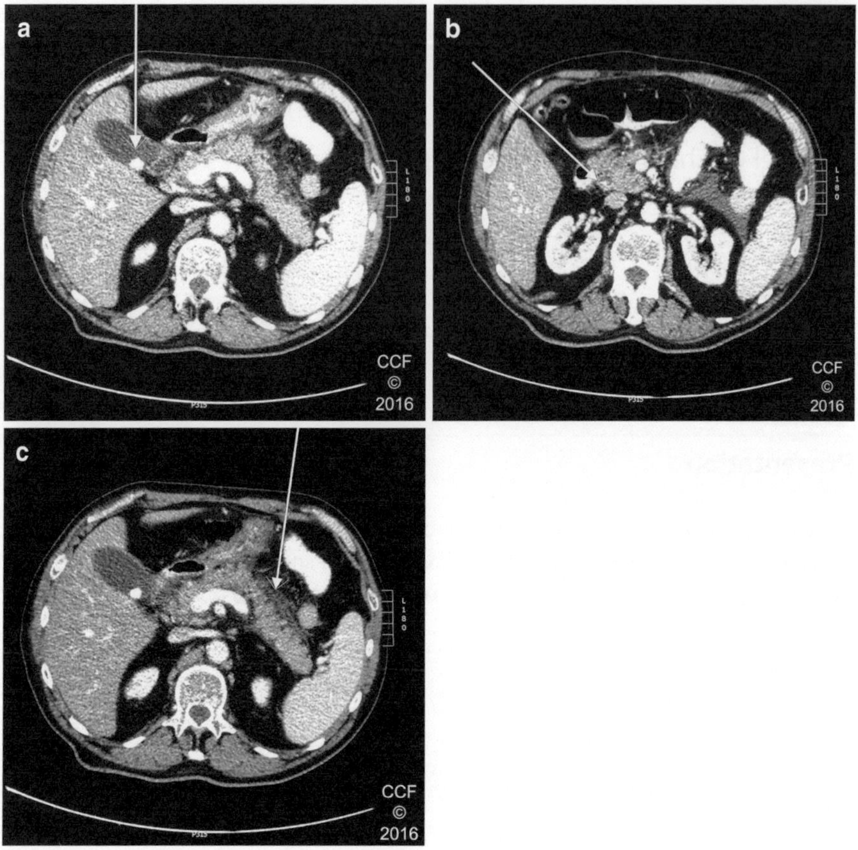

Fig. 232.1 Gallstone pancreatitis. (**a**) Gallstone in the gallbladder (arrow); (**b**) Gallstone within the distal common duct (arrow); (**c**) Pancreatic prominence and infiltration consistent with pancreatitis (arrow)

Comment

Management options for gallstone pancreatitis include procedures to remove the calculi [1, 2]. Pancreatic inflammation is associated with the development of splenic vein thrombosis which in turn can lead to left-sided portal hypertension with gastric varices due to lack of venous drainage from the short gastric veins [3]. An example of gastric varices secondary to gallstone pancreatitis is shown in Fig. 232.2.

In 1901, Opie described the relation of cholelithiasis to pancreatitis [4].

"The Relation of Cholelithiasis to Disease of the
Pancreas and to Fat-Necrosis
Dr. Opie.

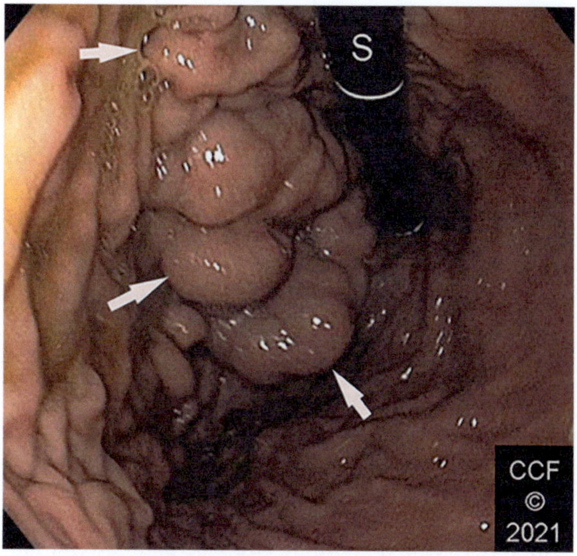

Fig. 232.2 Gastric varices (arrows) associated with pancreatitis-induced splenic vein thrombosis

"The patient whose history I shall relate was admitted to the service of Dr. Osler complaining of pain in the abdomen and fever. His family history is unimportant. He had suffered frequent attacks of indigestion characterized by pain after eating and, rarely, by nausea and vomiting. Six months before his fatal illness he had an attack of jaundice which lasted three weeks and was accompanied by severe abdominal pain and some fever. The jaundice disappeared and he remained in good health until the beginning of this illness. He was suddenly attacked about nine o'clock one night with very severe abdominal pain followed by nausea and vomiting. The vomiting continued throughout the night but subsequently was not severe. The pain was great for about four days but became less severe. On the seventh day of his illness, tenderness and swelling appeared in the right hypogastric region. Jaundice was not noticed previous to his admission to the hospital. His temperature ranged between 100° and 103°.

He was admitted to the hospital on the eighteenth day of his illness…. The patient was transferred to the surgical side where the diagnosis of acute pancreatitis was made by Dr. Bloodgood and an operation was performed. An abscess was entered through an incision in the great omentum between the stomach and the transverse colon. The cavity contained dark fluid, in which were necrotic particles. A drainage tube, packed about with gauze was inserted into the wound. There was a considerable amount of discharge from the wound. The patient did not rally from the operation and died at the end of four hours.

An autopsy was performed a few hours after death. The gall-bladder contained a large number of faceted calculi (about 100) of an average diameter of 1 cm. In the common duct, 1.5 cm from its origin, was a similar calculus. At this point the pancreatic duct was separated from the common bile-duct merely by a thin membranous septum, and it was upon this septum that the gall-stones lay.

Microscopic examination shows that the interstitial tissue of the pancreas is thickened and contains many cells in which are brownish-yellow pigment granules giving the reaction of iron. The necrotic material lying upon the surface of the pancreas is found to be changed blood.

> The changes in the pancreas show that hemorrhage had occurred into and about the pancreas sometime before death. In the common bile-duct was lodged a gall-stone in such a position that it might readily compress the pancreatic duct and give rise to changes in the pancreas."

In the same year, Opie, then an Instructor in Pathology at the Johns Hopkins University, concluded [5]:

> "The frequent association of cholelithiasis with hemorrhagic and gangrenous pancreatitis is the result of impaction of gall stones at the orifice of the diverticulum of Vater and penetration of bile into the pancreas."

Biographical Note

Eugene L. Opie (1873–1971) [6, 7]

Eugene Opie received his undergraduate degree in 1893 and the M.D. degree in 1897 from John's Hopkins University. He received training in pathology from Dr. William H. Welch at Johns Hopkins and worked both at the Johns Hopkins, the Rockefeller Institute, Columbia-Presbyterian Hospital, Washington University School of Medicine in St. Louis, the University of Pennsylvania School of Medicine, and Cornell University Medical College. In 1910, Opie was appointed Chair of Pathology at Washington University School of Medicine in St. Louis and served as Dean of the school from 1912 to 1915. During World War I, he served in France as a Colonel in the Medical Corps in association with the Barnes Hospital-Washington University Unit. In 1901, he established the relationship between obstruction of the ampulla of Vater by gallstones and the development of pancreatitis illustrated in this case. This was followed by the 1903 publication of *Disease of the Pancreas* [8].

References

1. Kaw M, Al-Antably Y, Kaw P. Management of gallstone pancreatitis: cholecystectomy or ERCP and endoscopic sphincterotomy. Gastrointest Endosc. 2002;56:61–5.
2. Vitale GC. Early management of acute gallstone pancreatitis. Ann Surg. 2007;245:18–9.
3. Butler JR, Eckert GJ, Zyromski NJ, Leonardi MJ, Lillemoe KD, Howard TJ. Natural history of pancreatitis-induced splenic vein thrombosis: a systematic review and meta-analysis of its incidence and rate of gastrointestinal bleeding. HPB. 2011;13:839–45.
4. Opie EL. The relation of cholelithiasis to disease of the pancreas and to fat necrosis. Johns Hopkins Hosp Bull. 1901;12:19–21.
5. Opie EL. The etiology of acute hemorrhagic pancreatitis. Johns Hopkins Hosp Bull. 1901;12:182–8.
6. Kidd JG. Eugene Lindsay Opie 1873-1971. Am J Pathol. 1971;65:483–92.
7. Eugene L. Opie, MD. American Association of Immunologists. www.aai.org. Accessed 24 Oct 2021.
8. Opie EL. Disease of the Pancreas, Its Cause and Nature. Philadelphia: JB Lippincott Company; 1903. Accessed from Internet Archive, archive.org, 30 Jun 2019.

233 Ileovesical Fistula

Victor W. Fazio, Gwendolyn A. Fuller, and James S. Wu

Presentation

A female developed fecaluria following treatment of ovarian cancer by surgery, chemotherapy, and pelvic irradiation. Cystogram revealed an ileovesical fistula as illustrated in Fig. 233.1.

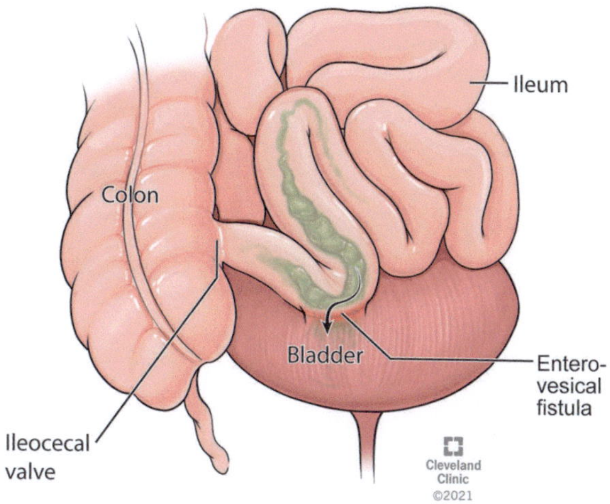

Fig. 233.1 Ileovesical fistula. The terminal ileum is directly connected to the bladder resulting in fecaluria. The enterovesical fistula, ileum, right colon and ileocecal valve are labelled

V. W. Fazio · J. S. Wu (✉)
Department of Colon and Rectal Surgery, Cleveland Clinic, Cleveland, OH, USA

G. A. Fuller
Medical Illustration Team, Enterprise Creative Services, Cleveland Clinic, Cleveland, OH, USA

J. S. Wu, M. D. Inkster (eds.), *Cleveland Clinic Colorectal Case Studies*, https://doi.org/10.1007/978-3-031-39880-3_233

Management

At surgery, a fistula between the terminal ileum and the bladder was found. The ileum was divided 10 cm proximal to the fistula. An anastomosis between the proximal end of the divided ileum and the ascending colon was made as illustrated in Fig. 233.2.

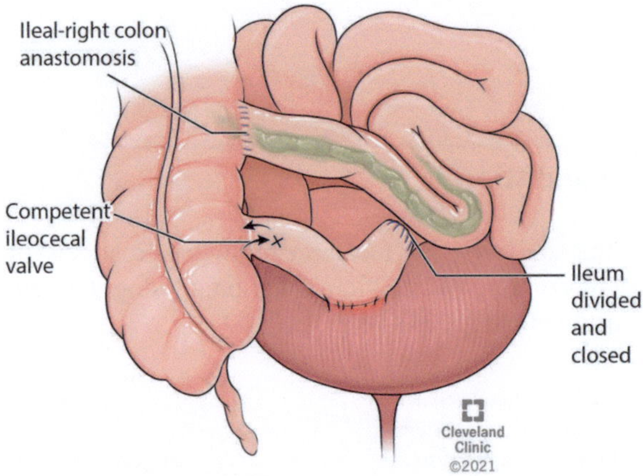

Fig. 233.2 The terminal ileum proximal to the fistula was divided. An anastomosis was made between the proximal end of the divided ileum and the ascending colon. The distal end of the divided ileum was closed. Contamination of the bladder from the ascending colon was prevented by ileocecal valve competence which allowed antegrade (arrow) but not retrograde (arrow x) passage of stool

Comment

In this case, ileovesical fistula was an adverse consequence of radiation injury to the terminal ileum and to the bladder that resulted in fecal contamination of the urinary tract. This operation was performed by Dr. Victor Fazio in 1995 with the third author assisting. Dr. Fazio noted that when the ascending colon was cross-clamped and pressure was applied to the cecum, there was no retrograde flow from the ascending colon into the terminal ileum.

Dr. Fazio reasoned aloud as follows:

1. Division of the ileum proximal to the fistula stops the inflow of succus entericus into the bladder.
2. The competent ileocecal valve prevents retrograde passage of stool from the colon to the bladder.
3. Anastomosis of the proximal end of the divided irradiated terminal ileum into colon distant from the irradiated pelvis ensures that one half of the ileocolic anastomosis would have a normal blood supply.
4. Best to leave the fistula between the irradiated bladder and ileum undisturbed.

War Wounds

234

James S. Wu

Presentation

Abdominal examination of an 80-year-old man showed scars. There was large stellate abdominal scar, a long midline incision, and a left-sided scar where a temporary colostomy had been created and later reversed. When I asked what caused them, his family spoke for him. He was a soldier, who as a young man went ashore on Omaha beach on D-Day, Tuesday, June 6, 1944. He took a single step onto the beach and fell. He was evacuated, had surgery, survived, and made it home.

I said, "thank you."

Comment

In his 1944 discussion of abdominal wounds encountered in war theatres, Major-General W. H. Ogilvie stated: [1]

> "The principle that all damaged parts of the large intestine must be excluded till the process of repair is complete applies to all injuries even suspected ones, and to all parts of the large bowel, particularly the extraperitoneal portion of the rectum."

Prior to D-day, the U.S. Army, instituted a policy, stated in Circular letter No. 178[1]:

[1]A copy of the original Circular Letter 178 from 1943 was kindly provided by Major Kenneth M. Koyle, AMEDD Office of Medical History, US Army Medical Department, Directorate of Strategic Communications, Falls Church, VA.

J. S. Wu (✉)
Department of Colon and Rectal Surgery, Cleveland Clinic, Cleveland, OH, USA

J. S. Wu, M. D. Inkster (eds.), *Cleveland Clinic Colorectal Case Studies*,
https://doi.org/10.1007/978-3-031-39880-3_234

ARMY SERVICE FORCES
Office of The Surgeon General
Washington 25, D. C.
23 October 1943.

CIRCULAR LETTER NO. 178
Subject: Care of the wounded in theaters of operation.

(5) Abdomen

(e) In large bowel injuries, the damaged segment will be exteriorized by drawing it out through a separate incision, preferably in the flank. In order to facilitate subsequent closure the two limbs of the loop should be approximated by suture for a distance of about 2 1/2 inches and then returned to the abdomen leaving the apex exteriorized with a short length of rubber tubing or other suitable material beneath it. If the segment cannot be mobilized the injury should be repaired and a proximal colostomy done.

(f) Penetrating injuries of the rectum should have exploratory laparotomy and posterior drainage by excision of the coccyx and incision of the fascia propria.

For The Surgeon General:
ROBERT J. CARPENTER
Lieut. Colonel, Medical Corps
Executive Officer.
DISTRIBUTION:
All officers of the Medical Corps, U. S. Army

The management of colonic injuries has evolved since World War II due to advances in transportation, antimicrobial therapy, and critical care [2].

References

1. Ogilvie WH. Abdominal wounds in the Western Desert. Surg Gynecol Obstet. 1944;78:225–38.
2. Sharpe JP, Magnotti LJ, Fabian TC, Croce MA. Evolution of the operative management of colon trauma. Trauma Surg Acute Care Open. 2017;2:1–7. https://doi.org/10.1136/tsaco-2017-000092.

Dr. Fazio's Operating Room Setup for Pelvic Surgery

235

Victor W. Fazio, Dawn M. Schultz, and James S. Wu

Presentation

Operations involving the rectum require long instruments that can reach deep into the pelvis. Figure 235.1 shows instruments located in the main table. Figure 235.2 shows a second tray containing instruments preferred by Dr. Fazio for deep pelvic dissection.

Figure 235.3 shows the positions of operating team members. The surgeon (usually right-handed) stands to the patient's left.

V. W. Fazio · J. S. Wu (✉)
Department of Colon and Rectal Surgery, Cleveland Clinic, Cleveland, OH, USA

D. M. Schultz
Department of Nursing, Cleveland Clinic, Cleveland, OH, USA

J. S. Wu, M. D. Inkster (eds.), *Cleveland Clinic Colorectal Case Studies*,
https://doi.org/10.1007/978-3-031-39880-3_235

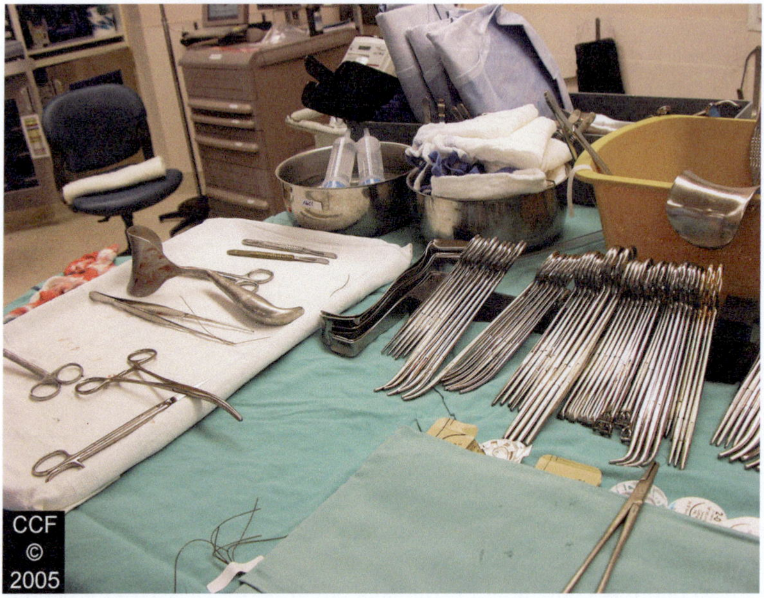

Fig. 235.1 The main table is elevated above the operative field. On it, featured here, are an array of long instruments suitable for work in the deep pelvis. Behind them are Mikulicz sponges, irrigating syringes, basins, and gowns. To the left are instruments for the opening including scalpels abdominal wall retractor, scissors, clamps, and forceps

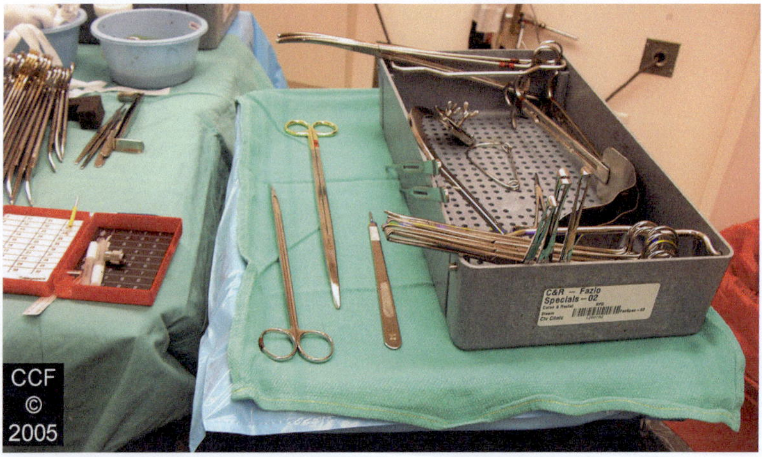

Fig. 235.2 A second elevated Mayo stand contains instruments preferred by Dr. Fazio (Fazio Specials) for deep pelvic dissection. The long scissors were passed down to Dr. Fazio from Dr. Rupert Turnbull who in turn received them from Dr. Thomas Jones

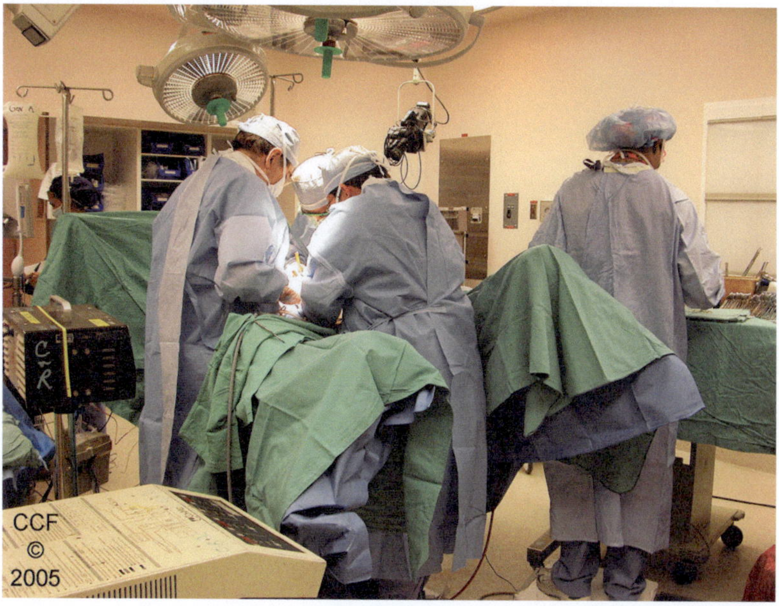

Fig. 235.3 The patient is positioned in stirrups. Dr. Fazio (on the patient's right) leads a right-handed fellow (on the patient's left) through the operation. The scrub nurse is located to the side of the operative field. A video camera is elevated opposite to Dr. Fazio. An intern (between the legs) holds a retractor and observes the operation that they might be privileged to do several years down the road

Correction to: Cleveland Clinic Colorectal Case Studies

James S. Wu and Michelle D. Inkster

Correction to:
J. S. Wu, M. D. Inkster (eds.), *Cleveland Clinic Colorectal Case Studies*, https://doi.org/10.1007/978-3-031-39880-3

An error in the production process unfortunately led to publication of this book prematurely, before incorporation of the final corrections. The version supplied here has been corrected and approved by the author [authors].

The errors have been corrected as listed below:

FM, TOC, Page xl: The chapter author Eric W. Wills' spelling was changed to Eric W. Willis

The chapter author Eric W. Willis' affiliation detail was changed to Department of Pathology, CORPath, Columbus, OH, USA, in the chapter opening pages of the chapters listed below:

Chapter 30, Chapter 32, Chapter 33, Chapter 37, Chapter 38, Chapter 41, Chapter 42, Chapter 43, Chapter 52, Chapter 54, Chapter 83, Chapter 88, Chapter 89, Chapter 92, Chapter 98, Chapter 100, Chapter 112, Chapter 114, Chapter 115, Chapter 118, Chapter 119, Chapter 128, Chapter 131, Chapter 132, Chapter 134, Chapter 136, Chapter 144, Chapter 146, Chapter 152, Chapter 154, Chapter 166, Chapter 167, Chapter 170, Chapter 172, Chapter 174, Chapter 187, Chapter 188, Chapter 193, Chapter 197, Chapter 198.

The updated version of the book can be found at https://doi.org/10.1007/978-3-031-39880-3

J. S. Wu, M. D. Inkster (eds.), *Cleveland Clinic Colorectal Case Studies*,
https://doi.org/10.1007/978-3-031-39880-3_236

Front Matter, Chinese Proverb, Page xix: The email address of contributor Jian Ma mamin@frontier.co, was changed to mamin@frontier.com

Chapter 18, Page 98: Figure 18.3 was replaced with the below figure:

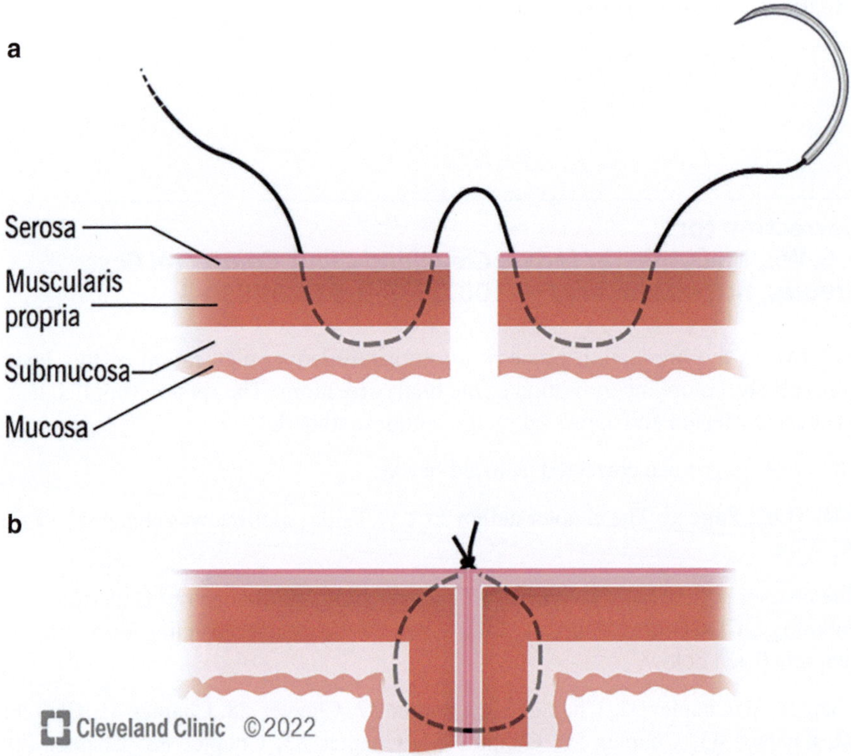

Fig. 18.3 Lembert's suture illustrated (after DeCosta, 1903). The suture on each side of the anastomosis picks up the submucosa because it is strong and will hold suture. When tied, the edges of the intestine are inverted

Chapter 46, Page 292: Fig. 46.2a was replaced with the below figure:

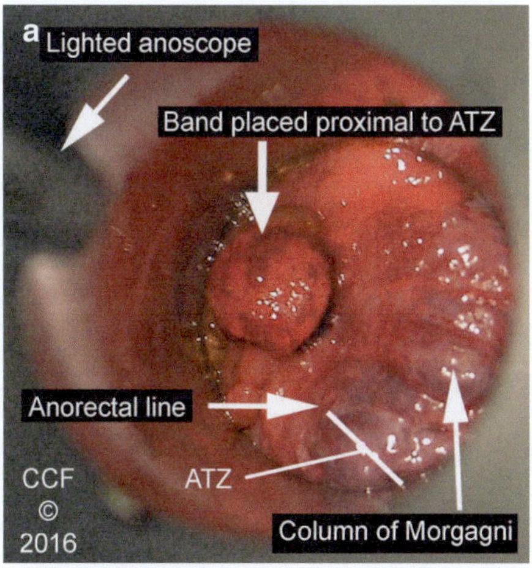

Fig. 46.2 (**a**, **b**) Photographs taken through a lighted beveled anoscope. The band is placed proximal to the sensate anal transitional zone (ATZ) whose borders are the anorectal line (the proximal border of the ATZ) and the dentate line. Within the ATZ are the internal hemorrhoids and the column/sinuses of Morgagni. Distal to the ATZ is the pecten

Chapter 48, Page 304: The caption of Fig. 48.1: Local anesthetic solution is injected peripheral to the external sphincter into the ischiorectal fat was changed to

Fig. 48.1: Local anesthetic solution is injected peripheral to the external sphincter into the ischiorectal fat **(after Nyström)**

Chapter 85, Page 511: The caption of Fig. 85.2: Ileal conduit (Bricker, 1950) after removal of the bladder, prostate, and rectum. A colostomy is seen in the left low quadrant was changed to

Fig. 85.2 Ileal conduit (Bricker, 1950) after removal of the bladder, prostate, and rectum. A colostomy is seen in the left low quadrant. **In this illustration, the colostomy has been drawn lateral to the rectus muscle. In practice, the colostomy is brought through the rectus muscle**

Chapter 191, Page 1074: Figure 191.5a was replaced with the below figure

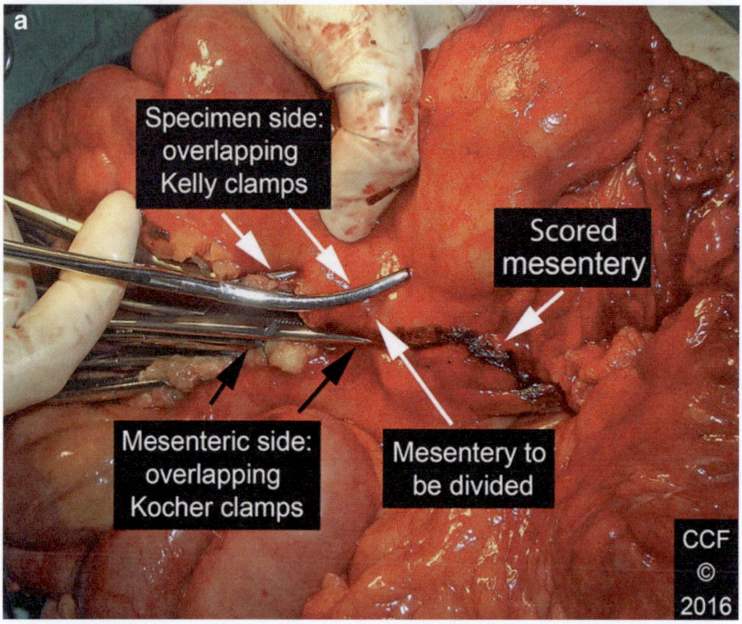

Fig. 191.5 (**a**, **b**) Starting at one end of the designated mesentery, the mesentery is divided between overlapping clamps. A Kocher clamp is used for the proximal side because it does not slip once placed. A Kelly clamp is used on the specimen side with the tips curved towards the specimen away from the line of resection. The mesentery to be divided is defined by the score on the mesentery

Chapter 192, Page 1081: Heineke was changed to Heinecke

Victor Warren Fazio, AO, MS: Recollections, Page 1315: End of paragraph 1: —complete with the pluses and minuses that we all have. Recollections of Victor Warren Fazio by Paula Erwin-Toth. Crina Floruta, was changed to —complete with the pluses and minuses that we all have. Crina Floruta

Index, Page 1339: left column, line 6 Heinecke-Mikulicz strictureplasties was changed to Heinecke-Mikulicz strictureplasty

Parting Thoughts

Parting Thought 1

There are no absolutes in medicine or surgery
Never say never or always

Parting Thought 2

Do good
Be good

Victor W. Fazio, AO, MS

J. S. Wu, M. D. Inkster (eds.), *Cleveland Clinic Colorectal Case Studies*,
https://doi.org/10.1007/978-3-031-39880-3

Move Forward with the Heart of a Novice

James S. Wu

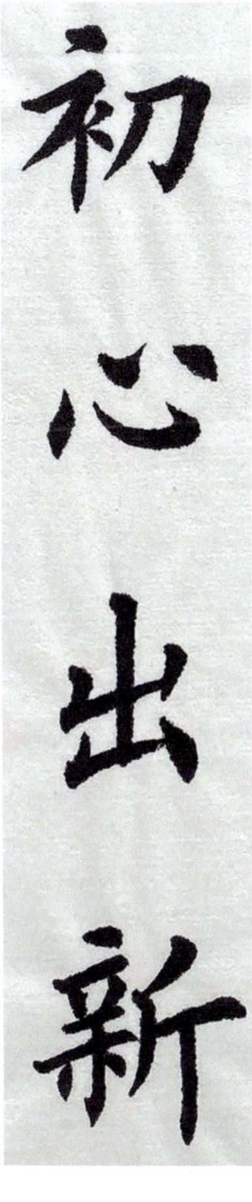

初心出新
Chū xīn chū xīn
Move forward with the heart of a novice
Calligraphy by: Jian Ma, mamin@frontier.com

J. S. Wu, M. D. Inkster (eds.), *Cleveland Clinic Colorectal Case Studies*,
https://doi.org/10.1007/978-3-031-39880-3

On Love

Being in love is total.
It challenges us forever.
We don't belong to ourselves anymore.
And we're not alone again ever.

History is full of stories of lovers.
Showing their devotion to all us others.
By dying for each other as the ultimate test,
When living for each other is harder and best.

The love in us all for universal mankind.
Should be a sumptuous banquet where all of us dined.
Sharing joys and all sorrows, through all of our tomorrows,
Giving and receiving for ourselves and all others.

Then love remains our most cherished gain.
Living in this shelter of everyone's pain,
And love now emerges in generous surges.
Triumphant and complete over all other urges.

Frank L. Weakley, MD.

Reproduced with permission from Mrs. Margaret Weakley

J. S. Wu, M. D. Inkster (eds.), *Cleveland Clinic Colorectal Case Studies*,
https://doi.org/10.1007/978-3-031-39880-3

Frank L. Weakley-A recollection

When first I interviewed at the Cleveland Clinic, candidates were seen one at a time, from a single seat facing the entire staff, collected in a single room, alphabetically. The process began early in the morning and proceeded until all had been scrutinized. My turn occurred in the late afternoon. When done, the department was empty. I had a plane to catch but had neglected to make arrangements to get to Hopkins airport. A gentle hand tapped me on the shoulder; and its voice said, "Do you need a lift?" It was Dr. Frank Weakley, who then drove me to the airport allowing me to make the flight with only minutes to spare. Years later, I operated on a patient that he had done surgery upon two and a half decades earlier. I reviewed the case, his operative report, and my plan with him before proceeding. When I needed an example of a skin grafted ileostomy for a presentation, Dr. Weakley invited me to his home to review his extensive slide collection. When he scrutinized an image using a hand-held viewing device, he told me the details of the case and the person with such clarity that I felt as if a canvas were being completed, each sentence, a brush stroke, retrieved from his memory of operations that he had performed years earlier. I still possess his personal copy of the 1967 *Atlas of Intestinal Stomas*. I remember him with fondness.

JSW

Victor Warren Fazio, AO, MS: Recollections

Recollections

The following are recollections of Dr. Fazio from those who knew him the best: his nurses, his secretaries, and his research associates. He had three secretaries and five office telephone extensions so that when you called, it was likely that you would speak to a human being. He had a team of nurses who were dedicated to his clinics and to his operating rooms. They knew his moves, his moods, and what had to be done to keep the service afloat. He maintained databases on everything so he could communicate his and the department's experience on all things colorectal.

Recollections

'There are so many fond memories I have of Dr. Fazio. He was brilliant, motivated, kind, humble, driven, supportive, loyal, and fun to work with. Working with Dr. Fazio in the operating room was an adventure and an education in more than surgical technique. Dr. Fazio could recall facts and figures from every article he read. He would teach and quiz the fellows and residents on anatomy and surgical technique through most of the operation. He was also a history buff, especially military history. One of his favorite sayings when he was getting to a point in surgery where there was no backing out was, "We are crossing the Rubicon." He would ask the residents what that meant and proceed to give them a lecture on ancient Roman history. Dr. Fazio's skills and reputation brought him the toughest operations and referrals. One of his former fellows said, "If you want a good operation go to Dr. ….. If you want a miracle, go to Dr. Fazio." Surgeons would send him their patients that they couldn't fix. Patients with complex surgical histories and miserable qualities of life came to him as their last chance, hoping he could help them. He helped the vast majority. Dr. Fazio had an amazing vocabulary. I would ask him what a word meant. If he didn't know, he would go home and look it up. This was before Google. He would always remember to explain the next day. One of his favorite words to use was *perspicacity*. When the fellows would be leaning over to see better and their heads would be in his way, Dr. Fazio would say, "Get me a sterile guillotine." Dr. Fazio never yelled, and he always treated everyone with respect, from his colleagues

J. S. Wu, M. D. Inkster (eds.), *Cleveland Clinic Colorectal Case Studies*,
https://doi.org/10.1007/978-3-031-39880-3

to the people in environmental services. Dr. Fazio would often say, "A picture is worth a thousand words." His drawings were excellent. He would draw pictures of patients' operations on the message boards in their rooms. Also, he had the fellows draw pictures of the operations for the patients. On rounds, he graded the drawings, with a letter on the board in red marker. Dr. Fazio appointed himself as "fashion police" and gave out citations to those who didn't meet up to his expectations. This was the same man who often had coffee stains on his lab coat; bagels, crackers, or rolls hanging out of his torn pocket; and his tie askew. I asked him once did he ever sleep, and his response was, "I shall have plenty of time to sleep when I am dead." He only slept 4 hrs a night. Dr. Fazio encouraged everyone around him to be the best they could be. Dr. Fazio loved his dog, *Sophie*. A patient had gifted the dog to Dr. Fazio just before her (the patient's) surgery. He brought the dog home. Years after she (the dog) died, he still had all her tags on his key ring. Dr. Fazio's patients loved and worshipped him. He saved many of their lives. A very special patient (who had many, many Crohn's surgeries with him) named her first daughter after him, Victoria. Dr. Fazio and his team were present for the deliveries of her first two children because the obstetrician was concerned about adhesions with her C-section. It was very moving to be there for her deliveries. Dr. Fazio was loyal to his employees and helped them if they needed help. He worked hard and long hours and expected his staff to do the same. If there was a problem or illness he always said, "Your family comes first." It was an honor and pleasure to work with Dr. Fazio, and I feel so blessed to have spent so many years working with him.'

Marlene Bambrick, RN
Operating room and office staff
1992–2021

'Dr. Fazio's favorite song was *American Pie* by Don McLean. He knew all the words. Every time I hear *American Pie,* I think about Dr. Fazio. (Me too, Marlene). Dr. Fazio's patients loved him. One named her stoma, "Victor." Not sure how he felt about that…. Dr. Fazio was rounding with one of his fellows one day, and the fellow was going to get the patient's chart (precomputer). The fellow sent him to the patient's room. When the fellow got to the nursing station, he realized Dr. Fazio's patient was one floor down. The fellow rushed back to the room to find Dr. Fazio sitting next to the patient on her bed. He had his hands on her belly and said, "You are very distended, and we shall have to take you to surgery today." The patient replied, "I don't understand, Doctor. I am 7 months pregnant!"'

Cheryl Cordell, RN
Operating room staff
1992–present

'I had the privilege and honor to work with Dr. Fazio my entire nursing career. I worked countless hours side-by-side with him in the operating room. He was an amazing surgeon, and also, he was an astonishing person who genuinely cared about his patients and staff. He was a gifted educationalist. In the OR, we would jokingly be amazed to see what letter of the alphabet he would create with the bowel, "J," "K," or "S." Dr. Fazio was truly a brilliant surgeon and wonderful person. He is greatly missed.'

Doreen Spence, RN
Operating room staff
1977–2012

'I had the honor and privilege of working with Dr. Fazio in surgery. He was fascinating, brilliant, and entertaining. Dr. Fazio had many sayings and quotes, including "*primum non nocere*." He would say it in Latin then translate it in English, "first do no harm." Dr. Fazio treated everyone with respect, and his patients admired and adored him. I feel very fortunate to have worked with him.'

Mary Kay Gilbride, RN
Operating room staff
1986–2020

'It is rare to remember the exact moment a person entered your life. It was 1982, and I was attending the R.B. Turnbull, Jr. *Enterostomal Therapy* course at the Cleveland Clinic. A disheveled man with a crop of black hair, white surgical scrubs, and a rumpled lab coat came barreling into the classroom. It was as if a full-blown hurricane had arrived. He introduced himself as "Vic Fazio" and asked us our names and a bit about our backgrounds. He had a great Australian accent and immediately put us at ease.

I was born with exstrophy of the bladder and had a urinary diversion created when I was 10 years old. As fate would have it, my "ET" at the time of my surgery was Ms. Norma Gill, the woman who along with Dr. Turnbull founded both the ET specialty and the first formal ET school in the world. Like Dr. Fazio, I remember exactly when I met Norma. As an ostomate herself, she immediately took control of the situation and fitted me with what were then archaic ostomy products. I saw her regularly for refitting as I grew and ostomy products improved. Having spent many of my early years in a hospital, I had always wanted to be a nurse. Once I met Norma, I knew what I wanted to do with my life. Dr. Fazio was a good friend of Norma's, and once he heard my story, he decided to take me under his wing.

A few years passed and I needed a revision of my ileal conduit. I elected to have a urinary Koch pouch. Dr. Fazio and Dr. Monte, a Cleveland Clinic urologist, performed my surgery. A few more years passed. I was working as an RN, ET in Akron, Ohio, and finishing up my Master of Science degree in nursing. As fate would have it, the combined position of Director of the ET school and manager of ET clinical services opened up. There was a rigorous search, and I was hired for the position. Since Vic and I developed a friendship over the years, he recused himself for most of the process. One question he did ask was whether I was ready to lead the ET school and ET clinical services at my relatively young age. I smiled and replied I would be the exact same age he was when he succeeded Dr. Turnbull. He burst out laughing. Over the years, Vic was my mentor, surgeon, boss, and my dear friend.

Somehow, we managed to keep all of those balanced in a professional manner. Before he became ill, Vic had boundless energy. Fellows and residents half his age could not keep up with his pace. He had an encyclopedic knowledge of everything from surgery to history to literature and Star Trek. The world became a smaller place after his passing, but his legacy lives on in his family, patients, and the scores of people he taught along the way. Mentor, Boss, Surgeon, Friend. Recollections of Victor Warren Fazio by Paula Erwin-Toth.

I had the privilege of working with Dr. Fazio for over 35 years. I have enjoyed working with him and learning from him. Through the years, I had the opportunity to watch Dr. Fazio interact with patients who came from all over the world. I have been impressed by his professional and personal demeanor and his attention to detail.

His clinics were always very busy. Many times he was late for the clinics, but his patients did not mind waiting to see him. He did not rush through their appointments. His patients appreciated his honesty, his concern, and the detailed explanation he gave about the disease process and the treatment options. It was not unusual to hear patients express their gratitude for the care they received from him. I heard many times comments like, "He is such a caring and wonderful doctor," or "Thank you for giving me my life back."

He had very unique traits. In those days, the clinic notes and the brief surgery notes were handwritten. I remember he always wrote in black ink and only used one type of ink pen. His penmanship was very unique. Only a handful of people who worked closely with him could read his handwriting. The diagrams he drew to show pre- and post-resection anatomy were specific to him, very detailed and helpful for future reference.

I remember being in the exam room while he and the fellow were doing an ileoscopy on a patient. He was closely observing the fellow doing the procedure. He looked out the window and asked the rest of us to name the clouds on the beautiful summer sky. Since we had difficulty with the answer, he proceeded to give us an overview of the types of clouds. He was one of the few people I knew that could multitask seamlessly, dictate a letter at the end of the visit, answer patient and family member questions, and watch one of us doing a dressing change while giving instructions.

The black ink pen was used many times to stir the coffee, the tie around his neck was off the straight line, tucked inside his shirt, the lab coat had few buttons missing—because he was human like the rest of us.

Dr. Fazio shared stories with all of us about his family, the places he has visited, the sports he enjoyed, and even his pets. Getting to know him on a personal level has made the working atmosphere more relaxed, pleasant, and congenial.

I felt confident that I could go to him with any question, ask for guidance, discuss patient issues, or make suggestions knowing that he would seriously consider them. I remember going to him with a personal problem, he asked his secretary to assist me, he made phone calls to his contacts, and, by the end of the day, he solved my problem.

He had a very unique way to let us know he cared. When he made rounds in the hospital, he sat on patient's bed and held their hand and listened. When I returned to work after losing my father, he passed by me and put his hand on my shoulder, did not say a word, but that touch said it all, and I still remember….

Through the years, he left us examples of dedication, compassion, thoughtfulness to patients and coworkers which we tried to emulate in our practices.

Dr. Fazio was a talented, understanding, and compassionate physician dedicated to his patients, but also a good colleague—complete with the pluses and minuses that we all have.'

Crina Floruta,
APRN, CNP
1976–2024

"Dr. Fazio was our celebrity chairman. He was a person of importance, influence, and a heavyweight in his field. Yet, when you interacted with him, you felt like family. His warmth, humor, and charm were ever present. I have to add that at conference no one touched the last cinnamon raisin bagel until Dr. Fazio had his. He'd sometimes eat it, but most of time he'd tuck it into his lab coat pocket. I always felt very grateful to have known him."

Kathrina Allen
Education Coordinator
Colorectal surgery
1995–present

'When Victor Fazio walked into a room, everything went quiet. When Victor Fazio walked out of a room, everything went quiet, all in anticipation of what he was going to say or what he was going to require to be accomplished for that period of time or that day. He had such a charisma about him. It just radiated off of him. He was not an individual that allowed mediocrity to enter his world. Neither in his administrative world nor in his patient care world. His patients idolized him. And rightly so. He was, after all, deemed a *Master of Surgery* in his field. *Best of the best.* But he was only asking for what he himself was willing to give in any situation. Dr. Fazio did not live his life with restrictions. There was always a solution to get things accomplished. His mind was constantly working. There was always something to achieve or something important that needed to be done (without delay). His productivity level was astounding. He required the same from his staff, but again, he was willing to give the same. You had to always expect the unexpected with him.

"Wait! What do you mean I have to dress into scrubs and come into the operating theater to take dictation?"

"Hold on! You want me to come to the Surgeon's lounge to ask all the questions I need answered and take notes for you?"

"Am I understanding correctly that you want me to start work at 7 o'clock in the morning each day so we can get more accomplished without interruptions?" (I commuted over an hour each way into work).

But my answer to all of these questions was, "Sure!" It was always an adventure. I kept pace with the best. He taught me so much about everything, including myself.

My accomplishments were numerous due to his guidance and belief in my abilities. It is a period of time I will never forget. After I was there for about 6 months, I was getting on the elevator at 6:50 in the morning when another physician/surgeon stepped on the elevator. I had no clue who he was. He looked at me and he said, "I know who you are. You're the one that works for Victor Fazio! I've heard about you!" I looked up at him and said, 'You're damn right I am!" I knew at that point, I had succeeded to the many and numerous challenges in front of me that were required to work for this amazing, gentle, talented, and magnificent man. Yes, I worked for Victor Fazio, and I was proud of it.'

Georgan Elizabeth Deka
Head Administrative Assistant to the Chairman
Division of Colorectal Surgery
Administrative Assistant to Editor and Chief
Digestive and Colorectal Publications

'Being asked to write a brief memory of the man I often referred to as the gentle bear is not an easy task. I remember interviewing in the conference room with Dr. Fazio for the position of word processor for the Department of Colon and Rectal Surgery. During the interview, Dr. Fazio had noted that I was coming from the Neurology Department as secretary to the Chairman and that I was applying for a word processing job. Dr. Fazio put his pen down, looked me in the eye, and said, "Bloody hell, why are you applying for this job when you're a Chairman's secretary?" I let him know that I was newly married and wanted to reduce my work stress, so the idea of typing all day seemed good. He said, "Ok, you're hired."

During my first few weeks, one Dr. Fazio's secretaries quit and the other just failed to show up to work one day. I was asked to fill in until a replacement was found. After a few weeks, I was walking to my car with Mary Iannone, the Administrator, and she happened to say, "It's a shame that you do not want to be a Chairman's secretary." I asked her why she said that. She then said that Dr. Fazio really wanted me to be his secretary. I took a few steps and stopped and said, "Ok, tell him I shall do it!"

This was the best decision of my career. I became enamored with his gentle bear demeanor. I watched him care for the sickest patients with the utmost compassion. During this time, I became pregnant with my first child. When it came time for me to return to work, I called Dr. Fazio to say I could not leave my daughter. He asked me to come back, even it is it only for a day or two a week, as "eight hours of you is equivalent to 40 hours of the average secretary." Dr. Fazio encouraged a work home balance and supported me as a new mother.

My lasting memory was when he had received a rug from an international patient. He called all of us into the conference room to see this beautiful gift. I walked in and unknowingly stepped onto the rug. Dr. Fazio bolted from his chair and said, "Oh, bloody, get her off the rug...it's a fertility rug." We all burst into laughter. I guess one child was enough (ha ha)....he did not want me to leave again.

My time was brief but full of fond memories and laughter working for my favorite boss!'

Lynne Daus
Secretary to the Chairman
1995–1998

'My memories of Dr. Fazio are still vivid, of a physician who could be said to have been "larger than life." I recall, when I began working for him, he had five phone numbers that rang into his office, all of them nonstop, much like his work ethic. It seemed strange at first that his medical secretaries managed a continuous stream of appointments and calls not just for his patients or from referring physicians, but also for those caregivers, fellows, residents, and other staff members, whom he encouraged to seek time with him. Eventually, it became strangely natural to see a long line outside his door on any day he was not traveling or in the OR. I often wondered at his ability to consistently function at a superior level no matter the day or circumstances. Many patients would come from across the globe for his expertise and healing hands. Many would wait hours to see him either knowing or hoping that he was the one who could make a difference. Many of them would return and bring him gifts of gratitude, often from their homeland, until his office was overflowing with objects of art. Regardless, if they were international, from another State or local, he would make time for them even if it meant skipping a decent meal or seeing them after a full day of surgery. Hence, the bit of food tucked away in a pocket that might later get the Vegemite treatment, a container of which he kept in his desk drawer. Not only could he perform successful, complex, seemingly miraculous surgeries, he would subsequently describe them effectively, in detail, in his letters to the referring physician. He could often be heard quoting a reference to a published paper, the journal, the author(s), and the year. Occasionally, he would recite poetry with aplomb. During the time I worked for him, I never witnessed an episode of him using his brilliance with arrogance, and he never raised his voice to me or anyone else in my presence. I especially loved hearing the eloquent manner in which he described the importance of medical research. It resonated with me to the extent that, following my tenure with Dr. Fazio, I went on to become and still am, a clinical research coordinator.'

Linda Libertini
Medical Secretary to the Chairman
2001–2004

'Dr. Fazio was not just my boss he was my dear friend and someone whom I considered family. He taught me so much about patients, their needs, and how to help them. I remember meeting Dr. Fazio when I worked at the Anesthesia Control Desk, and I was in total awe of this man who was a legend as I had heard so many stories (all good). I then moved up to the administrative area of Anesthesia to work with the Chairman at that time, and Dr. Fazio would come up there and get lost. I would always show him the way back to the ORs. One day he was up wandering the halls;

and I saw him; and we chatted as we walked and he said, "How would you like to work for me?" I was like sure! I couldn't believe this amazing surgeon wanted me to come and work with him and his team. That started the next 10 years of the best position here at Cleveland Clinic for me. I never saw working with Dr. Fazio as a job. It was such a pleasure and learning experience to be with him and our whole team. Dr. Fazio liked when I would make him spaghetti and meat sauce. He said it was his favorite meal, and he would always make sure he got me an Asiago cheese bagel in the morning. Even when I moved to Orthopedic Surgery, he would come up and find me with an Asiago cheese bagel in his pocket not in a bag but I wouldn't trade those bagels for anything. What I wouldn't give to have him walk up and hand me another one from his pocket. One of the most special gestures I remember with him was when he would be traveling before he left we would have a group hug as we were family and when you travel that is what families do. So many wonderful memories of such an amazingly wonderful man, surgeon, and friend.'

Jody Pucella
Secretary to the Chairman

'How do you condense 16 years of working with a person into one paragraph? I'm going to try. When I first started working for Dr. Fazio, I admit, I was scared of him. I rarely spoke unless I had to. You see he was a Giant of a man, confident, powerful, and respected by his colleagues. I never worked for anyone like that before, and I heard secretaries didn't last too long with him. When Georgann left, I became his primary secretary. Now I told you I was afraid of him. So I wrote him a letter and told him how I would not let him down, and I would keep his "ship afloat." After that, we bonded as a team. Dr. Fazio was a genius (I don't use that word lightly) and had a photographic memory so sharp that he would recall articles he wrote 10+ years ago. One day we got a call, and they wanted him to take on a patient who would not accept blood, didn't have insurance, and desperately needed surgery. Previous surgeries had failed him, and previous surgeons would not reengage. I just knew he was going to refuse the patient, but he didn't. He said, "Send him here" (in that loud Australian accented voice). I knew then, I would never leave him and give him my best. Now, he was a challenge to work for. One day, he gave me a crumpled piece of paper and said, "Here, type this!" Everyone is going to tell you how great he was, and what a great writer and surgeon he was. All is true but let me give you another side of him that I saw. He offered me tickets he had to a Browns game. On a Sunday morning, Dr. Fazio was at my side door personally delivering the tickets to me. He was that kind of a guy. When I had to talk to him, even in later years I would swing my arms. Well, he started mocking me and here was this WORLD FAMOUS SURGEON swinging his arms imitating me with this smile on his face. We could spend hours talking about old movies. He loved Chinese food and M&M's. I used to leave an M&M trail to guide him to documents for his signature. These are just a few snippets of what it was like working for Dr. Fazio. Dr. Wu describes me as the longest working secretary he had, and I'm proud to hold that position.'

Melonie Marshall
Secretary to the Chairman
1996–2010

"I was a 20 year plus employee in Colorectal Surgery. I started out as Dr. Fazio's medical administrative assistant. I just could not keep up the pace he kept, but I adored him and stayed for many, many years under his leadership working in other roles within the department. We were a family under his guidance, and I loved it. I have so many stories and plenty to raise a few chuckles but this brief synopsis of what happened to my family years ago is one I must share.

Dr. Fazio would travel around Christmas time for many years to spend some well-deserved time off with his family. At that time, my husband, Ray, had a diverticulitis attack and had surgery with another surgeon. Unfortunately, Ray ended up with an anastomotic leak. He was in the hospital for 31 days and endured two more surgeries due to complications. Upon Dr. Fazio's return a few weeks into his hospitalization, I requested that Dr. Fazio to perform the last surgery. To no surprise, the healing finally began. I came into visit my husband over the weekend after the final surgery and ran into Dr. Fazio in the parking garage. We sat on a bench on the walkway to the hospital as he pulled out an old napkin and borrowed a pen to draw a diagram of what Ray's colon presently looked like and what to expect. He looked me in the eyes and said it was going to be a long recovery but assured me, like no one else could, that it will be okay. For the first time in many weeks, I knew it would be.

Dr. Fazio was wonderful to work for. He was loved by his crew and respected worldwide. Visiting surgeons came to observe him in surgery throughout the years. There were hundreds; the proof is in a book they all signed. I hope his family has seen it. What a sacrifice for them as he spent many hours of his life healing patients. For one whose life he saved… we are forever grateful."

Marty Hodgson
Administrative secretary to the Chairman

"My first memories of Dr. Fazio occurred when I was in Enterostomal Therapy (as wound, ostomy, and continence (WOC) nurses were known back in the day) school in 1981. Dr. Fazio came in on a Friday morning to lecture to the class. He had no notes, and spent the next 3 h lecturing on a variety of topics, citing article upon article to support his ideas. He also had the most beautiful drawings to illustrate his content! I was in awe of him at this time, as I had never encountered anyone quite like him before. Once I began working at the Cleveland Clinic, these beliefs only increased as I saw the depth and breadth of his knowledge not only about colorectal surgery, but also a variety of other topics. I liked to think of him as a Renaissance man! I also found his before and after drawings following a surgical procedure most helpful. They allowed me to better understand what the person had been dealing with, as well as be clear in what was done. This allowed me to better educate my patients and our student WOC nursing students. I always missed those drawings when we went to an electronic charting system!

Dr. Fazio had a unique blend of confidence and caring that was evident from the very first meeting he had with an individual. It did not matter what the diagnosis was, how high the anxiety level, or whether bad/dire news needed to be delivered. Somehow when Dr. Fazio entered a person's room and began talking with the person, an instant trust developed, and they somehow managed to feel better. They knew he would give his very best (which was excellent indeed) and that he cared for them as an individual. This happened day in and day out. In my 42 years of nursing, I have never seen a physician have this effect on people in the way that Dr. Fazio did."

Barbara J. Hocevar, MSN, RN, CWOCN
Wound, Ostomy, and Continence Nurse (Retired)
Cleveland Clinic

"It was truly an honor to work alongside Dr. Fazio. He was not only a brilliant, compassionate surgeon; but also, he was an amazing man! He cared for his patients as though they were part of his own family and made a positive difference in so many lives! Dr. Fazio had a special place in his heart for Enterostomal Therapy (ET) nurses and he truly valued their dedication to colorectal patients. He was definitely, *the best of the best!*"

Coleen Potts, BSN, RN, CWOCN.

'As Chairman of Colorectal Surgery, Dr. Fazio was my boss for 20-plus years. He was also my most influential professional mentor, and he was my friend. He was an amazing pioneer, leader, and teacher in the colorectal surgery field, and yet he was humble, and always found a way to give credit and recognition to others. He knew that medicine was all about teamwork.

Dr. Fazio's patients loved him because he found a way to make their lives better. He treated each of his patients as special and unique. When we use the term "caregiver" in healthcare, Dr. Fazio instantly comes to mind as a "caregiver who genuinely cared for his patients, and his colleagues and employees."

What I remember most about Dr. Fazio was not a single event. Instead, it was his constant presence as a trusted leader and friend. He saw and embraced people in a whole sense. He knew my parents and my husband Don, whose poetry he read.

Dr. Fazio was a man of wisdom, who did his best in any given moment, but he saw the future, and knew how to create future generations of colorectal surgeons. When I think of Dr. Fazio, this Hippocrates quote comes to mind, "*Wherever the art of medicine is loved, there is also a love of humanity.*" Dr. Fazio's love of humanity made him one of the world's greatest surgeons.

Finally, Dr. Fazio was an amazing storyteller, and he had a great sense of humor. He loved to laugh and make others do the same. Sometimes humor is the best medicine.'

Mary Rothaermel Iannone
Administrator, Colorectal Surgery Department
Administrator, Digestive Disease Institute
1986–2007

'When I first interviewed for a computer science position at the Department of Colorectal Surgery, I recognized that I was talking to a great scientific mind. Dr. Fazio is well-known for shaping the world of colorectal surgery, but he was also one of the first surgeons who understood the pivotal power of data in surgery. Before the term "data science" even became popularized, Dr. Fazio inspired clinical researchers and computer scientists to build robust data-driven solutions. These digital solutions helped surgeons navigate challenging surgical procedures, helped patients understand complex genetic diseases, and helped young surgeons achieve better outcomes. The importance of Dr. Fazio's role in colorectal surgery is undeniable. As a computer science professor, I particularly admire his early vision of what has now become the field of Data Science. I was incredibly fortunate to know Dr. Fazio and was lucky to have worked with him.'

Elena Manilich
Professor of Computer Science
John Carroll University

'Upon meeting Dr. Fazio in 1983, I would never have imagined that one person would have been important to my career and building the volume of illustrations on colorectal surgery now owned by Cleveland Clinic. In fact, prolific is the one word I would use to describe work done in my 33-year association with Victor Fazio. Over the years, there was a regular stream of requests for artwork needed for publication, presentation, and video. Projects were usually presented to me as multiple thumbnail sketches using anything he could draw on. My favorite memory of one such project involves 39 tiny little sketches drawn on the front and back of a manila envelope. Fazio had called me to his office after returning from one of his many trips back to Australia. As he handed the envelope to me, he apologized for all the drawings he needed explaining, he was on the jet coming back to the States and "The muse just hit me."

As a young illustrator, just beginning my career, I appreciated the rough concept drawings he would provide always with a verbal explanation of the procedure. Back then, there were no Google images, e-mail, or fax, so my meetings with Victor Fazio were generally in person; and references he provided were always hand drawn by the man himself. I feel he fancied himself an artist; and, indeed, he did possess skills better than most physicians I've worked with in my career as a medical illustrator. Most importantly, Dr. Fazio took the time to meet with me, explain what was needed, and answer my questions. In that sense he was constantly educating, in the office, between patients in an exam room hallway, or even in the operating room where he would demonstrate a technique or provide an opportunity to view the *in situ* anatomy.

For Dr. Victor Fazio, his time as leader, colleague, and mentor, continues to provide lasting importance at Cleveland Clinic. His use of medical illustrations led many staff physicians, Fellows, and residents to incorporate our work in their own.'

Joseph A. Pangrace, CMI
Director,
Cleveland Clinic Department of Medical Art and Illustration

'As a photographer, I have great memories of working with Dr. Fazio covering calls to his OR and his clinic dating back to 1981 while working in the CCF Photography Department. In 1990, Dr. Fazio offered me a photography position with colorectal surgery. The transition afforded me the opportunity to incorporate other duties along with my photographic obligations. I once asked Dr. Fazio if he would explain the difference between a subtotal colectomy and a partial colectomy. He answered my question with a nicely drawn piece of artwork. When I asked him if he would autograph it he said, "I would have done a better job if I know you were going to ask me to sign it." I loved that drawing; so I had it framed. It hung in my office until I retired. Today my treasure resides with Mrs. Fazio.

I learned a lot from Dr. Fazio about colorectal procedures, diseases and what the contributing forefathers brought to this field of medicine from preparing his PowerPoint lectures. Dr. Fazio was a brilliant surgeon with an abundance of compassion for his patients. I remember him reminding the Colorectal Fellows, "Remember that you stand on the shoulders of those who came before you." Dr. Fazio was an extraordinary example for those he taught and served.'

Joyce Balliet
Photographer and
Administrative assistant
1981–2012

'I arrived in Cleveland the day before I was to begin working with Dr. Victor Fazio in the position of clinical associate staff, June 30, 1994. It was late in the afternoon. I went directly to the clinic offices on the 11th floor of the Crile building, A11. There I was met by Ms. Ellie Stanton, Dr. Fazio's secretary. It was 4:30 pm. "He's expecting you," she said. I then was led across the skyway to the change rooms, reattired in scrubs, and then guided to operating room 52. Dr. Fazio, looked over the ether screen and said, "Jim, I am glad you're here. Say hello to my nurses, Marlene Bambrick, Mary Kay Gilbride, Doreen Spence, and Cheryl Cordell. Next, introduce yourself to Tracy Hull in room 51. This is her last day as clinical associate. You take over tomorrow. Then, if you don't mind, scrub in." After getting the 30 second skinny from Tracy as she operated on a patient with Crohn's disease and being integrated into the surgical team, I looked at the wall clock. It was 7:30 pm. We then went on rounds: radiology, H50, H51, H52, up to G61, G81, and back to A11. It was

9:30 pm. "Jim, you look tired," Dr. Fazio said; "Why don't you take the rest of the day off." The next morning, I arrived at the office at six. Dr. Fazio was already there, standing at a counter, signing letters, and sorting through a pile of correspondence. "Do you like to write?" he queried? He handed me a list of topics from journals and books to which he had been asked to contribute. "Choose two to start with. You'll share an office with Ms. Joyce Balliet, next door to mine. Joyce keeps track of the photographs. Keep a camera with you and always take two shots. This way you can publish it twice. A drawing conveys an idea. A photograph shows it actually can be done." Prior to the electronic medical record at the Cleveland Clinic, a summary of each operation was entered into a patient's chart immediately following surgery. The green color of the paper, upon which this information was recorded, distinguished it from other notes. A brief description of the operation was written on the front side of the sheet. An illustration of the operation was hand-drawn on the back that clearly communicated the salient points of the surgery. Only once did Dr. Fazio give me an "A" for a drawing of sigmoid volvulus. When he saw my gleeful response, he added a "minus." When I queried why the demotion, he said that he didn't want success to go to my head. That was July, 1994. Now 28 years later, I recall Dr. Fazio as the teacher who shaped my surgical skills, judgment, and perspective more than any other individual. He led by showing us the way forward and enthusiastically supported our efforts to get there. When we won, he won. When we failed, he picked us up. He inspired us to perform at our highest level and then beyond. His presence made the Cleveland Clinic home.'

Jim Wu
Clinical associate, 1994–1998

Slides

Michelle D. Inkster and James S. Wu

Abstract

Digital educational presentations were preceded by 35 mm film slides and 3 × 4 in. glass lantern slides. Two examples of these slides are presented.

Keywords

35 mm slides; Glass-lantern slides

Presentation

In 2025, educational presentations and lectures are prepared using digital computer programs. Before this, the standard was 35 mm film slides, mounted in plastic or paper holders, loaded into a projector. Light, passing through the slide, projected an image on a screen. For the generation above us, the standard lecture tool was the glass-lantern slide composed of a positive transparent photograph attached to or sandwiched between 3 × 4 in. panes of glass. Examples of these are shown in Fig. E.1.

J. S. Wu, M. D. Inkster (eds.), *Cleveland Clinic Colorectal Case Studies*,
https://doi.org/10.1007/978-3-031-39880-3

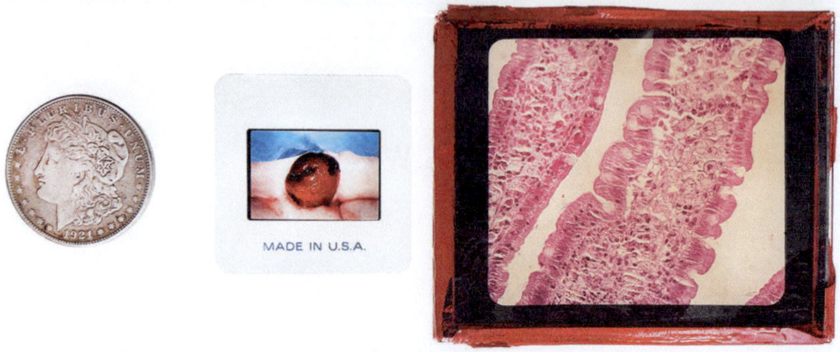

Fig. E.1 Left to right: 1921 Morgan silver dollar; 35 mm color film image sealed in a cardboard slide mount; median format color film image sealed in between two panes of glass. The 35 mm slide, showing rectal prolapse, was a gift from Robert D. Fry, MD. The glass-lantern slide showing Whipple's disease is from the Eugene I. Winkelman, MD collection in the Cleveland Clinic Archives

Postscript

In his twelfth-century work, *Metalogicon*, John of Salisbury, attributed to Bernard of Chartres the principle that we are allowed to advance because of the work of those who precede us.

Dicebat Bernardus Carnotensis nos esse quasi nanos, gigantium humeris incidentes, ut possimus plura eis et remotiora videre, non utique proprii visus acumine, aut eminentia corporis, sed quia in altum subvehimur et extollimur magnitudine gigantea Joannes Saresberiensis Metalogicus, III-4 [1]	Bernard of Chartres used to compare us to [puny] dwarfs perched on the shoulders of giants. He pointed out that we see more and farther than our predecessors, not because we have keener vision or greater height, but because we are lifted up and borne aloft on their gigantic stature John of Salisbury Metalogicon, III-4 [2]

Samuel Arbesman, in his book entitled, *The Half-Life of Facts. Why Everything We Know Has an Expiration Date*, writes:

> "Facts, in the aggregate, have half-lives: We can measure the amount of time for half of a subject's knowledge to be overturned." [3].

The preceding compilation of colorectal/GI cases represents a glimpse of the experiences of surgeons, physicians, and staff associated with one institution over a brief time period. The contributors realized during this work's preparation that a case approached in a certain way then might be handled differently later because of advances in surgical technique and medical therapeutics. We have attempted to select principles that have enduring value and that, hopefully, will serve as a foundation for future students.

Michelle D. Inkster
James S. Wu

J. S. Wu, M. D. Inkster (eds.), *Cleveland Clinic Colorectal Case Studies*,
https://doi.org/10.1007/978-3-031-39880-3

References

1. Ioannes Saresberiensis. Metalogicus. Liber Tertius, Cap. IV. Quae sit conceptio et utilitas Periermeniarum, vel rectius Periermenias; cited in Corpus Corporum, repositorium operum Latinorum apud universitem Turicensem, Universität Zürich[uzm].miat.uzh.ch.
2. Ioannes Saresberiensis. Metalogicvs. Paris, 1610. The Metalogicon of John of Salisbury: A Twelfth-Century defense of the Verbal and Logical Arts of the Trivium. Translated by Daniel D. McGarry. Mansfield Centre, CT: Martino Publishing; 2015. p. 167. Permission to reuse this text was generously granted by Mr. Maurizio Martino, Martino Fine Books; www.martinopublishing.com, August 2, 2021.
3. Arbesman S. The half-life of facts. Why everything we know has an expiration date. Current. New York: Penguin Group (USA) Inc.; 2012. p. 3. Permission to reuse this sentence was generously given by Mr. Christopher Aguirre of Penquinradomhousebooks; caquirre@penguinrandomhouse.com, August 4, 2021.

Editors' Statement

In 2005, Dr. Michelle Inkster conceived of a book on intestinal and anal diseases to educate students, trainees, and practitioners using a clinical case presentation format. Cases included in this work were contributed by physicians, surgeons, nurses, and staff associated with the Cleveland Clinic. Credit is given as far as is possible to sources of clinical material, medical illustration, authoritative references, and commentary. Drs. Michelle Inkster and James Wu are responsible for the design, drafting, revision, communication with authors, assessment of each case for intellectual content, copyright permissions, final approval of the version to be published, and agreement to be accountable for all aspects of the work in ensuring that questions related to any part of the work were appropriately investigated and resolved. We take full responsibility for any shortcomings that might be detected following publication.

Michelle D. Inkster
James S. Wu
Cleveland
January, 2025

J. S. Wu, M. D. Inkster (eds.), *Cleveland Clinic Colorectal Case Studies*,
https://doi.org/10.1007/978-3-031-39880-3

Index

J. S. Wu, M. D. Inkster (eds.), *Cleveland Clinic Colorectal Case Studies*,
https://doi.org/10.1007/978-3-031-39880-3

E

I

L

M

N

S

MIX
Papier aus verantwortungsvollen Quellen
Paper from responsible sources
FSC® C105338

If you have any concerns about our products,
you can contact us on
ProductSafety@springernature.com

In case Publisher is established outside the EU,
the EU authorized representative is:
Springer Nature Customer Service Center GmbH
Europaplatz 3, 69115 Heidelberg, Germany

Printed by Libri Plureos GmbH
in Hamburg, Germany